Brief Contents

MOSBY'S® TEXTBOOK FOR

NURSING ASSISTANTS

ELEVENTH EDITION

LEIGHANN N. REMMERT, MS, RN

SHEILA A. SORRENTINO, PhD, RN

ELSEVIER

Elsevier
3251 Riverport Lane
St. Louis, Missouri 63043

Notice

Previous editions copyrighted 2021, 2017, 2012, 2008, 2004, 2000, 1996, 1992, 1987, and 1984.

Director, Content Development: Laurie Gower
Executive Content Strategist: Sonya Seigafuse
Content Development Specialist: Brooke Kannady
Publishing Services Manager: Catherine Jackson
Book Production Specialist: Kristine Feeherty
Design Direction: Brian Salisbury

Printed in India

Last digit is the print number: 9 8 7 6 5 4 3 2 1

Working together
to grow libraries in
developing countries

www.elsevier.com • www.bookaid.org

In honor of all who…

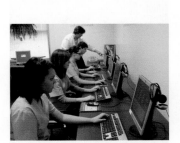
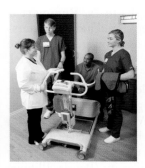

Teach how to assist with nursing care.

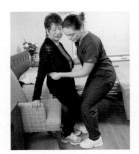

Learn how to assist with nursing care.

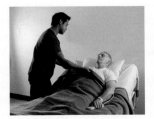

Assist with nursing care.

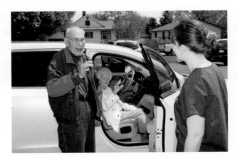

You change the lives of all who receive nursing care.

About the Authors

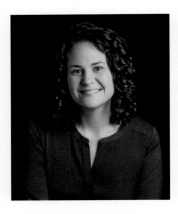

Leighann N. Remmert is a registered nurse and nursing assistant instructor. She has taught in high school, vocational, and community college nursing assistant programs in central Illinois.

Ms. Remmert has a Bachelor of Science degree in nursing from Bradley University (Peoria, Illinois) and a Master of Science degree in nursing education from Southern Illinois University Edwardsville (Edwardsville, Illinois).

Nursing practice for Ms. Remmert began at St. John's Hospital (Springfield, Illinois) as a nursing assistant/technician. As a registered nurse, Ms. Remmert concentrated in the area of emergency nursing at Memorial Medical Center (Springfield, Illinois). There, her roles included staff nurse, charge nurse, nurse preceptor, and trauma nurse specialist. As a clinical nursing instructor at Capital Area School of Practical Nursing (Springfield, Illinois), Ms. Remmert supervised, instructed, and evaluated student learning in various long-term care and acute care settings.

In her current focus on nursing assistant education, Ms. Remmert emphasizes the importance of professionalism and work ethics, safety, teamwork, communication, and accountability. She promotes the principles of valuing the role of the nursing assistant and treating the person with dignity, care, and respect.

Ms. Remmert is co-author of *Mosby's® Textbook for Nursing Assistants* (ed 8–11), *Mosby's® Essentials for Nursing Assistants* (ed 4–7), and *Mosby's® Textbook for Medication Assistants* (ed 1). She was a consultant on *Mosby's® Textbook for Long-Term Care Nursing Assistants* (ed 6) and served as a content adviser for *Mosby's® Nursing Assistant Video Skills* (version 4.0).

Ms. Remmert is a Basic Life Support instructor. She is a member of Sigma Theta Tau International, the Honor Society of Nursing, and the Certified Nursing Assistant Educator Association (Illinois, Central Region).

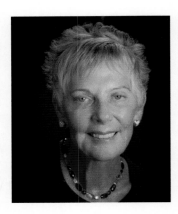

Sheila A. Sorrentino was instrumental in the development and approval of CNA-PN-ADN career-ladder programs in the Illinois community college system and has taught at various levels of nursing education—nursing assistant, practical nursing, associate degree nursing, and baccalaureate and higher degree programs. Her career includes experiences in nursing practice and higher education—nursing assistant, staff nurse, charge and head nurse, nursing faculty, program director, assistant dean, and dean.

A Mosby author and co-author of several nursing assistant titles since 1982, Dr. Sorrentino's titles include:
- *Mosby's® Textbook for Nursing Assistants*
- *Mosby's® Essentials for Nursing Assistants*
- *Mosby's® Textbook for Long-Term Care Nursing Assistants*
- *Mosby's® Textbook for Nursing Assistive Personnel*
- *Mosby's® Basic Skills for Nursing Assistants*
- *Mosby's® Textbook for Medication Assistants*

She was also involved in the development of an early version of *Mosby's® Nursing Assistant Video Skills* and *Mosby's® Nursing Video Skills*, winner of an AJN Book of the Year Award (electronic media).

Dr. Sorrentino has a Bachelor of Science degree in nursing, a Master of Arts degree in education, a Master of Science degree in nursing, and a PhD in higher education administration. Her past community activities include the Rotary Club of Anthem (Anthem, Arizona), the Provena Senior Services Board of Directors (Mokena, Illinois), the Central Illinois Higher Education Health Care Task Force, the Iowa-Illinois Safety Council Board of Directors, and the Board of Directors of Our Lady of Victory Nursing Center (Bourbonnais, Illinois).

She received an alumni achievement award from Lewis University for outstanding leadership and dedication in nursing education. She is also a member of the Illinois State University College of Education Hall of Fame.

Acknowledgments

Many individuals help to develop an accurate, up-to-date, and timely publication. With gratitude and appreciation, we acknowledge:

- MPS North America, LLC, for their talented artistry and prompt revisions.
- Graphic World for their copyediting services and proofreading efforts. The task requires attention to detail.
- The Elsevier staff involved:
  - Laurie Gower: Director, Content Development—for her planning, oversight, and prompt assistance as needs arose.
  - Sonya Seigafuse, Executive Content Strategist—for her management of this work and her attention to various author and instructor needs.
  - Brooke Kannady, Content Development Specialist—for her organization and communication during manuscript development.
  - Kristine Feeherty, Book Production Specialist—for her coordination during the production phase.
  - Brian Salisbury, Senior Book Designer—for his creativity and patience with revisions as we collaborated on the design.

To all of the individuals who contributed to this effort in any way, we are sincerely grateful.

Leighann N. Remmert and Sheila A. Sorrentino

Instructor Preface

The eleventh edition of *Mosby's® Textbook for Nursing Assistants* serves several purposes.
- Prepares students to function as nursing assistants in nursing centers, hospitals, and home care settings.
- Assists faculty in meeting educational goals.
- Serves as a resource when preparing for the competency evaluation.
- Serves as a resource for nursing assistants wanting to review or learn new information for safe care.

The following foundational principles and values are presented in specific chapters and integrated in content and key features (p. xiii–xvii) throughout the book.
- Patients and residents are *persons* with dignity having a past, a present, and a future. Such persons are physical, social, psychological, and spiritual beings with basic needs and protected rights.
- Nursing assistant roles, functions, and limitations are described in federal and state laws with dependence on effective delegation and good work ethics.
- Body structure and function, safe handling and positioning, preventing infection, and safety and comfort measures form an essential knowledge base.
- Communication skills enhance relationships with the nursing and health teams, patients and residents, and families and visitors.
- The nursing assistant has a key role in the nursing process.

CONTENT ISSUES

Content decisions are based on changes in laws or in guidelines and standards issued by federal and state governments, accrediting agencies, and national organizations. So are changes to state curricula and competency evaluations.

Student learning needs and abilities, instructor desires, work-related issues, course/program and book length, and student cost also are among the many factors considered.

New Content
Chapter 1: Health Care Agencies
- Staffing
- Box 1-3 HHS Agencies
- Workplace Safety
- Policies and Procedures

Chapter 2: The Person's Rights
- Protecting Rights

Chapter 3: The Nursing Assistant
- Employee Orientation

Chapter 4: Delegation
- Delegation Guidelines

Chapter 6: Student and Work Ethics
- Attention
- FOCUS ON COMMUNICATION: Planning Your Work
- Reporting Harassment

Chapter 7: The Person and Family
- Box 7-1 Meeting Basic Needs
- CARING ABOUT CULTURE: Culture
- Spirituality and Religion
- Gender Identity
- FOCUS ON COMMUNICATION: Gender Identity
- Health Care Beliefs and Practices
- FOCUS ON CHILDREN AND OLDER PERSONS: Behavior
- Family
- Box 7-5 Interacting With the Person's Family

Chapter 8: Health Team Communications
- FOCUS ON COMMUNICATION: Assessment
- Analysis
- FOCUS ON LONG-TERM CARE AND HOME CARE: Planning

Chapter 9: Medical Terminology
- Positional Terms

Chapter 11: Growth and Development
- Family Structure and the Caregiver Role
- PROMOTING SAFETY AND COMFORT: Family Structure and the Caregiver Role
- Electronic Media
- Box 11-1 Bullying: Types and Signs

Chapter 12: The Older Person
- Table 12-1 The Aging Process: Physical Changes and Care Measures (Immune System)

Chapter 13: The Person's Unit
- PROMOTING SAFETY AND COMFORT: The Person's Unit

Chapter 14: Safety
- Pandemics

Chapter 52: Urinary and Reproductive Disorders
- BODY STRUCTURE AND FUNCTION REVIEW: The Reproductive System
- Vaginitis
- Pelvic Inflammatory Disease
- Pelvic Organ Prolapse

Chapter 53: Mental Health Disorders
- FOCUS ON COMMUNICATION: Panic Disorder
- Box 53-9 Signs of Overdose
- PROMOTING SAFETY AND COMFORT: Care and Treatment

Chapter 55: Intellectual and Developmental Disabilities
- FOCUS ON COMMUNICATION: Down Syndrome
- ADHD

Chapter 58: Emergency Care
- Opioid Overdose
- Box 58-3 Stroke Emergency Care: FAST

Chapter 59: End-of-Life Care
- PROMOTING SAFETY AND COMFORT: Care of the Body After Death (Comfort)
- Caring for the Family

New Key Terms
- Advocate (Chapter 2)
- Analysis (Chapter 8)
- Anemia (Chapter 50)
- Avulsion (Chapter 41)
- Bath blanket (Chapter 22)
- Blanch (Chapter 42)
- Bloodborne pathogens (Chapter 17)
- Chain of command (Chapter 1)
- Consent (Chapter 5)
- Coping (Chapter 53)
- Deep (Chapter 9)
- Dignity (Chapter 2)
- Drug diversion (Chapter 5)
- Erythema (Chapter 42)
- Eupnea (Chapter 44)
- Exploitation (Chapter 5)
- Health system (Chapter 1)
- Hemiparesis (Chapter 49)
- Immobility (Chapter 35)
- Incident report (Chapter 14)
- Inferior (Chapter 9)
- Ischemic ulcer (Chapter 41)
- Mobility (Chapter 35)
- Occupied (Chapter 22)
- Paresis (Chapters 14)
- Preceptor (Chapter 3)
- Presbycusis (Chapter 47)
- Presbyopia (Chapter 47)
- Regulations (Chapter 1)

- Restraint (Chapter 16)
- Restraint alternative (Chapter 16)
- Risk factor (Chapter 7)
- Seclusion (Chapter 16)
- Suicidal ideation (Chapter 53)
- Superficial (Chapter 9)
- Superior (Chapter 9)
- Tolerance (Chapter 53)
- Unconscious (Chapter 14)
- Waterproof under-pad (Chapter 22)

New Key Abbreviations
- **ADHD** Attention-deficit/hyperactivity disorder
- **AFO** Ankle-foot orthosis
- **ANA** American Nurses Association
- **AUD** Alcohol use disorder
- **BiPAP** Bilevel positive airway pressure
- **BMI** Body mass index
- **CBT** Cognitive behavioral therapy
- **CPAP** Continuous positive airway pressure
- ***E. coli*** *Escherichia coli*
- **HHS** U.S. Department of Health & Human Services
- **PID** Pelvic inflammatory disease
- **PNS** Peripheral nervous system
- **POLST** Physician Orders for Life-Sustaining Treatment
- **SUD** Substance use disorder
- **TH** Thyroid hormone
- **WHO** World Health Organization

New Figures
- **Figure 8-7** 24-hour time. **A,** In 24-hour time, there are 4 digits. The first 2 are for the hours. The last 2 are for the minutes. A colon and AM and PM are not used.
- **Figure 8-8** From 1:00 PM to 11:00 PM, add 12 to the hours digit(s) to change from conventional time to 24-hour time. Remove the colon and PM.
- **Figure 9-2** A prefix is at the beginning of the word.
- **Figure 9-3** A root contains the basic meaning of the word.
- **Figure 9-4** A suffix is at the end of the word.
- **Figure 10-10** The nervous system is divided into the central nervous system and the peripheral nervous system.
- **Figure 11-10 B,** By 9 months, an infant sits without support.
- **Figure 16-13** Elbow splints (sleeves). **A,** Sleeve applied to an adult.
- **Figure 17-1** Bacteria vary in size and shape.
- **Figure 17-14** WHO's 5 Moments for Hand Hygiene.
- **Figure 17-15** How to read a disinfectant label.
- **Figure 17-18 A,** *BIOHAZARD* symbol.
- **Figure 18-2** Sample signs for Transmission-Based Precautions.
- **Figure 18-5** Applying (donning) gloves.

- **Figure 21-12 B,** Slide board. **C,** Air-assisted transfer device.
- **Figure 22-10** A hamper for used linens.
- **Figure 22-24** Occupied bed. **A,** The person is turned to the other side. Used linens are removed. (Gloves are removed and hand hygiene is performed before touching clean linens.) **B,** The clean bottom linens are pulled through and tucked in.
- **Figure 26-5** Applying a shirt that opens in the front with the person lying down.
- **Figure 27-12 C,** Commode with wheels.
- **Figure 27-17** A bladder scanner.
- **Figure 28-8** A leg bag.
- **Figure 28-18 A,** Condom catheter with an adhesive strip. **B,** Self-adhesive condom catheter.
- **Figure 31-1 D,** A "Nosey Cup."
- **Figure 32-5** Fractions measure parts of a whole.
- **Figure 32-6** Estimating intake using fractions.
- **Figure 34-1 D,** Non-contact infrared thermometer.
- **Figure 34-28** Blood pressure cuffs in different sizes.
- **Figure 39-1** A specimen is placed in a plastic bag with a *BIOHAZARD* label.
- **Figure 39-5** A 24-hour urine collection container and label.
- **Figure 42-1 B,** Healthy skin with dark pigment.
- **Figure 42-4** The forces of pressure and shear.
- **Figure 44-3 B,** O_2 concentration (SpO_2) is often measured with vital signs.
- **Figure 45-10** A CPAP device used for sleep apnea.
- **Figure 46-2 E,** Shoehorn.
- **Figure 48-8** Cellulitis
- **Figure 49-3** Major structures and lobes of the brain.
- **Figure 57-2** Some assisted living residents eat with other residents in the dining room. Others dine in their personal living areas.
- **Figure 58-21** Naloxone nasal spray is inserted into a nostril. The plunger is pressed to deliver the dose.

Body Structure and Function Review Boxes
Body Structure and Function Review boxes now include a section on *Changes With Aging*.

Review Questions
- True/False sections have been removed. Replacement questions are multiple choice.
- Questions have been added that evaluate the student's ability to apply knowledge.

FEATURES AND DESIGN
For features and design elements, see "Student Preface" on p. xii.

May this book serve you and your students well. We aim to provide current information for teaching and learning safe and effective care during a time of dynamic change in health care.

Leighann N. Remmert, BSN, MS, RN
Sheila A. Sorrentino, BSN, MA, MSN, PhD, RN

Student Preface

This book with special features (pp. xiii–xvii) was designed to help you learn. This preface gives study guidelines to help you use the book. To study effectively, remove distractions. Read in a quiet area. Allow yourself enough time to study thoroughly. Take breaks as you need them. Read the assignment *before* the information is presented in class.

Using a study system is helpful. The following steps can help you understand and retain (remember) more.
- Preview
- Question
- Read and record
- Review

PREVIEW

Preview the reading assignment for a few minutes. This gives an idea of what the assignment covers and how long it is. It also helps you recall what you already know about the subject. Preview the chapter title, objectives, key terms and abbreviations, and headings. (*Headings* are section titles.) Look at what boxes, tables, and figures are presented. Also, read through the review questions.

QUESTION

Questioning sets a purpose for reading. You consider what you should learn in the assignment. Questions should relate to how the information applies to care or possible test questions. Use the objectives, headings, and review questions as a guide.

READ AND RECORD

You read to:
- Gain new information.
- Connect new information to what you already know.
- Find answers to your questions.

As you read, we encourage you to underline or highlight important information. *Do not be afraid to write in this book.* Make notes in the margins, white (blank) spaces, or in a notebook. Taking notes as you read is very useful. You can organize important information in an outline or study guide. For example:

1 Main heading
  A Second level
  B Second level
    (1) Third level
    (2) Third level

You can also create diagrams or charts to show relationships or steps in a process. Also, note the boxes, tables, figures, or procedures to study again later. Add to your notes after the content is presented in class.

REVIEW

Finally, review. Reviewing is more about *when* to study rather than *what* to study. You decided *what* to study during your preview, question, and reading steps. It is best to study multiple times rather than all at once. For example, review the information right after the first study session, 1 week later, and before a quiz or test.

Review your notes (study guide) and ask questions until you are confident that you understand the information. Consider the "Question" step again. Did you learn what you were supposed to learn? For example:
- An objective is: "Explain how to protect the person's rights." A subheading in the section on resident rights is: "Personal Choice." Can you explain how to protect the person's rights related to personal choice?
- An objective is: "Perform the procedures described in this chapter." Are you comfortable performing the procedures? Or do you need more practice?
- Did you answer all of the review questions correctly?

Some students study well with another student or with a family member. Others prefer to study alone. If you review with another person, clearly communicate what you would like to review. You may need to write out the questions for the person to ask, if you have not already done so.

We hope you enjoy learning and your work. You and your work are important. You and the care you give make a difference in the person's life!

Leighann N. Remmert
Sheila A. Sorrentino

SPECIAL FEATURES

Chapter Openers

Each chapter contains a list of Objectives, Key Terms, and Key Abbreviations.
- *Objectives* are goals to accomplish while studying. The Objectives section lists what is presented in the chapter.
- *Key Terms* are important words and phrases used in the chapter. Each word or phrase is defined in the Key Terms section. In text, terms and definitions are identified with blue treatment. The term is *bold and italic.*
- *Key Abbreviations* are important abbreviations used in the chapter.

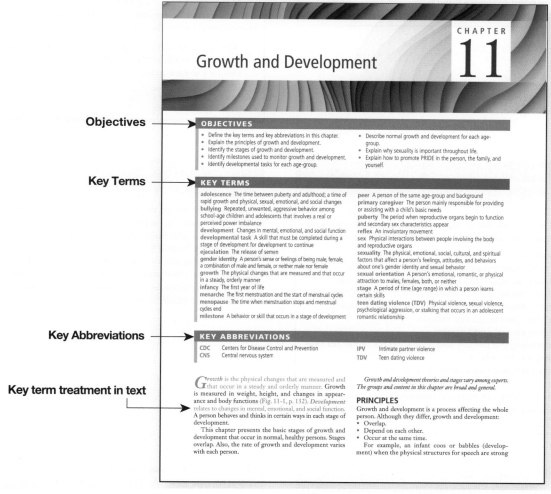

Focus Boxes

The following boxes highlight a certain part of the nursing assistant role. (See pp. xiv–xv for examples.)
- *Focus on Communication* boxes suggest what to say and questions to ask when interacting with patients, residents, visitors, and the nursing team.
- *Caring About Culture* boxes describe various cultural beliefs and practices that relate to health care.
- *Focus on Children and Older Persons* boxes identify needs and considerations of children and older persons (especially persons with Alzheimer's disease and other dementias).
- *Focus on Surveys* boxes list questions that surveyors may ask you or tasks they may observe you doing.
- *Focus on Long-Term Care and Home Care* boxes explain additional information needed to safely function in long-term care and home care settings.
- *Teamwork and Time Management* boxes suggest how to work with and help nursing team members.
- *Delegation Guidelines* boxes list information needed from the nurse and the care plan to perform a procedure. They also list the observations to report and record.
- *Promoting Safety and Comfort* boxes identify safety and comfort measures to consider when giving care.
- *Focus on Math* boxes explain math skills involved in various care measures and procedures.
- *Body Structure and Function Review* boxes review body systems as they relate to procedures and disorders. Boxes include a *Changes With Aging* section describing body system changes in older persons.

FOCUS ON COMMUNICATION
Emergency Care

Some illnesses and injuries are life-threatening. You may need to ask questions to find out what happened and the person's condition. For example:

- "Are you okay?"
- "Are you choking?"
- "Tell me what's wrong."
- "Where does it hurt?"
- "Can you point to where it hurts?"
- "Can you move your arms and legs?"

✿ CARING ABOUT CULTURE
Pain

Some people of *Mexico* and the *Philippines* may appear stoic in reaction to pain. In the *Philippines*, some people view pain as the will of God and believe that God will give strength to bear the pain.

In *Vietnam*, pain may be severe before some people request pain-relief measures. In *China*, showing emotion may be viewed as a weakness of character. If so, pain is often suppressed.

Non-English-speaking persons may have problems describing pain in English. The agency uses interpreters to communicate with the person.

Note: Each person is unique. A person may not follow all of the beliefs and practices of his or her culture. Follow the care plan.

Modified from D'Avanzo CE: Pocket guide to cultural health assessment, *ed 4, St Louis, 2008, Mosby.*

FOCUS ON CHILDREN AND OLDER PERSONS
Physical Restraint

Children
Cribs with raised rails are an age-appropriate safety measure for infants and toddlers. Cribs are not considered a restraint.

Older Persons
Dementia can affect behavior, mood, and personality. Symptoms such as aggression, agitation, delusions, and hallucinations can occur. Wandering is common. In Chapter 54 you will learn about causes and care measures for persons with dementia. Care measures include:

- Identifying causes and triggers
- Understanding the person and following his or her routine
- Providing a calm setting
- Using distraction or an activity that is meaningful to the person

Physical restraint can increase confusion and agitation. The person may try to get free. Serious injury and death are risks (p. 222).

FOCUS ON SURVEYS
Meeting Nutrition Needs

The health team develops a care plan to meet the person's nutrition needs. Surveyors may ask you:

- How food and fluid intake are observed and reported (Chapters 30 and 32).
- How eating ability is observed and reported.
- About the measures to prevent or meet changes in nutrition needs. Snacks and frequent meals are examples.
- About the goals for nutrition in the care plan.

FOCUS ON LONG-TERM CARE AND HOME CARE
Doors, Window Coverings, and Privacy Curtains

Long-Term Care
According to the CMS, each person has the right to full visual privacy. *Full visual privacy* is having the means to be completely free from public view while in bed. Ceiling-suspended privacy curtains help provide full visual privacy.

Home Care
Portable screens or room dividers help provide privacy in the home setting (Fig. 13-11). Decorated screens provide color and are pleasant to look at.

TEAMWORK AND TIME MANAGEMENT
Planning a Safe Move

Patients and residents are moved, turned, and re-positioned often. Some procedures are best done by at least 2 staff members.

Friendships are common among co-workers. And some working relationships are better than others. Do not just ask for help from or give help to friends or those with whom you work well. Include all co-workers. This includes new staff and those from other units.

DELEGATION GUIDELINES
Shaving

Facial shaving is a routine nursing task. Shaving mustaches and beards is not a routine nursing task. See "Caring for Mustaches and Beards" on p. 392. Shaving legs and underarms may be delegated to you.

To shave a person's face, you need this information from the nurse and the care plan.
- What shaver to use—safety razor or electric shaver
- If the person takes anticoagulant drugs
- When to shave the person
- What facial hair to shave
- If there are tender or sensitive areas on the person's face
- What observations to report and record:
  - Nicks (report at once)
  - Cuts (report at once)
  - Bleeding (report at once)
  - Irritation
- When to report observations
- What patient or resident concerns to report at once

PROMOTING SAFETY AND COMFORT
Hand Hygiene

Safety
Hand hygiene is very important. Your hands can pick up microbes from a person, place, or thing and transfer them to other people, places, or things. Know when to practice hand hygiene (see Box 17-3 and p. 246). Be careful and thorough.

Comfort
You will practice hand hygiene frequently during your shift. Hand lotions and hand creams help prevent chapping and dry skin. Use an agency-approved lotion or cream.

FOCUS ON MATH
Removing Indwelling Catheters

To remove indwelling catheters, you must know how to measure liquid using a syringe. Syringes are marked in milliliters (mL). An mL is a unit used to measure liquid. Read the syringe at the top of the plunger. See Figure 28-16.

The amount of water removed should equal the amount injected. The nurse tells you the amount used for balloon inflation. Subtract the amount removed from the amount injected. If there is a difference, tell the nurse before removing the catheter. For example:
- *An indwelling catheter balloon is filled with 10 mL. You remove 7 mL. The difference is 3 mL. Do not remove the catheter. Call for the nurse.*

$$10 \text{ mL} - 7 \text{ mL} = 3 \text{ mL}$$

- *An indwelling catheter balloon is filled with 10 mL. You remove 10 mL. The difference is 0 mL. You can safely remove the catheter.*

$$10 \text{ mL} - 10 \text{ mL} = 0 \text{ mL}$$

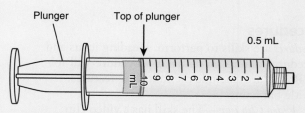

FIGURE 28-16 A syringe is read at the top of the plunger. This syringe measures 10 mL. Short lines mark 0.5 (one-half) mL measurements.

BODY STRUCTURE AND FUNCTION REVIEW
The Teeth and Gums

Structure and Function
The *teeth* cut, chop, and grind food into small bits for swallowing and digestion. A tooth has 3 main parts (Fig. 23-1):
- The *crown* is the outer part.
- The *neck* is surrounded by *gums (gingivae).*
- The *root* fits into the bone of the lower or upper jaw.

Teeth are covered with *enamel.* Enamel is a hard, outer coating. Below the enamel is a softer layer called *dentin.* The inner tooth contains nerves and blood vessels.

Changes With Aging
With age, *primary teeth* (baby teeth) are replaced with *permanent teeth* (adult teeth). Normally, adults have 32 permanent teeth.

Older persons may have decreased saliva production, loss of teeth, and difficulty chewing and swallowing. The number of taste buds decreases. Changes with aging can affect the person's appetite, eating, and speaking.

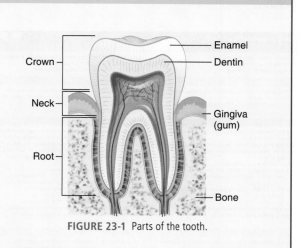

FIGURE 23-1 Parts of the tooth.

Boxes, Tables, and Figures

- *Boxes and tables* list rules, principles, guidelines, signs and symptoms, nursing measures, and other information useful for study.
- *Figures* include color illustrations (drawings) and photographs. They visually present key ideas, concepts, and procedure steps.
- Callouts for boxes, tables, and figures are in magenta font.

CHAPTER 9   Medical Terminology   107

Defining Medical Terms

Medical terms are formed by combining word elements. Remember, prefixes are at the beginning. Suffixes are at the end. A root can be combined with prefixes, roots, and suffixes. Some words have only a prefix or suffix.

The combining vowel of a root is usually used between roots and when the suffix begins with a consonant. When the suffix begins with a vowel (a, e, i, o, u), the combining vowel is not used.

To define a term, separate the word into its elements (Table 9-4). To read the meaning:
1 Begin with the suffix. Read the meaning of the suffix.
2 Go to the beginning of the word. Read the meaning of each word part up to the suffix.

For some terms with only a prefix and suffix, it is easier to read the meaning of the prefix first. Then read the meaning of the suffix.

← Table

TABLE 9-4	Defining Medical Terms	
Medical Term	Word Elements	Definition
Aphasia	*a-* (without, lack of) + *-phasia* (speaking) [prefix] [suffix]	Lack of speaking ability
Cyanosis	*cyan-* (blue) + *-osis* (condition) [prefix] [suffix]	Condition of having a bluish color
Dysphagia	*dys-* (difficult) + *-phagia* (swallowing) [prefix] [suffix]	Difficulty swallowing
Dyspnea	*dys-* (difficult, painful) + *-pnea* (breathing) [prefix] [suffix]	Difficult or painful breathing
Endocarditis	*endo-* (inner) + *card* (heart) + *-itis* (inflammation) [prefix] [root] [suffix]	Inflammation of the inner part of the heart
Gastrostomy	*gastr* (stomach) + *-ostomy* (creation of an opening) [root] [suffix]	A surgically created opening in the stomach
Mastectomy	*mast* (breast) + *-ectomy* (excision or removal) [root] [suffix]	Removal of a breast
Nephritis	*nephr* (kidney) + *-itis* (inflammation) [root] [suffix]	Inflammation of the kidney
Oliguria	*olig-* (scant, small amount) + *-uria* (urine) [prefix] [suffix]	A small amount of urine

ABDOMINAL REGIONS

The abdomen can be divided into 4 quadrants. *Quad* means 4. The quadrants are used to describe the location of body structures, pain, or discomfort. The quadrants are shown in Figure 9-5. They are:

Callouts in magenta font ⟶

- Right upper quadrant (RUQ)—contains much of the liver, the gallbladder, part of the pancreas, and parts of the small and large intestines
- Left upper quadrant (LUQ)—contains the rest of the liver, the stomach, the spleen, the rest of the pancreas, and parts of the small and large intestines
- Right lower quadrant (RLQ)—contains parts of the small and large intestines, the appendix, and part of the bladder
- Left lower quadrant (LLQ)—contains parts of the small and large intestines and part of the bladder

You will learn about the body structures found in these areas in Chapter 10.

Figure →

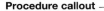

FIGURE 9-5   The 4 abdominal quadrants. (From Chabner D-E: *The language of medicine*, ed 12, St Louis, 2021, Elsevier.)

Procedures

Procedures are skills to perform. Heading icons and procedure callouts alert that a procedure will follow. Procedures include the following features.

- Title bar icons:
  - *Video Clip icon*—The skill has a video clip available on-line on *Evolve Student Learning Resources.*
  - *Video icon*—The skill has a procedure included in *Mosby's® Nursing Assistant Video Skills 4.0.*
- Procedures are divided into *Quality of Life*, *Pre-Procedure*, *Procedure*, and *Post-Procedure* sections. The *Quality of Life* section lists 6 simple courtesies that show respect for the person.

Heading icon ⟶   ▮▮▶ TRANSFER/GAIT BELTS

A *transfer belt (gait belt)* is a device applied around the waist and used to support a person who is unsteady or disabled (Fig. 15-10). It helps prevent falls and injuries.

- When used to transfer a person (Chapter 21), it is called a *transfer belt.*
- When used to help a person walk (Chapter 35), it is called a *gait belt.*

The belt goes around the waist. Grasp the belt from underneath for support. Use an upward grasp (see Fig. 15-10). A downward grasp at the top of the belt is not secure. If the belt has handles, grasp the belt by the handles (Fig. 15-11).

See *Promoting Safety and Comfort: Transfer/Gait Belts.*

Procedure callout ⟶ See procedure: *Using a Transfer/Gait Belt.*

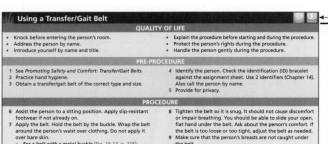

FIGURE 15-10   Transfer/gait belt. The buckle is off-center. Excess strap is tucked into the belt. The nursing assistant grasps the belt from underneath with an upward grasp.

Using a Transfer/Gait Belt

QUALITY OF LIFE

- Knock before entering the person's room.
- Address the person by name.
- Introduce yourself by name and title.
- Explain the procedure before starting and during the procedure.
- Protect the person's rights during the procedure.
- Handle the person gently during the procedure.

PRE-PROCEDURE

1 See *Promoting Safety and Comfort: Transfer/Gait Belts.*
2 Practice hand hygiene.
3 Obtain a transfer/gait belt of the correct type and size.
4 Identify the person. Check the identification (ID) bracelet against the assignment sheet. Use 2 identifiers (Chapter 14). Also call the person by name.
5 Provide for privacy.

PROCEDURE

6 Assist the person to a sitting position. Apply slip-resistant footwear if not already on.
7 Apply the belt. Hold the belt by the buckle. Wrap the belt around the person's waist over clothing. Do not apply it over bare skin.
  a For a belt with a metal buckle (Fig. 15-13, p. 216):
    1) Insert the belt's metal tip into the buckle. Pass the belt through the side with the teeth first (see Fig. 15-13, A).
    2) Bring the belt tip across the front of the buckle. Insert the tip through the buckle's smooth side (see Fig. 15-13, B).
  b For a belt with a quick release buckle, push the belt ends together to secure the buckle.
8 Tighten the belt so it is snug. It should not cause discomfort or impair breathing. You should be able to slide your open, flat hand under the belt. Ask about the person's comfort. If the belt is too loose or too tight, adjust the belt as needed.
9 Make sure that the person's breasts are not caught under the belt.
10 Place the buckle off-center in the front (see Fig. 15-13, C) or off-center in the back (see Fig. 15-12) for the person's comfort. A quick release buckle is in the back, out of the person's reach. The buckle is not over the spine.
11 Tuck any excess strap into the belt (see Fig. 15-13, C).
12 Complete the transfer (Chapter 21) or ambulation procedure (Chapter 35). Grasp the belt from underneath with 2 hands (see Fig. 15-10). Use an upward grasp. Or grasp the belt by the handles.

POST-PROCEDURE

13 Remove the belt after the procedure in step 12. The person is not left alone wearing the belt.
  a For a belt with a metal buckle:
    1) Bring the belt strap back through the buckle's smooth side.
    2) Pull the belt through the side with the teeth.
  b For a belt with a quick release buckle, push inward on the quick release buttons (see Fig. 15-12).
  c Remove the belt from the person's waist. Do not drag the belt across the back or waist.
14 Provide for comfort. (See the inside of the back cover.)
15 Place the call light and other needed items within reach.
16 Follow the care plan and the person's preferences for privacy measures to maintain. Leaving the privacy curtain, window coverings, and door open or closed are examples.
17 Complete a safety check of the room. (See the inside of the back cover.)
18 Return the transfer/gait belt to its proper place.
19 Practice hand hygiene.
20 Report and record your care and observations.

Title bar icons:
- *Video Clip*
- *Video*

Procedure sections:
- *Quality of Life*
- *Pre-Procedure*
- *Procedure*
- *Post-Procedure*

Focus on PRIDE: The Person, Family, and Yourself

This feature builds on chapter content to promote *pride* in the person, family, and yourself. The first letter of each section spells *PRIDE*.

- *Personal and Professional Responsibility*—how to have pride in yourself through personal and professional behaviors and development.
- *Rights and Respect*—how to promote the rights of others and respect them as persons with dignity and value.
- *Independence and Social Interaction*—ways to help the person retain or attain independence and interact socially with others.
- *Delegation and Teamwork*—how to work efficiently with and help nursing team members.
- *Ethics and Laws*—laws affecting nursing care and doing the right thing when dealing with patients, residents, and co-workers.

Each box ends with a *Focus on PRIDE: Application* section. Questions are intended for personal thought or classroom discussion. They relate to how you will apply the information in Focus on PRIDE.

Focus on PRIDE

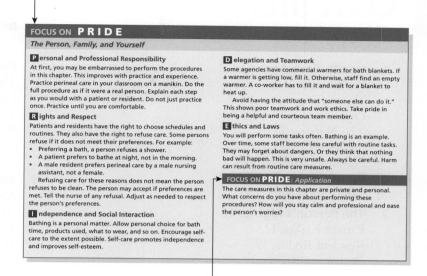

Focus on PRIDE: Application

Review Questions

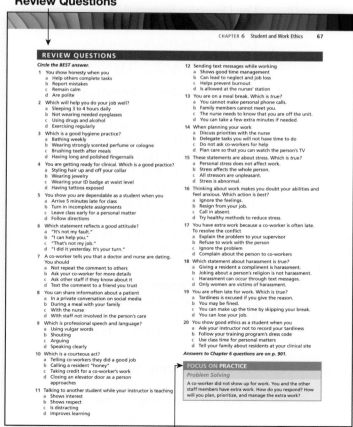

Focus on Practice: Problem Solving

Review Questions

Review Questions are multiple-choice questions at the end of every chapter. They are useful as study guides to review what you have learned. Use them to study for a test or for the competency evaluation. Answers are at the back of the book. See p. 901.

Each chapter ends with a *Focus on Practice: Problem Solving* scenario. A situation is presented that you may encounter as a student or in the work setting. For classroom discussion or self-study, questions relate to what you should do, how you should act, or how you can improve the situation.

Contents

Health Care Agencies

OBJECTIVES

- Define the key terms and key abbreviations in this chapter.
- Describe the purposes, types, and organization of health care agencies.
- Describe the health team and nursing team members.
- Describe the nursing service department.
- Describe 5 nursing care patterns.

- Describe the programs that pay for health care.
- Explain how government agencies and health care agencies ensure safe, quality care.
- Explain your role in meeting standards.
- Explain how to promote PRIDE in the person, the family, and yourself.

KEY TERMS

acute illness An illness of rapid onset and short duration; the person is expected to recover

admission The official entry of a person into a health care setting

assisted living residence (ALR) Provides housing, personal care, support services, health care, and social activities in a home-like setting to persons needing some help with daily activities

chain of command The order of authority in an agency

chronic illness A long-term health condition that may not have a cure; it can be controlled and complications prevented with proper treatment

discharge The official departure of a person from a health care setting

health system A coordinated network of health care agencies and services

health team The many health care workers whose skills and knowledge focus on the person's total care; interdisciplinary health care team

hospice A health care agency or program that promotes comfort and quality of life for the dying person and the person's family

licensed practical nurse (LPN) A nurse who has completed a practical nursing program and has passed a licensing test; called *licensed vocational nurse (LVN)* in California and Texas

licensed vocational nurse (LVN) See "licensed practical nurse (LPN)"

nursing assistant A person who has passed a nursing assistant training and competency evaluation program (NATCEP); performs delegated nursing tasks under the supervision of a licensed nurse

nursing team Those who provide nursing care—RNs, LPNs/LVNs, and nursing assistants

registered nurse (RN) A nurse who has completed a 2-, 3-, or 4-year nursing program and has passed a licensing test

regulations Rules made by government agencies

survey The formal review of an agency through the collection of facts and observations

surveyor A person who collects information by observing and asking questions

terminal illness An illness or injury from which the person will not likely recover; death is expected

KEY ABBREVIATIONS

ALR	Assisted living residence
APRN	Advanced practice registered nurse
DON	Director of nursing
HHS	U.S. Department of Health & Human Services
LPN	Licensed practical nurse

LVN	Licensed vocational nurse
OSHA	Occupational Safety and Health Administration
PPS	Prospective Payment Systems
RN	Registered nurse
SNF	Skilled nursing facility

The health care industry is one of the largest providers of jobs in the United States. Working in health care offers many opportunities. Nursing assistants are a valuable part of the health care team. You will learn about the roles and functions of nursing assistants in Chapter 3.

Persons of all ages need health care. The setting and reason for care vary. The *person* is always the focus of care.

PURPOSES

The purposes of health care are:

- *Health promotion and disease prevention.* The goal is to reduce the risk of physical or mental illness. People learn about life-style practices that affect health—diet, exercise, sleep needs, and risk behaviors such as smoking and alcohol use. *Screenings* check for diseases and health conditions before signs and symptoms are present. *Vaccines* prevent some infectious diseases (Chapter 17).
- *Detection and treatment of disease.* Physical exams and diagnostic tests are done. Treatment may involve life-style changes, drugs, surgeries, or other therapies. People learn how to manage and cope with health problems.
- *Rehabilitation and restorative care.* This involves returning persons to their highest desired level of physical and mental function and to independence. *Independence* means not relying on or needing care from others. The person learns or re-learns skills needed to live, work, and enjoy life. Maintaining function is important.

Student Learning

Agencies are often learning sites for students. Students assist in the purposes of health care. They are involved with and provide care.

TYPES OF AGENCIES

Health care agencies vary in services, size, and staff (Box 1-1). Some have a narrow focus. A certain health problem or age-group is the focus of care. Or a certain service is provided. Other agencies have many purposes and services.

Nursing assistants work in many settings. Most work in the following agencies.

BOX 1-1	Types of Health Care Agencies

- Doctors' offices and clinics—routine appointments, preventive care, treatment of minor injuries and illnesses, management of chronic illnesses.
- Acute care agencies—treatment of serious and urgent injuries and illnesses. Hospitals and urgent care centers are examples.
- Ambulatory surgery centers—surgical care not requiring an over-night stay.
- Rehabilitation and sub-acute care agencies—for persons who need rehabilitation or complex medical care when hospital care is no longer needed.
- Long-term care settings—for persons who cannot care for themselves at home. Nursing centers and assisted-living residences are examples.
- Home care agencies—services for persons living at home.
- Hospices—end-of-life care.
- Centers for persons with specific needs:
  - Centers for persons with mental health disorders
  - Centers for persons with intellectual and developmental disabilities
  - Memory care centers
  - Dialysis centers
  - Cancer treatment centers
  - Drug and alcohol treatment centers
  - Crisis centers for rape, abuse, suicide, and other emergencies

Hospitals

Hospitals provide emergency care, surgery, nursing care, x-ray procedures and treatments, and laboratory testing. Respiratory, physical, occupational, speech, and other therapies are provided.

A high level of medical and nursing care and close observation are needed. Care is costly. The length of stay is usually short.

Persons cared for in hospitals are called *patients*. Hospital care is either in-patient or out-patient.

- *In-patient care* is health care a person receives when admitted to an agency. *Admission* is the official entry of a person into a health care setting. At least 1 over-night stay is involved. See Figure 1-1.
- *Out-patient (ambulatory) care* includes medical or surgical care received when a person is not admitted to an agency. The person does not stay over-night.

People of all ages need hospital care. They have babies, surgery, physical and mental health disorders, and broken bones. Some are dying.

Hospitals are commonly divided into *units*. Each unit has a different focus. Surgical, medical, intensive (critical) care, pediatric, and mental health units are examples. Operating and recovery areas, emergency room, and maternity department are others. Some hospitals only treat certain illnesses, injuries, or age-groups.

Hospital patients have acute, chronic, or terminal illnesses.

- *Acute illness* is an illness of rapid onset and short duration. The person is expected to recover. A heart attack is an example.
- *Chronic illness* is a long-term health condition that may not have a cure. The illness can be controlled and complications prevented with proper treatment. Arthritis is an example.
- *Terminal illness* is an illness or injury from which the person will not likely recover. Death is expected (Chapter 59). Cancers not responding to treatment are examples.

Discharge occurs when the person can be treated in another setting safely. *Discharge* is the official departure of a person from a health care setting. The person returns home or goes to another agency after hospital care.

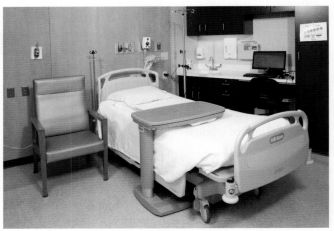

FIGURE 1-1 A hospital room.

Rehabilitation and Sub-Acute Care Agencies

After a hospital stay, some people are too sick or disabled to go home. Along with rehabilitation, complex equipment and care measures are often needed. Rehabilitation and sub-acute care agencies provide care for such persons. Afterward, some persons are able to return home. Others need long-term care.

Some hospitals and long-term care centers have rehabilitation and sub-acute care units. Others are separate agencies.

Long-Term Care Centers

Long-term care centers are designed to meet the needs of persons who cannot care for themselves at home. Care needs range from simple to complex.

Persons in long-term care centers are called *residents*. They are not *patients*. The center is their short- or long-term home. Short-term residents are usually recovering from illness or surgery after being in a hospital. They need care until able to return home. Other residents need care until the end of life (Chapter 59).

Most residents are older. Many have chronic diseases, poor nutrition, memory problems, or poor health. Not all residents are old. Some are disabled from birth defects, accidents, or disease.

Nursing Centers. A *nursing center (nursing facility, nursing home)* provides medical, nursing, dietary, recreation, and social services. Rehabilitation services (physical, occupational, speech-language) are also available.

Skilled care refers to nursing or rehabilitation services that must be provided by licensed nurses and therapists. Wound care, intravenous (IV) therapy, urinary catheter care, and physical therapy are examples. A *skilled nursing facility (SNF)* provides skilled care.

Memory Care Units. A memory care unit is designed for persons with Alzheimer's disease and other dementias (Chapter 54). Such persons suffer increasing memory loss and confusion. Over time, they cannot tend to simple personal needs. Wandering is common. The unit is usually closed off from other parts of the center. The closed unit provides a safe setting where residents can wander freely.

Assisted Living Residences. An *assisted living residence (ALR)* provides housing, personal care, support services, health care, and social activities in a home-like setting to persons needing some help with daily activities. (Chapter 57). Some ALRs are part of nursing centers or retirement communities (Chapter 12).

The person has a room, an apartment, or a cottage. Three meals a day and 24-hour supervision are provided. So are housekeeping, laundry, social, recreational, transportation, and some health care services. Help is given with personal care and drugs.

Mental Health Centers

Some persons have problems with life events. Others present dangers to themselves or others because of how they think and behave. Out-patient mental health care is common. Some need short-term or long-term in-patient care.

Home Care Agencies

Home care (home health care) agencies provide services to people where they live. Hospitals, health systems, public health departments, and private businesses offer home care. A variety of services are available. Health teaching, nursing care, physical therapy, supervision, and food services are examples.

People of all ages need home health care. Some persons need end-of-life care at home.

Hospices

A *hospice* is a health care agency or program that promotes comfort and quality of life for the dying person and the person's family. Hospice patients no longer respond to treatments aimed at cures. Usually they have less than 6 months to live.

The physical, emotional, social, and spiritual needs of the person and family are met. The focus is on comfort, not cure. Children and pets can visit. Family and friends can assist with care.

Hospice care is provided by hospitals, nursing centers, and home care and hospice agencies.

Health Systems

A *health system* involves a coordinated network of health care agencies and services. A system usually has hospitals, nursing centers, home care agencies, hospice settings, and doctors' offices (Fig. 1-2, p. 4). Surgery centers, ambulance services, and medical supply stores are other common parts. The system serves a community or larger region.

The goal is to meet all health care needs. A person uses system providers as needed. See Box 1-2 for an example.

BOX 1-2 **Using a Health System**

A local health system includes:

- 3 hospitals
- Doctors' offices
- A home care service
- An ambulance service
- A medical supply store
- A nursing center

A patient sees a hospital emergency room doctor because of sudden dizziness and right-sided weakness. Admitted to the hospital, the patient was having a stroke.

After 2 weeks of rehabilitation, the patient returns home by ambulance. The family obtains needed care items from the medical supply store—hospital bed, wheelchair, and other items.

The home care agency arranges for the patient's nursing needs. A nursing assistant will help with daily hygiene and grooming needs. A nurse will visit 3 times a week.

Because of another stroke, the patient is taken to the hospital by ambulance. After hospital care and rehabilitation, the patient and family agree to nursing center care.

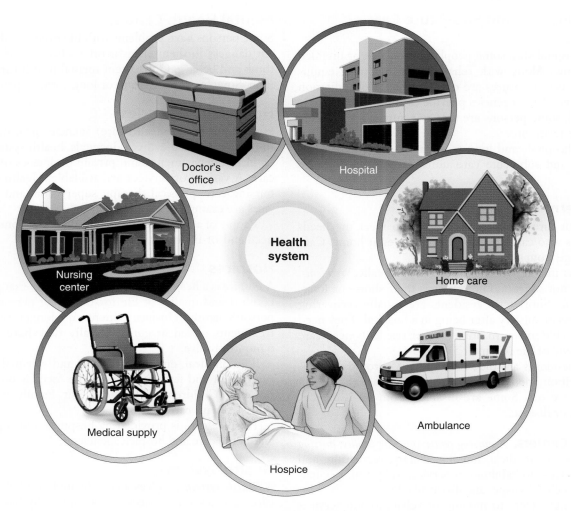

FIGURE 1-2 Common parts of a health system.

ORGANIZATION

Figure 1-3 shows a sample organizational chart for a health care agency. The chart outlines the agency's chain of command. *Chain of command* is the order of authority in an agency. It communicates the different levels of responsibility and oversight. It directs who makes decisions, who to report to, and who to ask for help.

An agency has a governing group called the *board of trustees* or *board of directors*. The board makes policies (p. 9). The focus is safe, quality care at the lowest possible cost. Local, state, and federal laws are followed.

An *administrator (president, chief executive officer [CEO])* manages the agency. This person reports directly to the board. Directors or department heads manage certain areas (departments). For example, a director of nursing (DON) manages the nursing department (p. 7). A human resources director handles personnel matters such as hiring staff. A social services director meets the social needs of the person and family. Department directors report to the administrator (president, CEO).

See *Focus on Long-Term Care and Home Care: Organization.*

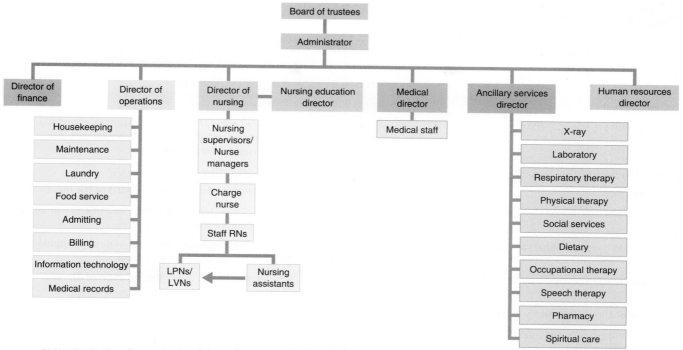

FIGURE 1-3 Sample organizational chart of a health care agency. Titles, departments, and structures vary among states and agencies.

The Health Team

The *health team* (*interdisciplinary health care team*) involves the many health care workers whose skills and knowledge focus on the person's total care. Many team members may be involved in the care of each person. See Table 1-1 (p. 6).

Coordinated care is needed. This means the team communicates and works together well. There is a common focus and goal. The person is the focus of care. The goal is to provide quality care.

See *Focus on Communication: The Health Team.*

FOCUS ON LONG-TERM CARE AND HOME CARE

Organization

Long-Term Care

Nursing centers are usually owned by an individual or a corporation. Some are owned by county or state health departments. The U.S. Department of Veterans Affairs (Veterans Administration; VA) also has nursing centers.

By law, nursing centers must have a doctor as a medical director. This doctor consults with the staff about medical problems not handled by a resident's doctor. Guidance is given about resident care policies and programs.

FOCUS ON COMMUNICATION

The Health Team

Team members have different roles. They communicate often. You may have questions or concerns about a person's care. A registered nurse (RN) usually coordinates care among team members. Tell the nurse. The nurse will communicate with other health team members.

TABLE 1-1	Health Team Members
Title	**Description**
Activities director/recreational therapist	Plans and directs recreation treatment programs to help maintain or improve a person's physical, social, and emotional well-being.
Audiologist	Treats hearing, balance, and ear problems.
Cleric (clergy)	Assists with spiritual needs.
Clinical nurse specialist (CNS)	Advanced practice registered nurse (APRN) who consults in a specialty. Geriatrics, critical care, diabetes, rehabilitation, and wound care are examples. Can prescribe drugs in some states.
Dental hygienist	Cleans teeth and provides preventive care.
Dentist	Treats problems with the teeth, gums, and related parts of the mouth.
Dietitian and nutritionist	Assesses and plans for nutritional needs to promote health and manage disease. Teaches about diet and healthy eating.
Home health aide/personal care aide	Assists persons in home settings with daily activities—laundry, bedmaking, grocery shopping, meals, hygiene, dressing, and grooming.
Licensed practical/vocational nurse (LPN/LVN)	Provides nursing care and gives drugs under the direction of RNs and doctors.
Medical or clinical laboratory technologist/technician	Collects specimens. Performs tests on blood, urine, and other body fluids.
Medical records specialist	Maintains the quality and security of medical records. Codes patient information for billing purposes.
Medication assistant-certified (MA-C)	Gives drugs as allowed by state law under the supervision of a licensed nurse.
Nurse practitioner (NP)	An APRN with specialized graduate education who diagnoses and treats common health problems. May prescribe some drugs and treatments.
Nursing assistant	Assists nurses and gives care. Supervised by a licensed nurse.
Occupational therapist (OT)	Assists persons to learn or retain skills needed for daily living and working.
Occupational therapy assistant	Performs tasks and services as directed by an OT.
Optometrist	Diagnoses and treats vision problems and eye disorders.
Pharmacist	Fills drug orders and advises about safe prescription use. Consults with doctors and nurses about drug actions and interactions.
Physical therapist (PT)	Assists ill and injured persons with movement, pain management, and rehabilitation.
Physical therapy assistant (PTA)	Performs tasks and services as directed by a PT.
Physician (doctor)	Diagnoses and treats diseases and injuries.
Physician's assistant (PA)	Performs exams, diagnoses, and provides treatments under a doctor's direction.
Podiatrist	Prevents, diagnoses, and treats foot, ankle, and lower leg problems.
Radiographer/radiologic technologist	Takes images using x-rays and other equipment.
Registered nurse (RN)	Provides and coordinates nursing care—assesses; analyzes data and identifies problems; and plans, implements, and evaluates nursing care. Supervises LPNs/LVNs and nursing assistants.
Respiratory therapist	Assists in treating disorders that affect the lungs. Gives respiratory treatments and therapies.
Social worker	Deals with social, emotional, and environmental issues affecting illness and recovery. Coordinates community agencies to assist the person and family.
Speech-language pathologist/speech therapist	Assesses and treats communication and swallowing disorders.

Modified from Bureau of Labor Statistics, U.S. Department of Labor: Occupational outlook handbook, *September 6, 2023.*

Nursing Service

Nursing service is a large department (see Fig. 1-3). The director of nursing (DON) is a registered nurse (RN). (*Director of nursing services, chief nurse executive, vice president of nursing,* and *vice president of patient services* are some other titles.) Usually a bachelor's or higher degree is required. The DON is responsible for the entire nursing staff and the nursing care given.

Nursing supervisors and nurse managers (usually RNs) over-see a nursing unit (p. 2) or certain nursing function. Staff development, infection control, and quality improvement are examples of nursing functions. Nursing supervisors (nurse managers) are responsible for all nursing care and the actions of nursing staff in their areas.

Nursing units usually have RN *charge nurses* for each shift. LPNs/LVNs can be charge nurses in some states. The charge nurse is responsible for all nursing care and nursing staff actions during that shift. Staff RNs report to the charge nurse. LPNs/LVNs report to staff RNs or to the charge nurse. You report to the nurse supervising your work.

Nursing education (staff development) is part of nursing service. Nursing education staff:
- Plan and present educational programs (in-service programs). This includes those that meet federal and state educational requirements.
- Provide new and changing information.
- Show how to use new equipment and supplies.
- Review policies and procedures on a regular basis.
- Educate and train nursing assistants.
- Conduct new employee orientation programs.

THE NURSING TEAM

The *nursing team* involves those who provide nursing care—RNs, LPNs/LVNs, and nursing assistants. All focus on the physical, social, emotional, and spiritual needs of the person and family.

Registered Nurses

A *registered nurse (RN)* has completed a 2-, 3-, or 4-year nursing program and has passed a licensing test.
- Community college programs—2 years
- Hospital-based diploma programs—2 or 3 years
- College or university programs—4 years

Graduates take a licensing test offered by their state board of nursing. They receive a license and become *registered* after passing the test. RNs must have a license recognized by the state in which they work.

RNs perform assessments, analyze data, and identify problems. Then they plan, implement, and evaluate nursing care (Chapter 8). They provide care and delegate (Chapter 4) nursing care and tasks to the nursing team.

RNs teach the person and family how to improve health and independence.

RNs receive and carry out (implement) the doctor's orders. They may delegate care to other nursing team members. RNs do not prescribe treatments or drugs. However, RNs can become *clinical nurse specialists* or *nurse practitioners.* Depending on state law, these RNs have limited diagnosing and prescribing functions.

RNs work as charge or staff nurses, nurse supervisors or managers, DONs, agency administrators, and instructors. Those and other career options depend on education, abilities, and experience.

Licensed Practical Nurses and Licensed Vocational Nurses

A *licensed practical nurse (LPN)* has completed a practical nursing program and has passed a licensing test. Hospitals, community colleges, vocational schools, and technical schools offer programs. Programs are 10, 12, or 18 months long. Some high schools offer 2-year programs.

Graduates take a licensing test for practical nursing. After passing the test, they have a license to practice and the title of *licensed practical nurse. Licensed vocational nurse (LVN)* is used in California and Texas. LPNs/LVNs must have a license recognized by the state where they work.

LPNs/LVNs are supervised by RNs and doctors. They have fewer responsibilities and functions than RNs do. They need less supervision when the person's condition is stable and care is simple. They assist RNs with acutely ill persons and complex procedures.

Nursing Assistants

A *nursing assistant* has passed a nursing assistant training and competency evaluation program (NATCEP). Nursing assistants perform delegated nursing tasks under the supervision of a licensed nurse. Nursing assistants are discussed in Chapter 3.

STAFFING

Agencies must provide enough nursing staff to safely provide care. *Nurse staffing* describes the number and type of nursing team members assigned to care for a group of patients or residents for a certain amount of time (work shift). Work shifts vary—8-, 10-, and 12-hour shifts are common. The DON and nursing supervisors (nurse managers) are responsible for ensuring safe staffing.

Agencies use different methods to plan nurse staffing. Decisions are usually based on the number of patients or residents needing care and the care needs or *acuity levels* of the persons needing care. *Acuity* relates to the severity of illness and the level of care required. Education and experience of staff, safety and quality goals, and cost are other factors.

NURSING CARE PATTERNS

Agencies organize and provide nursing care in different ways. Called *nursing care patterns* or *care delivery models*, the system used depends on how many persons need care, their care needs, staff abilities, and cost. The following are some patterns (models) used in different health care settings (Fig. 1-4).

- *Functional nursing* focuses on tasks and jobs. Each nursing team member has certain tasks and jobs to do. For example, 1 nurse gives all drugs. Another gives all treatments. Nursing assistants give baths, make beds, and serve meals.
- *Team nursing* involves a team of nursing staff led by an RN "team leader." The team leader delegates care to other nurses and nursing assistants. (Chapter 4 explains the delegation process.) Decisions about care depend on the person's needs and team member abilities. Team members report observations and the care given to the team leader.
- *Primary nursing* involves total care. The primary nurse (an RN) is responsible for the person's total care. The nursing team assists as needed. The RN gives nursing care and makes discharge plans. The RN teaches and counsels the person and family.

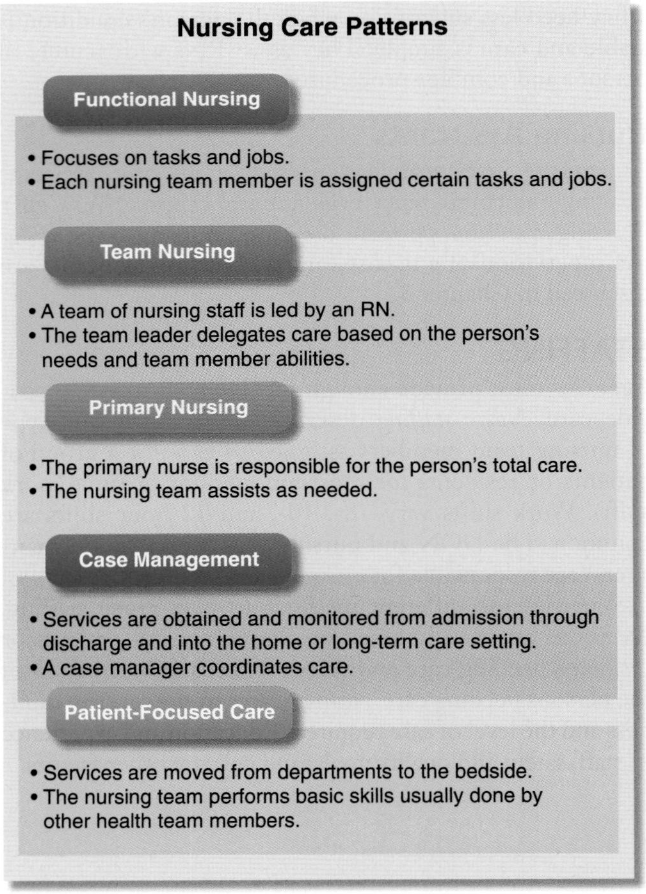

- *Case management* is when a nursing case manager coordinates care from admission through discharge and into the home or long-term care setting. The case manager communicates with the health team, insurance companies, and community agencies. Case managers work with certain doctors, certain age-groups, or persons with certain health problems. Heart disease, diabetes, and cancer are examples.
- *Patient-focused care* is when services are moved from departments to the bedside. Besides nursing care, the nursing team performs basic skills usually done by other health team members. For example, an RN draws a blood sample. This reduces the number of staff involved and the care costs.

PAYING FOR HEALTH CARE

Health care is costly. Some people avoid health care because they cannot pay. Others pay doctor bills but go without food or drugs. Health insurance covers some costs. Rarely are all costs covered.

These programs help pay for health care.
- *Private insurance* is bought by individuals and families.
- *Group insurance* is bought by groups or organizations for individuals. This is often an employee benefit.
- *Medicare* is a federal program for persons 65 years of age or older. Some younger people with certain disabilities qualify. Persons of any age with end-stage renal disease (kidney failure) also qualify (Chapter 52). Part A is for hospital, SNF, hospice, and home care costs. Part B is for doctors' services, preventive care, ambulance services, medical supplies, mental health care, and some drugs. Part B is voluntary. The person pays a monthly premium.
- *Medicaid* is jointly funded by the federal government and the states. People and families with low incomes usually qualify. It covers children and older, blind, and disabled persons.
- *Health Insurance Marketplace*® is a service that helps people shop for and enroll in affordable health insurance. The "Marketplace" or "exchange" began as part of the *Patient Protection and Affordable Care Act of 2010*. This act is commonly called the *Affordable Care Act (ACA)* or "Obamacare," after President Barack Obama. The federal government operates the Marketplace for most states. Some states run their own Marketplaces.

See *Promoting Safety and Comfort: Paying for Health Care.*

Nursing Care Patterns

Functional Nursing
- Focuses on tasks and jobs.
- Each nursing team member is assigned certain tasks and jobs.

Team Nursing
- A team of nursing staff is led by an RN.
- The team leader delegates care based on the person's needs and team member abilities.

Primary Nursing
- The primary nurse is responsible for the person's total care.
- The nursing team assists as needed.

Case Management
- Services are obtained and monitored from admission through discharge and into the home or long-term care setting.
- A case manager coordinates care.

Patient-Focused Care
- Services are moved from departments to the bedside.
- The nursing team performs basic skills usually done by other health team members.

FIGURE 1-4 Nursing care patterns.

PROMOTING SAFETY AND COMFORT
Paying for Health Care

Safety
Some conditions can be prevented with proper care. Medicare pays a lower rate for such conditions if they are acquired during a hospital stay. Pressure injuries (Chapter 42) and certain types of falls, trauma, and infections are examples. You must help prevent such conditions.

Prospective Payment Systems

The Centers for Medicare & Medicaid Services (CMS) uses Prospective Payment Systems (PPS). *Prospective* means before. The amount paid for services is determined before giving care. If costs are less than the amount paid, the agency keeps the extra money. If costs are greater, the agency takes the loss.

Different PPS are used for hospitals, home health care agencies, SNFs, rehabilitation centers, and other health care agencies. Each system determines the amount paid.

SAFETY AND QUALITY

The *U.S. Department of Health & Human Services (HHS)* is the government agency responsible for protecting the health and well-being of Americans. HHS has different divisions (agencies) that focus on certain areas of health care safety and quality. Box 1-3 lists some of the HHS agencies that over-see health care in the United States.

Regulations are rules made by government agencies. Regulations are based on standards that must be met. *Standards* identify what is expected for safety and quality of care. Health care agencies must meet the standards set by federal and state governments for:

- *Licensure*. A state license is required to operate and provide care.
- *Certification*. This is required to receive Medicare and Medicaid funds.

Accrediting agencies also have standards. *Accreditation* is voluntary. It signals quality and excellence. *The Joint Commission* is an example of an accrediting agency. The agency helps improve performance.

BOX 1-3	HHS Agencies

- *Agency for Healthcare Research and Quality (AHRQ)*—focuses on information (evidence) that promotes safety, quality, and reduced health care costs. The AHRQ gathers information, monitors outcomes, and provides resources to improve practice. This agency works with other HHS agencies to make sure information is understood and used.
- *Centers for Disease Control and Prevention (CDC)*—provides leadership and direction on the prevention and control of diseases. This agency responds to public health emergencies.
- *Centers for Medicare & Medicaid Services (CMS)*—oversees government-funded insurance programs such as Medicare, the federal part of the Medicaid program, and the Health Insurance Marketplace®.
- *Food and Drug Administration (FDA)*—regulates the safety of foods, drugs and vaccines (Chapter 17), medical devices, electronics that give off radiation, cosmetics, and tobacco products.
- *National Institutes of Health (NIH)*—conducts and supports medical research. The goal is to gain knowledge that helps prevent, detect, diagnose, and treat diseases and disabilities. The National Cancer Institute (NCI), National Institute on Aging (NIA), and the National Institute of Mental Health (NIMH) are examples of NIH institutes.

Modified from U.S. Department of Health & Human Services: HHS agencies & offices, *December 2, 2022.*

Workplace Safety

The *Occupational Safety and Health Administration (OSHA)* is the government agency responsible for ensuring safe working conditions. OSHA is part of the *United States Department of Labor*. OSHA sets and enforces standards for health and safety in the workplace. The agency provides information, training, and assistance to employers and workers.

There are health and safety risks for workers in health care settings. Infectious disease risks, injuries from handling and moving persons, workplace violence, and exposure to hazardous substances are examples. You will learn about safety measures related to your role in other chapters. Your employer must provide safety training.

Policies and Procedures

Policies are guides for staff conduct and daily operation. *Procedures* explain how to perform certain tasks or skills. Policies and procedures communicate what the health care agency expects. They promote compliance with regulations and accreditation requirements. *Compliance* means the agency is meeting the standards.

The Survey Process

Surveys are done to check for compliance. A *survey* is the formal review of an agency through the collection of facts and observations. Survey teams are made up of surveyors. A *surveyor* is a person who collects information by observing and asking questions.

A survey team will:

- Review policies, procedures, and medical records.
- Interview staff, patients and residents, and families.
- Observe how care is given.
- Observe if dignity and privacy are promoted.
- Check for cleanliness and safety.
- Make sure staff meet state requirements. (Are doctors and nurses licensed? Are nursing assistants on the state registry?)

If standards are met, the agency receives a license, certification, or accreditation. Sometimes problems *(deficiencies)* are found. The agency usually has 60 days or less to correct the problem. The agency can be fined for uncorrected or serious deficiencies. Or it can lose its license, certification, or accreditation.

Your Role

You have an important role in meeting standards and in the survey process. You must:

- Provide quality care.
- Protect the person's rights.
- Provide for the person's and your own safety.
- Help keep the agency clean and safe.
- Act in a professional manner.
- Have good work ethics.
- Follow agency policies and procedures.
- Answer questions honestly and completely.
  See *Focus on Surveys: Your Role*, p. 10.

FOCUS ON SURVEYS

Your Role

A surveyor may ask you questions. If so, be polite. Answer questions honestly and completely. If you do not understand a question, ask that it be re-phrased. Do not guess. Tell the surveyor where you can find the answer. You can say: "I will ask the nurse."

For example, a surveyor approaches you.

Surveyor: "May I ask you some questions?"

You: "Yes. I am happy to answer your questions."

Surveyor: "Thank you. First, what do you use for hand hygiene during routine patient care?"

You: "I use the hand sanitizer in the person's room."

Surveyor: "Thank you. Next, what are 2 appropriate patient identifiers?"

You: "I don't understand. Can you re-phrase the question?"

Surveyor: "Yes. Name 2 things you can use to identify a patient."

You: "Okay. Thank you. I can use the patient's full name and date of birth. I cannot use the room number."

Surveyor: "I have 1 last question. In a disaster, where would you find the Emergency Preparedness Plan?"

You: "I'm not sure. I will ask the charge nurse where to find it."

FOCUS ON PRIDE

The Person, Family, and Yourself

Personal and Professional Responsibility

Working in health care is rewarding. You provide care for a *person*. Your work affects the person's quality of care. Value the work that you do.

Focus on PRIDE is at the end of each chapter. The feature will help you promote pride in the person, the family, and yourself. Building on chapter content, it focuses on:

* *Personal and Professional Responsibility*—how personal and professional behaviors and development affect yourself and others.
* *Rights and Respect*—how to promote the rights of others and how to respect them as persons with dignity and value.
* *Independence and Social Interaction*—how to promote independence and positive interactions.
* *Delegation and Teamwork*—how to practice safe delegation (Chapter 4) and work well with and help other team members.
* *Ethics and Laws*—how to do the right thing when dealing with patients, residents, and co-workers. Laws affecting nursing care and real court cases are also presented.

For discussion purposes, each chapter ends with a *Focus on PRIDE: Application* section. The questions challenge you to think about your role and how you will value the person, family, or yourself.

Rights and Respect

Consider what type of agency would suit you. One person may prefer working in long-term care while another prefers a hospital setting. Careful career planning shows respect for employers, patients and residents, and yourself.

Independence and Social Interaction

You will interact with patients and residents, nursing staff, health team members, surveyors, and families. How you interact with others affects quality of care and job satisfaction.

Delegation and Teamwork

Health team members must work together to provide quality care. Offer to help others when you can. Helping others shows you value teamwork.

Ethics and Laws

Professional conduct is valued in all health care agencies. You will learn about ethical and legal aspects of care (Chapter 5) and student and work ethics (Chapter 6). As you study, consider how you will apply professional qualities as a student and in the workplace.

FOCUS ON PRIDE: Application

Why do you want to work in health care? Where do you want to work? What are your career goals?

REVIEW QUESTIONS

Circle the BEST answer.

1 The following are purposes of health care agencies. Which occurs *before* an illness?
   a Health promotion
   b Disease detection
   c Disease treatment
   d Rehabilitation

2 The purpose of rehabilitation is to
   a Prevent chronic illnesses
   b Detect terminal illnesses
   c Restore function and independence
   d Treat urgent illnesses

3 The length of stay in a hospital is usually short because
   a Care needs are simple
   b Patients heal quickly
   c Care is costly
   d The quality of care is poor

4 A person needs wound care and physical therapy after discharge from a hospital. Which agency would *best* meet the person's needs?
a An ambulatory surgery center
b A hospice agency
c An assisted living residence
d A skilled nursing facility

5 A person needs housing and some help with daily activities. Which agency would *best* meet the person's needs?
a A rehabilitation center
b An assisted living residence
c A hospital
d A home care agency

6 Home care agencies provide
a Home maintenance while a person is in a hospital
b Health care services to persons living at home
c Housing and personal care for persons unable to live at home
d A coordinated network of different types of health care agencies

7 A health care program for dying persons is called
a Hospice
b Sub-acute care
c Skilled care
d Assisted living

8 Who controls policy in a health care agency?
a The survey team
b The board of directors
c The health team
d Medicare and Medicaid

9 Which health team member helps the person retain skills needed for daily living and work?
a Respiratory therapist
b Social worker
c Occupational therapist
d Pharmacist

10 Who is responsible for the entire nursing staff and safe nursing care?
a The case manager
b The director of nursing
c The charge nurse
d The RN

11 The nursing team includes
a Doctors
b Pharmacists
c Physical and occupational therapists
d RNs, LPNs/LVNs, and nursing assistants

12 Nursing assistants are supervised by
a Licensed nurses
b Other nursing assistants
c The health team
d The medical director

13 Your hospital unit uses a team nursing care pattern. Your role is to
a Ask which task you are assigned for your work shift
b Report observations and the care you give to the nurse
c Perform tasks that are usually done by other departments
d Coordinate care with the case manager

14 Medicare is for persons who
a Are 65 years of age or older
b Need nursing center care
c Have group insurance
d Have low incomes

15 Which government agency over-sees government-funded insurance programs?
a Food and Drug Administration (FDA)
b Centers for Disease Control and Prevention (CDC)
c National Institutes of Health (NIH)
d Centers for Medicare & Medicaid Services (CMS)

16 Which is required for an agency to operate and provide care?
a Accreditation
b Certification
c A license
d An interview

17 Which is voluntary for health care agencies receiving Medicare or Medicaid funds?
a Licensure
b Certification
c Accreditation
d Surveys

18 Surveys are done to
a Reduce health care costs
b See if agencies meet set standards
c Educate the nursing team
d Determine the amount paid by insurers

19 A surveyor asks you some questions. You should
a Refer all questions to the nurse
b Answer as the DON tells you to
c Give as little information as possible
d Give honest and complete answers

20 Your role in any health care agency will involve
a Deciding which nursing care pattern to use
b Using the person's payment method to determine care quality
c Reporting directly to the agency's administrator
d Following agency policies and procedures

Answers to Chapter 1 questions are on p. 901.

FOCUS ON PRACTICE

Problem Solving

The nurse supervising you has not returned from a meal break. You have a question about a patient's care. Your nursing department is organized as shown in Figure 1-3. What will you do?

The Person's Rights

OBJECTIVES

- Define the key terms and key abbreviation in this chapter.
- Explain the purpose of *The Patient Care Partnership: Understanding Expectations, Rights, and Responsibilities.*
- Describe the purposes and requirements of the *Omnibus Budget Reconciliation Act of 1987 (OBRA).*
- Identify the person's rights under OBRA.
- Explain how to protect the person's rights.
- Explain the ombudsman role.
- Explain how to promote PRIDE in the person, the family, and yourself.

KEY TERMS

advocate Someone who acts or speaks on behalf of another person

dignity Having value and worth as a person

involuntary seclusion Separating a person from others against the person's will, keeping the person to a certain area, or keeping the person away from his or her room without consent

ombudsman Someone who supports or promotes the needs and interests of another person

representative Someone with the legal right to act on the patient's or resident's behalf when the person cannot do so alone

treatment The care provided to maintain or restore health, improve function, or relieve symptoms

KEY ABBREVIATION

OBRA Omnibus Budget Reconciliation Act of 1987

People want to know about their health problems and treatment. They want to understand and take part in treatment decisions. As patients and residents, they have certain rights.

PATIENT RIGHTS

The Patient Care Partnership: Understanding Expectations, Rights, and Responsibilities is from the American Hospital Association. The document explains the person's rights and expectations during hospital stays. The relationship between the doctor, health team, and patient is stressed. See Box 2-1.

RESIDENT RIGHTS

The *Omnibus Budget Reconciliation Act of 1987 (OBRA)* is a federal law. It applies to all 50 states. The law set minimum standards for quality of care in nursing centers. The Centers for Medicare & Medicaid Services (CMS) enforces OBRA through the survey process (Chapter 1).

OBRA requires that nursing centers provide care in a manner and in a setting that maintains or improves each person's quality of life, health, and safety. Nursing assistant training and competency evaluation are part of OBRA (Chapter 3). Resident rights are a major part of OBRA.

Residents have rights as United States citizens. For example, they have the right to vote. They also have rights relating to their every-day lives and care in a nursing center. These rights are protected by federal and state laws.

Nursing centers must protect and promote the person's rights. The center cannot interfere with a resident's rights. Some residents cannot exercise their rights. Then a representative (spouse, partner, adult child, court-appointed guardian) does so. A *representative* is someone with the legal right to act on the patient's or resident's behalf when the person cannot do so alone.

Nursing centers must inform residents of their rights—orally and in writing. Residents are also informed of the rules about their conduct and responsibilities in the center. Information is given before or during admission to the center, as needed during the person's stay, and when laws or center rules change.

BOX 2-1	The Patient Care Partnership: Understanding Expectations, Rights, and Responsibilities (A Summary)

High-Quality Care
- The hospital provides needed care with skill, compassion, and respect.
- The patient has the right to know the identities of:
  - Doctors, nurses, and other staff
  - Students and other trainees

Clean and Safe Setting
- There are policies and procedures to:
  - Avoid mistakes.
  - Prevent abuse and neglect.
- The patient is told of unexpected or significant events.
  - What happened
  - Needed changes in care

Involvement in Care
- The patient has the right to make informed decisions about treatment choices.
  - What are the benefits and risks of each treatment?
  - Is the treatment experimental or part of a research study?
  - What can be expected from treatment?
  - How might long-term effects of treatment affect quality of life?
  - What will the patient and family need to do after discharge?
  - What are the costs for uncovered services or providers?
- The patient has the right to consent to or refuse treatment. The person is told of the effects of refusing treatment.
- The patient is expected to give information about:
  - Past illnesses, surgeries, or hospital stays
  - Allergic reactions
  - Drugs or dietary supplements that are taken
  - Health insurance plan admission requirements
- The patient's health care goals, values, and spiritual beliefs are respected. The patient is responsible for sharing his or her wishes with the doctor, family, and health team.
- The patient is expected to communicate about who makes decisions when the patient is unable.
  - *Power of attorney, living will,* or *advance directive* documents are shared with the doctor, family, and health team (Chapter 59).
  - Help is provided with making difficult decisions. Counselors or chaplains are available.

Protection of Privacy
- The hospital protects the confidentiality of:
  - The patient's relationships with the doctor and health team
  - Information about the patient's health and care
- A "Notice of Privacy Practices" is provided describing:
  - How patient information is used, disclosed, and protected
  - How to obtain a copy of hospital records about patient care

Preparing to Leave the Hospital
- Sources for follow-up care are identified. The hospital's financial interest in any referrals is disclosed.
- Hospital activities are coordinated with community caregivers. The hospital requests permission to share care information.
- Information and training are given about self-care at home.

Help With Bills and Insurance Claims
- The hospital files insurance, Medicare, or Medicaid claims.
- Patients can contact the business office with billing questions.
- The hospital tries to find financial help or make other arrangements if the person is without health coverage. The patient provides needed information to obtain coverage or assistance.

Modified from American Hospital Association: The patient care partnership: understanding expectations, rights, and responsibilities, *Chicago, 2003.*

Resident rights and other information are given in the language and format the person uses and understands.

- An interpreter is used if the person speaks and understands a foreign language or communicates by sign language.
- Written translations are provided in the foreign languages common in the center's geographic area.
- Medical terms are avoided to the extent possible.
- Sign language and communication aids are used as necessary.
- Large-print texts are available for persons with vision problems.

Resident rights (Box 2-2) are posted throughout the center. Those affecting your role are described in this chapter.

See *Focus on Surveys: Resident Rights.*

FOCUS ON SURVEYS

Resident Rights

Resident rights are a major focus of surveys. Surveyors observe staff behaviors and actions. They listen to staff comments and remarks. Always assume they are doing so. What you say and do must promote quality of life, health, and safety. For example, a surveyor may observe:

- How you prevent exposure of the person's body
- How you help a person dress for the season and time of day
- How you label clothing
- If you knock on a person's door before entering the room
- If you change a person's music or TV without permission
- If you move personal items without permission
- How you address and speak to a person

You will learn how to protect the person's rights as you study this and other chapters. Always act and speak in a professional manner.

BOX 2-2	Resident Rights

- To be treated with respect and dignity. *Dignity* means having value and worth as a person.
- To receive quality care.
- To exercise rights as a center resident and as a United States citizen.
- To be informed orally and in writing of rights and center rules. This is done in a language the person understands.
- To access all of his or her records.
- To obtain copies of his or her records. This is at the resident's expense.
- To refuse treatment.
- To refuse to take part in experimental research. This is the development and testing of new treatments and drugs.
- To make advance directives (Chapter 59).
- To be informed of Medicare benefits and services. This includes costs covered and not covered.
- To be informed of center services and charges.
- To choose a doctor.
- To know the doctor's name, specialty, and contact information.
- To be informed of his or her health status and medical condition. Information is given in a language that the person understands. That language is used during care planning (Chapter 8).
- To be informed of:
  - Any accident or injury that may need medical attention.
  - A change in physical, mental, or psycho-social status.
  - The need to stop, change, or add a treatment.
  - A decision to transfer or discharge the person. *Transfer* means to move to a different setting. *Discharge* is when the person officially departs from the agency.
  - A room or roommate change.
  - A change in rights under federal or state law.
- To manage personal and financial affairs.
- To be informed in advance about care and treatment. This includes changes in care and treatment.
- To have privacy and confidentiality:
  - Of personal and medical records
  - Of treatment and care
  - Of written and phone communications
  - During visits with family and friends
  - When meeting with resident groups

- To voice grievances and have them solved promptly.
- To see the results of federal and state surveys and plans to correct problems or areas of weakness.
- To perform or refuse to perform services for the center.
- To send and receive un-opened mail. To buy supplies to send mail.
- To receive information about protecting persons with intellectual and developmental disabilities and mental health disorders.
- To have and use personal items and clothing.
- To take prescribed drugs without help if able.
- To refuse to change to a different room.
- To be free from restraints (Chapter 16).
- To be free from abuse (verbal, sexual, physical), bodily punishment, involuntary seclusion, and other abuse or mistreatment (Chapter 5).
- To file complaints with the appropriate state agency about abuse, neglect, and the mis-use of property.
- To be cared for in a manner and setting that maintains or enhances quality of life.
- To choose activities, schedules, and health care that meet his or her interests and needs.
- To interact with community members inside and outside the center.
- To make choices about his or her life in the center.
- To organize and take part in resident groups.
- To take part in social, religious, and community activities.
- To have a setting and services that consider his or her needs and choices.
- To have a clean, comfortable, and home-like setting. This includes temperature, lighting, and sound levels.
- To attain or maintain his or her highest desired level of function.
- To have closet space.
- To visit with a spouse or partner, family, and friends at any reasonable hour.

Information

The *right to information* means access to all records about the person. Medical records, contracts, incident reports, and financial records are included. The request can be oral or written.

The person has the right to be fully informed of his or her health condition. The person must also have information about his or her doctor. This includes the doctor's name, specialty, and contact information.

Report any information request to the nurse. You do not give the information described above to the person or family (Chapter 3).

See *Focus on Communication: Information*.

FOCUS ON COMMUNICATION

Information

You may be asked about a person's care. You must not give out information. This is the nurse's responsibility. You can say: "I am sorry. I am not allowed to give that information. I will report your request to the nurse."

Communicate the request promptly. You can tell the person: "I told the nurse about your question. The nurse will speak with you soon."

Refusing Treatment

The person has the *right to refuse treatment*. *Treatment* means the care provided to maintain or restore health, improve function, or relieve symptoms. A person cannot be treated without consent (Chapter 5).

The center must:
- Find out what the person is refusing and why.
- Explain the problems that can result from the refusal.
- Offer other treatment options.
- Continue to provide all other services.

Advance directives are part of the right to refuse treatment (Chapter 59). They include living wills and instructions about life support. *Advance directives* are written instructions about health care when the person is not able to make such decisions.

Report any treatment refusal to the nurse. The nurse may change the person's care plan (Chapter 8).

Privacy and Confidentiality

Residents have the *right to personal privacy*. Staff must maintain privacy of the person's body. Expose the person's body only as necessary. Only staff directly involved in care and treatment are present. Consent is needed for others to be present. For example, a person's consent is needed for a student to observe a treatment.

Privacy is maintained for all personal care measures. Bathing, dressing, and elimination are examples. To protect privacy:
- Close privacy curtains, doors, and window coverings.
- Remove residents from public view.
- Provide clothes or drape the person to prevent unnecessary exposure of body parts.

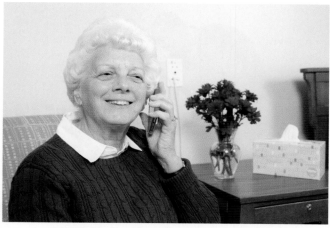

FIGURE 2-1 A resident talks privately on the phone.

Leaving the person without a gown, clothing, or bed covers violates the right to privacy. So does an open door when the person uses the bathroom, commode, urinal, or bedpan.

Residents have the right to visit in private—where others cannot see or hear them. If requested, the center must provide private space. Offices, chapels, dining rooms, and meeting rooms are options.

Residents have the right to make phone calls in private (Fig. 2-1). Calls must not be over-heard. Privacy is provided for phone calls in offices or at the nurses' station. Phones are at the correct height for use by persons in wheelchairs. Phones for hard of hearing persons are also available. Some residents use their own phones.

The person has the right to send and receive mail without others interfering. No one can open mail the person sends or receives without the person's consent. Un-opened mail is given to the person within 24 hours of delivery to the center. Out-going mail is delivered to the postal service within 24 hours on days of regular delivery or pick-up services.

Information about the person's care, treatment, and condition is kept confidential. So are medical and financial records. Consent is needed for their release to other agencies or persons.

You must provide privacy and protect confidentiality. Doing so shows respect and protects the person's dignity. See Chapters 5 and 6.

Personal Choice

The CMS uses the term *person-centered care* to describe the required care in nursing centers. With person-centered care, the person maintains control and is supported in making choices about his or her daily life. Staff try to understand the resident and the person's life before admission to the center. Staff identify what is important to the person regarding daily routines and preferred activities. Residents have the *right to make their own choices*.

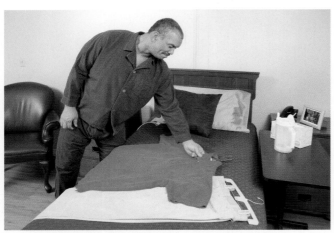

FIGURE 2-2 A resident chooses what clothing to wear.

Residents:
- Choose their doctors.
- Choose friends and visitors.
- Help plan their care and treatment.
- Choose activities, schedules, and care.
  - When to go to bed and when to get up
  - What to wear (Fig. 2-2)
  - How to spend time
  - What to eat

Personal choice promotes quality of life, dignity, and self-respect. Allow personal choice whenever safely possible.

Work

The person does not work for care, care items or other things, or privileges. The person is not required to perform services for the center.

However, the person has the *right to work or perform services if he or she desires.* Some people like to garden, repair or build things, clean, sew, mend, or cook. Other persons need work for rehabilitation or activity reasons. The care plan reflects the person's desire or need to work. Residents volunteer or are paid for their services.

Resident Groups

The person has the *right to form and take part in resident groups.* Families can meet with other families. These groups can plan activities, discuss concerns, take part in educational events, and suggest center improvements. They can support and comfort group members.

Residents have the right to take part in social, cultural, religious, and community events. They have the right to help in getting to and from such events.

Personal Items

Residents have the *right to keep and use personal items.* This includes clothing and some furnishings. The items

allowed depend on space needs and the health and safety of others.

Treat the person's property with care and respect. The items may lack value to you but have meaning to the person. They also relate to personal choice, dignity, a home-like setting, and quality of life.

The person's property is protected. Items are labeled with the person's name. The center must investigate reports of lost, stolen, or damaged items. Sometimes the police help. The person and family are advised to keep jewelry and costly items at home.

Protect yourself and the center from being accused of stealing. Do not go through a closet, drawers, purse, or other space without the person's knowledge and consent. Staff do not conduct searches unless the person or the person's representative understands the reason and agrees to a voluntary search. Staff do not act as law enforcement. The agency contacts the police for such concerns.

Freedom From Abuse, Mistreatment, and Neglect

Residents have the *right to be free from verbal, sexual, physical, and mental abuse* (Chapter 5). Abuse means:
- The willful infliction of injury, unreasonable confinement, intimidation, or punishment that results in physical harm, pain, or mental anguish. *Intimidation* means to make someone afraid with threats of force or violence.
- Depriving the person of the goods or services needed for well-being.

They also have the right to be free from *involuntary seclusion:*
- Separating a person from others against the person's will
- Keeping the person to a certain area
- Keeping the person away from his or her room without consent

No one can abuse, neglect, or mistreat a resident. This includes center staff, volunteers, and staff from other agencies or groups. It also includes other residents, family members, visitors, and legal representatives. Centers must investigate suspected or reported cases of abuse, neglect, or mistreatment. The person must be protected from harm during an investigation. A center cannot employ a person who:
- Has been found guilty of abusing, neglecting, or mistreating others by a court of law.
- Has a finding entered into a state's nursing assistant registry (Chapter 3) about abuse, neglect, mistreatment, or wrongful acts involving the person's money or property. A *finding* means that a state determined that the employee abused, neglected, mistreated, or wrongfully used the person's money or property.

Freedom From Restraint

Residents have the *right not to have body movements restricted.* Restraints and certain drugs restrict body movements. Some drugs are restraints because they affect mood, behavior, and mental function. Sometimes restraint use is needed for protection. Restraints are not used for staff convenience or to discipline a person. A doctor's order is needed for restraint use. Restraints are used only for a brief time to treat medical symptoms. Restraints are discussed in Chapter 16.

Quality of Life

Residents have the *right to quality of life.* They must be cared for in a manner and in a setting that promotes dignity and respect for self. Staff must provide care in a manner that maintains or enhances self-esteem and feelings of self-worth. Care must promote physical, mental, and social well-being. Protecting resident rights promotes quality of life. It shows respect for the person.

Be polite and courteous. Good, honest, and thoughtful care enhances quality of life. Box 2-3 lists OBRA-required actions that promote dignity and privacy.

See *Focus on Communication: Quality of Life.*

FOCUS ON COMMUNICATION

Quality of Life

Every person deserves to be addressed in a manner that shows dignity and respect. Address the person by title and last name. For example: Mr. Baker, Mrs. Harty, or Dr. Collins. Do not use a person's first name or another name unless the person requests it. Do not use terms like *sweetheart, honey, grandpa,* and *dear.*

BOX 2-3   OBRA-Required Actions to Promote Dignity and Privacy

Courteous and Dignified Interactions
- Use the right tone of voice.
- Use good eye contact.
- Stand or sit close enough as needed. Position yourself at the person's eye level. For example, sit to speak to a person who is seated.
- Use the person's proper name and title. For example: "Mrs. Crane." Or use the name the person prefers.
- Gain the person's attention before interacting with him or her.
- Explain the care you provide.
- Use touch if the person approves.
- Respect the person's social status.
- Listen with interest to what the person is saying.
- Do not yell at, scold, or embarrass the person.

Privacy and Self-Determination
- Knock on the door before entering. Wait to be asked in.
- Drape properly during care and procedures to avoid exposure and embarrassment.
- Use privacy curtains or screens during care and procedures.
- Close the room door during care and procedures. Also close window coverings.
- Close the bathroom door when the person uses the bathroom.
- Drape properly in a chair.

Personal Choice and Independence
- Person smokes in allowed areas.
- Person takes part in activities of his or her interest.
- Person takes part in scheduling activities and care.
- Person gives input into the care plan about preferences and independence.
- Person is involved in a room or roommate change.
- The person's items are moved or inspected only with the person's consent.

Courteous and Dignified Care
- Respond to requests for help in a timely manner.
- Assist with dressing in the right clothing for time of day and personal choice. The person wears his or her own clothing.
- Promote independence and dignity in dining.
- Respect private space and property. For example, change TV stations or music only with the person's consent.
- Assist with walking and transfers. Do not interfere with independence.
- Assist with hygiene and grooming preferences. Do not interfere with independence.
  - Appearance is neat and clean.
  - Hair is styled as the person prefers.
  - The person is clean shaven or has a groomed beard and mustache.
  - Nails are trimmed and clean.
  - Dentures, hearing aids, eyeglasses, and other devices are used correctly.
  - Clothing is clean.
  - Clothing fits and is properly fastened.
  - Shoes, hose, and socks are on properly and fastened.
  - Extra clothing is worn for warmth as needed. Sweaters and lap blankets are examples.

Environment. Residents have the *right to a safe, clean, comfortable, and home-like setting.* The person can have and use personal items to the extent possible. Doing so promotes personal choice and a home-like setting. See Figure 2-3.

The setting, services, and staff must meet the person's needs and preferences. They must promote independence, dignity, and well-being. The center must try to change schedules, call systems, and room arrangements to meet the person's desires and needs. For example, a person:

- Prefers a shower, not a tub bath.
- Wants a shower before breakfast.
- Is afraid of falling in the shower and elsewhere.
- Is uneasy about a staff member giving care.
- Cannot reach or use the call light.
- Cannot reach personal items.
- Does not like the food served.

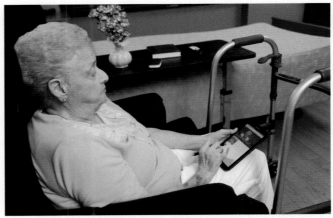

FIGURE 2-3 This resident's setting is safe, clean, and comfortable. Personal items are part of a home-like setting.

Activities. Residents have the *right to activities that enhance each person's physical, mental, and psycho-social well-being.* The center provides religious services for spiritual health. Activities are meaningful when they:

- Reflect the person's needs, interests, culture, background, and life-style.
- Are enjoyed by the person.
- Help the person feel useful or produce something useful.
- Provide a sense of belonging.

Activities involve large groups (bingo), small groups (a card game), or 2 people. The person may do something alone. Letter writing and computer games are examples.

See *Teamwork and Time Management: Activities.*

See *Focus on Communication: Activities.*

See *Focus on Surveys: Activities.*

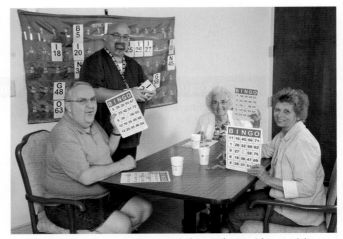

FIGURE 2-4 A nursing assistant helps residents with an activity.

TEAMWORK AND TIME MANAGEMENT

Activities

Know when an activity begins and ends. Before assisting residents to activities:

- Assist with elimination needs and hand hygiene.
- Assist with grooming such as brushing and combing hair. A person may want to apply perfume or make-up.
- Have the person wear the correct clothing and footwear for the activity.
- Provide needed adaptive (assistive) devices. Eyeglasses, hearing aids, canes, and walkers are examples.

Allow 15 to 20 minutes to assist residents to and from the activity. Help co-workers as needed.

Residents may need help with activities (Fig. 2-4). If not, use activity time wisely. Provide needed care and visit residents who cannot leave their rooms. You can clean and straighten rooms, bathrooms, shower rooms, and utility rooms.

Activities

You may need help assisting residents to and from activity programs. Politely ask a co-worker to help you. Share the following with your co-worker.
- What time you need help.
- How much of the co-worker's time you need.
- Which residents you need help with.
- If the person walks or uses a wheelchair.
- What adaptive (assistive) devices are used. Eyeglasses, hearing aids, canes, and walkers are examples.

   Always say "please" when asking for help. And thank the person for helping you. For example:

   Alex, can you please help me assist 2 residents to the concert? It starts at 2:00, so I'll need your help at 1:45. Mr. Harris needs his glasses, hearing aid, and walker. Mrs. Janz uses a wheelchair. She needs her glasses. The blanket for her lap is in the wheelchair. The concert is over at 3:00. Can you help me then, too? Thanks so much for helping me.

Activities

Surveyors may ask you about:
- Your role in getting residents ready for a group activity.
    - How do you make sure the person is dressed and ready for an activity?
    - How do you provide needed transportation?
- Your role in helping with activities of daily living during an activity. For example, does the person need to use the bathroom? Does the person need help eating?
- Your role in helping a person with an individual activity. For example, a person writes poetry. Does the person have needed supplies? Is the person properly positioned? Is the lighting good?
- How are activities provided when the activities staff members are not available?

Grievances

Residents have the *right to voice concerns, questions, and complaints about treatment and care*. The problem may involve another person. It may be about care that was given or not given. The center must promptly try to correct the matter. No one can punish the person in any way for voicing a grievance.

PROTECTING RIGHTS

An *advocate* is someone who acts or speaks on behalf of another person. Nurses act as advocates for their patients or residents. You also act as an advocate when you:
- Respect and protect the person's rights.
- Respect the person's decisions and choices.
- Treat the person with dignity.
- Are attentive to the person's needs, concerns, and requests.
- Promote a safe setting for the person.
- Tell the nurse about concerns.

Ombudsmen

The *Older Americans Act* is a federal law. It requires a long-term care ombudsman program in every state. An *ombudsman* supports or promotes the needs and interests of another person.

   Ombudsmen are advocates for residents. They protect a person's health, safety, welfare, and rights. They:
- Investigate and resolve complaints.
- Provide services to assist the person.
- Assist with hospital access or discharge concerns.
- Provide information about long-term care services.
- Monitor nursing care and conditions.
- Provide support to resident and family groups.
- Help the person and family resolve family conflicts.
- Help the center manage difficult problems.

   Nursing centers must post contact information for local and state ombudsmen. A resident or family may share a concern with you. Follow center policies and procedures for contacting an ombudsman. Ombudsman services are useful when:
- There is a concern about a person's care or treatment.
- Someone interferes with a person's rights, health, safety, or welfare.

FOCUS ON PRIDE

The Person, Family, and Yourself

Personal and Professional Responsibility

Nursing centers must plan for and provide person-centered care. A care plan (Chapter 8) that is specific to the person is developed. Personal choice and individual needs and preferences direct the plan of care. Your actions can promote person-centered care. For example, you:

- Ask questions to learn about the person's usual daily life.
- Listen to the person's needs and concerns and report them to the nurse.
- Ask what the person wants to do for himself or herself.
- Help the person to bed at a time the person prefers.
- Adjust the care schedule because the person has visitors coming.
These are just some examples of person-centered care. Each time you support personal choice and control, you promote person-centered care.

Rights and Respect

Seeing others as having value and worth affects your work and daily life. It guides your interactions with the person, visitors, and other staff. It affects how you view and care for yourself. It maintains and grows your personal relationships.

Everyone has a desire to be treated as valuable. Throughout this book, you will be taught ways to show dignity and respect. You must not overlook their importance. Embracing dignity and respect has powerful effects.

Independence and Social Interaction

Independence involves the person's ability to make decisions and to do as much for himself or herself as is safely possible. Independence promotes quality of life. As you learn how to assist with care, remember it is best to do tasks *with* the person rather than *for* the person. The task matters, but the person matters most.

Delegation and Teamwork

Schedules, care assignments, and room arrangements may need to change to meet the person's needs and preferences. Flexibility, good teamwork, and communication are required to provide quality care.

Ethics and Laws

Every person has the right to keep personal information private. This includes information about health care. The *Health Insurance Portability and Accountability Act of 1996 (HIPAA)* protects the privacy and security of a person's health information. HIPAA is discussed further in Chapter 5.

FOCUS ON PRIDE: Application

Do you believe that everyone has a desire to be treated as valuable? Identify ways to show dignity and respect to:

- Your instructor and other students
- The patient or resident
- The person's family or visitors
- Your co-workers

REVIEW QUESTIONS

Circle the BEST answer.

1 *The Patient Care Partnership: Understanding Expectations, Rights, and Responsibilities* is concerned with
   a Hospital care
   b Home care
   c Long-term care
   d All health care agencies and settings

2 The Omnibus Budget Reconciliation Act of 1987 (OBRA) is a federal law that
   a Requires health care agencies to limit treatment costs
   b Sets standards for quality of nursing center care
   c Restricts nursing center residents' rights
   d Provides affordable health insurance options

3 A son has the legal right to act on his mother's behalf. The son is his mother's legal
   a Ombudsman
   b Representative
   c Caregiver
   d Health care provider

4 Residents must be
   a Involved in resident groups
   b Able to provide some type of work for the center
   c Informed of rights orally and in writing
   d Willing to accept treatments ordered by their doctors

5 A resident says he does not want a shower. Which response is *best*?
   a "You smell badly and need a shower."
   b "You cannot refuse a shower."
   c "Why are you being difficult?"
   d "Why do you not want a shower?"

6 A daughter wants to read her father's medical record. What should you do?
   a Give her the medical record.
   b Ask the resident if she can read the record.
   c Tell the nurse.
   d Tell her that she cannot do so.

7 A resident asks about another resident's health. Which response is *best*?
   a "Mind your own business."
   b "The nurse can tell you."
   c "He had a heart attack."
   d "I cannot give information about another resident."

8 Which violates the person's right to privacy?
   a Closing the bathroom door when the bathroom is used
   b Opening window blinds when assisting with bathing
   c Covering the person for personal care
   d Asking the person's permission to observe a treatment

9 A resident has a phone and wants to make a call. What should you do?
  a Leave the room.
  b Tell the nurse.
  c Have the person use the phone at the nurses' station.
  d Stay in the room and finish your tasks.

10 Who decides how to style a person's hair?
  a The person
  b The nurse
  c You
  d The ombudsman

11 A resident would like to sleep later in the morning. You should
  a Explain why the agency has a set schedule
  b Tell the nurse why this is not convenient for you
  c Allow the person to sleep until the preferred time
  d Wake the person at a time best for you

12 Residents have the right to
  a Bring weapons into the center
  b Mistreat other residents
  c Use other residents' personal items
  d Voice complaints about care

13 Residents have the right to be free from
  a Disease
  b Grievances
  c Involuntary seclusion
  d Rules

14 A resident brought some items from home. They are
  a Kept at the nurses' station
  b Labeled with the person's name
  c Arranged as you prefer
  d Shared with the person's roommate

15 A resident carries a baby doll most of the day. You should
  a Ask the family to take the doll home
  b Remind the person that the doll is not allowed in the dining room
  c Threaten to take the doll away if the resident refuses care
  d Treat the doll with care and respect

16 A person found guilty of abuse
  a Cannot work in a nursing center
  b Can work in a nursing center with supervision
  c Can work as a nurse in a nursing center
  d Can work as a nursing assistant in a nursing center

17 Which action promotes dignity?
  a Restraining the person
  b Making clothing choices for the person
  c Scolding the person
  d Listening to the person

18 Which is the correct way to address a person?
  a "Hello, sweetie."
  b "Hello."
  c "Hello, Mrs. Smith."
  d "Hello, grandpa."

19 Which promotes privacy?
  a Entering a person's room without knocking
  b Closing the privacy curtain for a procedure
  c Leaving the door open during personal care
  d Looking through the person's belongings

20 A nursing center must provide
  a A safe, clean, and comfortable setting
  b An indoor smoking area
  c A bed near a window
  d A noise-free setting

21 Who selects activities for a resident?
  a The nurse
  b You
  c The activities director
  d The person

22 A long-term care ombudsman
  a Is employed by the nursing center
  b Investigates resident complaints
  c Grants a nursing center a license or certification
  d Is only contacted for legal matters

Answers to Chapter 2 questions are on p. 901.

FOCUS ON **PRACTICE**

Problem Solving

Before helping a resident change clothes, you ask what the person wants to wear. You ask if the person wants to change in the room or in the bathroom. You ask about other preferences. The resident thanks you for asking and says: "Some nursing assistants want to do it *their* way, not *my* way."

How will you respond? Explain how personal choice relates to independence and quality of life.

The Nursing Assistant

OBJECTIVES

- Define the key terms and key abbreviations in this chapter.
- Explain the history and trends affecting nursing assistants.
- Explain the laws that affect nursing assistants.
- Describe the training and competency evaluation requirements for nursing assistants.
- Identify what can cause a nursing assistant's certification (license, registration) to be denied, revoked, or suspended.
- Identify the information in the nursing assistant registry.
- Explain how to obtain certification, a license, or registration in another state.
- Describe what nursing assistants can do and their role limits.
- Describe the standards for nursing assistants.
- Explain why a job description is important.
- Explain employee orientation and why it is important.
- Explain how to promote PRIDE in the person, the family, and yourself.

KEY TERMS

certification Official recognition by a state that standards or requirements have been met

endorsement A state recognizes the certificate, license, or registration issued by another state; reciprocity or equivalency

equivalency See "endorsement"

job description A document that describes what an agency expects you to do

nursing task Nursing care or a nursing function, procedure, skill, or activity

preceptor An experienced staff member who mentors a new employee at the start of a job

reciprocity See "endorsement"

KEY ABBREVIATIONS

APRN	Advanced practice registered nurse
BON	Board of nursing
CNA	Certified nursing assistant; certified nurse aide
LNA	Licensed nursing assistant
LPN	Licensed practical nurse
LVN	Licensed vocational nurse
NATCEP	Nursing assistant training and competency evaluation program

NCSBN	National Council of State Boards of Nursing
OBRA	Omnibus Budget Reconciliation Act of 1987
RN	Registered nurse
RNA	Registered nurse aide
SRNA	State registered nurse aide
STNA	State tested nurse aide

Federal and state laws and agency policies combine to define your roles and functions. To give safe care, you need to know:

- What you can and cannot do
- Rules and standards of conduct affecting your work
- Your role limits

Laws, job descriptions, and the person's condition shape your work. So does the amount of supervision you need.

HISTORY AND CURRENT TRENDS

For decades, nursing assistants have helped nurses with basic nursing care. Often called nurse's aides, they helped with bathing, grooming, elimination, bedmaking, and other needs. Until the 1980s, training was not required by law. Nurses gave on-the-job training. Some hospitals, nursing centers, and schools offered courses.

In the 1980s, efforts to improve the quality of care in nursing centers led to the *Omnibus Budget Reconciliation Act of 1987 (OBRA)*. Among other standards, OBRA set training and competency evaluation requirements for nursing assistants. See "The Omnibus Budget Reconciliation Act of 1987."

Nursing assistants today care for patients and residents with complex needs. There is an aging population with chronic illnesses. Shorter hospital stays require recovery in long-term care and home care settings. New technology and equipment are being used. Many patients and residents have needs related to cognitive (thinking and memory) disorders such as Alzheimer's disease and other dementias (Chapter 54).

Nursing assistants are mainly employed by long-term care centers, hospitals, and home care agencies (Chapter 1). Employers need nursing assistants who value agency goals. Safety, quality, and cost goals are examples. Teamwork and time management goals are others.

The need for competent and skilled nursing assistants continues to grow. Many states and agencies offer advanced nursing assistant positions. Advanced nursing assistants, restorative aides, and medication assistants are examples.

FEDERAL AND STATE LAWS

The U.S. Congress makes federal laws for all 50 states to follow. State legislatures make state laws. You must know the federal and state laws affecting your work. The laws provide direction for what you can and cannot do.

Nurse Practice Acts

Each state has a nurse practice act. A nurse practice act describes:

- The different nursing levels and titles:
  - Advanced practice registered nurse (APRN)
  - Registered nurse (RN)
  - Licensed practical nurse/licensed vocational nurse (LPN/LVN)
- Education and licensing requirements for nurses
- Scope of practice (what nurses are allowed to do)
- Disciplinary actions for violations of the nurse practice act

A nurse practice act is enforced by the state's board of nursing (BON). The BON can deny, revoke, or suspend a nurse's license. The intent is to protect the public from harm. Reasons for discipline include:

- Unsafe nursing practice
- Mishandling or misusing drugs
- Violating professional boundaries (Chapter 5)
- Sexual misconduct (Chapter 5)
- Abuse (Chapter 5)
- Fraud (Chapter 5)
- Criminal conduct

Nursing Assistants. Some nurse practice acts regulate nursing assistant roles, functions, and education and certification requirements. Other states have separate laws for nursing assistants. The laws are enforced by the state's BON, health department, or other state agency.

If you do something beyond the legal limits of your role, you could be practicing nursing without a license. This means serious legal problems for you, your supervisor, and the agency. You must function with skill and safety within the limits of your role. See "Roles and Responsibilities" on p. 26.

The Omnibus Budget Reconciliation Act of 1987

The *Omnibus Budget Reconciliation Act of 1987 (OBRA)* is a federal law. It applies to all 50 states.

OBRA sets minimum requirements for nursing assistant training and evaluation. Each state must have a nursing assistant training and competency evaluation program (NATCEP). A nursing assistant must successfully complete a NATCEP to work in a nursing center, hospital long-term care unit, or home care agency receiving Medicare funds.

The Training Program. The training program (Fig. 3-1) includes the knowledge and skills needed to give basic nursing care. Areas of study include:

- Communication
- Infection control
- Safety and emergency procedures
- Promoting independence
- Respecting residents' rights
- Basic nursing skills and personal care skills—measuring vital signs, reporting abnormal observations, skin care, oral care, grooming, dressing, elimination, feeding, and so on
- Transferring, positioning, and turning methods
- Basic restorative care—use of adaptive (assistive) devices, range-of-motion exercises, bowel and bladder training
- Meeting mental health and social needs
- Caring for persons with confusion and dementia

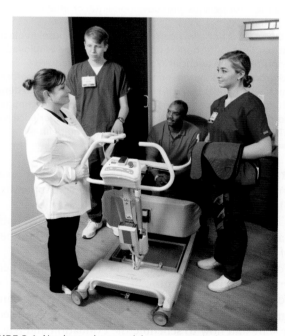

FIGURE 3-1 Nursing assistant training program. An instructor demonstrates a skill to students.

OBRA requires at least 75 hours of instruction. Some states require more hours. Classroom and at least 16 hours of supervised practical training are required. Practical training (clinical practicum or clinical experience) occurs in a laboratory or clinical setting. Students perform nursing tasks on another person. A nurse supervises this training.

See *Focus on Communication: The Training Program.*

See *Promoting Safety and Comfort: The Training Program.*

FOCUS ON COMMUNICATION

The Training Program

Student clinical experiences involve giving care to patients or residents. The patient or resident has the right to know who you are. Introduce yourself. Tell the person you are a student. For example:

Hello. My name is Jesse Smith. I am a nursing assistant student. I will be working with your nurse today.

PROMOTING SAFETY AND COMFORT

The Training Program

Safety

OBRA and other federal and state laws require background checks on individuals with direct patient or resident contact in long-term care agencies. This may include FBI (Federal Bureau of Investigation) fingerprint checks. Long-term care agencies include:

- Nursing centers and skilled nursing facilities
- Home care agencies
- Hospices
- Long-term care hospitals
- Assisted living residences
- Adult day-care centers
- Centers for persons with developmental or intellectual disabilities

OBRA does not allow persons convicted of abuse, neglect, mistreatment, or dishonest use of property to be employed in long-term care agencies. Your NATCEP may require a background check before enrolling in the program or before clinical experiences begin. Clinical sites have the right to deny a student's participation depending on the student's criminal record. Satisfactory completion of your clinical experience is a NATCEP requirement. Follow your NATCEP's guidelines.

Competency Evaluation. The competency evaluation has a written test and a skills test (Appendix A, p. 905).

- The written test has multiple-choice questions. Each has 4 choices. Only 1 answer is correct. The number of questions varies from state to state.
- For the skills test, you perform certain skills learned in your training program.

You take the competency evaluation after your training program. Your instructor knows the testing service used in your state and how to schedule the evaluation and pay the required fee. If working in a nursing center, the employer pays the fee. Otherwise you pay the fee.

Your training prepares you for the competency evaluation. If you listen, study hard, and practice safe care, you should do well. If the first attempt was not successful, you can re-test. OBRA allows at least 3 attempts to successfully complete the evaluation.

Each testing service has a candidate handbook. Review the handbook carefully as you prepare for the competency evaluation.

Certification. *Certification* is the official recognition by a state that standards or requirements have been met. After successfully completing your state's NATCEP, you have the title used in your state. Titles include:

- Certified nursing assistant (CNA) or certified nurse aide (CNA). CNA is used in most states.
- Licensed nursing assistant (LNA).
- Registered nurse aide (RNA).
- State registered nurse aide (SRNA).
- State tested nurse aide (STNA).

Nursing assistants can have their certifications (licenses, registrations) disciplined for actions that are harmful or dangerous to the public or a person's health. A state agency investigates complaints and may deny, revoke, or suspend a certification (license, registration).

Professional boundaries, ethics, and laws are discussed in Chapter 5. See "Roles and Responsibilities" on p. 26. Violations can affect your ability to work as a nursing assistant.

Nursing Assistant Registry. OBRA requires a nursing assistant registry in each state. It is the official record (listing) of persons who have successfully completed that state's approved NATCEP.

Before hiring a person as a nursing assistant, the employer must verify that the applicant has met competency requirements. The employer must also verify that the person is not disqualified for the position because of prior misconduct.

The registry must have at least the following information about each nursing assistant.

- Full name, including maiden name and any married names.
- Identifying information.
- Date the competency evaluation was passed.
- Information about findings of abuse, neglect, exploitation, or misappropriation. (*Exploitation* means to take advantage of for personal gain. *Misappropriation* is the dishonest use of property. See Chapter 5.) The nature of the offense and supporting evidence are documented. If a hearing was held, the date and its outcome are included. The person has the right to include a statement disputing the finding. All information stays in the registry unless the finding was made in error, the person is found not guilty, or the state is notified of the registrant's death.

The National Council of State Boards of Nursing (NCSBN) has a directory of nursing assistant registries. The directory lists contact information for who maintains the registry and who investigates complaints in each state. The directory is available on the NCSBN's website.

Any health care agency can access registry information. You also receive a copy of your registry information. The copy is sent when the first entry is made and when information is changed or added. You can correct wrong information.

If a nursing assistant has not worked in 24 months, OBRA requires that the person be removed from the registry. Entries remain for findings of abuse, neglect, mistreatment, or dishonest use of property.

Maintaining Competence. OBRA requires that agencies provide 12 hours of education to nursing assistants every year. Performance reviews also are required. That is, your work is evaluated. These requirements help ensure that you have the current knowledge and skills to give safe, effective care.

OBRA has requirements to ensure the competence of nursing assistants who have not worked for 24 months. It does not matter how long you worked as a nursing assistant before. What matters is how long you did *not* work. States can require:

- A new competency evaluation
- Both re-training and a new competency evaluation
  See *Teamwork and Time Management: Maintaining Competence.*
  See *Focus on Surveys: Maintaining Competence.*

TEAMWORK AND TIME MANAGEMENT

Maintaining Competence

Educational programs are commonly called *in-service programs* or *in-service training.* Some are required; others are optional. In-service announcements and schedules are often e-mailed or posted on nursing units, in staff locker rooms and lounges, by the time clock, or on websites. Know how the agency communicates in-service information. Check those areas often.

In-services are scheduled before, during, or after your shift. If before work, plan to arrive early. If after work, plan to stay late. Arrange for transportation and childcare as needed (Chapter 6).

If an in-service is during your shift, plan with your co-workers. Some staff stay on the unit while others attend the in-service. Staff on the unit tend to all patients and residents. After returning to the unit, thank your co-workers for helping you. Help your co-workers when they attend in-services.

FOCUS ON SURVEYS

Maintaining Competence

Surveyors make sure that nursing assistants are competent to give safe care. They will:

- Check if nursing assistants have completed a NATCEP.
- Ask nursing assistants:
  - Where they received their training
  - The length of their training
  - How long they have worked in the agency
- Observe if nursing assistants:
  - Maintain or improve the person's independent functioning
  - Perform range-of-motion exercises (Chapter 35)
  - Transfer the person from bed to a wheelchair safely (Chapter 21)
  - Observe, describe, and report the person's behavior and condition to the nurse (Chapter 8)
  - Practice safe delegation (Chapter 4)
  - Practice infection control (Chapters 17 and 18) and safety measures (Chapters 14 and 15)

Working in Another State

To work in another state, you must meet that state's NATCEP requirements. First, contact the state agency responsible for NATCEPs and the nursing assistant registry. The NCSBN has a directory on its website.

Then apply to the desired state agency for endorsement (reciprocity, equivalency) as a CNA (LNA, RNA, SRNA, STNA). *Endorsement (reciprocity, equivalency)* means that a state recognizes the certificate, license, or registration issued by another state. Your application is reviewed to see if you meet the state's requirements.

- Your certification (license, registration) is current and in good standing.
- You meet that state's education, work, and legal requirements.
  Follow the application instructions. Expect to:
- Complete required forms. You must be truthful. False or misleading information may result in:
  - Denial of certification (a license, registration)
  - Disciplinary action
  - A fine
- Provide proof of successfully completing a nursing assistant training program. If a school transcript, grade report, or completion certificate is needed, send a copy. Do not send the original.
- Request registry verification from the state in which you are currently certified (licensed, registered). Pay the required fee.
- Provide fingerprints.
- Pay the required application fee.
  Registry information is checked. A criminal background check is done. Both are used to identify disqualifying offenses. On a registry, substantiated findings of abuse,

neglect, exploitation, or misappropriation are disqualifying offenses. (*Substantiated findings* are those found to be true.) State laws for disqualifying convictions on a criminal background check are followed.

The application review results in 1 or more of the following.

- Being granted or denied certification (a license, registration).
- Having to take a NATCEP competency test. This may be the written test, the skills test, or both.
- Having to take the entire NATCEP in that state (training program and competency test).

ROLES AND RESPONSIBILITIES

OBRA, nurse practice acts and other state laws, and legal and advisory opinions direct what you can do. To protect persons from harm, you must understand what you can do, what you cannot do, and the legal limits of your role. This is called *scope of practice* or *range of functions*.

Licensed nurses supervise your work. You perform nursing tasks related to the person's care. A *nursing task is nursing care or a nursing function, procedure, skill, or activity.* (See Chapter 4.) Often you function without a nurse in the room. At other times you help nurses give care. The rules in Box 3-1 will help you understand your role.

The range of functions for nursing assistants varies among states and agencies. Before performing a nursing task make sure that:

- Your state allows nursing assistants to do so.
- It is in your job description.
- You have the education and training to do so.
- A nurse is available to answer questions and to guide and assist you as needed.

You perform nursing tasks to meet the person's hygiene, safety, comfort, nutrition, exercise, and elimination needs. You move and transfer persons and make observations. You measure temperatures, pulses, respirations, and blood pressures. And you help promote the person's mental comfort.

Box 3-2 describes the limits of your role—tasks that you should never do. State laws differ. Know what you can do in the state in which you are working. If you work in 2 states, you must know the laws for both states.

Your job description reflects your state's laws and rules. An agency can further limit what you can do. So can a nurse based on the person's needs. However, no agency or nurse can expand your range of functions beyond what your state's laws and rules allow.

See *Focus on Long-Term Care and Home Care: Roles and Responsibilities*.

BOX 3-1	Rules for Nursing Assistants

- You are an assistant to the nurse.
- A nurse assigns and supervises your work.
- You report observations about the person's physical and mental status to the nurse (Chapter 8). Report changes in the person's condition or behavior at once.
- The nurse decides what is done or not done for a person. You do not make these decisions.
- Review directions and the care plan (Chapter 8) with the nurse before going to the person.
- Perform only the nursing tasks that you are trained to do.
- Ask a nurse to guide and assist you if you are not comfortable performing a nursing task.
- Perform only the nursing tasks that your state and job description allow.

BOX 3-2	Role Limits

- ***Never give drugs.*** This includes drugs given:
  - Orally, rectally, vaginally, and by injection
  - By application to the skin, eyes, ears, and nose
  - Directly into the bloodstream or through an intravenous (IV) line

  Nurses give drugs. Many states allow nursing assistants to give some drugs after completing a state-approved medication assistant training program. The function must be in your job description. And you must have the necessary supervision.
- ***Never insert tubes or objects into body openings. Do not remove them from the body.*** You must not insert tubes into the person's bladder, esophagus, trachea, nose, ears, bloodstream, or surgically created body openings. Exceptions to this rule are the procedures you will study during your training. Giving enemas is an example. The task must be in your job description. And you must have the necessary supervision.
- ***Never take oral or phone orders from doctors.*** Politely give your name and title, and ask the doctor to wait for a nurse. Promptly find a nurse to speak with the doctor.
- ***Never tell the person or family the person's diagnosis or medical or surgical treatment plans.*** This is the doctor's responsibility. Nurses may clarify what the doctor has said.
- ***Never diagnose or prescribe treatments or drugs for anyone.*** Doctors, physician's assistants, and some advanced practice nurses diagnose and prescribe.
- ***Never supervise others, including other nursing assistants.*** This is a nurse's responsibility. You will not be trained to supervise others. Supervising others can have serious legal problems.
- ***Never ignore an order or request to do something.*** This includes nursing tasks that you can do, those you cannot do, and those beyond your legal limits. Promptly and politely explain to the nurse why you cannot carry out the order or request. The nurse assumes you are doing what you were told to do unless you explain otherwise. You cannot neglect the person's care.

Nursing Assistant Standards

All NATCEPs include the range of functions required by OBRA. Some states allow other functions. NATCEPs also prepare nursing assistants to meet standards for safe, quality care. See Box 3-3.

BOX 3-3	Nursing Assistant Standards

The nursing assistant:
- Performs nursing tasks within the range of functions allowed by the state and agency.
- Functions under the supervision of a licensed nurse.
- Practices safe delegation (Chapter 4).
  - Knows his or her role limits.
  - Asks questions to clarify what is expected.
  - Communicates when a task is unclear or unfamiliar.
  - Knows when to accept and refuse tasks.
  - Is responsible for his or her actions.
  - Communicates progress, problems, and changes in the person's status.
- Follows agency policies and procedures.
- Follows manufacturer instructions for equipment and supplies used.
- Protects the person, self, and others by practicing safety and infection prevention measures (Chapters 14 through 19).
- Respects the person's rights and dignity (Chapter 2).
- Protects confidential information (Chapter 5).
- Demonstrates ethical and professional behavior (Chapters 5 and 6).
- Communicates effectively with the person and health team (Chapters 7 and 8). Reporting and recording are accurate, concise, and timely.
- Follows the person's care plan (Chapter 8).
- Demonstrates and maintains competence in required skills and functions (p. 25).

Job Description

A *job description* is a document that describes what an agency expects you to do (Fig. 3-2, pp. 28-30). It also states educational requirements and your job title. (See "Nursing Assistant Job Titles.")

Always obtain a written job description when you apply for a job. Ask questions about it during your job interview (Chapter 60). Before accepting a job, tell the employer about:
- Functions you did not learn
- Functions you cannot do for moral or religious reasons

Clearly understand what is expected before taking a job. Do not take a job that requires you to:
- Act beyond the legal limits of your role.
- Function beyond your training limits.
- Perform acts that are against your morals or religion.

No one can force you to do something beyond the legal limits of your role. You must understand:
- Your roles and responsibilities
- What you can safely do
- The things you should never do
- Your job description
- The ethical and legal aspects of your role (Chapter 5)

See *Focus on Communication: Job Description.*

Nursing Assistant Job Titles. After successfully completing a NATCEP, you have the title used by law and the nursing assistant registry in your state (see "Certification"). For job purposes, agencies often use other titles. Your job title depends on the setting and your roles and functions in the agency. Examples include:
- Clinical technician
- Health care assistant (technician)
- Nurse technician
- Nursing care partner
- Nursing support technician
- Patient care assistant (attendant, monitor, technician, worker)
- Support partner

POSITION DESCRIPTION / PERFORMANCE EVALUATION

Job Title: LTC certified nursing assistant (CNA)   Supervised by: CNA coordinator, charge nurse
Prepared by: _____   Approved by: _____
Date: _____   Date: _____

Job summary: Provides direct and indirect resident care activities under the direction of an RN or LPN/LVN. Assists residents with activities of daily living, provides for personal care, comfort and assists in the maintenance of a safe and clean environment for an assigned group of residents.

DUTIES AND RESPONSIBILITIES:

        3 = Exceeds the standard   2 = Meets the standard   1 = Needs improvement

Demonstrates competency in the following areas:

	3	2	1
Assists in the preparation for admission of residents.	3	2	1
Assists in and accompanies residents in the admission, transfer and discharge procedures.	3	2	1
Provides morning care, which may include bed bath, shower or whirlpool, oral hygiene, combing hair, back care, dressing residents, changing bed linen, cleaning overbed table and bedside stand, straightening room and other general care as necessary throughout the day.	3	2	1
Provides evening care which includes hands/face washing as needed, oral hygiene, back rubs, peri-care, freshening linen, cleaning overbed tables, straightening room and other general care as needed.	3	2	1
Notifies appropriate licensed staff when resident complains of pain.	3	2	1
Provides postmortem care and assists in transporting bodies to the morgue.	3	2	1
Assists LPN/LVN in treatment procedures.	3	2	1
Provides general nursing care, such as positioning residents, lifting and turning residents, applying/utilizing special equipment, assisting in use of bedpan or commode and ambulating the residents.	3	2	1
Performs all aspects of resident care in an environment that optimizes resident safety and reduces the likelihood of medical/health care errors.	3	2	1
Supports and maintains a culture of safety and quality.	3	2	1
Takes and records temperature, pulse, respiration, weight, blood pressure and intake-output.	3	2	1
Makes rounds with outgoing shift; knows whereabouts of assigned residents.	3	2	1
Makes rounds with oncoming shift to ensure the unit is left in good condition.	3	2	1
Adheres to policies and procedures of the facility and the nursing department.	3	2	1
Participates in socialization activities on the unit.	3	2	1
Turns and positions residents as ordered and/or as needed, making sure no rough surfaces are in direct contact with the body. Lifts and turns with proper and safe body mechanics and with available resources.	3	2	1
Checks for reddened areas or skin breakdown and reports to RN or LPN/LVN.	3	2	1
Ensures residents are dressed properly and assists, as necessary. Ensures that used clothing is properly stored in bedside stand or on hangers in closet. Ensures that all residents are clean and dry at all times.	3	2	1
Checks unit for adequate linen. Folds neatly and arranges linen in linen closet. Cleans linen cart. Provides clean linen and clothing. Makes beds.	3	2	1
Treats residents and their families with respect and dignity.	3	2	1

FIGURE 3-2 Portions of a sample job description. Note that the job description is also a performance evaluation tool. (Modified from Medical Consultants Network, Inc., Englewood, Colo.)

Restrains residents properly, when ordered.	3	2	1
Accompanies residents to appointments, as directed.	3	2	1
Provides reality orientation in daily care.	3	2	1
Prepares residents for meals; serves and removes food trays and assists with meals or feeds residents, if necessary.	3	2	1
Distributes drinking water and other nourishments to residents.	3	2	1
Performs general care activities for residents in isolation.	3	2	1
Answers residents' call lights, anticipates residents' needs and makes rounds to assigned residents.	3	2	1
Assists residents with handling and care of clothing and other personal property (including dentures, glasses, contact lenses, hearing aids and prosthetic devices).	3	2	1
Transports residents to and from various departments, as requested.	3	2	1
Reports and, when appropriate, records any changes observed in condition or behavior of residents and unusual incidents.	3	2	1
Participates in and contributes to interdisciplinary care conferences.			
Must be able to follow directions, both oral and written, and work cooperatively with other staff members.	3	2	1
Must have the ability to acquire knowledge of and develop skills in basic nursing procedures and simple documenting.	3	2	1
Establishes and maintains interpersonal relationship with residents, family members and other facility staff while assuring confidentiality of resident information.	3	2	1
Attends in-service education programs, as assigned, to learn new treatments, procedures, developmental skills, etc.	3	2	1
Practices careful, efficient and nonwasteful use of supplies and linen and follows established charge procedure for resident charge items.	3	2	1
Maintains personal health in order to prevent absence from work due to health problems.	3	2	1
Possesses a genuine interest and concern for geriatric and disabled persons.	3	2	1

Professional requirements:

Adheres to dress code; appearance is neat and clean.	3	2	1
Completes annual education requirements.	3	2	1
Maintains regulatory requirements.	3	2	1
Maintains resident confidentiality at all times.	3	2	1
Reports to work on time and as scheduled, completes work within designated time.	3	2	1
Wears identification while on duty, uses computerized punch time system correctly.	3	2	1
Completes in-services and returns in a timely fashion.	3	2	1
Attends annual review and department in-services, as scheduled.	3	2	1
Attends at least _____ staff meetings annually, reads and returns all monthly staff meeting minutes.	3	2	1
Represents the organization in a positive and professional manner.	3	2	1

FIGURE 3-2, cont'd

Continued

Actively participates in performance improvement and continuous quality improvement (CQI) activities.	3	2	1
Complies with all organizational policies regarding ethical business practices.	3	2	1
Communicates the mission, ethics and goals of the facility.	3	2	1

Total points   _____ _____ _____

Regulatory requirements:

• High school graduate or equivalent.

• Current certified nursing assistant (CNA) certification in State of _____ for long-term care facilities.

• Current basic cardiac life support certification within three (3) months of hire date.

Language skills:

• Able to communicate effectively in English, both verbally and in writing.

• Additional languages preferred.

Skills:

• Basic computer knowledge.

Physical demands:

• For physical demands of position, including vision, hearing, repetitive motion and environment, see following description.

Reasonable accommodations may be made to enable individuals with disabilities to perform the essential functions of the position without compromising resident care.

- -

I have received, read and understand the Position description/Performance evaluation above.

_____   _____
Name/Signature   Date signed

FIGURE 3-2, cont'd

EMPLOYEE ORIENTATION

Employee orientation occurs at the start of a new job or with a job transition (change). Staff are introduced to their new workplace. Orientation usually includes the following:

• Agency-wide orientation:
  • Agency vision, mission, and goals
  • Completion of necessary paperwork
  • Tour of the agency
  • Payroll processes
  • Understanding and agreeing to the agency's code of conduct, dress code, and rules about privacy and confidentiality (Chapters 5 and 6)

• Role and unit-specific orientation:
  • Touring the unit
  • Meeting other staff
  • Training in:
    • Policies and procedures related to the role.
    • Safety, emergency, and infection control procedures.
    • Access and use of the medical record (Chapter 8). For electronic systems, a username and password are set up. Employees are taught to use the system.
    • Use of equipment related to the role.

The final step of orientation often includes time on the job with a preceptor. A *preceptor* is an experienced staff member who mentors a new employee at the start of a job. New employees work alongside their preceptors to gain comfort and confidence in performing the job on their own.

Orientation time varies. When interviewing for a job (Chapter 60), ask about the agency's new employee orientation program. Employee orientation is an important time to prepare you for your role as a nursing assistant in the agency.

FOCUS ON **PRIDE**

The Person, Family, and Yourself

Personal and Professional Responsibility

Personal and professional qualities allow you to do your job well. Communication skills, patience, compassion, and teamwork are examples. You will learn about other qualities when you study work ethics in Chapter 6.

Rights and Respect

Most NATCEPs involve practice in a clinical setting. Sometimes a patient or resident refuses to have a student. Or the person refuses to allow a student to watch a procedure. The person's right to refuse must be respected.

Independence and Social Interaction

You will practice many skills in the classroom or laboratory before going to the clinical setting. Practice as if you are with a real patient or resident. Practice what to say and how to act. Practice the skill many times. This will help you feel more comfortable and confident in the clinical setting.

Delegation and Teamwork

Delegation deals with what you are asked to do (Chapter 4). To safely assist the nurse, you must know what you can and cannot do. Do not be discouraged by what you *cannot* do. Value what you *can* do. Your attitude affects your work. Take pride in your role.

Ethics and Laws

Some nursing assistants work in more than 1 setting. Some are also emergency medical technicians (EMTs). EMTs give emergency care outside of health care settings. State laws and rules for EMTs and nursing assistants differ. For example, you work as an EMT and a nursing assistant. Your state laws allow EMTs to start intravenous (IV) lines. Nursing assistants do not start IVs.

The ability to do something does not give the right to do so in all settings. There are legal limits to your role. Be proud of the advanced skills and training you may have. But when working as a nursing assistant, follow your state's laws and rules for nursing assistants.

FOCUS ON **PRIDE**: *Application*

Your NATCEP involves a skills test. An evaluator will observe you performing certain skills. How will you prepare for the test?

REVIEW QUESTIONS

Circle the BEST answer.

1 The Omnibus Budget Reconciliation Act of 1987 (OBRA)
   a Made it easier to become a nursing assistant
   b Limited the roles and functions of nursing assistants
   c Set training and competency evaluation requirements for nursing assistants
   d Set fees for nursing assistant registry

2 What state law affects what nursing assistants can do?
   a Standards for nursing assistants
   b Medicaid
   c OBRA
   d Nurse practice act

3 Training programs for nursing assistants must include
   a At least 50 hours of instruction
   b Training in basic nursing and personal care skills
   c Practical training in a hospital setting
   d Training on how to take phone orders from doctors

4 You do not pass your state's competency evaluation on the first attempt. You
   a Are not allowed to re-test
   b Must repeat your training program to re-test
   c May re-take the test
   d Are not allowed to repeat a training program

5 OBRA requires a nursing assistant registry. You are placed on the registry after
   a Completing the classroom part of your training program
   b Working as a nursing assistant for 1 year
   c Paying a registration fee
   d Successfully completing a state-approved NATCEP

6 A nursing assistant has findings of abuse and neglect listed on a state's registry. OBRA
   a Does not allow the person to work as a nursing assistant in long-term care agencies
   b Allows the person to work as a nursing assistant in that state
   c Allows the person to work as a nursing assistant in a different state
   d Does not allow the person to dispute the findings

7 Your nursing assistant certification (license, registration) can be revoked for
   a Refusing a nursing task for moral reasons
   b Asking the nurse questions
   c Performing acts beyond your role
   d Keeping the person's information confidential

Continued

8   You have not worked as a nursing assistant for 3 years (36 months). You can work as a nursing assistant again if
   a   You meet your state's requirements for competency evaluation
   b   You worked as a nursing assistant for at least 5 years
   c   The agency waives your need for re-training
   d   You repeat a background check

9   As a nursing assistant, you
   a   Can explain the person's treatment plan to the family
   b   Report observations to the nurse
   c   Can remove tubes from the person's body
   d   Can ignore a nursing task if it is not in your job description

10   Giving drugs is outside of the nursing assistant range of functions. Which is *true*?
   a   Giving drugs can be included in your job description.
   b   The nurse can ask you to give a person's drugs.
   c   You cannot give drugs.
   d   The nurse is not responsible for knowing your range of functions.

11   Who assigns and supervises your work?
   a   A nurse
   b   The health team
   c   Another nursing assistant
   d   You

12   You are responsible for
   a   Supervising other nursing assistants
   b   Telling the person his or her diagnosis
   c   Knowing what you can safely do
   d   Deciding what treatments are needed

13   You perform a task not allowed by your state. Which is *true*?
   a   If a nurse asked you to do the task, there is no legal problem.
   b   You could be practicing nursing without a license.
   c   You can perform the task if it is in your job description.
   d   If you complete the task safely, there is no legal problem.

14   You show that you can meet standards when you
   a   Misuse equipment and supplies
   b   Pretend to be comfortable with an unfamiliar task
   c   Share confidential information
   d   Follow policies and procedures

15   Which describes what an agency expects you to do?
   a   Nurse practice act
   b   Range of functions
   c   Scope of practice
   d   Job description

16   Employee orientation
   a   Helps new employees prepare to do a job
   b   Is required as part of a state's NATCEP
   c   Occurs when staff have poor performance reviews
   d   Delays the start of a job and is a waste of time

Answers to Chapter 3 questions are on p. 901.

FOCUS ON PRACTICE

Problem Solving

You are practicing skills in the laboratory setting. How will you respond to the following situations?
- Other students are using equipment that you need in order to practice.
- Another student needs a partner in order to practice a skill.
- You have questions. Your instructor is helping other students.
- You practiced a skill once. You need more practice to feel confident.

Delegation

KEY TERMS

accountable To answer to one's self and others about one's choices, decisions, and actions

delegate To authorize or direct a nursing assistant to perform a nursing task

delegated nursing task
- A nursing task that is beyond the nursing assistant's usual work assignment
- Using the delegation process, the nurse transfers responsibility for completion of the task to the nursing assistant

delegation
- The process a nurse uses to direct a nursing assistant to perform a nursing task
- Allowing a nursing assistant to perform a nursing task that is beyond the nursing assistant's usual role and not routinely done by the nursing assistant

nursing task Nursing care or a nursing function, procedure, skill, or activity

routine nursing task A nursing task that is part of a nursing assistant's usual work assignment

KEY ABBREVIATIONS

ANA	American Nurses Association		NATCEP	Nursing assistant training and competency evaluation program
APRN	Advanced practice registered nurse		NCSBN	National Council of State Boards of Nursing
LPN	Licensed practical nurse		RN	Registered nurse
LVN	Licensed vocational nurse			

Nursing assistants function under the supervision of licensed nurses—advanced practice registered nurses (APRNs), registered nurses (RNs), or licensed practical nurses/licensed vocational nurses (LPNs/LVNs). Nurse practice acts give nurses the right to *assign* or *delegate* nursing tasks to nursing assistants.

Definitions and rules about delegation vary among state nurse practice acts, agency job descriptions, and national organizations. (The National Council of State Boards of Nursing [NCSBN] and the American Nurses Association [ANA] are examples.) You need to know the rules about delegation in your state and agency. The following definitions are used in this textbook.

- *Nursing task*—nursing care or a nursing function, procedure, skill, or activity
- *Delegate*—to authorize or direct a nursing assistant to perform a nursing task
- *Delegation*:
  - The process a nurse uses to direct a nursing assistant to perform a nursing task
  - Allowing a nursing assistant to perform a nursing task that is beyond the nursing assistant's usual role and not routinely done by the nursing assistant

Some tasks are part of the nursing assistant's routine work. The tasks are commonly assigned to nursing assistants. You will learn these routine nursing tasks in your training program. Feeding, moving and transfer procedures, hygiene and grooming measures, and how to measure weight and height are examples. Such tasks will be part of your usual work assignment.

Some states and agencies allow nurses to delegate tasks that are not routinely done by nursing assistants. The following guidelines outlined by the NCSBN and ANA are used for safe delegation of such tasks.

- The person delegating has the authority to do so. See "Who Can Delegate."
- The task is within the delegating nurse's scope of practice.
- The task is within the nursing assistant's range of functions and job description.
- The nursing assistant has the education and training to perform the task.
- The nursing assistant has shown competence in performing the task. *Competence* means having the ability to do something successfully.
- The task *does not* involve nursing judgment or critical decision making. Such tasks cannot be delegated.

DELEGATION GUIDELINES

Before performing a task, you need information. *Delegation Guidelines* boxes accompany the procedures in this book. The guidelines list the information you need from the nurse and care plan (Chapter 8) before performing a task. They also list the observations to record and report to the nurse.

Tasks are identified as routine nursing tasks or delegated nursing tasks.

- A *routine nursing task* is a nursing task that is part of a nursing assistant's usual work assignment. These tasks are learned in a basic nursing assistant training and competency evaluation program (NATCEP).
- A *delegated nursing task* is a nursing task that is beyond the nursing assistant's usual work assignment. Using the delegation process, the nurse transfers responsibility for completion of the task to the nursing assistant. The task must not require a nurse's professional knowledge or judgment. The nursing assistant must be competent to perform the task.

Examples of delegated nursing tasks may include procedures related to:

- Urinary catheters (Chapter 28)
- Enemas (Chapter 29)
- Nutritional support and IV therapy (Chapter 33)
- Measuring blood glucose (Chapter 39)
- Wound care (Chapter 41)
- Oxygen therapy (Chapter 44)

States and agencies differ on what nursing assistants can do. You must follow the rules in your state and agency. Before performing a delegated nursing task, make sure that:

- Your state allows you to perform the task.
- The task is in your job description (Chapter 3).
- You have the necessary education and training.
- The agency has determined that you are competent to perform the task safely.
- You review the procedure with the delegating nurse.
- The delegating nurse is available to answer questions and to guide and assist you as needed.

See *Promoting Safety and Comfort: Delegation Guidelines.*

PROMOTING SAFETY AND COMFORT

Delegation Guidelines

Safety

Delegated nursing tasks must be allowed by your state and in your job description. If not learned in your NATCEP, the agency must:

- Provide needed education and training.
- Evaluate your ability to perform the task safely.

Although delegated nursing tasks are beyond the nursing assistant's usual work assignment, such tasks should:

- Occur frequently within the regular care of the patient or resident population.
- Follow an established procedure.
- Require little or no variation each time the task is performed.
- Have a predictable outcome.

Some nursing responsibilities *cannot* be delegated to you. They include:

- Performing nursing tasks that require a nurse's professional knowledge and judgment.
- Making delegation decisions.
- The nursing process (Chapter 8).
  - Performing assessments
  - Developing care plans
  - Evaluating responses to care
- Providing education (teaching) to the person and family.
- Supervising others.
- Taking oral or phone orders from doctors or APRNs.
- Giving drugs.
- Inserting intravenous (IV) catheters (Chapter 33).

See "Your Role in Delegation" on p. 37.

WHO CAN DELEGATE

Licensed nurses can delegate.

- An APRN can delegate to RNs, LPNs/LVNs, and nursing assistants.
- An RN can delegate to LPNs/LVNs and nursing assistants.
- An LPN/LVN can delegate to nursing assistants if allowed by the state's nurse practice act.

A nurse's delegation decisions must result in the best care for the person. Otherwise the person's health and safety are at risk. The delegating nurse is accountable for safe delegation decisions. *Accountable* means to answer to one's self and others about one's choices, decisions, and actions. The nurse must make sure the task was completed safely and correctly. You are responsible for completing tasks safely.

Nursing assistants cannot delegate. You cannot assign or delegate any task to other nursing assistants or to any other worker. You can ask someone to help you. For example, you ask a co-worker to help you move a person in bed. But you cannot ask or tell someone to do your work. If you are unable to complete a task or need guidance, tell the delegating nurse. The nurse decides whether to re-assign or re-delegate the task.

See *Promoting Safety and Comfort: Who Can Delegate.*

DELEGATION PROCESS

For safe delegation, the person's needs, the nursing task, and the staff member doing the task must fit (Fig. 4-1). The nurse decides if the task is safe for you to do. The person's needs and the task may require a nurse's knowledge, judgment, and skill. You may be asked to assist.

Delegation is a process (Fig. 4-2) involving:

- Assessment of needs
- Communication
- Guidance and assistance
- Follow-up and feedback

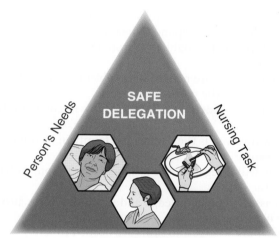

FIGURE 4-1 The nurse considers the person's needs, the task, and the staff member's abilities when making delegation decisions.

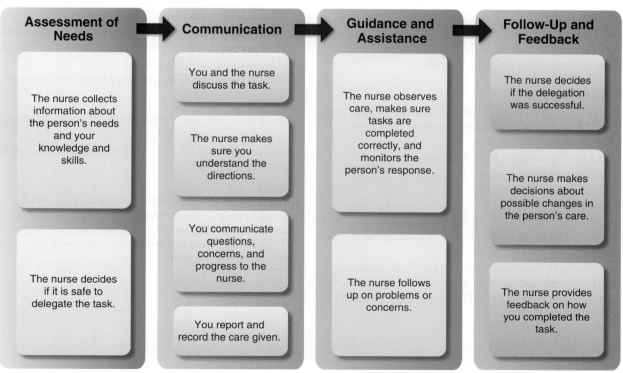

FIGURE 4-2 The delegation process.

Assessment of Needs

The nurse needs to understand the person's needs. And the nurse needs to know your knowledge, skills, and job description.

To assess the person's needs, the nurse answers these questions.

- What are the person's needs? How complex and urgent are they? How can they vary?
- What are the most important long-term and short-term needs?
- How much judgment is needed to meet the person's needs and give care?
- How predictable is the person's health status? How does the person respond to health care?
- What problems might arise from the task? How severe might they be?
- What actions are needed if a problem occurs? How complex are the needed actions?
- What emergencies might arise? How likely might they occur?
- How involved is the person and family in health care decisions?
- How will delegating the task help the person? What are the risks?

To assess your knowledge and skills, the nurse answers these questions.

- What knowledge and skills are needed to safely perform the task?
- What is in your job description?
- What are the conditions affecting the task?
- What is expected from the task?
- What problems might the person develop during the task?
- What problems can arise from the task?

The nurse decides if you can safely perform the task. It must be safe for the person and you. If unsafe, the nurse stops the delegation process. If safe for the person and you, the nurse continues the delegation process.

Communication

The communication step involves the nurse and you (Fig. 4-3). The nurse must give you clear and complete directions about:

- How to perform and complete the task
- What observations to report and record
- When to report observations
- What patient or resident concerns to report at once
- Priorities for tasks
- What to do if the person's condition changes or needs change

The nurse asks questions to make sure you understand. The nurse may ask you to explain what you will do. Do not be insulted by such questions. The intent is to protect the person and you.

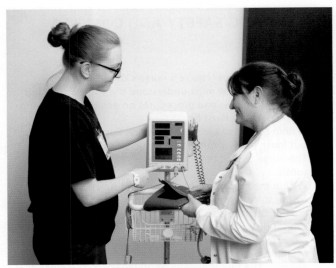

FIGURE 4-3 A nurse and nursing assistant discuss a nursing task.

Before performing a delegated task, discuss the task with the nurse. Make sure that you:

- Ask questions about the task and what you are expected to do.
- Tell the nurse if you have not done the task before or not often.
- Ask for needed training or supervision.
- Re-state what is expected of you.
- Re-state what patient or resident concerns to report to the nurse.
- Explain how and when you will report progress in completing the task.
- Know how to call the nurse for an emergency.
- Know what to do during an emergency.

After completing a task, report and record the care given. Also report and record your observations. See "Reporting and Recording" in Chapter 8.

See *Focus on Long-Term Care and Home Care: Communication*.

FOCUS ON LONG-TERM CARE AND HOME CARE

Communication

Home Care

The delegating nurse is often not with you during your home care visits. The nurse may be at the agency or in another home. You must know how to get help at once if you need it. Have a communication plan with the nurse before leaving the agency.

Guidance and Assistance

The nurse supervises your work. The nurse must be available to guide and assist you as needed. The nurse:

- Observes the care you give as needed.
- Makes sure that you complete the task correctly.
- Observes the person's condition and response to care. The frequency of the nurse's observations depends on:
  - The person's health status and needs
  - If the person's condition is stable or unstable
  - If the nurse can predict the person's responses and risks to care
  - The setting where the task occurs
  - The resources and support available
  - If the task is simple or complex

The nurse follows up on problems or concerns. For example, the nurse takes action if:

- You did not complete the task in a timely manner.
- The task did not meet expectations.
- There is a change in the person's condition.

The nurse is alert for possible changes in the person's condition. With your help, the nurse can act before the person's condition changes.

Depending on the person's needs, the nurse might need to assist you with the task. Or the nurse can decide to perform the task.

After you complete the task, the nurse may review and discuss what happened with you. This helps you learn. If something similar happens again, you have ideas about how to adjust.

Follow-Up and Feedback

Follow-up means to review and take needed action. The nurse decides if the delegation was successful. The nurse answers these questions.

- Was the task done correctly?
- Did the person respond as expected?
- Was the result (outcome) as desired? Was the result good or bad?
- Did you and the nurse have timely and effective communication?
- What went well? What were the problems?
- Does the care plan need to change (Chapter 8)?
- Did the nurse give feedback? *Feedback* means to respond. The nurse tells you what you did correctly and about any errors. Feedback helps you learn and improve the care you give.

YOUR ROLE IN DELEGATION

You must protect the person from harm. You have 2 choices when delegated a task. You either *accept* or *refuse* a task. Use the *Five Rights of Delegation* in Box 4-1 to guide your decision.

BOX 4-1 | **The *Five Rights of Delegation* for Nursing Assistants**

The Right Task
- Does your state allow you to perform the task?
- Is the task in your job description?
- Were you trained to do the task?

The Right Circumstance
- Do you have experience with the task given the person's condition and needs?
- Do you understand the purposes of the task for the person?
- Can you perform the task safely under the current circumstances?
- Do you have needed equipment and supplies?
- Do you know how to use the equipment and supplies?

The Right Person
- Are you comfortable performing the task?
- Do you have concerns about performing the task?

The Right Directions and Communication
- Did the nurse give clear directions and instructions?
- Did you review the task with the nurse?
- Do you understand what the nurse expects?
- Did you ask the nurse about questions you have?

The Right Supervision and Evaluation
- Is a nurse available to answer questions?
- Is a nurse available if the person's condition changes or if problems occur?
- Did the nurse evaluate the result?

Modified from National Council of State Boards of Nursing, Inc.: The five rights of delegation, as referenced in National guidelines for nursing delegation, Chicago, April 29, 2019, National Council of State Boards of Nursing and American Nurses Association.

Accepting a Task

When you agree to perform a task, you are responsible for your actions. What you do or fail to do can harm the person. *You must complete the task safely.* Ask for help if you are unsure or have questions. Report to the nurse what you did and your observations.

Refusing a Task

You have the right to refuse (not accept) a delegated task. You should refuse when:

- The task is beyond the range of functions for nursing assistants allowed by your state.
- The task is not in your job description.
- The task requires a nurse's professional knowledge, judgment, or skill.
- You were not trained to do the task.
- The task could harm the person.
- The person's condition has changed.
- You do not know how to use the supplies or equipment.
- Directions are not ethical or legal.
- Directions are against agency policies.
- Directions are not clear or complete.
- A nurse is not available to guide and assist you as needed.

Use common sense. This protects you and the person. Ask yourself if what you are doing is safe for the person.

Never ignore an order or a request to do something. Share your concerns with the nurse. For tasks within the legal limits of your role and in your job description, the nurse can help increase your comfort. The nurse can:

- Answer your questions.
- Demonstrate the task.
- Show you how to use supplies and equipment.
- Observe you doing the task.
- Help you as needed.
- Check on you often.
- Arrange for needed training.

Do not refuse a task because you do not like it or do not want to do it. You must have sound reasons. Otherwise, you place the person at risk for harm. You could lose your job.

See *Focus on Communication: Refusing a Task.*

FOCUS ON COMMUNICATION

Refusing a Task

A nurse may delegate a task that was not part of your NATCEP or is unfamiliar. The task is in your job description. You can say:

> *I know this task is in my job description, but I have not done it alone yet. Can you observe me doing it? That would really help me.*

A nurse may ask you to do something that is not in your job description. With respect, firmly refuse the nurse's request. For example, the nurse sets a cup of pills in the room and asks you to give them to the person when you finish brushing the person's teeth. You can say:

> *I'm sorry, but I cannot. I am not trained to give drugs, and the task is not in my job description. Would you like to give them now? Or would you like me to tell you when I am done?*

FOCUS ON PRIDE

The Person, Family, and Yourself

Personal and Professional Responsibility

You must maintain competence in the skills and functions required to do your job (Chapter 3). Even after meeting competency requirements, you will likely have questions or concerns about performing tasks. For example:

- This will be your first time collecting a specimen (Chapter 39) without an instructor or preceptor. You want to review the procedure.
- You just learned to use new equipment. You want to make sure you are using it properly.
- A resident's condition has changed. You do not think you can complete a task without help.

Never be afraid to ask questions or to ask for help. If uncertain about your ability to safely perform a task, tell the nurse. Take pride in protecting the person from harm.

Rights and Respect

Feedback helps you learn and improve in your role as a nursing assistant. Receive feedback in a respectful manner.

- Listen carefully.
- Have good eye contact.
- Consider ways you can improve.
- Avoid arguing or being defensive.
- Thank the nurse for the feedback.

Independence and Social Interaction

After completing your NATCEP and your agency's orientation program (Chapter 3), you should be prepared to perform routine nursing tasks independently. With training and practice, you will perform most delegated nursing tasks independently. Take pride in growing in confidence and independence. However, be alert to when you need help or should refuse a task.

Delegation and Teamwork

Good teamwork improves the delegation process. Staff interactions matter. The person and nursing team benefit when staff:

- Communicate openly.
- Trust each other.
- Help and encourage each other.
- Work toward a common goal.

Ethics and Laws

Nurses are legally responsible for making safe and ethical delegation decisions. You are responsible for your decision to accept or refuse a task and for completing the task safely.

FOCUS ON PRIDE: Application

How do staff interactions affect the delegation process? Explain how good teamwork benefits the nursing team and the person.

REVIEW QUESTIONS

Circle the BEST answer.

1 What can be delegated to you?
   a Teaching the person and family
   b Performing tasks in your job description
   c Evaluating responses to care
   d Giving drugs

2 Removing urinary catheters is done frequently in your work area. The task is not part of your usual work assignment, but it is in your job description. You are trained to do it. This task
   a Is a routine nursing task
   b Cannot be delegated to you
   c Can be delegated to you using the delegation process
   d Requires a nurse's judgment and skill

3 You are responsible for
   a Completing tasks safely
   b Assessing the person's needs
   c Supervising other nursing assistants
   d Assigning and delegating nursing tasks

4 Which statement about who can delegate is *correct*?
   a Nursing assistants can delegate to other nursing assistants.
   b LPNs/LVNs can delegate to RNs.
   c RNs can delegate to nursing assistants.
   d RNs can delegate to APRNs.

5 In the delegation process, communication involves
   a Observing care
   b Determining who should perform a task
   c Deciding if the task was successful
   d Asking questions about a task

6 Which statement about guidance and assistance is *true*?
   a The nurse must be with you when you give care.
   b The nurse must make sure you complete tasks correctly.
   c Simple tasks require more assistance than complex ones.
   d More guidance is needed when the person's condition is stable.

7 A patient begins having trouble swallowing. The nurse decides not to assign feeding to you. Why?
   a The task is beyond the legal limits of your role.
   b You are not trained to do the task.
   c The nurse does not trust you to do the task safely.
   d The person's circumstances have changed.

8 You do not have clear directions for a task the nurse asked you to do. Which is *best*?
   a Ask questions to clarify what is expected.
   b Ignore the request.
   c Ask another nursing assistant to do the task.
   d Complete the task.

9 You can refuse to perform a task if
   a The task is within the legal limits of your role
   b The task is in your job description
   c You do not like the task
   d The task requires a nurse's judgment

10 To protect the person from harm, you should
   a Accept a delegated task that requires using unfamiliar equipment
   b Avoid asking for help
   c Refuse a task that you have not been trained to do
   d Accept all delegated tasks without question

11 You think you need to refuse a delegated task. What should you do?
   a Communicate your concerns to the nurse.
   b Tell the nurse you are sick and leave work.
   c Delay doing it and tell the nurse you ran out of time.
   d Talk to the director of nursing.

12 The nurse gives you feedback after a task. Which response is *best*?
   a Pretend to listen so you can return to work quickly.
   b Listen carefully and thank the nurse.
   c Defend yourself if the nurse corrects your errors.
   d Argue about the best way to do the task.

Answers to Chapter 4 questions are on p. 901.

FOCUS ON PRACTICE

Problem Solving

A nurse delegates a task that you have not done many times. What must you do to safely accept the task? How can the nurse help increase your comfort?

Ethics and Laws

OBJECTIVES

- Define the key terms and key abbreviations in this chapter.
- Describe ethical conduct.
- Describe a code of conduct for nursing assistants.
- Explain how to maintain professional boundaries.
- Explain how standards of care relate to negligence.
- Give examples of unintentional and intentional torts.
- Describe how to protect the right to privacy.

- Explain the correct use of electronic communications.
- Explain the purpose of informed consent.
- Describe elder abuse, child abuse and neglect, and intimate partner violence.
- Explain your role in relation to wills.
- Explain how to promote PRIDE in the person, the family, and yourself.

KEY TERMS

abuse
- The willful infliction of injury, unreasonable confinement, intimidation, or punishment that results in physical harm, pain, or mental anguish
- Depriving the person (or the person's caregiver) of the goods or services needed to attain or maintain well-being

assault Intentionally attempting or threatening to touch a person's body without the person's consent

battery Touching a person's body without consent

boundary crossing A brief act or behavior of being over-involved with the person; the intent of the act or behavior is to meet the person's needs

boundary sign An act, behavior, or thought that warns of a boundary crossing or boundary violation

boundary violation An act or behavior that meets your needs, not the person's

child abuse and neglect The intentional harm or mistreatment of a child under 18 years old that:
- Involves any recent act or failure to act on the part of a parent or caregiver
- Results in death, serious physical or emotional harm, sexual abuse, or exploitation
- Presents a likely or immediate risk for harm

civil law Laws concerned with relationships between people

code of ethics Rules, or standards of conduct, for group members to follow

consent Permission

crime An act that violates a criminal law

criminal law Laws concerned with offenses against the public and society in general

defamation Injuring a person's name and reputation by making false statements to a third person

drug diversion Stealing drugs for personal use, sale, or distribution to others

elder abuse Any intentional act, or failure to act, by a caregiver or other trusted person that causes harm or risk of harm to an older adult

ethics Knowledge of what is right conduct and wrong conduct

exploitation To take advantage of for personal gain

false imprisonment Unlawful restraint or restriction of a person's freedom of movement

fraud Saying or doing something to trick, fool, or deceive a person

informed consent The process by which a person receives and understands information about a treatment or procedure and is able to decide to receive or refuse the treatment or procedure

intimate partner violence (IPV) Abuse or aggression that occurs in a romantic relationship

invasion of privacy Violating a person's right not to have his or her name, photo, or private affairs exposed or made public without giving consent

law A rule of conduct made by a government body

libel Making false statements in print, in writing (including e-mail and text messages), through pictures or drawings, through broadcast (radio, TV, video), posted on-line on websites, or through video sites and social media sites

malpractice Negligence by a professional person

misappropriation The dishonest use of property

neglect When a caregiver or responsible person fails to:
- Protect a vulnerable person from harm
- Provide food, water, clothing, shelter, health care, or basic activities of daily living to a vulnerable person

negligence An unintentional wrong in which a person did not act in a reasonable and careful manner and a person or the person's property was harmed

professional boundary That which separates helpful actions and behaviors from those that are not helpful

KEY TERMS—cont'd

professional sexual misconduct A violation of professional interactions with an act, behavior, or comment that is sexual in nature
protected health information Identifying information and information about the person's health care that is maintained or sent in any form (paper, electronic, oral)
self-neglect When a person's behaviors and way of living threaten the person's own health, safety, and well-being
slander Making false statements through the spoken word, sounds, sign language, or gestures

standard of care The skills, care, and judgments required by a health team member under similar conditions
tort A wrong committed against a person or the person's property
vulnerable adult A person 18 years old or older who has a disability or condition that causes the person to be at risk for harm
will A legal document of how a person wants property distributed after death

KEY ABBREVIATIONS

CDC Centers for Disease Control and Prevention
HIPAA Health Insurance Portability and Accountability Act of 1996

IPV Intimate partner violence
OBRA Omnibus Budget Reconciliation Act of 1987
TDV Teen dating violence

Nurse practice acts, your training and job description, and safe delegation serve to protect patients and residents from harm (Chapters 3 and 4). Protecting them from harm also involves laws, rules, and standards of conduct. They form the ethical and legal aspects of care.

ETHICAL ASPECTS

Ethics is knowledge of what is right conduct and wrong conduct. Ethics involves choices or judgments about what should or should not be done. An ethical person behaves and acts in the right way. The person does not harm others.

Ethical behavior also involves not being prejudiced or biased. To be *prejudiced* or *biased* means making judgments and having views before knowing the facts. Judgments and views often are based on one's values and standards. They are based on culture, religion, education, and experiences. The person's situation and yours may be very different. For example:

- Children think their mother needs nursing home care. In your culture, children care for older parents at home.
- An older man does not want life-saving measures. You believe that everything must be done to save a life.

Do not judge the person by your values and standards. Do not avoid persons whose standards and values differ from your own.

Ethical problems involve choices. You must decide what is the right thing to do.

Codes of Ethics

Professional groups have codes of ethics. A *code of ethics* has rules, or standards of conduct, for group members to follow. Also called *codes of conduct*, professional nursing organizations have codes of ethics for nurses.

BOX 5-1	Code of Conduct for Nursing Assistants

- Respect each person as an individual.
- Know the limits of your role and knowledge.
- Perform only the tasks within the legal limits of your role.
- Perform only the tasks that you have been trained to do.
- Perform no act that will harm the person.
- Take drugs only if prescribed and supervised by a health care provider (doctor, dentist, physician's assistant, advanced practice registered nurse).
- Follow the nurse's directions to your best possible ability.
- Follow agency policies and procedures.
- Follow the manufacturer's instructions for equipment and supplies used.
- Complete each task safely.
- Be loyal to your employer and co-workers.
- Act as a responsible citizen at all times.
- Respect the person's rights and dignity.
- Keep the person's information confidential.
- Protect the person's privacy.
- Protect the person's property.
- Consider the person's needs to be more important than your own.
- Report errors and incidents honestly and at once.
- Be responsible for your actions.

The rules of conduct in Box 5-1 can guide your thinking, actions, and behavior. See Chapter 6 for student and work ethics.

Professional Boundaries

As a nursing assistant, you enter into a helping relationship with patients or residents and families. In this relationship, you are trusted with the person's care and with private information. The proper focus is on meeting the needs of the person and family.

Professional Boundaries

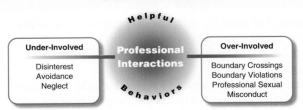

FIGURE 5-1 Professional boundaries guide your actions and behavior. Your focus is on helping the person. Being under-involved or over-involved is not helpful. (Modified from National Council of State Boards of Nursing, Inc.: *A nurse's guide to professional boundaries*, Chicago, 2018.)

A *boundary* limits or separates something. *Professional boundaries* separate helpful actions and behaviors from those that are not helpful. See Figure 5-1. Professional interactions involve helpful behaviors that meet the person's needs. Some behaviors are not helpful. They result in being *under-involved* or *over-involved* with the person.

If you are under-involved, the following can occur.

- Disinterest—You lack interest in the person.
- Avoidance—You avoid the person.
- Neglect—You do not properly care for the person (p. 47).

If you are over-involved, the following can occur.

- *Boundary crossing*—a brief act or behavior of being over-involved with the person. The intent of the act or behavior is to meet the person's needs. The act or behavior may be thoughtless or something you did not mean to do. Or it could have purpose if it meets the person's needs. For example, you give a crying patient a hug. The hug meets the person's needs at the time. If the hug meets your needs, the act is wrong. Also, it is wrong to hug the person every time you see each other.
- *Boundary violation*—an act or behavior that meets your needs, not the person's. The act or behavior is not ethical. It violates the code of conduct in Box 5-1. The person can be harmed. Boundary violations include:
  - Abuse (p. 46).
  - Giving a lot of information about yourself. You tell the person about your personal relationships or problems.
  - Keeping secrets with the person.
- *Professional sexual misconduct*—a violation of professional interactions with an act, behavior, or comment that is sexual in nature. It is sexual misconduct even if the person initiates it or gives *consent* (permission).

Some boundary violations and some types of professional sexual misconduct also are crimes. To maintain professional boundaries, follow the rules in Box 5-2. Be alert to boundary signs. *Boundary signs* are acts, behaviors, or thoughts that warn of a boundary crossing or boundary violation. See Box 5-2 for examples.

See *Focus on Communication: Professional Boundaries*.

BOX 5-2	Professional Boundaries

Maintaining Professional Boundaries

- Follow the code of conduct in Box 5-1. Maintain a professional relationship at all times.
- Talk to the nurse if you sense a boundary sign, crossing, or violation.
- Avoid caring for family, friends, and people you know. This may be hard to do in a small community. Tell the nurse if you know the person. The nurse may change your assignment.
- Do not make sexual comments or jokes.
- Do not use offensive language.
- Use touch correctly (Chapter 7). Touch or handle private areas only for needed care. The areas include the breasts, nipples, perineum, buttocks, thighs, and anus.
- Do not visit or spend extra time with someone who is not part of your assignment.
- The following apply to patients, residents, and families.
  - Do not flirt with or have a romantic relationship with them.
  - Do not discuss your romantic relationships with them.
  - Do not exchange (give or receive) gifts, loans, money, credit cards, or other valuables.
  - Do not borrow from them. This includes money, personal items, and transportation.
  - Do not develop a personal relationship with them.
  - Do not share personal or financial information with them.
  - Do not help with their finances.
  - Do not take a person home with you. This includes for holidays or other events.
- Ask yourself these questions before you date or marry a person whom you cared for. Be aware of the risk for professional sexual misconduct.
  - When were you involved with the person's care?
  - Was the person's care short-term or long-term?
  - What kind and how much information do you have about the person? How will that information affect your relationship with the person?
  - Will the person need more care in the future?
  - Does the relationship place the person at risk for harm?

Boundary Signs

- You think about the person when not at work.
- You visit with the person during breaks or when off duty.
- You trade assignments to provide the person's care.
- You prioritize the person's care over the care of others.
- You give the person more attention than others.
- You think no one else understands the person's needs.
- You give or receive gifts or money.
- You share personal information with the person.
- You notice more touch between you and the person.
- You flirt or make comments with a sexual message.
- You tell the person crude jokes.
- You use vulgar or offensive language when with the person.
- You and the person have secrets.
- You choose the person's side during disagreements.
- You select what to report and record. You do not give complete information.
- You do not like questions about your care or your relationship with the person.
- You change your appearance when you will see the person.
- You meet with the person after discharge from the agency.

FOCUS ON COMMUNICATION

Professional Boundaries

Some patients, residents, and families send thank-you cards and letters. Some offer thank-you gifts—candy, cookies, money, gift cards, flowers, and so on. Accepting gifts is a boundary violation. When offered a gift, you can say:

- "Thank you for thinking of me. It's very kind of you. However, it is against center policy to accept gifts. I do appreciate your offer."
- "Thank you for wanting me to have the flowers from your friend. They are lovely. However, it is against hospital policy to receive gifts. May I help you find a way to take them home?"

LEGAL ASPECTS

Ethics is about what you *should or should not do.* Laws tell you what you *can and cannot do.* A *law* is a rule of conduct made by a government body. The U.S. Congress and state legislatures make laws. Enforced by the government, laws protect the public welfare.

Criminal laws are concerned with offenses against the public and society in general. An act that violates a criminal law is called a *crime.* If found guilty of a crime, the person is fined or sent to prison. Murder, robbery, stealing (theft), rape, kidnapping, and abuse (p. 46) are crimes. Drug diversion is a form of theft. *Drug diversion* is stealing drugs for personal use, sale, or distribution to others. (*Diversion* means to use something in a way that it was not originally intended.)

Civil laws are concerned with relationships between people. Contracts and nurse practice acts are examples. A person found guilty of breaking a civil law usually has to pay a sum of money to the injured person.

Tort comes from the French word meaning *wrong.* Torts are part of civil law. A *tort* is a wrong committed against a person or the person's property. Some torts are *unintentional.* Harm was not intended. *Intentional* torts are done on purpose. Harm was intended. Some torts are also crimes.

What you do or do not do can lead to legal action if you harm a person or a person's property. You are legally responsible *(liable)* for your own actions. Sometimes refusing to follow the nurse's directions is your right and duty (Chapter 4).

Unintentional Torts

Health team members are expected to give care at a certain level. A *standard of care* refers to the skills, care, and judgments required by a health team member under similar conditions.

Standards of care come from laws, job descriptions (Chapter 3), agency policies and procedures (Chapter 1), and manufacturer's instructions for use of equipment and supplies. Approval (regulatory) agencies such as the Centers for Medicare & Medicaid Services (CMS) and accrediting agencies set standards (Chapter 1). Standards and guidelines also come from other government agencies like the Centers for Disease Control and Prevention (CDC). Textbooks, training programs, and employee orientation programs prepare students and workers to meet standards.

Negligence is a risk when standards of care are not met. *Negligence* is an unintentional wrong. The negligent person did not act in a reasonable and careful manner. A person or the person's property was harmed. The person causing the harm did not intend or mean to cause harm. The person failed to do what a reasonable and careful person *would have done.* Or the person did what a reasonable and careful person *would not have done.*

The following are examples of negligent acts.
- You fail to test the water temperature for a shower. The water is too hot. The person is burned.
- You do not answer a call light promptly. The person gets up without help. The person falls and breaks an arm.
- You do not follow the manufacturer's instructions for a mechanical lift. The person slips out of the lift and falls. The person fractures a hip.
- You do not tell the nurse about a patient's chest pain. The person has a heart attack and dies.
- You do not identify a person before a procedure. You perform the procedure on the wrong person. Both residents are harmed. One had a procedure that was not ordered. The other did not have a needed procedure.

Malpractice is negligence by a professional person. A person has professional status because of education and services provided. Nurses, doctors, dentists, and pharmacists are examples.

Intentional Torts

Intentional torts are meant to be harmful and may be crimes.

- *Defamation* is injuring a person's name and reputation by making false statements to a third person.
  - *Libel* is making false statements in print, in writing (including e-mail and text messages), through pictures or drawings, through broadcast (radio, TV, video), posted on-line on websites, or through video sites and social media sites. See "Wrongful Use of Electronic Communications."
  - *Slander* is making false statements through the spoken word, sounds, sign language, or gestures.
- *Fraud* is saying or doing something to trick, fool, or deceive a person. The act is fraud if it does or could harm a person or the person's property. Telling someone that you are a nurse is fraud. So is giving wrong or incomplete information on a job application.
- *False imprisonment* is the unlawful restraint or restriction of a person's freedom of movement. It involves:
  - Threatening to restrain a person
  - Restraining a person
  - Preventing a person from leaving the agency
- Invasion of privacy. See "Invasion of Privacy."
- *Assault* is intentionally attempting or threatening to touch a person's body without the person's consent. The person fears bodily harm. Threatening to "tie down" a person is an example of assault.
- *Battery* is touching a person's body without consent. The person must consent to any procedure, treatment, or other act that involves touching the body. The person has the right to withdraw consent at any time. See "Informed Consent."

See *Promoting Safety and Comfort: Intentional Torts.*

PROMOTING SAFETY AND COMFORT

Intentional Torts

Safety

To protect yourself from defamation, never make false statements about a patient, resident, family member, visitor, co-worker, or any other person. This includes:

- Through e-mails or text messages
- On websites, video sites, or social media sites
- In newspapers, magazines, or other print sources
- Through broadcasts (TV, radio, or film)
- With words, sounds, signs, gestures, or any form of communication

Examples of defamation include false statements about drug or alcohol use, mental illness, unprofessional conduct, criminal acts, negligence, and so on. The statement is false and is intended to damage a person's reputation. *Reporting a real concern is not defamation.*

You also must protect yourself from being accused of assault and battery. Explain to the person what you are going to do. Get the person's consent. Consent may be verbal—"yes" or "okay." Or it can be a gesture—a nod, turning over for a back massage, or holding out an arm for you to take a pulse.

Invasion of Privacy. Patients and residents have the right to personal privacy (Chapter 2). This involves privacy of the person's body, private affairs, and information about care, treatment, and condition. *Invasion of privacy* is violating a person's right not to have his or her name, photo, or private affairs exposed or made public without giving consent.

You must treat the person with respect and ensure privacy. See Box 5-3 for measures to protect privacy.

See *Focus on Communication: Invasion of Privacy.*

BOX 5-3   Protecting the Right to Privacy

- Keep all information about the person confidential.
- Cover the person when in hallways and elevators.
- Ask visitors to leave the room when care is given.
- Screen the person. Close the privacy curtain as in Figure 5-2. Close the room door and window coverings to give care.
- Close the bathroom door for elimination or hygiene.
- Expose only the body part involved in a task.
- Do not discuss the person or the person's treatment with anyone except the nurse supervising your work.
- Do not open the person's mail.
- Allow the person to visit with others in private.
- Allow the person to use the phone in private.
- Follow agency policies and procedures to protect privacy.

FOCUS ON COMMUNICATION

Invasion of Privacy

The *Health Insurance Portability and Accountability Act of 1996 (HIPAA)* protects the privacy and security of a person's health information. *Protected health information* refers to identifying information and information about the person's health care that is maintained or sent in any form (paper, electronic, oral). Failure to follow HIPAA rules can result in fines, penalties, and criminal actions including jail time.

To avoid HIPAA violations:
- Always follow agency policies and procedures.
- *Never take photos or videos of patients or residents or any person in the health care or home care setting.* Sharing photos or videos or posting them on video sites or social media sites is a very serious violation of HIPAA.
- *Never send an e-mail or text message or post anything on a website, video site, or social media site about a patient, resident, family member, or visitor.* Sharing information is a very serious violation of HIPAA.
- *Never write anything for a newspaper, magazine, or print source about a patient, resident, family member, or visitor.*
- *Never broadcast (through TV, radio, or video) anything about a patient, resident, family member, or visitor.*
- *Only discuss the person's health information with staff directly involved in the person's care.*
- See "Wrongful Use of Electronic Communications."

You may be asked questions about the person or the person's care. Direct such questions to the nurse. Also follow the rules for using computers and other electronic devices (Chapter 8).

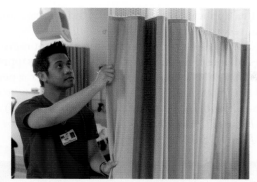

FIGURE 5-2 Pulling the privacy curtain around the bed helps protect the person's privacy.

Wrongful Use of Electronic Communications

Electronic communications include e-mail, text messages, faxes, websites, video sites, and social media sites. Video and social media sites include Facebook, LinkedIn, YouTube, Instagram, blogs and comments to blog postings, chat rooms, and so on. Other forms of electronic communications are expected in the future.

Correct use of electronic communications is essential in your personal life and as a nursing assistant. Follow the rules in Box 5-4. Do so whether using a computer, phone, camera, or other electronic device at home, at school, at work, or in any other setting. Wrongful use of electronic communications can result in job loss and loss of your certification (license, registration) for:

- Defamation
- Invasion of privacy
- HIPAA violations
- Violating the right to confidentiality (Chapter 6)
- Patient or resident abuse
- Unprofessional or unethical conduct

Wrongful use of electronic communications may be violations of federal and state laws that protect privacy and confidentiality. HIPAA is an example. Besides losing your certification (license, registration), wrongful use can result in:

- Civil action resulting in a fine
- Criminal action resulting in a fine or jail time

See *Focus on Communication: Wrongful Use of Electronic Communications.*

FOCUS ON COMMUNICATION

Wrongful Use of Electronic Communications

The following are examples of wrongful use of electronic communications.

- Laura is a nursing assistant student. On the last day of clinical, she asks 2 residents if she can take a photo with them. Laura posts the photo on a social media site with this comment: "Done with clinical! I'll miss my residents."
- Justin works in home care. He sends a text message to a friend that says: "I'll be done at 22 Third Street at noon. Want to get lunch?"

What did Laura and Justin do wrong?

Often wrongful use of electronic communications is not intentional. You must be very careful. Your communication must protect privacy and confidentiality at all times.

BOX 5-4   Electronic Communications

- Follow agency policies for using electronic communications.
- Remember that:
  - Anything you send or post electronically can be sent to or shared with someone other than the intended person.
  - Electronic communications last forever. They can be retrieved for legal purposes.
  - Private information shared with the intended person still violates the rights to privacy and confidentiality.
  - Referring to a person by nickname, room number, diagnosis, or other means but not by name still violates the rights to privacy and confidentiality.
- Protect privacy and maintain confidentiality at all times.
- Never take photos or videos of the person or any part of the person's body.
- Never send in any way information about the person or images (photos, videos, art) of the person.
- Never identify patients or residents by name.
- Never share information that can lead to the person being identified.
- Maintain professional boundaries. Avoid electronic contact with patients and residents, former patients and residents, and their family members.
- Do not use electronic communications to share or discuss workplace issues or co-workers.
- Tell the nurse at once if you may have violated the person's right to privacy or confidentiality. If you suspect that a co-worker has done so, also tell the nurse.
- See "Gossip" in Chapter 6.
- See "Unethical Student Behavior" in Chapter 6.
- See "Electronic Devices" in Chapter 8.

Modified from National Council of State Boards of Nursing: A nurse's guide to the use of social media, Chicago, 2018, Author.

Informed Consent

A person has the right to decide what will be done to his or her body and who can touch his or her body. The doctor is responsible for informing the person about all aspects of treatment. *Informed consent* is the process by which a person receives and understands information about a treatment or procedure and is able to decide to receive or refuse the treatment or procedure. (*Refuse* means to decline or not accept.) Consent is informed when the person clearly understands:

- The reason for a treatment, procedure, or care measure
- What will be done and how
- Who will do it
- The expected outcomes
- Other treatment, procedure, or care options
- The effects of not having the treatment, procedure, or care measure

Persons under legal age (usually 18 years) cannot give consent. Nor can persons who are mentally unable. This includes persons who are unconscious, sedated, or confused. Or they have certain mental health disorders. Informed consent is given by a responsible party—a spouse, parent, adult child, guardian, or legal representative.

A general consent to treatment is signed when the person enters the agency. Special consents are required for admission to secured memory care units (Chapter 54). Surgeries and some procedures performed by the doctor require special consents. The doctor informs the person about all aspects of the procedure. The nurse may have this responsibility.

You are never responsible for obtaining written consent. In some agencies, you can witness the signing of a consent. When a witness, you are present when the person signs the consent.

See *Focus on Communication: Informed Consent.*

FOCUS ON COMMUNICATION

Informed Consent

There are different ways to give consent.
- *Written consent.* The person signs a form agreeing to a treatment or procedure. You are not responsible for obtaining written consent.
- *Verbal consent.* The person states aloud that consent is given. "Yes" and "okay" are examples.
- *Implied consent.* For example, you ask if you can check a person's blood pressure. The person extends an arm. The movement implies consent.

Before any procedure or task, explain the steps to the person. This is how you obtain verbal or implied consent. Also explain each step during a procedure. This allows the person to refuse at any time.

REPORTING ABUSE

Some persons are mistreated or harmed on purpose. This is abuse. Abuse is a crime. *Abuse* is:
- The willful infliction of injury, unreasonable confinement, intimidation, or punishment that results in physical harm, pain, or mental anguish. *Intimidation* means to make afraid with threats of force or violence. Abuse includes involuntary seclusion (Chapter 2).
- Depriving the person (or the person's caregiver) of the goods or services needed to attain or maintain well-being.

Abuse can occur at home or in a health care agency. All persons must be protected from abuse. This includes persons in a coma (Chapter 7).

The abuser is often a family member or caregiver—spouse, partner, brother or sister, adult child, and others. The abuser can be a friend, neighbor, landlord, or other person. Both men and women are abusers. Both men and women are abused.

State laws, accrediting agencies, and the *Omnibus Budget Reconciliation Act of 1987 (OBRA)* do not allow agencies to employ persons who were convicted of abuse, neglect, or mistreatment. Before hiring, the agency must thoroughly check the applicant's work history, references, and any criminal records.

The agency also checks the nursing assistant registry for findings of abuse, neglect, exploitation, and misappropriation. *Exploitation* means to take advantage of for personal gain. *Misappropriation* is the dishonest use of property. Misappropriation is a form of financial abuse (p. 48).

See *Focus on Communication: Reporting Abuse.*
See *Focus on Surveys: Reporting Abuse.*

FOCUS ON COMMUNICATION

Reporting Abuse

Abused persons may confide in you. They may ask you to keep it a secret. For example, a person says: "If I tell you something, will you promise not to tell anyone?" Never promise to keep abuse a secret from the nurse. Be honest. Do not say you will keep a secret and then report it to the nurse. You can say: "For your safety, some things I must tell the nurse. What did you want to tell me?" If the person refuses to tell you, notify the nurse.

If you suspect abuse, tell the nurse. Give as much detail as you can. For example: "I am concerned about Ms. Sloan. She is very quiet today. When I asked about her visit with her family, she didn't answer. She refused her bath. And when I helped her to the bathroom, I saw bruises on her back."

FOCUS ON SURVEYS

Reporting Abuse

Abuse is a major focus during surveys. Surveyors look for signs of abuse through interviews, observations, and medical records.

Agencies must have procedures to:
- Screen staff applicants for a history of abuse, neglect, or mistreatment of residents. This includes information from:
  - Previous or current employers
  - Nursing assistant registries or licensing boards
- Train staff on how to prevent abuse.
- Identify and correct situations in which abuse is more likely to occur.
- Identify events, patterns, and trends that may signal abuse. Bruises, falls, and staff yelling are examples.
- Investigate abuse.
- Protect patients and residents from harm during an investigation.
- Report and respond to claims of abuse or actual abuse.

Vulnerable Persons

Vulnerable means at risk for harm. A *vulnerable adult* is a person 18 years old or older who has a disability or condition that causes the person to be at risk for harm. Such persons have problems caring for or protecting themselves due to:
- A mental, emotional, physical, intellectual, or developmental disability. See Chapter 55.
- Brain damage.
- Changes from aging.

All patients and residents, regardless of age or care setting, are vulnerable. Older persons and children (p. 50) are at risk for abuse and neglect.

Neglect is when a caregiver or responsible person fails to:
- Protect a vulnerable person from harm.
- Provide food, water, clothing, shelter, health care, or basic activities of daily living to a vulnerable person.

Some persons neglect themselves. *Self-neglect* is when the person's behaviors and way of living threaten the person's own health, safety, and well-being. Causes include declining health and chronic disease. Other causes are disorders that impair judgment or memory—Alzheimer's disease and other types of dementia, depression, substance use disorders, and other mental health disorders (Chapters 53 and 54). Some persons refuse care.

Persons at risk for self-neglect include those who:
- Live alone.
- Are women. More women live alone than men.
- Are depressed.
- Are confused.
- Are older.
- Have alcohol or drug problems.
- Have a history of poor hygiene or living conditions.

Report warning signs of neglect and self-neglect to the nurse. See Box 5-5.

Elder Abuse

The CDC defines *elder abuse* as any intentional act, or failure to act, by a caregiver or other trusted person that causes harm or risk of harm to an older adult. (An *older adult* is identified as a person age 60 or older.) Table 5-1 describes the common types of elder abuse.

See *Focus on Long-Term Care and Home Care: Elder Abuse,* p. 48.

BOX 5-5	Warning Signs of Neglect or Self-Neglect

The Setting
- Not enough food, drinking water, heat, or other necessities. Other necessities include indoor plumbing, running water, working toilet, electricity, and so on.
- Safety hazards in the home. See Chapter 14.
- Unclean living conditions—filth, odors (urine, feces, trash, food), soiled bedding or clothing, human or animal urine or feces, pests (mice, rats, ants, fleas, and other insects), and so on.
- Needed home repairs.
- Hoarding—saving, hiding, or storing things. For example, the person saves newspapers, magazines, food containers, shopping bags, and so on. The hoarding can present safety hazards—fires, pest problems (mice, rats, ants, fleas, other insects), and other hazards.

The Person
- Dehydration (Chapter 32)—poor urinary output, dry skin, dry mouth, confusion.
- Weight loss.
- Poor hygiene. The person has dirty hair, nails, or skin. The person smells of urine or feces.
- Skin rashes or pressure injuries (Chapter 42).
- Not wearing the correct clothing for the weather. Wearing dirty or torn clothing.
- Not having dentures, eyeglasses, hearing aids, walkers, wheelchairs, commodes, or other needed devices.
- Signs of confusion, disorientation, hallucinations, or delusions (Chapters 53 and 54).
- Mis-using drugs or alcohol. (See "Substance Use Disorder" in Chapter 53.)
- Untreated health problems.
- Refusing to seek medical treatment for serious illnesses.
- Failing to take needed drugs.

TABLE 5-1	Elder Abuse	
Type	**Description**	**Examples**
Physical abuse	The intentional use of physical force that results in: - Illness - Injury - Pain - Impaired function - Distress - Death	- Biting - Burning - Choking - Corporal punishment—punishment inflicted directly on the body (beatings, lashings, whippings, and so on) - Force-feeding - Grabbing, pinching, scratching - Hair-pulling - Hitting, kicking, stomping, punching, slapping - Pushing, shaking, shoving - Restraint—physical or chemical (Chapter 16) - Scratching - Striking—with or without an object - Suffocation
Sexual abuse	Forced or unwanted sexual interaction of any kind with an older adult or an incapacitated person. (*Incapacitated* means being unconscious or lacking awareness.) The interaction may: - Be completed or attempted. - Involve touching or non-touching.	- Unwanted sexual contact or penetration - Forced nudity - Forced watching of sexual acts - Harassing a person about sex or sexuality - Taking sexually oriented photos or videos

Continued

TABLE 5-1	Elder Abuse—cont'd	
Type	Description	Examples
Emotional or psychological abuse	Any verbal (oral or written) or nonverbal behavior that causes mental pain, anguish, fear, or distress.	• Yelling, screaming, or shouting at the person • Insults or name-calling • Scolding or criticizing • Threats of punishment or harm • Humiliation, harassment, or ridicule • Treating or talking to the person like an infant or child • Not speaking to the person • Unkind gestures • Saying things to frighten the person • Confining the person to a certain area • Isolation (seclusion) or control (with-holding needed resources) • Threatening to with-hold care
Neglect	Failure of a caregiver or responsible person to: • Protect a vulnerable person from harm. • Provide food, water, clothing, shelter, health care, or basic activities of daily living to a vulnerable person.	• Dirty clothing • Poor hygiene • Leaving the person lying or sitting in urine or feces • Failing to answer call lights and respond to needs • Lacking appropriate clothing for the weather • Cluttered or dirty home • Hoarding • Home in need of repairs • Fire or safety hazards in the home • Lacking needed utilities—water, electricity, plumbing, heating/cooling
Financial abuse	Improper use of an older person's money, benefits, belongings, property, or assets for someone else's personal benefit.	• Forging a person's signature • Theft of money or possessions • Using a person's money or possessions without permission or for a different purpose than permission was given for • Deceiving (tricking, manipulating), intimidating, or threatening a person to use money or possessions for someone else's personal gain • Changing names on a will, bank account, insurance policy, deed, or other financial or legal document
Abandonment	Deserting or leaving a vulnerable adult alone without someone being responsible for the person's care. Involves 4 points: • Accepting an assignment to care for a person or group of persons • Accepting the assignment for a certain time period • Removing yourself from the care setting— home, hospital, nursing center, or other agency • Failing to report off to a staff member who will assume responsibility for care	• Leaving the agency before your shift ends without telling the nurse • Failing to report to a home care assignment • Leaving without completing a home care assignment • Sleeping on the job

FOCUS ON LONG-TERM CARE AND HOME CARE

Elder Abuse

Home Care

Abandonment is always serious. However, it is most serious in home care. Unlike in hospitals and nursing centers, often you are the only caregiver in the home. If you leave before completing your assignment, there is no one to give care. The person is left alone without needed care. Serious harm could result. You could have your certification (license, registration) revoked or suspended for abandonment in any setting.

Reporting Elder Abuse. Federal and state laws require the reporting of elder abuse. If abuse is suspected, it must be reported. (To *suspect* means to think that it may have happened.) Be alert for signs of elder abuse (Box 5-6). A person may only show some signs.

Where and how to report abuse varies among states. If you suspect abuse, share your concerns and observations with the nurse. Be as detailed as possible. The nurse contacts health team members as needed.

The nurse also contacts community agencies that investigate elder abuse. They act at once if the problem is life-threatening. Sometimes the police or courts are involved.

BOX 5-6	Signs of Elder Abuse

- The person reports mistreatment.
- Living conditions are not safe, clean, or adequate. See Box 5-5.
- Personal and oral hygiene are lacking (Chapters 23 and 24). The person is not clean. Clothes are dirty.
- Weight loss—signs of poor nutrition and poor fluid intake.
- Adaptive (assistive) devices are missing or broken— eyeglasses, hearing aids, dentures, cane, walker, and so on.
- The person cannot reach toilet facilities, food, water, and other needed items.
- Medical needs are not met.
- Drugs are not taken properly. Drugs are not bought. Or too much or too little of the drug is taken.
- Frequent injuries—injuries are strange or seem impossible.
- Old and new injuries—bruises, pressure marks, welts, scars, fractures, punctures, and so on (Fig. 5-3).
- Burns on the feet, hands, buttocks, or other parts of the body. Cigarettes and cigars cause small circle-like burns.
- Problems walking or sitting.
- Bleeding, bruising, irritation, itching, or pain around the breasts, inner thighs, or genital or anal area.
- Torn, stained, or bloody under-garments.
- Pressure injuries (Chapter 42) or contractures (Chapter 35).

- Emotional problems (Chapter 53):
  - Panic attacks
  - Post-traumatic stress disorder
  - Quiet; withdrawn from others and normal activities
  - Does not want to talk or answer questions
  - Depression
  - Suicide thoughts or attempts
  - Fear, anxiety, or agitation
  - Inappropriate, unusual, or aggressive sexual behavior
- Sudden changes in alertness.
- Sudden changes in finances.
- The person is restrained. Or the person is locked in a certain area for long periods.
- Private conversations are not allowed. The caregiver is present during all conversations.
- Strained or tense relationships with a caregiver.
- Frequent arguments with a caregiver.
- The person seems anxious to please the caregiver.
- Emergency room visits may be frequent.
- The person may change doctors often. Some people do not have a doctor.

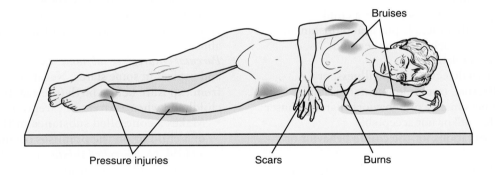

Pressure injuries   Scars   Burns   Bruises

Helping abused older persons is not always easy or possible. Some abuse is not recognized or reported. Or investigators cannot gain access to the person. A victim may want to protect the abuser, especially if the abuser is a spouse, partner, or adult child. Some victims are embarrassed or believe abuse is deserved. A victim may fear what will happen. The person may think that the present situation is better than no care at all. Some people fear not being believed if they report the abuse themselves.

In select chapters in this book, the "Ethics and Laws" section of the *Focus on PRIDE: The Person, Family, and Yourself* box presents a real reported case. Cases involve negligence, neglect, or abuse (physical, emotional, sexual, or financial). Reported cases are investigated. An investigation can lead to 1 or more of the following if the offense is *substantiated* (found to be true).

- Job loss
- Loss of certification (license, registration)
- Being convicted of a crime

See *Focus on Long-Term Care and Home Care: Reporting Elder Abuse.*

FOCUS ON LONG-TERM CARE AND HOME CARE

Reporting Elder Abuse

Long-Term Care

OBRA requires these actions if abuse is suspected within the center.

- The matter is reported at once to:
  - The administrator
  - Other investigative agencies as required by federal and state laws
- All claims of abuse are thoroughly investigated.
- The center must prevent further potential for abuse while the investigation is in progress.
- Investigation results are reported to the center administrator and required agencies within 5 days of the incident.
- Corrective actions are taken if the claim is found to be true.

Child Abuse and Neglect

Child abuse and neglect is the intentional harm or mistreatment of a child under 18 years old. It:
- Involves any recent act or failure to act on the part of a parent or caregiver.
- Results in death, serious physical or emotional harm, sexual abuse, or exploitation.
- Presents a likely or immediate risk for harm.

Child abuse and neglect occur in low-, middle-, and high-income families. The abuser's education level may be low or high. Often the abuser is a household member or caregiver—parent, parent's partner, brother or sister, foster parent, nanny, babysitter. Usually an abuser is someone the family knows. Risk factors for abusing children include:
- Stress
- Family crisis—divorce, unemployment, low income, moving, crowded living conditions, intimate partner violence
- Single-parenting
- Teenage parenting
- Several young children under 5 years of age
- Physical or mental illness, including depression and substance use disorder (Chapter 53)
- Abuser history of abuse or neglect as a child
- Discipline beliefs that include physical punishment
- Lack of emotional attachment to the child
- Poor parent-child relationships
- A child with birth defects, chronic illness, or a physical, intellectual, or developmental disability
- A child with a personality or behaviors that the abuser considers "different" or not acceptable
- Unrealistic expectations for the child's behavior or performance
- Lack of understanding about children's needs, child development, and parenting skills
- Families that move often and do not have family or friends nearby

Types of Child Abuse and Neglect.
Child abuse and neglect have many forms. Often more than 1 type is present.
- *Physical abuse* is injuring the child on purpose. It can cause bruising, wounds, fractures, or death. The examples in Table 5-1 also apply to child abuse.
- *Neglect* is failing to provide for a child's basic needs.
  - *Physical neglect*—failure to provide food, shelter, or supervision.
  - *Medical neglect*—failure to provide needed medical or mental health treatment. (Some religious beliefs do not allow medical care. State laws vary on what is considered medical neglect.)
  - *Educational neglect*—failure to educate a child or provide special education needs.
  - *Emotional neglect*—failure to meet the child's needs for affection and attention. It includes letting a child use alcohol or other drugs.

- *Sexual abuse* is pressuring or forcing a child to engage in or be exposed to sexual acts.
  - *Rape or sexual assault*—forced sexual acts against the child's will.
  - *Molestation*—sexual advances toward a child. It includes kissing, touching, or fondling sexual areas. The abuser kisses, touches, or fondles the child. Or the child is forced to kiss, touch, or fondle the abuser.
  - *Incest*—sexual activity between family members.
  - *Child pornography*—taking photos or videos of a child involved in sexual acts or poses.
  - *Child prostitution*—forcing a child to engage in sexual acts for money. Usually the child is forced to have many sexual partners.
- *Emotional abuse* is injuring the child mentally or lowering the child's sense of self-worth. The abuser constantly criticizes, threatens, or rejects the child. The abuser may with-hold love, support, or guidance. The child has changes in behavior, emotional responses, thinking, reasoning, learning, and so on. The child may show anxiety, depression, withdrawal, or aggressive behaviors. Emotional abuse is almost always present with other forms of abuse.
- *Parental or caregiver substance use* is part of child abuse and neglect in some states. Negative effects occur from exposure before birth (pre-natal) or during childhood when a parent or caregiver:
  - Makes a controlled substance in the presence of a child or on the premises occupied by a child. (A *controlled substance* is a drug or chemical substance whose possession and use are controlled by law.)
  - Allows a child to be where there are chemicals or equipment used to make or store a controlled substance.
  - Sells, distributes, or gives drugs or alcohol to a child.
  - Uses a controlled substance that impairs the ability to care for the child.
  - Exposes the child to equipment and supplies for using, selling, or distributing drugs.
  - Exposes the child to other drug-related activities.
- *Abandonment* is when the parent's identity or whereabouts are unknown. The child is left in circumstances that cause serious harm. Or the parent fails to maintain contact with the child or provide support for the child.

Reporting Child Abuse and Neglect.
Table 5-2 lists the signs of child abuse and neglect. Report any changes in the child's body or behavior. Child and parent behaviors may alert to something wrong.

TABLE 5-2	Signs of Child Abuse and Neglect	
Type and Description	**Signs of Abuse—Child**	**Signs of Abuse—Parent or Parent and Child**
General behaviors—may be present with any type of mistreatment	**The Child** • Reports bad treatment or abuse by a parent or caregiver. • Has sudden changes in behavior. • Has sudden changes in school performance. • Has learning problems or problems concentrating. The problem is not caused by a physical or mental health disorder. • Has untreated health problems. • Seems watchful; seems to wait for something bad to happen. • Lacks adult supervision. • Is overly agreeable or obedient. • Is quiet, withdrawn, or uninvolved. • Arrives early at school or stays late. • Does not want to go home from school, activities, or someone's house. • Fears a parent or certain person; does not want to be around a parent or certain person.	**The Parent** • Denies that the child has problems at school or home. • Blames the child for problems at school or home. • Asks teachers or caregivers to use harsh discipline. • Describes the child as bad, worthless, or a burden. • Demands physical or academic performance above the child's abilities. • Shows little concern for the child. • Relies on the child for care, attention, or emotional satisfaction. **The Parent and Child** • Rarely touch or look at each other. • View their relationship as poor or bad. • State that they do not like each other.
Physical abuse—injuring the child on purpose	**The Child** • Has injuries that are not explained—burns, bites, bruises, broken bones, black eyes. • Has fading bruises or other marks after being gone from school. • Is scared, anxious, depressed, withdrawn, or aggressive. • Fears parents and does not want to go home. • Shrinks (cowers) when an adult approaches. • Has changes in eating and sleeping habits. • Reports injury by a parent or caregiver. • Abuses animals or pets.	**The Parent** • Gives different or confusing stories about an injury. Or does not give an explanation. • Uses harsh discipline. • Has a history of abusing animals or pets.
Neglect—failing to provide for the child's basic needs (food, clothing, shelter, supervision, health care, education, affection and attention)	**The Child** • Begs or steals food or money. • Is dirty or has a severe body odor. • Lacks the correct clothing for the weather. • Abuses alcohol or drugs. • States that no one is at home to provide care. • Is often absent from school. • Lacks medical or dental care. Does not have needed eyeglasses.	**The Parent** • Seems to have little interest in the child. • Shows little or no emotion or is depressed. • Has behaviors that are bizarre or not logical. • Abuses alcohol or drugs.
Sexual abuse—using, persuading, or forcing the child to engage in any sexual contact, activity, or behavior or exposing the child to sexual acts	**The Child** • Has trouble walking or sitting. • Has bleeding, bruising, or swelling in sexual areas. • Refuses to go to school. • Has nightmares or wets the bed. • Has a sudden change in appetite. • Has sexual knowledge or behavior that is unusual or does not fit with the child's age. • Is pregnant or has a sexually transmitted disease (Chapter 52), especially under age 14. • Runs away. • Reports sexual abuse. • Attaches to strangers or new adults quickly.	**The Parent** • Tries to be the child's friend instead of a parent. • Makes up excuses to be alone with the child. • Tells the child about personal problems or relationships.

Continued

TABLE 5-2	Signs of Child Abuse and Neglect—cont'd	
Type and Description	Signs of Abuse—Child	Signs of Abuse—Parent or Parent and Child
Emotional abuse—injuring the child mentally or damaging the child's sense of self-worth	**The Child** • Has extremes in behavior—overly agreeable or demanding, quiet and withdrawn, or aggressive. • Acts much younger or older than the child's actual age. For example, the child shows infant-like behaviors (rocking, head-banging). Or the child acts like a parent to other children. • Has physical or emotional developmental delays. • Is depressed. • Has suicidal thoughts. • Has trouble bonding with others.	**The Parent** • Blames, criticizes, or scolds the child often. • Describes the child negatively. • Rejects the child.

Modified from Child Welfare Information Gateway: What is child abuse and neglect: recognizing the signs and symptoms, *Washington, DC, April 2019, Children's Bureau.*

Child abuse is complex. Many more behaviors, signs, and symptoms are present than discussed here. You must be alert for signs and symptoms of child abuse. All states require the reporting of suspected child abuse. Remember, making a false claim to damage someone's reputation is defamation. Reporting a real concern is necessary.

If you suspect child abuse, share your concerns with the nurse. Give as much detail as you can. The nurse contacts the health team and child protection agencies as needed.

Intimate Partner Violence

The CDC describes *intimate partner violence (IPV)* as abuse or aggression that occurs in a romantic relationship. An *intimate partner* may be a current or former spouse, dating partner, or sexual partner. Also known as domestic violence, IPV includes dating violence and teen dating violence (Chapter 11).

In IPV, a partner has power and control over the other through abuse. The abuse may range from 1 event to chronic, severe violence over several years. The CDC describes 4 main types of IPV.

- *Physical violence*—A person hurts or tries to hurt a partner using physical force (hitting, kicking, and so on).
- *Sexual violence*—A person forces or attempts to force a partner to take part in a sex act, sexual touching, or a non-physical sexual event. (Sexting is an example of a non-physical event. *Sexting* [Chapter 6] involves the sending of sexual messages, photos, or videos using technology.) With sexual violence, the act occurs (or is attempted) *without the victim's consent*. The victim does not or cannot give consent. Being asleep, unconscious, or incapacitated by alcohol or drugs are some reasons a person cannot give consent. Alcohol or drug use may be voluntary or involuntary.

- *Psychological aggression*—A person uses verbal and nonverbal communication to harm a partner mentally or emotionally. The intent may be to control the partner.
- *Stalking*—There is a pattern of repeated, unwanted attention and contact that causes fear or concern for one's safety or the safety of someone close to the victim (family, friend). Examples include:
  - Watching or following the victim
  - Showing up in places (home, workplace, school) when the victim does not want to see the person
  - Using global positioning system (GPS) technology to monitor or track the victim's location
  - Sneaking into the victim's home or car
  - Leaving strange or threatening items for the victim to find
  - Leaving unwanted cards, letters, flowers, presents, or other items
  - Using technology (camera, computer) to spy on the victim from a distance
  - Making unwanted phone calls (including voice messages and hanging up)
  - Sending unwanted messages or photos through text messaging or on-line

Both men and women can be victims of IPV. However, women are victims more often. There is no set age, race, culture, religion, educational level, income level, or marital status for IPV. Patients and residents can suffer from IPV. You, yourself, may be a victim.

See Box 5-7 for warning signs of IPV. Having 1 or 2 warning signs in a relationship may indicate IPV.

State laws vary about reporting IPV. However, the health team has an ethical duty to give information about safety and community resources. If you suspect IPV, tell the nurse. The nurse gathers information to help the person.

See *Focus on Children and Older Persons: Intimate Partner Violence.*

See *Focus on Long-Term Care and Home Care: Intimate Partner Violence.*

See *Promoting Safety and Comfort: Intimate Partner Violence.*

BOX 5-7	**Warning Signs of Intimate Partner Violence**

A partner:
- Says the victim never does anything right.
- Shows extreme jealousy of the victim's friends or time away.
- Prevents or discourages the victim from spending time with friends or family.
- Insults, demeans (lowers the dignity of), or shames the victim (especially in front of others).
- Prevents the victim from making decisions, including decisions about working or attending school.
- Controls the victim's finances without discussion, including:
  - Taking the victim's money
  - Refusing to provide money for necessary expenses
- Pressures the victim to have sex or perform sexual acts that the victim is not comfortable with.
- Pressures the victim to use drugs or alcohol.
- Intimidates the victim with threatening expressions or actions.
- Insults the victim's parenting.
- Threatens to harm or take away the victim's children or pets.
- Intimidates the victim with weapons (guns, knives, bats, mace).
- Destroys the victim's belongings or home.

Modified from National Domestic Violence Hotline: Warning signs of abuse: know what to look for, *Austin, TX.*

FOCUS ON **CHILDREN AND OLDER PERSONS**

Intimate Partner Violence

Children
Teenagers can be victims of dating violence (Chapter 11). *Teen dating violence (TDV)* is a type of IPV. The CDC reports that TDV affects millions of young people in the United States. As with IPV, dating violence can include physical violence, sexual violence, psychological aggression, or stalking. TDV can occur:
- In person or electronically
- With a current or former dating partner

Victims of teen dating violence are at risk for depression and anxiety, unhealthy behaviors (tobacco, drug, and alcohol use), and antisocial behaviors (Chapter 53). Suicide thoughts and attempts are other risks.

FOCUS ON **LONG-TERM CARE AND HOME CARE**

Intimate Partner Violence

Long-Term Care
Under OBRA, the resident has the right to be free from abuse, mistreatment, and neglect. If a resident is abused by anyone, the abuse must be reported. This includes abuse by a partner.

PROMOTING SAFETY AND COMFORT

Intimate Partner Violence

Safety
Resources and services are available for victims of abuse. See *Focus on PRIDE: The Person, Family, and Yourself* on p. 54. A personalized *safety plan* can help a victim of IPV:
- Improve safety in a relationship.
- Respond to an emergency.
- Prepare to leave an abusive situation.
- Plan what to do after leaving an abusive relationship.

WILLS

A *will* is a legal document of how a person wants property distributed after death. You can ethically and legally witness a will signing. Or you can refuse without fear of legal action.

You cannot prepare wills. Politely refuse if asked to do so. Explain that you do not have the legal knowledge or ability to prepare a will. Report the request to the nurse. The nurse will discuss contacting a lawyer with the person or family.

Do not witness a will signing if you are named in the will. Doing so prevents you from getting what was left to you. As a witness, be prepared to testify that:
- The person was of sound mind when the will was signed.
- The person stated that the document was his or her last will.

Many agencies do not let staff witness wills. Know your agency's policy before you agree to witness a will. If you have questions, ask the nurse. If you witness a will, tell the nurse.

FOCUS ON PRIDE
The Person, Family, and Yourself

Personal and Professional Responsibility

States have laws about who must report abuse and neglect. Such persons are called *mandatory reporters. Mandatory* means required. For example, most states require that health care providers report suspected abuse or neglect of children, vulnerable adults, and elders. Tell the nurse if you suspect abuse or neglect.

Some states require that all persons report suspected mistreatment. Other states allow voluntary reporting. You or someone you know may be in danger. Or you suspect abuse or neglect.

- For dangerous or life-threatening situations—Call 911.
- For child abuse or neglect—Contact your local child protective services office or the police. Call the Childhelp National Child Abuse Hotline at 1-800-4-A-CHILD (1-800-422-4453).
- For intimate partner violence—The National Domestic Violence Hotline has resources and information. You can call 1-800-799-SAFE (1-800-799-7233) or visit www.thehotline.org.
- For sexual violence—Call the National Sexual Assault Hotline at 1-800-656-HOPE (1-800-656-4673).
- For elder abuse, neglect, or exploitation—Visit the National Center on Elder Abuse's website.

Rights and Respect

Abuse and neglect can take many forms. For example:
- A person constantly crying out for help is left alone with the door closed.
- A person is told to be nice or care will not be given.
- A person is turned in a rough and hurried manner.
- A person lies in a wet and soiled bed all night.
- A person uses the call light a lot. It is removed from the room.
- A person's belongings are stolen.
- A person is told that family does not visit because the person is mean.

The person has the right to be free from abuse and neglect. Practice safe, ethical care. Be alert for signs of mistreatment.

Independence and Social Interaction

You will interact closely with patients, residents, and families. You may begin to know them well. Social and professional relationships differ. Use good judgment when interacting with patients, residents, and families. Maintain professional boundaries (p. 41).

Delegation and Teamwork

Working within the limits of your role protects persons from harm. You must understand your roles and responsibilities to know when a task is outside these limits. Accepting a task beyond the legal limits of your role can lead to negligence.

Ethics and Laws

The following is a real account of an intentional tort committed by a nursing assistant.

A licensed nursing assistant (LNA) worked at a nursing center. Her license was suspended for using a resident's credit card without the resident's knowledge or consent. The LNA signed the resident's name to charges for about $1490. The LNA also took and used a nurse's credit card. Criminal charges of false impersonation were filed against the LNA.

The LNA was charged with:
- *Failing to comply with federal or state laws and rules*
- *Abusing or neglecting a patient*
- *Misappropriating patient property (p. 46)*
- *Being unfit or incompetent to function as a nursing assistant by reason of any cause*
- *Engaging in conduct of a character likely to deceive, defraud, or harm the public*

The LNA's license was suspended indefinitely. This means that the LNA:
- *Had to give her license to the Board.*
- *Could ask the Board to re-instate her license, but she had to prove that:*
  - *She posed no danger to the public or the practice of nursing.*
  - *She would safely and competently perform an LNA's duties.*
  - *She meets the requirements for license renewal and re-instatement.*

(State of Vermont Board of Nursing, 2004.)

FOCUS ON PRIDE: *Application*

A code of conduct guides your thinking and behavior. Write a personal code of conduct stating what you expect of yourself as a nursing assistant.

REVIEW QUESTIONS

Circle the BEST answer.

1 Ethics is
   a Making judgments before you have the facts
   b Knowledge of right and wrong conduct
   c A behavior that meets your needs, not the person's
   d A health team member's skill, care, and judgment

2 Which is ethical behavior?
   a Sharing information about a resident with a friend
   b Accepting gifts from a resident's family
   c Reporting errors
   d Calling your family before answering a call light

3 On your days off, you call the agency to check on a patient. This is a
   a Professional boundary
   b Tort
   c Boundary violation
   d Boundary sign

4 To maintain professional boundaries, focus on
   a Helping the person
   b Meeting your needs
   c Being biased
   d Showing that you care

5 You help with a friend's hospital care. This is a
  a Professional boundary
  b Boundary crossing
  c Tort
  d Crime

6 If a harmful act was intentional, it was
  a Attempted but not completed
  b Done by a professional person
  c Accidental
  d Done on purpose

7 These statements are about negligence. Which is *true?*
  a It is an intentional tort.
  b The negligent person acted in a reasonable manner.
  c The person or the person's property was harmed.
  d A prison term is likely.

8 Threatening to touch a person's body without the person's consent is
  a Assault
  b Battery
  c Defamation
  d False imprisonment

9 Restraining a person's freedom of movement is
  a Neglect
  b Invasion of privacy
  c Defamation
  d False imprisonment

10 Sharing a resident's photo on a social media site is
  a Fraud
  b Allowed with the family's consent
  c A violation of HIPAA
  d Allowed if you obtain informed consent

11 You tell others that you are a nurse. This is
  a Negligence
  b Fraud
  c Libel
  d Slander

12 Which is an example of defamation?
  a Telling a co-worker that a nurse steals drugs
  b Lying on a job application
  c Slapping a co-worker
  d Sharing a patient's private information with a friend

13 Informed consent is when the person
  a Fully understands all aspects of treatment
  b Signs a consent form
  c Is admitted to the agency
  d Agrees to a procedure

14 Self-neglect is when
  a A caregiver harms a person
  b The person's behaviors put him or her at risk for harm
  c A person is deprived of food, clothing, hygiene, and shelter
  d The person does not receive attention or affection

15 You scold an older person for not eating lunch. This is
  a Physical abuse
  b Neglect
  c Battery
  d Emotional or psychological abuse

16 A home care nursing assistant keeps the person's money after shopping for groceries. This is
  a Allowed as a tip for services
  b A boundary crossing
  c Unprofessional but legal
  d Financial abuse

17 Which is a sign of elder abuse?
  a Stiff joints and joint pain
  b Weight gain
  c Poor personal hygiene
  d Forgetfulness

18 An older adult has a black eye and bruises on the face. These are signs of
  a Physical abuse
  b Sexual abuse
  c Neglect
  d Normal aging

19 A child is consistently dirty and has a severe body odor. These are signs of
  a Physical abuse
  b Sexual abuse
  c Neglect
  d Normal childhood appearance

20 Bruising around a child's genitalia is a sign of
  a Physical abuse
  b Sexual abuse
  c Neglect
  d Self-neglect

21 A person feels intimidated by a partner in a dating relationship. This is
  a Normal in many relationships
  b Not abuse if there is no physical harm
  c Neglect
  d A sign of intimate partner violence

22 You suspect a resident was abused. You should
  a Tell the nurse
  b Call the police
  c Tell the family
  d Ask the person about the abuse

Answers to Chapter 5 questions are on p. 901.

FOCUS ON PRACTICE

Problem Solving

You finish giving nail care to a resident. The resident offers you money as a tip. How will you respond? How do you know if an act is a boundary violation?

Student and Work Ethics

OBJECTIVES

- Define the key terms and key abbreviations in this chapter.
- Describe the qualities and traits of a successful nursing assistant.
- Describe good health and hygiene practices.
- Explain how to look professional.
- Explain how to prepare for school and work.
- Explain how to function as a safe and effective member of a team.
- Explain how to manage stress.

- Explain how to problem solve and deal with conflict.
- Explain the aspects of harassment and what to do if it occurs.
- Explain how to resign from a job.
- Identify the common reasons for losing a job.
- Explain the reasons for drug testing.
- Describe unethical student behavior and possible consequences.
- Explain how to promote PRIDE in the person, the family, and yourself.

KEY TERMS

burnout A job stress resulting in being physically or mentally exhausted, having doubts about your abilities, and having doubts about the value of your work

confidentiality Trusting others with personal and private information

conflict A clash between opposing interests or ideas

courtesy A polite, considerate, or helpful comment or act

gossip To spread rumors or talk about the private matters of others

harassment To trouble, torment, offend, or worry a person by one's behavior or comments

priority The most important thing at the time

professionalism Following laws, being ethical, having good work ethics, and having the skills to do your work

stress The response or change in the body caused by any emotional, psychological, physical, social, or economic factor

stressor The event or factor that causes stress

teamwork Staff members work together as a group; everyone does their part to give safe and effective care

work ethics Behavior in the workplace

KEY ABBREVIATIONS

ID Identification

NATCEP Nursing assistant training and competency evaluation program

As a student and as a nursing assistant, you must act and function in a professional manner. *Professionalism* involves following laws, being ethical, having good work ethics, and having the skills to do your work.

Laws and ethics are discussed in Chapter 5. *Laws* are rules of conduct made by government bodies. *Ethics* deals with right and wrong conduct. It involves choices and judgments about what to do or what not to do. An ethical person does the right thing.

Work ethics deals with behavior in the workplace. Certain behaviors (conduct), choices, and judgments are expected. Work ethics involves:

- How you look
- What you say
- How you behave
- How you treat and work with others
- The qualities and traits shown and described in Figure 6-1.

In this chapter, *work ethics* applies to you as a student. For student success, practice good work ethics in the classroom and clinical setting and with instructors and fellow students.

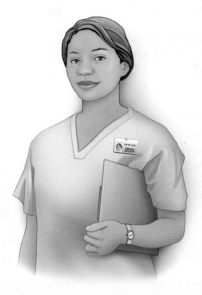

Caring—having concern for the person; making the person's life happier, easier, or less painful

Cheerful—greeting and talking to others in a pleasant manner

Conscientious—being careful, alert, and exact in following instructions; giving thorough care; protecting the person's property

Considerate—respecting the person's physical and emotional feelings; being kind to patients, residents, families, and the health team

Cooperative—helping and working with others willingly; willing to do more during busy and stressful times

Courteous—being polite to patients, residents, families, and the health team

Dependable—reporting to work on time and as scheduled; completing assignments; keeping obligations and promises

Empathy—seeing things from the person's point of view; putting yourself in the person's place

Enthusiastic—being eager, interested, and excited about your work

Honest—reporting the care given, your observations, and any errors accurately

Patient—coping with problems and delays; staying calm rather than getting upset, annoyed, or angry; not rushing the person or a co-worker

Respectful—treating the person with respect and dignity at all times; respecting the person's rights, values, beliefs, and feelings; showing respect for the health team

Self-aware—knowing your feelings, strengths, and weaknesses; understanding yourself so you can understand patients and residents

Trustworthy—keeping information confidential; not gossiping about patients, residents, families, or the health team

FIGURE 6-1 Good work ethics involves these qualities and traits.

HEALTH, HYGIENE, AND APPEARANCE

Your health, hygiene, and appearance need careful attention. If you do not look professional, people wonder if you give good care. Schools and employers have expectations. Patients, residents, and their families and visitors do as well.

Your Health

To learn and give safe and effective care, you must be physically and mentally healthy. The following affect your health.

- *Diet.* You need a balanced diet for good nutrition (Chapter 30). Eat a good breakfast. To maintain your weight, balance calorie intake with your energy needs. To lose weight, have fewer calories than your energy needs. Avoid foods high in fat and sugar. Also avoid salty foods and "crash" diets.
- *Sleep and rest.* Most adults need 7 to 8 hours of sleep daily. Fatigue, lack of energy, and being irritable mean you need more rest and sleep.
- *Body mechanics.* You will bend, carry heavy objects, and move and turn persons. Use your muscles correctly and avoid stress and strain on your body (Chapter 19).
- *Exercise.* Exercise promotes muscle tone, circulation, and weight control. Walking, running, swimming, and hiking are good forms of exercise. Regular exercise promotes physical and mental health. Do something you enjoy. Consult your doctor before starting a vigorous exercise program.

- *Your eyes.* You must read instructions and measurements correctly. Wrong readings and measurements can harm the person. Have your eyes checked. Wear needed eyeglasses or contact lenses. Have good lighting for reading and fine work.
- *Smoking.* Smoke odors stay on your breath, hands, clothing, and hair. Hand-washing and good hygiene are needed.
- *Drugs.* Some drugs affect thinking, feeling, behavior, and function. Working under the influence of drugs affects the person's safety and yours. Take only prescribed drugs in the prescribed way.
- *Alcohol.* Alcohol is a drug that affects thinking, balance, coordination, and alertness. Never go to work under the influence of alcohol. Do not drink alcohol while working. Alcohol affects the person's safety and yours.

Your Hygiene

Your hygiene needs careful attention. Bathe daily. Use a deodorant or antiperspirant to prevent body odors. Brush your teeth often. Brushing upon awakening, before and after meals, and at bedtime are common times (Chapter 23). Use mouthwash to prevent breath odors. Shampoo often. Keep fingernails clean, short, and smoothly and neatly shaped.

Menstrual hygiene is important. Change tampons or sanitary pads often, especially for heavy flow. Wash your genital area with soap and water at least once a day. Also practice good hand-washing.

Foot care prevents odors and infection. Wash your feet daily. Dry thoroughly between the toes. Cut toenails straight across after bathing or soaking them.

Your Appearance

How you look affects what people think about you and the agency. If staff or students are clean and neat, people think the agency is clean and neat. If staff or students are messy and unkempt, people may question the agency's cleanliness and quality of care.

You need to look clean, neat, and professional. See Box 6-1 and Figure 6-2.

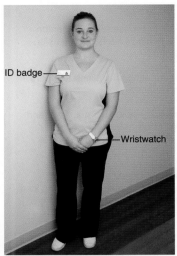

FIGURE 6-2 The nursing assistant is well groomed. The uniform and shoes are clean. Hair has a simple style—away from the face and off of the collar. An ID badge and wristwatch are worn. Jewelry is not worn.

BOX 6-1   Professional Appearance

- Practice good hygiene.
- Follow the dress code of your agency or training program for:
  - Uniforms
  - Jewelry
  - Shoes
  - Hair
  - Nails, make-up, and fragrances

Uniforms
- Wear required uniforms. Do not wear home or social attire at work or as a student in the clinical setting. This includes tight, revealing, or sexual clothing. Halter tops, tank tops, low-cut tops, tops with arm slits, jeans, shorts, short skirts, low-rise pants, leggings, yoga pants, or high-cut pants are not worn.
- Uniforms fit well and are modest in length and style. Do not wear tight, revealing, or sexual-looking uniforms.
  - Women—Do not show cleavage, tops of breasts, or upper thighs.
  - Men—Do not wear tight pants. Do not expose your chest. Open just the top button of your shirt.
- Keep uniforms clean, pressed, and mended. Sew on buttons. Repair zippers, tears, and hems.
- Wear a clean uniform and clean under-garments daily.
- Wear appropriate under-garments for your body shape and uniform.
  - Under-garments are clean and fit properly.
  - Under-garments are the correct color for your skin tone.
  - Colored (red, pink, blue, and so on) and patterned under-garments are not worn. They can be seen through white and light-colored uniforms.
- Wear clean socks or stockings that fit well. Change them daily.
- Wear your name badge or photo ID (identification) according to the dress code. The badge or ID is usually worn above the waist where it can be seen by others (see Fig. 6-2). Agencies may use first and last names or only first names. Your student ID will have your school's name.
- Cover tattoos (body art) with your uniform. Tattoos (body art) may offend others.

Jewelry
- Wear only allowed jewelry.
  - Wedding and engagement rings may be allowed. Do not wear rings that can scratch a person.
  - Bracelets are not allowed. They can scratch a person.
  - Necklaces and dangling earrings are not allowed. Confused or combative persons and young children might pull on them.
  - One set of small, simple earrings is usually allowed.
- Do not wear jewelry in visible piercings—eyebrows, nose, lips, cheek, tongue, or other sites.
- Wear a wristwatch with a second (sweep) hand (Fig. 6-3).

Shoes
- Wear shoes that fit, are comfortable, give needed support, and have slip-resistant soles.
  - Do not wear sandals or open-toed shoes.
- Wear clean shoes. Wash or replace shoes and laces as needed.

Hair
- Have a simple, attractive hair-style.
  - Hair is off your collar and away from your face. This includes men with long hair.
- Use simple pins, barrettes, hair ties, clips, bands, or other devices to keep long hair up and in place. This includes men with long hair.
- Keep beards and mustaches clean and trimmed.

Nails, Make-Up, and Fragrances
- Keep fingernails clean, short, and smoothly and neatly shaped. Long or jagged nails can scratch a person.
- Do not wear nail polish. Chipped nail polish may provide a place for microbes to grow.
  - If nail polish is allowed, wear only a light-colored polish.
- Do not wear non-natural nails. Fake and artificial nails and nail extenders are examples. Nails must be natural.
- Use make-up that is modest in amount and moderate in color. Avoid a painted and severe look.
- Do not wear perfume, cologne, or after-shave lotion. The scents (fragrances) may offend, nauseate, or cause breathing problems in patients and residents.

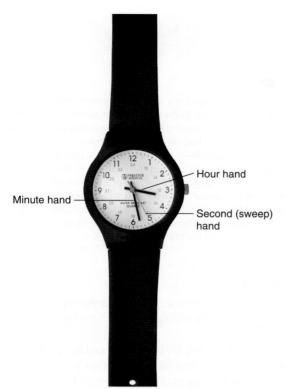

FIGURE 6-3 A watch with a second (sweep) hand. (Courtesy Prestige Medical, Northridge, Calif.)

PREPARING FOR SCHOOL OR WORK

Being dependable is important as a student and as an employee. As a student, you are preparing yourself for work. The classroom and clinical settings help you develop dependable behaviors.

To be dependable as a student:
- Arrive on time for class and clinical experiences. Arrive early to store your things, use the restroom, and gather needed items for class or clinical. Be ready for class or clinical to start.
- Complete and turn in assignments on time.
- Pay attention and follow directions.
- Stay for the entire class or clinical experience.
To be dependable in the work setting, you must:
- Work when scheduled.
- Get to work on time. See "Attendance" on p. 60.
- Stay the entire shift.

Absences and tardiness (being late) can affect your success in school. Your state's nursing assistant training and competency evaluation program (NATCEP) requires a certain number of hours. You must complete the required number of hours.

Absences and tardiness are also common reasons for losing a job. Childcare and transportation issues often interfere with getting to school and work. You need to plan carefully.

Childcare

Someone needs to care for your children when you leave for school or work, while you are at school or work, and before you get home. Also plan for emergencies.
- Your childcare provider is ill or cannot care for your children that day.
- A child becomes ill or injured while you are at school or work.
- You will be late getting home from school or work.

Transportation

Plan for getting to and from school or work. If you drive, keep your car in good working order. Keep enough gas in the car. Or leave early to get gas.

Carpooling is an option. Carpoolers depend on each other. If the driver is late, everyone is late for school or work. If 1 person is not ready, everyone is late for school or work. Carpool with people you trust to be ready on time. Be on time as a driver and as a passenger.

Know bus or train schedules. Know what bus or train to take if delays occur. Always carry enough money for fares to and from school or work.

Have a back-up transportation plan. Your car may not start, the carpool driver may not be going that day, or public transportation may not run.

TEAMWORK

Teamwork means that staff members work together as a group. Everyone does their part to give safe and effective care. Teamwork involves:
- Working when scheduled.
- Having a good attitude.
- Completing assignments.
- Helping others willingly.
- Being kind to others.

You are an important member of the health and nursing teams. Quality of care is affected by how you work with others and how you feel about your job. Some days it might seem that you are doing more than others. Other days, your co-workers may feel that you are not doing enough. Avoid comparing your assignments to what others are doing. Each staff member has a role individually and as a team member.

Attendance

Report to work when scheduled and on time. The entire unit is affected when just 1 person is late. Call the agency if you will be late or cannot go to work. Follow the attendance policy in your employee handbook. Poor attendance can cause you to lose your job.

You must be dependable. Be *ready to work* when your shift starts.

- Store your things before your shift starts.
- Use the restroom when you arrive at the agency.
- Arrive on your nursing unit a few minutes early. Greet others and settle yourself.

You must stay the entire shift. Watching the clock for your shift to end gives a bad image. You may need to work over-time. Prepare to stay longer if necessary. When it is time to leave, report off duty to the nurse.

See *Focus on Communication: Attendance.*

See *Teamwork and Time Management: Attendance.*

See *Focus on Long-Term Care and Home Care: Attendance.*

FOCUS ON COMMUNICATION

Attendance

Illness, a family death, and other emergencies may require an absence. You must tell your instructor or the agency about your absence. Otherwise you could have an unexcused absence from your NATCEP. If working, you could lose your job. To report an absence:

- *Call well before class, clinical, or your shift begins.* See the attendance policy in your student or employee handbook for when to call. At least 2 hours ahead is common.
- *Know who to call.* Students call their instructors. Charge nurses, nurse managers, or supervisors handle absences in the work setting. You may need your call transferred. For example: "Hello. This is Terry Jones. Please transfer me to the charge nurse." You must give information to the right person.
- *Give the reason for your absence.* Be honest. You can say: "I am sorry. I will be absent from work (class, clinical) today. I have a fever and a cough."
- *Give the length of your absence.* People often miss 1 or 2 days for illness or a family emergency. Longer absences require more communication.

TEAMWORK AND TIME MANAGEMENT

Attendance

A staff member may be late for work. Or someone is absent from work. Until a replacement arrives, you and other staff have extra work. Patient and resident care cannot suffer.

To promote teamwork and manage your time:

- Ask the nurse how you can help.
- Do not complain about not having enough staff.
- Ask the nurse to list the most important tasks and care measures.

FOCUS ON **LONG-TERM CARE AND HOME CARE**

Attendance

Home Care

You must complete home care assignments. Never leave in the middle of an assignment or before someone from the next shift arrives. Leaving before completing an assignment is *abandonment* (Chapter 5).

Sometimes problems occur in the home setting. Try to finish the assignment. Explain the problem to the nurse who will try to make needed changes. Do not walk out on (abandon) the person. Walking out (abandonment) is abuse, unsafe for the person, and very unethical behavior (Chapter 5).

See "Workplace Violence" in Chapter 14 for how to handle violent or threatening situations.

Your Attitude

You need a good attitude. Show that you enjoy your work. Listen to others. Be willing to learn. Stay busy and use your time well.

You and your work are important and have value. Nurses, patients, residents, and families rely on you for good care. They want you to be pleasant and respectful.

Always think before you speak. These statements signal a bad attitude.

- "That's not my resident (patient)."
- "I can't. I'm too busy."
- "I didn't do it."
- "I don't feel like it."
- "It's not my fault."
- "Don't blame me."
- "It's not my turn. I did it yesterday."
- "Nobody told me."
- "That's not my job."
- "You didn't say that you needed it right away."
- "I did more than they did."
- "I work harder than anyone else."
- "No one appreciates what I do."
- "I'm tired of this place."
- "Is it time to leave yet?"
- "Good luck. I had a horrible day."

Speech and Language

Your speech and language must be professional. Some words used in home and social settings are not proper in class, the clinical setting, and at work. Such words may offend others. Remember:

- Do not swear or use foul, vulgar, slang, sexual, or abusive language.
- Speak softly and gently.
- Speak clearly. Hearing problems are common.
- Do not shout or yell.
- Do not argue with a patient or resident, family member, visitor, co-worker, your instructor, or a fellow student.

Gossip

To *gossip* means to spread rumors or talk about the private matters of others. Gossiping is unprofessional and hurtful. To avoid gossip:

- Remove yourself from where people are gossiping.
- Do not make or repeat any comment that can hurt a person—patient or resident, family member, visitor, co-worker, fellow student, instructor, the school or agency, and so on.
- Do not make or write false statements about another person. See Chapter 5.
- Do not talk about patients, residents, family members, visitors, co-workers, fellow students, instructors, the school or agency, or others at home or in social settings.
- Do not send or post comments about others or the school or agency by e-mail, instant messaging, text messaging, video sites, social media, or other electronic means. This is especially true of hurtful, false, or private comments. See "Wrongful Use of Electronic Communications" in Chapter 5.

Courtesies

A *courtesy* is a polite, considerate, or helpful comment or act. Courtesies take little time or energy. Even the smallest kind act can brighten someone's day.

- Address others by Miss, Mrs., Ms., Mr., or Doctor. Or use the name the person prefers. Do not call your instructor by his or her first name.
- Say "please." Begin or end each request with "please."
- Say "thank you" when someone does something for you or helps you.
- Apologize. Say "I'm sorry" when you make a mistake or hurt someone. Even little things—like bumping someone in the hallway—need an apology.
- Be thoughtful. Compliment others. Wish others a happy birthday, day or weekend off, or holiday.
- Wish the person and family well when they leave the agency. "Stay well" and "stay healthy" are examples.
- Hold doors and elevator doors open for others. If you are at the door first, open the door and let others pass through.
- Let patients, residents, families, and visitors enter elevators first.
- Stand to greet families and visitors.
- Help others willingly when asked.
- Give praise. When a co-worker or student does something that impresses you, tell that person. Also tell your co-workers or other students.
- Do not take credit for another person's deeds. Give the person credit for the action.

Confidentiality

The person's information is private and personal. *Confidentiality* means trusting others with personal and private information. The person's information is shared only among staff involved in the person's care. The person has the right to privacy and confidentiality. Agency, family, co-worker, and student information also is confidential.

Share information only with the nurse or your instructor. Do not talk about patients, residents, families, the agency, or co-workers when others are present. Do not talk about them in hallways, elevators, dining areas, or outside the agency. Others may over-hear you and eavesdrop. To *eavesdrop* means to listen in or over-hear what others are saying. It invades a person's privacy.

Patients, residents, and visitors are very alert to comments. They think you are talking about them or their loved ones. This leads to wrong information and wrong impressions about the person's condition. You can easily upset or hurt the person or family. Be very careful about what, how, when, and where you say things.

Many agencies have intercom systems. They allow for communication between the bedside and the nurses' station (Chapter 13). The person uses the intercom to call for help. The intercom is answered at the nurses' station. The nursing team may also use the intercom to communicate with each other. Be careful what you say. The intercom is like a loud speaker. Others nearby can hear what you are saying.

See *Focus on Communication: Confidentiality*.

FOCUS ON **COMMUNICATION**

Confidentiality

Your family and friends may ask about patients, residents, families, or staff. For example, your mother says: "I heard my neighbor is in your nursing home. Do you know what's wrong?"

Do not share any information with your family and friends. Doing so violates the person's right to privacy and confidentiality (Chapters 2 and 5). You can say:

I'm sorry, but I can't tell you about anyone in the center. It is unprofessional and against center policies. And it violates the person's right to privacy and confidentiality. Please don't ask me about anyone in the center.

Attention

Your attention (focus) matters. At work, distractions can affect quality of care and safety. You must focus on your work. See "Personal Matters."

As a student, being distracted affects your ability to learn. Distracting (disruptive) behaviors also interfere with other students' learning. Such behaviors do not show respect for your instructor or other students. The following are examples of distracting (disruptive) behaviors.

- Talking while the instructor or another student is talking.
- Talking while other students are finishing an assignment or examination.
- Making unnecessary noises (tapping or clicking an object, sighing, and so on).
- Fidgeting or moving a lot.
- Not participating in learning activities. Or doing something other than what is expected.
- Bringing children to class.
- Sleeping in class.
- Arriving late or leaving early.
- Using electronic devices during class.

Listen well, participate (be involved), and take notes in class. When you take notes, you write about what is read or presented. Ask questions about what you do not understand. These actions help you focus and learn.

Personal Matters

Personal matters must not interfere with your training or job. To keep personal matters out of school and the workplace:

- Make phone calls during meals and breaks.
- Do not let family and friends visit you at school or on the unit. If they must see you, meet during a break.
- Make appointments (doctor, dentist, lawyer, and others) for your days off.
- Do not use school or agency computers, printers, fax machines, copiers, or other equipment for your personal use.
- Do not take the school's or agency's supplies (pens, paper, and others) for your personal use.
- Do not discuss personal problems.
- Control your emotions. If you need to cry or express anger, do so in private. Get yourself together quickly and return to your work.
- Do not borrow money from or lend it to fellow students or co-workers. This includes meal money and bus or train fares. Borrowing and lending can lead to problems with students and co-workers.
- Do not sell things or engage in fund-raising. For example, do not sell your child's candy or raffle tickets to other students or co-workers.
- Turn off personal phones and other electronic devices.
- Do not send or check e-mails, text messages, or other electronic messages during class or work.

Meals and Breaks

Meal breaks are usually 30 minutes. Other breaks are usually 15 minutes. Meals and breaks are scheduled so that some staff are always on the unit. Staff on the unit cover for the staff away on break.

Staff members depend on each other. Leave for and return from breaks on time. Other staff need their turn. Do not take longer than allowed. Tell the nurse when you leave and return to the unit.

Student or staff break rooms usually have tables and chairs, a microwave, a refrigerator, and a sink. Some have coffee makers, cups, and utensils. Do not leave a mess. Clean up after yourself before leaving the break room. Follow school or agency policies for keeping food and drinks in the refrigerator. Discard or take home food and food containers daily.

Job Safety

You must protect patients, residents, families, visitors, co-workers, and yourself from harm. Negligent acts affect the safety of others (Chapter 5). Safety practices are presented throughout this book. These guidelines apply to everything you do.

- Understand the roles, functions, and responsibilities in your job description.
- Follow agency rules, policies, and procedures.
- Know what is right and wrong conduct.
- Know what you can and cannot do.
- Develop the desired qualities and traits in Figure 6-1.
- Follow the nurse's directions and instructions.
- Question unclear directions and things you do not understand.
- Help others willingly when asked.
- Ask for any training you might need.
- Report accurately—measurements, observations, the care given, the person's complaints, and any errors (Chapters 8 and 14).
- Be responsible for your actions. Admit when you are wrong or make mistakes. Do not blame others. Do not make excuses. Learn what you did wrong and why. Try to learn from your mistakes.
- Handle the person's property carefully and prevent damage.
- Follow the safety measures in Chapter 14 and throughout this book. Also see the *Promoting Safety and Comfort* boxes throughout this book.

Planning Your Work

Some care measures and nursing unit tasks are done at certain times. Others are done at the end of the shift. Deciding what to do and when is called *priority setting*. A *priority* is the most important thing at the time. To set your priorities, decide:

- Who has the greatest or most life-threatening needs.
- What task the nurse or person needs done first.
- What tasks need to be done at a certain time.
- What tasks need to be done when your shift starts and at the end of your shift.
- How long it takes to complete a task.
- How much help you need to complete a task.
- Who can help you and when.

Priorities change as the person's needs change. A person's condition can improve or worsen. New patients and residents are admitted. Others are transferred to other nursing units or discharged. These and many other factors can change priorities.

Setting priorities becomes easier with experience. Plan your work to give safe, thorough care and to use your time well (Box 6-2).

See *Focus on Communication: Planning Your Work.*

BOX 6-2	Planning Your Work

- Discuss priorities with the nurse.
- Know the routine of your shift and nursing unit.
- Follow unit policies for shift reports. In an *end-of-shift report*, the nurse gives a report to the on-coming shift (Chapter 8).
- List tasks that are on a schedule. For example, some persons are turned or offered the bedpan every 2 hours. Or a person's vital signs are to be measured every 4 hours.
- Judge how much time you need for each person and task.
- Identify tasks to do while patients and residents are eating, visiting, or involved with activities or therapies.
- Plan care around meal times, visiting hours, and therapies. Also consider recreation and social activities.
- Identify when you will need help from a co-worker. Ask a co-worker to help you. Give the time when you will need help and for how long.
- Schedule equipment or rooms for the person's use. The shower room is an example.
- Review your assignment sheet (Chapter 8). Gather needed supplies ahead of time.
- Do not waste time. Stay focused on your work.
- Leave a clean work area. Make sure rooms and utility areas are neat and orderly.
- Be a self-starter. Have initiative. Ask others if they need help. Follow unit routines, stock supply areas, and clean utility rooms. Stay busy.

FOCUS ON COMMUNICATION
Planning Your Work

You can ask your instructor or the nurse to help you set priorities. Communicate what you know—what you need to do and which tasks are time-sensitive (must be done at a certain time). Ask your instructor or the nurse to help you plan. For example, you say to the nurse:

I have 2 showers to give after breakfast—Mr. Lim's and Ms. Parker's. I also need to measure Ms. Parker's vital signs. Mr. Lim needs to be ready for his appointment at 9:30 AM. Do you need Ms. Parker's vital signs by a certain time? Would you like me to check them before giving Mr. Lim's shower?

STRESS

Stress is the response or change in the body caused by any emotional, psychological, physical, social, or economic factor. Stress is normal. It occurs every day and in every area of life.

A *stressor* is the event or factor that causes stress. Many stressors are pleasant—getting married, buying a house, starting a new job, planning a party. Some are not pleasant—illness, injury, family problems, death of loved ones, divorce, money concerns. School and some parts of your job are stressful.

Stress affects the whole person (Chapter 7).

- Physically—sweating, rapid heart rate, faster and deeper breathing, increased blood pressure, dry mouth
- Mentally and emotionally—fear, anger, apprehension, irritability, sadness, use of defense mechanisms (Chapter 53)
- Socially—changes in relationships, avoiding others, needing others, blaming others
- Spiritually—changes in beliefs about life's meaning and purpose, changes in values, strengthening or questioning one's beliefs in God or a higher power

Prolonged or frequent stress that is not managed threatens physical and mental health. Headaches, nausea, sleep problems, muscle tension, anxiety, and depression can occur. Life-threatening problems can occur—high blood pressure, heart attack, stroke, and ulcers.

School, job, and personal stresses can affect your family, friends, studies, and work. Stress affects you, the care you give, the person's quality of life, and how you relate to co-workers.

Burnout

Burnout is a job stress resulting in:

- Being physically or mentally exhausted
- Having doubts about your abilities
- Having doubts about the value of your work

Burnout occurs over time. Causes, signs, and symptoms are listed in Box 6-3, p. 64. Burnout can cause physical and mental health problems. They include fatigue, sleep problems, depression, anxiety, misuse of alcohol, drug use, heart disease, diabetes, stroke, and weight gain. Problems can develop at home and with personal relationships.

BOX 6-3	Burnout: Causes, Signs, and Symptoms

Causes of Burnout
- Schedules, assignments, or workloads that you find difficult
- Not being comfortable with your supervisor or co-workers
- Being harassed or heavily criticized by your supervisor or a co-worker
- Conflicts with how problems and grievances are handled
- Not liking your job or the agency
- Having skills that are greater than or lesser than what the job requires
- Lacking emotional support at work, at home, or socially
- Lacking balance between work and home, family, and social life

Signs and Symptoms of Burnout
- Lack of energy
- Sense of dread about going to work, not wanting to go to work, calling in sick, going to work late
- Sleep problems
- Problems concentrating, forgetfulness
- Frequent illness—infection, cold, influenza
- Physical symptoms:
  - Chest pain
  - Rapid or irregular heartbeat
  - Shortness of breath
  - Gastro-intestinal pain
  - Dizziness, fainting
  - Headaches
  - Loss of appetite
- Anxiety, depression
- Anger, irritability
- Wanting to be alone

Managing Stress

To reduce or cope with (manage) stress:
- Exercise regularly. Physical and mental benefits include cardiovascular health, weight control, tension release, emotional well-being, and relaxation.
- Get enough rest and sleep.
- Eat healthy.
- Plan personal and quiet time for you. Read, take a bath, go for a walk, meditate, or listen to music. Do what you enjoy.
- Use common sense about what you can and cannot do. Do not try to do everything that others ask you to do. Consider the amount of time and energy that you have.
- Do 1 thing at a time. You may feel overwhelmed with demands. List each thing to do. Set priorities.
- Do not judge yourself harshly. Do not try to be perfect or expect too much from yourself.
- Give yourself praise. You do good and wonderful things every day.
- Have a sense of humor. Laugh at yourself. Laugh with others. Spend time with those who make you laugh.
- Have a social life that does not include co-workers.
- Talk to your supervisor if your work or a person is causing too much stress. Your supervisor can help you deal with the matter.

Dealing With Conflict

People bring their values, attitudes, opinions, experiences, and expectations to school and work settings. Differences often lead to conflict. *Conflict* is a clash between opposing interests or ideas. People disagree and argue. There are misunderstandings and unrest.

Conflicts arise over issues or events. Work schedules, absences, and the amount and quality of work are examples. The problems must be resolved (settled, worked out, solved). Otherwise, unkind words or actions may occur. The learning or work setting becomes unpleasant. Care is affected.

Resolving Conflict. *Problem solving* steps are used to resolve conflict.
- Step 1: Define the problem. *A nurse ignores me.*
- Step 2: Collect information about the problem. Do not include unrelated information. *The nurse does not look at me. The nurse does not talk to me. The nurse does not respond when I ask for help. The nurse does not ask me to help with tasks that require 2 people. The nurse talks to other staff members.*
- Step 3: Identify possible solutions. *Ignore the nurse. Talk to my supervisor. Talk to co-workers about the problem. Change jobs.*
- Step 4: Select the best solution. *Talk to my supervisor.*
- Step 5: Carry out the solution. *See below.*
- Step 6: Evaluate the results. *See below.*

Communication and good work ethics help prevent and resolve conflicts. Identify and solve problems before they become major issues. To deal with conflict:
- Ask your instructor or supervisor for time to talk privately. Explain the problem. Give facts and specific examples. Ask for advice to solve the problem.
- Approach the person with whom you have the conflict. Ask to talk privately. Be polite and professional.
- Agree on a time and place to talk.
- Talk in a private setting. No one should hear you or the other person.
- Explain the problem and what is bothering you. Give facts and specific behaviors. Focus on the problem. Do not focus on the person.
- Listen to the person. Do not interrupt.
- Identify ways to solve the problem. Offer your thoughts. Ask for the other person's ideas.
- Set a date and time to review the matter.
- Thank the person for meeting with you.
- Carry out the solution.
- Review the matter as scheduled.

See *Focus on Communication: Resolving Conflict.*

Resolving Conflict

Dealing with conflict is hard for many people. However, letting the problem continue will make the matter worse. The following may help you start talking to the person. Always ask the person involved if you can talk privately.

- "You say 'no' when I ask you to help me. I help you when asked. Can we talk about this privately for a few minutes?"
- "I heard you tell Sam that I was sitting in a resident's room. You seemed angry when you said it. Can we talk privately? I want to explain why I was sitting. If it bothers you, you can tell me why."
- "The new schedule shows me working every weekend this month. Please tell me why. The employee handbook says that we work every other weekend."
- "We were late for class 2 times this week when you drove. How can I help so that we are not late?"

HARASSMENT

Harassment means to trouble, torment, offend, or worry a person by one's behavior or comments. Harassment can involve age, race, ethnic background, gender identity (Chapter 11), sexuality, religion, or disability. Respect others. Do not offend others with gestures, remarks, use of touch, or through electronic communications. Do not offend others with jokes, photos, or other images (pictures, drawings, cartoons, and so on). Harassment is not legal.

You have the right not to be harassed. No student (in your NATCEP or otherwise) should be allowed to harass or bully you. The same applies to instructors and other school staff, clinical staff, and co-workers. See "Reporting Harassment."

Sexual Harassment

Sexual harassment involves unwanted sexual behaviors by another. The behavior may involve sexual advances, requests for sexual favors, or unwanted comments or touching. The behavior affects work (school) and comfort. In extreme cases, a job (or grade) is threatened if sexual favors are not granted.

Sexual harassment can take the form of sexting. *Sexting* combines the words *sex* and *texting*. Sexting involves creating, sending, and posting sexual text messages, photos, or videos of oneself or others. Phones and other electronic devices are used.

Victims of sexual harassment may be any gender. The harasser's gender may be the same or different. Offensive comments about groups of people are also considered harassment.

Sexual harassment in the workplace is not legal. Employers must not allow harassment to occur. They must take action to stop it if they know it is happening.

Be careful about what you say or do. Even innocent remarks and behaviors can be viewed as sexual harassment.

You might not be sure about your own or another person's remarks or behaviors. If so, talk to your instructor or supervisor.

Bullying

Bullying is a form of youth violence that occurs among school-aged children and adolescents. With bullying there is repeated, unwanted, aggressive behavior that involves a real or perceived power imbalance. A bully tries to gain power and control over a target. Bullying can happen in school or social settings. It also occurs through the use of technology (electronic bullying, cyberbullying). See Chapter 11.

Reporting Harassment

If you believe that you are being harassed or bullied, take action. If you are able, ask the person to stop. Follow the school's or agency's policies for reporting misconduct. As a student, tell your instructor or school counselor. At work, tell your supervisor or contact the human resources department.

You may need to write down details about the misconduct. Be specific. Include dates, times, locations, names, what was said or done, and what you said or did. Record who else was present. You cannot be punished for reporting harassment.

See *Focus on Communication: Reporting Harassment.*

Reporting Harassment

You have the right to feel safe and not threatened. If comments make you uncomfortable, you can say: "Please don't say things like that. It's unprofessional." If someone's actions make you uneasy, you can say: "Please don't do that. It's unprofessional." Leave the area. Report the person's statements or actions to your instructor or supervisor.

RESIGNING FROM A JOB

A job closer to home, better pay, or new opportunities may prompt you to leave your job. School, children, and illness are other reasons. Whatever your reason for resigning, tell your employer. Agency policy may require:

- A written notice
- A resignation letter
- Completing a form in the human resources department

A 2-week notice is a good practice. Do not leave without notice. Include the following in your notice.

- Reason for leaving
- The last date you will work
- Comments thanking the employer for the opportunity to work in the agency

An exit interview (on or before your last day) or an exit survey is common practice. You are asked about the agency, your job, and how the agency can improve.

LOSING A JOB

You must perform your job well and protect patients and residents from harm. Poor performance can result in the with-holding of a pay raise or termination (job loss). Failing to follow agency policy is often grounds for termination. So is failing to get along with others. Box 6-4 lists the many reasons why you can lose your job. To protect your job, function at your best. Always practice good work ethics.

DRUG TESTING

Drug and alcohol use affects patient, resident, and staff safety. Quality of care suffers. Being late to or absent from work is more common. Many agencies have drug testing policies. Review your agency's policy for when and how you might be tested.

UNETHICAL STUDENT BEHAVIOR

Your NATCEP and school will likely have a code of conduct (Chapter 5). Violating the code of conduct is unethical behavior. Many of the reasons listed in Box 6-4 are violations of your school's and NATCEP's code of conduct. As a result, your school and NATCEP may take 1 or more of the following actions.

- Dismiss you from the school or NATCEP
- Issue a failing grade
- Not recommend that you take the competency evaluation (written and skills tests)

Act in an ethical manner at all times. Always try to do the right thing. If you do, you will be a successful nursing assistant.

BOX 6-4	Common Reasons for Losing a Job

- Poor attendance—not going to work or excessive tardiness (being late).
- Abandonment—leaving the job during your shift.
- Falsifying a record—job application or a person's record.
- Violent behavior in the workplace.
- Weapons in the workplace—guns, knives, explosives, or other dangerous items.
- Having, using, or distributing alcohol or drugs in the work setting. This excludes having or using drugs ordered by your doctor.
- Taking a person's drugs for your own use or giving them to others.
- Harassment.
- Offensive speech and language.
- Stealing or destroying the agency's or a person's property.
- Disrespect to patients, residents, families, visitors, co-workers, or supervisors.
- Abusing or neglecting a person.
- Invading a person's privacy.
- Failing to maintain patient, resident, family, agency, or co-worker confidentiality.
- Wrongful use of electronic communications (Chapter 5).
- Using the agency's supplies and equipment for your own use.
- Defamation—see Chapter 5 and "Gossip" (p. 61).
- Abusing meal breaks and break time.
- Sleeping on the job.
- Violating the agency's dress code.
- Violating any agency policy or care procedure.
- Tending to personal matters while on duty.

FOCUS ON **PRIDE**

The Person, Family, and Yourself

Personal and Professional Responsibility

Your job as a nursing assistant is important. How you act makes a difference. You can help persons feel safe, secure, and cared for. Through good work ethics, you can make others' lives happier, easier, and less painful. Take pride in your work ethics. Your work affects quality of life.

Rights and Respect

Conflict with other students and co-workers will arise. Do not gossip, put others down, or talk about people behind their backs. These behaviors are disrespectful and not professional. Deal with conflict in a respectful and mature way.

Independence and Social Interaction

Smile and greet patients and residents by name. Politely introduce yourself. Display a caring and friendly manner all the time. Remain calm and helpful in stressful situations. These actions promote good relationships and reflect well on you and the agency.

Delegation and Teamwork

Your work ethics affect the team. Greet co-workers pleasantly. Help others willingly. After completing tasks, ask if you can help with anything else. Be someone others enjoy working with.

Ethics and Laws

As a student and as a nursing assistant, you are responsible for following the ethical guidelines in this chapter. Patients, residents, families, visitors, and co-workers depend on you for safe and effective care.

FOCUS ON **PRIDE**: Application

Think of a person you enjoy working with. What qualities do you value in a co-worker? How will you apply these qualities in your work?

REVIEW QUESTIONS

Circle the BEST answer.

1 You show honesty when you
   a Help others complete tasks
   b Report mistakes
   c Remain calm
   d Are polite

2 Which will help you do your job well?
   a Sleeping 3 to 4 hours daily
   b Not wearing needed eyeglasses
   c Using drugs and alcohol
   d Exercising regularly

3 Which is a good hygiene practice?
   a Bathing weekly
   b Wearing strongly scented perfume or cologne
   c Brushing teeth after meals
   d Having long and polished fingernails

4 You are getting ready for clinical. Which is a good practice?
   a Styling hair up and off your collar
   b Wearing jewelry
   c Wearing your ID badge at waist level
   d Having tattoos exposed

5 You show you are dependable as a student when you
   a Arrive 5 minutes late for class
   b Turn in incomplete assignments
   c Leave class early for a personal matter
   d Follow directions

6 Which statement reflects a good attitude?
   a "It's not my fault."
   b "I can help you."
   c "That's not my job."
   d "I did it yesterday. It's your turn."

7 A co-worker tells you that a doctor and nurse are dating. You should
   a Not repeat the comment to others
   b Ask your co-worker for more details
   c Ask other staff if they know about it
   d Text the comment to a friend you trust

8 You can share information about a patient
   a In a private conversation on social media
   b During a meal with your family
   c With the nurse
   d With staff not involved in the person's care

9 Which is professional speech and language?
   a Using vulgar words
   b Shouting
   c Arguing
   d Speaking clearly

10 Which is a courteous act?
   a Telling co-workers they did a good job
   b Calling a resident "honey"
   c Taking credit for a co-worker's work
   d Closing an elevator door as a person approaches

11 Talking to another student while your instructor is teaching
   a Shows interest
   b Shows respect
   c Is distracting
   d Improves learning

12 Sending text messages while working
   a Shows good time management
   b Can lead to neglect and job loss
   c Helps prevent burnout
   d Is allowed at the nurses' station

13 You are on a meal break. Which is *true?*
   a You cannot make personal phone calls.
   b Family members cannot meet you.
   c The nurse needs to know that you are off the unit.
   d You can take a few extra minutes if needed.

14 When planning your work
   a Discuss priorities with the nurse
   b Delegate tasks you will not have time to do
   c Do not ask co-workers for help
   d Plan care so that you can watch the person's TV

15 These statements are about stress. Which is *true?*
   a Personal stress does not affect work.
   b Stress affects the whole person.
   c All stressors are unpleasant.
   d Stress is abnormal.

16 Thinking about work makes you doubt your abilities and feel anxious. Which action is *best?*
   a Ignore the feelings.
   b Resign from your job.
   c Call in absent.
   d Try healthy methods to reduce stress.

17 You have extra work because a co-worker is often late. To resolve the conflict
   a Explain the problem to your supervisor
   b Refuse to work with the person
   c Ignore the problem
   d Complain about the person to co-workers

18 Which statement about harassment is *true?*
   a Giving a resident a compliment is harassment.
   b Joking about a person's religion is not harassment.
   c Harassment can occur through text messages.
   d Only women are victims of harassment.

19 You are often late for work. Which is *true?*
   a Tardiness is excused if you give the reason.
   b You may be fined.
   c You can make up the time by skipping your break.
   d You can lose your job.

20 You show good ethics as a student when you
   a Ask your instructor not to record your tardiness
   b Follow your training program's dress code
   c Use class time for personal matters
   d Tell your family about residents at your clinical site

Answers to Chapter 6 questions are on p. 901.

FOCUS ON **PRACTICE**

Problem Solving

A co-worker did not show up for work. You and the other staff members have extra work. How do you respond? How will you plan, prioritize, and manage the extra work?

The Person and Family

- Define the key terms and key abbreviation in this chapter.
- Identify the parts that make up the whole person.
- Explain Abraham Maslow's theory of basic needs.
- Explain the importance of understanding the person's cultural and spiritual beliefs and practices.
- Explain how to properly address the person.
- Identify the factors that influence health care beliefs and practices.
- Describe the persons cared for in health care agencies.
- Explain how to care for persons with special needs.

- Identify the elements needed for good communication.
- Describe how to use verbal and nonverbal communication.
- Explain the methods and barriers to good communication.
- Describe how behavior is a form of communication.
- Identify ways to manage difficult behaviors.
- Explain why family is important to the person.
- Describe how to interact with the person's family and visitors.
- Explain how to promote PRIDE in the person, the family, and yourself.

bariatrics The field of medicine focused on the treatment and control of obesity

body language Messages sent through facial expressions, gestures, posture, hand and body movements, gait, eye contact, and appearance

comatose Being unable to respond to stimuli; unconscious

communication The exchange of information—a message sent is received and correctly interpreted by the intended person

culture The characteristics of a group of people—language, values, beliefs, habits, likes, dislikes, customs—passed from 1 generation to the next

disability Any lost, absent, or impaired physical or mental function

esteem The worth, value, or opinion one has of a person

gender identity A person's sense or feelings of being male, female, a combination of male and female, or neither male nor female

geriatrics The field of medicine concerned with the problems and diseases of old age and older persons

holism A concept that considers the whole person; the whole person has physical, psychological, social, and spiritual parts that are woven together and cannot be separated

need Something necessary or desired for maintaining life and mental well-being

nonverbal communication Communication that does not use words

obesity Having a weight that is higher than what is healthy for a given height

obstetrics The field of medicine concerned with the care of women during pregnancy, labor, and childbirth and for 6 to 8 weeks after birth

optimal level of function A person's desired level of ability

paraphrasing Re-stating the person's message in your own words

pediatrics The field of medicine concerned with the growth, development, and care of children—newborns to teenagers

psychiatry The field of medicine concerned with mental health disorders

religion An organized system of spiritual beliefs and practices

risk factor Something that increases the chance of illness or injury

self-actualization Experiencing one's potential

self-esteem Thinking well of oneself and seeing oneself as useful and having value

sexuality The physical, emotional, social, cultural, and spiritual factors that affect a person's feelings, attitudes, and behaviors about one's gender identity and sexual behavior

verbal communication Communication that uses written or spoken words

BMI Body mass index

Each person is unique and has value. The person is someone who thinks, acts, feels, and makes decisions. Each has needs, fears, rights, abilities, talents, and interests. Each has suffered losses—loss of home, family, friends, body functions, independence. And each has desires for life—meaning, purpose, belonging, worth.

Your care becomes more personal (individualized) as you better understand the person. This chapter explains the different aspects of the *whole person* and how to apply this understanding to your interactions with the person and family.

THE WHOLE PERSON

Holism means whole. *Holism* is a concept that considers the whole person. The whole person has physical, psychological, social, and spiritual parts. These parts are woven together and cannot be separated (Fig. 7-1). Each part relates to and depends on the others.

- *Physical* involves the person's body.
- *Psychological* relates to the person's mental abilities and emotional and behavioral responses.
- *Social* involves relational aspects of the person's life.
- *Spiritual* relates to meaning, connection, and purpose in the person's life. Spirituality is broader than religion (p. 71).

To consider only the physical part is to ignore the person's ability to think, make decisions, and interact with others. It also ignores experiences, life-style, culture, beliefs, joys, sorrows, and needs.

Disability and illness affect the whole person. The health team plans care to address the person's physical, mental and emotional, social, and spiritual needs. The person is helped to regain or maintain his or her *optimal level of function*—the person's desired level of ability.

BASIC NEEDS

A *need* is something necessary or desired for maintaining life and mental well-being. According to psychologist Abraham Maslow, basic needs must be met for a person to survive and function. The needs are arranged from the lowest level to the highest level (Fig. 7-2). Lower-level needs are basic survival needs. As those needs are met, higher-level needs can be met.

From the lowest level to the highest level, basic needs are:

- *Physical needs.* Oxygen, food, water, shelter, elimination, rest, and activity are needed for survival and health.
- *Safety and security needs.* The person needs to feel safe from harm, danger, and fear.
- *Love and belonging needs.* These needs relate to love, closeness, affection, and meaningful relationships with others. Family and friends meet love and belonging needs. The health team can also provide meaningful interaction.
- *Self-esteem needs.* *Esteem* is the worth, value, or opinion one has of a person. *Self-esteem* means to think well of oneself and to see oneself as useful and having value. Illness, injury, disability, and aging can affect self-esteem.
- *The need for self-actualization.* *Self-actualization* means experiencing one's potential. It involves learning, understanding, and creating to the limit of a person's ability. This is the highest need. Rarely, if ever, is it totally met. Most people constantly try to learn and understand more. This need can be postponed and life will continue.

See Box 7-1 (p. 70) for examples of how the nursing assistant meets basic needs.

See *Focus on Long-Term Care and Home Care: Basic Needs*, p. 70.

See *Focus on Communication: Basic Needs*, p. 70.

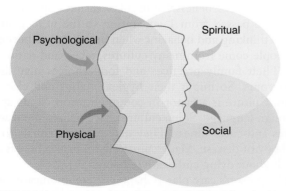

FIGURE 7-1 A person is a physical, psychological, social, and spiritual being. The parts over-lap and cannot be separated.

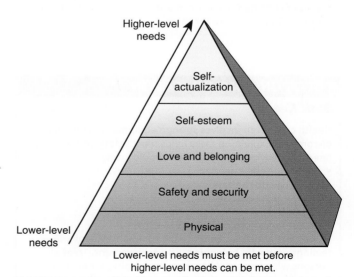

FIGURE 7-2 Basic needs for life as described by Maslow. (Adapted from Maslow AH, Frager RD, editor, Fadiman J, editor: *Motivation and personality*, ed 3. © 1987.)

BOX 7-1	Meeting Basic Needs

Physical Needs
- Meet oxygen needs (Chapter 44).
  - Assist with breathing exercises.
  - Position the person upright for easier breathing.
  - Report signs of altered respiratory function.
  - Assist with oxygen therapy as directed.
- Meet food and fluid needs (Chapters 31 and 32).
  - Prepare persons for meals. Assist with feeding as needed.
  - Provide fresh drinking water. Keep water within reach.
- Meet elimination needs (Chapters 27 and 29).
  - Assist persons to the bathroom or with the bedpan, urinal, or commode. Keep devices in reach if they can be used alone.
  - Change soiled incontinence products and linens promptly. Provide skin care.
  - Follow the person's bowel or bladder training program.
- Meet rest and activity needs (Chapters 35 and 36).
  - Provide a quiet, restful setting.
  - Report pain promptly. Meet comfort needs as directed.
  - Avoid interrupting sleep.
  - Perform turning and re-positioning, range-of-motion exercises, and ambulation (walking) activity as directed.

Safety and Security Needs
- Maintain a safe, clean, and comfortable setting (Chapters 13 and 14).
- Explain procedures.
- Keep needed items within reach.
- Respond to call lights promptly.
- Protect the person's belongings.
- Provide privacy.

Love and Belonging Needs
- Respect the person's time with family and visitors.
- Encourage social activities.
- Do not seem rushed.
- Treat the person with dignity and respect. Be kind.
- Use touch appropriately (p. 77).
- Respect the person's sexuality needs (Chapter 12).

Self-Esteem Needs
- Call the person by name. Use the name the person prefers.
- Promote independence and personal choice.
- Praise the person's effort and ability.
- Meet the person's grooming needs (Chapter 25).
- Show interest in the person. Ask questions. Listen.

Self-Actualization Needs
- Encourage involvement in activities and events that the person enjoys. Assist persons to activities and events as needed.
- Provide good lighting and other needed items for activities the person enjoys alone. Reading or listening to audiobooks are examples.
- Encourage the person's unique creative abilities—art, music, writing, scrapbooking, gardening, knitting, and so on.
- Ask about what is meaningful to the person, what the person enjoys doing, or what the person still wants to try to do in life. Share anything learned with the nurse for care planning (Chapter 8).

FOCUS ON LONG-TERM CARE AND HOME CARE

Basic Needs

Long-Term Care
Some people feel safe and secure in a nursing center. They have help when needed and staff to protect them. Others feel scared or confused. They are in a strange place with strange routines. Strangers care for them.

Show new residents their setting. Listen to their concerns. Explain all routines and tasks. You may have to repeat information often—sometimes for days or weeks until the person feels safe and secure. Be patient, kind, and understanding.

FOCUS ON COMMUNICATION

Basic Needs

Health care often involves strange equipment, pain, and discomfort. Explaining tasks helps meet safety and security needs. For each task, the person should know:
- Why the task is needed
- Who will do the task
- How it will be done
- What the person needs to do
- What sensations or feelings to expect

Respect and independence increase self-esteem and feelings of worth, belonging, and achievement. Treat all persons with respect. Allow personal choice. While it takes more time, encourage them to do as much for themselves as possible. Compliment effort and accomplishments. Give adults praise with sincerity and maturity, as speaking to an adult and not a child.

CULTURE

Culture is the characteristics of a group of people—language, values, beliefs, habits, likes, dislikes, and customs. They are passed from 1 generation to the next. Culture affects thinking and behavior when health care is needed.

People come from many cultures, races, and nationalities. Their family practices and food choices may differ from yours. So might their hygiene habits and clothing styles. Culture is a factor in communication. Some speak a foreign language. Some cultures have beliefs about what causes and cures illness. They may perform rituals to rid the body of disease. Many cultures have health beliefs and rituals about dying and death (Chapter 59).

The person's care plan (Chapter 8) communicates what is important to the person. Show interest in the person's culture.

See *Caring About Culture: Culture.*
See *Focus on Long-Term Care and Home Care: Culture.*

✿ CARING ABOUT CULTURE

Culture

The following guidelines will help you communicate with persons from different cultures.

- Determine your own beliefs and practices. Do not let your own ideas, attitudes, beliefs, or values negatively affect care.
- Learn about the person's culture. You can ask the nurse and the person. The person's family may be another valuable source.
- Remember that each person is unique. *A person may not follow all of the beliefs and practices of his or her culture.*
- Consider how culture affects communication. Modify your approach to meet the person's needs. For example, it is important to learn how listening (p. 78) is communicated in the person's culture.
- Be alert to signs of fear, anxiety, or confusion.
- Be kind and attentive to needs.
- Have an attitude of interest, respect, and flexibility.
- Be patient and develop trust. Listen well and allow time for the person to respond. If the person gives "extra" information, listen with interest. Give the person your full attention.
- See "Verbal Communication" on p. 75 for communicating with persons who speak a foreign language.

Modified from Giger JN, Haddad L: Transcultural nursing: assessment and intervention, ed 8, St Louis, 2021, Elsevier.

FOCUS ON **LONG-TERM CARE AND HOME CARE**

Culture

Home Care

Culture is reflected in the home. Homes vary in size, neatness, furnishings, and price. Whether rich or poor, treat each person and family with respect, kindness, and dignity. Do not judge the person's life-style, habits, religion, or culture.

SPIRITUALITY AND RELIGION

Spirituality is a broad term that involves the person's source of meaning, connection, and purpose in life. Spiritual health can promote:

- Connection to what the person considers "ultimate"—a higher being, nature, a greater purpose, oneself
- Assurance that the person's life has value, meaning, and purpose
- Healthy coping—endurance (resilience), peace, hope
- Self-awareness—the person's understanding of his or her values, motives, behaviors, strengths, weaknesses, desires, reactions to thoughts and feelings, and other "internal" characteristics

Spirituality is unique for each person. Beliefs differ. The ways people discover and live out their spiritual beliefs and values also differ.

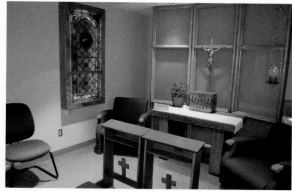

FIGURE 7-3 A hospital chapel provides a quiet area for prayer. (Courtesy Gene Vogelgesang, Illinois Valley Community Hospital, Peru, Ill.)

Religion is an organized system of spiritual beliefs and practices. Religions provide a framework and community for meeting spiritual needs. Common practices include:

- Gatherings, services, and events
- Meditation, prayer, or solitude
- Reading religious texts
- Listening to or singing to music
- Following a certain diet
- Having or wearing items with spiritual significance

Many people find comfort and strength from their spirituality during illness. They may want to pray and observe religious practices. Hospitals and nursing centers offer religious services and have areas for prayer or meditation (Fig. 7-3). Assist the person to attend services as needed.

A person may want to see a cleric (clergy) (Chapter 1). If so, tell the nurse. Make sure the room is neat and orderly. Have a chair ready for the cleric. Provide privacy during the visit.

The person's care plan (Chapter 8) includes the practices that are important to the person. Show interest in the person's beliefs and practices. This helps you understand the person and give better care.

A person may not follow all of the beliefs and practices of his or her religion. Some people do not practice a religion. Each person is unique. Do not judge the person by your standards. And do not force your ideas on the person.

See *Focus on Communication: Spirituality and Religion.*

FOCUS ON **COMMUNICATION**

Spirituality and Religion

Show interest in the person's spirituality. Respect the person's practices. For example:

- A person's necklace has a religious symbol. You say: "Your necklace is pretty. Does it have special meaning for you?"
- A person wants quiet time for meditation. You say: "How much time would you like? I will make sure you are not disturbed."
- A person likes to pray before meals. You wait patiently and listen before feeding the person.
- A person asks: "Will you read to me from my journal?" You take time to read to the person.

SEXUALITY

Sexuality is the physical, emotional, social, cultural, and spiritual factors that affect a person's feelings, attitudes, and behaviors about one's gender identity and sexual behavior. In this book, sexuality is explained further within the context of growth and development (Chapter 11) and the changes that occur with aging (Chapter 12). See "Gender Identity."

ADDRESSING THE PERSON

How you address the person matters. Too often a person is referred to as a room number. For example: "12A needs the bedpan" rather than "Mrs. Olson in 12A needs the bedpan." To address patients and residents with dignity and respect:

- Greet the person by title—Mrs. Jones, Mr. Wills, Miss Parker, Ms. Norris, or Dr. Gonzalez. Then ask what name the person prefers.
- Do not use their first names or any other name unless they ask you to.
- Do not call them grandma, papa, sweetheart, honey, or other names.

Gender Identity

Gender identity refers to a person's sense or feelings of being male, female, a combination of male and female, or neither male nor female. Sometimes a person's gender identity differs from the person's biological sex. There may be name and pronoun changes. For example, Jamie and "she" and "her" are used instead of James and "he" and "him." Or Allison is changed to Allen with pronoun changes.

Use the person's preferred name and pronouns. These are included in the person's care plan (Chapter 8).

See *Focus on Communication: Gender Identity.*

FOCUS ON COMMUNICATION

Gender Identity

If you do not yet know a person's preferred name or pronouns:

- Avoid using gender terms or pronouns until this information is known. For example: say "May I help you?" instead of "May I help you, sir?"
- Never refer to a person as "it."
- Ask how the person would like to be addressed. Do not assume. You can say: "I want to be respectful. What name and pronouns would you like me to use?"
- Apologize for mistakes. You can say: "I'm sorry for using the wrong name. I meant no disrespect."

HEALTH CARE BELIEFS AND PRACTICES

Many factors affect a person's health care beliefs and practices. Age, gender, culture, and religion are some. Family and work roles, education, income, family and social support, and community resources are others. Past health problems and family history of illness also shape a person's thoughts and behaviors.

These and other factors influence the person's:

- Life-style choices
- Thoughts about risk
- Practices to promote health and prevent illness and injury
- Decisions about treatment
- Access to care
- Ability to follow through with a treatment plan

The nurse asks questions to better understand the person's beliefs and practices.

The nurse teaches the person about risk factors. A *risk factor* is something that increases the chance of illness or injury. Some risk factors can be controlled. Others cannot. For example, a person has a family history of heart disease. The nurse teaches the person about diet, exercise, and not smoking. The goal is to promote health and decrease the risk of illness and injury.

See *Caring About Culture: Health Care Beliefs and Practices.*

CARING ABOUT CULTURE

Health Care Beliefs and Practices

Culture can influence beliefs about the cause of illness and how to treat illness. The following are examples.

Some *Chinese* cultures believe in a balance of 2 forces—*yin* and *yang*. The opposite force is used for treatment. For example, a person believes an infection (caused by yang forces) can be treated with green vegetables and fruits (foods with yin qualities). Some believe spatial arrangements (the practice of *feng shui*), colors, and numbers affect health and life.

In *Mexican* culture, some believe that outside forces (luck or God) control health. Some relate health and illness to a balance of forces (hot, cold, wet, dry). The opposite force is used to cure. Older adults may not seek treatment if aging is considered the cause. Seeking care from a family member or folk healer is common. An herbalist (*yerbero, herbero*) uses herbs and spices to prevent or cure disease. A healer (*curandero, curandera*) may give care for serious illness.

NOTE: *Each person is unique. A person may not follow all of the beliefs and practices of his or her culture. Follow the care plan.*

Modified from Giger JN, Haddad L: Transcultural nursing: assessment and intervention, ed 8, St Louis, 2021, Elsevier.

PERSONS NEEDING HEALTH CARE

People of all ages need health care. They are often grouped by their problems, needs, and age (Table 7-1). Goals are set to meet the person's various needs (Chapter 8).

TABLE 7-1	Persons Needing Health Care
Group	Description
Mothers and newborns	• *Obstetrics*—the field of medicine concerned with the care of women during pregnancy, labor, and childbirth and for 6 to 8 weeks after birth. • Pre-natal (before birth) care is given in clinics and doctors' offices. • Mothers are admitted to hospital obstetric (maternity) units for labor and delivery. • Problems can occur during and after pregnancy and childbirth. • See Chapter 56.
Children	• *Pediatrics*—the field of medicine concerned with the growth, development, and care of children—newborns to teenagers. • Pediatric units are designed and equipped for the needs of children (usually up to age 16) and parents.
Adults with medical problems	• The focus is on illnesses, diseases, and injuries not needing surgery. • Health problems are acute, chronic, or terminal (Chapter 1).
Persons having surgery	• Care is given before, during, and after surgery. • Surgeries are simple (removal of an appendix) to complex (heart surgery). • See Chapter 40.
Persons with mental health disorders	• *Psychiatry*—the field of medicine concerned with mental health disorders. • Problems range from mild to severe (Chapter 53). • Some persons need help coping with life stresses. Others present dangers to self and others.
Persons needing bariatric care	• *Bariatrics*—the field of medicine focused on the treatment and control of obesity. • *Obesity*—having a weight that is higher than what is healthy for a given height. The person has excess body fat. • *Body mass index (BMI)* is used to screen for weight problems. BMI is calculated using the person's weight and height. A high BMI indicates obesity. • The person is at high risk for many serious health problems.
Persons in special care units	• Special care units are designed to treat and prevent life-threatening problems. • Emergency rooms and intensive care, coronary (cardiovascular) care, burn, and kidney dialysis units are examples.
Persons needing rehabilitation or sub-acute care	• The person needs rehabilitation or more recovery time than hospital care allows. • See Chapter 46.
Older persons	• *Geriatrics*—the field of medicine concerned with the problems and diseases of old age and older persons. • See Chapter 12.
Persons needing long-term care	• *Alert, oriented persons*—know who and where they are. Care needs depend on their physical problems. • *Confused and disoriented persons*—are mildly to severely confused and disoriented. This may be a short-term or long-term problem. See Chapter 54. • *Persons needing complete care*—cannot meet their own needs. Require total help with all activities of daily living (ADL). Some cannot say what they need or want. • *Short-term residents*—are recovering from fractures or other injuries, acute illness, or surgery. May need tube feedings, wound care, or other treatments or therapies (physical, occupational, speech, language, respiratory). The goal is optimal level of function and to return home. • *Persons needing respite care*—respite means rest or relief. The person living at home goes to a nursing center for a short stay. Caregivers get relief for a vacation, business, or rest. Respite care can be a few days to several weeks. • *Life-long residents*—may have disabilities from birth defects or childhood or adult diseases or injuries. There may be physical impairments, intellectual impairments, or both. Life-long assistance, support, and special devices are needed. • *Persons with mental health disorders*—have problems with behaviors and function. Self-care and independent living may be impaired. Some persons have both physical and mental health disorders. • *Persons who are terminally ill*—the goal is quality end-of-life care for persons who are dying. See Chapter 59.

Persons With Special Needs

Each person is unique. Special knowledge and skills may be required to meet the person's needs.

Persons With Disabilities. A *disability* is any lost, absent, or impaired physical or mental function. Temporary or permanent, a disability can develop at any age.

Children can develop hearing problems from ear infections. Head injuries can impair cognitive function. Spinal cord injuries can affect movements. And loud noise (music, machines) is linked to hearing loss.

To communicate with persons who have disabilities, see persons:

- Who have speech disorders—Chapter 47
- Who are hard of hearing—Chapter 47
- Who are blind—Chapter 47
- Who are confused—Chapter 54
- With Alzheimer's disease and other dementias—Chapter 54

Common courtesies and manners (*etiquette*) apply to any person with a disability. See Box 7-2 for disability etiquette.

BOX 7-2	Disability Etiquette

- Show the same courtesies to the person as you do to anyone else.
- Provide for privacy.
- Touch or handle the person's wheelchair only with consent.
- Do not hang on or lean on a person's wheelchair.
- Treat adults as adults. Use the person's first name only when asked to do so. Do the same for others present.
- Do not pat a person who is in a wheelchair on the head.
- Speak directly to the person. Do not direct questions for the person to a companion.
- Do not be embarrassed for using words that relate to the disability. For example, you say: "See you later" to a person with a vision problem.
- Sit or squat to talk to a person in a wheelchair or in a chair. You and the person are at eye level.
- Ask if help is needed before acting. If the answer is "no," respect the person's wishes. If the person wants help, ask what to do and how to do it.
- Think before giving directions to a person in a wheelchair. Think about distances, weather conditions, stairs, curbs, steep hills, and other obstacles.
- Let the person set the pace in walking, talking, or other activities.
- See Chapter 47 for persons with hearing or vision problems.

Modified from Easter Seals, Disability etiquette, 2024.

The Person Who Is Comatose. *Comatose (unconscious)*
means being unable to respond to stimuli. (A *stimulus* is something that causes the person to change, react, or respond.) The person is not alert (awake). The person cannot respond to others. Often the person can hear and can feel touch and pain. Pain may be shown by grimacing or groaning. Assume that the person hears and understands you. Use touch and give care gently. Practice these measures.

- Knock before entering the person's room.
- Tell the person your name, the time, and the place every time you enter the room.
- Follow the same schedule every day.
- Explain what you are going to do. Explain care measures step-by-step as you do them.
- Use touch to communicate care, concern, and comfort (p. 77).
- Tell the person when you are completing care.
- Tell the person what time you will return.
- Tell the person when you are leaving the room.

EFFECTIVE COMMUNICATION

Good communication is needed to give effective care. *Communication* is the exchange of information—a message sent is received and correctly interpreted by the intended person.

You communicate with the person every time you give care. You give information to the person. The person gives information to you. For effective communication between you and the person, follow the rules in Box 7-3.

See *Focus on Children and Older Persons: Effective Communication.*

BOX 7-3	Communicating With the Person

- Use words that have the same meaning for you and the person.
- Avoid medical terms and words not familiar to the person.
- Communicate in a logical and orderly manner. Do not wander in thought.
- Give facts and be specific.
- Be brief and concise.
- Understand and respect the patient or resident as a person. Your interactions are not just task-oriented. You are building a trusting relationship.
- View the person as a physical, psychological, social, and spiritual human being.
- Appreciate the person's problems and frustrations.
- Respect the person's rights, religion, and culture.
- Give the person time to understand the information that you give.
- Repeat information as often as needed. Repeat what you said. Use the exact same words. Do not give the person a new message to process. If the person does not seem to understand after repeating, re-phrase the message. This is very important for persons with hearing problems.
- Ask questions to see if the person understood you.
- Be patient. People with memory problems may ask the same question many times. Do not say that you are repeating information.
- Include the person in conversations when others are present. This includes when a co-worker is assisting with care.

FOCUS ON CHILDREN AND OLDER PERSONS

Effective Communication

Older Persons

Communicating with persons who have dementia can be hard. The Alzheimer's and Related Dementias Education and Referral Center (ADEAR) recommends the following.

- Gain the person's attention before speaking. Say the person's name. Make eye contact.
- Be aware of your voice tone and body language (p. 77).
- Choose simple words and short sentences. Give simple, step-by-step instructions.
- Use a gentle, calm voice. Show a caring manner.
- Do not talk to the person as you would a baby.
- Do not talk about the person as if he or she is not there.
- Keep distractions and noise to a minimum.
- Repeat instructions as needed. Be patient.
- Give the person time to respond. Do not interrupt.
- Try to provide the word the person is struggling to find.
- State questions and instructions in a positive way. For example, "please do this" instead of "don't do that."

You will learn more about how to communicate with persons with Alzheimer's disease and other types of dementia in Chapter 54.

Verbal Communication

Verbal communication uses written or spoken words. Most verbal communication involves the spoken word. Follow these rules.

- Face the person. Look at the person.
- Position yourself at the person's eye level. Sit or squat by the person as needed.
- Control the loudness and tone of your voice.
- Speak clearly, slowly, and distinctly.
- Do not use slang or vulgar words.
- Repeat information as needed.
- Ask 1 question at a time. Wait for an answer.
- Do not shout, whisper, or mumble.
- Be kind, courteous, and friendly.

You use the written word when the person cannot speak or hear but can read. The nurse and care plan tell you how to communicate with the person (Fig. 7-4). The person may have poor vision. When writing messages:

- Keep them simple and brief.
- Use a black felt pen on white paper.
- Print in large letters.
- Use black and a large font (print size) if using a computer or other electronic device.

Some persons cannot speak or read. Ask questions that have "yes" or "no" answers. The person can nod, blink, or use other gestures for "yes" and "no." Follow the care plan. Picture boards or cards may be used (Fig. 7-5). Persons who are deaf may use sign language. See Chapter 47.

See *Caring About Culture: Verbal Communication.*

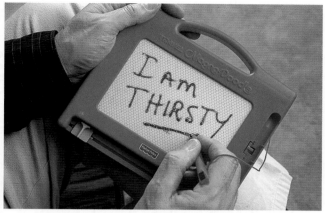

FIGURE 7-4 A written message is used to communicate.

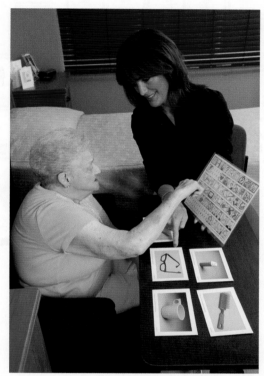

FIGURE 7-5 A therapist helps a resident use a picture board and picture cards to communicate.

✿ CARING ABOUT CULTURE

Verbal Communication

Persons from different cultures may speak a language you do not understand. The following are helpful when communicating with a person who speaks a different language.

- Convey comfort by your voice tone and body language (p. 77).
- Speak slowly and clearly. Do not speak loudly or shout.
- Keep messages short and simple.
- Use words that you know the person understands. Avoid using medical terms and abbreviations.
- Use a language dictionary or a list of common words and phrases. See *Evolve Student Learning Resources* for a "Spanish Vocabulary and Phrases Audio Glossary."

- Use gestures, pictures, or communication boards to communicate (Fig. 7-6, p. 76).
- Be alert for signs that the person does not understand. A confused or concerned look is an example. Or the person may pretend to understand. Nodding and answering "yes" to all questions may signal that the person does not understand.
- Repeat the message as often as needed. Say the message in another way if needed.

When health care staff cannot speak the person's language, a translator (interpreter) is used. If used, speak as if speaking to the person, not the translator. Digital translators (electronic language translators) offer another means of communication.

Modified from Giger JN, Haddad L: Transcultural nursing: assessment and intervention, *ed 8, St Louis, 2021, Elsevier.*

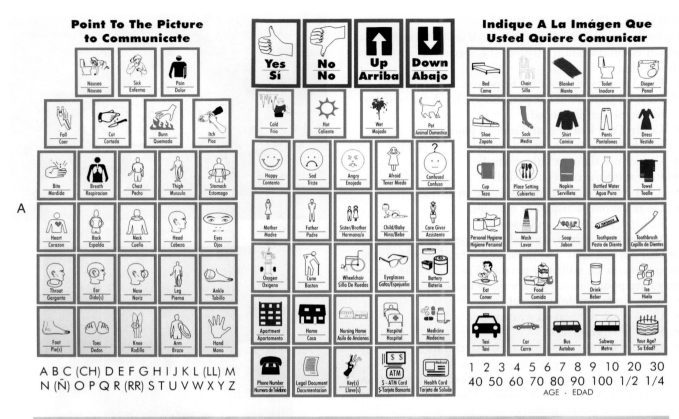

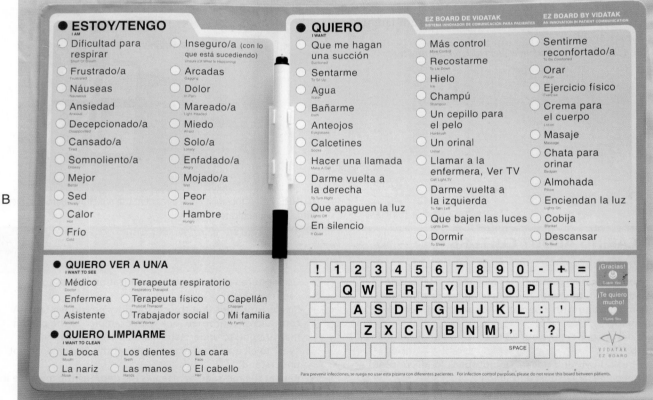

FIGURE 7-6 A, Picture board in English and Spanish. **B,** Communication board in Spanish.

Nonverbal Communication

Nonverbal communication does not use words. Gestures, facial expressions, posture, body movements, touch, and smell are used. Nonverbal messages more accurately reflect a person's feelings than words do. They are usually involuntary and hard to control. A person may say one thing but act another way. Watch the person's eyes, hand movements, gestures, posture, and other actions. They may tell you more than words.

Touch. Touch is an important form of nonverbal communication. It conveys comfort, caring, love, affection, interest, trust, concern, and reassurance. Touch means different things to different people. The meaning depends on age, gender, experiences, and culture.

Some people do not like being touched. However, touching an arm or shoulder or holding a hand can comfort a person. Touch should be gentle—not hurried, rough, or sexual. To use touch, follow the person's care plan. Remember to maintain professional boundaries.

See *Caring About Culture: Touch.*

See *Focus on Children and Older Persons: Touch.*

Many messages are sent through body language. Slumped posture may mean the person is not happy or not feeling well. A person may deny pain but stand, sit, or lie in a certain way to protect a body part.

Your actions, movements, and facial expressions send messages. Your body language should show interest, caring, respect, and enthusiasm.

Often you will need to control your body language. Control reactions to odors from body fluids or the person's body. The person cannot control some odors. Embarrassment increases if you react to odors.

See *Caring About Culture: Body Language.*

❀ CARING ABOUT CULTURE

Touch

Touch practices vary among cultural groups. The following are examples.

- For *Americans,* hugs are common among family and friends. A pat on the shoulder is often a gesture of friendship. A firm handshake can show good character and be a sign of strength.
- In some *American Indian* groups a firm, lengthy handshake may be seen as aggressive and offend the person. Instead, there is a light touch, grasp, or just the passing of hands.
- In the *East Indian Hindu* culture, showing public affection is usually considered disrespectful. A common greeting is to bow with clasped hands and say the word *namaste* ("I bow to thee").
- In *Japanese* culture, touch is often minimal, especially among adults. Likewise, in *Chinese* culture, people do not usually touch each other while speaking. Touching a person's head is very rude.
- Touch is often used in *Mexican* cultures. A hug or hand-holding while walking is common among close friends.

  Note: *Each person is unique. A person may not follow all of the beliefs and practices of his or her culture. Follow the care plan.*

Modified from Giger JN, Haddad L: Transcultural nursing: assessment and intervention, ed 8, St Louis, 2021, Elsevier.

FOCUS ON **CHILDREN AND OLDER PERSONS**

Touch

Children

Touch soothes and comforts infants and young children. They like to be held, stroked, rocked, patted, and cuddled. Older children and teenagers like to give and receive hugs.

Contact must be professional, casual, and with consent. It must not be sexual or involve sexual areas.

Body Language. With *body language*, messages are sent through facial expressions, gestures, posture, hand and body movements, gait, eye contact, and appearance. Appearance includes clothing, hygiene, jewelry, perfume, cosmetics, body art and piercings, and so on.

❀ CARING ABOUT CULTURE

Body Language

Facial Expressions

Through facial expressions, *Americans* may communicate:

- *Coldness*—there is a constant stare. Face muscles do not move.
- *Fear*—eyes are wide open. Eyebrows are raised. The mouth is tense with the lips drawn back.
- *Anger*—eyes are fixed in a hard stare. Upper lids are lowered. Eyebrows are drawn down. Lips are tightly compressed.
- *Tiredness*—eyes are rolled upward.
- *Disapproval*—eyes are rolled upward.
- *Disgust*—eyes are narrowed. The upper lip is curled. There are nose movements.
- *Embarrassment*—eyes are turned away or down. The face is flushed. Pretending to smile; rubbing the eyes, nose, or face; or touching the hair, beard, or mustache are common.
- *Surprise*—the person has a direct gaze with raised eyebrows.

  Italian, Jewish, African American, and *Hispanic* persons are known to smile readily. They may use many facial expressions and gestures for happiness, pain, or displeasure. *Irish, English,* and *Northern European* persons tend to have less facial expression.

  In some cultures, facial expressions mean the opposite of what the person feels. For example, *Asians* may conceal negative emotions with a smile.

Eye Contact

In the *American* culture, eye contact usually signals a good self-concept. It also shows openness, interest in others, attention, honesty, and warmth. Lack of eye contact can have different meanings—shyness, lack of interest, humility, guilt, embarrassment, low self-esteem, rudeness, dishonesty.

For some *Asian* and *American Indian* cultures, eye contact is impolite. It is an invasion of privacy. In certain *Indian* cultures, eye contact is avoided with persons of higher or lower socio-economic class. Long, direct eye contact may be avoided in *African American* cultures.

  Note: *Each person is unique. A person may not follow all of the beliefs and practices of his or her culture. Follow the care plan.*

Modified from Giger JN: Transcultural nursing: assessment and intervention, ed 8, St Louis, 2021, Elsevier.

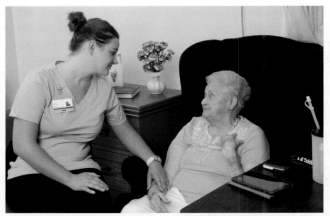

FIGURE 7-7 This nursing assistant faces the person, leans forward, and uses eye contact and touch while listening.

Communication Methods

Certain methods help you communicate with others. They result in better relationships. More information is gained about the person.

Listening. Listening (active listening) means to focus on verbal and nonverbal communication. You use sight, hearing, touch, and smell. You focus on what the person is saying. You observe nonverbal clues. They can support or not support what the person says. For example, a person says: "I want to stay here so my family won't have to care for me." You see tears. The person looks away from you. The person's verbal says *happy*; nonverbal shows *sadness*.

Listening requires that you care and have interest. Follow these guidelines.

- Face the person (Fig. 7-7).
- Look at the person. Make eye contact as appropriate. (Consider the cultural meanings of eye contact.)
- Lean toward the person. Do not sit back with your arms crossed.
- Respond to the person. Nod your head. Say: "Uh huh," "mmm," and "I see." Ask questions. Repeat what you heard. See "Paraphrasing."
- Avoid communication barriers. See "Communication Barriers."

See *Caring About Culture: Listening*.

> ### 🌸 CARING ABOUT CULTURE
> #### Listening
> Communicating respect is important in all cultural groups. This can be shown in how you listen. Giving the person your attention and showing kindness and interest communicate respect. In some cultures, eye contact communicates listening. In others, the listener turns an ear to listen.
>
> *Modified from Giger JN, Haddad L: Transcultural nursing: assessment and intervention, ed 8, St Louis, 2021, Elsevier.*

Paraphrasing. *Paraphrasing* is re-stating the person's message in your own words. You use fewer words than the person did. Paraphrasing:

- Shows you are listening.
- Lets the person see if you understand the message.
- Promotes more communication.

The person usually responds to your statement. For example:

Mrs. Hayes: I grew up on a farm. I never liked having to get up so early in the morning. The days were long and tiring.
You: You like to sleep in?
Mrs. Hayes: Yes, I would much rather stay up later and sleep until the sun rises.

Direct Questions. Direct questions focus on certain information. You ask what you need to know. Some direct questions have "yes" or "no" answers. Others require more information. For example:

You: Mr. Walker, do you want to shower this morning?
Mr. Walker: Yes.
You: Mr. Walker, when would you like to do that?
Mr. Walker: Could we start in 15 minutes? I want to call my son first.
You: Yes, we can start in 15 minutes. You said you didn't eat much breakfast. What did you eat?
Mr. Walker: I had toast and coffee. I didn't feel like eating.

Open-Ended Questions and Statements. Open-ended questions and statements lead or invite the person to share thoughts, feelings, or ideas. The topic is broad. The person controls the information given. Answers require more than a "yes" or "no." For example:

- "What do you like about living with your son?"
- "Tell me about your grandchildren."
- "What do you like about being retired?"

Clarifying. Clarifying helps you understand the message. You can ask the person to repeat the message, say you do not understand, or re-state the message. For example:
- "Could you say that again?"
- "I'm sorry. I don't understand what you mean."
- "Are you saying that you want to go home?"

Focusing. Focusing deals with a certain topic. It is useful when a person rambles or wanders in thought. For example, a person talks at length about places to eat. You need to know why the person did not eat much breakfast. To focus on breakfast you say: "Let's talk about breakfast. You said you didn't feel like eating."

Silence. Silence is a powerful way to communicate. Sometimes you do not need to say anything. This is true during sad times. Just being there shows you care.

At other times, silence gives time to think, organize thoughts, or choose words. It also helps when the person is upset and needs to gain control. Silence on your part shows caring and respect for the person's situation and feelings.

Pauses or long silences may seem uncomfortable. You do not need to talk when the person is silent. The person may need silence.

Communication Barriers

Communication barriers prevent the sending and receiving of messages. Communication fails.
- *Unfamiliar language.* You and the person may speak different languages. Or you use words the person does not understand. Slang, medical terms, and abbreviations are examples.
- *Cultural differences.* The person may attach different meanings to verbal and nonverbal communication.
- *Changing the subject.* Someone changes the subject when the topic is uncomfortable.
- *Giving your opinion.* Opinions involve judging values, behaviors, or feelings. Let others express feelings and concerns without adding your opinion. Do not make judgments or jump to conclusions.
- *Talking a lot when others are silent.* Talking too much is usually because of nervousness and discomfort with silence.
- *Failure to listen.* Do not pretend to listen. It shows lack of interest and caring. This causes poor responses. You miss important information or symptoms to report to the nurse.
- *Pat answers.* "Don't worry." "Everything will be okay." "Your doctor knows best." These show a lack of caring about the person's concerns, feelings, and fears.
- *Illness and disability.* Speech, hearing, vision, cognitive function, and body movements are often affected. Verbal and nonverbal communication is affected.
- *Age.* Values and communication styles vary among age-groups.
See *Focus on Communication: Communication Barriers.*

FOCUS ON COMMUNICATION

Communication Barriers

Some persons who need a translator may normally have a family member translate. However, in health care settings, the nurse may prefer to use a translator from the agency. Trained translators know medical terms. Family or friends may state something other than what was meant. Receiving wrong information is a risk.

Having family or friends translate also violates the right to privacy. The *Health Insurance Portability and Accountability Act of 1996 (HIPAA)* protects the right to privacy and security of a person's health information (Chapter 5). Privacy is protected when using the agency's translator.

The *Patient Protection and Affordable Care Act of 2010* requires health care agencies to provide access to language assistance services. Qualified interpreters and written information in other languages are examples.

BEHAVIOR

Behaviors communicate needs. Understanding some of the causes of the following behaviors can help you give better care.

- *Anger.* Causes include fear, pain, and dying and death. Loss of function and loss of control over health and life are causes. Anger is a symptom of some diseases that affect thinking and behavior. Verbal outbursts, shouting, raised voices, and rapid speech are common. Some people are silent. Others are not cooperative. Nonverbal signs include rapid movements, pacing, clenched fists, and a red face. Glaring and getting close to you when speaking are other signs. Violent behaviors can occur.
- *Demanding and self-centered behavior.* Nothing seems to please the person. The person is impatient, critical, and wants care at a certain time and in a certain way. The person thinks others' needs are less important. The person expects time and attention from others. Loss of independence, loss of health, and loss of control of life are causes. So are unmet needs.
- *Aggressive behavior.* The person may swear, bite, hit, pinch, scratch, or kick. Fear, anger, pain, and dementia are causes. Protect the person, others, and yourself from harm (Chapter 14).
- *Withdrawal.* There is little or no contact with others. The person spends time alone and does not take part in social or group events. This may signal physical illness or depression. Some people are not social. They prefer to be alone.
- *Inappropriate sexual behavior.* Some people make inappropriate sexual remarks. Or they touch others in the wrong way. Some undress or masturbate in public. These behaviors may be on purpose. Or they are caused by disease, confusion, dementia, or drug side effects.

Such behaviors can be difficult to manage. You cannot avoid the person or lose control. You cannot punish the person. Good communication is needed. Behaviors are addressed in the care plan. The care plan may include some of the guidelines in Box 7-4.

See *Focus on Communication: Behavior.*
See *Focus on Children and Older Persons: Behavior.*
See *Teamwork and Time Management: Behavior.*

FOCUS ON COMMUNICATION

Behavior

Anger is a common response to illness and disability. The person may be angry with the situation. You might have problems dealing with anger directed at you. Act professionally. Stay calm. Listen to the person's concerns. Give needed care. Try not to take angry statements personally. If a person says hurtful things, you can kindly say: "Please don't say those things. I'm trying to help you." Tell the nurse about the person's behavior.

Caring for demanding or angry persons can be hard. Ask the nurse or co-workers to help if needed.

FOCUS ON CHILDREN AND OLDER PERSONS

Behavior

Older Persons

Changes in the brain with Alzheimer's disease and other forms of dementia can affect communication and judgment. Unable to communicate needs as usual, the brain uses other methods. *Caregivers and staff must remember that behaviors communicate needs.* For example, a person is hot. Instead of saying "I am hot," the person begins taking off clothes in the dining room. You will learn about behavior changes and how to provide for the person's needs in Chapter 54.

TEAMWORK AND TIME MANAGEMENT

Behavior

Persons showing demanding behavior can take a lot of time. A simple task, such as filling a water mug, can take several minutes. The mug may be too full or not full enough. The water may be too warm or too cold. Or the person may have a list of other care needs.

Learn to recognize these situations. Offer to help co-workers with the person or other tasks. Hopefully they also will help you.

BOX 7-4	Managing Difficult Behavior

- Recognize frustrating and frightening situations. Put yourself in the person's situation. How would you feel? How would you want to be treated?
- Treat the person with dignity and respect.
- Answer questions clearly and thoroughly. Ask the nurse to answer questions you cannot answer.
- Keep the person informed. Tell the person what you are going to do and when.
- Anticipate (expect) needs.
- Do not keep the person waiting. Answer call lights promptly. If you tell the person that you will do something, do it promptly.

- Explain the reason for long waits. Ask if you can get or do something to increase the person's comfort.
- Stay calm and professional, especially if the person is angry or hostile. Do not take the person's negative comments personally. Often the person is angry at another person or situation, not at you.
- Do not argue with the person.
- Listen and use silence. The person may feel better if able to express his or her feelings.
- Protect yourself from violent behaviors (Chapter 14).
- Report the person's behavior to the nurse. Discuss how to help the person.

FAMILY

The person's family often includes individuals related by birth, marriage, or adoption. Family may also include persons who share a deep feeling of closeness and connection without being related. Some persons consider friends or neighbors as family when the person lacks living relatives or connection with relatives.

Family structures vary (Chapter 11). The nurse asks questions in order to understand the person's family and the effect on health care needs. For example:

- Who lives with you?
- Who do you consider to be your family?
- Do you feel safe at home?
- What is your role in the family?
- Who makes decisions?
- Do you have someone who helps you understand your health care? If yes, who?
- Do you want your family involved in your care? If yes, how?

The presence or absence of family affects the person's quality of life. Relationships are stronger among some families than others. A supportive family:

- Helps meet safety, security, love, and belonging needs.
- Provides comfort, help, and encouragement.
- Relieves loneliness.
- Helps with difficult decisions while respecting the person's independence.
- Acts as caregivers as the need arises.

Nursing assistants commonly have contact with members of the person's family. See Box 7-5 for ways to promote positive interactions with family.

See *Focus on Long-Term Care and Home Care: Family*.

FOCUS ON LONG-TERM CARE AND HOME CARE

Family

Home Care

Family personalities and attitudes affect the mood in the home. Families may have good or poor relationships. Mental or physical illness, substance use disorder, unemployment, and delinquency (illegal conduct) may affect the family. Some families have problems coping with or accepting the person's illness or disability.

Your supervisor explains family problems to you. Do not get involved. Be professional and have empathy. Do not give advice, take sides, or make judgments about family conflicts. Maintain professional boundaries at all times.

BOX 7-5	Interacting With the Person's Family

- Learn the names of the person's family members. Greet them by their preferred names.
- Be welcoming.
- Show kindness and respect.
- Use effective communication (p. 74).
- Provide privacy and a clean, comfortable setting for visits. See "Visitors."
- Learn family routines and preferences. Be attentive to their needs as you are able.
- Encourage the family's support and involvement in care (if the person consents).
- Show empathy when the family expresses emotion—sadness, anger, fear. When you show *empathy*, you relate to what the person feels without pitying the person.
- Avoid getting involved in family affairs.
- Listen to complaints with patience and understanding. Tell the person that you will follow-up with the nurse. Follow-up promptly. Never say you will do something and not do it.
- Refer questions about care to the nurse.

Visitors

The person has the right to visit with family or friends in private and without unneeded interruptions. You may need to give care when visitors are there. Protect the right to privacy. Do not expose the person's body in front of others. Politely ask them to leave the room. Show them where to wait. Tell them how much time you need. Promptly tell them when they can return. A partner or family member may want to help you. If the patient or resident consents (gives permission), you can let the person stay.

Treat visitors with courtesy and respect. They have concerns about the person's condition and care. They need support and understanding. However, do not discuss the person's condition with them. Refer their questions to the nurse.

Visiting rules depend on agency policy and the person's condition. Parents can usually visit with children whenever they want. Dying persons usually can have family present all the time. Know your agency's visiting policies and what is allowed for the person.

Visitors may have questions about the chapel, gift shop, lounge, or cafeteria. Know the location, special rules, and hours of these areas.

A visitor may upset or tire a person. Report your observations to the nurse. The nurse will speak with the visitor about the person's needs.

FOCUS ON PRIDE

The Person, Family, and Yourself

Personal and Professional Responsibility

Improving communication is on-going. You may be uncomfortable interacting with the person or family at first. To develop communication skills:

- Use methods such as listening and clarifying.
- Pay attention to the nonverbal messages you send.
- Avoid communication barriers.
- Learn from your mistakes.

With practice, you will communicate more effectively. This is a valuable skill.

Rights and Respect

Some persons seem demanding and self-centered when needs are not met properly. When needs are met, they can be grateful and kind. Ask about the person's preferences. Say that you want to do the task the way the person wants it done. Listen and follow the person's preferences as much as is safely possible.

Showing respect can develop rapport. *Rapport* means you have a trusting relationship. You communicate well and have positive interactions. This can lessen or stop demanding and self-centered behaviors.

Independence and Social Interaction

Normal, daily activities bring pleasure, worth, and contact with others. With illness and disability, such activities may be hard or impossible. The person may feel angry and useless when help is needed with routine functions. The need for hospital or long-term care can bring feelings of isolation and loneliness. Self-esteem is affected.

To provide a sense of identity, worth, and belonging:

- Greet the person by name. Smile and show that you are happy to see the person.
- Talk to the person while giving care.
- Take an extra minute to talk or just listen.
- Encourage as much independence as possible. This often takes more time. Plan and be patient. Encouragement and independence improve self-esteem.
- Focus on the person's abilities, not the disabilities.
- Allow private time with visitors.

Delegation and Teamwork

Your co-workers are valuable resources. If you have questions or need advice, ask. For example, a resident shows anger when told it is time to shower. You ask the nurse if the task is difficult for other nursing assistants. The nurse shares advice about timing of the shower, words to say and avoid, and distraction techniques. You try, and the person is calmer.

Value your co-workers. Thank them for helpful advice.

Ethics and Laws

You will care for persons with different ideas, values, and life-styles. These shape the person's character and identity. Each person is unique and has value. Do not insult the person or force your views or beliefs on the person. Respect the person as a whole.

FOCUS ON PRIDE: Application

Imagine yourself as a patient or resident. What would you want the staff to know about you? Ask 1 or 2 others what would be important to them. How does understanding the person help you give better care?

REVIEW QUESTIONS

Circle the BEST answer.

1 You apply holism when you focus on
  a What the family thinks the person needs
  b What you think the person needs
  c The person's physical, psychological, social, and spiritual needs
  d The person's health care problems

2 Which basic need is the *most* essential?
  a The need to feel safe
  b The need to feel valued
  c The need for affection
  d The need for food

3 A person says: "I'm falling!" Which needs are *most* important at the time?
  a Self-actualization needs
  b Safety and security needs
  c Love and belonging needs
  d Self-esteem needs

4 A person has a garden behind the nursing center. This relates to
  a Self-actualization
  b Physical needs
  c Love and belonging
  d Safety and security

5 A patient is talking about her culture. You should
a Listen with interest
b Change the subject
c Give your opinion
d Pretend to listen

6 Which statement about spirituality is *correct*?
a You can ignore a person's spiritual needs.
b Everyone practices a religion.
c People discover and live out spirituality in different ways.
d You should argue with the person about spiritual beliefs.

7 When addressing a person
a Use "dear" or "honey" if you forget the person's name
b Say "it" if you do not know which pronoun to use
c Do not greet the person by title
d Use the name the person prefers

8 A person has risk factors for illness. The nurse teaches about risk factors to
a Help the person form healthy practices
b Control the person's decisions
c Show that the person has been making bad choices
d Earn the person's trust

9 Which description is *correct*?
a Obstetrics focuses on the treatment of obesity.
b Geriatrics focuses on the care of older persons.
c Pediatrics focuses on the treatment of mental health disorders.
d Psychiatry focuses on the care of sick children.

10 A person uses a wheelchair. You should
a Lean on the wheelchair
b Pat the person on the head
c Direct questions to the companion
d Sit or squat next to the person

11 A person is comatose. You should
a Assume that the person cannot hear
b Explain what you are going to do
c Listen and use silence to communicate
d Enter the room without knocking

12 Which statement about communication is *correct*?
a Nonverbal communication uses the written or spoken word.
b Verbal communication is the truest reflection of a person's feelings.
c Body language cannot be controlled.
d Eye contact communicates different things to different people.

13 When talking with the person, you should
a Repeat information as needed
b Use slang
c Use medical words and phrases
d Shout

14 You touch a person on the forearm and smile. Which response shows the touch was received well?
a The person pulls the arm away.
b The person moves your hand off of the arm.
c The person pats your hand and smiles back.
d The person says "ouch" and grabs the arm.

15 Which shows that you are listening?
a You stand with your arms crossed.
b You sit and face the person.
c You avoid asking questions.
d You change the subject.

16 Which is an open-ended question?
a "What hobbies do you enjoy?"
b "Do you want to wear your red sweater?"
c "Would you like eggs and toast for breakfast?"
d "Do you want to sit in your chair?"

17 You ask: "What name do you prefer?" This is
a A communication barrier
b A direct question
c Paraphrasing
d An open-ended question

18 Which statement promotes communication?
a "Don't worry."
b "Everything will be fine."
c "In my opinion, you shouldn't do it."
d "Go ahead. I'm listening."

19 Which is a barrier to communication?
a Focusing
b Asking questions
c Talking a lot when others are silent
d Using familiar language

20 A person wants care given at a certain time and in a certain way. Nothing seems to please the person. Which response is *best*?
a "Please stop being so picky."
b "I don't have time for this."
c "Please tell me what you would like done."
d "You are never happy with what I do."

21 A person is angry. You should
a Put yourself in the person's situation
b Ignore the behavior
c Ask the person to be nicer
d Avoid the person

22 Which statement about family is *correct*?
a Friends and neighbors cannot be considered family.
b Family does not affect the person's quality of life.
c Family helps meet love and belonging needs.
d Family is limited to who lives with the person.

23 Which shows you understand the importance of the person's family?
a You avoid contact with them.
b You leave the room messy before a visit.
c You complain about them to co-workers.
d You are welcoming.

24 A visitor seems to tire a person. What should you do?
a Ask the person to leave.
b Tell the nurse.
c Stay in the room to observe the person and visitor.
d Find out the visitor's relationship to the person.

Answers to Chapter 7 questions are on p. 901.

FOCUS ON PRACTICE

Problem Solving

A resident was admitted to your nursing center 2 weeks ago. The resident is withdrawn, impatient, and angry toward the staff. Explain possible reasons for the behaviors. How will you manage the behaviors and provide quality care?

Health Team Communications

- Define the key terms and key abbreviations in this chapter.
- Explain why health team members need to communicate.
- Describe the rules for good communication.
- Explain the purpose, parts, and information found in the medical record.
- Describe the legal and ethical aspects of medical records.
- Describe the 5 steps in the nursing process.
- Explain your role in the nursing process.
- Explain the difference between objective and subjective data (signs and symptoms).

- List the observations and information you need to report to the nurse.
- List the rules for recording.
- Explain how electronic devices are used in health care.
- Explain how to protect the right to privacy when using electronic devices.
- Describe how to answer phones.
- Use the 24-hour clock.
- Explain how to promote PRIDE in the person, the family, and yourself.

KEY TERMS

analysis Interpreting data and identifying problems; see "nursing process"

assessment Collecting information about the person; see "nursing process"

care plan See "nursing care plan"

chart See "medical record"

electronic health record (EHR) An electronic version of a person's medical record; electronic medical record

electronic medical record (EMR) See "electronic health record"

end-of-shift report A report that the nurse gives at the end of the shift to the on-coming shift; change-of-shift report

evaluation To measure if goals in the planning step were met; see "nursing process"

implementation To carry out nursing interventions in the care plan; see "nursing process"

medical record The legal account of a person's condition and response to treatment and care; chart

nursing care plan A written guide about the person's nursing care; care plan

nursing intervention An action or measure taken by the nursing team to help the person reach a goal; nursing action, nursing measure, nursing task

nursing process The method nurses use to plan and deliver nursing care; it includes assessment, analysis, planning, implementation, and evaluation

objective data Information that is seen, heard, felt, or smelled by an observer; signs

observation Using the senses of sight, hearing, touch, and smell to collect information

planning Setting priorities and goals; see "nursing process"

progress note Describes the care given and the person's response and progress

recording The written account of care and observations; charting, documentation

reporting The oral account of care and observations

signs See "objective data"

subjective data Things a person tells you about that you cannot observe through your senses; symptoms

symptoms See "subjective data"

KEY ABBREVIATIONS

ADL	Activities of daily living	EMR	Electronic medical record
BM	Bowel movement	EPHI; ePHI	Electronic protected health information
CAA	Care Area Assessment	MDS	Minimum Data Set
CMS	Centers for Medicare & Medicaid Services	OASIS	Outcome and Assessment Information Set
EHR	Electronic health record	PHI	Protected health information

Communication is needed for coordinated and effective care. Health team members share information about:

- What was done for the person
- What needs to be done for the person
- The person's response to treatment

For example, a patient needs comfort measures. The nurse plans to give a pain-relief drug and asks you to position the person. The nurse explains the plan to you and the patient. The nurse tells you when the drug is given and evaluates the person's response. You position the person. The nurse records about pain. You report and record the care you gave. The nurse reports observations and care to the next nurse on duty.

Communication and care were coordinated. The person knew what to expect. Care was reported and recorded so team members know what was done.

You need to practice the aspects and rules of communication. Then you can communicate effectively with the nursing and health teams. For good communication, see Box 8-1.

BOX 8-1	**Communication Rules**

- Use words that have the same meaning for you and the message receiver. Avoid words with more than 1 meaning. Does "far" mean 50 feet or 100 feet?
- Ask about messages you do not understand. You will learn medical terms (Chapter 9). If you do not know a term, ask what it means. Or use a dictionary. You must understand the message for communication to occur.
- Be brief and concise. Do not add unrelated or unnecessary information. Stay on the subject. Do not wander in thought or get wordy.
- Give information in a logical and orderly way. Organize your thoughts. Present them step-by-step.
- Give facts and be specific. Reporting a pulse rate of 110 is more specific than "the pulse is fast."

THE MEDICAL RECORD

The *medical record (chart)* is the legal account of a person's condition and response to treatment and care. Medical records are written on paper forms or electronically with computers or other electronic devices. An *electronic health record (EHR)* or *electronic medical record (EMR)* is an electronic version of a person's medical record. Most agencies use EHRs (EMRs) (Fig. 8-1).

The health team uses the medical record to communicate information about the person. The record is a permanent legal document. Often it is used months or years later if the person's health history is needed. It can be used in court as legal evidence of the person's problems, treatment, and care.

Government and accrediting agencies review medical records to see if license, certification, or accrediting standards have been met. The record is also used to determine the amount paid for services (Chapter 1).

The record has different parts (Table 8-1, p. 86). Each part has the person's name, identification (ID) number, room and bed number, and other identifying information. The record tells about care provided and the person's response.

See *Focus on Long-Term Care and Home Care: The Medical Record*, p. 87.

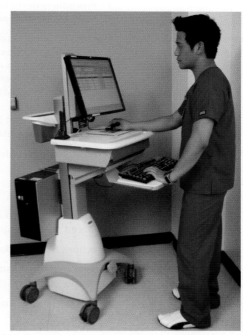

FIGURE 8-1 A nursing assistant uses an electronic health record (electronic medical record).

TABLE 8-1	Parts of a Medical Record
Part	**Description**
Admission record	Completed on admission (entry) into the agency. Contains personal and identifying information—legal name, birth date, age, biological sex (male or female), address, insurance information, marital status, nearest relative and legal representative, religion, place of worship, employer, diagnoses, date and time of admission, doctor's name. A signed general consent for treatment is included.
Advance directives	A document stating a person's wishes about end-of-life care (Chapter 59).
Health history	A record of the person's medical history. • Chief complaint—reason for seeking health care • History of current illness—onset (time, sudden or gradual) and signs and symptoms • Past health problems, surgeries, and injuries • Childhood illnesses • Allergies and type of reaction • Current drugs • Vaccinations • Family health history • Life-style—habits, diet, sleep, hobbies • Adaptive (assistive) devices used—dentures, eyeglasses, contact lenses, hearing aids, cane, walker, wheelchair, and so on • Ability to perform *activities of daily living (ADL)*—the activities usually done during a normal day in a person's life • Education and occupation
Nursing assessment	Data collected during the nurse's physical assessment (p. 89).
Nursing care plan; care plan	A guide about the person's nursing care (p. 91).
Nursing progress notes	*Progress notes* describe the care given and the person's response and progress (Fig. 8-2). For example, the nurse records: • Signs and symptoms • Information about treatments and drugs • Information about teaching and counseling • Procedures performed • Visits by health team members
Flow sheets and graphic sheets	Used for frequent care measures, measurements, and observations (Fig. 8-3). • Hygiene and grooming measures • Activity and positioning • Vital signs—temperature, pulse, respirations, blood pressure, and pulse oximetry (Chapters 34 and 44) • Weight • Intake and output (Chapter 32) • Urinary and bowel elimination
Medication administration record (MAR); electronic medication administration record (eMAR)	A record of drugs ordered, given, and not taken.
Physical examination	Information collected during the physical examination. The examination is done by a doctor, advanced practice registered nurse (APRN), or physician's assistant (PA).
Orders	Directions from the doctor, APRN, or PA about tests and care measures to be performed.
Progress notes (health team)	Reports from the health team—medical (doctor, APRN, PA); physical, occupational, speech-language, and recreational therapies; dietary; social services; and others.
Laboratory results	Results of tests done on blood, urine, and other body fluids and tissues.
X-ray reports	Results of x-ray tests.
Therapy records	Records for intravenous (IV), respiratory, wound care, and other therapies.
Consultation reports	Reports from other health care providers consulted by the person's doctor.
Special consents	Signed permissions for surgeries and procedures needing informed consent (Chapter 5).
Discharge summary	Information and instructions for the person when leaving the agency—wound care; drug prescriptions and changes; rest, activity, and exercise; diet; signs and symptoms to report; follow-up appointments.

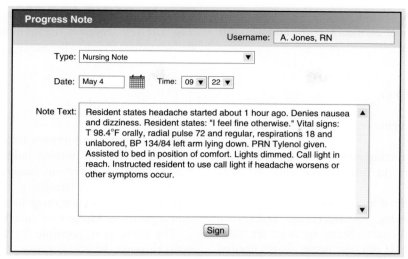

FIGURE 8-2 A sample progress note.

		06/16 12:00	06/16 13:00	06/16 13:10	06/16 13:20	06/16 15:00	06/16 15:10	06/16 15:15			
Vital Signs	Temperature	98.4									
	Pulse	72									
	Respiration	18									
	Blood Pressure	118/76									
	O2SAT	99									
	O2 L/M										
Intake/Output	P.O. ORAL	240									
	New Intake										
	VOIDED URINE			250			200				
	New Output										
	NUTRITION:	SELF									
	ELIMINATION:			TOILET			TOILET				
Activity	ACTIVITY:	CHAIR	CHAIR	BATH	BED	AMBUL	BATH	BED			
	POSITIONING:	SELF			BACK			RIGHT			
	HYGIENE:		ORAL	PERI			PERI				
Safety	SAFETY:	CALL	CALL	BELT	CALL	BELT	BELT	CALL			

Ready   Interface CHART MENU   Reflex Completed Room: 274-1 Exit

FIGURE 8-3 A sample flow sheet. (Courtesy Abraham Lincoln Memorial Hospital, Lincoln, Ill.)

FOCUS ON LONG-TERM CARE AND HOME CARE
The Medical Record

Long-Term Care
The Centers for Medicare & Medicaid Services (CMS) requires that nursing center medical records communicate each resident's condition and progress toward meeting care plan goals. (See "Planning" on p. 91.) The record must include the resident's condition, plan of care, care provided, response to treatment, and any changes in condition.

Home Care
A weekly record has sections for each day and for care activities. There are sections for personal care, activity, measurements, nutrition, household services, and procedures. You record on the day care was given.

Legal and Ethical Aspects

Agencies have policies about medical records and who can see them. Policies address:

- Who records
- When to record
- Ink color (paper charting)
- Abbreviations
- How to make and sign entries
- How to correct errors

Some agencies allow nursing assistants to record observations and care. Others do not. Follow your agency's policies.

Professional staff involved in a person's care can review charts. Cooks and laundry, housekeeping, and office staff do not need to read charts. Some agencies let nursing assistants read charts. If not, the nurse shares needed information.

You have an ethical and legal duty to keep information confidential. If not involved in the person's care, you have no right to read the person's chart. Doing so is an invasion of privacy.

Patients and residents have the right to the information in their medical records. The person or the person's legal representative may ask to see the chart. Tell the nurse. The nurse handles the request.

CARE SUMMARIES

Some agencies use a care summary to summarize information in the medical record—drugs, treatments, diagnoses, routine care measures, equipment, and special needs. Sometimes called a *Kardex*, the summary is a quick, easy source of information about the person. It may be electronic or on paper as a card file. Some types are not part of the permanent medical record.

THE NURSING PROCESS

The *nursing process* is the method nurses use to plan and deliver nursing care. The nursing process includes:

- Assessment
- Analysis
- Planning
- Implementation
- Evaluation

Nurses gather and process information about a person's care needs and use nursing judgment to make decisions. Nurses plan and carry out measures to meet the person's needs. Then they determine if the outcome is what was expected. The process is on-going (Fig. 8-4). New information is gathered. The person's needs may change at any time.

The nurse is responsible for the nursing process. You assist through the observations you make and the care you give.

See *Focus on Communication: The Nursing Process.*

FOCUS ON COMMUNICATION

The Nursing Process

The person and nursing team need good communication. With good communication, nursing care is organized and has purpose. All nursing team members do the same things for the person. They focus on the same goals for the person.

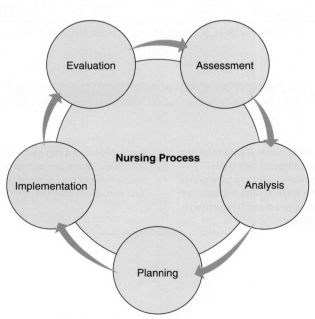

FIGURE 8-4 The nursing process is continuous.

Assessment

Assessment involves collecting information about the person. The nurse takes a health history about current and past health problems. The family's health history is important. Information from the doctor is reviewed. So are test results and past medical records.

The nurse assesses the person's body systems and mental status. You assist with assessment. You make observations as you give care and talk to the person.

Observation is using the senses of sight, hearing, touch, and smell to collect information.

- You *see* how the person lies, sits, or walks. You see flushed or pale skin. You see red and swollen body areas.
- You *listen* to the person breathe, talk, and cough. You use a stethoscope to measure blood pressure.
- Through *touch*, you feel if the skin is hot or cold, or moist or dry. You use touch to take a pulse.
- *Smell* is used to detect body, wound, and breath odors. You also smell odors from urine and bowel movements (BMs).

The word *data* relates to information that is collected and used for decision making. *Objective data (signs)* are seen, heard, felt, or smelled by an observer. You can feel a pulse. You can see urine color. *Subjective data (symptoms)* are things a person tells you about that you cannot observe through your senses. You cannot feel or see the person's pain, fear, or nausea.

Box 8-2 lists observations to report at once (right away). You will also learn about signs and symptoms of conditions that require emergency care in Chapter 58. Box 8-3 (p. 90) lists the basic observations to make and report to the nurse. Note observations as you make them. Use your notes when reporting to the nurse (p. 95).

You do not assess. The nurse performs the assessment step of the nursing process. However, what you observe helps the nurse with assessment.

See *Focus on Communication: Assessment.*

See *Focus on Long-Term Care and Home Care: Assessment.*

FOCUS ON **COMMUNICATION**

Assessment

The phrases "complains of" and "complaints of" are not intended to label the person as a complainer. The intent is to communicate abnormal symptoms (things the person must tell you about). The health team may understand this intent, but the person may not. The following are examples of other ways to communicate abnormal symptoms.

- Instead of saying "Mr. West complains of fatigue," use the person's exact words. You say: "Mr. West said, 'I get tired walking from my chair to the bathroom.'"
- Instead of writing in the medical record "Ms. Snow complained of nausea," you say she reported the feeling. You write: "Ms. Snow reported nausea."

BOX 8-2	Observations to Report at Once

- A change in the person's ability to respond
  - A responsive person no longer responds.
  - A non-responsive person now responds.
- A change in the person's mobility
  - The person cannot move a body part.
  - The person can now move a body part.
- A new or worsening area of weakness or numbness
- Facial changes—drooping eyelid, uneven smile, drooling
- Sudden onset of confusion (Chapter 54)
- Complaints of sudden, severe pain
- A sore or reddened area on the skin
- Complaints of a sudden change in vision
- Complaints of painful or difficult breathing
- Abnormal respirations (Chapter 44)
- Complaints of or signs of difficulty swallowing (Chapter 31)
- Vomiting
- Bleeding
- Dizziness
- Vital signs above or below normal ranges—temperature, pulse, respirations, blood pressure, and pulse oximetry (Chapters 34 and 44)

FOCUS ON **LONG-TERM CARE AND HOME CARE**

Assessment

Long-Term Care

The CMS requires the *Minimum Data Set (MDS)* for nursing center residents (Appendix B, p. 906). The MDS is an assessment tool. It is used to gather information about the person. Examples include memory, communication, hearing and vision, physical function, and activities.

The MDS is started when the person is admitted to the center. A new MDS is done once a year and for a significant change (decline or improvement) in the person's health status. Quarterly assessments (every 3 months) are also required.

Home Care

Medicare-certified home health agencies use the *Outcome and Assessment Information Set (OASIS)*. It is used for adult home care patients. Besides assessment, OASIS is used for planning care.

BOX 8-3	Basic Observations

Ability to Respond
- Is the person easy or hard to wake up?
- Can the person give his or her name, the time, and location when asked?
- Does the person identify others correctly?
- Does the person answer questions correctly?
- Does the person speak clearly?
- Are instructions followed correctly?
- Is the person calm, restless, or excited?
- Is the person conversing, quiet, or talking a lot?

Movement
- Can the person squeeze your fingers with each hand?
- Can the person move arms and legs?
- Are movements shaky or jerky?
- Does the person complain of stiff or painful joints?
- Are there areas of weakness?
- Does the person complain of fatigue (feeling tired)?

Pain or Discomfort
- Where is the pain located? (Have the person point to the pain.)
- Does the pain go anywhere else?
- How does the person rate the severity of the pain—mild, moderate, severe?
- How does the person rate the pain on a scale of 0 to 10 (Chapter 36)?
- When did the pain begin?
- What was the person doing when the pain began?
- How long does the pain last?
- How does the person describe the pain?
  - Sharp
  - Severe
  - Stabbing
  - Dull
  - Burning
  - Aching
  - Comes and goes
  - Depends on position
- Was a pain-relief drug given?
- Did the pain-relief drug relieve pain? Is pain still present?
- Can the person sleep and rest?
- What is the position of comfort?

Skin
- Is the skin pale or flushed?
- Is the skin cool, warm, or hot?
- Is the skin moist or dry?
- Does the skin appear mottled (blotchy, spotted with color)?
- What color are the lips and nail beds?
- Is the skin intact? Are there broken areas? If so, where?
- Are sores or reddened areas present? If yes, where?
- Are bruises present? If yes, where?
- Does the person complain of itching? If yes, where?

Eyes, Ears, Nose, and Mouth
- Is there drainage from the eyes? Drainage color?
- Are the eyelids closed? Do they stay open?
- Are the eyes reddened?
- Does the person complain of spots, flashes, or blurring?
- Is the person sensitive to bright lights?
- Is there drainage from the ears? Drainage color?
- Can the person hear? Is repeating necessary? Are questions answered correctly?
- Is there drainage from the nose? Drainage color?

Eyes, Ears, Nose, and Mouth—cont'd
- Can the person breathe through the nose?
- Is there breath odor?
- Does the person complain of a bad taste in the mouth?
- Does the person complain of painful gums or teeth?
- Do the person's gums bleed with oral hygiene (Chapter 23)?
- Does the person with dentures say that dentures are loose or do not fit well?

Respirations
- Do both sides of the chest rise and fall with respirations?
- Is breathing noisy?
- Does the person complain of pain or difficulty breathing?
- What is the amount and color of sputum?
- How often does the person cough? Is the cough dry or productive?

Bowels and Bladder
- Is the abdomen firm or soft?
- Does the person complain of gas?
- Which does the person use: toilet, commode, bedpan, or urinal?
- What are the amount, color, and consistency of bowel movements (BMs)?
- What is the frequency of BMs?
- Can the person control BMs?
- Does the person have pain or difficulty urinating?
- What is the amount of urine?
- What is the color of urine?
- Is the urine clear? Are there particles in the urine?
- Does urine have a foul smell?
- Can the person control the passage of urine?
- What is the frequency of urination?

Appetite
- Does the person like the food served?
- How much of the meal is eaten?
- What foods does the person like?
- Can the person chew food?
- What is the amount of fluid taken?
- What fluids does the person like?
- How often does the person drink fluids?
- Can the person swallow food and fluids?
- Does the person cough when swallowing?
- Does the person complain of nausea?
- What is the amount and color of vomitus?
- Does the person have hiccups?
- Is the person belching?

Activities of Daily Living
- Can the person perform personal care without help?
  - Bathing?
  - Brushing teeth or caring for dentures?
  - Combing and brushing hair?
  - Shaving?
- Does the person need help with feeding?
- Can the person walk?
- What amount and kind of help is needed?
- Does the person have problems using adaptive (assistive) devices? Examples include devices for mobility (walker, cane, wheelchair), devices for hygiene and grooming (Chapters 24 and 25), and devices for eating (Chapter 31).

Bleeding
- Is the person bleeding? If yes, from where and how much?

Analysis

Gathered data must be analyzed. *Analysis* involves interpreting data and identifying problems. The nurse uses nursing judgment to make decisions on what is normal and abnormal. For example, a person's vital signs are measured. The measurements are given to the nurse. The nurse compares the values to normal values and decides if there is a problem that needs to be addressed.

Agencies use different methods to describe and communicate identified problems. One method is to use nursing diagnoses. A *nursing diagnosis* describes a health problem that can be treated by nursing measures. Nursing diagnoses are not the same as medical diagnoses. A medical diagnosis is the identification of a disease or condition by a doctor. Doctors use drugs, therapies, and surgery to treat medical diagnoses such as cancer, stroke, and diabetes. Nurses use nursing interventions to address various physical, mental and emotional, social, and spiritual needs. (See "Planning.")

The person's condition and needs can change at any time. New problems are identified. The nurse works with the health team to make decisions about care.

See *Focus on Long-Term Care and Home Care: Analysis.*

FOCUS ON LONG-TERM CARE AND HOME CARE

Analysis

Long-Term Care
The CMS uses a *Care Area Assessment (CAA)* process to make decisions about the information gathered in the MDS. If an area is "triggered" as a potential problem on the MDS, the CAA process begins. Appendix C (p. 908) shows a summary of the different areas that may be triggered. The intent is to identify problem areas, assess those areas more fully, and determine what to include in the care plan (see "Planning").

Planning

Planning involves setting priorities and goals.
- *Priorities*—what is most important for the person.
- *Goals*—what is desired for or by a person as a result of nursing care. Also called *outcomes* or *objectives*, goals are aimed at the person's highest level of well-being and function.

Nursing interventions are chosen after goals are set. An *intervention* is an action or measure. A *nursing intervention* (*nursing action, nursing measure, nursing task*) is an action or measure taken by the nursing team to help the person reach a goal. A nursing intervention does not need a doctor's order. Actions to prevent falls, provide hygiene, and promote comfort are examples.

The *nursing care plan (care plan)* is a written guide about the person's nursing care. It has the person's

identified problems and goals. It also has the nursing measures or actions for each goal. A communication tool, the care plan:
- Communicates what care to give
- Helps ensure that nursing team members give the same care

The care plan is found in the written or electronic medical record (Fig. 8-5, p. 92). The plan is carried out. It changes as the person's needs change.

See *Focus on Surveys: Planning.*

See *Focus on Long-Term Care and Home Care: Planning.*

FOCUS ON SURVEYS

Planning

During a survey, you may be asked about the person's care plan. Give honest and complete answers. You may be asked about:
- The person's goals
- Nursing interventions
- How the nursing interventions are carried out
- How you give input about the person's care needs and your observations

FOCUS ON LONG-TERM CARE AND HOME CARE

Planning

Long-Term Care
The CMS requires a *comprehensive care plan*. It is a guide about the person's care. The care plan must be person-centered (Chapter 2). It includes the person's problems, goals, and actions to take. The person's strengths and preferences are also included.

Through the care planning process, staff work with the resident and family to understand the person's needs and meet the person's goals. The resident's goals guide decisions about care. Goals vary. For example, one resident desires to perform ADL independently in order to return home. Another resident desires to perform ADL as independently as possible while receiving help with what cannot be done alone. Another resident's goal is pain relief and comfort for end-of-life.

The person's goals and abilities determine to what extent staff assist. For some, staff fully provide needed care.

Care Conferences. Care conferences are held to share information and ideas about the person's care. The purpose is to develop or revise the nursing care plan. Effective care is the goal. Nursing assistants may take part in conferences.

See *Focus on Communication: Care Conferences*, p. 92.

See *Focus on Long-Term Care and Home Care: Care Conferences*, p. 93.

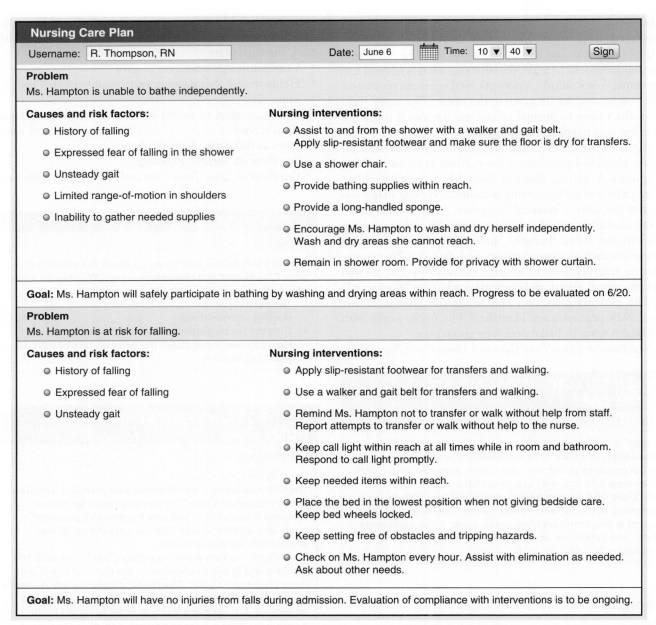

Nursing Care Plan

Username: R. Thompson, RN   Date: June 6   Time: 10 ▼ 40 ▼   Sign

Problem

Ms. Hampton is unable to bathe independently.

Causes and risk factors:

- History of falling
- Expressed fear of falling in the shower
- Unsteady gait
- Limited range-of-motion in shoulders
- Inability to gather needed supplies

Nursing interventions:

- Assist to and from the shower with a walker and gait belt. Apply slip-resistant footwear and make sure the floor is dry for transfers.
- Use a shower chair.
- Provide bathing supplies within reach.
- Provide a long-handled sponge.
- Encourage Ms. Hampton to wash and dry herself independently. Wash and dry areas she cannot reach.
- Remain in shower room. Provide for privacy with shower curtain.

Goal: Ms. Hampton will safely participate in bathing by washing and drying areas within reach. Progress to be evaluated on 6/20.

Problem

Ms. Hampton is at risk for falling.

Causes and risk factors:

- History of falling
- Expressed fear of falling
- Unsteady gait

Nursing interventions:

- Apply slip-resistant footwear for transfers and walking.
- Use a walker and gait belt for transfers and walking.
- Remind Ms. Hampton not to transfer or walk without help from staff. Report attempts to transfer or walk without help to the nurse.
- Keep call light within reach at all times while in room and bathroom. Respond to call light promptly.
- Keep needed items within reach.
- Place the bed in the lowest position when not giving bedside care. Keep bed wheels locked.
- Keep setting free of obstacles and tripping hazards.
- Check on Ms. Hampton every hour. Assist with elimination as needed. Ask about other needs.

Goal: Ms. Hampton will have no injuries from falls during admission. Evaluation of compliance with interventions is to be ongoing.

FIGURE 8-5 Sample portion of a nursing care plan. Problems are identified. Goals are set. There are nursing interventions listed to reach each goal.

FOCUS ON COMMUNICATION

Care Conferences

You see what patients and residents like and do not like and what they can and cannot do. They talk to you. They tell you about their families and interests. You make observations when you are with them. Share this information during care conferences. Also share ideas about care.

For example, you can say:

- "Mr. Antonio misses the fresh tomatoes and broccoli from his garden. Can we ask the family to bring those more often?"
- "Mrs. Clark can propel her wheelchair with her feet. Why do we push her wheelchair?"
- "Miss Walsh never talks when her family visits. She talks to her roommate often."

Care Conferences

Long-Term Care
Nursing center care plans are prepared and then reviewed and revised after each assessment (on admission, quarterly and yearly, and for a significant change). An *interdisciplinary team* is involved—doctor, nursing staff (including a nursing assistant), dietary staff, the resident and any representatives (such as family), and other staff as determined by the person's needs.

The person and family have the right to take part in planning conferences. The agency must facilitate their involvement if possible. This includes holding care conferences at times that the resident and family can attend and giving advance notice. Video conferencing or conference calls are an option.

The resident has the right to participate in setting goals and making decisions about care. The resident can refuse actions suggested by the health team.

Implementation

To *implement* means to do, carry out, or perform. In the *implementation* step, nursing interventions in the care plan are carried out. Care is given.

Nursing care ranges from simple to complex. The nurse assigns tasks within your legal limits and job description. The nurse may delegate (Chapter 4) or ask you to assist with complex measures.

Assignment Sheets. An assignment sheet is used to communicate the tasks the nurse has assigned to you (Fig. 8-6). The assignment sheet tells you about:
- Each person's care.
- What nursing interventions and tasks to do.
- Which nursing unit tasks to do. Cleaning utility rooms and stocking shower rooms are examples.

Talk to the nurse about an unclear assignment. Also check the care plan for more information.

See *Focus on Communication: Assignment Sheets*, p. 94.
See *Teamwork and Time Management: Assignment Sheets*, p. 94.

Assignment Sheet

Date: 9–10
Shift: Day
Nursing assistant: J. Reed
Supervisor: M. Garcia, RN

Breaks: 1000   1400
Lunch: 1230
Unit Tasks: Pass drinking water at 0900
Clean utility room at 1430

Check the care plan for other care measures and information

Room # 501A Name: Mrs. Ann Lopez ("Annie")	Functional status/care measures and procedures
ID Number: S1514491530 Date of birth: 11/04/1940	Total assist with ADL
VS: Daily at 0700	Full-sling mechanical lift transfer
T____ P____ R____ BP____	Uses wheelchair with footplates
Wt: Weekly (Monday at 0700)	Incontinent of bowel and bladder – uses briefs
Intake____ Output____ BM____	Passive ROM exercises to extremities twice daily
Bath: Complete bed bath	Turn and re-position q2h when in bed
Shampoo Bed rails	Wears eyeglasses and dentures / Diet: High fiber (dependent)
Room # 510B Name: Mr. Mark Lee	Functional status/care measures and procedures
ID Number: D4468947762 Date of birth: 12/29/1946	Independent with ADL
VS: 2 times daily, at 0700 and 1500	Ambulates with a walker
0700: T____ P____ R____ BP____	Attends exercise group every morning
1500: T____ P____ R____ BP____	Continent of bowel and bladder – q4h bathroom schedule to maintain continence
Wt: Daily at 0700	Wears eyeglasses
Intake____ Output____ BM____	Coughing and deep-breathing exercises q4h
Bath: Shower	Diet: Sodium-controlled (independent)

FIGURE 8-6 A sample assignment sheet. NOTE: This assignment sheet is a computer printout.

Evaluation

Evaluate means to measure. The *evaluation* step involves measuring if the goals in the planning step were met. Assessment information is used to evaluate progress. Goals may be met totally, in part, or not at all. Changes to the care plan may result.

Your Role

You have key roles in the nursing process. Your observations are used for planning. You may help develop care plans. In the implementation step, you perform tasks in the care plan. Your assignment sheet tells you what to do. Your observations are used for the evaluation step.

REPORTING AND RECORDING

The health team communicates by reporting and recording. *Reporting* is the oral account of care and observations. *Recording* (*charting, documentation*) is the written account of care and observations.

Reporting and Recording Time

The 24-hour clock (military time or international time) has 4 digits (Fig. 8-7, *A*). The first 2 digits are for the hours. The last 2 digits are for the minutes. A colon and AM and PM are not used.

The 24-hour clock is shown in Figure 8-7, *B*. The clock begins at midnight. After the noon hour (1200), the hours keep counting up (13, 14, and so on) instead of starting over at 1 (as done with conventional time). When midnight is reached (2400 or 0000), a new day begins. Follow agency policy for whether to use 2400 or 0000 for midnight. Box 8-4 shows how conventional time is written in 24-hour time.

See *Focus on Math: Reporting and Recording Time.*
See *Focus on Communication: Reporting and Recording Time.*

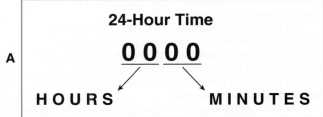

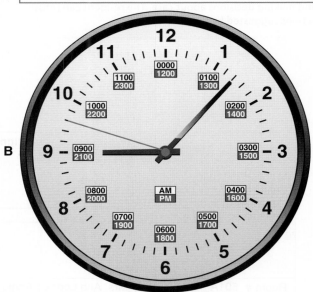

FIGURE 8-7 24-hour time. **A,** In 24-hour time, there are 4 digits. The first 2 are for the hours. The last 2 are for the minutes. A colon and AM and PM are not used. **B,** The 24-hour clock. NOTE: 12:00 AM (midnight) is 0000 (or 2400 in some agencies); 12:00 PM (noon) is 1200.

BOX 8-4   24-Hour Time

AM		PM	
Conventional Time	24-Hour Time	Conventional Time	24-Hour Time
12:00 MIDNIGHT	0000 or 2400	12:00 NOON	1200
1:00 AM	0100	1:00 PM	1300
2:00 AM	0200	2:00 PM	1400
3:00 AM	0300	3:00 PM	1500
4:00 AM	0400	4:00 PM	1600
5:00 AM	0500	5:00 PM	1700
6:00 AM	0600	6:00 PM	1800
7:00 AM	0700	7:00 PM	1900
8:00 AM	0800	8:00 PM	2000
9:00 AM	0900	9:00 PM	2100
10:00 AM	1000	10:00 PM	2200
11:00 AM	1100	11:00 PM	2300

FOCUS ON MATH

Reporting and Recording Time

A *digit* is any number from 0 to 9. With conventional time, 3 or 4 digits are used with a colon and AM or PM (7:30 AM, 7:45 PM, 10:15 PM). With 24-hour time, 4 digits are used without a colon and without AM or PM (0730, 1945, 2215).

When changing from conventional time to 24-hour time, the hours from 1:00 PM to 11:00 PM require math. Twelve (12) is added to the hours digit(s). The minutes digits do not change. See Figure 8-8.

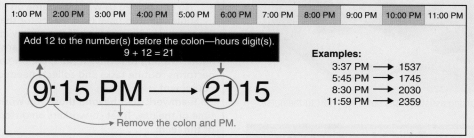

FIGURE 8-8 From 1:00 PM to 11:00 PM, add 12 to the hours digit(s) to change from conventional time to 24-hour time. Remove the colon and PM.

FOCUS ON COMMUNICATION

Reporting and Recording Time

Reading and saying 24-hour time is different than conventional time.
- When a 24-hour time begins with zero (0), read or say the "0" as "zero" or "oh."
- When the last 2 digits (minutes) end in "00," read or say the numbers as "hundred" or "hundred hours."
  When the last 2 digits are numbers other than 2 zeros (00), read or say the first 2 numbers (hours) and the last 2 numbers (minutes).

The following are examples of how to say 24-hour times.
- 0200: "zero two hundred (hours)" or "oh two hundred (hours)"
- 1700: "seventeen hundred (hours)"
- 0620: "zero six twenty" or "oh six twenty"
- 1215: "twelve fifteen"

Reporting

Report care and observations to the nurse.
- When there is a change from normal or a change in the person's condition. Report these changes at once.
- When the nurse asks you to do so.
- Before leaving the unit for meals, breaks, or other reasons.
- Before the end-of-shift report (p. 96).
- After the end-of-shift report and before reporting off duty.
  When reporting, follow the rules in Box 8-5.
  See *Teamwork and Time Management: Reporting*, p. 96.

BOX 8-5	Rules for Reporting

- Be prompt, thorough, and accurate.
- Give the person's name and room and bed number.
- Give the time you made the observations or gave care. Use 24-hour time or conventional time (AM or PM) according to agency policy.
- Report only what you observed and did yourself.
- Report care measures that the person might need. For example, the person may need the bedpan during your meal break.
- Report expected changes in the person's condition. For example, the person may be tired after lunch.
- Report refusals of care. For example, the person refuses a shower.
- Give reports as often as the person's condition requires. Also give them when the nurse asks you to.
- Report at once any changes from normal or changes in the person's condition.
- Use your written notes for a specific, concise, and clear report (Fig. 8-9, p. 96).

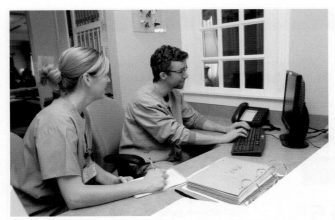

FIGURE 8-9 The nursing assistant uses notes to report to the nurse.

TEAMWORK AND TIME MANAGEMENT

Reporting

The nurse needs your full attention when reporting. If distracted, you could leave out important information.

Nurses must give their full attention when receiving reports. While a nurse is receiving a report, do not interrupt unless the matter is urgent. Do not distract the nurse.

End-of-Shift Report. An *end-of-shift report (change-of-shift report)* is a report that the nurse gives at the end of the shift to the on-coming shift. The nurse reports about:

- The care given
- The care to give during other shifts
- The person's current condition
- Likely changes in the person's condition
- New or changed orders

Some agencies have the entire nursing team hear the end-of-shift report as they come on duty. In other agencies, only nurses hear the report. After the report, nursing assistants receive needed information.

See *Teamwork and Time Management: End-of-Shift Report.*

See *Promoting Safety and Comfort: End-of-Shift Report.*

Recording

When recording (documenting, charting), you must communicate clearly and thoroughly. Follow the rules in Box 8-6. Anyone reading your charting should know:

- What you observed
- What you did
- The person's response

See *Focus on Communication: Recording.*

TEAMWORK AND TIME MANAGEMENT

End-of-Shift Report

The end of shift requires good teamwork. Your attitude is important. Greet your co-workers politely. If going off duty, avoid saying or thinking:

- "I'm ready to go home. Let them do it."
- "It's their turn. I've been here all day (evening, night)."
- "No one helped us when we came on duty."

Some agencies have clear duties for the 2 shifts. For example, those going off duty know about the patients or residents. They continue to answer call lights. Waiting to receive report, the on-coming shift performs routine tasks and collects needed supplies and equipment.

Teamwork goes beyond those you work with at a certain time of the day. Treat co-workers on different shifts as part of the team.

PROMOTING SAFETY AND COMFORT

End-of-Shift Report

Safety

You may answer call lights and give care before receiving report (being given information for your shift from the nurse). For safe care:

- Check the care plan before granting a request. The person's condition or care plan may have changed. There may be new orders.
- Ask a nurse about the care needs of new patients or residents. If the need is urgent, politely interrupt the end-of-shift report to ask your questions.
- Do not take directions or orders from another nursing assistant. Remember, nursing assistants cannot supervise or delegate to other nursing assistants.

You may answer call lights during the end-of-shift report as you go off duty. Be sure to report observations, care measures, requests, and so on before you leave. For example, you assist a resident onto the bedpan before going home. The nursing team of the on-coming shift needs to know so they can check on the person. Otherwise the person could be left on the bedpan for a long time, causing the person harm.

FOCUS ON COMMUNICATION

Recording

"Small," "moderate," "large," "long," and "short" mean different things to different people. Measurements and descriptions like "dime-sized" or "quarter-sized" are clearer. If not sure how to describe something, ask the nurse for help.

BOX 8-6	Rules for Recording

General Rules

- Follow agency policies and procedures for recording. Ask for needed training.
- Check the name and identifying information on the chart. You must record on the correct chart.
- Include the date and time for each recording. Use 24-hour time or conventional time (AM or PM) according to agency policy.
- Use only agency-approved abbreviations (see "Abbreviations" in Chapter 9).
- Use correct spelling, grammar, and punctuation.
- Do not use ditto (") marks.
- Record only what you observed and did yourself. Do not record for another person.
- Never chart a procedure, treatment, or care measure until after it is completed.
- Be accurate, concise, and factual. Do not record judgments or interpretations. For example, "The person felt sad" is a judgment. "The person was crying" is factual.
- Record in a logical manner and in sequence.
- Be descriptive. Avoid terms with more than 1 meaning.
- Use the person's exact words when possible. Use quotation marks ("…") for a direct quote.
- Chart changes from normal or changes in the person's condition. Also chart that you told the nurse (include the nurse's name), what you said, and the time you made the report.
- Do not omit (leave out) information.
- Record safety measures. Examples include placing the call light within reach, assisting the person when up, or reminding a person not to get up without help.
- Sign or save all entries as required by agency policy.

On Computer

- Log in (sign in) using your username and password (Fig. 8-10). Do not use another person's username.
- Check the time your entry is made. Make sure it is the right time.
- Check for accuracy. Review your entry before saving.
- Save your entries. Un-saved data will be lost. You click an icon or button to save the entry. If you forget, most systems have a reminder. You can choose to log off without saving (delete the entry) or save the entry.
- Follow the manufacturer's instructions to change or un-chart a mistaken entry. Most electronic systems keep a record of original entries and changes.
- Log off after charting. This prevents others from charting under your username.
- See "Electronic Devices" on p. 98.

On Paper

- Make sure each form and page has the person's name and other identifying information.
- Always use ink. Use the ink color required by the agency.
- Make sure writing is readable and neat.
- Follow agency policy for correcting errors. Never erase or use correction fluid (white out). Draw a line through the incorrect part. Date and initial the line. Write "mistaken entry" over it if this is agency policy. Then re-write the part. See Figure 8-11.
- Sign your entry. Include your name and title at the end (see Fig. 8-11).
- Do not skip lines. Draw a line through the blank space of a partially completed line or to the end of the page (see Fig. 8-11). This prevents others from recording in a space with your signature.

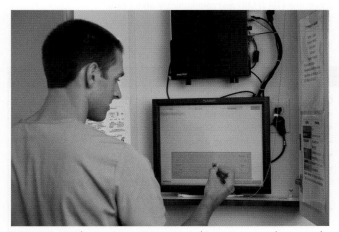

FIGURE 8-10 The nursing assistant enters his username and password to log in to a medical record.

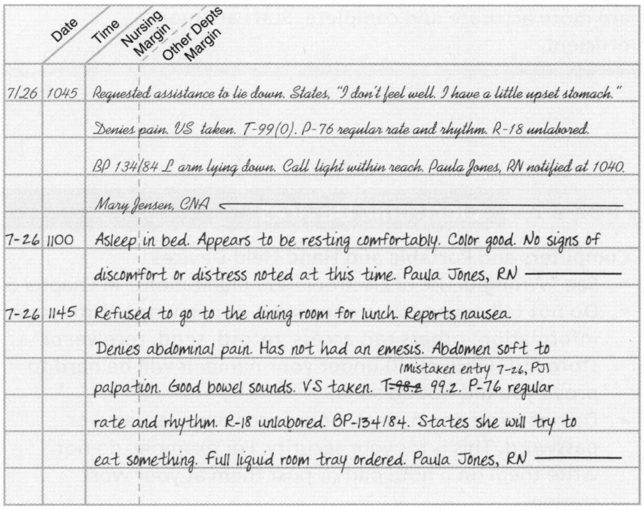

Date	Time	Nursing Margin	Other Depts Margin
7/26	1045	Requested assistance to lie down. States, "I don't feel well. I have a little upset stomach."	
		Denies pain. VS taken. T-99(0). P-76 regular rate and rhythm. R-18 unlabored.	
		BP 134/84 L arm lying down. Call light within reach. Paula Jones, RN notified at 1040.	
		Mary Jensen, CNA	
7-26	1100	Asleep in bed. Appears to be resting comfortably. Color good. No signs of	
		discomfort or distress noted at this time. Paula Jones, RN	
7-26	1145	Refused to go to the dining room for lunch. Reports nausea.	
		Denies abdominal pain. Has not had an emesis. Abdomen soft to	
		palpation. Good bowel sounds. VS taken. T-~~98.2~~ 99.2. P-76 regular *(mistaken entry 7-26, PJ)*	
		rate and rhythm. R-18 unlabored. BP-134/84. States she will try to	
		eat something. Full liquid room tray ordered. Paula Jones, RN	

FIGURE 8-11 Progress note on paper. A mistaken entry is corrected by drawing a single line through the incorrect part.

Electronic Recording. Electronic health (medical) records improve access to medical records. Recording may be done in patients' or residents' rooms, in hallways, at the nurses' station, or on portable or hand-held devices (Fig. 8-12).

Users log in (sign in) to access or record on the person's medical record. You will be trained to use your agency's system.

ELECTRONIC DEVICES

Electronic devices are used to store and send information to the health team. Computers and portable and hand-held devices are common (Fig. 8-13). Fax machines are used to send and receive paper documents.

Follow agency policies when using electronic devices. Use only your username and password. You must keep protected health information (PHI) and electronic protected health information (EPHI; ePHI) confidential.

Follow the rules in Box 8-7 and the ethical and legal rules about privacy, confidentiality, and defamation (Chapters 5 and 6) when using electronic devices.

See *Teamwork and Time Management: Electronic Devices*.

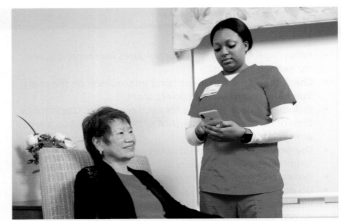

FIGURE 8-12 A nursing assistant uses an agency's hand-held device to record on a person's medical record.

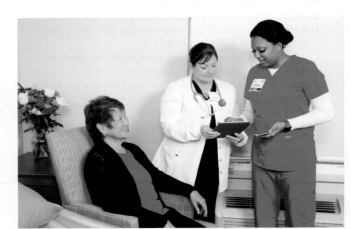

FIGURE 8-13 A nurse and nursing assistant use electronic devices to access the EHR (EMR) and communicate about care.

TEAMWORK AND TIME MANAGEMENT

Electronic Devices

Electronic devices are often used for measurements such as blood pressures, temperatures, and heart rates. Some electronic devices for measuring vital signs (Chapter 34) send measurements directly to the EHR (EMR). The system alerts the nursing staff to abnormal vital signs.

Such systems save time and reduce recording errors. Quality care and safety are increased. Records are more accurate and complete. Staff are more efficient.

BOX 8-7	Electronic Devices

Computers and Portable and Hand-Held Devices
- See "Wrongful Use of Electronic Communications" in Chapter 5.
- Do not tell anyone your username or password. With your information, others can access, record, send, receive, or store PHI (EPHI; ePHI) under your name. It will be hard to prove you did not do so.
- Do not write down, post, or expose your username or password. This is for your security. For example, do not write them on a note pad or post them at your work station.
- Change your password often. Follow agency policy.
- Do not use another person's username or password.
- Prevent others from seeing the screen.
  - Place the screen so it cannot be seen by others.
  - Be aware of anyone standing behind you.
  - Stand or sit with your back to the wall if using a mobile computer.
  - Do not leave a device unattended.

Computers and Portable and Hand-Held Devices—cont'd
- Follow the rules for recording (see Box 8-6).
- Enter data carefully. Double-check your entries.
- Log off after making an entry.
- Do not leave printouts where others can read or pick them up.
- Shred or destroy printouts, assignment sheets, or worksheets. Place such documents in a wastebasket marked *CONFIDENTIAL INFORMATION* for shredding. Follow agency policy.
- Send e-mail and messages only to those needing the information.
- Do not e-mail information or messages that require immediate reporting. Give the report in person. The person may not read the e-mail in a timely manner.
- Do not use e-mail or messages to report confidential information. This includes addresses, phone numbers, and Social Security numbers. The computer system may not be secure.

BOX 8-7 | Electronic Devices—cont'd

Computers and Portable and Hand-Held Devices—cont'd
- Remember that any communication can be read or heard by someone other than the intended person.
- Remember that deleted communications can be retrieved by authorized staff.
- Do not use agency devices for personal use. Do not:
  - Send personal e-mail messages.
  - Send or receive e-mail or messages that are offensive, not legal, or sexual.
  - Send or receive e-mail for illegal activities, jokes, politics, gambling (including football and other pools), chain letters, or other non-work activities.
  - Post information, opinions, or comments on websites or video or social media sites.
  - Upload, download, or send materials containing a copyright, trademark, or patent.
- Remember that the agency has the right to monitor your use of electronic devices. This includes Internet use.
- Do not open another person's e-mail or messages.
- Follow agency policy for mis-directed e-mails.

Faxes
- See "Wrongful Use of Electronic Communications" in Chapter 5.
- Use the agency's "cover sheet." The sheet has instructions about:
  - The confidentiality of PHI (EPHI; ePHI)
  - The receiver's responsibilities about PHI (EPHI; ePHI)
  - The receiver's responsibilities for a fax received in error (mis-directed fax)
- Complete the "cover sheet" according to agency policy. The following are common.
  - Name of the person to receive the fax
  - Receiver's fax number
  - Date
  - Number of pages being faxed
  - Department name
  - Name and phone number of the person sending the fax
- Follow agency policy for a mis-directed fax.
- Do not leave sent or received faxes unattended in the fax machine or lying around.

PHONE COMMUNICATIONS

You will answer phones at the nurses' station or in the person's room. Use good communication skills. Your tone of voice, speech clarity, and attitude are important. Be professional and courteous. Also practice good work ethics. Follow the agency's policy and the guidelines in Box 8-8.

See *Focus on Long-Term Care and Home Care: Phone Communications*, p. 100.

BOX 8-8 | Answering Phones

- Answer the call after the first ring if possible. Be sure to answer by the fourth ring.
- Do not answer in a rushed or hasty manner.
- Give a courteous greeting. Identify the agency or nursing unit and give your name and title. For example: "Good morning, 3 center. Pat Wills, nursing assistant."
- Follow agency policy for answering phones in patient or resident rooms.
- Note this information to take a message.
  - The caller's name and phone number (include the area code and extension number)
  - The date and time
  - Who the message is for
- Repeat the message and phone number back to the caller.
- Ask the caller to "Please hold" if necessary. First find out who is calling and the caller's number. Then ask if the caller can hold. Do not put callers with an emergency on hold.
- Do not lay the phone down or cover the receiver with your hand when not speaking to the caller. The caller may over-hear confidential conversations.
- Return to a caller on hold within 30 seconds. Ask if the caller can wait longer or if the call can be returned.
- Do not give confidential information to any caller. Patient, resident, and employee information is confidential. Refer such calls to the nurse.
- Transfer the call if appropriate.
  - Tell the caller that you are going to transfer the call.
  - Give the name of the department or the name of the person who should answer the phone if appropriate.
  - Get the caller's name and number in case the call gets disconnected.
  - Give the caller the phone number to call in case the call gets disconnected or the line is busy.
- End the conversation politely. Thank the person for calling and say good-bye.
- Give the message to the appropriate person.

FOCUS ON LONG-TERM CARE AND HOME CARE

Phone Communications

Home Care

If you need to answer a phone in a patient's home, answer with "hello." This is to protect the person, family, and you. Too much information is shared when you give the person's name ("Price residence") or your name and title.

People call homes for many reasons. Some make sales calls or ask for donations. Others have criminal intent. Some criminals target vulnerable people. Saying that you are a home health assistant means that an ill, older, or disabled person is in the home.

Do not give your name or the person's name until you know who is calling and why. Make sure it is someone you or the person wants to talk to—the person's family or friend, your supervisor, or a caller expected by the person.

FOCUS ON PRIDE

The Person, Family, and Yourself

Personal and Professional Responsibility

You are responsible for what you report and record. It must be accurate and timely. Remember:

- Document what you did. If you do not, it is assumed that the task was not done.
- Never document that something *was* done when it really *was not* done.
- Record a task *after* completing it, not before.

Rights and Respect

The intent of care planning is to communicate how the person's individual goals, needs, and preferences will be met. The care plan must be specific to the person. The person has input on desired outcomes. Goals must be measurable with an identified timeframe for evaluation. The person has the right to take part in care planning.

Independence and Social Interaction

Health team communications are not limited to reporting and recording. You interact in the nurses' station, patient and resident rooms, hallways, break room, cafeteria, parking lot, and so on. Treat co-workers with kindness and respect. Have a good attitude. Be someone others enjoy working with!

Delegation and Teamwork

Assignment sheets communicate the nursing tasks and unit tasks assigned to you. If you have a problem with an assignment, share your reason with the nurse. Not liking a task is not a good reason. The nurse will decide if a change is needed.

Ethics and Laws

Legal action can be taken against persons who record false information. For example:

A licensed nursing assistant (LNA) worked at a home health and hospice agency. On November 9, she recorded on a time sheet that she was in a patient's home for about 30 minutes. However, the patient was in the hospital from November 8 through November 14.

The LNA admitted to unprofessional conduct. Her conduct violated Administrative Rules of the Board of Nursing for:
- *Making inaccurate or misleading entries*
- *Failing to comply with federal or state laws or rules*

The LNA was given a reprimand by the Board.
(State of Vermont Board of Nursing, 2003.)

A *reprimand* means that the Board considered the nursing assistant's conduct to be improper. However, the Board did not limit her ability to work as an LNA.

FOCUS ON PRIDE: Application

Explain why accurate and timely reporting and recording are important. What problems may occur from incorrect or delayed reporting or recording?

REVIEW QUESTIONS

Circle the BEST answer.

1 To communicate well, you should
   a Use terms with many meanings
   b Give long descriptions
   c Use unfamiliar terms
   d Give facts and be specific

2 A person is discharged from the agency. The medical record is
   a Destroyed
   b Sent home with the family
   c Permanent
   d No longer private

3 You help with Mr. Hild's care. If you record on his medical record, you have
   a Violated his right to privacy
   b Provided a record of what care was given
   c The right to access his wife's medical records too
   d To give him your username so he can read what you wrote

4 You measured a person's vital signs and re-positioned the person. You should
   a Only record if there is something abnormal
   b Record your care on the flow sheet in the person's medical record
   c Not record because these are routine care measures
   d Ask the nurse to record it in the health history part of the chart

5 Which statement about the nursing process is *correct?*
   a Assessment involves gathering information.
   b Analysis involves measuring if goals have been met.
   c Implementation involves planning goals and priorities.
   d The person is discharged when the evaluation step is reached.

6 You measured a person's temperature and pulse. You have
   a Performed an assessment
   b Completed the nursing process
   c Collected subjective data
   d Collected objective data

7 Which is a symptom?
   a Skin redness
   b Vomiting
   c Pain
   d Yellow urine

8 Which should you report at once?
   a The person can no longer move a body part.
   b The person answers questions correctly.
   c The person has a breath odor.
   d The person walked to the dining room.

9 The care plan
   a Is written by the doctor
   b Communicates what care to give
   c Is the same for all persons
   d Does not change after it is developed

10 To communicate assigned tasks to you, the nurse uses
   a The care plan
   b The Minimum Data Set
   c An assignment sheet
   d Care conferences

11 Your role in the nursing process involves
   a Reporting observations
   b Interpreting assessment data
   c Writing the care plan
   d Evaluating if goals are met

12 In the evening, the clock shows 9:26. In 24-hour clock time this is
   a 9:26 PM
   b 1926
   c 0926
   d 2126

13 In the morning, the clock shows 7:45. In 24-hour clock time this is
   a 0745
   b 1945
   c 745
   d 7:45 AM

14 Which is a safe recording practice?
   a Recording a task at 1330 that you plan to do at 1400
   b Checking the identifying information on the chart before recording
   c Asking another nursing assistant to chart something for you
   d Using a co-worker's username and password to log in

15 Which entry is descriptive and concise?
   a "Mrs. Jones ate some of her breakfast."
   b "Mrs. Jones ate fairly well."
   c "Mrs. Jones ate half of her oatmeal and half of her fruit."
   d "Mrs. Jones ate as much as she usually eats."

16 You type a correct entry into an electronic medical record. You click the button to log off. A message pops up asking "Do you want to save your entry?" You should
   a Try to log off again
   b Turn off the computer
   c Click "No"
   d Click "Yes"

17 You have access to the agency's computer. Which is *true?*
   a The agency can monitor your computer use.
   b E-mail is used for reports the nurse needs at once.
   c You can post your username and password in your work area.
   d You can use the computer for your personal needs.

18 A phone rings at the nurses' station. Which greeting is *best?*
   a "Good morning. This is Joey."
   b "North hall."
   c "Good morning, North hall. Joey Wilson, nursing assistant, speaking."
   d "Hello."

Answers to Chapter 8 questions are on p. 901.

FOCUS ON **PRACTICE**

Problem Solving

You measure a patient's vital signs. You continue with other tasks before reporting and recording them. An hour later, the nurse asks for the measurements. You say: "They were fine." What problems do you notice? Can harm result? How can communication be improved?

Medical Terminology

OBJECTIVES

- Define the key terms in this chapter.
- Identify the word parts that make up medical terms.
- Explain how to define medical terms.
- Locate the 4 abdominal quadrants.
- Identify the directional terms used to describe the locations of body parts.
- Identify the terms used to describe the position of the body when lying down.
- Define common abbreviations and health care terms.
- Explain how to promote PRIDE in the person, the family, and yourself.

KEY TERMS

abbreviation A shortened form of a word or phrase
anterior At or toward the front of the body or body part; ventral
deep Below the surface
distal The part farthest from the center or from the point of attachment
dorsal See "posterior"
inferior Below another structure
lateral Away from the mid-line; at the side of the body or body part
medial At or near the middle or mid-line of the body or body part
posterior At or toward the back of the body or body part; dorsal

prefix A word element at the beginning of a word; it changes the meaning of the word
proximal The part nearest to the center or to the point of attachment
root A word element that contains the basic meaning of the word
suffix A word element at the end of a word; it changes the meaning of the word
superficial On the surface
superior Above another structure
ventral See "anterior"
word element A part of a word

Medical terms and abbreviations are used in health care. Understanding the basics of medical terminology is important for your training and work.

If you do not understand a word, phrase, or abbreviation, ask a nurse for its meaning. Otherwise, communication does not occur. A medical dictionary is useful to learn new words.

MEDICAL TERMS

Like all words, medical terms are made up of parts of words called *word elements*—prefixes, roots, and suffixes. Most are from Greek or Latin. Word elements are combined to form medical terms (Fig. 9-1).

Prefixes, Roots, and Suffixes

A *prefix* is a word element at the beginning of a word. It changes the meaning of the word. For example, the prefix *hemi-* (half) is placed before *-plegia* (paralysis) to make *hemiplegia*. It means paralysis on half of the body. Prefixes

are used with other word elements. Prefixes are not used alone.

The *root* is the word element that contains the basic meaning of the word. It is combined with another root, a prefix, or a suffix. A vowel (an *o* or an *i*) may be added when 2 roots are combined or when a suffix that begins with a consonant is added to a root. (A consonant is any letter other than a vowel.) The vowel (*combining vowel*) makes the word easier to pronounce.

A *suffix* is a word element at the end of a word. It changes the meaning of the word. Suffixes are not used alone. For example, *colonoscopy* means examination of the large intestine using a scope. It is formed by combining the root *colon (o)* (colon, large intestine) and the suffix *-scopy* (examination using a scope).

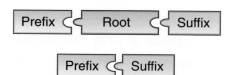

FIGURE 9-1 Prefixes, roots, and suffixes are combined to form medical terms. (Modified from Leonard PC: *Building a medical vocabulary with Spanish translations*, ed 11, St Louis, 2022, Elsevier.)

Learning Word Elements. Studying word elements will help you understand the meanings of medical terms.

- See Table 9-1 for a list of common prefixes. The prefixes in the table are followed by a hyphen. For example: *hyper-*.
- See Table 9-2 (p. 105) for a list of common roots. Each root is followed by its combining vowel in parentheses. For example: *hem (o)*.
- See Table 9-3 (p. 106) for a list of common suffixes. The suffixes in the table are written with a hyphen at the beginning. For example: *-itis*.

TABLE 9-1	Word Elements: Prefixes		
Prefix	**Meaning**	**Prefix**	**Meaning**
a-, an-	without, no, not, lack of	intra-	within
ab-	away from	intro-	into, within
ad-	to, toward, near	leuko-	white
ante-	before, forward, in front of	macro-	large
anti-	against	mal-	bad, illness, disease
auto-	self	meg-	large
bi-	double, two (2), twice	micro-	small
brady-	slow	mono-	one (1), single
circum-	around	neo-	new
contra-	against, opposite	non-	not
cyan-	blue	olig-	small, scant
de-	down, from, off, opposite	para-	beside, beyond, after
dia-	across, through, apart	per-	by, through
dis-	apart, free from	peri-	around
dys-	bad, difficult, abnormal, painful	poly-	many, much
ecto-	outer, outside	post-	after, behind
en-	in, into, within	pre-	before, in front of, prior to
endo-	inner, inside	pro-	before, in front of
epi-	on, upon, over (Fig. 9-2, p. 104)	re-	again, backward
erythro-	red	retro-	backward, behind
eu-	normal, good, well, healthy	semi-	half
ex-	out, out of, from, away from	sub-	beneath, under (see Fig. 9-2)
hemi-	half	super-	above, over, excess
hyper-	excessive, too much, high	supra-	above, over
hypo-	under, decreased, less than normal	tachy-	fast, rapid
in-	in, into, within, not	trans-	across
inter-	between	uni-	one (1)

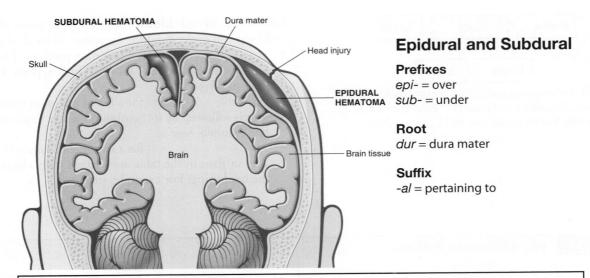

Epidural and Subdural

Prefixes

epi- = over
sub- = under

Root

dur = dura mater

Suffix

-al = pertaining to

A *prefix* is at the beginning of the word.
Changing the prefix changes the meaning of the word.

epi- + *dur* + *-al* = pertaining to <u>over</u> the dura mater (outer lining of the brain and spinal cord)

sub- + *dur* + *-al* = pertaining to <u>under</u> the dura mater (outer lining of the brain and spinal cord)

FIGURE 9-2 A prefix is at the beginning of the word. This figure shows hematomas in 2 areas of the brain. *Hematoma* means a mass of blood (*hemat* + *-oma*). *Epidural* and *subdural* describe the locations. Changing the prefix changes the meaning of the word. (Modified from Chabner D-E: *Medical terminology: a short course,* ed 8, St Louis, 2018, Elsevier.)

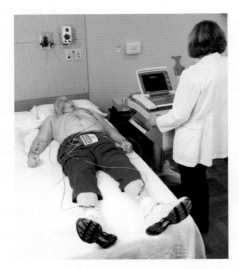

Electrocardiogram

Roots

electr (o) = electricity
cardi (o) = heart

Suffix

-gram = record

A *root* contains the basic meaning of the word.
A word can have more than 1 root.

electr (o) + ***cardi (o)*** + *-gram* = A record of the electricity in the heart

---

FIGURE 9-3 A root contains the basic meaning of the word. A word can have more than 1 root. *Electrocardiogram* has the roots *electr (o)* (meaning electricity) and *cardi (o)* (meaning heart). An electrocardiogram is a test that records the heart's electrical activity.

TABLE 9-2	Word Elements: Roots		
Root (Combining Vowel)	**Meaning**	**Root (Combining Vowel)**	**Meaning**
abdomin (o)	abdomen	men (o)	menstruation
aden (o)	gland	my (o)	muscle
adren (o)	adrenal gland	myel (o)	spinal cord, bone marrow
angi (o)	vessel	necr (o)	death
arteri (o)	artery	nephr (o)	kidney
arthr (o)	joint	neur (o)	nerve
bronch (o)	bronchus, bronchi	ocul, ophthalm (o)	eye
carcino (o)	cancerous, cancer	onc (o)	tumor
card, cardi (o)	heart (Fig. 9-3)	oophor (o)	ovary
cephal (o)	head	orth (o)	straight, normal, correct
cerebr (o)	cerebrum (largest part of the brain)	oste (o)	bone
chole, chol (o)	bile	ot (o)	ear
chondr (o)	cartilage	path (o)	disease
col, colon (o)	colon, large intestine	ped (o)	child, foot
cost (o)	rib	pharyng (o)	pharynx (throat)
crani (o)	skull	phleb (o)	vein
cyst (o)	bladder, cyst	pneum (o)	lung, air, gas
cyt (o)	cell	pod (o)	foot
dent (i)	tooth	proct (o)	rectum
derm, dermat (o)	skin	psych (o)	mind
duoden (o)	duodenum (part of the small intestine)	pulmon (o)	lung
dur (o)	dura mater (outer lining of the brain and spinal cord) (see Fig. 9-2)	py (o)	pus
		rect (o)	rectum
electr (o)	electricity (see Fig. 9-3)	ren (o)	kidney
encephal (o)	brain	rhin (o)	nose
enter (o)	intestines	salping (o)	eustachian tube, fallopian tube
fibr (o)	fiber, fibrous	splen (o)	spleen
gastr (o)	stomach	stern (o)	sternum
gloss (o)	tongue	stomat (o)	mouth
gluc (o)	sweetness, glucose (Fig. 9-4, p. 106)	therm (o)	heat
glyc (o)	sugar	thorac (o)	chest
gyn, gyne, gynec (o)	woman	thromb (o)	clot, thrombus
hem, hema, hem (o), hemat (o)	blood	thyr (o)	thyroid
hepat (o)	liver	toxic (o)	poison, poisonous
hydr (o)	water	trache (o)	trachea (windpipe)
hyster (o)	uterus	urethr (o)	urethra
ile (o)	ileum (part of the small intestine)	urin (o)	urine
ili (o)	ilium (part of the hip bone)	ur (o)	urine, urinary tract, urination
jejun (o)	jejunum (part of the small intestine)	uter (o)	uterus
lapar (o)	abdomen, loin, flank	vas (o)	blood vessel, vas deferens
laryng (o)	larynx (voice box)	vascul (o)	blood vessel
lith (o)	stone	ven (o)	vein
mamm, mast (o)	breast, mammary gland	vertebr (o)	spine, vertebrae

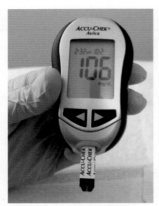

Glucometer

Root
gluc (o) = glucose

Suffix
-meter = measuring instrument

A *suffix* is at the end of the word.

gluc (o) + *-meter* = a measuring instrument for glucose

FIGURE 9-4 A suffix is at the end of the word. The suffix *-meter* means measuring instrument. A *glucometer* is a device used to measure blood glucose.

TABLE 9-3	Word Elements: Suffixes		
Suffix	**Meaning**	**Suffix**	**Meaning**
-ac, -al	pertaining to (see Fig. 9-2)	-oma	tumor, mass
-algia	pain	-opsy	to view
-asis	condition, usually abnormal	-osis	condition
-cardia	heart action or location	-pathy	disease
-cele	hernia, herniation, pouching	-penia	lack, deficiency
-centesis	surgical puncture to remove fluid	-phagia	to eat or consume, swallowing
-cyte	cell	-phasia	speaking, speech
-ectasis	dilation, stretching	-phobia	an exaggerated fear
-ectomy	excision, removal of	-plasty	surgical repair or re-shaping
-emesis	vomiting	-plegia	paralysis
-emia, emic	blood condition	-pnea	breathing, respiration
-genesis	development, production, creation	-ptosis	falling, sagging, dropping down
-genic	producing, causing	-rrhage, rrhagia	excessive flow
-gram	record (see Fig. 9-3)	-rrhaphy	stitching, suturing
-graph	a diagram, a recording instrument	-rrhea	flow, discharge
-graphy	making a recording	-sclerosis	hardening
-iasis	condition of	-scope	examination instrument
-ic	pertaining to	-scopy	examination using a scope
-ism	a condition	-stasis	maintenance, maintaining a constant level, controlling, stopping
-itis	inflammation		
-logy	the study of	-stenosis	narrowing
-lysis	breakdown, destruction of, decomposition	-stomy, -ostomy	creation of an opening
-megaly	enlargement	-tomy, -otomy	incision, cutting into
-mentia	condition of the mind	-trophy	growth, development, nourishment
-meter	measuring instrument (see Fig. 9-4)	-uria	urine

Defining Medical Terms

Medical terms are formed by combining word elements. Remember, prefixes are at the beginning. Suffixes are at the end. A root can be combined with prefixes, roots, and suffixes. Some words have only a prefix and suffix.

The combining vowel of a root is usually used between roots and when the suffix begins with a consonant. When the suffix begins with a vowel (a, e, i, o, u), the combining vowel is not used.

To define a term, separate the word into its elements (Table 9-4). To read the meaning:

1 Begin with the suffix. Read the meaning of the suffix.
2 Go to the beginning of the word. Read the meaning of each word part up to the suffix.

For some terms with only a prefix and suffix, it is easier to read the meaning of the prefix first. Then read the meaning of the suffix.

TABLE 9-4	Defining Medical Terms	
Medical Term	**Word Elements**	**Definition**
Aphasia	*a-* (without, lack of) + *-phasia* (speaking) [prefix] [suffix]	Lack of speaking ability
Cyanosis	*cyan-* (blue) + *-osis* (condition) [prefix] [suffix]	Condition of having a bluish color
Dysphagia	*dys-* (difficult) + *-phagia* (swallowing) [prefix] [suffix]	Difficulty swallowing
Dyspnea	*dys-* (difficult, painful) + *-pnea* (breathing) [prefix] [suffix]	Difficult or painful breathing
Endocarditis	*endo-* (inner) + *card* (heart) + *-itis* (inflammation) [prefix] [root] [suffix]	Inflammation of the inner part of the heart
Gastrostomy	*gastr* (stomach) + *-ostomy* (creation of an opening) [root] [suffix]	A surgically created opening in the stomach
Mastectomy	*mast* (breast) + *-ectomy* (excision or removal) [root] [suffix]	Removal of a breast
Nephritis	*nephr* (kidney) + *-itis* (inflammation) [root] [suffix]	Inflammation of the kidney
Oliguria	*olig-* (scant, small amount) + *-uria* (urine) [prefix] [suffix]	A small amount of urine

ABDOMINAL REGIONS

The abdomen can be divided into 4 quadrants. *Quad* means 4. The quadrants are used to describe the location of body structures, pain, or discomfort. The quadrants are shown in Figure 9-5. They are:

- Right upper quadrant (RUQ)—contains much of the liver, the gallbladder, part of the pancreas, and parts of the small and large intestines
- Left upper quadrant (LUQ)—contains the rest of the liver, the stomach, the spleen, the rest of the pancreas, and parts of the small and large intestines
- Right lower quadrant (RLQ)—contains parts of the small and large intestines, the appendix, and part of the bladder
- Left lower quadrant (LLQ)—contains parts of the small and large intestines and part of the bladder.

You will learn about the body structures found in these areas in Chapter 10.

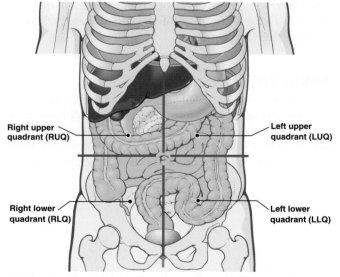

FIGURE 9-5 The 4 abdominal quadrants. (From Chabner D-E: *The language of medicine*, ed 12, St Louis, 2021, Elsevier.)

DIRECTIONAL TERMS

Certain terms describe the location of 1 body part in relation to another. These terms give the direction of the body part when a person is standing and facing forward. The arms are stretched out with the thumbs pointing outward. See Figure 9-6.

- *Anterior (ventral)*—at or toward the front of the body or body part
- *Posterior (dorsal)*—at or toward the back of the body or body part
- *Proximal*—the part nearest to the center or to the point of attachment
- *Distal*—the part farthest from the center or from the point of attachment
- *Lateral*—away from the mid-line; at the side of the body or body part
- *Medial*—at or near the middle or mid-line of the body or body part
- *Superior*—above another structure
- *Inferior*—below another structure
- *Superficial*—on the surface
- *Deep*—below the surface

POSITIONAL TERMS

These terms describe the position of the body when lying down (Chapter 19).

- *Supine*—lying flat and facing up
- *Prone*—lying flat and facing down
- *Semi-prone*—lying on the side of the abdomen
- *Lateral*—lying on the side
- *Fowler's*—lying on the back with the head of the bed raised

In Fowler's position, the head of the bed is raised between 45 and 60 degrees. Variations of Fowler's include *semi-Fowler's* (the head of the bed is only raised 30 degrees) and *high-Fowler's* (the head of the bed is raised 60 to 90 degrees). See Chapter 19.

ABBREVIATIONS

Abbreviations are shortened forms of words or phrases. They save time and space when recording. Each agency has a list of allowed abbreviations. Obtain the list when you are hired. Use only those on the list. If not sure about an abbreviation, write the term out in full. This promotes clear communication.

See Table 9-5 for a list of common abbreviations that you may see. Chapters containing important abbreviations have a "Key Abbreviations" list at the beginning of the chapter. See p. 930 for a full list of all of the Key Abbreviations used in the book.

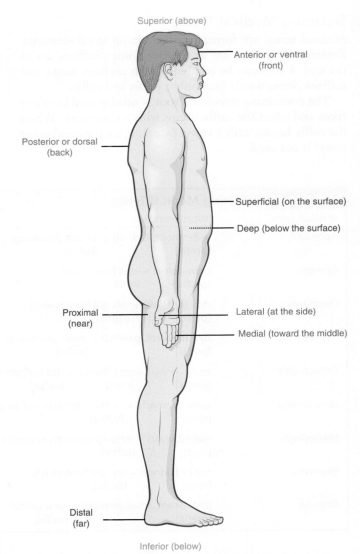

FIGURE 9-6 Directional terms describe the location of 1 body part in relation to another. (Modified from Chabner D-E: *The language of medicine*, ed 12, St Louis, 2021, Elsevier.)

TABLE 9-5   Common Abbreviations

Abbreviation	Meaning	Abbreviation	Meaning
abd	abdomen	lt; L	left
AC; a.c.	before meals	meds	medications
ADL	activities of daily living	mid noc	midnight
ad lib	as desired	min	minute
AED	automated external defibrillator	mL	milliliter
AIDS	acquired immunodeficiency syndrome	neg	negative
AM	morning	noc	night
AMB; amb	ambulate (to walk); ambulatory (able to walk)	NPO; npo	nothing by mouth (nil per os)
amt	amount	O_2	oxygen
ap; AP	apical	OOB	out of bed
bid; b.i.d.	2 times a day	OR	operating room
BM; bm	bowel movement	os	mouth
BP	blood pressure	OT	occupational therapy
BRP	bathroom privileges	oz; OZ	ounce
c̄	with	PC; p.c.	after meals
C	centigrade; Celsius	per	by, through
cal	calories	PM	afternoon
cath	catheter	PO; po	by mouth; orally
CBR	complete bed rest	prep	preparation
C/O; c/o	complains of	prn	when necessary
CPR	cardiopulmonary resuscitation	Pt; pt	patient
CS	central service; central supply	PT	physical therapy
drsg	dressing	q	every
Dx	diagnosis	qh	every hour
ECG; EKG	electrocardiogram	q2h, q3h, etc.	every 2 hours, every 3 hours, and so on
ER; ED	emergency room; emergency department	qid; q.i.d.	4 times a day
F	Fahrenheit	R	rectal temperature, respiration
fl; fld	fluid	R/O	rule out
Fx	fracture	ROM	range of motion; range-of-motion
GI	gastro-intestinal	rt; R	right
h; hr	hour	s̄	without
H_2O	water	Spec; spec	specimen
HIV	human immunodeficiency virus	stat	at once, immediately
ht	height	tbsp	tablespoon
hx	history	tid; t.i.d.	3 times a day
ICU	intensive care unit	TPR	temperature, pulse, and respirations
I&O	intake and output	tsp	teaspoon
IV	intravenous	UA; U/A; u/a	urinalysis
L	liter	UTI	urinary tract infection
Lab	laboratory	VS; vs	vital signs
lb	pound	w/c	wheelchair
LOC	level of consciousness	Wt; wt	weight

COMMON TERMS AND PHRASES

Some terms and phrases apply to basic care, safety, or the person's condition. Because they are used throughout this book, they are defined in Table 9-6. Some are presented as key terms in other chapters.

TABLE 9-6	Common Health Care Terms and Phrases
Term	Definition
abnormal	Different from what is normal or usual
activities of daily living (ADL)	The activities usually done during a normal day in a person's life
adaptive (assistive) device	Any item used by the person or staff to promote the person's function or safety (hand rails, grab bars, mechanical lifts, canes, walkers, wheelchairs, devices for eating or dressing, and so on)
aphasia	The total or partial loss (a) of the ability to use or understand language (phasia)
atrophy	The decrease (a) in size or the wasting away of tissue (trophy)
biological sex	Male or female
call light	Part of the call system allowing the person to signal the nurses' station for help
care plan	A written guide about the person's care
chronic	An on-going illness that is slow or gradual in onset; it has no known cure; it can be controlled and complications prevented with proper treatment
cognitive function	Involves memory, thinking, reasoning, ability to understand, judgment, and behavior
contracture	The lack of joint mobility caused by abnormal shortening of a muscle
dementia	The loss (de) of cognitive function (mentia) that interferes with daily life and activities; it is caused by changes in the brain (Chapter 54)
dependent	Relying on others to meet one's needs
drug	A substance taken by mouth, injected, or applied to treat or prevent a disease or condition; medication, medicine
dysphagia	Difficulty (dys) swallowing (phagia)
dyspnea	Difficult, labored, or painful (dys) breathing (pnea)
feces	The semi-solid mass of waste products in the colon that is expelled through the anus; stool or stools
fever	Elevated body temperature
immobility	The inability to move
incontinence	Not being able to control urination (urinary incontinence) or bowel movements (fecal incontinence)
independent	Not relying on others; able to meet one's own needs
mobility	The ability to move
orientation; oriented	Awareness of one's self and others, one's location, and the time; or awareness of one's surroundings
perineal	The genital and anal areas
pressure injury	Localized damage to the skin and underlying soft tissue; the injury is usually over a bony prominence or related to a medical or other device and results from pressure or pressure in combination with shear
range of motion (ROM)	The movement of a joint to the extent possible without causing pain
stool, stools	Excreted feces
unconscious	Being unaware of one's setting and being unable to react or respond to people, places, or things
vital signs	Temperature, pulse, respirations, and blood pressure (and pulse oximetry [Chapter 44] and pain in some agencies)
voiding	Emptying urine from the bladder; urinating, urination

FOCUS ON **PRIDE**

The Person, Family, and Yourself

Personal and Professional Responsibility

To communicate in health care you must learn medical terms. You may feel overwhelmed at first. Start by learning the word elements. Study a little at a time. Use a medical dictionary for words you do not understand and to learn new words. You will understand more as you study body structure, care measures, and disorders.

Rights and Respect

The person must be given information in understandable language. The person may not know medical terms. Use familiar words when talking to the patient or resident.

Independence and Social Interaction

Only use abbreviations allowed by your agency. Social media and texting abbreviations are not used in your work.

Delegation and Teamwork

Assignment sheets often include medical terms and abbreviations. (See "Assignment Sheets" in Chapter 8.) Review the assignment sheet example on p. 93. Do you understand the sheet better? Take pride in learning.

Ethics and Laws

Never be afraid to ask for a term or abbreviation to be explained. You must know the meaning to provide safe care. A careful person asks for needed help. Negligence results when reasonable care is not taken and the person is harmed.

FOCUS ON **PRIDE**: *Application*

Identify ways to study word elements and medical terms. How do you plan to study? Do you study better alone or with someone? Ask other students how they plan to learn.

REVIEW QUESTIONS

Circle the BEST answer.

1 To define a medical term, what do you do *first?*
a Read the meaning of the root.
b Read the meaning of the suffix.
c Separate the word into its parts.
d Read the meaning of the prefix.

2 A suffix is
a Placed at the beginning of a word
b Placed at the end of a word
c A shortened form of a word or phrase
d The main meaning of the word

3 The prefix *hypo-* means
a Less than normal
b Difficult
c Large
d Half

4 The root *vascul (o)* means
a Vertebrae
b Air
c Blood vessel
d Heat

5 The suffix *-algia* means
a Paralysis
b Pain
c Disease
d Removal of

6 Which word means a blood condition involving too much sugar?
a Hepatitis (hepat-itis)
b Tachycardia (tachy-cardia)
c Hyperglycemia (hyper-glyc-emia)
d Hemolysis (hemo-lysis)

7 Which word means an excessive flow of blood?
a Hemiplegia (hemi-plegia)
b Cyanosis (cyan-osis)
c Laparoscopy (laparo-scopy)
d Hemorrhage (hemo-rrhage)

8 Which word means examination of the bladder using a scope?
a Ileostomy (ileo-stomy)
b Colonoscopy (colono-scopy)
c Tracheostomy (tracheo-stomy)
d Cystoscopy (cysto-scopy)

9 The stomach is located in the
a RUQ (right upper quadrant)
b LUQ (left upper quadrant)
c RLQ (right lower quadrant)
d LLQ (left lower quadrant)

10 Which description is *correct?*
a Proximal means far away.
b Inferior means inside.
c Anterior means toward the back.
d Lateral means at the side.

11 You are studying the heart. A structure is described as "superior." This means it is
a Below another structure
b Above another structure
c More important than other structures
d Inside another structure

12 Which is *true?*
a The shoulder is proximal and the wrist is distal.
b The toes are posterior.
c The brain is superficial.
d The thumb is on the medial side of the hand.

13 You are told to place a person in the lateral position. You
a Help the person lie flat
b Raise the head of the bed
c Turn the person onto the side
d Move the person to the side of the bed

14 You must complete a task *stat.* "Stat" means
a At once, immediately
b As desired
c Without moving the person
d When necessary, as needed

Continued

15 What are ADL?
a The activities a person does daily
b Devices used to assist with care
c Foods allowed on the person's diet
d Drugs a person takes daily

16 You see I&O on your assignment sheet. I&O means
a Inside and outside
b Intervention and outcome
c Intake and output
d Inspect and observe

17 Your assignment sheet says VS q4h. You will
a Refuse the task because it involves giving drugs
b Have the person void 4 times during your shift
c Do a visual safety check 4 times an hour
d Measure vital signs every 4 hours

18 Moving a person's joints to the extent possible without causing pain is called
a Physical therapy (PT)
b Range of motion (ROM)
c Cardiopulmonary resuscitation (CPR)
d Occupational therapy (OT)

19 A person with dementia has
a Difficulty swallowing
b Painful or difficult breathing
c Damage to the skin and tissues
d Loss of cognitive and social function

20 Which definition is *correct*?
a *Contracture* is the decrease in size or wasting away of tissue.
b *Perineal* is the genital and anal areas.
c *Feces* is an elevated body temperature.
d *Pressure injury* is a lack of joint mobility caused by shortening of a muscle.

21 Incontinence is a term meaning
a Inability to control urination or bowel movements
b Lack of awareness of surroundings
c Damage to the skin and tissues
d Inability to use or understand language

22 A care plan lists care measures for aphasia and dysphagia. You know that
a These mean the same thing
b *a-* means with and *dys-* means without
c *-phasia* means speaking and *-phagia* means swallowing
d *-phasia* means breathing and *-phagia* means speaking

Answers to Chapter 9 questions are on p. 901.

Answers to Chapter 9 questions are on p. 901.

FOCUS ON PRACTICE

Problem Solving

You are training in the clinical setting. A person has an *NPO* sign above the bed. You do not remember what "NPO" means. What will you do? Why is it important for you to know?

Body Structure and Function

OBJECTIVES

- Define the key terms and key abbreviations in this chapter.
- Explain the organization of the body.
- Identify the basic structures of the cell.
- Describe how cells divide.

- Describe 4 types of tissues.
- Identify the structures and functions of each body system.
- Explain how to promote PRIDE in the person, the family, and yourself.

KEY TERMS

artery A blood vessel that carries blood away from the heart

capillary A very tiny blood vessel; nutrients, oxygen, and other substances pass from capillaries into the cells

cell The basic unit of body structure

digestion The process that breaks down food physically and chemically so it can be absorbed for use by the cells

hemoglobin The substance in red blood cells that carries oxygen and gives blood its red color

hormone A chemical substance secreted by the endocrine glands into the bloodstream

immunity Protection against a disease or condition; the person will not get or be affected by the disease

joint The point at which 2 or more bones meet to allow movement

menstruation The process in which the lining of the uterus (endometrium) breaks up and is discharged from the body through the vagina

metabolism How the body uses nutrients to provide energy and maintain body functions

organ Groups of tissue that function together

peristalsis The alternating contraction and relaxation of muscles that moves food through the digestive system

reflex The body's response to a stimulus that does not require conscious thought

respiration The process of supplying cells with oxygen and removing carbon dioxide from them

stimulus Anything that causes a body part to respond

system Organs that work together to perform certain functions

tissue A group of cells with similar functions

vein A blood vessel that returns blood to the heart

KEY ABBREVIATIONS

CNS	Central nervous system		**O$_2$**	Oxygen
CO$_2$	Carbon dioxide		**PNS**	Peripheral nervous system
GI	Gastro-intestinal		**RBC**	Red blood cell
mL	Milliliter		**WBC**	White blood cell

Ideally, the human body is in *homeostasis*—a steady state. (*Homeo* means sameness. *Stasis* means maintenance.) Various body functions and processes work to promote health and survival. Homeostasis is affected by illness, disease, and injury.

Knowing the body's normal structure (*anatomy*) and function (*physiology*) will help you understand signs, symptoms, and the reasons for care and procedures. You will give safe and more effective care.

See Chapter 12 for the changes in body structure and function that occur with aging.

ORGANIZATION OF THE BODY

Cells are the most basic structure in the body. Groups of cells form *tissues*. Groups of tissue form *organs*. Organs that work together form *body systems*. See Figure 10-1, p. 114.

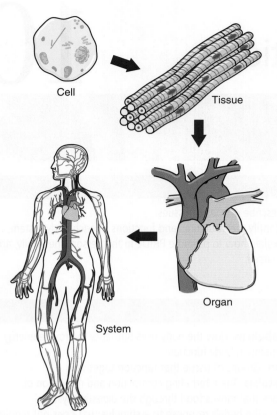

FIGURE 10-1 Organization of the body.

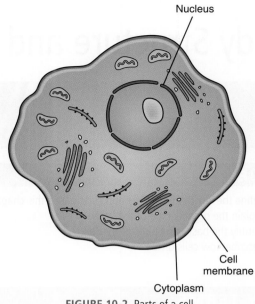

FIGURE 10-2 Parts of a cell.

Cells

The basic unit of body structure is the *cell*. Cells have the same basic structure. Function, size, and shape may differ. Cells are very small. You need a microscope to see them. Cells need water, oxygen (O_2), and nutrients to live and function. Nutrients include proteins, fats, carbohydrates, vitamins, and minerals (Chapter 30).

Figure 10-2 shows the cell and its structures. The *cell membrane* is the outer covering. It encloses the cell and helps hold the cell's shape. The *nucleus* is the control center of the cell. It directs the cell's activities. The nucleus is in the center of the cell. The *cytoplasm* is a gelatin-like substance much like an egg white that surrounds the nucleus. Cytoplasm contains small structures *(organelles)* that perform cell functions.

Chromosomes are thread-like structures in the nucleus. Each cell has 46 chromosomes. Chromosomes contain *genes*. Genes control the traits children inherit from their parents. Height, eye color, and skin color are examples.

The nucleus controls cell reproduction. Cells reproduce by dividing in half. The process of cell division is called *mitosis* (Fig. 10-3). It is needed for tissue growth and repair. During mitosis, the 46 chromosomes arrange themselves in 23 pairs. As the cell divides, the 23 pairs are pulled in half. The 2 new cells are identical. Each has 46 chromosomes.

Tissues

Cells are the body's building blocks. Groups of cells with similar functions combine to form *tissues*.

- *Epithelial tissue* covers internal and external body surfaces. Tissue lining the nose, mouth, respiratory tract, stomach, and intestines is epithelial tissue. So are the skin, hair, nails, and glands. *Glands* secrete (release) substances that perform specific functions in the body.
- *Connective tissue* anchors, connects, and supports other tissues. It is in every part of the body. Bones, tendons, ligaments, and cartilage are connective tissue. Blood is a form of connective tissue.
- *Muscle tissue* stretches and contracts to let the body move.
- *Nerve tissue* receives and carries impulses to the brain and back to body parts.

A *membrane* is a thin sheet of epithelial or connective tissue. Membranes cover body surfaces and organs and line body cavities (areas that contain organs). *Mucous membranes* are 1 type of membrane. These membranes line areas of the body that open to the outside. The linings of the ears, nose, and mouth are examples. Mucous membranes secrete *mucus*—a watery substance that coats and protects cells. In some areas, mucus helps trap contaminants.

Organs and Body Systems

Groups of tissue that function together form *organs*. An organ has 1 or more functions. Examples of organs are the heart, brain, liver, lungs, and kidneys. *Systems* are formed by organs that work together to perform certain functions (see Fig. 10-1). This chapter explains the basic structure and function of the body's systems.

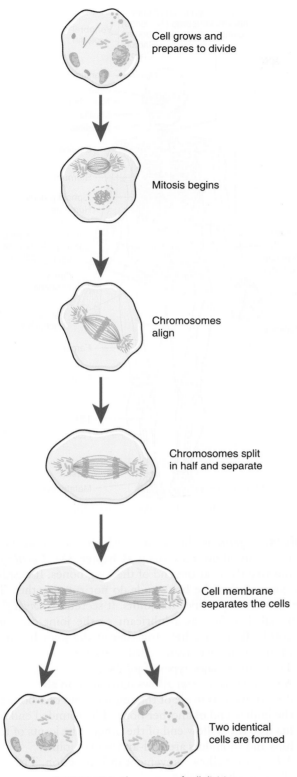

FIGURE 10-3 The process of cell division.

Cell grows and prepares to divide

Mitosis begins

Chromosomes align

Chromosomes split in half and separate

Cell membrane separates the cells

Two identical cells are formed

THE INTEGUMENTARY SYSTEM

The *integumentary system*, or *skin*, is the largest system. *Integument* means covering. The skin covers the body. It has epithelial, connective, and nerve tissue. It also has oil glands and sweat glands. There are 2 skin layers (Fig. 10-4).

- The *epidermis* is the outer layer. It has living cells and dead cells. The dead cells were once deeper in the epidermis. They were pushed upward as the cells divided. Dead cells constantly flake off. They are replaced by living cells. Living cells die and flake off. Living cells of the epidermis contain *pigment*. Pigment gives skin its color. The epidermis has no blood vessels and few nerve endings.
- The *dermis* is the inner layer. It is made up of connective tissue. Blood vessels, nerves, sweat glands, and oil glands are found in the dermis. So are hair roots.

The epidermis and dermis are supported by *subcutaneous tissue*. The subcutaneous tissue is a thick layer of fat and connective tissue.

Oil glands and *sweat glands*, *hair*, and *nails* are skin appendages.

- Hair—covers the entire body, except the palms of the hands and the soles of the feet. Hair in the nose and ears and around the eyes protects these organs from dust, insects, and other foreign objects.
- Nails—protect the tips of the fingers and toes. Nails help fingers pick up and handle small objects.
- Sweat glands *(sudoriferous glands)*—help the body regulate temperature. Sweat consists of water, salt, and a small amount of waste. Sweat is secreted through pores in the skin. The body is cooled as sweat evaporates.
- Oil glands *(sebaceous glands)*—lie near the hair shafts. They secrete an oily substance into the space near the hair shaft. Oil travels to the skin surface. This helps keep the hair and skin soft and shiny.

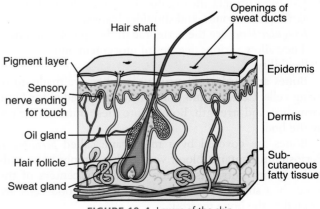

Hair shaft

Openings of sweat ducts

Pigment layer

Sensory nerve ending for touch

Oil gland

Hair follicle

Sweat gland

Epidermis

Dermis

Sub-cutaneous fatty tissue

FIGURE 10-4 Layers of the skin.

Functions of the Skin

The skin has many functions.

- It is the body's protective covering.
  - It prevents microorganisms and other substances from entering the body.
  - It is waterproof. It prevents excess amounts of water from leaving the body.
  - It protects organs from injury.
  - It helps protect the body from the sun's harmful rays.
- Nerve endings in the skin sense both pleasant and unpleasant stimulation. Nerve endings are over the entire body. They sense cold, pain, touch, and pressure to protect the body from injury.
- It helps regulate body temperature. Blood vessels *dilate* (widen) when temperature outside the body is high. More blood is brought to the body surface for cooling during evaporation. When blood vessels constrict (narrow), the body retains heat. This is because less blood reaches the skin.
- It excretes (rids the body of) waste substances through sweat.
- It is involved in the body's production of vitamin D.

THE MUSCULO-SKELETAL SYSTEM

The *musculo-skeletal system* provides the framework for the body. It lets the body move. This system also protects internal organs and gives the body shape.

Bones

The human body has 206 *bones* (Fig. 10-5). There are 4 types of bones.

- *Long bones* bear the body's weight. Leg bones are long bones.
- *Short bones* allow skill and ease in movement. Bones in the wrists, fingers, ankles, and toes are short bones.
- *Flat bones* protect the organs. They include the ribs, skull, pelvic bones, and shoulder blades.
- *Irregular bones* are the vertebrae in the spinal column. They allow various degrees of movement and flexibility.

Bones are hard, rigid structures. They are made up of living cells. Calcium and phosphorus are needed for bone formation and strength. Bones store these minerals for use by the body.

Bones are covered by a membrane called *periosteum*. Periosteum contains blood vessels that supply bone cells with O$_2$ and nutrients. Inside the hollow centers of the bones is a substance called *bone marrow*. Blood cells are formed in the bone marrow.

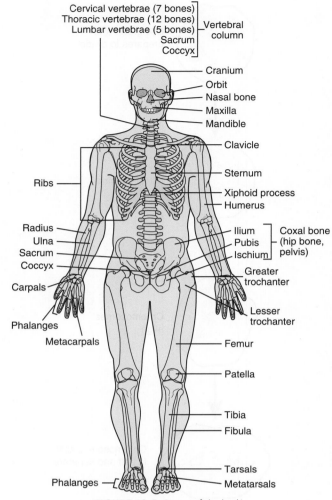

FIGURE 10-5 Bones of the body.

Joints. A *joint* is the point at which 2 or more bones meet. Joints allow movement (Chapter 35). *Cartilage* is connective tissue at the end of the long bones. It cushions the joint so that the bone ends do not rub together. The *synovial membrane* lines the joints. It secretes *synovial fluid*. Synovial fluid acts as a lubricant so the joint can move smoothly. Bones are held together at the joint by strong bands of connective tissue called *ligaments*.

There are 3 major types of joints (Fig. 10-6).

- A *ball-and-socket joint* allows movement in all directions. It is made of the rounded end of 1 bone and the hollow end of another bone. The rounded end of 1 fits into the hollow end of the other. The joints of the hips and shoulders are ball-and-socket joints.
- A *hinge joint* allows movement in 1 direction. The elbow is a hinge joint.
- A *pivot joint* allows turning from side to side. A pivot joint connects the skull to the spine.

Some joints cannot move. They connect the bones of the skull.

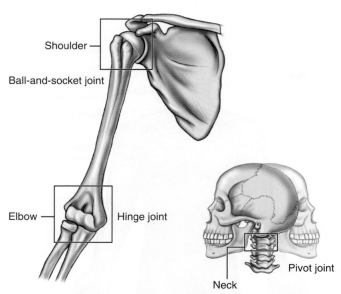

FIGURE 10-6 Types of joints. (Modified from Herlihy B: *The human body in health and illness,* ed 7, St Louis, 2022, Elsevier.)

Muscles

The body has over 500 *muscles* (Figs. 10-7 and 10-8). Some are voluntary. Others are involuntary.

- *Voluntary muscles* can be consciously controlled. Muscles attached to bones *(skeletal muscles)* are voluntary. Arm muscles do not work unless you move your arm; likewise for leg muscles. Skeletal muscles are *striated.* That is, they look striped or streaked.
- *Involuntary muscles* work automatically. You cannot control them. They control the action of the stomach, intestines, blood vessels, and other body organs. Involuntary muscles also are called *smooth muscles.* They look smooth, not streaked or striped.
- *Cardiac muscle* is in the heart. It is an involuntary muscle. However, it appears striated like skeletal muscle.

  Muscles have 3 functions.
- Movement of body parts
- Maintenance of posture or muscle tone
- Production of body heat

Strong, tough connective tissues called *tendons* connect muscles to bones. When muscles *contract* (shorten), tendons at each end of the muscle cause the bone to move. The body has many tendons. See the Achilles tendon in Figure 10-8. Some muscles constantly contract to maintain posture. When muscles contract, they use energy. Heat is produced. The more muscle activity, the greater the amount of heat produced. Shivering is how the body produces heat when exposed to cold. Shivering is from rapid, general muscle contractions.

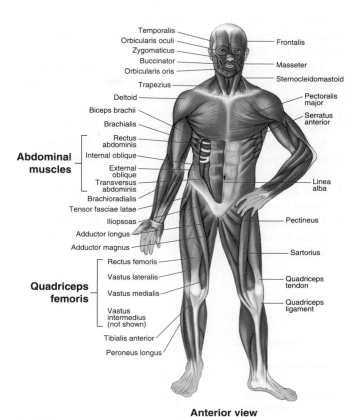

Anterior view

FIGURE 10-7 Anterior view of the muscles of the body. (Modified from Herlihy B: *The human body in health and illness,* ed 7, St Louis, 2022, Elsevier.)

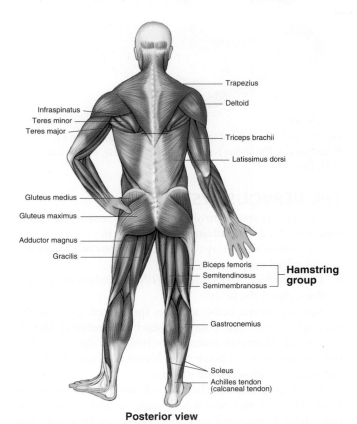

Posterior view

FIGURE 10-8 Posterior view of the muscles of the body. (From Herlihy B: *The human body in health and illness,* ed 7, St Louis, 2022, Elsevier.)

Sphincters are circular bands of muscle fibers. They *constrict* (narrow) a passage. Or they close a natural body opening. For example:

- The *lower esophageal sphincter* (Fig. 10-9) is between the esophagus and the stomach. It prevents food from moving back up into the esophagus.
- The *pyloric sphincter* (see Fig. 10-9) is an opening from the stomach into the small intestine. Closed, it holds food in the stomach for partial digestion. It opens to allow partially digested food to enter the small intestine.
- The *anal sphincter* keeps the anus closed. It opens for a bowel movement.
- *Urethral sphincters* seal off the bladder. This allows urine to collect in the bladder. The sphincters open for urination.

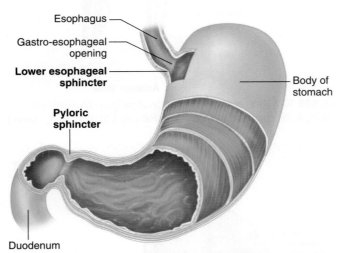

FIGURE 10-9 Examples of sphincters. (Redrawn from Patton KT, Thibodeau GA: *The human body in health and disease*, ed 7, St Louis, 2018, Elsevier.)

THE NERVOUS SYSTEM

The *nervous system* controls, directs, and coordinates body functions. Its 2 main divisions are shown in Figure 10-10.

- The *central nervous system (CNS)* consists of the brain and spinal cord.
- The *peripheral nervous system (PNS)* involves the nerves throughout the body.

Neurons (nerve cells) are the specialized cells in the nervous system that conduct (send and receive) signals (impulses). *Neurotransmitters* are chemicals that allow signals to pass between nerve cells. Nerve cells can also transmit signals to muscles and glands.

Nerves are groupings (bundles) of nerve cells. Nerves are easily damaged and take a long time to heal. Some nerve fibers have a protective covering called a *myelin sheath*. The myelin sheath also insulates the nerve fiber. Nerve fibers covered with myelin conduct impulses faster than those fibers without it.

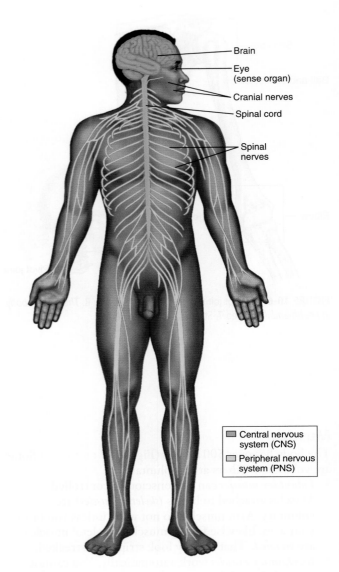

FIGURE 10-10 The nervous system is divided into the central nervous system and the peripheral nervous system. (Modified from Patton KT, Bell F, Thompson T, et al: *Anatomy and physiology*, ed 11, St Louis, 2022, Elsevier.)

The Central Nervous System

The *brain* and *spinal cord* make up the CNS (Fig. 10-11). The brain is covered by the skull. The 3 main parts of the brain are the *cerebrum*, the *cerebellum*, and the *brainstem* (Fig. 10-12).

The *cerebrum* is the largest part of the brain. It is the center of thought and intelligence. The outside of the cerebrum is called the *cerebral cortex*. It controls the highest functions of the brain. These include reasoning, memory, consciousness, speech, voluntary muscle movement, vision, hearing, sensation, and other activities.

The cerebrum is divided into 2 halves called *right* and *left hemispheres*. The right hemisphere controls movement and activities on the body's left side. The left hemisphere controls the right side. The hemispheres are connected by a pathway that allows communication between them. Each hemisphere is divided into 4 major sections, called *lobes—frontal, parietal, temporal,* and *occipital*. Different areas are responsible for different functions.

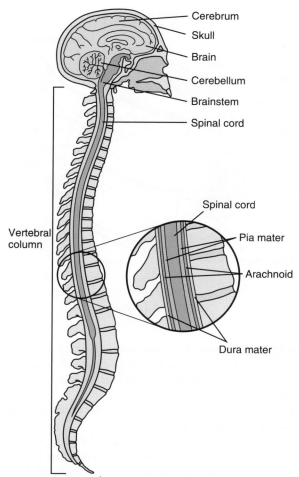

FIGURE 10-11 Central nervous system.

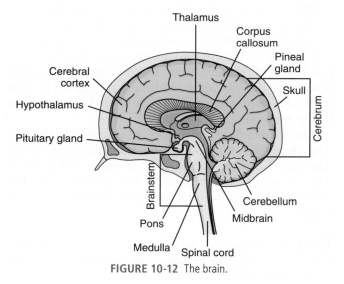

FIGURE 10-12 The brain.

The *cerebellum* regulates and coordinates body movements. It controls balance and the smooth movements of voluntary muscles. Injury to the cerebellum results in jerky movements, loss of coordination, and muscle weakness.

The *brainstem* connects the cerebrum to the spinal cord. The brainstem contains the *midbrain, pons,* and *medulla.* The midbrain and pons relay messages between the medulla and the cerebrum. The medulla controls heart rate, breathing, blood vessel size, swallowing, coughing, and vomiting. The brain connects to the spinal cord at the lower end of the medulla.

The spinal cord lies within the spinal column. The cord is 17 to 18 inches long. It has 2 main functions.

- It contains pathways that conduct messages to and from the brain. Sensory impulses travel to the brain. Motor impulses travel from the brain to cause movement or function of a body part.
- It serves as a reflex center. A *reflex* is the body's response to a stimulus that does not require conscious thought. A *stimulus* is anything that causes a body part to respond. Reflexes are fast and involuntary. For example, you immediately pull your hand away (reflex) when it touches a hot object (stimulus).

The brain and spinal cord are covered and protected by 3 layers of connective tissue called *meninges* (see Fig. 10-11).

- The outer layer is a tough covering called the *dura mater.*
- The middle layer is the *arachnoid.*
- The inner layer is the *pia mater.*

The space between the middle layer (arachnoid) and inner layer (pia mater) is the *arachnoid space.* The space is filled with *cerebrospinal fluid.* It circulates around the brain and spinal cord. Cerebrospinal fluid protects the central nervous system. It cushions shocks that could easily injure brain and spinal cord structures.

The Peripheral Nervous System

Peripheral relates to the outer part or surrounding area of something. The nerves that spread throughout the body make up the peripheral nervous system.

- *Cranial nerves* conduct impulses between the brain and the head, neck, chest, and abdomen. They conduct impulses for smell, vision, hearing, taste, pain, touch, temperature, and pressure. They also conduct impulses for voluntary and involuntary muscles. There are 12 pairs of cranial nerves.
- *Spinal nerves* carry impulses from the skin, extremities, and internal structures not supplied by the cranial nerves. There are 31 pairs of spinal nerves, named for where they come out of the vertebral column. See Figure 10-13, p. 120.

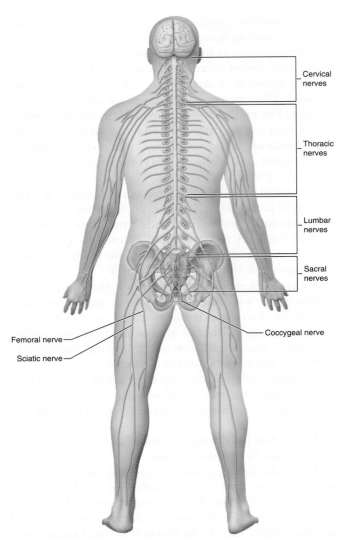

FIGURE 10-13 Spinal nerves and major nerve branches of the peripheral nervous system. (Modified from Solomon EP: *Introduction to human anatomy and physiology*, ed 4, St Louis, 2016, Saunders.)

The Autonomic Nervous System. The *autonomic nervous system* is part of the peripheral nervous system. This system controls involuntary muscles and certain body functions. The functions include the heartbeat, blood pressure, intestinal contractions, and glandular secretions. These functions occur automatically.

The autonomic nervous system is divided into the *sympathetic nervous system* and the *parasympathetic nervous system*. They balance each other. The sympathetic nervous system speeds up functions. The parasympathetic nervous system slows functions. When you are angry, scared, excited, or exercising, the sympathetic nervous system is stimulated. The parasympathetic system is activated when you relax or when the sympathetic system is stimulated for too long.

The Sense Organs

The 5 senses are *sight, hearing, taste, smell,* and *touch*. Receptors for taste are in the tongue. They are called *taste buds*. Receptors for smell are in the nose. Touch receptors are in the dermis, especially in the toes and fingertips.

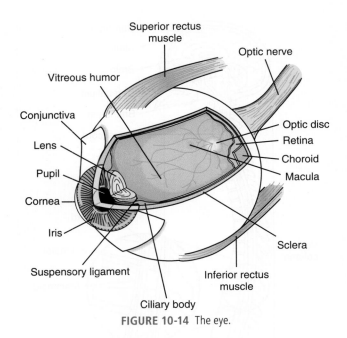

FIGURE 10-14 The eye.

The Eye. Receptors for vision are in the eyes (Fig. 10-14). The eye is easily injured. Bones of the skull, eyelids and eyelashes, and tears protect the eyes from injury.

The eye has 3 layers.
- The *sclera*, the white of the eye, is the outer layer. It is made of tough connective tissue.
- The *choroid* is the second layer. Blood vessels, the *ciliary muscle*, and the *iris* make up the choroid. The iris gives the eye its color. The opening in the middle of the iris is the *pupil*. Pupil size varies with the amount of light entering the eye. The pupil constricts (narrows) in bright light. It dilates (widens) in dim or dark places.
- The *retina* is the inner layer. It has receptors for vision and the nerve fibers of the *optic nerve*. The *macula* is a portion of the retina responsible for central vision.

Light enters the eye through the *cornea*. It is the transparent part of the outer layer that lies over the eye. Light rays pass to the *lens*, which lies behind the pupil. The light is then reflected to the retina. Light is carried to the brain by the optic nerve.

The *aqueous chamber* separates the cornea from the lens. The chamber is filled with a fluid called *aqueous humor*. The fluid helps the cornea keep its shape and position. The *vitreous humor* is behind the lens. It is a gelatin-like substance that supports the retina and maintains the eye's shape.

The Ear. The *ear* is a sense organ (Fig. 10-15). It functions in hearing and balance. The ear has 3 parts—the *external ear, middle ear,* and *inner ear*.

The external ear (outer part) is called the *pinna* or *auricle*. Sound waves are guided through the external ear into the *auditory canal*. Glands in the auditory canal secrete a waxy substance called *cerumen*. The auditory canal extends about 1 inch into the *eardrum*. The eardrum *(tympanic membrane)* separates the external and middle ear.

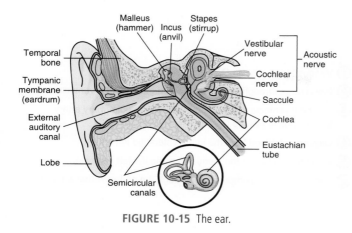

FIGURE 10-15 The ear.

The middle ear contains the *eustachian tube* and 3 small bones called *ossicles*. The eustachian tube connects the middle ear and the throat. Air enters the eustachian tube so there is equal pressure on both sides of the eardrum. The ossicles amplify sound received from the eardrum and transmit the sound to the inner ear. The 3 ossicles are:

- The *malleus*—looks like a hammer.
- The *incus*—looks like an anvil.
- The *stapes*—shaped like a stirrup.

The inner ear consists of *semicircular canals* and the *cochlea*. The cochlea contains fluid. The fluid carries sound waves from the middle ear to the *acoustic nerve*. The acoustic nerve then carries messages to the brain.

The 3 semicircular canals are involved with balance. They sense the head's position and changes in position. They send messages to the brain.

THE CIRCULATORY SYSTEM

The *circulatory system (cardiovascular system)* is made up of the *blood*, *heart*, and *blood vessels*. The heart pumps blood through the blood vessels. The circulatory system has many functions.

- Blood carries nutrients, hormones, and other substances to the cells.
- Blood transports (carries) the gases of respiration (p. 124). It brings O_2 to the cells.
- Blood removes waste products from cells.
- Blood plays a role in maintaining the body's fluid balance.
- Blood and blood vessels help regulate body temperature. The blood carries heat from muscle activity to other body parts. Blood vessels in the skin dilate to cool the body. They constrict to retain heat.
- The system produces and carries cells that defend the body from microbes that cause disease.

The Blood

The *blood* consists of blood cells and *plasma*. Plasma is mostly water. It carries blood cells to other body cells. Plasma also carries substances that cells need to function. This includes nutrients, hormones (p. 127), and chemicals.

Red blood cells (RBCs) are called *erythrocytes*. **Hemoglobin** is a substance in RBCs that carries oxygen and gives blood its red color. As RBCs circulate through the lungs, hemoglobin picks up O_2. Hemoglobin carries O_2 to the cells. When blood is bright red, hemoglobin in the RBCs is filled with O_2. As blood circulates through the body, O_2 is given to the cells. Cells release carbon dioxide (CO_2, a waste product). It is picked up by the hemoglobin. RBCs filled with CO_2 make the blood look dark red.

The body has about 25 trillion (25,000,000,000,000) RBCs. About 4½ to 5 million cells are in a cubic millimeter of blood (the size of a tiny drop). RBCs live for 3 to 4 months. They are destroyed by the liver and spleen as they wear out. New RBCs are formed in the bone marrow. About 1 million RBCs are produced every second.

White blood cells (WBCs) are called *leukocytes*. They have no color. They protect the body against infection. There are about 5,000 to 10,000 WBCs in a cubic millimeter of blood. At the first sign of infection, WBCs rush to the infection site and multiply rapidly. The number of WBCs increases when there is an infection. Formed by the bone marrow, WBCs live for about 9 days.

Platelets (thrombocytes) are needed for blood clotting. They are formed by the bone marrow. There are about 200,000 to 400,000 platelets in a cubic millimeter of blood. A platelet lives for about 4 days.

The Heart

The *heart* is a muscle. It pumps blood through the blood vessels to the tissues and cells. The heart lies in the middle to lower part of the chest cavity toward the left side (Fig. 10-16).

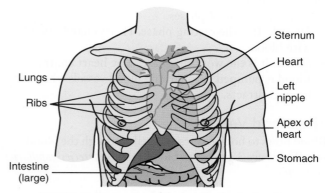

FIGURE 10-16 Location of the heart in the chest cavity.

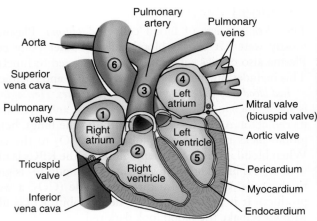

① Venous blood, poor in O$_2$, enters the right atrium.

② Blood flows through the tricuspid valve into the right ventricle.

③ The right ventricle pumps blood through the pulmonary artery to the lungs to pick up O$_2$.

④ Oxygen-rich blood from the lungs enters the left atrium.

⑤ Blood flows through the mitral valve into the left ventricle.

⑥ The left ventricle pumps blood through the aorta to other arteries.

FIGURE 10-17 Structures of the heart and blood flow through the heart.

The heart is hollow with 3 layers (Fig. 10-17).
- The *pericardium* is the outer layer. It is a thin sac covering the heart.
- The *myocardium* is the second layer. It is the thick, muscular part of the heart.
- The *endocardium* is the inner layer. A membrane, it lines the inner surface of the heart.
  The heart has 4 chambers (see Fig. 10-17).
- Upper chambers receive blood and are called *atria*. The *right atrium* receives blood from body tissues. The *left atrium* receives blood from the lungs.
- Lower chambers are called *ventricles*. Ventricles pump blood. The *right ventricle* pumps blood to the lungs for O$_2$. The *left ventricle* pumps blood to all parts of the body.

Valves are between the atria and ventricles. The valves allow blood flow in 1 direction. They prevent blood from flowing back into the atria from the ventricles. The *tricuspid valve* is between the right atrium and the right ventricle. The *mitral valve (bicuspid valve)* is between the left atrium and left ventricle.

Heart action has 2 phases.
- *Diastole.* It is the resting phase. Heart chambers fill with blood.
- *Systole.* It is the working phase. The heart contracts. Blood is pumped through the blood vessels when the heart contracts.

The Blood Vessels

Blood flows to body tissues and cells through the blood vessels. There are 3 groups of blood vessels: *arteries, capillaries,* and *veins.*

Arteries are blood vessels that carry blood away from the heart. Arterial blood is rich in O$_2$. The *aorta* is the largest artery. It receives blood directly from the left ventricle. The aorta branches into other arteries that carry blood to all parts of the body (Fig. 10-18). These arteries branch into smaller parts within the tissues. The smallest branch of an artery is an *arteriole*.

Arterioles connect to capillaries. *Capillaries* are very tiny blood vessels. Nutrients, oxygen, and other substances pass from capillaries into the cells. The capillaries pick up waste products (including CO$_2$) from the cells. Veins carry waste products back to the heart.

Veins are blood vessels that return blood to the heart. They connect to the capillaries by *venules*. Venules are small veins. Venules branch together to form veins. The many veins also branch together as they near the heart to form 2 main veins—the *inferior vena cava* and the *superior vena cava* (see Fig. 10-18). Both empty into the right atrium. The inferior vena cava carries blood from the legs and the trunk (torso—chest and abdomen). The superior vena cava carries blood from the head and the arms. Venous blood is dark red. It has little O$_2$ and a lot of CO$_2$.

Blood flow through the heart is shown in Figure 10-17. From there:
1 Arterial blood is carried to the tissues by arterioles and to the cells by capillaries.
2 Cells and capillaries exchange O$_2$ and nutrients for CO$_2$ and waste products.
3 Capillaries connect with venules. Venules carry blood that has CO$_2$ and waste products.
4 Venules form veins.
5 Veins return blood to the heart.

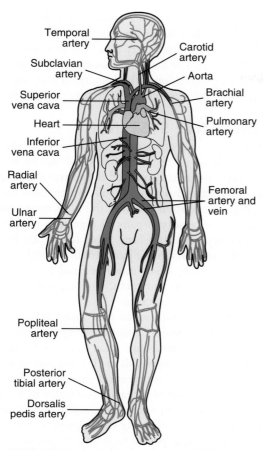

FIGURE 10-18 Arterial *(red)* and venous *(blue)* systems.

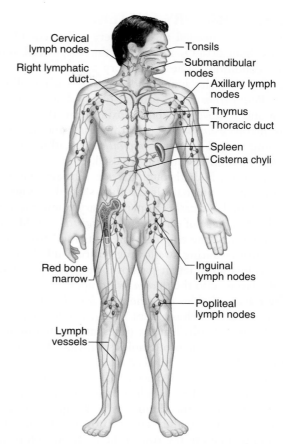

FIGURE 10-19 Lymphatic system. (From Patton KT, Thibodeau GA: *The human body in health and disease,* ed 7, St Louis, 2018, Elsevier.)

THE LYMPHATIC SYSTEM

The lymphatic (lymph) system is a complex network that transports lymph throughout the body (Fig. 10-19). *Lymph* is a clear, thin, watery fluid. Lymph contains proteins and fats from the intestines. Lymph also contains WBCs.

The lymphatic system:

- Collects extra lymph from the tissues and returns it to the blood. This helps maintain fluid balance. Water, proteins, and other substances normally leak out of the capillaries. The lymphatic system drains the extra fluid from the tissues. Otherwise, the tissues swell.
- Defends the body against infection by producing lymphocytes. *Lymphocytes* are a type of WBC that defends the body against microorganisms that cause infection (Chapter 17).
- Absorbs fats from the intestines and transports them to the blood.

Lymph is formed in the tissues. Lymph is transported by *lymphatic vessels*—lymphatic capillaries to lymphatic venules to the right lymphatic duct and the thoracic duct. Lymph then enters the blood in veins near the neck.

- The *right lymphatic duct* collects lymph from the right arm and from the right side of the head, neck, and chest. It empties into a vein on the right side of the neck.
- The *thoracic duct (left lymphatic duct)* collects lymph from the pelvis, abdomen, lower chest, and the rest of the body. It empties into a vein on the left side of the neck.

Lymph nodes are shaped like beans. They range from the size of a pinhead to as large as a lima bean. They are found in the neck, underarm, groin area, chest, abdomen, and pelvis. Usually, you cannot see or feel lymph nodes. They swell when producing more lymphocytes to fight infection.

Lymph enters lymph nodes through the lymphatic vessels. The lymph nodes filter bacteria, cancer cells, and damaged cells from the lymph. This prevents such substances from circulating throughout the body.

See Figure 10-19 for the location of the *thymus (thymus gland)*. Certain lymphocytes—T lymphocytes (T cells)—develop in the thymus. Such lymphocytes are important for immune system function (p. 128). The thymus reaches full growth at puberty. Then thymus tissue is slowly replaced by fat and connective tissue. By age 80, it is usually gone.

The *tonsils* are in the back of the throat. *Adenoids* are behind the nose. These structures trap microorganisms in the mouth and nose to help prevent infection.

The *spleen* is the largest structure in the lymphatic system. It is about the size of a fist. The spleen has a rich blood supply—about 500 milliliters (mL) (1 pint) of blood. The spleen:

- Filters and removes bacteria and other substances.
- Destroys old RBCs.
- Saves the iron found in hemoglobin when RBCs are destroyed.
- Stores blood. When needed, the blood is returned to the circulatory system.

THE RESPIRATORY SYSTEM

Oxygen (O_2) is needed to live. Every cell needs O_2. Air contains about 21% O_2. This meets the body's needs under normal conditions. The respiratory system (Fig. 10-20) brings O_2 into the lungs and removes carbon dioxide (CO_2). *Respiration* is the process of supplying cells with oxygen and removing carbon dioxide from them. Respiration involves *inhalation* (breathing in) and *exhalation* (breathing out). The terms *inspiration* (breathing in) and *expiration* (breathing out) also are used.

Air enters the body through the *nose*. The air then passes into the *pharynx* (throat). It is a tube-shaped passage-way for air and food. Air passes from the pharynx into the *larynx* (voice box). A piece of cartilage, the *epiglottis*, acts like a lid over the larynx. The epiglottis prevents food from entering the airway during swallowing. During inhalation the epiglottis lifts up to let air pass over the larynx. Air passes from the larynx into the *trachea* (windpipe).

The trachea divides into the *right bronchus* and the *left bronchus*. Each bronchus enters a lung. Upon entering the lungs, the bronchi divide many times into smaller branches called *bronchioles*. The bronchioles subdivide. They end up in tiny 1-celled air sacs called *alveoli*.

Alveoli look like small clusters of grapes. They are supplied by capillaries. The alveoli and capillaries exchange O_2 and CO_2. Blood in the capillaries picks up O_2 from the alveoli. Then the blood is returned to the left side of the heart and pumped to the rest of the body. Alveoli pick up CO_2 from the capillaries for exhalation.

The lungs are filled with alveoli, blood vessels, and nerves. Each lung is divided into lobes. The right lung has 3 lobes; the left lung has 2. The lungs are separated from the abdominal cavity by a muscle called the *diaphragm*.

Each lung is covered by a 2-layered sac called the *pleura*. One layer is attached to the lung and the other to the chest wall. The pleura secretes a very thin fluid that fills the space between the layers. The fluid prevents the layers from rubbing together during inhalation and exhalation. A bony framework made up of the ribs, sternum, and vertebrae protects the lungs.

THE DIGESTIVE SYSTEM

Digestion is the process that breaks down food physically and chemically so it can be absorbed for use by the cells. The digestive system is also called the gastro-intestinal (GI) system. The system also removes solid wastes from the body.

The digestive system involves the *alimentary canal (GI tract)* and the accessory organs of digestion (Fig. 10-21). The alimentary canal is a long tube. It extends from the mouth to the anus. Its major parts are the mouth, pharynx, esophagus, stomach, small intestine, and large intestine. Accessory organs are the teeth, tongue, salivary glands, liver, gallbladder, and pancreas.

Digestion begins in the *mouth (oral cavity)*. It receives food and prepares it for digestion. Using chewing motions, the *teeth* cut, chop, and grind food into small particles for digestion and swallowing. The *tongue* aids in chewing and swallowing. *Taste buds* on the tongue's surface contain nerve endings. Taste buds allow sweet, sour, bitter, and salty tastes to be sensed. *Salivary glands* in the mouth secrete *saliva*. Saliva moistens food particles to ease swallowing and begin digestion. During swallowing, the tongue pushes food into the *pharynx*.

The pharynx (throat) is a muscular tube. Swallowing continues as the pharynx contracts. Contraction of the pharynx pushes food into the *esophagus*. The esophagus is a muscular tube about 10 inches long. It extends from the pharynx to the *stomach*. Movement of food through the GI tract occurs because of *peristalsis*—the alternating contraction and relaxation of muscles that moves food through the digestive system.

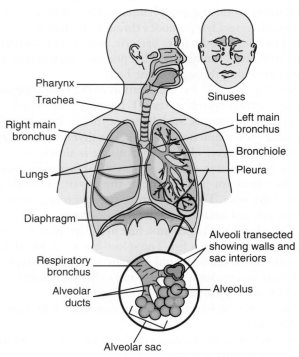

FIGURE 10-20 Respiratory system.

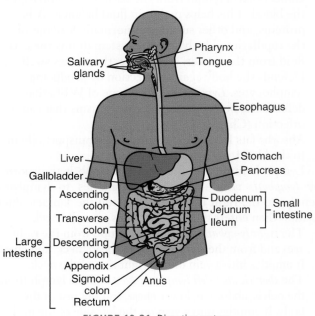

FIGURE 10-21 Digestive system.

The stomach is a muscular, pouch-like sac. It is in the upper left part of the abdominal cavity. Strong stomach muscles stir and churn food to break it up into even smaller particles. A mucous membrane lines the stomach. It contains glands that secrete *gastric juices*. Food is mixed and churned with the gastric juices to form a semi-liquid substance called *chyme*. Through peristalsis, the chyme is pushed from the stomach into the small intestine.

The *small intestine* is about 20 feet long. It has 3 parts. The first part is the *duodenum*. There, more digestive juices are added to the chyme. One is called *bile*. Bile is a greenish liquid made in the *liver*. Bile is stored in the *gallbladder*. Juices from the *pancreas* and small intestine are added to the chyme. Digestive juices chemically break down food into nutrients to be absorbed.

Peristalsis moves the chyme through the 2 other parts of the small intestine: the *jejunum* and the *ileum*. Tiny projections called *villi* line the small intestine. Villi absorb nutrients into the capillaries. Most nutrient absorption takes place in the small intestine.

Undigested chyme passes from the small intestine into the *large intestine* (*large bowel* or *colon*). The colon absorbs most of the water from the chyme. The remaining semi-solid material is called *feces*. Feces contain a small amount of water, solid wastes, and some mucus and germs. These are the waste products of digestion. Feces pass through the colon into the *rectum* by peristalsis. Feces pass out of the body through the *anus*.

THE URINARY SYSTEM

The digestive system rids the body of solid wastes. The lungs rid the body of CO_2. Water and other substances leave the body through sweat. There are other waste products in the blood.

The urinary system (Fig. 10-22):

- Removes waste products from the blood.
- Maintains water balance within the body.
- Maintains electrolyte balance. *Electrolytes* are substances that dissolve in water—sodium, potassium, calcium, and magnesium.
  - Sodium is needed for fluid balance. The body retains water if sodium levels are high. Loss of sodium (through vomiting, diarrhea, some drugs, and other causes) can result in dehydration.
  - Potassium is needed for the proper function of skeletal and cardiac muscles.
  - Calcium and magnesium are needed for normal nerve and muscle function and for bone and teeth formation.
- Maintains acid-base balance. A pH scale measures if a substance is acidic, neutral, or basic. A pH of 7 is neutral. Anything below 7 is acidic. Anything above 7 is basic. The blood must remain within a certain pH range (7.35–7.45) for normal body function.

The *kidneys* are 2 bean-shaped organs in the upper abdomen. Protected by the lower edge of the ribs, the kidneys lie against the back muscles on each side of the spine.

Each kidney has over a million tiny *nephrons* (Fig. 10-23). Each nephron is the basic working unit of the kidney. Each

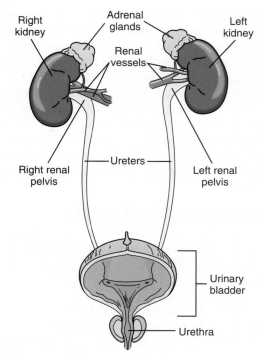

FIGURE 10-22 Urinary system.

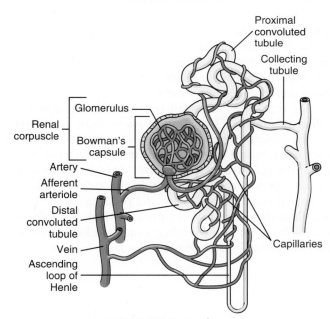

FIGURE 10-23 A nephron.

nephron has a *convoluted tubule*, which is a tiny coiled tube. Each convoluted tubule has a *Bowman's capsule* at 1 end. The capsule partly surrounds a cluster of capillaries called a *glomerulus*. Blood passes through the glomerulus and is filtered by the capillaries.

The fluid part of the blood is squeezed into the Bowman's capsule. The fluid then passes into the tubule. Most of the water and other needed substances are re-absorbed by the blood. The rest of the fluid and the waste products form *urine* in the tubule. Urine flows through the tubule to a *collecting tubule*. All collecting tubules drain into the *renal pelvis* in the kidney.

A tube called the *ureter* is attached to the renal pelvis of the kidney. Each ureter is about 10 to 12 inches long. The ureters carry urine from the kidneys to the *bladder*. The bladder is a hollow, muscular sac. It lies toward the front in the lower part of the abdominal cavity.

Urine is stored in the bladder until the need to urinate is felt. This usually occurs when there is about a half pint (250 mL) of urine in the bladder. Urine passes from the bladder through the *urethra*. The opening at the end of the urethra is called the *meatus*. Urine passes from the body through the meatus. Urine is a clear, yellowish fluid.

THE REPRODUCTIVE SYSTEM

Human reproduction results from the union of a male sex cell and a female sex cell. The male and female reproductive systems are different. This allows for the process of reproduction.

The Male Reproductive System

The male reproductive system is shown in Figure 10-24. The *testes (testicles)* are the male sex glands. Sex glands also are called *gonads*. The 2 testes are oval or almond-shaped glands. Male sex cells *(sperm)* are produced in the testes.

Testosterone, the male hormone, is produced in the testes. This hormone is needed for reproductive organ function. It also is needed for the development of the male secondary sex characteristics. There is facial hair; pubic and axillary (underarm) hair; and hair on the arms, chest, and legs. Neck and shoulder sizes increase.

The testes are suspended between the thighs in a sac called the *scrotum*. The scrotum is made of skin and muscle.

The *epididymis* is a coiled tube on top and to the side of each testis. Sperm travel from the testis to the epididymis. From the epididymis, sperm travel through a tube called the *vas deferens*. Each vas deferens joins a *seminal vesicle*. The 2 seminal vesicles store sperm and produce *semen*. Semen is a fluid that carries sperm from the male reproductive tract. The ducts of the seminal vesicles unite to form the *ejaculatory duct*. It passes through the *prostate gland*.

The prostate gland lies just below the bladder. It is shaped like a donut. The gland secretes fluid into the semen. As the ejaculatory ducts leave the prostate, they join the *urethra*. The urethra runs through the prostate gland. The urethra is the outlet for urine and semen. The urethra is contained within the *penis*.

The penis is outside of the body. The *glans* is at the end of the penis. The urethra opens at the end of the glans. A fold of skin (*prepuce* or *foreskin*) is at the end of the penis (Chapter 24).

The penis has *erectile* tissue. When a man is sexually excited, blood fills the erectile tissue. The penis enlarges and becomes hard and erect. The erect penis can enter a female's vagina. *Cowper's glands* are 2 pea-sized glands under the prostate. They produce a clear, colorless fluid before ejaculation (release of semen). The fluid cleanses the urethra, protects sperm from damage, and provides some lubrication for intercourse. With ejaculation, semen—containing sperm—is released into the vagina.

The Female Reproductive System

Figure 10-25 shows the female reproductive system. The female gonads are 2 almond-shaped glands called *ovaries*. An ovary is on each side of the uterus in the abdominal cavity.

The ovaries contain eggs called *ova*. Ova are the female sex cells. One ovum (egg) is released monthly during the woman's reproductive years. Release of an ovum is called *ovulation*.

The ovaries secrete the female hormones *estrogen* and *progesterone*. These hormones are needed for reproductive system function. They also are needed for the development of female secondary sex characteristics. These include increased breast size, pubic and axillary (underarm) hair, slight deepening of the voice, and widening and rounding of the hips.

When an ovum is released from an ovary, it travels through a *fallopian tube*. There are 2 fallopian tubes, 1 on each side. The tubes are attached at 1 end to the *uterus*. The ovum travels through the fallopian tube to the uterus.

The uterus is a hollow, muscular organ shaped like a pear. It is in the center of the pelvic cavity behind the bladder and in front of the rectum. The main part of the uterus is the *fundus*.

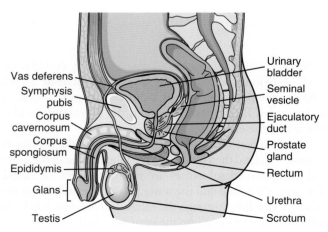

FIGURE 10-24 Male reproductive system.

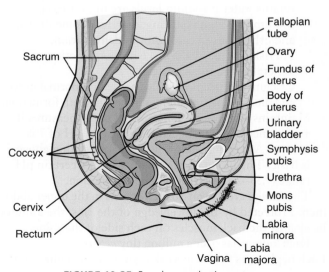

FIGURE 10-25 Female reproductive system.

The neck or narrow section of the uterus is the *cervix.* Tissue lining the uterus is the *endometrium.* The endometrium has many blood vessels. If sex cells from the male and female unite into 1 cell, that cell implants into the endometrium. There, the cell grows into a *fetus* (unborn baby) and receives nourishment.

The cervix of the uterus projects into a muscular canal called the *vagina.* The vagina opens to the outside of the body. It is just behind the urethra. The vagina receives the penis during intercourse. It also is part of the birth canal. Glands in the vaginal wall keep it moistened with secretions. The external vaginal opening is partially closed by a membrane called the *hymen.* The hymen can stretch or tear (rupture) from intercourse, injury, or surgery.

The external female genitalia are called the *vulva* (Fig. 10-26).

- The *mons pubis* is a rounded, fatty pad over a bone called the *symphysis pubis.* The mons pubis is covered with hair in the adult female.
- The *labia majora* and *labia minora* are 2 folds of tissue on each side of the vaginal opening.
- The *clitoris* is a small organ composed of erectile tissue. It becomes hard when sexually stimulated.

Menstruation. The endometrium is rich in blood to nourish the cell that grows into a fetus. If pregnancy does not occur, menstruation begins. *Menstruation* is the process in which the lining of the uterus (endometrium) breaks up and is discharged from the body through the vagina. It occurs about every 28 days. Therefore it is called the *menstrual cycle.*

The first day of the menstrual cycle begins with menstruation. Blood flows from the uterus through the vaginal opening. Menstrual flow usually lasts 3 to 7 days. Ovulation occurs during the next phase. An ovum matures in an ovary and is released. Ovulation usually occurs on or about day 14 of the cycle.

Meanwhile, estrogen and progesterone (the female hormones) are secreted by the ovaries. These hormones cause the endometrium to thicken for pregnancy. If pregnancy does not occur, the hormones decrease in amount. This causes the blood supply to the endometrium to decrease. The endometrium breaks up. It is discharged through the vagina. Another menstrual cycle begins.

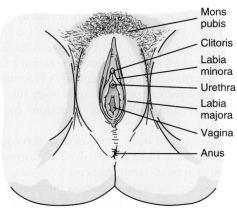

FIGURE 10-26 External female genitalia.

Mons pubis

Clitoris

Labia minora

Urethra

Labia majora

Vagina

Anus

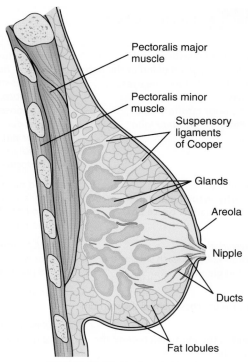

FIGURE 10-27 The female breast.

Pectoralis major muscle

Pectoralis minor muscle

Suspensory ligaments of Cooper

Glands

Areola

Nipple

Ducts

Fat lobules

Mammary Glands. The *mammary glands (breasts)* secrete milk after childbirth. Breasts are made up of glandular tissue and fat (Fig. 10-27). The milk *(breast-milk)* drains into ducts that open onto the *nipple.*

Fertilization

To reproduce, a male sex cell (sperm) must unite with a female sex cell (ovum). The uniting of the sperm and ovum into 1 cell is called *fertilization.* A sperm has 23 chromosomes. An ovum has 23 chromosomes. When the 2 cells unite, the fertilized cell has 46 chromosomes.

During intercourse, millions of sperm are deposited into the vagina. Sperm travel up the cervix, through the uterus, and into the fallopian tubes. If a sperm and an ovum unite in a fallopian tube, fertilization results. Pregnancy occurs. The fertilized cell travels down the fallopian tube to the uterus. After a short time, the fertilized cell implants into the thick endometrium and grows during pregnancy.

THE ENDOCRINE SYSTEM

The endocrine system is made up of glands called the *endocrine glands.* The endocrine glands secrete chemical substances called *hormones* into the bloodstream. Hormones regulate the activities of other organs and glands in the body. See Table 10-1 and Figure 10-28 (p. 128).

TABLE 10-1	Endocrine System
Gland	**Hormones and Actions**

Pituitary gland (master gland):
• Small, cherry-sized gland at the base of the brain behind the eyes
• 2 parts:
  • *Anterior pituitary lobe*
  • *Posterior pituitary lobe*
	Anterior pituitary lobe secretes:
	• *Growth hormone (GH)*—stimulates the growth of muscles, bones, and organs.
	• *Thyroid-stimulating hormone (TSH)*—stimulates thyroid gland function.
	• *Adrenocorticotropic hormone (ACTH)*—stimulates adrenal gland function.
	• Hormones regulating growth, development, and function of the male and female reproductive systems.
	Posterior pituitary lobe secretes:
	• *Antidiuretic hormone (ADH)*—prevents the kidneys from excreting too much water.
	• *Oxytocin*—causes uterine contractions during childbirth.

Thyroid gland: • Butterfly-shaped gland in the neck below the larynx (voice box)	*Thyroid hormone (TH)* regulates *metabolism*—how the body uses nutrients to provide energy and maintain body functions. • Too little TH causes slow body processes, slow movements, and weight gain. • Too much TH causes increased metabolism, excess energy, and weight loss.
Parathyroid glands: • 4 total—2 lie on each side of the thyroid gland	*Parathormone* regulates calcium use. Calcium is needed: • For nerve and muscle function • To prevent *tetany*—a state of severe muscle contraction and spasm that can lead to death
Thymus: • Gland in the chest behind the sternum	*Thymosin*—needed for development and function of the immune system.
Pancreas: • Gland in the abdomen behind the stomach	*Insulin*—regulates the amount of sugar in the blood available for use by the cells. Without insulin, sugar cannot enter the cells. Excess sugar builds up in the blood, causing *diabetes*.

Adrenal glands:
• 2 glands—1 on top of each kidney
• Each gland has 2 parts:
  • *Adrenal medulla* (inner part)
  • *Adrenal cortex* (outer part)
	Adrenal medulla secretes:
	• Epinephrine and norepinephrine—stimulate the body to quickly produce energy during emergencies. Heart rate, blood pressure, muscle power, and energy increase.
	Adrenal cortex secretes:
	• Glucocorticoids—regulate metabolism of carbohydrates and control the body's response to stress and inflammation.
	• Mineralocorticoids—regulate the amount of salt and water absorbed and lost by the kidneys.
	• Small amounts of male and female sex hormones.

Gonads: • Testes—male sex glands • Ovaries—female sex glands	• Male glands (testes) secrete testosterone. • Female glands (ovaries) secrete estrogen and progesterone.

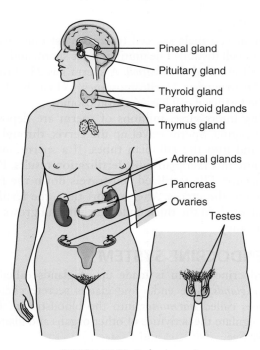

Pineal gland
Pituitary gland
Thyroid gland
Parathyroid glands
Thymus gland
Adrenal glands
Pancreas
Ovaries
Testes

FIGURE 10-28 Endocrine system.

THE IMMUNE SYSTEM

The immune system protects the body from disease and infection. Abnormal body cells can grow into tumors. Sometimes the body produces substances that cause the body to attack itself. Microorganisms (bacteria, viruses, and other germs) can cause an infection. The immune system defends against threats inside and outside the body.

The immune system gives the body immunity. *Immunity* means that a person has protection against a disease or condition. The person will not get or be affected by the disease. *Specific immunity* is the body's reaction to a certain threat. *Non-specific immunity* is the body's reaction to anything it does not recognize as a normal body substance.

Special cells and substances function to produce immunity.

- *Antibodies*—normal body substances that recognize other substances. They are involved in destroying abnormal or unwanted substances.
- *Antigens*—substances that cause an immune response. Antibodies recognize and bind with unwanted antigens. This leads to the destruction of unwanted substances and the production of more antibodies.

- *Phagocytes*—WBCs that digest and destroy microorganisms and other unwanted substances (Fig. 10-29).
- *Lymphocytes*—WBCs that produce antibodies. Lymphocyte production increases as the body responds to an infection.
  - *B lymphocytes (B cells)*—cause the production of antibodies that circulate in the plasma. The antibodies react to specific antigens.
  - *T lymphocytes (T cells)*—destroy invading cells. *Killer T cells* produce poisons near the invading cells. Some T cells attract other cells. The other cells destroy the invaders.

When the body senses an antigen from an unwanted substance, the immune system acts. Phagocyte and lymphocyte production increases. Phagocytes destroy the invaders through digestion. The lymphocytes produce antibodies that identify and destroy the unwanted substances.

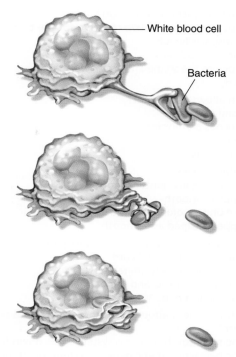

FIGURE 10-29 A phagocyte digests and destroys a microorganism. (Barbara Cousins; from Patton KT, Thibodeau GA: *Structure and function of the body*, ed 15, St Louis, 2016, Mosby.)

FOCUS ON **PRIDE**
The Person, Family, and Yourself

Personal and Professional Responsibility

Taking care of yourself is a personal and professional responsibility. A healthy diet, exercise, and rest are needed. To care for others, you need a strong and healthy body.

Rights and Respect

Patients and residents have the right to make decisions about their bodies. You may not agree with those decisions. But you must respect the person's choices. If the decision will cause no harm, comply with the request. For example, a person does not want to wear a sweater today.

If the person's decision may cause harm, tell the nurse at once. For example, a person refuses to eat. You tell the nurse. The person cannot be forced to eat. But the nurse can talk with the person about the decision, the consequences, and possible solutions.

Independence and Social Interaction

The body does not always work right. People become ill or injured. Sometimes the health team cannot prevent loss of function. Take pride in helping each person regain or maintain the highest level of function possible.

Delegation and Teamwork

The body works like a team. Each system has independent functions. But all systems interact and depend on each other. When a person has a problem with 1 body system, other systems are affected. Understanding each system and how the systems interact helps you provide better care.

Ethics and Laws

Sometimes a person is not able to make health care decisions. Spouses, parents, family members, or legal representatives may make decisions. Some persons have an advance directive (Chapter 59). Sometimes the court appoints a guardian for a short time. Finally, the agency's ethics committee may address complex issues. The person's safety and best interests must guide care decisions.

FOCUS ON **PRIDE**: *Application*

Body systems interact for normal function. Explain how the circulatory and respiratory systems interact. How might a problem in 1 system affect the other?

REVIEW QUESTIONS

Circle the BEST answer.

1 The basic unit of body structure is the
   a Cell
   b Neuron
   c Nephron
   d Ovum

2 The process of cell division is called
   a Physiology
   b Mitosis
   c Homeostasis
   d Metabolism

Continued

3 Which is a function of the skin?
a Provides the protective covering for the body
b Transports lymph
c Forms blood cells
d Provides the shape and framework for the body

4 Which allows movement?
a Bone marrow
b Mucous membranes
c Joints
d Ligaments

5 Skeletal muscles
a Are under involuntary control
b Appear smooth
c Are under voluntary control
d Appear striped and smooth

6 The central nervous system is made up of
a The brain and spinal cord
b Cranial nerves and spinal nerves
c Cervical, thoracic, and lumbar nerves
d The midbrain, pons, and medulla

7 Which statement about the autonomic nervous system is correct?
a The sympathetic nervous system slows down functions.
b The parasympathetic nervous system speeds up functions.
c It controls voluntary actions.
d It is part of the peripheral nervous system.

8 The ear is involved with
a Regulating body movements
b Balance
c Smoothness of body movements
d Controlling involuntary muscles

9 Which statement about the phases of heart action is correct?
a Diastole is the working phase.
b Systole is the resting phase.
c The heart contracts (pumps) during systole.
d Diastole and systole occur at the same time.

10 Which part of the heart pumps blood to the body?
a Right atrium
b Left atrium
c Right ventricle
d Left ventricle

11 Which carry blood away from the heart?
a Capillaries
b Veins
c Venules
d Arteries

12 Which statement about the lymphatic system is correct?
a The tonsils are the largest structures in the lymphatic system.
b Lymph transports oxygen and nutrients to cells.
c The spleen filters and removes bacteria.
d Extra lymph from the blood is moved to the tissues.

13 Oxygen and carbon dioxide are exchanged
a In the bronchi
b Between the alveoli and capillaries
c Between the lungs and pleura
d In the trachea

14 Digestion begins in the
a Mouth
b Stomach
c Small intestine
d Colon

15 Most nutrient absorption takes place in the
a Stomach
b Small intestine
c Colon
d Large intestine

16 Urine is formed by the
a Jejunum
b Kidneys
c Bladder
d Liver

17 Urine passes from the body through the
a Ureters
b Urethra
c Anus
d Nephrons

18 Which statement about the reproductive system is correct?
a The prostate is the male sex gland.
b The uterus is the female sex gland.
c Male sex cells are called sperm.
d Female sex cells are called ovaries.

19 The discharge of the lining of the uterus is called
a The endometrium
b Ovulation
c Fertilization
d Menstruation

20 The endocrine glands secrete
a Hormones
b Mucus
c Semen
d Antibodies

21 The pancreas
a Has digestive and endocrine functions
b Secretes thyroid hormone
c Is a gland in the brain
d Regulates calcium use

22 The immune system protects the body from
a Low blood sugar
b Disease and infection
c Loss of fluid
d Stunted growth

Answers to Chapter 10 questions are on p. 901.

FOCUS ON PRACTICE

Problem Solving

A patient has a disorder that affects the immune system. How does this affect body function? How will you provide care in a way that protects the person?

Growth and Development

OBJECTIVES

- Define the key terms and key abbreviations in this chapter.
- Explain the principles of growth and development.
- Identify the stages of growth and development.
- Identify milestones used to monitor growth and development.
- Identify developmental tasks for each age-group.

- Describe normal growth and development for each age-group.
- Explain why sexuality is important throughout life.
- Explain how to promote PRIDE in the person, the family, and yourself.

KEY TERMS

adolescence The time between puberty and adulthood; a time of rapid growth and physical, sexual, emotional, and social changes

bullying Repeated, unwanted, aggressive behavior among school-age children and adolescents that involves a real or perceived power imbalance

development Changes in mental, emotional, and social function

developmental task A skill that must be completed during a stage of development for development to continue

ejaculation The release of semen

gender identity A person's sense or feelings of being male, female, a combination of male and female, or neither male nor female

growth The physical changes that are measured and that occur in a steady, orderly manner

infancy The first year of life

menarche The first menstruation and the start of menstrual cycles

menopause The time when menstruation stops and menstrual cycles end

milestone A behavior or skill that occurs in a stage of development

peer A person of the same age-group and background

primary caregiver The person mainly responsible for providing or assisting with a child's basic needs

puberty The period when reproductive organs begin to function and secondary sex characteristics appear

reflex An involuntary movement

sex Physical interactions between people involving the body and reproductive organs

sexuality The physical, emotional, social, cultural, and spiritual factors that affect a person's feelings, attitudes, and behaviors about one's gender identity and sexual behavior

sexual orientation A person's emotional, romantic, or physical attraction to males, females, both, or neither

stage A period of time (age range) in which a person learns certain skills

teen dating violence (TDV) Physical violence, sexual violence, psychological aggression, or stalking that occurs in an adolescent romantic relationship

KEY ABBREVIATIONS

CDC	Centers for Disease Control and Prevention	IPV	Intimate partner violence
CNS	Central nervous system	TDV	Teen dating violence

*G*rowth is the physical changes that are measured and that occur in a steady and orderly manner. Growth is measured in weight, height, and changes in appearance and body functions (Fig. 11-1, p. 132). *Development* relates to changes in mental, emotional, and social function. A person behaves and thinks in certain ways in each stage of development.

This chapter presents the basic stages of growth and development that occur in normal, healthy persons. Stages overlap. Also, the rate of growth and development varies with each person.

Growth and development theories and stages vary among experts. The groups and content in this chapter are broad and general.

PRINCIPLES

Growth and development is a process affecting the whole person. Although they differ, growth and development:
- Overlap.
- Depend on each other.
- Occur at the same time.

For example, an infant coos or babbles (development) when the physical structures for speech are strong

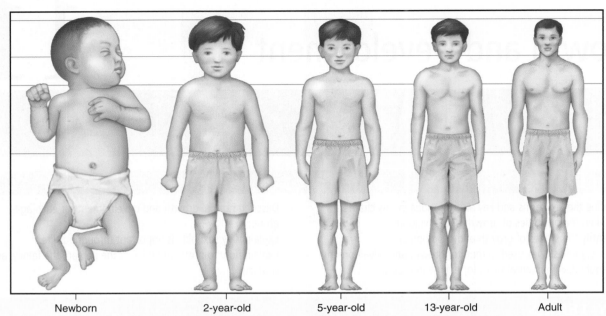

FIGURE 11-1 Changes in appearance from birth to maturity. (From Patton KT, Thibodeau GA: *The human body in health and disease,* ed 7, St Louis, 2018, Elsevier.)

Newborn 2-year-old 5-year-old 13-year-old Adult

enough (growth). Basic principles of growth and development are:

- The process starts at fertilization and continues until death.
- The process proceeds from the simple to the complex. A baby sits before standing, stands before walking, and walks before running.
- The process occurs in certain directions.
  - From head to foot. Babies hold their heads up before sitting. They sit before standing.
  - From the center of the body outward. Babies control shoulder movements before controlling hand movements.
- The process occurs in a sequence, order, and pattern. A *stage* is a period of time (age range) in which a person learns certain skills. A stage cannot be skipped. Each stage is the basis for the next stage.
- *Milestones* track progress. A *milestone* is a behavior or skill that occurs in a stage of development. Milestones involve:
  - Physical growth and movement.
  - Language and communication.
  - Social and emotional changes.
  - Cognitive changes (learning, thinking, and problem solving).
- The rate of the process is uneven. It is not at a set pace. Growth is rapid during infancy. Some children develop fast. Others develop slowly.
- Each stage has its own characteristics and developmental tasks. A *developmental task* is a skill that must be completed during a stage of development for development to continue. For example, an infant must learn to walk in order to become less dependent as a toddler.

Family Structure and the Caregiver Role

Family structures vary. The following are examples:

- *Two-parent families*—2 parents and 1 or more children related by birth, marriage, or adoption. Foster children may be a part. Parents may or may not be married and may be any gender combination. A *blended family* includes children from previous relationships.
- *Single-parent families*—1 parent and 1 or more children. Divorce, death of a partner, and choosing single-parenting commonly result in a single-parent family structure.
- *Extended families*—other relatives (grandparents, aunts, uncles, cousins, and so on) are part of the family structure.

The *primary caregiver* is the person mainly responsible for providing or assisting with a child's basic needs. Who fills this role depends on the family's structure. A mother, father, partner, relative, or court-appointed guardian may have this role. *Parent* and *parents* are used in this chapter. However, another primary caregiver may have the parent role.

See *Promoting Safety and Comfort: Family Structure and the Caregiver Role.*

PROMOTING SAFETY AND COMFORT

Family Structure and the Caregiver Role

Safety

From birth, children rely on parents to meet their basic needs. Having a safe and loving home and proper nutrition, sleep, and exercise are important factors in a child's growth and development. The Centers for Disease Control and Prevention (CDC) identifies these positive parenting practices to support healthy development.

- Responding to children in a predictable way
- Showing warmth and sensitivity
- Having routines and household rules
- Reading to and talking with children
- Supporting health and safety
- Using appropriate discipline without harshness

INFANCY (BIRTH TO 1 YEAR)

Infancy is the first year of life. Growth and development are rapid during this time. During this stage infants:

- Learn to walk.
- Learn to eat solid foods.
- Begin to talk and communicate with others.
- Learn to trust.
- Begin to have emotional relationships with parents, brothers, and sisters.
- Develop stable sleep and feeding patterns.

A baby is called a *neonate* or *newborn* from birth to 1 month (Fig. 11-2). (*Neo* means new; *nate* means born.) The average newborn weighs 6 to 9 pounds and is about 20 inches long. At 1 year the infant is about 29 inches.

Newborns have certain ***reflexes*** (involuntary movements). These reflexes decline and then disappear as the central nervous system (CNS) develops.

- *Rooting reflex*—occurs when the cheek is touched near the mouth (Fig. 11-3). The mouth opens and the head turns toward the touch. This reflex is needed for feeding. It guides the baby's mouth to the nipple.
- *Sucking reflex*—occurs when the lips are touched.
- *Moro reflex (startle reflex)*—occurs when the baby is startled by a loud noise, a sudden movement, or the head falling back. The arms are thrown apart. The legs extend and then flex. A brief cry is common. See Figure 11-4.
- *Palmar grasp reflex*—occurs when the palm is stroked. The fingers close firmly around the object (Fig. 11-5).
- *Stepping reflex*—occurs when the baby is held upright and the feet touch a surface. The feet move up and down and in stepping motions (Fig. 11-6).

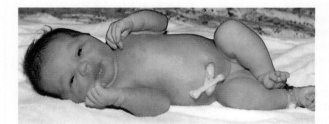

FIGURE 11-2 A newborn. (Courtesy Marjori M. Pyle for LifeCircle, Costa Mesa, Calif.)

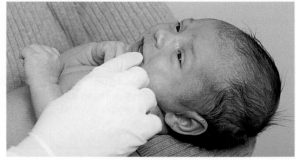

FIGURE 11-3 Rooting reflex. (From Seidel HM, Ball J, Dains J, Benedict GW: *Mosby's guide to physical examination,* ed 7, St Louis, 2011, Mosby.)

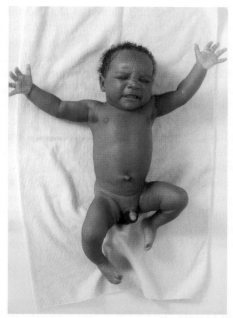

FIGURE 11-4 Moro reflex. (Courtesy Paul Vincent Kuntz, Texas Children's Hospital, as found in Hockenberry MJ, Wilson D, Rodgers CC: *Wong's nursing care of infants and children,* ed 11, St Louis, 2019, Elsevier.)

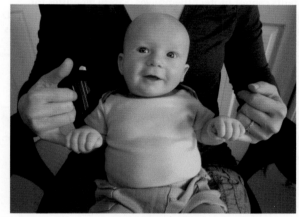

FIGURE 11-5 The palmar grasp reflex. (Courtesy Anne Skowronski, Mount Juliet, Tenn.)

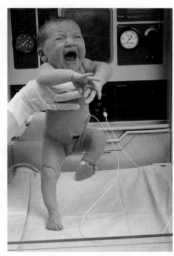

FIGURE 11-6 Stepping reflex. (From McKinney E, James S, Murry S, Nelson K, Ashwill J: *Maternal-child nursing,* ed 6, St Louis, 2022, Elsevier.)

See Table 11-1 for the milestones that normally occur by 2 months, 4 months, 6 months, 9 months, and 1 year.

Infants are bottle-fed (formula-fed) or breast-fed. Solid foods are given at 4 to 6 months. Rice cereal mixed with breast-milk or formula is given first. Fruits, vegetables, and meats are introduced slowly. Foods are pureed and thin at first. Thicker and chunkier foods are given as more teeth erupt and chewing and swallowing skills increase. Teething often begins with the bottom front teeth. Weaning (stopping bottle-feeding or breast-feeding) may begin at the end of infancy.

With consistent care, the infant develops a sense of trust. Physical and safety needs (feeding, comfort, warmth, touch, stimulation, and caring) must be met for the infant to learn to trust.

See *Promoting Safety and Comfort: Infancy (Birth to 1 Year)*.

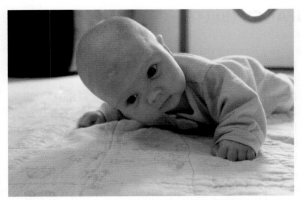
FIGURE 11-7 By 2 months, an infant can hold the head up.

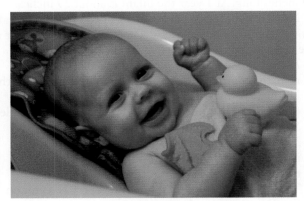
FIGURE 11-8 A 2-month-old smiles in response to others.

PROMOTING SAFETY AND COMFORT

Infancy (Birth to 1 Year)

Safety
Infants cannot protect themselves. Safety measures for infants are presented in Chapters 14 and 56 and Appendix D (p. 909). Also see *Focus on Children and Older Persons* boxes throughout this book.

TABLE 11-1	Milestones: Infancy (Birth to 1 Year)		
Movement/Physical	Language and Communication	Social and Emotional	Learning, Thinking, Problem Solving
By 2 months • Can hold head up (Fig. 11-7) • Moves both arms and both legs • Opens the hands briefly	• Makes sounds other than crying • Reacts to loud sounds	• Calms down when spoken to or picked up • Looks at faces • Seems happy when a parent approaches • Begins to smile at others (Fig. 11-8)	• Watches a parent move • Looks at a toy for several seconds
By 4 months • Holds head steady without support while being held • Can hold a toy • Swings at dangling toys • Brings hands to mouth • Pushes up to elbows when on stomach (Fig. 11-9)	• Makes cooing sounds (oooo, aahh) • Makes sounds back when talked to • Turns head toward the sound of a voice	• Smiles to get a person's attention • Chuckles (not yet a full laugh) when a person tries to make the infant laugh • Looks at, makes sounds at, or moves to get or keep a person's attention	• Opens the mouth when the breast or bottle is seen when hungry • Looks at own hands with interest
By 6 months • Rolls front to back • Pushes up with straight arms when on stomach • Begins to sit by leaning on the hands for support (Fig. 11-10, A)	• Takes turns making sounds with a parent • Sticks tongue out and blows (blows "raspberries") • Makes squealing noises	• Knows familiar faces • Laughs • Likes looking at self in a mirror	• Puts things in the mouth to explore them • Reaches to grab a wanted toy • Closes the lips to show that no more food is wanted

TABLE 11-1	Milestones: Infancy (Birth to 1 Year)—cont'd		
Movement/Physical	Language and Communication	Social and Emotional	Learning, Thinking, Problem Solving
By 9 months • Can get into a sitting position without help • Sits without support (Fig. 11-10, *B*) • Moves things from 1 hand to the other hand • Uses the fingers to "rake" food toward self	• Makes different sounds (mamamama, bababab) • Lifts the arms up to be picked up	• Is shy, clingy, or fearful around strangers • Shows different facial expressions (happy, sad, angry, surprised) • Looks when parent calls the infant's name • Reacts when parent leaves (looks, reaches for the parent, cries) • Smiles or laughs at peek-a-boo	• Looks for objects when dropped out of sight • Bangs 2 things together
By 1 year • Pulls up to stand • Uses thumb and index finger to pick up little things (pincer grasp) (Fig. 11-11) • Walks holding on to furniture (Fig. 11-12) • Drinks from a cup without a lid while a parent holds it	• Waves "bye-bye" • Calls a parent "mama," "dada," or other special name • Understands "no" (pauses briefly or stops when the parent says it)	• Plays games like "pat-a-cake"	• Puts things in a container (like a block in a cup) • Looks for hidden items after seeing them be hidden (like a toy under a blanket)

Modified from Centers for Disease Control and Prevention: Milestone checklists.

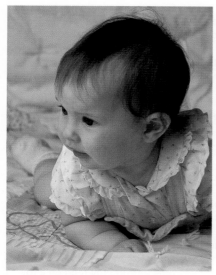

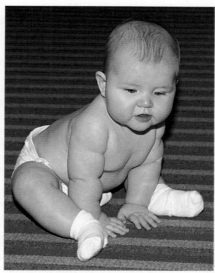

FIGURE 11-9 By 4 months, an infant can push up to the elbows when lying on the stomach.

FIGURE 11-10 A, A 6-month-old begins to sit by leaning on the hands for support. **B,** By 9 months, an infant sits without support. (A, From James SR, Nelson KA, Ashwill JW: *Nursing care of children: principles and practices,* ed 4, St Louis, 2013, Saunders.)

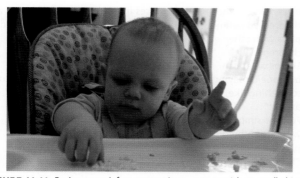

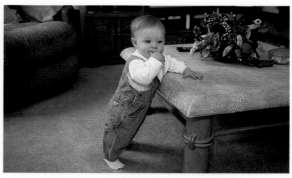

FIGURE 11-11 By 1 year, an infant uses a pincer grasp to pick up small objects.

FIGURE 11-12 By 1 year, an infant can walk while holding on to furniture.

TODDLERHOOD (1 TO 3 YEARS)

Growth rate in toddlerhood is slower than during infancy. Toddlers learn to:

- Tolerate separation from parents.
- Gain control of bowel and bladder function.
- Use words to communicate.
- Become less dependent on parents.

See Table 11-2 for the milestones that normally occur during the toddler years.

Toddlers learn to walk well. They are curious and get into everything and anything. They touch, taste, smell, and climb to explore their settings. They go farther away from parents. They learn to do some things without help. Safety measures and supervision are very important, as toddlers lack the judgment to make safe decisions on their own. (See Appendix D on p. 909.)

Computer play often begins in toddlerhood. Toddlers like to push keys and play with levers and buttons on computer toys. Such actions help develop fine motor skills and hand-eye coordination.

Toilet training begins in toddlerhood. Bowel and bladder control is related to CNS development. Children must be mentally and physically ready for toilet training. Some are ready at 2 years. Others are ready at 2½ to 3 years of age.

Play skills increase. Toddlers play alongside other children. Sometimes they play with other children. Toddlers are possessive and do not understand sharing.

Temper tantrums and saying "no" are common. Toddlers kick and scream to express anger and frustration. That is how they object when independence is challenged. The child saying "no" can frustrate parents. Almost every request may be answered "no," even if the child follows the request.

Toddlers learn separation from parents. With discomfort, frustration, fear, or injury, they return to a parent or cry for attention. If parents are consistently present when needed, children learn security. They learn to tolerate brief periods of separation.

TABLE 11-2	Milestones: Toddlerhood (1 to 3 Years)		
Movement/Physical	**Language and Communication**	**Social and Emotional**	**Learning, Thinking, Problem Solving**
By 1½ years • Walks alone • Scribbles • Drinks from a cup without a lid (may spill sometimes) • Feeds self with fingers • Tries to use a spoon (Fig. 11-13) • Climbs on and off a couch or chair without help	• Tries to say 3 or more words besides "mama" or "dada" • Follows 1-step directions without any gestures (giving a parent a toy when the parent says: "Give it to me.") • Shakes head "no" • Points to show what is wanted	• Moves away from a parent but looks to see if the parent is close by • Points to show something of interest • Puts hands out for them to be washed • Looks at a few pages in a book with someone • Helps with dressing by pushing an arm through a sleeve or lifting up a foot	• Copies someone doing chores (sweeping with a broom) • Plays with toys in a simple way (pushing a toy car)
By 2 years • Kicks a ball • Runs • Walks up a few stairs with or without help • Eats with a spoon	• Points to pictures or things when asked ("Where is the bear?" when looking at a book) • Says at least 2 words together ("More milk") • Points to at least 2 body parts when asked • Uses more gestures than waving and pointing (blowing a kiss, nodding yes)	• Notices when others are hurt or upset (looks sad when someone is crying) • Looks at a parent's face to see how to react in a new situation	• Holds an item in 1 hand while using the other hand (holding a container and taking off the lid) • Tries to use switches, knobs, or buttons on a toy • Plays with more than 1 toy at a time (putting toy food on a toy plate)
By 2½ years • Uses hands to twist things (turning doorknobs, unscrewing lids) • Takes off some clothes without help (loose pants, open jacket) • Jumps off the ground with both feet • Turns book pages 1 at a time when read to	• Says about 50 words • Says 2 or more words together with 1 action word ("Doggie run") • Names items in a book when someone points and asks, "What is this?" • Says words like "I," "me," or "we"	• Plays next to other children; sometimes plays with other children • Shows what can be done by saying something like, "Look at me!" • Follows simple routines when told (helping to pick up toys when told, "It's clean-up time.")	• Uses items to pretend (feeding a block to a doll as if it were food) • Shows simple problem-solving skills (standing on a stool to reach something) • Follows 2-step instructions ("Put the toy down and close the door.") • Can identify at least 1 color (points to a red crayon when asked, "Which one is red?")

TABLE 11-2	Milestones: Toddlerhood (1 to 3 Years)—cont'd		
Movement/Physical	**Language and Communication**	**Social and Emotional**	**Learning, Thinking, Problem Solving**
By **3 years** • Strings items together (large beads or macaroni) • Puts on some clothes without help (loose pants, a jacket) • Uses a fork	• Talks in conversation with at least 2 back-and-forth exchanges • Asks "who," "what," "where," or "why" questions ("Where is mommy?") • Says what action is happening in a picture or book when asked (running, eating, playing) • Says first name when asked • Talks well enough for others to understand most of the time	• Calms down within 10 minutes after a parent leaves (childcare drop-off) • Notices other children and joins them to play	• Draws a circle when shown how • Avoids dangers when warned (touching a hot stove)

Modified from Centers for Disease Control and Prevention: Milestone checklists.

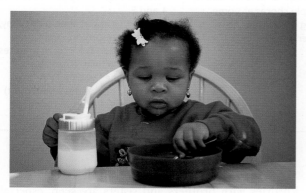

FIGURE 11-13 A toddler learns to use a spoon.

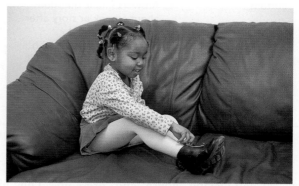

FIGURE 11-14 This preschool child can put on her shoes.

PRESCHOOL (3 TO 6 YEARS)

Preschool children grow 2 to 3 inches per year. They gain about 5 pounds a year. Preschoolers are thinner, more coordinated, and more graceful than toddlers. Preschoolers:

• Increase their ability to communicate and understand others.
• Perform self-care.
• Learn gender differences and develop sexual modesty.
• Learn right from wrong and good from bad.
• Learn to play with others.
• Develop family relationships.

See Table 11-3 (p. 138) for the milestones that normally occur in the preschool years.

Personal care skills increase. Preschool children put on clothes and shoes and manage buttons (Fig. 11-14). They wash their hands, brush their teeth, feed themselves, and help with chores (setting the table).

Play is important. Preschool children enjoy crayons, cutting paper, pasting, and painting (Fig. 11-15). Imaginary friends and imitating adults are common. They like computer and board games, TV, riding toys (wagons, tricycles,

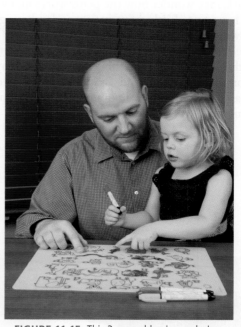

FIGURE 11-15 This 3-year-old enjoys coloring.

TABLE 11-3	Milestones: Preschool (3 to 6 Years)		
Movement/Physical	Language and Communication	Social and Emotional	Learning, Thinking, Problem Solving
By 4 years • Catches a large ball most of the time • Can pour water and serve food for self with supervision • Unbuttons some buttons • Holds a crayon or pencil between the fingers and thumb (not a fist)	• Says sentences with 4 or more words • Says some words from a song, story, or nursery rhyme • Talks about at least 1 thing that happened during the day • Answers simple questions ("What is a coat for?")	• Pretends to be something else when playing (teacher, dog, superhero) • Asks to go play with children if none are around • Comforts others who are hurt or sad (hugging a crying friend) • Avoids danger (not jumping from tall heights) • Likes to help • Changes behavior based on the location (library, playground, place of worship)	• Names some colors of items • Draws a person with 3 or more body parts • Says what will happen next in a well-known story
By 5 years • Hops on 1 foot • Buttons some buttons	• Tells a story that was heard or made up with at least 2 events • Answers simple questions about a book or story after it was read or told • Talks in conversation with more than 3 back-and-forth exchanges • Uses or recognizes simple rhymes (bat/cat, ball/tall)	• Follows rules or takes turns when playing with others • Sings, dances, or acts for others • Does simple chores at home (matching socks, clearing a table after a meal)	• Counts to 10 • Identifies some letters • Identifies some numbers between 1 and 5 • Uses words about time (yesterday, tomorrow, morning, night) • Pays attention for 5 to 10 minutes during an activity (story, craft; "screen time" with a TV or an electronic device does *not* count) • Writes some letters in his or her name

Modified from Centers for Disease Control and Prevention: Milestone checklists.

bicycles), and playing "house" and "dress-up." They play with other children and learn to share (Fig. 11-16).

Differences between males and females are noticed. Three-year-olds know that there are "boys" and "girls." Little girls may wonder how the penis works and why they do not have one. Little boys may wonder how girls can urinate without a penis.

Preschool children tend to tease, tattle, and tell fibs. When they have done something wrong, they may blame others or an imaginary friend. Bragging, telling tales about family, and showing off are common. They are proud of achievements but have mood swings.

Rivalries with brothers and sisters are seen, especially when another child takes the child's things. Rivalries also occur when older children have more and different privileges. The family is often the focus of the child's frustrations. They enjoy doing things with parents (Fig. 11-17). Cooking, housekeeping, shopping, yard work, and sports are examples.

Five-year-olds learn to follow rules and be responsible. They are eager to do things right. They learn about manners, independence, and honesty. Fears lessen, but nightmares and dreams are common.

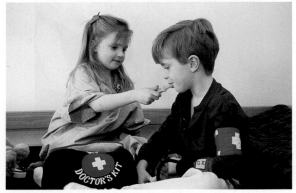
FIGURE 11-16 These 4-year-olds play "doctor and nurse" together.

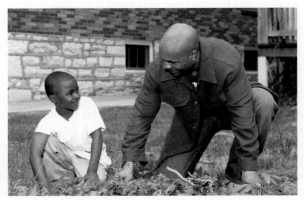
FIGURE 11-17 This 5-year-old does yard work with his father.

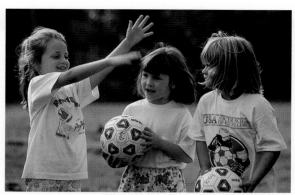

FIGURE 11-18 These 6-year-old girls enjoy soccer.

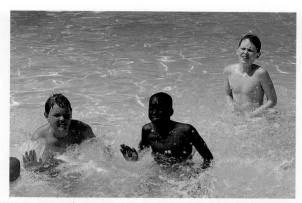

FIGURE 11-19 Belonging to a peer group is important to school-age children.

SCHOOL AGE (6 TO 9 OR 10 YEARS)

School-age children grow 2 to 3 inches a year. They gain 4½ to 6½ pounds a year. They:

- Develop the social and physical skills needed for playing games.
- Learn to get along with persons of the same age-group and background.
- Learn behaviors and attitudes common for one's gender.
- Learn basic reading, writing, and math skills.
- Develop a conscience and morals.
- Develop a good feeling and attitude about oneself.

Baby teeth are lost and permanent teeth erupt. This starts around age 6.

School-age children can run, jump, skip, hop, and ride a 2-wheeled bike. They can swim, skate, dance, and jump rope. Learning to play in groups, they can take part in team sports. Soccer, T-ball, baseball, football, and volleyball are examples (Fig. 11-18). They learn teamwork and sportsmanship and follow rules. Quiet play involves collections, board games, video games, and crafts.

Reading, writing, grammar, and math skills develop. Sentences are longer and more complex. As reading skills increase, so do language skills. Children like to read and be read to.

Play activities have purpose and involve "work." School-age children can help with household tasks—cleaning, cooking, yard work. They like crafts, building things, and scout groups. Rewards are important—good grades, trophies, payment for chores, scouting badges.

At about age 7, usually boys prefer playing with boys. Girls usually prefer playing with girls. From 8 to 9 years, play may involve boys and girls. Some show an interest in boy-girl relationships at about 8 to 9 years. However, children may deny such interest.

Peer groups develop. *Peers* are persons of the same age-group and background. Peer groups are important for love, belonging, and self-esteem needs (Fig. 11-19). These children get along well with and need adults. However, they prefer peer group fads, opinions, and activities.

Electronic Media

Children use electronic media for learning and for entertainment. Computers and tablets are often used for schoolwork. Computers, tablets, TVs, video game consoles, and phones are used for games, for watching videos and shows, and for social media.

"Screen time" is a term used for the amount of time spent using electronic devices. The more screen time a child has, the less time there is for exercise, play, time with friends and family, schoolwork, and sleep. Too much screen time can affect a child's school performance, sleep, mood, self-image, and weight. The risk of obesity increases because screen time is a sedentary activity. *Sedentary* means it involves very little physical activity.

Healthy use of electronic media includes limits. Current guidelines recommend no more than 1 to 2 hours per day for a child's entertainment screen time. Parents also need to monitor content. Certain video games, videos, and Internet content are not age-appropriate. Children risk exposure to sexual content, violence, promotion of dangerous activities, substance use, misleading information, cyber-bullying (p. 140), and on-line interaction with persons seeking to harm children.

LATE CHILDHOOD (9 OR 10 TO 12 YEARS)

Late childhood *(pre-adolescence)* is the time between childhood and adolescence. Developmental tasks are like those for school-age children. In addition, pre-adolescents are expected to:

- Become independent of adults and learn to depend on oneself.
- Develop and keep friendships with peers.
- Understand physical, psychological, and social changes.
- Develop moral and ethical behavior.
- Develop greater muscular strength, coordination, and balance.
- Learn how to study.

Many permanent teeth erupt. Girls have a growth spurt. By age 12 years, they are taller and heavier than boys. Both boys and girls are more graceful and coordinated.

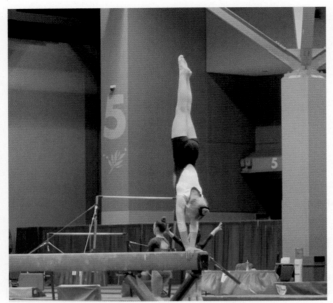

FIGURE 11-20 Physical skills and coordination increase in late childhood. (Courtesy Melissa Remmert, Mt. Pulaski, Ill.)

Muscle strength and physical skills increase (Fig. 11-20). Participation in individual and team sports is common.

Math and language skills increase. These children read for information and pleasure. They enjoy books and stories about mystery, adventure, friendship, and science fiction.

The onset of puberty nears. *Puberty* is the period when reproductive organs begin to function and secondary sex characteristics appear. In girls, the hips widen and breast buds appear. Some 9-, 10-, and 11-year-old girls begin puberty. Boys show fewer signs of maturing sexually. Genital organs begin to grow. There is concern about body image.

Factual sex information is important. If parents avoid the subject, children get information elsewhere. Information shared by friends is often not complete and not accurate. Information gained on-line may not be age-appropriate. When a child asks questions, answers must be honest, complete, and in terms that the child understands.

Peer groups are the center of activities. The group affects attitudes and behavior. Friends are loyal and share problems. A "best friend" is common. Interest in and feeling attraction to others begins.

These children are aware of the mistakes and faults of adults. Adult rules and standards are questioned. It is common to rebel against adults and test limits. Parents and children disagree. However, parents are needed for the child's development.

Bullying

Bullying is repeated, unwanted, aggressive behavior among school-age children and adolescents that involves a real or perceived power imbalance. Bullying is a form of youth violence. See Box 11-1 for the different types of bullying and the signs of bullying.

BOX 11-1 Bullying: Types and Signs

Types
- *Verbal bullying* is saying or writing mean things. It includes:
  - Teasing
  - Name calling
  - Inappropriate sexual comments
  - Taunting
  - Threatening to cause harm
- *Social bullying (relational bullying)* involves hurting someone's reputation or relationships. It includes:
  - Leaving someone out on purpose
  - Telling others not to be friends with someone
  - Spreading rumors about someone
  - Embarrassing someone in public
- *Physical bullying* involves hurting a person's body or possessions. It includes:
  - Hitting, kicking, pinching
  - Spitting
  - Tripping, pushing
  - Taking or breaking someone's things
  - Making mean or rude hand gestures

Signs That a Child Is Being Bullied
- Unexplained injuries
- Lost or destroyed clothing, books, electronics, jewelry
- Frequent headaches, stomach aches, or feeling sick
- Faking illness
- Changes in eating habits—skipping meals, binge eating (Chapter 53), coming home hungry (from not eating at school)
- Problems sleeping
- Frequent nightmares
- Declining grades, loss of interest in schoolwork, not wanting to go to school
- Sudden loss of friends
- Avoidance of social situations
- Feeling helpless
- Having decreased self-esteem
- Self-harm behaviors—running away from home, harming oneself, talking about suicide

Signs That a Child Is Bullying Others
- Getting into physical or verbal fights
- Having friends who bully others
- Showing increasing aggression
- Getting disciplined at school frequently—sent to the principal's office, detention
- Having unexplained extra money or new belongings
- Blaming others
- Not accepting responsibility for actions
- Being competitive and worried about reputation or popularity

Modified from U.S. Department of Health and Human Services: What is bullying, last reviewed August 1, 2023, and Warning signs for bullying, last reviewed November 10, 2021. https://www.stopbullying.gov.

Most reported bullying occurs in school. It also happens on the playground, on the school bus, on the way to or from school, and in the community. Bullying also occurs electronically (cyber-bullying).

Bullying causes distress and harm to the victim. It can result in injury, social and emotional distress, self-harm, and even death. Victims are at risk for depression, anxiety, sleep problems, and poor school performance. Those who bully are at risk for substance use, school problems, and violence as a teenager and adult.

ADOLESCENCE (12 TO 18 YEARS)

Adolescence is the time between puberty and adulthood. There is rapid growth and physical, sexual, emotional, and social changes. The stage begins with puberty. Girls reach puberty between 9 and 16 years. Boys reach puberty between 13 and 15 years. Developmental tasks in adolescence include:

* Accepting changes in the body and appearance.
* Developing appropriate relationships with others and beginning to attract partners.
* Becoming independent from parents and adults.
* Establishing a sense of personal identity.
* Preparing for a career.
* Developing the morals, attitudes, and values needed to function in society.

Boys and girls have a growth spurt. Both gain height and weight. They need about 9½ hours of sleep because of such rapid growth. Girls usually complete physical development by age 17. Boys usually stop growing between 18 and 21 years.

Active oil glands lead to acne. Sweat glands are more active. Good hygiene is needed. Deodorants or antiperspirants prevent body odors.

Menarche marks the onset of puberty in girls. *Menarche is the first menstruation and the start of menstrual cycles* (Chapter 10). *Pregnancy can now occur*. Secondary sex characteristics appear. They include:

* Increase in breast size
* Pubic, axillary (underarm), and leg hair
* Slight deepening of the voice
* Widening and rounding of the hips

Ejaculation (the release of semen) signals the onset of puberty in boys. *Nocturnal emissions* ("wet dreams") occur. During sleep *(nocturnal)* the penis becomes erect. Semen is released *(emission)*. *The male can father children*. Other secondary sex characteristics include:

* Facial, pubic, and axillary (underarm) hair
* Hair on the chest, arms, and legs
* Deepening of the voice
* Increases in neck and shoulder sizes

Accepting body changes and appearance occurs over time. Girls worry about weight gain. Breast development can embarrass girls, especially if breasts are large or small. Some do not like wearing a bra. Others wear clothes that show off the breasts. Boys may worry about genital size. Height is a concern for boys and girls. Being small limits play in some sports. Boys do not like being shorter than their peers. Tall girls may be embarrassed about being taller than other girls and boys.

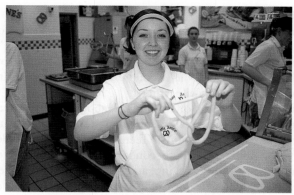

FIGURE 11-21 This teenager has a part-time job.

Mood swings occur. Emotional reactions are hard to predict. They control emotions better later in this stage. Sometimes 14- to 18-year-olds are sad and depressed. However, they have more control over the time and place of emotional reactions.

Adolescents need to become independent of parents and other adults. They must learn to function, make decisions, and act responsibly without adult supervision. Many teenagers (teens) have part-time jobs or babysit (Fig. 11-21). They go to dances and parties, shop without an adult, and stay home alone. Many take part in school clubs and organizations.

Judgment and reasoning are not always sound. They still need guidance, discipline, and emotional and financial support from parents. Teens and parents often disagree about behavior and activity restrictions and limits. Teens prefer doing things with their peers rather than with family. They tend to confide in and seek advice from adults other than their parents.

Teens like parties, dances, and other social events. Appearance is important (clothing, hair-styles). Teens experiment with make-up and hair-styles. They spend time talking to friends on the phone, texting, on social media sites, listening to music, and reading teen magazines.

Interests and activities also reflect the need to develop intimate relationships. See "Teen Dating" on p. 142. See "Sexuality" on p. 143.

Thoughts about careers and what to do after high school become a focus. Interests, skills, talents, and money are some factors that influence college or job choices.

Teens need to develop morals, values, and attitudes for living in society. Parents, peers, culture, religion, the media, and school are influencing factors. Substance use, unwanted pregnancy, criminal acts, and suicide are risks for troubled teens.

Establishing a sense of personal identity is an important developmental task of adolescence. Identity develops as teens explore interests, gain independence, develop values, and respond to changes in adolescence. Sexuality (p. 143), spirituality (Chapter 7), and the influence of family and peers are factors.

Teen Dating

The age for dating varies. At first, dating involves school events, such as dances or football games. "Group dating" is common. The same group of girls is with the same group of boys. "Pairing off" as a couple replaces group dating. Couples may be sexual partners.

Parents and teens often disagree about dating. Parents worry about sexual activities, pregnancy, and sexually transmitted diseases (infections). Teens usually do not understand or appreciate these concerns. Dating helps meet security, love and belonging, and self-esteem needs. Teens may have problems controlling sexual urges and considering the results of sexual activity.

See *Promoting Safety and Comfort: Teen Dating.*

PROMOTING SAFETY AND COMFORT

Teen Dating

Safety

Intimate partner violence (IPV) (Chapter 5) can start with teen dating. *Teen dating violence (TDV)* is physical violence, sexual violence, psychological aggression, or stalking that occurs in an adolescent romantic relationship. The CDC describes these types of behaviors that can occur with TDV.

- *Physical violence*—hurting or trying to hurt a partner by hitting, kicking, or another type of force.
- *Sexual violence*—forcing or attempting to force a partner to take part in a sex act or sexual touching without the partner's consent. Non-physical behaviors like sharing sexual pictures of a partner without consent or sexting someone without the person's consent are other forms.
- *Psychological aggression*—using verbal and nonverbal communication to harm a partner mentally or emotionally. The intent may be to control the partner.
- *Stalking*—there is repeated, unwanted attention and contact that causes fear or concern for one's safety or the safety of someone close to the victim.

TDV can occur in person, electronically, and with a current or former dating partner. Behavior may begin as teasing and name-calling. Serious violence such as assault and rape can result.

TDV has short-term and long-term effects. Teens who experience dating violence are more likely to have symptoms of depression and anxiety. They are more likely to use tobacco, drugs, and alcohol; have antisocial behaviors (lying, theft, bullying, hitting); and think about suicide (Chapter 53). Victims are at higher risk for IPV after high school (Chapter 5).

Violence is preventable. Learning healthy relationship skills is an essential part of prevention. The following resources are available for teens experiencing dating violence.

- National Teen Dating Abuse Helpline
- National Sexual Assault Hotline
- National Sexual Violence Resource Center
- National Domestic Violence Hotline

YOUNG ADULTHOOD (18 TO 40 YEARS)

Mental and social development continue during young adulthood. There is little physical growth. Adult height has been reached. Body systems are fully developed. Young adulthood involves:

- Choosing education and a career.
- Selecting a partner (if desired).
- Learning to live with a partner.
- Developing a satisfactory sex life.
- Becoming a parent and raising children (if desired).

Most jobs require certain knowledge and skills. The education needed depends on career choice. Education usually increases job choices. Employment is needed for economic independence and to support a family.

Many adults marry at least once (Fig. 11-22). Others choose to have a long-term relationship without marriage. Some young adults choose to remain single. They may live alone or with friends.

Many factors affect partner selection. They include age, culture, religion, interests, education, social status, personality, and love. Desires regarding children and family is another factor. Partners must work together to build a relationship based on trust, respect, caring, and friendship.

Partners must learn to live together. Habits, routines, meals, and pastimes are changed or adjusted to "fit" the other person's needs. They learn to solve problems and make decisions together. They need to work toward the same goals. Open and honest communication is needed. Some relationships are happy and successful. Others are not.

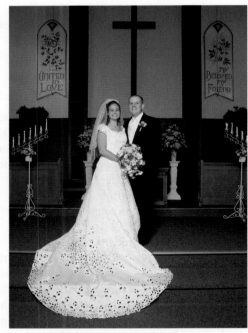

FIGURE 11-22 A wedding celebrates a couple's marriage. (Courtesy Dean Williams Photography, Springfield, Ill.)

Sexual frequency, desires, practices, and preferences vary. For a satisfying and intimate relationship, partners must understand and accept the other's needs. See "Sexuality."

Many young adults become parents. Birth control methods allow couples to plan when to have children and how many to have. Some pregnancies are not planned. Some couples choose adoption or foster parenting. Some require assisted reproduction (medical treatments and procedures for fertilization and pregnancy). Other couples choose not to have children.

Parents must agree on child-rearing practices and discipline methods. They need to adjust to the child and to the child's needs for parental time, energy, and attention.

MIDDLE ADULTHOOD (40 TO 65 YEARS)

This stage of life becomes more stable and comfortable. Children grow up and move away. Partners have time together. Worries about children and money are fewer.

Middle-age adults:

- Adjust to physical changes.
- Adjust to having grown children.
- Develop leisure-time activities.
- Adjust to aging parents.

Physical changes occur. Many are gradual and are not noticed. Others are seen early. Energy and endurance begin to slow down. So do metabolism and physical activities. Therefore weight control becomes a problem. Facial wrinkles and gray hair appear. Needing eyeglasses is common. Hair loss may begin. Menstruation stops and menstrual cycles end *(menopause)*. It occurs between the ages of 45 and 55 years. Ovaries stop secreting hormones. The woman cannot have children.

Many diseases and illnesses can develop. Some disorders are chronic. Some threaten life.

Children leave home for college, marry, move to their own homes, and start families. Adults have to let children go and adjust to being in-laws and grandparents (Fig. 11-23). Parents must let children lead their own lives. However, they provide support when needed.

Spare time (free time) increases as parenting demands decrease. Hobbies and pastimes bring pleasure. Examples include gardening, fishing, painting, golfing, volunteer work, and being part of clubs and organizations (Fig. 11-24). These activities are even more important after retirement and during late adulthood.

Some middle-age adults have aging parents in poor health. Responsibility for aging parents may begin during this stage. Many middle-age adults deal with the death of parents.

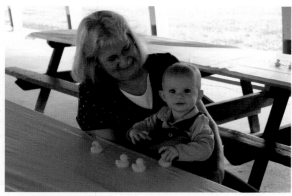

FIGURE 11-23 This woman enjoys time with her grandchild.

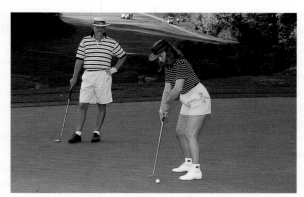

FIGURE 11-24 Middle-age adults usually have more time for leisure activities.

LATE ADULTHOOD (65 YEARS AND OLDER)

Chapter 12 describes the many changes that occur in older persons. Older persons:

- Adjust to decreased strength and loss of health.
- Adjust to retirement and reduced income.
- Cope with a partner's death.
- Develop new friends and relationships.
- Prepare for one's own death.

SEXUALITY

NOTE: *Definitions and descriptions related to sexuality vary. Some are very complex. Terms used in society continue to change over time as more information becomes known. Those used in this section are broad and dictionary-based.*

Sexuality is the physical, emotional, social, cultural, and spiritual factors that affect a person's feelings, attitudes, and behaviors about one's gender identity and sexual behavior. Sexuality is more than *sex*—the physical interactions between people involving the body and reproductive organs. Sexuality involves the whole person (Chapter 7)—physical, mental and emotional, social, and spiritual. The personality and the body reflect a person's sexuality—how a person behaves, thinks, dresses, and responds to others.

Sexuality development begins when a baby's biological sex—male or female—is known. Biological sex is based on reproductive organs and structures. Some parents choose names, clothing, decorations, and toys to represent male or female. For example, blue clothing for boys and pink clothing for girls. Other parents prefer gender-neutral names and items. By the age of 3, children can identify males and females. They learn usual male and female behaviors, practices, and roles from adults. Gender identity is a specific part of the adolescent's development of personal identity.

As children develop and grow older, interest increases about the body and how it works. Adolescents are more aware of their bodies. Their bodies respond to stimulation. They may begin to feel or show a sexual orientation. They may engage in sexual behaviors. They kiss, embrace, pet, or have intercourse. Pregnancy and sexually transmitted diseases (infections) (Chapter 52) are risks.

Sex and sexuality have more meaning as young adults mature. Partners are selected. Decisions are made about sexual practices and parenting. Attitudes, feelings, and needs are important. Needs relate to love, affection, sexual intimacy, desires for family, and a sense of well-being.

Sexuality is important throughout life. Attitudes and needs change with aging (Chapter 12). They are affected by life events. These include bodily changes from aging, death or loss of a partner, injury, illness, and surgery.

Sexual Orientation

Sexual orientation refers to a person's emotional, romantic, or physical attraction to males, females, both, or neither. Attraction may be to persons of the opposite sex (*heterosexual, straight*), the same sex (*gay, lesbian*), or both (*bisexual*). Some persons have no sexual attraction (*asexual*).

Gender Identity

Gender identity refers to a person's sense or feelings of being male, female, a combination of male and female, or neither male nor female. *Cisgender* is the term used when a person's gender identity is the same as the person's biological sex. *Transgender* is the term used when a person's gender identity differs from the person's biological sex. Neither term implies any specific sexual orientation.

People can express gender identity by their behaviors, clothing, hair-style, grooming, voice, and so on. Gender identity is also expressed by a preferred name and preferred pronouns (Chapter 7). Hormone and surgical measures are options for transgender persons desiring body changes.

FOCUS ON PRIDE

The Person, Family, and Yourself

Personal and Professional Responsibility

Development affects your approach to care. Care measures and procedures change. Safety concerns differ. The person's level of trust and fears vary. *Focus on Children and Older Persons* boxes explain how to adjust care for the different stages of development. As you study, consider how development affects the care you give.

Rights and Respect

Bullying can affect multiple age-groups. It can even occur in the workplace (Chapter 6). Respect for others is needed to prevent bullying. Parents, teachers, students, co-workers, and communities must work together to promote healthy and supportive relationships.

Independence and Social Interaction

Developmental screening is done to monitor development. For example, does the child move, play, learn, and behave as expected? Is the child learning independence? Does the child communicate and interact normally? Delays may indicate an intellectual or developmental disability (Chapter 55).

Delegation and Teamwork

For children, the primary caregiver is an important part of the health team. The nurse teaches the person how to help with care. When interacting with caregivers:
- Be polite. Treat them with kindness and respect.
- Thank them for helping with care.
- Praise actions that are done well.
- Remind them of care measures taught by the nurse.
- Tell the nurse about any questions or concerns.

Ethics and Laws

State laws determine the age of adulthood for making legal and health care decisions. This age varies, but age 18 is common. *Minors* are under the age to legally make decisions. A parent or legal guardian makes decisions for a minor.

FOCUS ON PRIDE: *Application*

Select 2 developmental stages. Describe normal development for the 2 stages. Explain how developmental level affects your approach to care.

REVIEW QUESTIONS

Circle the BEST answer.

1 Changes in mental, emotional, and social function are called
 a Growth
 b Development
 c A reflex
 d A stage

2 Which statement about growth and development is *correct?*
 a They occur from complex to simple.
 b They occur at a set pace.
 c There is no order or pattern.
 d Each stage has its own characteristics.

3 Which reflexes does the infant need for feeding?
 a The Moro and startle reflexes
 b The rooting and sucking reflexes
 c The grasping and Moro reflexes
 d The rooting and palmar grasp reflexes

4 Which occurs *first* in infants?
 a Holding the head up
 b Rolling from front to back
 c Sitting without support
 d The pincer grasp

5 A 6-month-old can
 a Say 3 to 5 words
 b Understand simple instructions
 c Make sounds and squealing noises
 d Respond to "no"

6 By 1½ years a child can usually
 a Identify body parts
 b Walk alone
 c Name colors
 d Put on clothes and shoes

7 Toilet training begins
 a During infancy
 b During the toddler years
 c When children say they are ready
 d At the age of 4 years

8 The toddler can
 a Use a spoon and cup
 b Count items
 c Identify letters
 d Hop on 1 foot

9 Learning to perform self-care
 a Begins during infancy
 b Is complete during toddlerhood
 c Is a developmental task in the preschool years
 d Begins during the school-age years

10 Losing baby teeth usually begins at the age of
 a 2 years
 b 4 years
 c 6 years
 d 8 years

11 Peer groups become important to
 a Toddlers
 b Preschool children
 c School-age children
 d Young adults

12 A school-age child plays video games and watches TV 4 hours a day. This
 a Promotes normal growth and development
 b Is healthy if it is done with a peer
 c Lowers the child's risk of obesity
 d Is not a healthy amount of screen time

13 Reproductive organs begin to function. Secondary sex characteristics appear. This is called
 a Late childhood
 b Puberty
 c Adolescence
 d Adulthood

14 An 11-year-old fears going to school and has lower self-esteem than last school year. The child has frequent stomach aches and trouble sleeping. These
 a May be signs that the child is being bullied
 b Are normal, age-related changes
 c Are signs that puberty has begun
 d Indicate a developmental disability

15 Dating usually begins
 a During late childhood
 b Before puberty
 c With "pairing off"
 d During adolescence

16 Teen dating violence
 a Can occur electronically or in person
 b Does not include stalking
 c Does not have long-term effects
 d Is not preventable

17 Young adulthood normally involves
 a Caring for aging parents
 b Making career choices
 c Physical growth and changes in body appearance
 d Adjusting to having grown children

18 Middle adulthood is a time when
 a Parenting demands increase
 b Physical energy increases
 c Adults develop leisure activities
 d People need to prepare for death

19 Late adulthood involves
 a Retirement
 b Menopause
 c Stable health
 d Few changes

20 When is sexuality important?
 a Starting at puberty
 b When dating begins
 c During marriage
 d Throughout life

Answers to Chapter 11 questions are on p. 901.

FOCUS ON **PRACTICE**

Problem Solving

You are caring for a toddler. You take the child away from the mother for a weight measurement. You ask the child to stand on the scale. The child resists and says, "No." You try to place the child on the scale. The child cries and runs from you. Is this response normal? What could have been done to avoid this?

The Older Person

Late adulthood ranges from 65 years of age and older. The oldest-old are 85 years of age and older. *Gerontology* is the study of the aging process. Normal changes occur in body structure and function. Psychological and social changes also occur. Often changes are slow.

The risk for illness, injury, and disability increases with aging. *Geriatrics* is the care of aging people. Many older persons have 1 or more chronic diseases and disabilities. Disabilities can become more severe with aging and as the disease progresses. Quality of life is affected when disabilities interfere with every-day activities. They include:

- Managing money
- Shopping
- Preparing meals
- Taking prescribed drugs
- Tending to personal hygiene
- Dressing and undressing
- Feeding oneself
- Toileting (elimination)
- Moving about (mobility) in or outside the home
- Enjoying family and friends
- Enjoying leisure and recreational activities

Despite common myths, most older people adjust well and lead happy, meaningful lives. A *myth* is a widely believed story that is not true. See Box 12-1 for some common myths and truths about aging and older persons. Knowing the facts is important to give good care.

PSYCHOLOGICAL AND SOCIAL CHANGES

Older persons experience a variety of life changes. Work and social roles change. Losses occur. Living arrangements may change. Some changes are pleasant. Others are not. People adjust to change in their own way. How they adjust depends on:

- Health status
- Life experiences
- Personality
- Coping ability and stress management (Chapter 53)
- Education and finances
- Social support systems

Social isolation, loneliness, and depression are risks. Mental health and social interaction are important for healthy aging and quality of life.

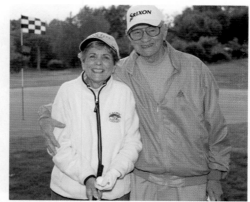
FIGURE 12-1 A retired couple enjoys golf as a leisure-time activity.

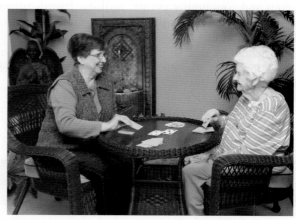
FIGURE 12-2 This retired woman is a nursing center volunteer.

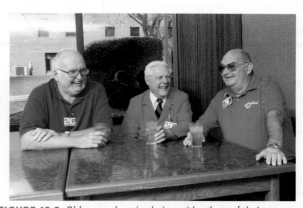
FIGURE 12-3 Older people enjoy being with others of their own age.

Retirement

Retirement is when a person stops working. People usually retire between ages 62 and 66. Some retire earlier. Others work longer. Retirement allows time to relax and enjoy life (Fig. 12-1). Travel, leisure, and doing what one wants are retirement "benefits." Many people enjoy retirement. For others, poor health, disability, and medical bills can make retirement very hard.

Some retired people work part-time or do volunteer work (Fig. 12-2). Work helps meet belonging and self-esteem needs. The person feels useful and forms friendships.

Reduced Income. Retirement often means reduced income. Social Security may provide the only income. House or rent payments continue. Food, clothing, utility bills, and taxes are other expenses. Car expenses, home repairs, drugs, and health care are other costs.

Reduced income may force life-style changes. Examples include:

- Limiting social and leisure events
- Buying cheaper food, clothes, and household items
- Moving to cheaper housing
- Living with children or other family
- Avoiding health care or needed drugs
- Relying on children or other family for money or needed items

Money problems can result. Some people have income from savings, investments, retirement plans, and insurance.

Social Relationships

Social relationships change throughout life. Children grow up, leave home, and have families. Some live far away. Family members and friends die, move away, or are disabled. Yet many older people have regular contact with children, grandchildren, family, and friends. Companionship with people their own age is important (Fig. 12-3).

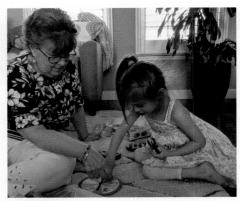

FIGURE 12-4 An older woman plays a game with her grandchild.

Many older people adjust to social changes. Hobbies, religious and community events, and new friends provide enjoyment. Some community groups sponsor bus trips to ball games, shopping, plays, and concerts.

Grandchildren and family times can bring great love and joy (Fig. 12-4). They help the older person feel useful and wanted.

See *Caring About Culture: Social Relationships.*

See *Focus on Long-Term Care and Home Care: Social Relationships.*

 CARING ABOUT CULTURE

Social Relationships

Some older persons speak and understand a foreign language. Communication is with family and friends who speak the same language. They also share cultural values and practices. If family and friends move away or die, the person may not have anyone to talk to. The person may feel lonely and isolated.

FOCUS ON LONG-TERM CARE AND HOME CARE

Social Relationships

Long-Term Care
The social changes of aging can cause loneliness. With nursing center care, the loneliness can seem greater. Staff and other residents do not replace family and friends. However, you can help the person feel less lonely. To provide social contact, you can:

• Suggest calling a family member or friend. Offer to help with phone numbers and dialing. Many residents have their own phones.
• Keep the phone within reach. Calls or text messages can be placed or answered with greater ease.
• Suggest reading cards and letters. Offer to assist.
• Visit with the person a few times during your shift.
• Introduce new residents to other residents and staff.
• Encourage e-mailing or video calls with family and friends. Some residents have electronic devices with center-provided Internet access.

Children as Caregivers

Sometimes parents and children change roles. The child cares for the parent. The older person may feel more secure or unwanted, in the way, and useless. Some lose dignity and self-esteem. Tensions may occur among the child, parent, and other household members. Lack of privacy and loss of independence are causes. So are disagreements and criticisms about housekeeping, raising children, meals, and friends.

Death and Grieving

A person may try to prepare for a loss, but death and grief are still devastating. Feelings of loneliness and emptiness are common after the death of a partner. As people live longer, some out-live their adult children. Parents of any age experience grief when a child dies. Emotional needs are great. Life changes and physical and mental health problems are common.

A surviving spouse or partner may live alone. Others need to decide on housing options (p. 155). Some people re-marry or have new partners.

PHYSICAL CHANGES

Physical changes of aging happen to everyone. See Table 12-1. Body processes slow. Energy level and body efficiency decline. The rate and degree of changes vary with each person. They depend on diet, health, exercise, stress, environment, heredity, and other factors. Changes are slow over many years. Often they are not seen for a long time.

SEXUALITY AND OLDER PERSONS

Reproductive organs change with aging (see Table 12-1). Appearance changes. Strength decreases. Partners are lost through death, divorce, and relationship break-ups. Or a partner needs hospital or nursing center care. Health problems and housing changes are other factors. Changes can affect a person's:
• Thoughts and feelings about being attractive
• Ways of expressing affection
• Sexual function

Sexuality is important throughout life. See "Sexuality Needs" on p. 152.

Frequency of sex may decrease with aging. Some older people do not have intercourse. This does not mean loss of sexual needs or desires. Often needs are expressed in other ways. They hold hands, touch, caress, and embrace. These bring closeness and intimacy.

TABLE 12-1	The Aging Process: Physical Changes and Care Measures
Physical Changes	**Care Measures**

Nervous System

- Brain and spinal cord lose nerve cells
- Nerve cells send messages at a slower rate
- Reflexes slow
- Reduced blood flow to the brain
- Abnormal structures can form in the brain
- Brain tissue may shrink (*atrophy*)
- May experience cognitive changes
  - Forgetfulness
  - Trouble with short-term memory (recall of recent events); long-term memory (recall of events long ago) is affected less
  - Slower reaction time (response time)
  - Trouble with multi-tasking
  - Reduced problem-solving ability
  - Slower learning than when younger (the person can still learn new skills)
- Dizziness
- Sleep patterns change
  - Difficulty falling asleep
  - Waking during the night
  - Going to sleep early and waking early are common
- Reduced sensitivity to temperature, pressure, and pain
- Smell and taste decrease
- Eyes and vision change
  - Eyelids thin and wrinkle
  - Less tear secretion
  - Pupils less responsive to light
  - Decreased vision at night or in dark rooms
  - Problems seeing green and blue colors
  - Poor vision; problems focusing on close objects
- Hearing loss
  - Changes in acoustic nerve
  - Eardrums atrophy
  - Earwax hardens and thickens; impacted earwax (earwax wedged in the ear) can cause hearing loss
  - High-pitched sounds are hard to hear

- Practice safety measures to prevent injuries and falls.
- Remind the person to get up slowly from bed or chair.
- Follow the care plan to assist with memory or mental changes.
- Prevent skin tears and pressure injuries.
- Check for signs of skin breakdown and pressure injuries.
- Give good skin care.
- Follow safety measures for heat and cold.
- Follow the care plan to promote sleep. Day-time naps and rest may be needed.
- Have the person wear eyeglasses, contact lenses, and hearing aids as needed.
- Provide good room lighting and night-lights.
- See the following chapters for care measures.
  - Chapters 14 and 15—safety and preventing falls
  - Chapter 20—turning and moving
  - Chapter 21—getting in and out of bed or chair
  - Chapter 36—sleep
  - Chapter 41—skin tears
  - Chapter 42—pressure injuries
  - Chapter 43—heat and cold
  - Chapter 47—eyeglasses, contact lenses, and hearing aids
  - Chapters 53 and 54—mental changes and confusion

Integumentary System

- Skin becomes less elastic
- Skin thins and sags
- Skin loses strength
- Skin is fragile and easily injured or burned
- Brown spots (*age spots* or *liver spots*) on the wrists and hands
- Fewer nerve endings affect temperature, pressure, and pain sensation
- Fewer blood vessels
- Blood vessels become more fragile
- Fatty tissue layer thins
- Folds, lines, and wrinkles appear
- Decreased secretion of oil and sweat glands
- Dry, itchy skin
- More sensitive to cold
- Nails become thick and tough
- Whitening or graying hair
- Facial hair in some women
- Loss or thinning of hair
- Drier hair

- Protect from drafts and cold.
- Provide sweaters, lap blankets, socks, and extra blankets.
- Check thermostat settings. Higher settings are helpful.
- Provide for hygiene—shower or bath 2 times a week; partial baths on other days.
- Use mild soaps or soap substitutes to clean the underarms, genitals, and under the breasts. Soap may be avoided on the face, arms, legs, back, chest, and abdomen.
- Apply lotions and creams to prevent drying and itching.
- Provide nail and foot care.
- Prevent burns. Do not use hot water bottles or heating pads on the feet.
- Brush and shampoo hair as needed for hygiene and comfort. Shampoo frequency often decreases with age.
- Protect from prolonged sun exposure.
- See the following chapters for care measures.
  - Chapter 14—preventing burns
  - Chapters 24 and 25—hygiene, skin care, and grooming
  - Chapter 41—skin tears
  - Chapter 42—pressure injuries

Continued

TABLE 12-1	The Aging Process: Physical Changes and Care Measures—cont'd
Physical Changes	**Care Measures**
Musculo-Skeletal System	
• Muscles shrink *(atrophy)* • Muscle strength, tone, and contractility decrease • Bone mass decreases • Bones become weaker • Bones become brittle; can break easily • Vertebrae shorten • Joints become stiff and painful • Hip and knee joints become flexed (bent) • Gradual loss of height; trunk (torso) becomes shorter • Decreased mobility	• Promote exercise and activity as ordered to prevent atrophy and loss of strength. • Assist with range-of-motion exercises as ordered (Chapter 35). • Encourage a diet high in protein, calcium, and vitamins as ordered. • Practice safety measures to prevent injuries and falls (Chapters 14 and 15). • Turn and move the person gently and carefully. • Assist the person in getting out of bed or chair as needed. • Provide support when walking as needed (Chapter 35).
Circulatory System	

• Heart pumps with less force
• Heart valves thicken and become stiff
• Heart rate may slow
• Abnormal heart rhythms may occur
• Heart may enlarge slightly
• Heart walls thicken
• Arteries narrow and become stiffer
• Less blood flows through narrowed arteries
• Weakened heart works harder to pump blood through narrowed vessels
• Number of red blood cells decreases
• Fatigue
	• Follow the person's activity limits.
	  • Promote exercise as ordered. Encourage the person to be as active as possible. Moderate daily exercise helps maintain health and well-being.
	  • Assist with range-of-motion exercises as ordered.
	  • Avoid over-exertion. The person should not walk far, climb many stairs, or carry heavy things. Encourage rest periods.
	  • Follow orders for bed rest if it is needed (Chapter 35). *Bed rest* means being confined to bed.
	• Keep personal care items, TV controls, phone, and other needed items within reach.

Respiratory System	
• Respiratory muscles weaken • Some lung tissue is lost • Lung tissue becomes less elastic • Chest is less able to expand and contract to breathe • Difficulty breathing *(dyspnea)* • Decreased strength for coughing and clearing the airway	• Promote normal breathing (Chapter 44). • Position the person for easier breathing. Semi-Fowler's or Fowler's position (Chapter 19) may be preferred. • Assist with coughing and deep-breathing exercises as ordered (Chapter 44). • Avoid heavy bed linens over the chest. • Turn and position the person according to the care plan. Persons on bed rest are re-positioned often. • Encourage activity as ordered. Allow for periods of rest. Observe for difficulty breathing with exertion (activity) and at rest.
Digestive System	
• Decreased saliva production • Loss of teeth • Difficulty chewing • Difficulty swallowing *(dysphagia)* • Decreased number of taste buds • Decreased appetite • Decreased secretion of digestive juices • Difficulty digesting fried and fatty foods • Indigestion • Decreased peristalsis causing *flatulence* (gas) and constipation	• Provide oral hygiene and denture care to improve taste (Chapter 23). • Encourage diet as ordered (Chapter 30). Dry, fried, fatty, and hard-to-chew foods are avoided. The person may need food ground, chopped, or pureed. • Promote fluid intake as ordered (Chapter 32). Thickened liquids may be needed for persons with swallowing problems. • Follow the care plan to prevent *flatulence* (gas) and constipation (Chapter 29). High-fiber foods help prevent constipation. Some are hard to chew and irritate the intestines. Apricots, celery, and fruits and vegetables with skins and seeds are avoided.
Urinary System	
• Kidney function decreases • Reduced blood supply to kidneys • Kidneys atrophy • Bladder tissues less able to stretch • Bladder muscles weaken • Bladder may not empty completely • Urinary tract infections (UTIs) may occur • Urinary frequency, urgency, incontinence (loss of bladder control), or night-time urination may occur • Prostate gland enlarges (men)	• Answer call lights promptly (Chapter 13). • Promote normal urination (Chapter 27). Provide the bedpan, urinal, or commode as needed. • Follow the care plan to manage incontinence (Chapter 27). • Provide catheter care according to the care plan (Chapter 28). • Encourage fluids as ordered to prevent UTIs. Most fluids should be taken before 5:00 PM (1700) to reduce the need to urinate at night. • Follow the person's bladder training program (Chapter 27).

TABLE 12-1	The Aging Process: Physical Changes and Care Measures—cont'd
Physical Changes	**Care Measures**
Immune System	

• Fewer immune cells
• Immune response slows
  • Increased risk for infection
  • Different signs of infection than usual
• Healing slows
• Ability to detect and correct cell defects (problems) declines
  • Increased cancer risk
	• Practice measures to prevent infection (Chapters 17 and 18).
	• Monitor closely for signs of infection.
	  • Usual signs are lessened or absent. The person may have only a slight *fever* (elevated body temperature) or no fever.
	  • Confusion, mood changes, a change in level of consciousness, or a recent fall may signal infection.
	• Prevent injuries and falls (Chapters 14 and 15).
	• Promote exercise (Chapter 35) and a healthy diet (Chapter 30) as ordered. Exercise and good nutrition strengthen the immune system.
	• Follow the care plan for wound care measures and pressure injury prevention (Chapters 41 and 42).
	• The nurse teaches about healthy life-style choices and illness prevention.
	  • Smoking slows healing and weakens the immune system.
	  • Vaccines may prevent certain infections. Influenza and pneumonia are examples (Chapter 50).

Reproductive System	

• Men
  • Testosterone decreases slightly
  • Erections take longer
  • Longer phase between erection and orgasm
  • Less forceful orgasms
  • Erections lost quickly
  • Longer time between erections
• Women
  • *Menopause*—the time when menstruation stops and menstrual cycles end; there has been at least 1 year without a menstrual period
  • Estrogen and progesterone decrease
  • Uterus, vagina, and genitalia atrophy
  • Thinning of vaginal walls
  • Vaginal dryness
  • Arousal takes longer
  • Less intense orgasms
  • Quicker return to pre-excitement state
	• Follow the care plan for the person with reproductive changes (Chapter 52).
	• See "Sexuality Needs" on p. 152.

Altered Sexual Function

Injury, illness, and surgery can affect sexual function. Sometimes the nervous, circulatory, and reproductive systems are involved. Sexual ability may change. Most chronic illnesses affect sexual function. Heart disease, stroke, diabetes, and chronic obstructive pulmonary disease are examples. Some drugs affect sexual desire or performance.

Reproductive system surgeries have physical and mental effects. Removal of the uterus, ovaries, or a breast affects women. Prostate or testes removal affects erections.

Erectile dysfunction (ED) (impotence) is the inability of the male to have or maintain an erection. The many causes include diabetes, spinal cord injuries, prostate problems, substance use disorder, cardiovascular disorders, and psychological factors. Some drugs for high blood pressure cause ED. So do other drugs. Some drugs treat ED.

Changes in sexual function greatly affect the person. Emotional changes are common in men and women. A person may feel unwhole, unattractive, or mutilated. The person may feel unfit for closeness and love. Fear, anger, worry, and depression are seen in behaviors and comments. The person's feelings are normal and expected. Time and understanding are helpful. So is a caring partner. Some persons need counseling.

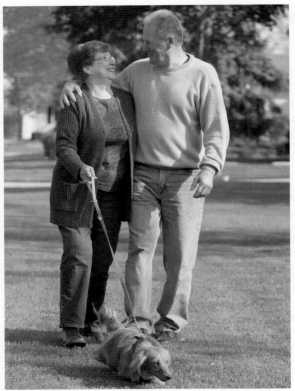

FIGURE 12-5 Love and affection are important to persons of all ages.

Sexuality Needs

Loving relationships and affection are important to older persons (Fig. 12-5). Feeling attractive promotes self-esteem. Having privacy and time for intimacy are needed. The measures in Box 12-2 show respect for the person's sexuality needs.

See *Focus on Long-Term Care and Home Care: Sexuality Needs.*

Inappropriate Sexual Behavior

Patients and residents may have inappropriate sexual behaviors. Such behaviors may be innocent and non-aggressive. Others are aggressive.

Some persons flirt or make sexual advances or comments. Some expose themselves or touch staff. Often there are reasons for the person's behavior. Understanding this helps you deal with the matter.

Inappropriate sexual behaviors have many causes. They include:
- Nervous system disorders
- Confusion, disorientation, and dementia
- Drug side effects
- Infection
- Poor vision

Some behaviors are innocent. The person may mistake another person as a partner. Or the person cannot control the behavior. The healthy person controls sexual urges. Changes in the brain and mental function make control difficult.

Sometimes touch is used to gain attention. For example, a person cannot speak or move the right side. Your buttocks are within reach. To get your attention, the person touches your buttocks. The behavior is not sexual.

Touching the genitals may signal a health problem or a need. Urinary or reproductive system disorders can cause genital soreness and itching. So can poor hygiene and being wet or soiled from urine or feces. Some persons touch or grab at their clothing to communicate an elimination need. Such behaviors are not sexual. They communicate needs.

Sexually aggressive behaviors—touching, grabbing, offensive comments—may be about power, control, or fears about sexual function. For example, a person wants to prove attractiveness and the ability to perform sexually. You must be professional about the matter.

- Ask the person not to touch you. State the places where you were touched.
- Stand back from the person.
- Tell the person what you will not do.
- Tell the person what behaviors make you uncomfortable. Politely ask the person not to act that way.
- Tell the person how to address you. For example, tell the person your name. Ask the person not to call you honey, sweetheart, and so on.
- Allow privacy if the person is becoming aroused. Provide for safety. Complete a safety check of the room (see the inside of the back cover). Tell the person when you will return.
- Discuss the matter with the nurse. The nurse can help you understand the behavior.
- Follow the care plan. It has measures to deal with sexually aggressive behaviors. They are based on the cause of the behavior.

See *Focus on Communication: Inappropriate Sexual Behavior.*

Protecting the Person

The person must be protected from unwanted sexual comments and advances. This is sexual abuse (Chapter 5). Tell the nurse right away. No one is allowed to sexually abuse another person. This includes staff members, patients, residents, family members or other visitors, and volunteers.

FOCUS ON COMMUNICATION

Inappropriate Sexual Behavior

Dealing with sexually inappropriate behavior is hard for new and experienced staff alike. Consider:

- Does the person have a health problem that affects impulse control? If yes, the behavior may not have a sexual purpose.
- Is the person's behavior on purpose? Is the intent sexual? If yes, you must confront the behavior. Be direct and matter-of-fact. For example, you can say:
  - "You brushed your hand across my breast (or other body part) twice this morning. Please don't do that again."
  - "No, I cannot kiss you. It would be unprofessional."
  - "You exposed yourself to me again today. Please do not do that again."

The sexually aggressive person needs the nurse's attention. Report what happened and when. Also report what you said and did. The nurse must deal with the problem. If other staff report such behaviors, the problem is viewed in a broader way.

HOUSING

A person's home is more than a place to live. A home has family memories. It is a link to neighbors and the community. A home can represent a person's independence, social status, and personal identity. It brings pride and self-esteem.

Most older people live in their own homes. Many function without help. Others need help from family, home care, or community-based services for daily living and safety (Box 12-3). Bathing, dressing, meals, housekeeping, shopping, and transportation are examples. Many services also provide social contact.

Some older persons choose smaller homes when children have left home. Others retire to warmer climates or move closer to children and family. Some choose other housing (p. 155). Reduced income, taxes, home repairs, and yard work are factors. Some people require other housing when they can no longer care for themselves.

See *Focus on Long-Term Care and Home Care: Housing,* p. 154.

BOX 12-3	In-Home and Community-Based Services

- *Adult day care*—a safe setting for those who cannot be alone during the day. Services may include personal care, social and recreational activities, meals, drug reminders, counseling, and home health aide services. See p. 155.
- *Adult protective services*—a state agency, it provides help to vulnerable adults and elders to stop or prevent abuse (Chapter 5).
- *Caregiver programs*—for older adults and for grandparents raising grandchildren. Programs offer information about available services, help obtaining support services, counseling, support groups, and other services.
- *Case management*—a case manager assesses the needs of the older person and family. Arrangements are made for needed services.
- *Companionship services*—volunteers provide supervision and support services as needed.

- *Emergency response systems*—in-home 24-hour alarm systems to call for emergency help. The person wears a necklace or bracelet with a button to push if help is needed. An operator responds and sends help.
- *Financial counseling*—help with checking accounts, paying bills, taxes, and insurance claims and forms. Counseling is available about Social Security benefits, prescription drug programs, food stamps, and other programs.
- *Home health care*—nursing and physical, occupational, and speech therapies. The person may need help with such things as taking drugs, changing dressings, or catheter care.
- *Housekeeping services*—help with household tasks. Cleaning, changing linens, laundry, shopping, and preparing meals are examples.

Continued

BOX 12-3	In-Home and Community-Based Services—cont'd

- *Home repair and modification*—programs to keep the house in good repair. Roofing and plumbing are examples. See *Focus on Long-Term Care and Home Care: Housing* for home changes.
- *Hospice care*—end-of-life care (Chapter 59).
- *Legal assistance*—advice for some legal matters. Wills, advance directives (Chapter 59), renters' rights, and consumer problems are examples. A lawyer may represent the person in court.
- *Meal programs*—meals in-home or at a senior center, nutrition site, or other group setting.
- *Personal care*—help with eating, bathing, oral care, grooming, and dressing.
- *Rehabilitation*—therapies to assist the person to regain or maintain the person's desired level of functioning.

- *Respite care*—relieves caregivers of daily care for a short time.
- *Senior centers*—offer many social and recreational activities. Classes, day trips, travel groups, performing arts, and nature activities are examples. Services also include meals, counseling, legal help, health screenings, and transportation.
- *Phone reassurance*—regular phone contact with the person. The person is called at various times. If the person does not answer, someone is sent to the person's home. Also, the older person can call the service when help is needed.
- *Transportation*—rides to and from doctor visits, appointments, shopping, religious services, and other places.
- *Wellness programs*—blood pressure, blood sugar, and other tests are done to promote health. Sessions are held about fitness, nutrition, and other health topics.

FOCUS ON LONG-TERM CARE AND HOME CARE

Housing

Home Care
Simple changes can make a home safe, easy to use, and promote independence. The nurse discusses needed changes with the patient and family.

The Bathroom
- Non-slick flooring
- Slip-resistant surfaces in showers and tubs (bath mats, slip-resistant bath strips)
- Grab bars by showers, tubs, and toilets
- Rugs have non-slip backing and are secured to the floor outside the tub and shower and in front of the toilet; no throw rugs
- Hand-held shower nozzle or adjustable shower head
- Shower chair for shower or bathtub
- Transfer bench
- Lever-handle faucets
- Water controls close to the shower or tub entrance
- Anti-scald devices on faucets and shower heads
- Storage area for liquid soap and hair products is attached to the wall for easy access
- Towel bars or hooks raised or lowered for the person's reach
- Comfort-height toilet, elevated toilet seat, or a toilet seat riser
- Chair placed in front of the sink for sitting
- Knee space under the sink for the person who sits
- Bright, non-glare lighting

The Bedroom
- Clear walking path in the room and to the bathroom; un-wanted and un-used furniture and items are removed
- Loose flooring is repaired
- Area rugs and cords are removed
- Phone on a nightstand
- Flashlight and extra batteries on a nightstand
- Remotes for the TV, fans, and lamps on a nightstand
- Bed rails if needed
- Night-lights
- Lit path to the bathroom
- Closet rods that adjust for height
- Lowered shelves or pull-down shelves
- Pull-out drawers, bins, and baskets in closets
- A commode chair near the bed for night-time use (Chapter 27)

The Kitchen
- Appliances within reach and accessible
- Stove controls on the front of the stove
- Stove controls clearly marked and easy to see
- Lowered shelves or pull-down or pull-out shelves
- Height of sink and countertops adjusted for the person's needs (lowered for wheelchair use; raised for the person who cannot bend easily)
- Anti-scald devices on faucets
- Lever-handle faucets
- Spray attachment to the sink

Other
- Lever door handles on all doors
- Easy-to-grasp cabinet and drawer handles
- Hand rails on both sides of stairways and outside steps
- Keyless locking system
- Security system
- Shelves near outside doors—items can be set down to open the door
- Bright lights inside and outside entry-ways
- Motion-activated entrance lights
- Slip-free walk-ways and entry-ways
- House numbers that are easy to see from the street
- Automatic garage door opener
- Rocker light switches that turn on and off with a push
- Electrical outlets 18 inches above the floor
- Peepholes or view panels in doors at the correct height for the person
- Washer and dryer on the main floor
- Wall-mounted, fold-down ironing board
- Stair or platform lifts
- No scatter or throw rugs
- Thick carpeting replaced with low pile carpeting
- Furniture arranged for wheelchair use
- Phones in all rooms, including the bathroom
- Chairs throughout the home so the person can sit when tired, weak, dizzy, and so on
- Smoke alarms as required by local fire code
- Carbon monoxide alarms
- For poor eyesight—see Chapter 47
- For hearing loss—see Chapter 47
- For other safety measures—see Chapter 14
- For fall prevention—see Chapter 15

Housing Options

People respond differently to the need to relocate (change housing). The new setting may maintain, improve, or lower the person's quality of life. The person's response depends on many factors. The person's level of choice and control, the amount of time to prepare, and the number and kind of losses associated with the move are examples.

There are many housing options available to meet the needs of older people. Having a safe and home-like setting is important.

Living With Family. Sometimes older brothers, sisters, and cousins live together. They provide companionship and help during illness or disability. Living expenses are shared.

Some older persons live with their adult children. The older parent (parents) moves in with the child. Or the child moves to the parent's home. The parent may be healthy, may need some help, or may be ill or disabled. Some children give needed care or arrange for home care. Many community and religious groups have volunteers who help give care.

Living with family is a social change. Everyone in the home must adjust. Schedules, meals, and room and sleeping arrangements may change. An adult child's family needs time alone. Other family members may help give care. Respite care is an option. *Respite care* gives the family relief from the person's care for a short period of time. It may be provided at home, in a health care facility, or at an adult day care center.

Adult Day Care. Adult day-care centers provide supervision, meals, and activities for adults needing day-time care. Transportation, rehabilitation (Chapter 46), and dementia care (Chapter 54) are common. Requirements vary. Most require some self-care abilities and the ability to be mobile (by walking or with a wheelchair).

Some centers are inter-generational. Children and older persons are in the same center. They eat, play, and work together on activities. Young children bring much joy to older persons. They give older persons purpose, love, and affection. In turn, children learn about aging and receive attention and affection.

Elder Cottage Housing Opportunity and Accessory Dwelling Units. *Elder Cottage Housing Opportunity (ECHO)* homes are small homes designed for older and disabled persons. The portable home is placed in the yard of a single-family home. Some ECHO homes attach to a house as a home addition. Government funding may be available.

An *accessory dwelling unit (ADU)* is a separate living area in a home or yard. It can be over a garage, in the basement, an addition to the house, or in a side or back yard. It has a kitchen, bedroom, and bathroom. Some have a small living room.

ADUs are also called "in-law apartments," "granny flats," "accessory apartments," "second units," and other names. ECHO homes and ADUs allow older persons to live independently but near family and friends.

Rental Options. Rental options include a single-family home, an apartment, a condo, a mobile home, or a room in a house. The renter pays rent and utility bills. The benefits of renting include:

- The renter does not have the responsibilities of home ownership.
- The owner (landlord) provides maintenance, yard work, snow removal, and repairs.
- The older person remains independent.
- The older person can keep personal items.
  Downsides to renting include:
- Restrictions about having pets
- Relying on the landlord for repairs and maintenance
- Rent increases
- Ending rental agreements before the person wants to move
- Lack of gardening or yard work opportunities

Senior Citizen Housing. In many areas, state and federal funds support apartment complexes for older and disabled persons. Such persons have low to moderate incomes. Monthly rents depend on the person's monthly income.

Home-Sharing. Two or more people share a house or apartment. They share living spaces—kitchen, bathroom, living room. They share household chores and expenses. Or cooking, cleaning, and yard work are exchanged for rent.

Shared housing is a way to avoid living alone. It provides companionship. Some people feel safer when living with another person.

Residential Care Facilities and Assisted Living. These settings provide housing and services for groups of residents. Staff are available 24 hours a day. Services vary. Some provide only housing, meals, and housekeeping. Many provide social activities and services to support personal care and independent living.

Residential Care Facilities. Residential care facilities (board and care homes; group homes) are small, private facilities. They house older persons or people with certain problems. Dementia, mental health disorders, and intellectual and developmental disabilities are examples.

These settings usually house fewer than 20 residents. Rooms are private or shared. Personal care and meals are provided. Nursing and medical care are usually not provided on-site.

Assisted Living. Assisted living residences are for persons needing some help with daily living. Residents usually have their own room or apartment and share common areas with other residents. Services include meals, help with personal care and drugs, and housekeeping and laundry services. Staff are available on-site for supervision and security at all times. Social and recreational activities are provided. See Chapter 57.

Continuing Care Retirement Communities.
Continuing care retirement communities (CCRCs; life care communities) offer different levels of service for a person's changing needs. Independent living units (house or apartment), assisted living residences, and nursing center care are available in 1 location.

When in an independent living unit, residents perform self-care and take their own drugs. Food service is provided. Help is nearby if needed. Many people travel or drive their own cars. Rides are provided for those who need them.

Services are added as the person's needs change. Over time, some persons need home care, assisted living, or nursing center care. The nursing center is within the CCRC. Many older couples find comfort in this plan. One partner needs nursing care. The other is close by and can visit often.

Nursing Centers.
Nursing centers serve to meet the needs of older and disabled persons who cannot care for themselves (Chapter 1). Aging changes and safety needs are considered in the center's design. Programs and services are provided to meet basic needs. Some people stay in nursing centers until death. Others return home.

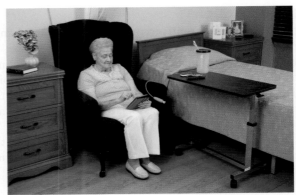

FIGURE 12-6 A nursing center is as home-like as possible. Some centers allow residents to bring their own bed and furniture from home.

The person needing nursing center care may suffer some or all of these losses.
* Loss of identity as a productive member of a family and community
* Loss of possessions—home, household items, car, and so on
* Loss of independence
* Loss of real-world experiences—shopping, traveling, cooking, driving, hobbies, and so on
* Loss of health and mobility

Feeling useless, powerless, and hopeless are common emotions. The health team helps the person cope with loss and improve quality of life.

To receive Medicare or Medicaid funds, nursing centers must meet OBRA requirements. OBRA protects the person's rights and promotes quality of life. The Centers for Medicare & Medicaid Services (CMS) has rules and regulations for OBRA. Chapter 13 discusses the requirements for the person's living space. The setting must be safe, clean, and comfortable. It is as home-like as possible (Fig. 12-6). Resident needs and preferences are planned for and met (Chapter 8). Box 12-4 lists the features of a quality nursing center.

BOX 12-4   Features of a Quality Nursing Center

Basic Information
* The center is Medicare-certified.
* The center is Medicaid-certified.
* The center and administrator are licensed by the state.
* The center provides the level of care needed. Rehabilitation, dementia, ventilator, and hospice services are examples.
* The center is located close enough for family and friends to visit.
* The center gives information in writing about policies, services, extra charges, and fees. For example, is there an extra charge for beauty shop services?

Living Spaces
* The center is free from strong, unpleasant odors.
* The center appears clean and well-kept.

Living Spaces—cont'd
* The temperature is comfortable for the residents.
* The center has good lighting.
* Noise levels in the dining room and in common areas are comfortable.
* Furnishings in rooms and lounges are sturdy, comfortable, and attractive.
* Exits are clearly marked.
* The center has quiet areas where residents can visit with family and friends.
* All common areas, resident rooms, and doorways are designed for wheelchair use.
* The center has hand rails in the hallways.
* The center has grab bars in bathrooms.
* The center has smoke alarms and sprinklers.

BOX 12-4	Features of a Quality Nursing Center—cont'd

Menus and Food

- Residents have food choices at meal times.
- The center provides for special dietary needs.
- Nutritious snacks are available.
- Staff help residents eat and drink if needed.

Staff

- The relationship between the staff and residents appears to be warm, polite, and respectful.
- Staff knock on the person's door before entering the room.
- Staff refer to residents by name.
- The center offers a training and continuing education program for all staff.
- The center does background checks to make sure staff are not hired who:
  - Have been found guilty of abuse, neglect, or mistreatment of residents.
  - Have a finding of abuse, neglect, or mistreatment of residents in the state nurse aide registry.
- The center has licensed nurses 24 hours a day. An RN (registered nurse) is present as required by federal standards.
- The center posts information about the number of nursing staff working. This includes the number of nursing assistants.
- Nursing assistants help plan the person's care.
- The center has a staff member to meet the social needs of residents.
- The center will call the person's doctor for medical needs.
- The center's management team has worked together for at least 1 year. This includes the administrator and director of nursing.
- The resident's primary language is spoken by the staff. If not, an interpreter is available for the resident to communicate needs.

Residents' Rooms

- Residents may have personal belongings and furniture in their rooms.
- Residents have personal storage space (closet and drawers) in their rooms.
- Residents have a window in their rooms.
- Residents have access to a personal phone, TV, the Internet, and a computer.
- Residents have a choice of roommates.
- The center has policies and procedures to protect resident possessions. Cabinets and closets that lock are examples.

Activities

- Residents may choose a variety of activities. This includes residents who stay in their rooms.
- The center has outdoor areas for resident use. Staff help residents go outside.
- The center has an active volunteer program.
- Residents help plan or choose activities.
- The resident chooses when to get up, go to sleep, and bathe.
- Residents can have visitors at any time. This includes during early or late hours.
- The center has procedures for when a resident wants to leave the center for a few hours or days.
- The center provides or arranges for a resident's religious and cultural needs.

Safety and Care

- The center takes action to protect residents from abuse, neglect, mistreatment, and exploitation. Policies and procedures prohibit abuse and neglect. Reporting is required. There is information about how to report a concern and how the center responds.
- The center has no citations related to abuse in the last 2 years. (*Citations* are violations of regulations found during a survey [Chapter 1]. A required standard was not met.)
- Residents are clean and well-groomed.
- Residents are dressed correctly for the season or time of day.
- Residents may see their personal doctors.
- The center has an arrangement with a nearby hospital.
- Care plan meetings are held with residents and family members. Meetings are held at times that are convenient and flexible for the resident and family when possible.
- The center has inspection reports—quality care, health, fire—available for residents to see.
- The center has corrected all problems on its last state inspection report.
- The center has policies and procedures related to the care of persons with dementia. This includes non-drug-based approaches.
- The center takes part in efforts to reduce the use of antipsychotic drugs.

Modified from Centers for Medicare & Medicaid Services: Your guide to choosing a nursing home or other long-term services & supports, CMS product no. 02174, revised October 2019.

FOCUS ON PRIDE

The Person, Family, and Yourself

P ersonal and Professional Responsibility

All older persons are not the same. Each person is unique. Treat each person as an individual.

R ights and Respect

Simple actions can promote dignity and respect for the older person. For example:

- Knock before entering the room.
- Greet the person by name. Make eye contact and smile. Be pleasant.
- Treat the person as an adult, not a child.
- Speak to the person, not just to a caregiver or family member.
- Listen to the person.
- Promote independence and a sense of control. Offer choices. Follow the person's preferences.

I ndependence and Social Interaction

Physical changes of aging can affect a person socially. For example:

- A person has trouble hearing conversations when there is background noise. The person decides not to attend social events.
- A person has vision changes and slowed responses. No longer feeling safe to drive, the person remains at home more.
- Mobility problems and incontinence prevent a person from doing desired activities.

Social isolation and loneliness are risks. Depression and other health problems are linked to isolation and loneliness. Staying active and connected are important. Meaningful activities and social interaction can prevent isolation and loneliness.

D elegation and Teamwork

Co-workers often work together to assist older persons. A co-worker may be closer to your age, share your interests, relate to your work, share your native language, and so on. You must not ignore the person or speak in a foreign language. Focus on the person, not on others. This promotes a sense of belonging and self-worth.

E thics and Laws

Older persons may need help from family or caregivers. Watch for signs of abuse.

- The person is treated like an infant or child.
- The person is not spoken to.
- The person is insulted, scolded, or criticized.
- Threats to with-hold care are made.
- Mis-use or theft of money or possessions is suspected.
- The person lacks needed care or has poor hygiene.
- The person has signs of physical abuse—bruises, scars, burns, and so on.

See "Elder Abuse" in Chapter 5. If you suspect abuse, tell the nurse. The person must be protected from mistreatment.

FOCUS ON PRIDE: *Application*

List 5 changes that occur with aging. Describe how each affects the person. How would you modify care to meet the person's needs?

REVIEW QUESTIONS

Circle the BEST answer.

1 The care of aging people is called
   a Geriatrics
   b Dysphagia
   c Gerontology
   d Dyspnea

2 Retirement usually results in
   a Lowered income
   b Nursing center care
   c Less free time
   d Financial security

3 Which causes loneliness in older persons?
   a Having hobbies
   b Children moving away
   c Attending community events
   d Contact with other older persons

4 Which statement about a partner's death is *true*?
   a The surviving partner's life will not likely change.
   b Preparing for the event lessens grief.
   c Grief cannot cause physical problems.
   d Feelings of loss and emptiness occur.

5 Aging causes changes in the nervous system. Which is *true*?
   a Sleep patterns change.
   b Recent memories are easier to recall than past memories.
   c Sensitivity to pressure increases.
   d Confusion occurs in all older persons.

6 Changes can occur in the eyes with aging. Which is *true*?
   a Tear secretion increases.
   b There is no change in seeing colors.
   c There is more trouble focusing on far objects.
   d Vision is poor at night and in dark rooms.

7 Which is *true* of hearing loss in older persons?
   a Low-pitched sounds are hard to hear.
   b Acoustic nerve changes affect hearing.
   c Earwax cannot affect hearing.
   d Ear infections often cause hearing loss.

8 Skin changes occur with aging. Care should include
   a Keeping the room cool
   b A daily bath with soap
   c Applying lotion
   d Bathing in hot water

9 An older person complains of cold feet. You should
  a Provide socks
  b Apply a hot water bottle
  c Soak the feet in hot water
  d Apply a heating pad

10 Musculo-skeletal changes occur with aging. Which is *true?*
  a Bones become firm.
  b Exercise promotes muscle atrophy.
  c Joints become stiff and painful.
  d Bed rest prevents loss of strength.

11 An older person has circulatory changes. Which care measure would you question?
  a Keep needed items nearby.
  b Get a moderate amount of daily exercise.
  c Avoid over-exertion.
  d Take long walks.

12 Respiratory changes occur with aging. Which is *true?*
  a Heavy bed linens are used.
  b The person is turned often if on bed rest.
  c The side-lying position is best for breathing.
  d Deep breathing is avoided.

13 Older persons should avoid dry foods because of
  a Decreases in saliva and difficulty swallowing
  b Appetite changes
  c Increased amounts of digestive juices
  d Increased peristalsis

14 Changes occur in the digestive system. Older persons should eat
  a Fruits and vegetables with skins and seeds
  b Dry and fatty foods
  c Raw apricots and celery
  d High-fiber foods

15 Changes occur in the urinary system. Which is *true?*
  a Kidneys increase in size.
  b Bladder muscles weaken.
  c The prostate gland in men shrinks.
  d Blood flow to the kidneys increases.

16 An older person is at risk for a urinary tract infection (UTI). The doctor ordered increased fluid intake. You should
  a Give most of the fluid before 1700 (5:00 PM)
  b Question the order
  c Give thickened liquids
  d Insert a catheter

17 Erectile dysfunction
  a Occurs in men and women
  b Results from a lack of interest in sex
  c Affects sexual performance
  d Is an inappropriate sexual behavior

18 Which shows respect for the older person's sexuality needs?
  a Leaving the door open after the person asked for privacy
  b Staying in the room while a spouse visits
  c Styling a person's hair as the person prefers
  d Saying a person is too old to wear a certain outfit

19 Which response is appropriate?
  a A resident makes sexually offensive comments. You laugh.
  b A resident touches you sexually. You ask the person not to touch you.
  c A resident is masturbating in the dining room. You scold the person.
  d A resident keeps grabbing at his pants. You do nothing.

20 An older person and family are discussing housing. Which *best* supports the person's desire for independent living?
  a The family makes housing decisions for the person.
  b The family insists that the person move in with them.
  c The family refuses to get involved.
  d The family offers to modify the person's home for safety.

21 A husband needs 24-hour nursing care. His wife needs an independent living unit. Which would meet their needs?
  a Respite care
  b Home health care
  c A continuing care retirement community
  d An assisted living residence

22 An older person needs nursing center care. Which signals quality?
  a The center appears clean and well-kept.
  b Staff refer to residents by room number.
  c The center has had 3 different administrators in the last year.
  d Personal belongings are not allowed to prevent theft of items.

Answers to Chapter 12 questions are on p. 901.

FOCUS ON **PRACTICE**

Problem Solving

A person has urinary incontinence and swallowing problems due to changes from aging. A co-worker uses the term "diaper" to describe incontinence products and "bib" for clothing protectors. The co-worker threatens to with-hold privileges if the person does not finish meals.

Why should you treat the person as an adult and not a child? Describe ways to provide age-appropriate care. How will you respond to your co-worker's statements and actions?

The Person's Unit

OBJECTIVES

- Define the key terms and key abbreviations in this chapter.
- Explain how to maintain the person's unit.
- Describe the CMS requirements for resident rooms.
- Describe how to control the person's setting for comfort.
- Describe the basic bed positions.
- Identify the 7 hospital bed system entrapment zones.
- Identify the persons at risk for bed entrapment.

- Explain how to use the furniture and equipment in the person's unit.
- Explain how to safely use the call system.
- Describe how a bathroom is equipped for the person's use.
- Describe how to promote safety, privacy, and comfort in the person's unit.
- Explain how to promote PRIDE in the person, the family, and yourself.

KEY TERMS

entrapment Getting caught, trapped, or entangled in spaces created by the bed rails, the mattress, the bed frame, the head-board, or the foot-board

full visual privacy Having the means to be completely free from public view while in bed

hospital bed system The bed frame and its parts—mattress, bed rails, head- and foot-boards, and bed attachments

person's unit The space, furniture, and equipment used by the person in the agency

KEY ABBREVIATIONS

CMS	Centers for Medicare & Medicaid Services	F	Fahrenheit

The *person's unit* is the space, furniture, and equipment used by the person in the agency (Fig. 13-1). The person's unit is designed for comfort, safety, and privacy. In nursing centers, the person's unit is as personal and home-like as possible. Always treat the person's unit with respect.

A private room is for 1 person. Semi-private rooms have 2 units. The person's unit is kept clean, neat, safe, and comfortable. See Box 13-1.

See *Focus on Long-Term Care and Home Care: The Person's Unit.*
See *Promoting Safety and Comfort: The Person's Unit*, p. 162.

BOX 13-1 Maintaining the Person's Unit

- Keep the following within the person's reach. Arrange them as the person prefers.
  - Call light (p. 171). The call light is within reach at all times.
  - Over-bed table and bedside stand (p. 170).
  - Phone, TV, bed, and light controls.
  - Tissues.
  - Other items as requested.
- Meet the needs of persons who cannot use the call system (p. 171).
- Adjust lighting, temperature, and ventilation for the person's comfort.
- Handle equipment carefully to prevent noise.
- Explain the causes of strange noises.

- Prevent odors. See p. 162.
- Use room deodorizers according to agency policy.
- Empty wastebaskets at least daily and when full. In some agencies, they are emptied every shift.
- Respect the person's belongings. An item may not be important to you. Yet even a scrap of paper can have great meaning to the person.
- Do not discard any items belonging to the person.
- Do not move furniture or the person's belongings. Persons with poor vision rely on memory or feel to find items.
- Straighten bed linens and towels as often as needed.
- Complete a safety check before leaving the room. (See the inside of the back cover.)

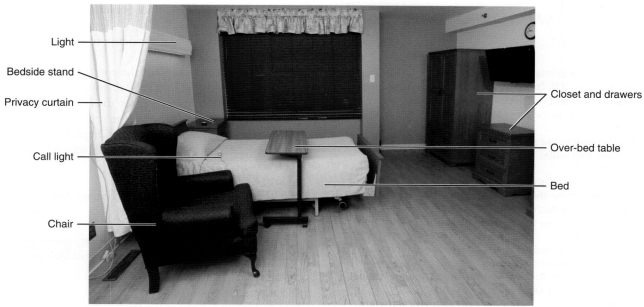

Light

Bedside stand

Privacy curtain

Call light

Chair

Closet and drawers

Over-bed table

Bed

FIGURE 13-1 Furniture and equipment in a resident's unit.

FOCUS ON LONG-TERM CARE AND HOME CARE

The Person's Unit

Long-Term Care

The Centers for Medicare & Medicaid Services (CMS) has requirements for residents' living space.

- The setting is clean, in good condition, and free of clutter. The setting is safe and comfortable for residents, staff, and visitors.
- Rooms are designed for 1 or 2 persons. (Some older facilities are allowed up to 4.)
- Rooms have a direct access to an exit hallway.
- Rooms have at least 1 window to the outside.
- Rooms are designed or equipped for full visual privacy (p. 170).
- Each person has closet space with accessible racks and shelves. Each person's clothing is stored separately.
- Each room has its own bathroom with at least a toilet and sink. Bathing facilities are in the bathroom or nearby. (Some older facilities are allowed to have toilet and bathing facilities nearby.)
- Rooms, bathrooms, and bathing areas have a functioning call system.
- The person has a bed of proper height and size.
- The person has a clean, comfortable mattress.
- Bed and bath linens (towels and washcloths) are clean, dry, and in good condition.
- Bed linens are correct for the weather and climate.
- The room has furniture for clothing, personal items, and a chair for visitors.
- There is space for wheelchair or walker use.

- Rooms, drawers, and shelves are clean and orderly.
- Room temperature levels are between 71°F (Fahrenheit) and 81°F.
- Water temperatures are comfortable and at a safe level in resident rooms and in bathrooms and bathing areas.
- Ventilation, humidity, and odor levels are acceptable.
- Sound levels are comfortable.
- Lighting is adequate and comfortable with little glare.
- The room is free of pests and rodents.
- Hand rails are in good repair. Residents can access the hand rails.
- Care equipment is in good repair and functions safely.
- The person's room is home-like. Personal belongings are allowed.
- Items are within reach for use in bed or the bathroom.
- The person's setting accommodates the person's individual needs and preferences. (Accommodations are reasonable and do not interfere with the health or safety of other residents.)

Resident units must be as personal and home-like as possible. Residents can bring and use some furniture and personal items from home. This promotes dignity and self-esteem.

As space allows, the person chooses where to place personal items. However, a resident cannot take or use another person's space. Doing so violates the other person's rights.

PROMOTING SAFETY AND COMFORT

The Person's Unit

Comfort

Admission is the official entry of a person into a health care setting (Chapter 37). On admission to an agency, the nurse may have you orient the person and family to the area.

- Identify items in the person's unit. Explain the purpose of each.
- Explain how to use room furniture and equipment.
  - Over-bed table
  - Call light
  - Bed, TV, and light controls
- Show the person the bathroom. Explain how to use the call light in the bathroom (p. 173).
- Explain how to use the agency's phone. Place the phone within reach.
- Explain how to connect to the Internet and show where to charge electronic devices.
- Explain where to find the nurses' station, lounge, chapel, dining room, and other areas.
- Identify staff—housekeeping, dietary, physical therapy, and others. Also identify students who are in the agency.
- Explain when meals and snacks are served.
- Explain visiting hours and policies.
  Do not rush. Treat the person and family as guests. Be polite. Tell them good things about the agency. Introduce other nurses and nursing assistants. Help the person adjust to a new setting.

COMFORT

Comfort is a state of well-being (Chapter 36). Age, illness, and activity affect comfort. So do temperature, ventilation, noise, odors, and lighting. These factors are controlled to meet the person's needs.

See *Focus on Communication: Comfort.*

FOCUS ON COMMUNICATION

Comfort

What is comfortable for 1 person may not be for another. Ask about the person's comfort. You can say:
- "How is the temperature? Is it too hot or too cold?"
- "Is the noise level okay?"
- "Please let me know if you notice any bad odors."
- "How is the lighting? Is it too bright or too dark?"
- "Are you comfortable?"

Temperature and Ventilation

Most healthy people are comfortable with room temperatures between 68°F and 74°F. This range may be too hot or too cold for others. Persons who are older or ill may need higher temperatures for comfort. The CMS requires that nursing centers maintain a temperature of 71°F to 81°F.

Less active persons may not like cool areas. They need warm clothing and warm room temperatures.

Stale room air and lingering odors affect comfort and rest. Ventilation systems provide fresh air and move room air, causing drafts. Infants, older persons, and those who are ill are sensitive to drafts.

To protect patients and residents from cool areas and drafts:
- Have them wear enough of the correct clothing.
- Offer lap coverings (blankets, throws) to those in chairs and wheelchairs to cover the legs.
- Provide enough blankets for warmth.
- Cover them with bath blankets (Chapter 22) when giving care. A bath blanket provides warmth and privacy during care measures.
- Move them from drafty areas.

See *Focus on Children and Older Persons: Temperature and Ventilation.*

FOCUS ON CHILDREN AND OLDER PERSONS

Temperature and Ventilation

Older Persons
Poor circulation and loss of the skin's fatty tissue layer occur with aging. Therefore older persons are sensitive to cold (Chapter 12). They may wear extra clothing for warmth. Many wear sweaters or jackets in warm weather. Respect the person's wishes and choices.

Odors

Odors occur in health care settings and in home care. Bowel movements and urine have embarrassing odors. So do draining wounds and vomitus. Body, breath, and smoke odors may offend others.

Some people are very sensitive to odors. They may become nauseated. Good nursing care, ventilation, and housekeeping practices help prevent odors. To reduce odors:
- Empty, clean, and disinfect bedpans, urinals, commodes, and kidney basins promptly.
- Make sure toilets are flushed.
- Check incontinent persons often (Chapters 27 and 29).
- Clean persons who are wet or soiled from urine, feces (stools), vomitus, or wound drainage.
- Change wet or soiled linens and clothing promptly.
- Follow agency policy for where to place wet or soiled linens and clothing.
- Keep laundry containers closed.
- Dispose of incontinence and ostomy products promptly (Chapters 27 and 29).
- Provide good hygiene to prevent body and breath odors (Chapters 23 and 24).
- Use room deodorizers as needed and allowed by agency policy. Do not use sprays around persons with breathing problems. Ask the nurse if you are unsure.

Smoke odors present special problems. If you smoke, follow the agency's policy. Practice hand-washing after smoking, after handling smoking materials, and before giving care. Pay attention to your uniform, hair, and breath because of smoke odors.

Noise

According to the CMS, a "comfortable" sound level:
- Does not interfere with a person's hearing.
- Promotes privacy when privacy is desired.
- Allows the person to take part in social activities.

Common health care sounds can be disturbing. Examples include:
- Clanging and clattering equipment, dishes, and meal trays
- Loud voices, TVs, music, and so on
- Ringing phones
- Intercom systems and call lights
- Equipment or wheels needing repair or oil
- Cleaning and housekeeping equipment

People want to know the cause and meaning of new sounds. This relates to safety and security needs. Some sounds seem dangerous, frightening, or irritating. Patients and residents may become upset, anxious, and uncomfortable. What is noise to one person may not be noise to another. For example, some people enjoy loud music. It disturbs others.

Health care agencies are designed to reduce noise. Window and floor coverings absorb noise. Plastic items make less noise than metal equipment (bedpans, urinals, wash basins). To decrease noise levels:
- Control your voice.
- Handle equipment carefully.
- Keep equipment in good working order.
- Answer phones, call lights, and intercoms promptly.

See *Focus on Communication: Noise.*
See *Focus on Children and Older Persons: Noise.*
See *Focus on Surveys: Noise.*

FOCUS ON COMMUNICATION

Noise

All staff must try to reduce noise. To reduce noise:
- Do not talk loudly in the hallways or nurses' station.
- Ask others to speak more softly if necessary. Ask politely.
- Avoid unnecessary conversation. Be professional. Do not discuss inappropriate topics at work. Others may overhear and become offended.

FOCUS ON CHILDREN AND OLDER PERSONS

Noise

Older Persons

Persons with dementia may not understand what is happening around them. Common, every-day sounds can disturb them. For example, a person has an extreme reaction to a ring tone on a phone (Chapter 54). The reaction may be more severe at night. This is likely if the sound startles or suddenly awakens the person. A dark, strange room can make the problem worse.

FOCUS ON SURVEYS

Noise

Surveyors will observe for comfortable sound levels.
- Do background noises affect the person's ability to be heard or take part in activities?
- Do staff raise their voices to be heard?
- Are sound levels comfortable in the evening and during the night?

Do your best to decrease noise and provide comfortable sound levels.

Lighting

Safe and comfortable lighting:
- Lessens glares.
- Lets the person control the brightness, location, and direction of light.
- Lets visually impaired persons maintain or increase independent functioning.

Glares, shadows, and dull lighting can cause falls, headaches, and eyestrain. A bright room is cheerful. Dim light is better for relaxing and rest.

Adjust window coverings and lighting to meet the person's needs. The over-bed and ceiling lights provide soft, medium, or bright lighting.

Persons with poor vision need bright lighting. This is very important at meal time and when moving about in the room and agency. Bright lighting also helps the staff perform procedures.

Always keep light controls within the person's reach. This protects the right to personal choice.

See *Focus on Children and Older Persons: Lighting.*

FOCUS ON CHILDREN AND OLDER PERSONS

Lighting

Older Persons

Persons with dementia may become agitated or aggressive at times. There is often a reason for the reaction (Chapter 54). Lighting may be a factor. Adjust lighting for the person's needs. Soft, non-glare lights are relaxing. Brighter lighting lets the person see more clearly. This may improve orientation.

ROOM FURNITURE AND EQUIPMENT

Rooms are furnished and equipped for safety and to meet basic needs—comfort, sleep, elimination, nutrition, hygiene, and activity. There is equipment to communicate with staff. The right to privacy is considered.

The Bed

Beds have controls to:

- Raise and lower the whole bed (Fig. 13-2).
  - The bed is raised to give care and reduce bending and reaching.
  - The bed is lowered to let the person get out of bed with ease and to prevent injury from falls.
- Adjust the head and foot of the bed for comfort. The person is told of any position limits or restrictions. For example, lowering the head of the bed fully causes shortness of breath *(dyspnea)*. The care plan includes keeping the head of the bed raised at least 30 degrees.

Beds are manual or electric. Manual beds are controlled with cranks at the foot of the bed (Fig. 13-3). The cranks are turned to raise and lower the whole bed or the head or foot of the bed. Electric beds are controlled with buttons. Electric beds are common.

Electric controls may be hand-held or on the bed rail (Fig. 13-4). Sometimes controls are on the foot-board. Some beds have pedals near the floor that can be controlled with the foot.

Bed rail controls are often different on the inner and outer parts of the bed rail.

- Controls on the inner part are for patient or resident use (see Fig. 13-4, *B*). These controls are limited. This prevents the person from placing the bed in a dangerous position.
- Controls on the outer part are for staff use (see Fig. 13-4, *C*). These control all of the bed's functions.

See *Focus on Long-Term Care and Home Care: The Bed.*
See *Promoting Safety and Comfort: The Bed.*

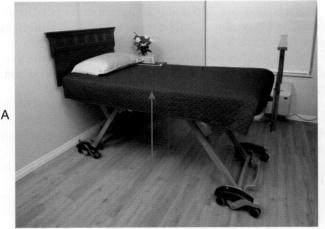 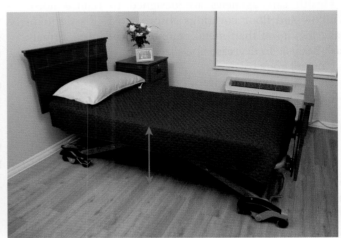

FIGURE 13-2 A, The bed is in a high position. **B,** The bed is in a low position.

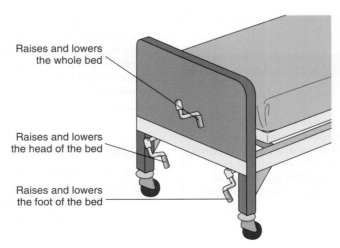

Raises and lowers the whole bed

Raises and lowers the head of the bed

Raises and lowers the foot of the bed

FIGURE 13-3 A manual bed has cranks at the foot of the bed.

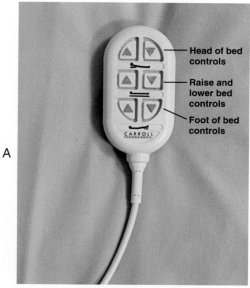

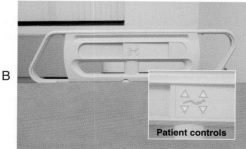

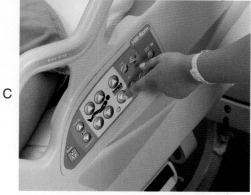

FIGURE 13-4 Electric bed controls. **A,** A hand-held bed control. **B,** Bed controls on the inner part of a bed rail. **C,** Bed controls on the outer part of a bed rail. (C, Courtesy © Hill-Rom Services, Inc. Reprinted with permission. All rights reserved.)

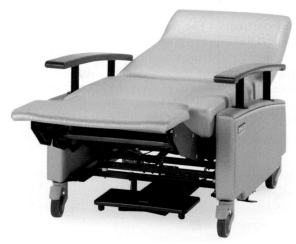

FIGURE 13-5 A medical (patient) recliner. (Courtesy © Hill-Rom Services, Inc. Reprinted with permission. All rights reserved.)

FOCUS ON LONG-TERM CARE AND HOME CARE

The Bed

Home Care

Some home care patients have hospital beds or medical (patient) recliners instead of a bed (Fig. 13-5). Others use their regular beds. You cannot raise recliners or regular beds to give care. You will bend more when giving care. To avoid injury, follow the principles of body mechanics and safe handling. See Chapter 19.

PROMOTING SAFETY AND COMFORT

The Bed

Safety

Most electric beds lock into any position. The person cannot adjust the bed to unsafe positions. Beds may be locked for persons restricted to certain positions and for persons with confusion or dementia.

Bed wheels (Chapter 15) are locked (braked) at all times except when moving the bed. They must be locked to:

* Give bedside care.
* Transfer the person to and from the bed. The person can be injured if the bed moves. You could be injured too.

If using a manual bed, the cranks are pulled up for use. Cranks in the "up" position are safety hazards. Anyone walking past may bump into them. Return cranks to the "down" position after use.

Many people touch bed controls. Plan your care and use careful judgment to prevent the transmission of microbes to the person and others. Follow the guidelines for hand hygiene in Chapter 17. You need to remember to:

* Practice hand hygiene *before* tasks involving contact with mucous membranes, non-intact skin, or invasive medical devices. (Hand hygiene occurs just before the task, after contact with bed controls.)
* Practice hand hygiene *after* tasks that expose the hands to blood or body fluids. (Hand hygiene occurs before contact with bed controls.)

Bed rails are discussed in Chapter 15. Use bed rails as the nurse and care plan direct. Otherwise, the person could suffer injury or harm.

Before leaving a person's room, check that the whole bed is lowered to a safe level. Follow the care plan for the correct height.

Comfort

Adjust the bed to meet the person's needs. Tell the nurse if the bed or mattress is causing discomfort.

Bed Positions. The bed is often positioned flat for sleeping. The basic bed positions in Table 13-1 may be used for comfort or to treat a health problem. See Chapter 19 for proper alignment and positioning.

Some beds are able to convert into a chair position. See "Bariatric Beds" on p. 169.

See *Focus on Long-Term Care and Home Care: Bed Positions.*

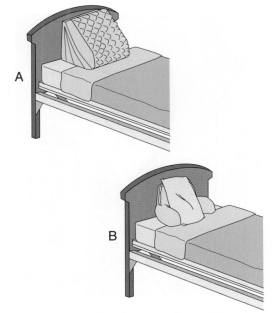

FIGURE 13-6 Backrests for regular beds. **A,** Wedge pillow. **B,** Study pillow (dorm pillow) with armrests. A pillow provides added support.

FOCUS ON LONG-TERM CARE AND HOME CARE

Bed Positions

Home Care

Backrests are used with regular beds for the various Fowler's positions (Fig. 13-6). Large, sturdy sofa pillows are another option. Check the head-board to make sure it is sturdy. It needs to provide support when the person leans against the backrest.

TABLE 13-1	Bed Positions	
Position	**Description**	**Example**
Semi-Fowler's position	The head of the bed is raised 30 degrees. In some agencies, the knee (foot) portion is also raised 15 degrees.	30°
Fowler's position	The head of the bed is raised 45 to 60 degrees.	45°

TABLE 13-1	Bed Positions—cont'd	
Position	**Description**	**Example**
High-Fowler's position	The head of the bed is raised 60 to 90 degrees.	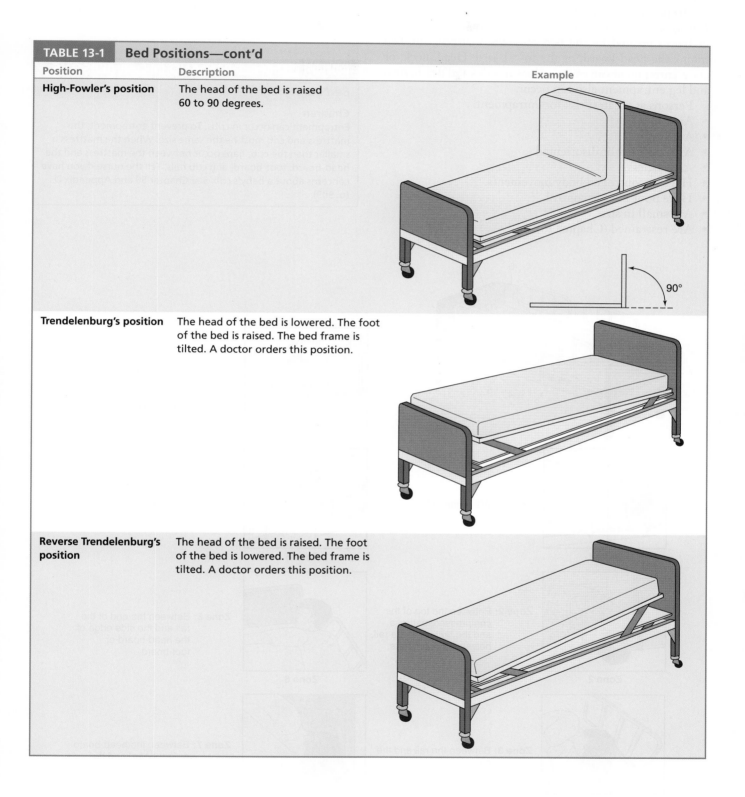
Trendelenburg's position	The head of the bed is lowered. The foot of the bed is raised. The bed frame is tilted. A doctor orders this position.	
Reverse Trendelenburg's position	The head of the bed is raised. The foot of the bed is lowered. The bed frame is tilted. A doctor orders this position.	

Bed Safety. Bed safety involves the *hospital bed system*—the bed frame and its parts. The parts include the mattress, bed rails, head- and foot-boards, and bed attachments.

Hospital bed systems have 7 entrapment zones (Fig. 13-7). *Entrapment* means getting caught, trapped, or entangled in spaces created by the bed rails, the mattress, the bed frame, the head-board, or the foot-board. Head, neck, or chest entrapment can cause serious injuries and death. Arm and leg entrapment also can occur.

Persons at greatest risk for entrapment:
- Are older.
- Are frail.
- Are confused or disoriented.
- Are restless.
- Have uncontrolled body movements.
- Have poor muscle control.
- Are small in size.
- Are restrained (Chapter 16).

Always check the person for entrapment. If a person is caught, trapped, or entangled in the bed or any of its parts, try to release the person. Also call for the nurse at once.

See *Focus on Children and Older Persons: Bed Safety.*

FOCUS ON CHILDREN AND OLDER PERSONS

Bed Safety

Children

Entrapment can occur in cribs. To prevent entrapment, the mattress and crib must be the same size. When the mattress is smaller than the crib, gaps occur between the mattress and the head-board, foot-board, and crib rails. Tell the nurse if you have concerns about a baby's crib. See Chapter 56 and Appendix D (p. 909).

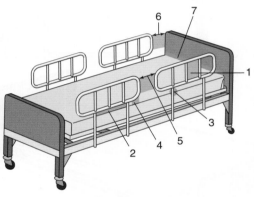

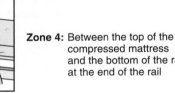

Zone 4: Between the top of the compressed mattress and the bottom of the rail, at the end of the rail

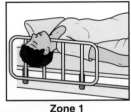

Zone 1: Within the rail

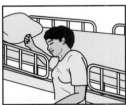

Zone 5: Between the split bed rails

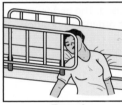

Zone 2: Between the top of the compressed mattress and the bottom of the rail, between the supports

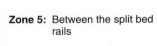

Zone 6: Between the end of the rail and the side edge of the head-board or foot-board

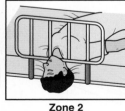

Zone 3: Between the rail and the mattress

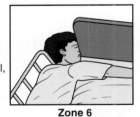

Zone 7: Between the head-board or foot-board and the mattress end

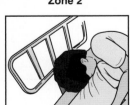

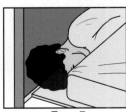

FIGURE 13-7 Hospital bed system entrapment zones. (Redrawn from Food and Drug Administration: *Hospital bed system dimensional and assessment guidance to reduce entrapment,* March 10, 2006, content current as of August 23, 2018.)

Bariatric Beds. Bariatric beds may have these and other features.

- A wide frame with a weight capacity from 500 to 1000 pounds. Some frames adjust for the person's height. For example, the bed length is shortened so the person's feet touch the foot-board. The person does not slide down in bed. Or the frame is made longer for a taller person.
- A chair position. The bed can become a chair without moving the person (Fig. 13-8, *A*). The foot-board becomes a footrest.
- Front and side egress positions. *Egress* means to go out or leave. Moving the foot-board out of the way allows a lying to sitting to standing position (Fig. 13-8, *B*). Or the person can get out of bed on the side.

- Power transport to move the bed. The person is not transferred to a stretcher (Chapter 21) for transport to other areas.
- A pressure-relief surface to prevent pressure injuries. The surface allows turning the person for care measures.
- A trapeze to use for re-positioning (Chapter 20).
- A built-in scale.

Bariatric beds vary depending on the model. Follow the manufacturer's instructions for safe use.

See *Focus on Communication: Bariatric Beds.*

FOCUS ON COMMUNICATION

Bariatric Beds

Comments about weight or size may offend some persons. Use other words. For example, do not say: "The nurse is getting a bed big enough for you." Instead, you can say: "The nurse is getting a bed that will be comfortable for you."

Be aware of your verbal and nonverbal communication. Your words and actions must show dignity and respect.

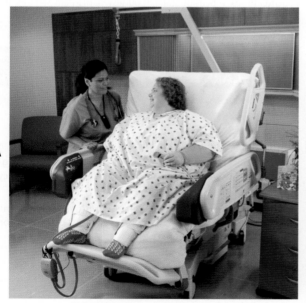
A

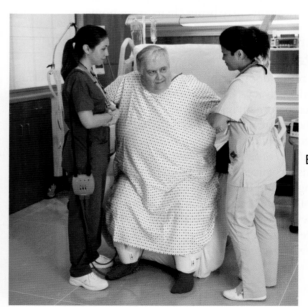
B

FIGURE 13-8 A, Bariatric bed converted to a chair. **B,** The bariatric bed allows the person to get out of bed from the chair position. (Courtesy © Hill-Rom Services, Inc. Reprinted with permission. All rights reserved.)

Over-Bed Tables and Bedside Stands

The over-bed table (Fig. 13-9) is moved over the bed by sliding the base under the bed. The table is raised or lowered for bed or chair use and to prevent bending when used as a work surface. Use the handle, crank, or lever to adjust the table's height.

The person uses the over-bed table for meals, writing, reading, and other activities. The nursing team uses the over-bed table as a work area. Some over-bed tables have a vanity area with a mirror and storage for beauty, hair care, shaving, or other personal items.

The bedside stand is used for personal items and personal care equipment (Fig. 13-10).

- Stand top—used for tissues, clock, photos, phone, flowers, cards, and so on.
- Top drawer—used for eyeglass case, books, kidney basin with oral hygiene items.
- Middle drawer or shelf—stores the wash basin with personal care items (soap, lotion, washcloth and towels, and so on).
- Bottom drawer or lower shelf—stores the bedpan, urinal, and toilet paper.

Only place clean items on the over-bed table and bedside stand. Never place bedpans, urinals, or soiled linens on the top. Clean the over-bed table or bedside stand after use as a work surface. Clean the over-bed table before serving meal trays and after removing them.

Chairs

The person's unit has at least 1 chair (see Fig. 13-1). It must be comfortable, sturdy, and not move or tip during transfers. The person should be able to get in and out of the chair with ease. It should not be too low or too soft. Bariatric chairs are wider and have expanded capacity. Nursing center residents may bring chairs from home.

Doors, Window Coverings, and Privacy Curtains

The room door, bathroom door, and window coverings provide privacy. Close doors and window coverings as needed before giving care.

The privacy curtain (see Fig. 13-1) is pulled around the bed to provide privacy. *Always pull the curtain completely around the bed before giving care.* Privacy curtains do not block sounds or voices. Others in the room can hear sounds or talking behind the curtain.

Follow the care plan and the person's preferences for privacy measures to maintain after giving care.

See *Focus on Long-Term Care and Home Care: Doors, Window Coverings, and Privacy Curtains.*

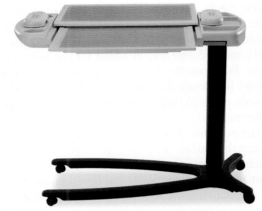

FIGURE 13-9 An over-bed table. (Courtesy © Hill-Rom Services, Inc. Reprinted with permission. All rights reserved.)

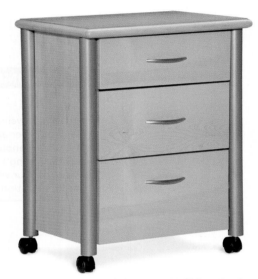

FIGURE 13-10 A bedside stand. (Courtesy © Hill-Rom Services, Inc. Reprinted with permission. All rights reserved.)

FOCUS ON **LONG-TERM CARE AND HOME CARE**

Doors, Window Coverings, and Privacy Curtains

Long-Term Care
According to the CMS, each person has the right to full visual privacy. *Full visual privacy* is having the means to be completely free from public view while in bed. Ceiling-suspended privacy curtains help provide full visual privacy.

Home Care
Portable screens or room dividers help provide privacy in the home setting (Fig. 13-11). Decorated screens provide color and are pleasant to look at.

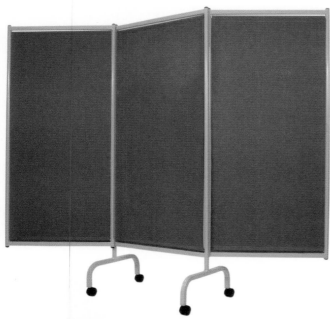

FIGURE 13-11 A portable screen provides privacy in the home. (Copyright Medicus Health.)

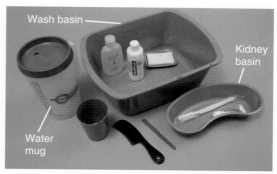

FIGURE 13-12 Personal care items.

Personal Care Items

Personal care items are used for hygiene and elimination (Fig. 13-12). A bedpan, urinal, or commode is provided as needed (Chapter 27). The agency also provides a wash basin, kidney basin, and water mug (see Fig. 13-12). Linens (Chapter 22) are provided.

Hygiene items are available. Some persons have their own oral and personal hygiene equipment and supplies. Respect the person's choices in personal care products.

The Call System

Whether in the room, bathroom, or bathing area, the person must be able to contact the staff. The call system lets the person signal for help. The call light is at the end of a long cord (Fig. 13-13, *A*). It connects to a wall panel and attaches to the bed or chair with a clip. To get help, the person presses the button on the device. A light above the room door turns on (Fig. 13-13, *B*). A computer, light panel, or intercom system at the nurses' station notifies staff that the person needs help.

An intercom system lets the person communicate with staff at the nurses' station. The person says what is needed. Staff reply through the intercom. Persons who are hard of hearing may have problems using an intercom. Also, remember confidentiality. Persons nearby can hear what is said through an intercom.

Always keep the call light within the person's reach—in the room, bathroom, and shower or tub room. (See "The Bathroom" on p. 173 for call lights in bathrooms and shower and tub rooms.)

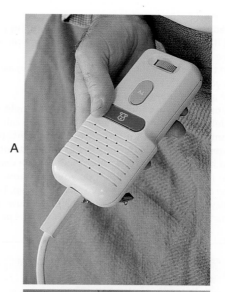

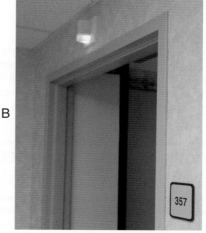

FIGURE 13-13 The call system. **A,** The call light button is pressed when help is needed. **B,** A light above the room door turns on. (NOTE: There are different types of call systems.)

Some persons have limited hand movement and need a call light that is turned on with a tap of the hand or fist (Fig. 13-14). Some people cannot use call lights. Examples are persons who are confused or unconscious. The care plan lists special communication measures. Check these persons often. Make sure their needs are met.

See *Focus on Communication: The Call System*.

See *Focus on Long-Term Care and Home Care: The Call System*.

See *Teamwork and Time Management: The Call System*.

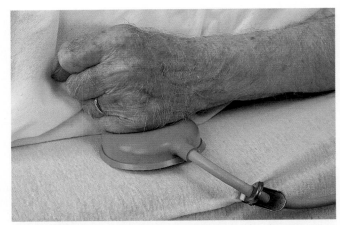

FIGURE 13-14 Call light for a person with limited hand movement.

FOCUS ON **COMMUNICATION**

The Call System

You will answer call lights for patients and residents not assigned to you. The following examples of what to say promote safe care, quality of life, and teamwork.
- "My name is Chris Hines. I'm a nursing assistant. How can I help you?"
- "I need to check your care plan before bringing you more salt. I'll be right back. Is there anything else I can do before I leave?"
- "I can take your meal tray. I'll tell your nursing assistant what you ate."
- "I can assist you onto the bedpan."

Sometimes patients and residents signal for help often. Do not delay in meeting their needs. Never take call lights away from them. This is not safe. Avoid statements that make a person feel like a burden. For example, do *not* say:
- "I just helped you to the bathroom. Can't you wait?"
- "I was just in your room. What do you want now?"

Do not discourage the person from asking for help. The person may try to do something alone. This could cause injury. Tell the nurse. Your co-workers can help you meet the person's needs.

FOCUS ON **LONG-TERM CARE AND HOME CARE**

The Call System

Home Care
Some home care patients stay in bed or in a certain part of the home. They need a way to call for help. Tap bells, dinner bells, baby monitors, and other devices are useful (Fig. 13-15). Children's toys with bells, horns, and whistles are other options. Smart speakers can be used as intercoms in homes.

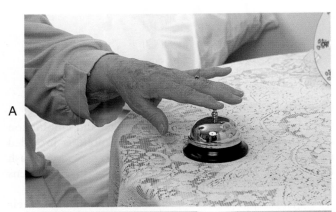

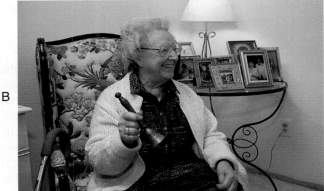

FIGURE 13-15 **A,** Tap bell. **B,** Dinner bell.

TEAMWORK AND TIME MANAGEMENT

The Call System

A person may use a call light for help when you are with another person. The same may happen to other staff. If staff answer call lights for each other, lights are answered promptly. Patients and residents receive quality care. Everyone is responsible for answering call lights even if not assigned to the person.

Call System Safety. The phrase "call light" is used in this book when referring to the call system. You must:

- Keep the call light within the person's reach. Even if the person cannot use the call light, keep it within reach for use by visitors and staff. They may need to call for help.
- Place the call light on the person's strong (unaffected) side if the person has a weak (affected) side from illness or injury.
- Remind the person to signal when help is needed.
- Answer call lights promptly. For example, the person may have an urgent elimination need. Respond promptly to prevent embarrassing problems and complications from incontinence (Chapters 27 and 29). Infection, skin breakdown, pressure injuries, and falls are examples.
- Answer bathroom and shower or tub room call lights at once.

The Bathroom

A toilet, sink, call light, and mirror are standard equipment in bathrooms (Fig. 13-16). Some bathrooms have showers.

Grab bars (safety bars) are by the toilet for getting on and off the toilet. Some bathrooms have higher toilets or elevated (raised) toilet seats. They make wheelchair transfers easier and are helpful for persons with joint problems.

Towel racks, toilet paper, soap, paper towel dispenser, and a wastebasket are in the bathroom. They are within the person's reach.

The call light is a button or pull cord next to the toilet. The bathroom call light flashes red above the room door and at the nurses' station. To alert staff of bathroom use, the sound at the nurses' station is different from room call lights. Someone must respond at once when a person needs help in the bathroom.

Closet and Drawer Space

Closet and drawer space are provided (see Fig. 13-1). The CMS requires that nursing centers provide each person with closet space with shelves and a clothes rack. The person must be able to reach and have free access to the closet and its contents (Fig. 13-17).

See *Promoting Safety and Comfort: Closet and Drawer Space.*

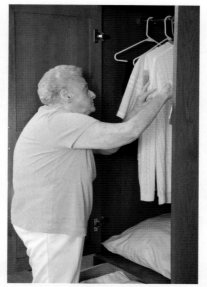

FIGURE 13-17 The resident can reach items in her closet.

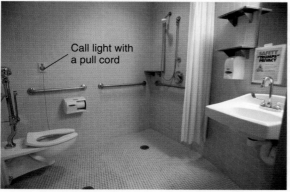

FIGURE 13-16 Bathroom in a person's room.

Call light with a pull cord

PROMOTING SAFETY AND COMFORT
Closet and Drawer Space

Safety
Closets and drawers contain the person's property. Ask the person's permission before opening them.

Sometimes people hoard items—drugs, napkins, straws, food, sugar, salt, pepper, and so on. Hoarding causes safety and health risks (Chapter 14). Tell the nurse if hoarding is suspected. Consent is required for a search of the person's belongings (Chapter 2). Follow agency policies and procedures for inspecting a person's closet, drawers, or personal items. Having the person (or the person's representative) and a witness present protects you if the person claims that something was stolen or damaged.

Other Equipment

Many agencies furnish rooms with a TV, radio, and clock. Many rooms have a phone and Internet access.

Other equipment in the room depends on the care setting. Blood pressure equipment may be mounted on walls. In hospital settings there are wall outlets for oxygen and suction and a pole for intravenous (IV) infusions and feeding bags (Chapter 33). See Figure 13-18. Oxygen equipment and portable suction equipment are common in nursing centers and home care settings.

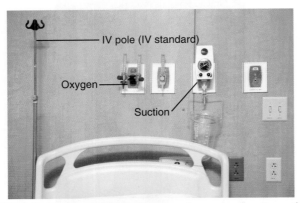

FIGURE 13-18 This room has an IV pole and oxygen and suction outlets.

Personal Belongings

Nursing center residents had furniture, appliances, and many belongings and treasures at home. Leaving one's home and living in a new place can be hard. The center is now the person's home. A home-like setting is important for quality of life.

Residents can bring personal items and some furniture from home. Photos, TVs, radios, books, religious items, and plants are examples. A chair, footstool, lamp, and small table are often allowed.

You can help the person choose the best place for personal items. Allow personal choice. Make sure the person's choices:
- Are safe.
- Will not cause falls or other accidents.
- Do not interfere with the rights of others.

FOCUS ON PRIDE

The Person, Family, and Yourself

Personal and Professional Responsibility

Reducing noise requires cooperation from all staff. It is not your responsibility alone. But you can help. Do your part to reduce noise. Politely remind others to speak softly if needed. Take pride in providing a quiet and comfortable setting.

Rights and Respect

You will need to move items in the person's setting when giving care. For example, you need to use the over-bed table as a work area. The person has items on the table. Ask permission to move personal items aside and use the table. Return items to their proper place before leaving the room. Ask if the placement meets the person's preferences. These actions show respect for the person.

Independence and Social Interaction

People want to be independent. Often accidents and injuries occur when the person tries to get needed items. The person has to reach too far and falls. Or the person tries to get up without help.

To promote independence and safety:
- Keep needed personal items within reach.
- Place adaptive (assistive) devices nearby. Walkers and canes are examples.
- Place the call light within the person's reach. Answer call lights and tend to the person's needs promptly.

Delegation and Teamwork

Some nursing units check on the person at regular times. For example, every hour staff ask about needs, positioning, comfort, and needed personal items. Needs are met. The person is reminded that staff will return in 1 hour. Nursing staff sign a form or record in the medical record each time. The person uses the call light for urgent needs.

If your unit uses this practice:
- Be prompt. Check on the person at the correct time.
- Be honest. Do not sign the form or record in the medical record if you did not check on the person. Also, do not sign or record before completing the check.
- Have a good attitude. Do not complain. Reasons for the practice may be to improve care, decrease call light use, or help nurses with time management.

Ethics and Laws

This chapter focuses on how objects and surroundings in the person's unit affect comfort and well-being. You are a part of that setting. Your words and actions are heard and seen by others. Your conduct affects quality of care. Always provide care in a way that promotes comfort, safety, and quality of life.

FOCUS ON PRIDE: *Application*

What makes your living space comfortable and personal? How would this change if you lived in a nursing center? What would change in a hospital setting? Why is it important to provide privacy, safety, and comfort?

REVIEW QUESTIONS

Circle the BEST answer.

1 To maintain the person's unit
a Throw away items that do not look important
b Remove cards from the bedside stand
c Place personal items as you choose
d Straighten bed linens as needed

2 Which temperature range is required by the CMS?
a 61°F to 66°F
b 66°F to 71°F
c 71°F to 81°F
d 80°F to 85°F

3 To protect a person from drafts
a Adjust the room temperature to 68°F
b Use a bath blanket during a bed bath
c Dress the person in light-weight clothing
d Position the person near an open window

4 You get hot while giving a person a shower. You should
a Open the bathroom door to cool off the room
b Adjust the room temperature for your comfort
c Bring a fan in the bathroom
d Ask if the person is comfortable

5 To prevent odors
a Place flowers in the room
b Empty commodes at the end of your shift
c Keep laundry containers open
d Clean persons who are wet or soiled

6 To control noise
a Answer phones after the third ring
b Use the intercom system when possible
c Handle equipment carefully
d Talk with others in the hallway

7 Mr. Tanner is hard of hearing. He listens to the TV loudly. Residents playing cards nearby complain about the noise. You should
a Ask Mr. Tanner to turn off his TV
b Tell the residents playing cards to play somewhere else
c Ask to close Mr. Tanner's door and ask if the noise level improved
d Listen to the complaints but do nothing

8 The whole bed is raised to
a Prevent bending and reaching when giving care
b Promote the person's comfort
c Prevent falls
d Lock the bed in position

9 The head of the bed is raised 30 degrees. This is called
a Semi-Fowler's position
b Fowler's position
c Trendelenburg's position
d Reverse Trendelenburg's position

10 Which shows you understand how to safely use the person's bed?
a You leave the room with the whole bed in the high position.
b You follow the care plan for bed rail use.
c You leave manual bed cranks in the up position.
d You touch the bed controls with soiled gloves.

11 Which statement about hospital bed system entrapment is *true*?
a Bed rails present the only risk for entrapment.
b Serious injury and death can occur.
c A person must be small in size for entrapment to occur.
d Frail older persons have a lower risk of entrapment.

12 A person has right-sided weakness. You complete a safety check. Which do you need to correct before leaving the room?
a The call light is on the right side of the bed.
b The over-bed table is on the left side of the bed within reach.
c The bed is in the low position.
d Bed wheels are locked (braked).

13 You see the following on the person's over-bed table. Which should be moved?
a A water mug
b A TV remote control
c A urinal (container for urine)
d A crossword puzzle

14 Which action is *correct* when using the over-bed table as a work surface?
a You raise the table to a comfortable working height.
b You place soiled linens on the table.
c You replace personal items after use without cleaning it.
d You place the bedpan on the table.

15 The privacy curtain is pulled around the bed
a To prevent others from hearing conversations
b To remind the person to stay in bed
c To block sounds from the hallway
d To prevent others from seeing the person

16 Call lights are answered
a When you have time
b At the end of your shift
c Promptly
d When you are near the person's room

Answers to Chapter 13 questions are on p. 901.

FOCUS ON **PRACTICE**

Problem Solving

Since your shift began an hour ago, a resident has called for help 6 times. You just left the room and are helping another resident. The call light is used again. What do you do?

The resident uses the call light more often at night, after family visits, and when not checked on regularly. How might this information be helpful for the nurse in care planning?

Safety

OBJECTIVES

- Define the key terms and key abbreviations in this chapter.
- Describe accident risk factors.
- Explain why you identify a person before giving care.
- Explain how to correctly identify a person.
- Describe the safety measures to prevent burns, poisoning, and suffocation.
- Identify the signs and causes of choking.
- Explain how to prevent equipment accidents.
- Explain how to handle hazardous chemicals.

- Describe how agencies prepare for disasters.
- Describe fire prevention measures and oxygen safety.
- Explain what to do during a fire.
- Explain how to protect yourself from workplace violence.
- Describe your role in risk management.
- Perform the procedures described in this chapter.
- Explain how to promote PRIDE in the person, the family, and yourself.

KEY TERMS

coma A prolonged state of unconsciousness

dementia The loss of cognitive function that interferes with daily life and activities

disaster A harmful event that can affect the agency, patient or resident population, community, or larger geographic area

electrical shock When electrical current passes through the body

elopement When a patient or resident leaves the agency without staff knowledge

ground That which carries leaking electricity to the earth and away from an electrical item

hazard Anything in the person's setting that could cause injury or illness

hazardous chemical Any chemical that is a physical hazard or a health hazard

incident Any event that has harmed or could harm a patient, resident, visitor, or staff member; adverse event

incident report Documentation of the details about a harmful or potentially harmful event

paralysis Loss of muscle function

paresis Weak or impaired muscle function without complete paralysis; partial paralysis

poison Any substance harmful to the body when ingested, inhaled, injected, or absorbed through the skin

suffocation When breathing stops from the lack of oxygen; asphyxia

unconscious Being unaware of one's setting and being unable to react or respond to people, places, or things

workplace violence Violent acts (including assault or threat of assault) directed toward persons at work or while on duty

KEY ABBREVIATIONS

AED	Automated external defibrillator	ID	Identification
CDC	Centers for Disease Control and Prevention	MRN	Medical record number
CMS	Centers for Medicare & Medicaid Services	NFPA	National Fire Protection Association
CO	Carbon monoxide	OSHA	Occupational Safety and Health Administration
CPR	Cardiopulmonary resuscitation	PASS	*Pull* the safety pin, *aim* low, *squeeze* the lever, *sweep* back and forth
DOB	Date of birth		
EMS	Emergency Medical Services	PPE	Personal protective equipment
F	Fahrenheit	RACE	Rescue, alarm, confine, extinguish or evacuate
FBAO	Foreign-body airway obstruction	RRS	Rapid Response System
HCS	Hazard Communication Standard	SDS	Safety data sheet

Safety is a basic need. Patients and residents are at great risk for accidents and falls. (See Chapter 15 for information on falls.) Some accidents and injuries cause death. You must protect patients, residents, visitors, co-workers, and yourself from harm.

The goal is to prevent accidents and injuries without limiting the person's mobility and independence. Safety measures must not interfere with the person's rights (Chapter 2).

This chapter covers general safety. The care plan lists specific safety measures for the person. Common sense and safety measures can prevent most accidents. The safety measures in this chapter apply to all health care settings and daily life.

See *Focus on Surveys: Safety*.

FOCUS ON **SURVEYS**
Safety

A survey team will observe the agency setting and patient or resident rooms. Surveyors look for:

- Potential or actual hazards. A *hazard* is anything in the person's setting that could cause injury or illness. Examples include spills, loose hand rails, unanswered call lights, burnt-out bulbs, unsafe equipment, and other safety issues described in this chapter and other chapters.
- How staff respond to potential or actual hazards.
- If the care plan was followed on each shift for persons at risk.
- How staff supervise persons at risk.
- If a hazard was changed or removed.
  During staff interviews, a surveyor may ask:
- About measures in the person's care plan to reduce the risk for an accident.
- When and how you report risks and hazards.
- When and how you correct an immediate hazard. A spill is an example.
- The agency's procedures for removing or reducing a hazard.
  Always provide for safety. Know what to do if you find a hazard. Remember to give surveyors complete and honest answers. Surveys protect patients and residents.

A SAFE SETTING

In a safe setting, there is little risk of illness or injury. The setting is free of hazards to the extent possible. The person has enough room and light to move about safely. The person and property are safe from fire and intruders. The person receives the correct care and treatments. The person feels safe and secure physically and mentally. The person is not afraid and has few worries and concerns.

See *Teamwork and Time Management: A Safe Setting*.

TEAMWORK AND TIME MANAGEMENT
A Safe Setting

The health team works together to provide a safe setting. You may see something unsafe. Correct the matter right away if it is something you can do. For example:

- Wipe up spills right away. Do so even if you did not cause the spill.
- A person is sliding out of a wheelchair. Position the person correctly. Do so even if a co-worker is responsible for the person's care.
- A person has problems holding a coffee cup. Offer to help the person.
  Follow agency policy to report problems that you cannot correct. They include:
- Electrical outlets or switches that do not work or are coming out of the wall
- Water leaks from windows, doors, ceilings, pipes, faucets, tubs, showers, toilets, water heaters, and other sources
- Toilets that do not work properly
- Water from faucets that does not warm up or is very hot
- Broken or damaged windows or furniture
- Windows, doors, knobs, or handles that are broken or do not work properly
- Hand rails and grab bars that are loose or need repair
- Odd smells, odors, and sounds
- Signs of rodents, flies, ants, or other pests
- Lights and lamps that do not work or have burnt-out bulbs
- Flooring (carpeting, tiles, hardwood flooring) needing repair

---

ACCIDENT RISK FACTORS

Some people cannot protect themselves. They present dangers to themselves and others. Certain factors increase the risk of accidents and injuries.

- *Awareness of surroundings and ability to respond.* Confused and disoriented persons may not understand what is happening to and around them. A *disoriented* person lacks awareness of 1 or more of the following—the self or others, time, location, or surroundings. Changes in level of consciousness can occur from illness or injury.
  - *Unconscious*—being unaware of one's setting and being unable to react or respond to people, places, or things
  - *Coma*—a prolonged state of unconsciousness
- *Agitated and aggressive behaviors.* Pain can cause these behaviors. So can confusion, decreased awareness of surroundings, and fear of what may happen.
- *Vision loss.* Persons with poor vision can fall or trip over toys, rugs, equipment, furniture, and cords. Some cannot read container labels. Poisoning can result. Taking the wrong drug or the wrong dose can be harmful.

- *Hearing loss.* Persons with hearing loss may not hear warning signals or fire alarms. Some cannot hear approaching meal carts, drug carts, stretchers, or wheelchairs. They do not know to move to safety.
- *Impaired smell and touch.* Illness and aging affect smell and touch. The person may not detect smoke or gas odors. Burns are a risk from impaired touch. The person has problems sensing heat and cold. Some people have a decreased sense of pain. They may be unaware of injury. For example, a person does not feel a blister from shoes. Leg and foot circulation is poor. The blister can become a serious wound.
- *Impaired mobility. Mobility* is the ability to move (Chapter 35). Some diseases and injuries affect mobility. The person may not be able to move to safety. Some persons cannot walk or propel wheelchairs. Some persons are paralyzed. *Paralysis* means loss of muscle function. Loss of sensation can also occur. Paralysis may involve just the lower body (*paraplegia*), the upper and lower body (*quadriplegia* or *tetraplegia*), or 1 side of the body (*hemiplegia*). Some persons have *paresis (partial paralysis).* There is weak or impaired muscle function without complete paralysis. *Hemiparesis* is paresis on 1 side of the body.
- *Drugs.* Drug side effects may include loss of balance, drowsiness, and poor coordination. Reduced awareness, confusion, and disorientation may occur.
- *Age.* Children and older persons are at risk for injuries.
  See *Focus on Children and Older Persons: Accident Risk Factors.*

IDENTIFYING THE PERSON

Each person has different treatments, therapies, and activity limits. The wrong care can threaten life and health.

The person may receive an identification (ID) bracelet when admitted to the agency (Fig. 14-1). The bracelet has the person's name, ID number, room and bed number, date of birth (DOB), age, and doctor. Other identifying information and numbers are included. A medical record number (MRN)—used to identify the person's medical record—is an example.

You use the ID bracelet to identify the person before giving care. Your assignment sheet states what care to give. To identify the person:

- Compare identifying information on the assignment sheet with that on the ID bracelet (Fig. 14-2). Carefully check the information. Some people have the same first and last names. For example, John Smith is a common name.
- Use at least 2 identifiers. Some agencies require the person to state and spell his or her name and give his or her birth date. Others require checking the person's ID number. You cannot use the person's room or bed number. Always follow agency policy.
- Call the person by name when checking the ID bracelet. This is a courtesy as you touch the person and before giving care. Just calling the person by name is not enough for identification. Confused, disoriented, drowsy, hard of hearing, or distracted persons may answer to any name.
  See *Focus on Communication: Identifying the Person.*
  See *Focus on Long-Term Care and Home Care: Identifying the Person.*
  See *Promoting Safety and Comfort: Identifying the Person.*

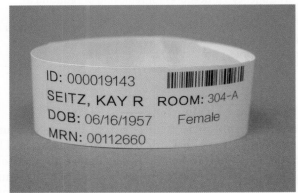

FIGURE 14-1 ID bracelet (ID–identification; DOB–date of birth; MRN–medical record number).

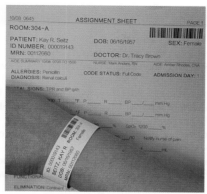

FIGURE 14-2 The ID bracelet is checked against the assignment sheet to accurately identify the person.

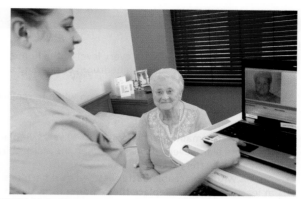

FIGURE 14-3 The nursing assistant uses the photo to identify the person.

FOCUS ON COMMUNICATION

Identifying the Person

To identify the person, call the person by name. Ask to see the ID bracelet. For example: "Hello, Mr. Hall. May I see your ID bracelet?" Then ask for 2 identifiers. You can say: "Please tell me your full name and birth date." Compare the identifiers with the information on the ID bracelet and your assignment sheet.

Identifying oneself over and over again can be annoying. The person may say: "Do I have to say it again? You know who I am." Be polite. Explain why you check identity. You can say: "It is important to check so I give care to the right person. It is for your safety." Thank the person. Use the person's title and name or preferred name. For example: "Thank you, Mr. Hall."

FOCUS ON LONG-TERM CARE AND HOME CARE

Identifying the Person

Long-Term Care
Alert and oriented residents may not wear ID bracelets. This is noted on the person's care plan. Follow center policy and the care plan to identify the person.

Some nursing centers use photo ID systems (Fig. 14-3). The person's photo is taken on admission for the medical record. If your center uses such a system, learn to use it safely.

PROMOTING SAFETY AND COMFORT

Identifying the Person

Safety
Always identify the person before giving care. Do not identify the person and then leave the room for supplies and equipment. You could go to the wrong room and give care to the wrong person. The person needing care would not receive it. Harm could result.

Water, spilled food and fluids, and every-day wear and tear can damage ID bracelets. If you cannot read the information on the ID bracelet, tell the nurse. The nurse can have a new bracelet made.

Comfort
Make sure ID bracelets are not too loose or too tight. You should be able to slide 1 or 2 fingers under a bracelet. If it is too loose or too tight, tell the nurse.

PREVENTING BURNS

Smoking, spilled hot liquids, children playing with matches, grills, fireplaces, stoves, electrical items, and very hot water (sinks, tubs, showers) are common causes of burns. Burns from hot water can occur in seconds. The safety measures in Box 14-1 (p. 180) can prevent burns. See Chapter 58 for the emergency care of burns.

See *Focus on Children and Older Persons: Preventing Burns.*

FOCUS ON CHILDREN AND OLDER PERSONS

Preventing Burns

Older Persons
Older persons are at risk for burns. Risk factors include decreased skin thickness, decreased sensitivity to heat, reduced reaction time, decreased mobility, communication problems, confusion, and dementia. Many of the measures in Box 14-1 for children apply to persons who are confused or have dementia.

BOX 14-1   Preventing Burns

Smoke Alarms
- Have working smoke alarms on every level of the home, in each bedroom, and outside each bedroom or sleeping area.
- Test alarms every month.
- Follow the manufacturer's instructions on when to replace batteries and the alarm.
  - Alarms with non-replaceable 10-year batteries are designed to remain effective for up to 10 years. Replace the entire alarm every 10 years or when the alarm chirps with a low-battery warning.
  - Alarms with replaceable batteries need new batteries at least once a year. Replace them sooner if the alarm chirps with a low-battery warning. Replace the alarm every 10 years.
- Use alarms with flashing strobe lights for hard of hearing persons.

Children
- Do not leave children home alone.
- Supervise young children at all times.
- Do not leave children alone in the kitchen, bathroom, or a room with a fireplace.
- Secure fireplaces with door guards or heat-resistant gates.
- Install barriers around fireplaces, ovens, and furnaces. Avoid glass screens that can become very hot and take a long time to cool down.
- Store matches, lighters, lamp oils, or other flammable materials in locked cabinets.
- Do not let children near stoves, space heaters, fireplaces, grills, radiators, registers, oil lamps, candles, curling irons, and other heat sources.
- Do not carry or hold a child while cooking.
- Keep space heaters and materials that can catch fire away from children.
- Teach children fire safety and fire prevention measures. Also teach the dangers of fire.
- Check metal playground equipment. Metal surfaces exposed to sunlight can heat to high temperatures. They can burn a child's face, hands, arms, legs, and buttocks.
- Check car seats, seat belts, and seat-belt buckles. If hot, they can burn children.
- Cover car seats with towels if you park in the sun. Also use a sun visor for the windshield.
- Protect children from sun exposure.
  - Use sunscreen.
  - Cover exposed areas.
  - Limit time in the sun.

Kitchen and Cooking
- Do not let children help you cook.
- Use the back stove burners when cooking.
- Point pot and pan handles inward, toward the back. They point away from where people stand and walk.
- Stay in the kitchen when cooking. Turn off the stove if you have to leave the kitchen.
- Use a timer when baking, roasting, or simmering food. Check the food regularly.

Kitchen and Cooking—cont'd
- Do not leave cooking utensils in pots and pans.
- Do not wear long-sleeved or loose-fitting clothes while cooking.
- Keep things that can catch fire away from stoves. Examples include towels and paper towels, oven mitts, pot-holders, food packages, and curtains.
- Do not put wet food into frying pans or deep-fryers. Water causes the oil to splatter.
- Use dry oven mitts and pot-holders. Water conducts heat.
- Stay by the stove, oven, microwave oven, or grill when cooking. Do not leave cooking unattended.
- Open or uncover microwaved foods slowly. Steam can burn your fingers, hands, or face.
- Turn the oven and stove burners off when not in use.

Eating and Drinking
- Assist with eating and drinking as needed. Spilled hot food or liquids can cause burns.
- Be careful when carrying hot foods and liquids.
- Keep hot food and liquids away from counter and table edges. Use the center of the counter or table.
- Do not pour hot liquids near a person.

Water
- Set the water heater temperature no higher than 120°F (Fahrenheit).
- Have anti-scald devices on faucets and shower-heads.
- Turn on cold water first, then hot water (for a 2-handled faucet). Turn off hot water first, then cold water.
- Measure bath or shower water temperature (Chapter 24). Check it before bathing a baby or before a person gets into the tub or shower.
- Check for "hot spots" in bath water. Move your hand back and forth in the water.

Appliances and Other Electrical Equipment
- See "Preventing Equipment Accidents" on p. 191.
- Avoid using space heaters. If used, they must be at least 3 feet away from items that can burn. Turn off and unplug the heater before leaving the room or going to sleep.
- Avoid heating pads and electric blankets during sleep.
- Turn off and unplug irons, curling irons, electric rollers, and hair dryers when not in use.

Smoking
- Be sure patients and residents smoke only in areas designated for smoking.
- Do not leave smoking materials at the bedside.
- Supervise the smoking of persons who cannot protect themselves.
- Do not allow smoking in bed.
- Do not allow smoking where oxygen is used or stored (Chapter 44).
- Be alert to ashes that may fall onto a person.

Other
- See "Fire Safety" on p. 195.
- Follow safety guidelines when applying heat and cold (Chapter 43).

PREVENTING POISONING

A *poison* is any substance harmful to the body when ingested, inhaled, injected, or absorbed through the skin. If too much is taken, any substance can be poisonous. Poisonings are unintentional or intentional.

- *Unintentional*—The person takes or gives a substance without intending to cause harm. This includes drugs or chemicals in excess amounts—an "overdose."
- *Intentional*—The person takes (suicide) or gives (assault or homicide) a substance to cause harm.

Poisoning can cause illness, brain damage, coma, and death. Children and older persons are at risk. Drugs and household products are common poisons. Poisoning in adults may be from carelessness, confusion, or poor vision when reading labels. As a result, a person may take too much of a drug or ingest a harmful substance.

Common poisons include:

- Drugs (legal and illegal) and vitamins
- Household products—detergents, soaps, sprays, furniture polish, window cleaners, bleach, paint, paint thinner, toilet bowl and other cleaners, gasoline, kerosene, glue, and so on
- Personal care products—soaps, shampoos, hair conditioners, bath oils, powders, lotions, nail polish removers, sprays, make-up, perfumes, after-shave, deodorants, mouthwashes, and so on
- Fertilizers, insecticides, bug sprays, and so on
- Lead (p. 183)
- House plants
- Wild mushrooms
- Lamp oil
- Alcohol
- Liquid nicotine
- Carbon monoxide (p. 185)

The measures in Box 14-2 can prevent poisoning. Poisoning is an emergency. The Poison Control Center provides free 24-hour guidance for poison emergencies. The number is 1-800-222-1222. See Chapter 58 for the emergency care for poisoning.

See *Focus on Long-Term Care and Home Care: Preventing Poisoning*, p. 182.

See *Promoting Safety and Comfort: Preventing Poisoning*, p. 183.

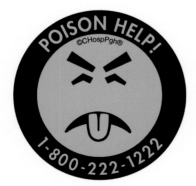

FIGURE 14-4 The Mr. Yuk symbol has been used to teach children about poison prevention. The symbol promotes Poison Control Center awareness. (Courtesy Children's Hospital, Pittsburgh Poison Center, Pittsburgh, Pa.)

BOX 14-2 | **Preventing Poisoning**

Children

- Teach children about the dangers of harmful products and about poison prevention (Fig. 14-4).
- Teach children not to eat plants and unknown foods. Teach them not to eat leaves, stems, seeds, berries, nuts, or bark.
- Practice safe drug use.
  - Do not call drugs or vitamins "candy."
  - Do not take drugs in front of children.
  - Do not put a dose on a counter or table where a child can reach it.
  - Do not leave drugs unattended when taking them.
  - Secure child-safety caps on every drug.
  - Put drugs away after taking them. Put them out of the sight and reach of children.
  - Be aware that guests (including family and friends) may bring legal or illegal drugs into a home. Do not let children have access to purses, handbags, briefcases, backpacks, coat pockets, or similar items.
- Supervise children when visiting family and friends. Look for harmful products in and on counters, tables, bathrooms, and other areas and surfaces.
- Prevent lead poisoning (p. 183).

All Ages

- Keep drugs and harmful products in high, locked areas (Fig. 14-5, p. 182). Children and confused persons cannot see or reach them.
- Use prescription drugs correctly.
  - Only take drugs prescribed by a licensed health care professional.
  - Take drugs as prescribed. Do not take larger or more frequent doses. This is especially important for pain-relief drugs.
  - Do not share or sell drugs.
  - Read and follow all directions and warning labels. Have good lighting.
  - Keep drugs in their original bottles or containers.
- Buy products with child-resistant packaging.
- Keep child-resistant caps on all harmful products.
- Keep harmful products in their original containers. Do not use food containers.
- Leave the original label on harmful products.
- Store personal care items according to agency policy. Soap, mouthwash, lotion, deodorant, and shampoo are examples. These products are harmful when swallowed.
- Use and store harmful products according to the manufacturer's instructions.
- Do not sniff chemical containers.
- Read all labels carefully before using the product.
- Do not leave harmful products unattended when in use.
- Do not mix cleaners or other household products together.
- Turn on fans and open windows when using cleaners and other household products.
- Point spray nozzles away from your face and other people.
- Do not store harmful products near food.
- Dispose of out-dated, unwanted, and un-used drugs and products. See *Focus on Long-Term Care and Home Care: Preventing Poisoning*, p. 182.
- Use safety latches on kitchen, bathroom, utility, garage, basement, and workshop cabinets and drawers.
- Discard poisonous household plants. Or place them where persons at risk cannot reach them.
- Prevent carbon monoxide poisoning (p. 185).

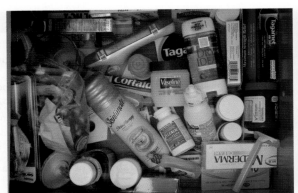
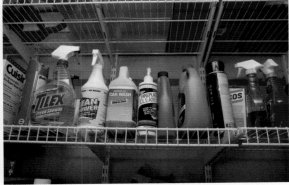

A

B

FIGURE 14-5 Harmful products must be kept in locked areas and out of the reach of children and persons who are confused. **A,** Bathroom drawers and cabinets hold many harmful products. **B,** Household cleaners can be harmful.

FOCUS ON LONG-TERM CARE AND HOME CARE

Preventing Poisoning

Home Care

Provide good lighting when patients take their drugs. Make sure they read prescription labels correctly and are taking the correct drug and dosage (Chapter 57).

Some products and drugs are out-dated, unwanted, or un-used. The nurse may have you check bathroom medicine cabinets, drawers, and counters for such items. The kitchen and bedrooms are checked too.

For safe disposal, obtain permission from the person and the nurse. Follow agency policy for disposal. For drugs, agency policy may involve 1 of these disposal methods.

- The disposal instructions on the label.
- Take-back programs.
  - National Prescription Drug Take-Back events are hosted by the U.S. Drug Enforcement Administration (DEA). Collection sites are set up in areas across the country.
  - Local law enforcement agencies sponsor take-back programs.
- Local waste management agency disposal options and guidelines.
- Household trash (Fig. 14-6).
  1. *Mix* the drugs with an unpalatable substance. (*Palatable* means to have a good taste. *Unpalatable* means to have an unpleasant or disagreeable taste.) Dirt, cat litter, and used coffee grounds are examples. Do not crush tablets or capsules.
  2. *Place* the mixture in a container. A sealed plastic bag is suggested.
  3. *Throw* the container in the household trash.
  4. *Scratch* out all personal information on the prescription label. Make it unreadable. Discard the empty bottle or package into the trash.
- Flushing. The nurse tells you what drugs can be flushed.

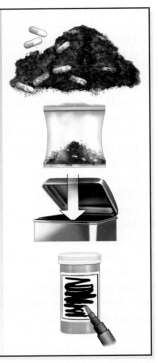

Follow these simple steps to dispose of drugs in the household trash

MIX
Mix drugs (do not crush tablets or capsules) with a bad tasting, unpleasant substance such as dirt, cat litter, or used coffee grounds.

PLACE
Place the mixture in a container such as a sealed plastic bag.

THROW
Throw the container in your household trash.

SCRATCH OUT
Scratch out all personal information on the prescription label of your empty bottle or empty drug packaging to make it unreadable. Then dispose of the container.

FIGURE 14-6 Steps for drug disposal in the household trash. (Redrawn from Food and Drug Administration: *Drug disposal: dispose "non-flush list" medicine in trash,* Silver Spring, Md.)

PROMOTING SAFETY AND COMFORT
Preventing Poisoning

Safety

Keep emergency numbers by the phone or stored in your phone. If you call 911 or the Poison Control Center (1-800-222-1222), give the following information.

- Your location, name, phone number, and distance to the nearest hospital
- The person's signs and symptoms, condition (breathing; not breathing), and health problems
- The person's age and weight
- The substance, containers, or bottles involved
- How you think the substance entered the body— swallowed, inhaled or smelled, injected, skin contact, splashed into the eyes
- When you think the substance entered the body
- If the person has vomited
- Emergency care given (Chapter 58)
  Follow the rules for basic emergency care in Chapter 58. Follow the directions given by the Poison Control Center.

Lead Poisoning

Lead is a metal. It can be found in all parts of the environment. When in the body, it affects normal body functions. A very strong poison, it can injure the brain, nervous system, red blood cells, kidneys, liver, teeth, and bones. It can lower intelligence and cause learning and behavior problems.

See Box 14-3 (p. 184) for sources of lead. Lead enters the body through:

- *Inhaling dust.* Windows may have lead-based paint. When windows are opened and closed, dust is created. Dust from soil may contain lead.
- *Ingestion.* Young children can eat, chew, and suck on non-food items containing lead. Toys and lead-painted surfaces—window sills and railings—are examples. Children may eat paint chips. Water is a source of lead if plumbing materials contain lead.

Children under 6 years are at risk for lead poisoning. Lead can affect almost every body system. Signs and symptoms are usually gradual in onset. They are often not obvious. See Box 14-3 for signs, symptoms, and safety measures. Children at risk for lead exposure need to be tested. A blood test is used to diagnose lead poisoning.

See *Caring About Culture: Lead Poisoning.*

See *Focus on Long-Term Care and Home Care: Lead Poisoning.*

CARING ABOUT CULTURE
Lead Poisoning

Lead has been found in some traditional medicines used by *East Indian, Indian, Middle Eastern, West Asian, Chinese,* and *Hispanic cultures.* Lead and other metals have been found in powders and tablets used for arthritis, upset stomach, colic, vomiting, diarrhea, constipation, fertility problems, menstrual cramps, and other illnesses. Some are used for teething babies or to calm young children. Lead may also get into a medicine accidentally during grinding or coloring or from the package.

Modified from Centers for Disease Control and Prevention: Childhood lead poisoning prevention, *Atlanta, Ga., page reviewed May 17, 2022.*

FOCUS ON LONG-TERM CARE AND HOME CARE
Lead Poisoning

Home Care

Homes built before 1986 may have lead pipes and fixtures that are corroded—water taps, pipes in the house, pipes from the street to the house. *Corrosion* is when the metal dissolves or wears away from a chemical reaction between the water and plumbing. Lead can enter the water, especially hot water.

High levels of lead in tap water can cause health problems. Because of their size, unborn babies, infants, and young children are at greater risk than adults. Infants who drink formula are at high risk when formula is made with tap water containing lead.

Community water systems are required to provide a water quality report to customers every year. Water quality from a private well is the responsibility of the homeowner. If there is a concern about lead in drinking water, the water should be tested. The following can reduce exposure to lead in drinking water.

- Flush the pipes before using water for drinking and cooking. Run tap water, take a shower, do laundry, or do a load of dishes to flush the pipes. Contact the public water utility for the recommended time to flush pipes.
- Use *cold* water for drinking and cooking and making baby formula. Warm or hot tap water can have higher lead levels. Boiling water does not remove lead.
- Clean the faucet's screen (aerator) regularly. Sediment, debris, and lead particles can collect in the screen.
- Use filters properly. Make sure the filter is certified to remove lead. Change the filter as often as directed by the manufacturer.
- Use bottled water instead of tap water if needed.

BOX 14-3   Lead Poisoning

Sources of Lead Poisoning

- House paint before 1978. Children can swallow peeling paint and paint chips. When paint is stripped or sanded, lead dust is released into the air.
- Painted and plastic toys and decorations, especially old toys and those made outside of the United States.
- Toy jewelry made of lead.
- Some imported candies (includes candy wrappers).
- Certain water pipes. Lead can be found in drinking water if plumbing, pipes, or faucets contain lead.
- Contaminated soil. Exposure may be from swallowing or breathing in soil particles. Young children often put contaminated hands in their mouths. Soil may be brought indoors on shoes, clothing, or pets.
- Jobs and hobbies that involve lead products and supplies. Welding, making lead-glazed pottery, stained glass work, home building and repair, fishing, hunting, and automotive repair are examples.

Lead Poisoning in Children: Signs and Symptoms

Lead poisoning can occur without any obvious signs or symptoms. Signs and symptoms may include:

- Abdominal pain; cramping
- *Anemia* (low amount of red blood cells)
- Appetite: poor or loss of
- Attention and learning problems
- Behavior problems; aggressive behavior; irritability
- Coma (with very high lead levels)
- Constipation
- Development: regression (loss of skills)
- Fatigue
- Growth: slowed
- Headaches
- Hearing loss
- Joint pain
- Muscle weakness
- Seizures (with very high lead levels)
- Sensations: reduced
- Sleep problems
- Vomiting

Safety Measures

- Prevent or discourage children from eating, chewing, or sucking on non-food items. They include the lead sources listed in this box.
- Do not let children play in dirt. Have them play in grassy or sandy areas.
- Assist the child with hand-washing before eating, after playing outside, and before going to bed.
- Use doormats at entryways and remove shoes to avoid tracking soil into the home.

Safety Measures—cont'd

- Keep the home as dust-free as possible. Use a wet mop and wet cloths to clean floors, furniture, window sills, and dusty surfaces. (A wet method controls dust.)
- Keep play areas clean. Wash toys, bottles, pacifiers, and stuffed animals regularly.
- Prevent exposure to lead-based plumbing. See *Focus on Long-Term Care and Home Care: Lead Poisoning.*
- Prevent exposure to lead-based paint.
  - Get your home tested for lead by a professional if the home was built before 1978.
  - Keep painted surfaces in excellent condition. Paint is not cracked, damaged, peeling, or chipped.
  - Repair damaged paint surfaces. Consult a professional who is certified in lead-safe practices to remove paint hazards.
  - Keep children away from paint chips and dust contaminated with lead paint.
  - Do not bump into walls or furniture that may contain lead-based paint.
  - Do not open and close windows that have lead-based paint. This prevents dust and paint chips.
  - Use a wet mop and wet cloths to clean up dust and paint chips. Do not sweep or vacuum lead-based paint dust or paint chips.
- Prevent exposure to food and drinks contaminated with lead.
  - Do not use lead-glazed pottery for cooking, serving, or storing food or drinks.
  - Do not eat foods that are canned outside the United States. (In 1995 the Food and Drug Administration [FDA] banned the use of lead solder in food cans, including imported products.)
  - Do not store wine, alcohol, or vinegar-based salad dressings in lead crystal decanters for long periods. Lead can get into the liquid.
- Prevent children from having contact with work or hobby materials that may contain lead.
  - Store lead-based products where children cannot see or reach them.
  - Take shoes off before entering the home.
  - Shower and change clothes before contact with children.
  - Wash and store clothes contaminated with lead separately from others.
- Do not let children handle or play with old newspapers, magazines, or books. The ink may contain lead.
- Ensure a low-fat diet that is high in iron, calcium, and vitamin C (Chapter 30). A healthy diet can protect against the harmful effects of lead.

Carbon Monoxide Poisoning

Carbon monoxide (CO) is a deadly colorless, odorless, and tasteless gas. It is produced by the burning of fuel—gasoline, oil, kerosene, propane, wood, charcoal (Fig. 14-7). Fuel-burning devices must work properly and be used correctly. Otherwise, dangerous levels of CO can build up in closed or semi-closed areas. Instead of breathing in oxygen, the person breathes in air filled with CO. Red blood cells pick up CO faster than oxygen. Oxygen does not get into the body. CO can kill quickly or slowly. If not fatal, brain and nervous system damage can result.

People and animals are at risk for CO poisoning. Sleeping or intoxicated persons can die before having symptoms. CO poisoning may be unintentional or intentional as a suicide attempt. See Box 14-4 for the signs and symptoms of CO poisoning and safety measures.

BOX 14-4   Carbon Monoxide Poisoning

Signs and Symptoms
- Breathing problems
- Chest pain
- Confusion
- Consciousness: loss of
- Dizziness
- Headache
- Nausea
- Sleepiness
- Vomiting
- Weakness

Safety Measures
- Get outside into fresh air immediately if CO poisoning is suspected. Call 911.
- Have CO alarms installed on every level of the home and outside sleeping areas. Also install them near any major gas-burning appliances (furnace, water heater).
- Follow the manufacturer's instructions when using fuel-burning devices. Use the correct fuel for the device. Ensure that devices are vented properly.
- Have the home's heating system (including chimneys and vents) and water heater inspected and serviced every year by a qualified technician. Do so for any other fuel-burning appliances as well.
- Have an odor from a gas refrigerator inspected by a qualified technician.
- Never use a portable generator inside a house, basement, or garage. Use it outside, far away from the home (at least 20 feet away from any window, door, or vent).
- Never use a charcoal grill or portable gas camp stove indoors, in a tent, or in a garage. Do not burn charcoal indoors.
- Never use a gas stove, oven, or dryer to heat a home or room.
- Do not put foil on the bottom of a gas oven.
- Open the fireplace damper before lighting a fire. Keep it open until ashes are cool.
- Have vehicle exhaust systems checked regularly.
- Do not leave a vehicle running in a garage (even with the garage door open).

Examples of Carbon Monoxide Sources
- Fireplaces (wood and gas)
- Furnaces
- Gas clothes dryers
- Gas stoves and ovens
- Wood-burning stoves
- Gas water heaters
- Generators (portable)
- Grills and camp stoves used indoors (gas, charcoal)
- Lanterns
- Lawn mowers; weed trimmers
- Snow blowers
- Motor vehicles
- Space heaters (gas, kerosene)

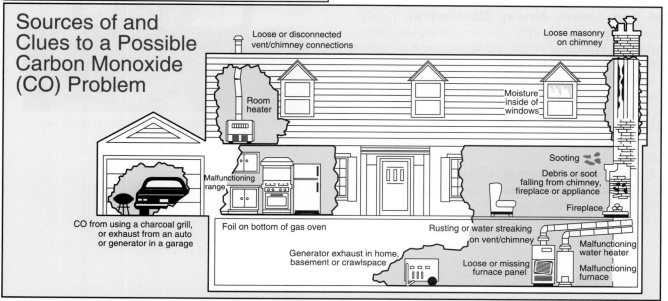

FIGURE 14-7 Sources of and clues to possible carbon monoxide problems. (Bottom image from U.S. Consumer Product Safety Commission: *The invisible killer*, CPSC-464, Washington, DC.)

PREVENTING SUFFOCATION

Suffocation (asphyxia) is when breathing stops from the lack of oxygen. Death occurs if the person does not start breathing. Common causes include choking, drowning, inhaling gas or smoke, strangulation, and electrical shock (p. 191). (See "Altered Respiratory Function" in Chapter 44.)

Measures to prevent suffocation are listed in Box 14-5. Clear the airway if the person is choking.

Choking

A foreign body (food or object) can obstruct (block) the airway. This is called *choking* or *foreign-body airway obstruction (FBAO)*. Air cannot pass through the airways into the lungs. The body does not get enough oxygen. Death can result.

Choking often occurs during eating. A large, poorly chewed piece of meat is a common cause. Laughing and talking while eating also are common causes. So is excessive alcohol intake.

Unconscious persons can choke. Common causes are aspiration of (breathing in) vomitus and the tongue falling back into the airway.

See *Focus on Children and Older Persons: Choking.*

FOCUS ON CHILDREN AND OLDER PERSONS

Choking

Children
Children under age 4 are at a high risk for choking while eating. Children must be supervised while eating. Foods served must be safe (see Box 14-5). Cook hard foods until soft. Cut foods into thin slices, strips, or small pieces (no larger than ½ inch).

Older Persons
Older persons are at risk for choking. Weakness, dentures that fit poorly, *dysphagia* (difficulty swallowing), and chronic illness are common causes.

Mild and Severe Airway Obstruction. Foreign bodies can cause mild (partial) or severe (complete) airway obstruction. With *mild airway obstruction*, some air moves in and out of the lungs. The person is conscious and usually can speak. Often forceful coughing can remove the object. Breathing may sound like wheezing between coughs. For mild airway obstruction:

- Stay with the person.
- Encourage the person to keep coughing to expel the object.
- Do not interrupt the person's efforts to clear the airway. If the person is breathing and coughing, abdominal thrusts are not needed.
- If the obstruction persists, call for help.

A person with *severe airway obstruction* has difficulty breathing. Air does not move in and out of the lungs. The person may not be able to breathe, speak, or cough. If able to cough, the cough is of poor quality. When the person tries to inhale (breathe in), there is either no noise or a high-pitched noise. The person may appear pale and *cyanotic* (bluish color). Severe airway obstruction is an emergency.

Relieving Choking. When choking, the conscious person usually clutches at the throat (Fig. 14-8). Clutching at the throat is often called the *universal sign of choking*. The conscious person is very frightened. If the obstruction is not removed, the person will die.

Abdominal thrusts are used to relieve severe airway obstruction. Abdominal thrusts are quick, upward thrusts to the abdomen. Also known as the *Heimlich maneuver,* the thrusts force air out of the lungs and create an artificial cough. They are done to try to expel the foreign body from the airway.

You may observe a person choking. And you may perform emergency measures to relieve choking. Relief of choking occurs when the foreign body is removed. Or it occurs when you feel air move and see the chest rise and fall when giving breaths during emergency care (Chapter 58).

If you assist a choking person, report and record what happened. Include what you did and the person's response.

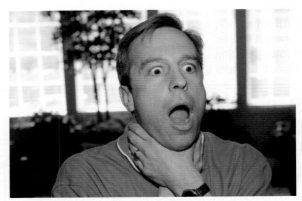

FIGURE 14-8 A choking person clutches at the throat.

BOX 14-5 Preventing Suffocation

All Age-Groups
- Make sure dentures fit properly and are in place.
- Report loose teeth or dentures.
- Check the care plan for swallowing problems before serving food (including snacks) or fluids. The person may have special food (fluid) orders (Chapter 31). Make sure the person is able to chew and swallow what is served.
- Cut foods into small, bite-sized pieces for persons who cannot do so themselves.
- Tell the nurse at once if the person has swallowing problems.
- Do not give oral foods or fluids to persons with feeding tubes (Chapter 33).
- Follow aspiration precautions (Chapter 31). Aspiration precautions prevent *aspiration*— breathing in fluid, food, vomitus, or an object into the lungs.
- Do not leave a person unattended in a bathtub or shower.
- Remove the key from a gas fireplace. Store it out of reach.
- Move all persons from the area if you smell smoke.
- Position the person in bed properly.
- Prevent entrapment in the bed system (Chapter 13).
- Use bed rails correctly (Chapter 15).
- Practice safe use of restraints if they must be used for protection. Restraints can cause strangulation. See Chapter 16.
- Do not use power strips for care equipment.
- See "Preventing Equipment Accidents" on p. 191.

Children
- Electrical safety:
  - Use safety plugs in outlets with caution (p. 192). Children can remove and choke on them. And they can be misplaced when removed to use the outlet.
  - Keep electrical cords and electrical items out of the reach of children.
- Sleep safety:
  - Position infants on their backs for sleep. This reduces the risk for sudden infant death syndrome (SIDS) (Chapter 56).
  - Practice crib safety (Chapter 56 and Appendix D). Use a firm, flat sleep surface that meets federal safety standards. The surface is covered only by a fitted sheet.
  - Keep soft bedding (blankets, pillows), bumper pads, and soft toys out of a baby's sleeping area. Do not let babies sleep on soft surfaces (beds, sofas, chairs), recliners, bouncy chairs, or swings.
  - Do not let babies or young children sleep with an adult or older child. Children can be rolled over or be caught between the mattress and wall.
  - Do not let children under the age of 6 sleep on a top bunk bed.
- Practice safe swaddling for babies. To *swaddle* means to wrap snugly in a thin blanket or garment for safety and warmth.
  - Use a sleep sack for warmth. A sleep sack is a wearable blanket. Make sure the baby's head and face are not covered.
  - Check that zippers or other fasteners are securely attached.
  - Avoid over-heating. Sweating, damp hair, flushed cheeks, rash, and rapid breathing are signs that the baby is too hot.
  - Stop swaddling if the baby can roll.

Children—cont'd
- Food safety:
  - Do not prop a bottle for a baby to drink while lying down. Do not leave a baby alone when drinking from a bottle. The baby could aspirate (breathe in) fluid and choke.
  - Have children sit when they eat. They should not eat or suck on anything while lying down or playing.
  - Do not give infants and young children small (marble-sized), hard, or sticky foods. Examples include chunks of cheese; chewing gum and hard candy; dried fruit; gummy fruit snacks; ice cubes; marshmallows; nuts and seeds; pretzels; popcorn; spoonfuls of peanut butter; uncut round or tube-shaped foods like grapes, cherry tomatoes, cherries, hot dogs, and sausages; and raw, hard vegetables and fruit (carrots, apples).
  - Remove pits, seeds, and small bones from fruits, vegetables, fish, chicken, and so on.
  - Give infants soft foods that do not require chewing.
  - Offer fluids to children while they are eating.
  - Do not let children play with dried beans or dried peas.
- Balloon safety:
  - Use Mylar balloons instead of latex ones.
  - Store latex balloons where children cannot see or reach them.
  - Do not let children inflate or deflate latex balloons.
  - Deflate and discard latex balloons after use.
  - Pick up and discard broken balloon pieces at once. Do not let children near them.
- Small object and toy safety:
  - Make sure toys are intact. They should not be broken, have cracks or chips, sharp or rough edges, need repair, and so on.
  - Give the child age-appropriate toys.
  - Check floors for small objects—buttons, coins, beads, marbles, pins, tacks, nails, screws, jewelry, and so on. Keep them out of a child's reach. Pick up and store or discard such objects. Children can choke on them. When checking floors, it is best to get on the floor on your hands and knees—the child's eye level.
  - Keep refrigerator magnets out of reach.
  - Remove rubber knobs or tips from door stops.
  - Check toys for removable parts.
  - Do not let babies play with small toys or toys with small parts.
- Cord, string, and ribbon safety:
  - Do not string or hang any object on or near a crib. This includes a mobile, toy, or diaper bag. The child can get caught in it and strangle.
  - Never tie pacifiers or teethers around a child's neck.
  - Do not use bibs; clothes with ribbons, ties, or cords; or necklaces whenever the child is put in a crib or playpen.
  - Make sure dangling cords are not within a baby's reach. This includes cords from drapes, shades, and blinds.
- Other:
  - Keep appliance doors closed—ovens, refrigerators, clothes dryers, washing machines, freezers, dishwashers, coolers, and so on.
  - Keep plastic bags away from children. This includes grocery bags, garment bags, and dry-cleaning bags. Tie the bags in knots. Then discard them.
  - See Chapter 56 for other child safety measures.

Older Persons
- Report signs and symptoms of weakness.
- Report signs or symptoms of difficulty swallowing *(dysphagia).*
- Be aware of chronic illnesses.

Chest thrusts are used for obese or pregnant persons (Fig. 14-9). If you are alone and choking, perform self-administered abdominal thrusts. See Box 14-6.

See *Focus on Children and Older Persons: Relieving Choking.*

See procedure: *Relieving Choking—Adult or Child (1 Year of Age and Older).*

See procedure: *Relieving Choking—In the Infant (Less Than 1 Year of Age),* p. 190.

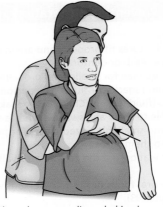

FIGURE 14-9 Chest thrusts to relieve choking in a pregnant woman.

BOX 14-6	Relieving Choking: Special Situations

Chest Thrusts for Obese or Pregnant Persons
1 Stand behind the person.
2 Place your arms under the person's underarms. Wrap your arms around the person's chest.
3 Make a fist. Place the thumb side of the fist on the middle of the sternum (breastbone).
4 Grasp the fist with your other hand.
5 Give chest thrusts until the object is expelled or the person becomes unresponsive.
6 If the person becomes unresponsive, have someone activate the Emergency Medical Services (EMS) system or the agency's Rapid Response System (RRS) if not already done. An RRS is a team that quickly responds to give care in life-threatening situations. Start cardiopulmonary resuscitation (CPR). See Chapter 58.

Self-Administered Abdominal Thrusts
1 Make a fist with 1 hand.
2 Place the thumb side of the fist above your navel and below the lower end of the sternum.
3 Grasp your fist with your other hand.
4 Press inward and upward quickly.
5 Press the upper abdomen against a hard surface if the thrust did not relieve the obstruction. Use the back of a chair, a table, or a railing.
6 Use as many thrusts as needed.

FOCUS ON CHILDREN AND OLDER PERSONS

Relieving Choking

Children
Respiratory infections can cause airway obstruction in infants and children. Airway structures become swollen. The airway narrows or becomes completely blocked. Air cannot enter the airway. The child needs emergency care at once.

The procedures that follow will not relieve airway obstruction caused by an infection. Do not try them if the child has a fever, rash, congestion, hoarseness, or other signs and symptoms of respiratory infection. You will waste precious time. Activate the EMS system or the agency's RRS. Give rescue breaths if the child is not breathing but has a pulse. Start CPR if the child is not responding, not breathing or not breathing normally (gasping), and has no pulse. You will learn about giving rescue breaths and CPR in Chapter 58.

Abdominal thrusts are not given to infants. They can damage the liver and other organs. Back slaps (back blows) and chest thrusts are used for infants (p. 190).

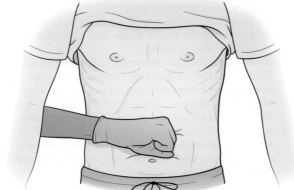
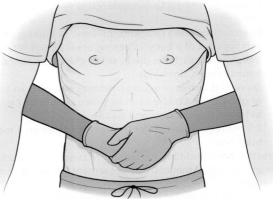
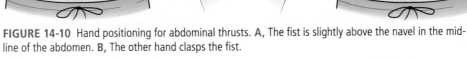

A   B

FIGURE 14-10 Hand positioning for abdominal thrusts. **A,** The fist is slightly above the navel in the midline of the abdomen. **B,** The other hand clasps the fist.

Guidelines for emergency care are updated as new information becomes available. You are responsible for following current guidelines. Updates can be found on-line at the American Heart Association's website.

Relieving Choking—Adult or Child (1 Year of Age and Older)
PROCEDURE

1 Ask the person: "Are you choking?"
  a *If the person can cough or talk,* see p. 186 for mild airway obstruction.
  b *If the person is unresponsive,* you may not know the cause. Call for help and begin CPR. See Chapter 58.
  c *If the person nods "yes" and cannot talk,* continue to step 2.
2 Have someone call for help if another person is available. If not, continue to step 3.
  a *In a public area,* have someone call 911 to activate the EMS system. Send someone to get an automated external defibrillator (AED) (Chapter 58).
  b *In an agency,* have someone call the agency's RRS and get a defibrillator (AED).
3 Give abdominal thrusts.
  a Stand or kneel behind the person.
  b Wrap your arms around the person's waist.
  c Make a fist with 1 hand.
  d Place the thumb side of the fist against the abdomen. The fist is slightly above the navel in the middle of the abdomen and well below the end of the sternum (breastbone). See Figure 14-10, *A.*
  e Grasp your fist with your other hand (Fig. 14-10, *B*).
  f Press your fist into the abdomen with a quick, upward thrust (Fig. 14-11).
  g Repeat thrusts until the object is expelled or the person becomes unresponsive. Each thrust is a separate, distinct movement.
4 *If the object is dislodged,* encourage hospital care. Injuries can occur from abdominal thrusts.

5 *If the person becomes unresponsive:*
  a Lower the person to the floor or ground. Position the person supine (lying flat on the back).
  b Make sure the EMS or RRS was called.
    1) *If alone with a phone,* call while giving care.
    2) *If alone without a phone,* give about 2 minutes of CPR first. Then call the EMS or RRS and get an AED.
  c Start CPR. See Chapter 58. Do not check for a pulse.
    1) Give 30 chest compressions.
    2) Open the airway with the head tilt–chin lift method (Fig. 14-12). Open the person's mouth wide. Look for an object. Remove the object if you can see it and can remove it easily.
    3) Give 2 breaths.
    4) Continue cycles of 30 compressions followed by 2 breaths. Look for an object every time you open the airway.
  d *If choking is relieved,* check for a response, breathing, and a pulse. (NOTE: Choking is relieved when you feel air move and see the chest rise and fall when giving breaths.)
    1) *If no response, no normal breathing, and no pulse*—Continue CPR. Use the AED as soon as possible (Chapter 58).
    2) *If no response and no normal breathing but there is a pulse*—Give rescue breaths. For an adult, give 1 breath every 6 seconds. For a child, give 1 breath every 2 to 3 seconds. Check for a pulse about every 2 minutes. If no pulse, begin CPR.
    3) *If the person has normal breathing and a pulse*—Place the person in the recovery position if there is no response (Chapter 58). Continue to check the person until help arrives. Encourage hospital care.

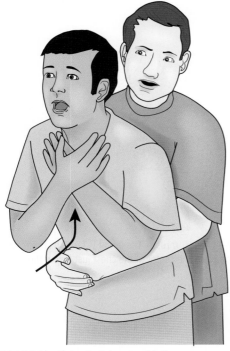

FIGURE 14-11 Abdominal thrusts with the person standing.

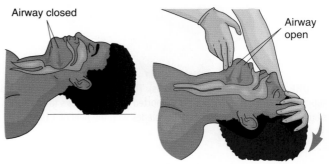

Airway closed

Airway open

FIGURE 14-12 The head tilt–chin lift method opens the airway. One hand is on the person's forehead. Pressure is applied to tilt the head back. The chin is lifted with the fingers of the other hand.

Guidelines for emergency care are updated as new information becomes available. You are responsible for following current guidelines. Updates can be found on-line at the American Heart Association's website.

Relieving Choking—In the Infant (Less Than 1 Year of Age)

PROCEDURE

1 Have someone call for help if another person is available. If not, continue to step 2.
   a *In a public area,* have someone call 911 to activate the EMS system. Send someone to get an AED. See Chapter 58.
   b *In an agency,* have someone call the agency's RRS and get a defibrillator (AED).
2 Sit or kneel with the infant in your lap.
3 Hold the infant face down over your forearm. (Support your arm on your thigh or lap.) The infant's head is lower than the chest. Support the head and jaw with your hand.
4 Give up to 5 forceful back slaps (back blows) (Fig. 14-13). Use the heel of your hand. Give the back slaps between the shoulder blades. (Stop the back slaps if the object is expelled.)
5 Turn the infant as a unit.
   a Continue to support the infant's face, jaw, head, neck, and chest with 1 hand.
   b Support the back and the back of the infant's head with your other hand. Your palm supports the back of the head.
   c Turn the infant as a unit. The infant is face up on your forearm. Your forearm rests on your thigh. The infant's head is lower than the chest.
6 Give up to 5 chest thrusts (Fig. 14-14).
   a Place 2 fingers in the center of the chest just below the nipple line.
   b Give chest thrusts at a rate of about 1 every second. The thrusts are quick and downward.
   c Stop chest thrusts if the object is expelled.

7 Continue giving 5 back slaps followed by 5 chest thrusts until the object is expelled or the infant becomes unresponsive.
8 *If the infant becomes unresponsive:*
   a Make sure the EMS or RRS was called.
      1) *If alone with a phone,* call while giving care.
      2) *If alone without a phone,* give about 2 minutes of CPR first. Then call the EMS or RRS and get an AED.
   b Place the infant on a firm, flat surface.
   c Start CPR. Do not check for a pulse. Give 30 chest compressions. (See Chapter 58 for infant CPR.)
   d Open the airway. Use the head tilt–chin lift method. Open the infant's mouth. Look for an object. Remove the object if you see it and can remove it easily. Use your fingers.
   e Give 2 breaths.
   f Continue cycles of 30 compressions followed by 2 breaths. Look for an object every time you open the airway. Use your fingers to remove it if you see it and can remove it easily.
   g Continue CPR until help takes over or until choking is relieved.

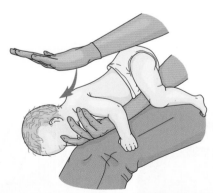

FIGURE 14-13 Back slaps (back blows). The infant is held face down and supported with 1 arm. The arm is supported on the rescuer's thigh. Back slaps are given between the shoulder blades with the heel of 1 hand.

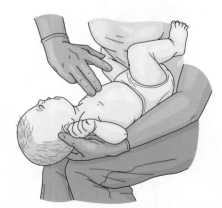

FIGURE 14-14 Chest thrusts. The infant is face up. The rescuer uses 2 fingers to compress the center of the chest just below the nipple line.

PREVENTING EQUIPMENT ACCIDENTS

All equipment is unsafe if broken, not used correctly, not working properly, or in need of repair. This includes hospital beds. Inspect equipment before use. Check all items for cracks, chips, and sharp or rough edges. They can cause cuts, stabs, or scratches. (See "Bloodborne Pathogen Standard" in Chapter 17 for blood exposure precautions.)

Bariatric-Safe Equipment

Beds, chairs, wheelchairs, stretchers, toilets, commodes, and other equipment usually have a weight capacity of 250 to 350 pounds. Bariatric patients and residents can weigh from 250 pounds to over 1000 pounds. Bariatric equipment is labeled:

- "Bariatric"
- "EC" for "expanded capacity"
- With the weight limit suggested by the manufacturer

Do not use the item if the person's weight is greater than the item's weight capacity. Follow the nurse's directions and the care plan.

Wheelchair and Stretcher Safety

Wheelchairs are useful for people who cannot walk or who have severe problems walking. Stretchers are used to transport persons who cannot sit up or must lie down. Stretchers are used in hospitals and by emergency medical personnel.

The person can fall from the wheelchair or stretcher. Or the person can fall during transfers to and from the wheelchair or stretcher. See Chapter 21 for wheelchair and stretcher safety.

Electrical Equipment

Frayed cords (Fig. 14-15, *A*) and over-loaded electrical outlets (Fig. 14-15, *B*) can cause fires, burns, and electrical shocks. *Electrical shock* is when electrical current passes through the body. It can burn the skin, muscles, nerves, and other tissues. It can affect the heart and cause death.

Three-pronged outlets and three-pronged plugs are designed to protect against electrical shock (Fig. 14-16). Two prongs carry electrical current. The third prong is a safety feature called a *ground*. A *ground* carries leaking electricity to the earth and away from an electrical item. Without a ground, leaking electricity can be conducted to the person. It can cause electrical shocks and possible death.

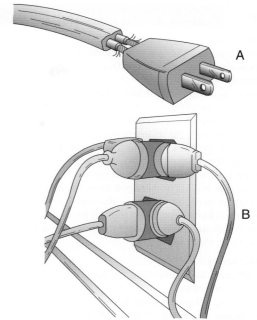

FIGURE 14-15 A, A frayed electrical cord. **B,** An over-loaded electrical outlet.

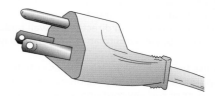

FIGURE 14-16 A 3-pronged plug.

Warning signs of a faulty electrical item include:

- Shocks
- Loss of power or a power surge
- Dimming or flickering lights
- Sparks
- Sizzling or buzzing sounds
- Burning odor
- Loose plugs

Report a problem at once. Do not use the item.

Practice the electrical safety measures in Box 14-7 (p. 192). Complete an incident report (p. 204) for an equipment-related accident. The *Safe Medical Devices Act* requires that agencies report equipment-related illnesses, injuries, and deaths.

BOX 14-7	Preventing Equipment Accidents

General Safety
- Follow agency policies and procedures.
- Follow the manufacturer's instructions. Use equipment correctly.
- Read all caution and warning labels.
- Do not use an unfamiliar item. Ask for training. Also ask a nurse to supervise you the first time you use the item.
- Use an item only for its intended purpose.
- Make sure the item works before you begin.
- Have all needed equipment before you begin.
- Do not use broken or damaged items.
- Do not give broken or damaged items to patients or residents.
- Do not try to repair broken or damaged items.
- Show a broken or damaged item to the nurse. Follow the nurse's instructions and agency policies for discarding items or sending them for repair.

Electrical Safety
- Check cords and equipment for damage. Make sure they are in good repair.
- Never alter a 3-pronged plug (see Fig. 14-16). Make sure all prongs are intact. Do not use a plug with a cracked prong.
- Avoid using extension cords. If you must use an extension cord, use it for only 1 device. This prevents over-loading a circuit.
- Follow agency policy for use of power strips. Do not use power strips for care equipment.
- Connect a bed power cord directly to a wall outlet. Do not connect a bed power cord to an extension cord or power strip.
- Do not use the person's electrical items until they have been approved for safety by maintenance staff.
- Do not cover or run any cord under rugs, carpets, linens, or other materials.

Electrical Safety—cont'd
- Keep electrical items away from water.
- Keep work areas clean and dry. Wipe up spills right away.
- Do not touch electrical items if you are wet, if your hands are wet, if you are in water (tub, pool), or if you are standing in water. This includes using a phone when it is plugged into a charger.
- Do not put a finger or any other item (coin, paperclip, fork, and so on) into an outlet. To protect children and confused persons:
  - Use tamper-resistant outlets. Tamper-resistant outlets block items from being inserted into the outlet.
  - If necessary, use outlet safety covers or plates over standard electrical outlets (Fig. 14-17, A).
  - Use safety plugs with caution (Fig. 14-17, B). Children can remove and choke on outlet plugs or stick their fingers or small objects into outlet openings.
  - Use power strip covers for power strips and attached cords.
- Do not give showers or tub baths during storms. Lightning can travel through pipes.
- Do not use electrical items or phones during storms.
- Do not use water to put out an electrical fire. If possible, turn off or unplug the item. Call 911 at once.
- Do not touch a person who is having an electrical shock. If possible, turn off or unplug the item. Call 911 or the RRS.
- Keep electrical cords away from heating vents and other heat sources.
- Turn off the device when done using the item.
- Turn off equipment before unplugging it. Sparks occur when electrical items are unplugged while turned on.
- Unplug all devices when not in use.
- Hold on to the plug (not the cord) when removing it from an outlet (Fig. 14-18).

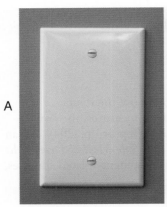 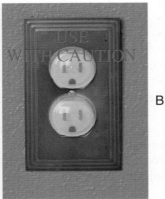

A   B

FIGURE 14-17 Outlet safety. **A,** Outlet safety cover. **B,** Outlet plugs. Use plugs with caution.

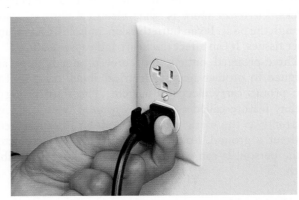

FIGURE 14-18 Hold on to the plug to remove it from the outlet.

HAZARDOUS CHEMICALS

A *hazardous chemical* is any chemical that is a physical hazard or a health hazard. *Physical hazards* can cause fires or explosions. *Health hazards* can cause health problems. Health hazards can:

- Cause cancer.
- Affect blood cell formation and function.
- Damage the kidneys, nervous system, lungs, skin, eyes, or mucous membranes.
- Cause birth defects, miscarriages, and fertility problems.

Exposure to hazardous chemicals can occur from equipment failures, container ruptures, or the release of a hazard into the workplace. Workplace hazards include:

- Equipment containing latex (Chapter 18)
- Thermometers and blood pressure equipment containing mercury (Chapter 34)
- Cleaners and disinfectants (Chapter 17)

The *Hazard Communication Standard (HCS)* is a policy of the Occupational Safety and Health Administration (OSHA). It requires container labeling, safety data sheets (SDSs), and employee training. Eyewash and total body wash stations are required where hazardous chemicals are used.

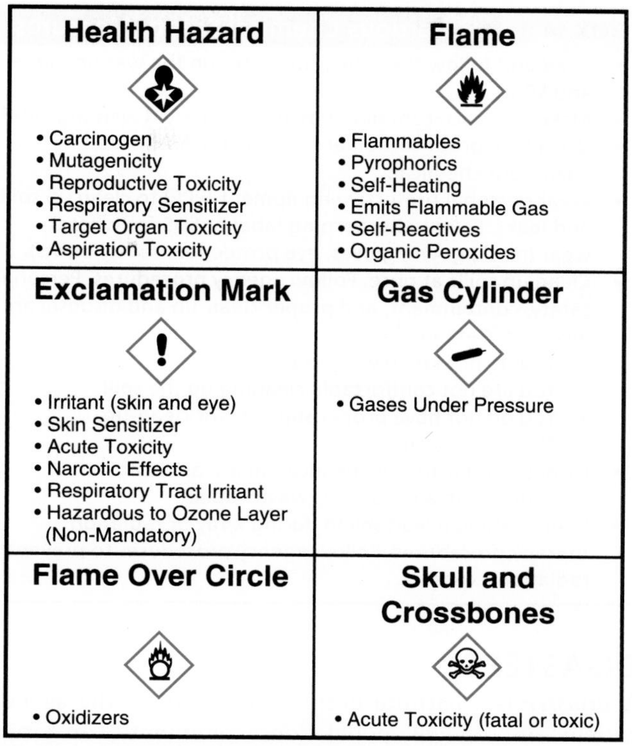

Labeling

Hazardous chemical containers have warning labels. The warning labels contain *pictograms*—symbols used to communicate specific information about a chemical hazard. See Figure 14-19 for examples.

If a warning label is removed or damaged, do not use the substance. Show the container to the nurse and explain the problem. Do not leave the container unattended.

Safety Data Sheets

Every hazardous chemical has a *safety data sheet (SDS)*. Some agencies use the term *material safety data sheet (MSDS)*. Information provided includes:

- Name and common names
- Hazards about the chemical
- Chemical ingredients
- Emergency measures
- Fire-fighting measures
- Accidental release measures
- Safe handling and storage measures
- Personal protection measures

Check the SDS before using a hazardous chemical, cleaning up a leak or spill, or disposing of the substance. Call for the nurse about a leak or spill right away. Do not leave a leak or spill unattended.

FIGURE 14-19 Some pictograms from the Occupational Safety and Health Administration. Depending on the chemical, the warning label contains the necessary pictograms and associated hazards. (Redrawn from OSHA Quick Card, OSHA Occupational Safety and Health Administration, U.S. Department of Labor, Washington, DC.)

Employee Training

Your employer provides hazardous chemical training. You learn about hazards, exposure risks, and protection measures. You learn to read and use warning labels and the SDS.

Each hazardous chemical requires certain protection measures. See the safety measures in Box 14-8 (p. 194).

BOX 14-8	Hazardous Chemical Safety Measures

- Read and follow the safety measures on the warning label and SDS.
- Make sure each container has an undamaged warning label.
- Use a leak-proof container to carry or transport a hazardous chemical.
- Wear personal protective equipment (PPE) to clean up spills and leaks. Follow the warning label or SDS for what to wear (mask, gown, gloves, eye protection, safety boots).
- Clean up spills at once. Follow agency procedures. Personal safety, containment, and proper clean-up and disposal are involved. Get help if:
  - You do not know what was spilled.
  - You are not comfortable cleaning up the spill.
  - You do not have proper supplies for clean-up.
  - The spill is large.
- Dispose of hazardous chemicals in a sealed bag or container with a hazardous waste label.
- Stand behind a lead shield during x-ray or radiation therapy procedures. Follow agency procedures to prevent radiation exposure.
- Do not enter a room while a person is having x-rays or radiation therapy.
- Wash your hands after handling hazardous chemicals.
- Work in well-ventilated areas to avoid inhaling gases.
- Use cleaning products safely.
  - Read and follow warnings and label directions.
  - Keep products in their original containers.
  - Make sure the area is well-ventilated.
  - Do not mix products. Mixing products can cause dangerous gases. For example, do not mix ammonia and bleach.
  - Close containers properly.
  - Put cleaning products away after use.
  - Do not store cleaning products near food.
  - Empty buckets, pails, basins, and other containers with cleaning solutions.
  - Do not use an empty container for other purposes or things.
- Dispose of or store a hazardous chemical according to the SDS.

DISASTERS

A *disaster* is a harmful event that can affect the agency, patient or resident population, community, or larger geographic area. The following are examples.

- Natural disasters—tornadoes, hurricanes, blizzards, earthquakes, volcano eruptions, floods, some fires
- Human-made disasters—auto, bus, train, and airplane accidents; fires; bombings; power plant accidents; gas or chemical leaks; explosions; wars
- Power failures
- Communication failures and cyber-attacks (criminal activity involving information systems)
- Infectious disease threats (see "Pandemics" on p. 200)
- Missing residents (see "Elopement" on p. 200)

Communities and fire and police departments have disaster plans. The Centers for Medicare & Medicaid Services (CMS) requires that health care agencies have an *emergency preparedness program* in place. The program describes the agency's approach to meeting health, safety, and security needs of patients or residents, staff, and the community before, during, and after a disaster.

Planning for disasters includes development of an *emergency plan*.

- Potential hazards are identified.
- Policies and procedures are formed and implemented (carried out).
- A communication plan is developed.
- Staff are trained and the plan is tested.

Your agency provides training on policies and procedures and your role in responding in an emergency.

See *Focus on Long-Term Care and Home Care: Disasters.*
See *Focus on Surveys: Disasters.*

FOCUS ON LONG-TERM CARE AND HOME CARE

Disasters

Home Care

A severe storm may occur when you are in a patient's home. For safety:

- Stay informed through local TV and radio stations. Satellite services may not have a signal during heavy storms.
- Keep a flashlight with you for power outages.
- Move the patient, family, and yourself to a "safe room."
  - Basement
  - Room on the ground floor
  - Interior room away from outside walls, windows, and doors
  - Center hallway
  - Bathroom
  - Closet

Bomb Threats

Follow agency procedures for a bomb threat or if you find an item that looks or sounds strange. Bomb threats can be sent by phone, mail, e-mail, text message, messenger, or other means. Or the person can leave a bomb in the agency. If you see a stranger or strange item or package in the agency, tell the nurse at once. You cannot be too safe.

Fire Safety

Faulty electrical equipment and wiring, over-loaded electrical circuits, and smoking are major causes of fires. The health team must prevent fires and act quickly during a fire. See Box 14-9.

See *Focus on Long-Term Care and Home Care: Fire Safety,* p. 196.

BOX 14-9	Fire Prevention Measures

- Follow the safety measures:
  - For oxygen use (p. 197)
  - To prevent equipment accidents (p. 191)
  - To prevent burns (p. 179)
- Practice smoking and ashtray safety.
  - Smoke only where allowed to do so. Do not smoke in patients' homes.
  - Supervise persons who smoke. This is very important for persons who are confused or disoriented.
  - Follow the manufacturer's instructions for electronic cigarette use and care. Do not leave an electronic cigarette unattended while charging.
  - Provide ashtrays. Deep, wide, and sturdy ashtrays are best. Keep ashtrays away from anything that can burn.
  - Empty ashtrays only when sure that all ashes, cigars, cigarettes, and other smoking materials are out (extinguished).
  - Empty ashtrays into a metal container partially filled with sand or water. Do not empty ashtrays into plastic containers or wastebaskets lined with paper or plastic bags.
  - Do not smoke or light matches or lighters around flammable liquids or materials or oxygen equipment (Chapter 44). Alcohol-based hand sanitizer (Chapter 17) is flammable (it can catch on fire).
- Keep smoking materials, matches, lighters, candles, incense, flammable liquids and materials, and other fire sources away from children and confused or disoriented persons.
- Light matches carefully.
  - Be alert for sparks when lighting a match. Sparks can start a fire.
  - Keep your hair, clothing, and anything that will burn away from the match and flame.

- Do not leave cooking unattended on stoves, in ovens, in microwave ovens, or on grills.
- Practice safety measures for candles.
  - Do not use candles in bedrooms or other sleeping areas.
  - Use sturdy candle holders that will not tip over.
  - Place candle holders on sturdy, clutter-free surfaces.
  - Light candles carefully. Keep your hair and loose clothing away from the flame.
  - Do not burn a candle all the way down. Blow it out before it gets close to the holder.
  - Do not use candles where oxygen is used.
  - Keep candles at least 12 inches away from anything that can burn. This includes window coverings.
  - Blow out candles when you leave the room or go to bed.
  - Do not use candles during power outages. Use flashlights and battery-operated lighting.
  - Keep candles away from flammable liquids and materials.
- Store flammable liquids outside in their original containers. Keep containers where children and confused or disoriented persons cannot reach them.
- Keep materials that will burn away from heat sources. Stacked newspapers, magazines, books, and paint rags are examples. Heat sources include space heaters, fireplaces, radiators, registers, candles, incense, and oil lamps.
- Use clothes dryers safely.
  - Clean the lint filter before and after each use.
  - Use the correct plug and outlet.
  - Turn the dryer off when you leave the home.
  - Do not run dryers when people are sleeping.
- Follow the safety measures in this box when using incense.

FOCUS ON LONG-TERM CARE AND HOME CARE

Fire Safety

Home Care

According to the National Fire Protection Association (NFPA):

- Cooking fires are the leading cause of home fires. Unattended cooking is the main cause of kitchen fires. Most kitchen fires involve the stove.
- Smoking materials are the leading cause of fire deaths. The victim who dies in a fire may not be the one whose cigarette started the fire. The risk of dying in a home fire caused by smoking materials increases with age.
- Many fire deaths happen in homes with no smoke alarms or alarms that do not work.
- Most home heating fire deaths involve space heaters. Fires often occur when heating equipment is too close to items that can burn (furniture fabrics, clothing, mattresses, bedding).
- Home candle fires occur most often in December. Many candle fires start in bedrooms. Most start when candles are too close to items that can burn.
- Many fires result because children can reach matches and lighters. All children are at risk from the unsafe use of fire.

Fire and the Use of Oxygen

Home care patients may need oxygen therapy. Remind the patient, family, and visitors about safety measures. See Chapter 44.

Smoke Alarms

Smoke alarms save lives, prevent injuries, and lessen property damage. Always locate them in a patient's home. They should be outside every sleeping area, in every bedroom, and on every floor. Make sure they are working. Tell the nurse, patient, and family if a smoke alarm does not work.

Special smoke alarms are available for persons who are deaf or hard of hearing. The following examples activate when a special smoke alarm sounds.

- Strobe lights that flash
- A pillow or bed shaker
- An alert device that has a loud, mixed, low-pitched sound

Preventing Fires

Practice safety measures to prevent burns (p. 179) and for the safe use of fuel-burning devices (p. 185) and electrical equipment (p. 191).

Space heaters present fire hazards. Electric and fuel-burning heaters are common. Practice these safety measures.

- Follow the manufacturer's instructions. Use the correct fuel.
- Light a gas space heater correctly. Strike the match first. Then turn on the gas.
- Do not use extension cords with space heaters.
- Keep heaters at least 3 feet away from any person and from window coverings, furniture, and anything that will burn.
- Place heaters on a solid, flat surface. Do not place heaters on stairs, in doorways, or where people walk.
- Make sure the heater can automatically shut off if it tips over.
- Protect yourself and others from burns. Heaters are hot. Do not touch them. Keep them away from children and persons who cannot protect themselves.

Preventing Fires—cont'd

- Prevent electrocution (being injured or killed by electrical shock). Keep electric heaters away from water. (Water conducts electricity.) Make sure the cord is in good repair.
- Do not leave heaters unattended. Turn off and unplug heaters before leaving the room or going to sleep.
- Store fuel in the original container. Keep the fuel container outside.
- Refill the fuel container outside.
- Do not add fuel while the heater is running or hot. Do not over-fill the heater.

Hoarding

Hoarding is a disorder in which a person has difficulty discarding or getting rid of things. The person has a great need to save the items that might have little or no value. The home or living space becomes filled with stacks or piles of clutter. Often there are only narrow pathways from 1 room to another. Doors may be blocked.

The NFPA explains why hoarding increases danger for the person, others in the home, and firefighters.

- Items that can burn are close to the stove or oven.
- A heat source may be too close to things that can burn.
- Heat sources may be on unstable surfaces.
- Electrical wiring may be old or worn from heavy piles. Pests and rodents can chew on wires.
- Flames from smoking materials or candles may be close to clutter.
- Narrow and blocked pathways and doors may prevent escaping from a fire.
- Firefighters have difficulty moving through a home with clutter.
- Blocked windows and doors may trap firefighters.
- Falling objects can injure firefighters.
- The building can collapse on firefighters. Water to fight the fire increases the weight of the clutter.
- Clutter can block the way for firefighters to search for people and pets.

Fire Exits and Escape Plans

Know 2 exits from each room and 2 exits from the building. Do not use elevators. Keep exits clear. Keep furniture and heavy items away from doors and windows. Doors and windows should open easily.

Have an escape plan. Discuss the plan with everyone in the home. Map out the exits from each room. Designate an outside meeting place. Practice the escape plan twice a year. Practice the different ways to exit. Close doors as you exit. A closed door may slow the spread of smoke, heat, and fire.

In an apartment building, know how to alert others. Manual fire alarms are usually near exits. Pull the bar or handle. Call 911 or the fire department when out of the building. Do not go back into the building.

A quick exit is important. Once a smoke alarm sounds, you may have only a few minutes to get out safely.

Fire Extinguishers

Locate fire extinguishers in the patient's home. Read the manufacturer's instructions. Make sure the device works. Tell the nurse, patient, and family if a fire extinguisher does not work. See p. 198 for how to use a fire extinguisher.

Fire and Oxygen. Three things are needed for a fire—a spark or flame, a material that will burn, and oxygen. Air has some oxygen. However, some people need extra oxygen (Chapter 44). Safety measures are needed where oxygen is used and stored.

- *NO SMOKING* signs are on the door and near the bed.
- No one can smoke in the room.
- Smoking materials (cigarettes, electronic cigarettes, cigars, and pipes), matches, and lighters are removed from the room.
- Safety measures to prevent equipment accidents are followed (see Box 14-7).
- Wool blankets and synthetic fabrics that cause static electricity are removed from the room.
- The person wears a cotton gown or pajamas.
- Lit candles, incense, and other open flames are not allowed.
- Materials that ignite easily are removed from the room—oil, grease, nail polish remover, and so on.

Know and follow agency policies on smoking. Know which areas are designated as smoking areas (where smoking is allowed). Follow the agency's safety practices for patients or residents who smoke.

See *Focus on Communication: Fire and Oxygen.*

What to Do During a Fire. You must know your agency's fire emergency and evacuation procedures. (*Evacuation* is the removal of people from a dangerous area.) Know your role. Know where to find fire alarms, fire extinguishers, and emergency exits. Fire drills are held to practice emergency fire procedures.

The word *RACE* is used as a reminder of what to do (Fig. 14-20).

- *R*—for *rescue.* Rescue persons in immediate danger. Move them to a safe place.
- *A*—for *alarm.* Sound the nearest fire alarm. Call 911 or activate the agency's fire response system.
- *C*—for *confine.* Close doors and windows to confine (contain) the fire.
- *E*—for *extinguish* or *evacuate.* If the fire is small and confined to a small area (such as a wastebasket), a fire extinguisher may be used. Spreading, uncontained fires require evacuation (p. 199). (See "Using a Fire Extinguisher" on p. 198.)

Procedures for turning off oxygen, other gases, and electrical equipment are part of the agency's emergency plan. *Do not use elevators if there is a fire.* All normal and emergency exits need to be clear (not blocked by equipment or other items).

See *Promoting Safety and Comfort: What to Do During a Fire,* p. 198.

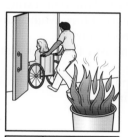

Rescue

Rescue persons in immediate danger.

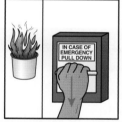

Alarm

Sound the fire alarm.

Call 911 or activate the agency's fire response system.

IN CASE OF EMERGENCY PULL DOWN

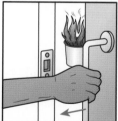

Confine

Close doors to contain the fire.

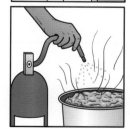

Extinguish or Evacuate

Use a fire extinguisher only on a small, contained fire.

Evacuate immediately if the fire is not small, is spreading, or cannot be extinguished.

FIGURE 14-20 During a fire, remember *RACE: Rescue, Alarm, Confine, Extinguish. Evacuate* if the fire is spreading or cannot be extinguished.

PROMOTING SAFETY AND COMFORT

What to Do During a Fire

Safety

Touch doors before opening them. Do not open a hot door. Use another exit from the room or building. If your clothing is on fire, do not run. Drop to the floor or ground. Cover your face. Roll to smother flames. If another person's clothing is on fire, get the person to the floor or ground. Roll the person or cover the person with a blanket, bedspread, or coat to smother the flames.

For smoke, cover your nose and mouth with a damp cloth. Do the same for patients, residents, visitors, and other staff. Have everyone crawl to the nearest exit.

Do the following if you cannot exit the building because of flames or smoke.

- Call 911 or the fire department. Tell the operator (dispatcher) where you are. Give exact information: agency name and address or the home care patient's name, address, phone number, and where you are in the building or home.
- Cover your nose and mouth with a damp cloth. Do the same for patients, residents, visitors, and other staff.
- Move away from the fire. Go to a room with a window. Close the room door. Stuff wet towels, blankets, sheets, or bedspreads at the bottom of the door.
- Open the window.
- Hang something from the window (towel, sheet, blanket, clothing). This helps firefighters find you.

Using a Fire Extinguisher. Different extinguishers are designed for different kinds of fires. Multi-purpose extinguishers can be used for fires involving:

- Ordinary materials that burn easily like paper, cloth, and wood (Type A fires)
- Flammable liquids like oil and grease (Type B fires)
- Electrical sources (Type C fires)

Only use a fire extinguisher on a *small, contained* fire. Immediate evacuation is needed if:

- There is any doubt about the ability to extinguish the fire.
- The fire is spreading.
- The extinguisher is empty and the fire is not out.
A general procedure for using a fire extinguisher follows.
See procedure: *Using a Fire Extinguisher.*

Using a Fire Extinguisher

PROCEDURE

1. Pull the fire alarm.
2. Get the nearest fire extinguisher.
3. Take it to the fire. Carry it upright.
4. Position yourself so you can exit safely. Do not allow the fire, smoke, or heat to block your exit path.
5. Follow the word *PASS* (Fig. 14-21).
   a. *P*—for *pull the safety pin* (see Fig. 14-21, *A*). This unlocks the handle.
   b. *A*—for *aim low* (see Fig. 14-21, *B*). Direct the hose (nozzle) at the base of the fire. Do not try to spray the tops of the flames.
   c. *S*—for *squeeze the lever* (see Fig. 14-21, *C*). Squeeze or push down on the lever, handle, or button to start the stream. Release the lever, handle, or button to stop the stream.
   d. *S*—for *sweep back and forth* (see Fig. 14-21, *D*). Sweep the stream back and forth (side to side) at the base of the fire.
6. Evacuate immediately if the fire is spreading or cannot be extinguished.

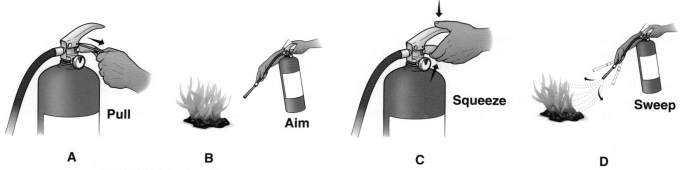

FIGURE 14-21 Using a fire extinguisher. **A,** *Pull* the safety pin. **B,** *Aim* the hose at the base of the fire. **C,** *Squeeze* the top handle down. **D,** *Sweep* back and forth.

Evacuating. Agencies have evacuation procedures. Patients or residents closest to the fire go out first. A staff member takes them to a safe place. Those who are able to walk do so. Wheelchairs and stretchers (Chapter 21) are used for persons unable to walk. Other devices used for transfers (Chapter 21) are used as needed. Life-saving carrying techniques may be required. See Figures 14-22 and 14-23. Once firefighters arrive, they direct rescue efforts.

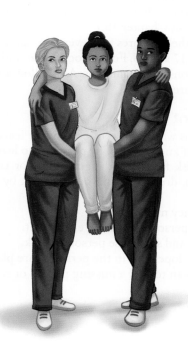

FIGURE 14-22 Two-rescuer swing-carry. Two rescuers lock arms at the person's back and below the person's knees. (The rescuers create a "swing" with their arms.) The person's arms are over the rescuers' shoulders.

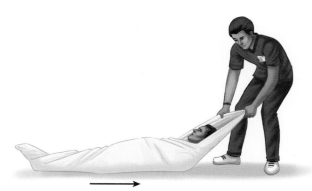

FIGURE 14-23 One-rescuer carry using a blanket. A large blanket is placed on the floor next to the lowered bed. The person is lowered to the blanket. The blanket is wrapped around the person. The person is pulled to a safe area.

Pandemics

An *epidemic* occurs when a disease spreads within a large number of people in a community or region at the same time. A *pandemic* occurs when the disease spreads over several countries or continents. The CMS includes infectious disease threats among the hazards to be considered when preparing for disasters and emergencies.

The Centers for Disease Control and Prevention (CDC), CMS, and OSHA have plans and guidance for managing pandemics. Proper hand hygiene and infection control practices (Chapters 17 and 18) and social distancing help reduce the spread of infection. Measures for *social distancing (physical distancing)* limit person-to-person contact and maintain a distance of at least 6 feet from others. Screening measures for persons within and entering the agency and personal protective equipment (PPE) requirements are other safety practices. (See "Personal Protective Equipment" in Chapter 18.)

Practice the measures to prevent the spread of infection in Chapters 17 and 18. Follow local, state, and federal guidance in response to a pandemic. Also follow agency policies and procedures.

Elopement

Elopement is when a patient or resident leaves the agency without staff knowledge. The person who leaves a safe setting is at risk for many dangers. Heat or cold exposure, dehydration, drowning, and being struck by a vehicle are examples.

The agency must:
- Identify persons at risk for elopement.
- Monitor and supervise persons at risk.
- Address elopement in the person's care plan.
- Have a plan to find a missing patient or resident.

WORKPLACE VIOLENCE

Workplace violence is violent acts (including assault or threat of assault) directed toward persons at work or while on duty. It includes:
- Murders
- Beatings, stabbings, and shootings
- Rapes and sexual assaults
- Use of weapons—firearms, bombs, knives, and so on
- Kidnapping
- Robbery
- Threats—obscene phone calls; threatening oral, written, or body language
- Harassment of any kind (Chapter 6)—including being followed, sworn at, or shouted at

Staff in health care settings are at risk for workplace violence. The nursing staff has regular contact with patients, residents, and visitors. See Box 14-10 for risk factors in the health care setting.

OSHA has guidelines for preventing workplace violence. Work-site hazards are identified. Prevention measures are followed. Also, staff receive safety and health training. Box 14-10 has some safety measures to prevent or control workplace violence. See Appendix E on p. 916 for personal safety practices. You need to:
- Follow your agency's workplace violence prevention program.
- Follow safety and security measures.
- Voice safety and security concerns.
- Report suspicious persons right away.
- Report violent incidents promptly and accurately. Complete an incident report (p. 204).
- Serve on committees that review workplace violence.
- Attend training programs to recognize and manage agitation, assaultive behavior, and criminal intent.

Restraints may be ordered if patients or residents are a threat to themselves or others (Chapter 16). Restraints are a last resort for protection. Security officers deal with agitated, aggressive, and disruptive persons.

See *Focus on Long-Term Care and Home Care: Workplace Violence*, p. 202.

| BOX 14-10 | Workplace Violence: Risk Factors and Safety Measures |

Risk Factors
- Being with persons (or family members) who have a history of violence, have substance use disorders (Chapter 53), or are gang members
- Transporting patients and residents
- Working alone
- Working in a setting where a staff member cannot see the escape route or be able to escape from danger
- Poorly lit hallways, rooms, parking lots, and other areas
- Lacking a way to communicate an emergency situation
- People having access to firearms, knives, and other weapons
- Working in areas with high crime rates
- Lacking policies and training to recognize and manage hostile and assaultive behaviors from patients, residents, visitors, and staff
- Low staff levels during meal times and visiting hours
- High staff turn-over rates
- Not enough security and mental health staff
- Long waits for patients or residents
- Over-crowded and uncomfortable waiting rooms
- Visitors being able to go anywhere in the agency
- A sense that violence is tolerated and that victims cannot contact the police or press charges

Safety Measures
Agitated or Aggressive Persons
- Stand away from the person. Judge the length of the person's arms and legs. Stand far enough away that the person cannot hit or kick you.
- Be able to exit the room. Do not become trapped in the room.
- Identify items in the room that can be used as weapons. Move away from such objects. Vases, phones, radios, letter openers, paper weights, and belts are examples.
- Know where to find and how to use panic buttons, call lights, alarms, closed-circuit monitors, and other security devices.
- Keep your hands free.
- Stay calm. Talk to the person in a calm manner. Do not raise your voice or argue, scold, or interrupt the person.
- Be aware of your body language. Do not point a finger or glare at the person. Do not put your hands on your hips.
- Do not touch the person.
- Say that you will get the nurse to speak to the person.
- Leave the room as soon as you can. Make sure the person is safe.
- Tell the nurse and security officer about the matter at once. Report items in the room that can be used as weapons.

Security Devices
- Alarm systems, paging systems, closed-circuit video monitors (inside and outside), panic buttons, hand-held alarms, phones, 2-way radios, and phone systems are installed (Fig. 14-24, p. 202). These systems have a direct line to security staff or the police.
- Staff wear personal alarm devices.
- Metal detectors are at entrances to identify guns, knives, or other weapons.
- Curved mirrors are in hallways and hard-to-see areas.
- Bullet-resistant, shatter-proof glass is at nurses' stations.

Security Devices—cont'd
- Doors have glass panels.
- Door alarms remain on.
- Staff do not share security codes with anyone.

Weapons
- Jewelry and scarves are not worn. They can be used as weapons. For example, a person can grab earrings and bracelets. Or a person can strangle someone with a necklace or scarf.
- Long hair is worn up and off the collar (Chapter 6). A person can pull long hair and cause head injuries.
- Keys, scissors, pens, or other items that could be used as weapons are not within the person's reach.
- Pictures, vases, and other items that could be used as weapons are limited (few in number).
- Tools or items left by maintenance staff or visitors are removed if they could be used as weapons.

Family and Visitors
- Visitors sign in and receive a pass to access patient and resident areas.
- Visiting hours and policies are enforced.
- A list of "restricted visitors" is made for patients and residents with a history of violence or who are victims of violence.
- Waiting rooms and lounges are comfortable and reduce stress.
- Family and visitors are informed in a timely manner.

Building Safety and Security
- Un-used doors are locked.
- Bright lights are inside and outside buildings.
- Broken lights, windows, and door locks are replaced or repaired.
- Staff restrooms lock and prevent access to visitors.
- Access to the pharmacy and drug storage areas is controlled.
- Furniture is placed for a clear exit route. This includes furniture in patient and resident rooms and in therapy areas, dining rooms, and lounges.
- Furniture and other items are secured so they cannot be used as weapons.
- Keys are always attended and secure.

Staff Safety Measures
- Staff receive an update about a person's violent history or an incident.
- Staff work together when caring for persons with agitated or aggressive behaviors. Staff do not work alone.
- Staff wear ID badges that prove employment. IDs do not have last names or addresses.
- Staff use a "buddy system" when using elevators, stairways, restrooms, and low traffic areas.
- Uniforms fit well. Tight uniforms limit running. An attacker can grab loose uniforms.
- Shoes are slip-resistant and fit well. Shoes that cause slipping limit running.
- Staff do not wear expensive jewelry or carry large sums of money.
- Vehicles are locked and in good repair.
- Security escort services are used for walking to vehicles, bus stops, or train stations.
- Staff have a "safe room" for emergencies.

Risk factors modified from Occupational Safety and Health Administration: Guidelines for preventing workplace violence for healthcare and social service workers, U.S. Department of Labor, OSHA publication 3148.

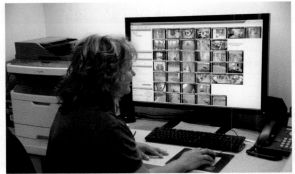

FIGURE 14-24 People entering and leaving the agency are monitored on a closed-circuit TV.

FOCUS ON LONG-TERM CARE AND HOME CARE

Workplace Violence

Home Care

More measures are needed for home safety.

- Follow log-in and log-out procedures. Contact the agency when you arrive at the home, when you are leaving, and when you arrive at your next destination (another patient's home, the agency, your own home, or other destination).
- Have tracking applications on your phone and car.
- Know how to use the agency's communication system and a personal panic button.
- Keep your phone with you and on.
- Know at least 2 exit routes out of the home.
- Make sure the device you carry for supplies and equipment has a working lock.
- Always keep doors locked.
- Do not let strangers into the home or building.
- Do not give information over the phone (Chapter 8).
- Do not let any stranger know that you are with a child or an older, ill, or disabled person.

Child abuse, elder abuse, intimate partner violence, and workplace violence can occur in home settings. If you feel uncomfortable or threatened, tell the nurse. Give as much information as you can. Failing to report the matter does not help you or the patient. Follow agency policy for what to do if you are threatened or feel threatened. You may need to leave the home, ask for back-up help from the agency, or call the police.

The following can threaten your safety. Report these and other threats to the nurse.

- Sexual abuse or harassment by the patient or any person in the home.
- Hitting, kicking, slapping, spitting, biting, scratching, pinching, pushing, or other attacks by the patient or anyone in the home.
- Attacks or threatened attacks with a weapon or an item that can be used as a weapon—knife, gun, bat, rope, tool (hammer, screwdriver, and so on), razor, scissors, self-defense spray, pot, pan, cane, chair, and so on.
- Denial of meal breaks, water, bathroom use, toilet paper, or hand-washing facilities.
- Denial of adequate sleeping conditions for a live-in situation.
- Poor heating or ventilation.
- Name calling, obscene language, or racial or cultural slurs.
- Exposure to unsafe conditions—blocked fire escapes, broken stairways, hoarding, pest infestations, and so on.

RISK MANAGEMENT

Risk management involves identifying and controlling risks and safety hazards affecting the agency. The intent is to:

- Protect all in the agency—patients, residents, visitors, and staff.
- Protect agency property from harm or danger.
- Protect the person's valuables.
- Prevent accidents and injuries.

Risk management deals with these and other safety issues.

- Accident and fire prevention
- Negligence, malpractice, and abuse (Chapter 5)
- Workplace violence
- Federal and state requirements

Risk managers look for patterns and trends in incidents (p. 204), complaints (patients, residents, staff, visitors), and accident and injury investigations. Unsafe situations are corrected. Policy, procedure, and training changes are made as needed.

Color-Coded Wristbands

Color-coded wristbands promote the person's safety and prevent harm. They quickly communicate an alert or warning (Fig. 14-25). The type of alert is printed on the band. The printing is useful in dim lighting and for persons who are color blind.

These colors are common.

- Red—for an "allergy alert." Red is a warning to "stop." A red wristband warns of allergies to food, drugs, treatment supplies such as tape or latex gloves, and so on. Allergies are not listed on the wristband.
- Yellow—for a "fall risk." Yellow implies "caution." Yellow wristbands are used for persons with a history of falls. Or they are used for persons at risk for falls because of dizziness, balance problems, confusion, and so on.
- Purple—for a "Do Not Resuscitate" (DNR) order. See Chapter 59.

Some agencies have colors for other alerts. For example, pink is for a "limb alert." This means that an arm or leg is not used for blood pressure measurements, blood draws, or intravenous infusions.

To safely use color-coded wristbands:

- Know the colors used in your agency. Colors may vary among agencies.
- Check the care plan and your assignment sheet when you see a color-coded wristband. You need to know the reason for the wristband and the care measures needed. Ask the nurse if you have questions.
- Do not confuse "social cause" bands with your agency's color-coded wristbands.
- Check for wristbands on persons transferred from another agency. That agency may use different colors. Or the meanings may differ from those in your agency. The nurse needs to remove wristbands from another agency.
- Tell the nurse if you think a person needs a color-coded wristband.

Personal Belongings

The person's belongings must be kept safe. Often valuables are sent home with the family. A personal belongings list is completed. Each item is listed and described. The staff member and the person sign the completed list.

A valuables envelope is used for jewelry and money. Each jewelry item is listed and described on the envelope. Describe what you see. For example, describe a ring as having a white stone with 4 prongs in a yellow setting. Do not assume the stone is a diamond in a gold setting. For valuables:

- Count money with the person.
- Put money and each jewelry item in the envelope. Have the person watch. Seal and sign the envelope like a personal belongings list.
- Give the envelope to the nurse. Have a witness. The nurse takes it to the safe or sends it home with the family.

Dentures, eyeglasses, hearing aids, watches, some jewelry, radios and music players, phones, and other electronic devices are kept at the bedside. Items kept at the bedside are listed in the person's record. Some people keep money for newspapers and personal items. The amount kept is noted in the person's record.

See *Focus on Long-Term Care and Home Care: Personal Belongings.*

FOCUS ON LONG-TERM CARE AND HOME CARE

Personal Belongings

Long-Term Care
Nursing center residents have the right to have and use personal possessions (Chapter 2). The center must take reasonable care to protect resident property from loss and theft. Labeling items helps to identify personal property. Clothing and shoes are labeled in a way that respects dignity. For example, labels are placed on the inside of clothing and shoes. Or a color-coded system is used. Follow center procedures to label personal items.

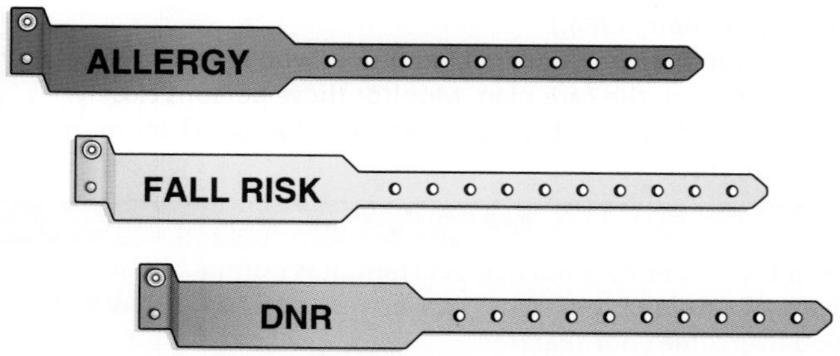

FIGURE 14-25 Color-coded wristbands. The alert is printed on the band.

Reporting Incidents

An *incident (adverse event)* is any event that has harmed or could harm a patient, resident, visitor, or staff member. The event is usually unexpected. Examples include:

- Accidents involving patients, residents, visitors, or staff.
- Errors in care—giving the wrong care, giving care to the wrong person, not giving care, giving poor quality of care, inadequate monitoring.
- Broken or lost items owned by the person. Dentures, hearing aids, and eyeglasses are examples.
- Lost money or clothing.
- Hazardous chemical incidents.
- Workplace violence incidents.
- Infections that should have been prevented (Chapter 17).

Incidents that *could have* caused harm are commonly called "near misses." Such incidents pose a risk for future harm and must be reported. For example, you test water temperature before a bath. The water is very hot. It could burn the person. You add cold water and check the temperature again before giving the bath. Report the problem to the nurse.

Report incidents at once. Complete an incident report as soon as possible. An *incident report* is documentation of the details about a harmful or potentially harmful event. The agency has a paper or electronic form to use.

Incident reports are reviewed by a risk management committee. They look for immediate problems and patterns and trends. Information gained signals areas for improvement. The committee plans how to correct problems and monitor results. There may be new policies and procedures to prevent future incidents.

FOCUS ON **PRIDE**

The Person, Family, and Yourself

Personal and Professional Responsibility

Always do your best to give safe care. When errors or accidents happen, be responsible. Tell the nurse. Complete an incident report. Incident reports are used to improve systems and promote safety. They are not intended to be punitive (for punishment). Take pride in doing the right thing by honest reporting.

Rights and Respect

If you value safety and respect others' well-being, you will perform safety measures. For example, you will:

- Identify the person before giving care.
- Check water temperature before bathing.
- Use and store harmful products safely.
- Observe for swallowing problems and signs of choking.
- Use equipment correctly.
- Know what to do during a fire or disaster.
- Report concerns and incidents.

Independence and Social Interaction

Children and older persons are at increased risk for injury. Children often try to show independence before they are able to judge safety. Older persons often want to maintain independence but may need help to do some tasks safely.

Listen to the person. Let the person do as much as is safely possible. Kindly communicate safety limits. Discuss doing the task with help if help is needed. Tell the nurse about safety concerns.

Delegation and Teamwork

Work as a team for the safety of all staff arriving at and leaving the agency.

- Wait for a person finishing work a few minutes late.
- Walk with others to and from the parking area.
- Do not leave the parking area until your co-workers are safely in their vehicles. Have them do the same for you.
- Offer to call security escort services for a co-worker going to a different location (for example, a bus stop).

Ethics and Laws

Some persons are at risk for choking. Persons with developmental and intellectual disabilities (Chapter 55), young children, and older persons are examples. The following case shows what can occur when safety measures are neglected.

A 32-year-old man had an intellectual disability and epilepsy (a seizure disorder). He was a patient at a developmental center since the age of 25. According to the facts reported in the court case, the following occurred.

- *He had a dinner of beef and noodles. The pieces of beef were about ½ inch wide and ¾ inch long.*
- *While eating, he stood up, coughed out his milk, reached for his throat, and collapsed.*
- *Efforts were made to revive him.*
- *He was transported to the hospital where he died a short while later.*
  The lawsuit claimed negligence because:
- *His swallowing was affected by the dosage of a drug.*
- *He was not given a soft diet.*
- *He was not properly supervised at meal time.*
  In the Court's opinion, negligent care resulted in the patient's death.
  (B. Szydelko v. The Department of Mental Health of the State of Illinois, 1984.)

You can help prevent choking. Know who is at risk. Ask the nurse or check the care plan. Monitor those persons closely. Check that they have the right diet. See Chapter 31 for more precautions.

FOCUS ON **PRIDE**: *Application*

As a student or new nursing assistant, it is normal to have fears of causing harm. What concerns do you have? How will you overcome your fears?

REVIEW QUESTIONS

Circle the BEST answer.

1 Safety measures are meant to prevent accidents and injuries while
  a Protecting rights
  b Limiting mobility
  c Limiting independence
  d Saving staff time

2 Which is *safe?*
  a Not wearing needed eyeglasses
  b Having hearing problems
  c Being disoriented
  d Being able to sense pain

3 An unconscious person
  a Has suffered an electrical shock
  b Has dementia
  c Is unaware of surroundings
  d Has stopped breathing

4 Dementia increases the risk for accidents and injuries because it affects
  a Vision and hearing
  b Thinking and reasoning
  c Pain sensation
  d Muscle function

5 Persons with
  a Quadriplegia cannot move to safety alone
  b Hemiparesis cannot read a warning label
  c Hemiplegia cannot smell smoke odors
  d Paraplegia cannot signal that they are choking

6 To identify a person, you
  a Call the person by his or her first name
  b Ask the person for his or her ID number
  c Compare information on the ID bracelet against your assignment sheet
  d Check that you entered the correct room number

7 To prevent burns
  a Keep smoking materials at the person's bedside
  b Pour hot liquids near a person
  c Turn on hot water first
  d Check water temperature before the person enters the shower

8 Which helps to prevent poisoning?
  a Keeping harmful products in low storage areas
  b Keeping harmful products in their original containers
  c Removing product labels
  d Storing harmful products near food

9 Who is most at risk for lead poisoning?
  a An adult who works in health care
  b A teenager who plays paintball
  c A toddler who lives in a house built in 1970
  d An older woman who knits as a hobby

10 A home has lead-based plumbing. You should
  a Boil water for cooking and drinking
  b Use hot tap water to make baby formula
  c Flush the pipes before using water for cooking
  d Avoid using water filters

11 A carbon monoxide alarm sounds. You should
  a Go to an interior room or basement
  b Go outside into fresh air and call 911
  c Turn off oxygen that is in use
  d Turn on a fan

12 Which can cause suffocation?
  a Checking for loose teeth or dentures
  b Using electrical items that are in good repair
  c Cutting food into small, bite-sized pieces
  d Restraints

13 If severe airway obstruction occurs, the person usually
  a Clutches at the throat
  b Can speak, cough, and breathe
  c Is calm
  d Has a seizure

14 These statements are about FBAO. Which is *true?*
  a A person is coughing forcefully. Give abdominal thrusts.
  b A person is pregnant. Give abdominal thrusts.
  c Injuries can occur from abdominal or chest thrusts.
  d Unconscious persons cannot choke.

15 How do you know that a new resident's electric shaver is safe to use?
  a You turn the device on.
  b The maintenance staff checks and approves the device.
  c You check the SDS.
  d You ask the resident if it is working properly.

16 You are using an electrical device. Which measure is *unsafe?*
  a Unplugging the item while it is turned on
  b Keeping the item away from water and spills
  c Holding on to the plug (not the cord) when unplugging it
  d Following the manufacturer's instructions

17 Which is *unsafe?*
  a A chair's weight capacity exceeds the person's weight.
  b A person's weight exceeds a wheelchair's weight capacity.
  c A person who cannot walk uses a wheelchair.
  d A person who cannot sit up is transported by stretcher.

18 You spilled a hazardous substance. Which action is *correct?*
  a Follow the instructions on the safety data sheet.
  b Let it air dry.
  c Wipe up the spill with paper towels.
  d Leave the spill for housekeeping.

19 You work in a nursing center. In a severe weather alert, you should
  a Go home
  b Follow the center's emergency plan
  c Make sure your family is safe
  d Pull the fire alarm

20 The fire alarm sounds. Which action is *correct?*
  a Do not respond if it is a drill.
  b Use elevators.
  c Open doors and windows.
  d Move residents to a safe place.

21 Your clothing is on fire. What should you do *first?*
  a Run to get help.
  b Drop to the floor and roll to smother the flames.
  c Use a fire extinguisher.
  d Call 911.

Continued

22 Which shows you know how to use a fire extinguisher *correctly*?
   a You try to use it on a large, spreading fire.
   b You leave the safety pin in place.
   c You aim the nozzle at the tops of the flames.
   d You sweep the stream back and forth at the base of the fire.

23 Social distancing is a safety measure used during
   a A pandemic
   b Workplace violence
   c Elopement
   d A fire

24 A person is agitated and aggressive. Which is *unsafe*?
   a Standing away from the person
   b Standing so the person does not block your exit
   c Using touch to show you care
   d Talking to the person without raising your voice

25 Risk managers
   a Look for patterns or trends in accidents and errors
   b Prevent legal problems when injuries occur
   c Are only responsible for staff safety
   d Are the same as surveyors

26 You see a resident with a color-coded wristband. You should
   a Remove it
   b Ask the person what it means
   c Check the person's care plan for more information
   d Apply wristbands to the other residents

27 A resident brought items from home. Which action *best* promotes use of and protection of personal property?
   a Sending the items home with family
   b Labeling the items with the person's name
   c Putting the items in a safe
   d Storing the items at the nurses' station

28 A resident fell in the bathroom. Which action is *correct*?
   a Report the fall at the end of the shift.
   b Report the fall only if the person was injured.
   c Do not report the fall if you did something wrong.
   d Call the nurse and complete an incident report.

Answers to Chapter 14 questions are on p. 902.

FOCUS ON PRACTICE

Problem Solving

A person begins to cough loudly during a meal. The person can speak a few words. You hear wheezing between breaths. What do you do? The person is suddenly unable to cough, speak, or breathe. What do you do?

Preventing Falls

- Define the key terms and key abbreviations in this chapter.
- Identify the causes and risk factors for falls.
- Describe the safety measures that prevent falls.
- Explain how to use position change alarms safely.
- Explain how to use bed rails safely.
- Explain the purpose of hand rails and grab bars.
- Explain how to use wheel locks (brakes) safely.
- Describe how to use transfer/gait belts.
- Explain how to help the person who is falling.
- Perform the procedures described in this chapter.
- Explain how to promote PRIDE in the person, the family, and yourself.

KEY TERMS

bed rail A device that serves as a guard or barrier along the side of the bed; side rail

gait belt See "transfer belt"

position change alarm Any physical or electronic device that monitors a person's movement and alerts staff of movement

transfer belt A device applied around the waist and used to support a person who is unsteady or disabled; gait belt

KEY ABBREVIATIONS

CDC	Centers for Disease Control and Prevention	ID	Identification
CMS	Centers for Medicare & Medicaid Services		

The risk of falling increases with age. Persons 65 years and older are at risk. A history of falls increases the risk of falling again. Falls are the most common accidents in nursing centers.

According to the Centers for Disease Control and Prevention (CDC):

- Each year, over a quarter (¼) of adults age 65 and older fall.
- Falls are the main cause of injuries and injury-related deaths in older adults.
- Falls can cause serious injuries.
  - Broken bones. Wrist, arm, ankle, and hip fractures are common. Hip fractures are very serious. Recovery can be hard. Many people are not able to live on their own afterward.
  - Head injuries. Head injuries are very serious, especially if the person takes anticoagulant drugs (drugs that slow blood clotting).
- A fall often causes a fear of falling again, even if the person was not injured. The person may limit daily activities to prevent falling. Less active, the person becomes weaker. This increases the risk of falling. See *Focus on Surveys: Preventing Falls.*

FOCUS ON SURVEYS

Preventing Falls

The Centers for Medicare & Medicaid Services (CMS) defines a *fall* as:

- Unintentionally coming to rest on the ground, floor, or other lower level. Force, such as being pushed, was not involved.
- When a person loses balance and would have fallen if staff did not act to prevent the fall.
- When a person is found on the floor unless matters suggest otherwise.
- When a person falls but is not injured. A fall without injury is still a fall.

The survey team will observe and interview staff about:

- Fall risk factors described in this chapter.
- The hazards described in this chapter and in Chapter 14.
- Safety measures to prevent falls.
- The safe use of bed rails, hand rails and grab bars, and wheel locks (brakes).
- The safe use of adaptive (assistive) devices. Canes, walkers, and transfer/gait belts (p. 214) are examples.
- Safe transfer and ambulation (walking) procedures. See Chapters 21 and 35.
- Answering call lights promptly.
- Following the person's care plan and meeting care needs.

CAUSES AND RISK FACTORS FOR FALLS

Most falls are caused by many risk factors. The more risk factors present, the greater the risk of falling. The accident risk factors described in Chapter 14 can lead to falls. The problems listed in Box 15-1 increase a person's risk of falling.

See *Focus on Long-Term Care and Home Care: Causes and Risk Factors for Falls*.

See *Teamwork and Time Management: Causes and Risk Factors for Falls*.

BOX 15-1	Fall Risk Factors

Care Setting
- Bed height: too low or too high
- Care equipment: IV (intravenous) poles, drainage tubes and bags, and others
- Floors: cluttered, wet, slippery, or uneven
- Furniture out of place
- Lighting: poor or glares
- No hand rails or grab bars
- Restraint use
- Setting: new, strange, and unfamiliar
- Throw rugs or other tripping hazards
- Wet and slippery bathtubs and showers
- Wheelchairs, walkers, canes, and crutches: improper use or fit

The Person
- Age: 65 years and older
- Alcohol: over-use
- Balance problems
- Blood pressure: low or high
- Confusion; disorientation
- Depression
- Dizziness or light-headedness; dizziness on standing
- Drug side effects
  - Confusion and disorientation
  - Coordination: poor
  - Diarrhea
  - Dizziness
  - Drowsiness
  - Fainting
  - Low blood pressure when standing or sitting
  - Unsteadiness
  - Urination: frequent
- Elimination: incontinence (urinary or fecal), frequency, urgency, urinating at night (*nocturia*)
- Falls: history of; fear of falling
- Foot problems; foot pain
- Gait: unsteady
- Joint pain and stiffness
- Judgment: poor
- Memory problems
- Mobility: impaired
- Reaction time: slow
- Shoes that fit poorly; no shoes or shoes without slip-resistant surfaces
- Sleep problems
- Vision problems
- Weakness; leg weakness

FOCUS ON LONG-TERM CARE AND HOME CARE

Causes and Risk Factors for Falls

Long-Term Care
Nursing center residents are at increased risk for falls. Weakness and walking problems are common causes. Care setting hazards are other causes—poor lighting, wet floors, incorrect bed height. Other risk factors are transfer problems (Chapter 21), shoes that fit poorly, and improper use or fit of wheelchairs, walkers, canes, and other devices. See Box 15-1.

Home Care
In the home, many factors increase fall risk. Hazards include:
- Cluttered rooms, stairways, and hallways
- Objects on the floor and stairways—wires, cords, shoes, books, magazines, blankets, and so on
- Throw rugs
- Pets
- Flooring problems—loose tiles and floor boards, raised linoleum, frayed carpet
- Wet floors and slippery bathtub or shower floors
- Ice or snow on driveways, steps, and sidewalks
- Loose or missing hand rails and grab bars (p. 213)
- Poor lighting
- No footwear or unsafe footwear—slippers, shoes without slip-resistant surfaces, shoes that do not fit well, and shoes with long shoelaces
- Adaptive (assistive) devices that need repair—walkers, canes, wheelchairs
- Having to climb or reach for objects

TEAMWORK AND TIME MANAGEMENT

Causes and Risk Factors for Falls

The health team must protect the person. If you see something unsafe, tell the nurse at once. Do not assume the nurse knows or that the matter is being corrected.

Answer call lights promptly. This includes the call lights of patients and residents assigned to co-workers.

During shift changes, staff are busy going off and coming on duty. Confusion can occur about who gives care and answers call lights. Falls can result. Know your role during shift changes. Nursing staff must work together to prevent falls.

FALL PREVENTION PROGRAMS

Agencies have fall prevention programs. Nurses assess fall risk and identify interventions to minimize the risk of falls and injuries. The nursing staff implements the planned interventions.

Meeting the person's basic needs is an essential part of fall prevention. Make sure that:

- Food and fluid needs are met.
- Needed items are within reach.
- Help is given with elimination needs. Assist the person to the bathroom or with the bedpan, urinal, or commode.
- The bedpan, urinal, or commode is kept within reach if the person can use the device without help.
- A warm drink, soft lights, or a back massage is used to calm the person who is agitated.
- The person is properly positioned in bed or in a chair or wheelchair. Use pillows or other positioning devices as the nurse and care plan direct (Chapters 19 and 35).
- Correct procedures and equipment are used for transfers and ambulation (walking). See Chapters 21 and 35. Follow the care plan. Explain tasks before and while performing them.
- The person is involved in meaningful activities.
- Exercise programs are followed. They help improve balance, strength, walking, and physical function.
- The person's setting is safe. Complete a safety check before leaving the room. (See the inside of the back cover.)

The measures listed in Box 15-2 (p. 210) may be part of the agency's program and the person's care plan. The care plan also lists measures for the person's specific risk factors. Many measures also apply to home settings.

Common sense and simple safety measures can prevent many falls. The health team works with the person and family to reduce fall risk factors. The goal is to prevent falls without decreasing quality of life.

See *Focus on Communication: Fall Prevention Programs*.

See *Focus on Long-Term Care and Home Care: Fall Prevention Programs*.

See *Promoting Safety and Comfort: Fall Prevention Programs*.

FOCUS ON COMMUNICATION

Fall Prevention Programs

A person can fall when reaching for needed items. The person reaches too far and falls. Or the person tries to get up without help. To prevent falls, ask the person:

- "What things would you like near you?"
- "Can I move this closer to you?"
- "Can you reach the call light?"
- "Can you reach your cane?" (Walker and wheelchair are other examples.)
- "Do you need to use the bathroom?"
- "Do you need anything else before I leave the room?"

FOCUS ON LONG-TERM CARE AND HOME CARE

Fall Prevention Programs

Home Care

People of all ages fall in home settings. Older persons are at risk. Simple changes can prevent falls (Chapter 12). So can some of the measures in Box 15-2.
For example:

- Place furniture to allow clear walking paths.
- Remove throw and area rugs.
- Keep objects off of the floor and stairs.
- Use night-lights in bedrooms, hallways, and bathrooms.
- Place a lamp by the bed if bedroom lights are hard to reach.
- Keep often-used items within easy reach. In kitchens, move items to lower shelves.
- Place slip-resistant bath mats or self-stick strips in showers and tubs.
- Install hand rails on both sides of stairs.

PROMOTING SAFETY AND COMFORT

Fall Prevention Programs

Safety

Some people have vision and hearing problems. Be sure eyeglasses and hearing aids are worn as needed. Reading glasses are not worn when up and about. Besides the measures in Box 15-2, other safety measures may be needed to prevent falls. See Chapter 47.

BOX 15-2	Measures to Prevent Falls and Injuries

Bathrooms and Shower/Tub Rooms
- Showers and tubs have slip-resistant surfaces or slip-resistant bath mats.
- The person uses grab bars (safety bars) in bathrooms and showers (p. 213).
- Shower chairs are used (Chapter 24).
- Safety measures for tub baths and showers are followed (Chapter 24).

Floors, Stairs, and Hallways
- Carpeting (if used) is wall-to-wall or tacked down.
- Scatter, area, and throw rugs are not used.
- Flooring is 1 color. Bold designs can cause dizziness in older persons.
- Floors have non-glare, slip-resistant surfaces.
- Non-skid wax is used on hardwood, tiled, or linoleum floors.
- Slip-resistant strips are on the floor next to the bed and in the bathroom. They are intact.
- Loose floor boards and tiles are reported. So are frayed rugs and carpets.
- Floors and stairs are free of clutter, cords, and other items that can cause tripping.
- Floors are free of spills. Wipe up spills at once. Put a *WET FLOOR* sign by the wet area.
- Floors are free of excess furniture and equipment.
- Electrical and extension cords are out of the way. This includes power strips.
- Equipment and supplies are kept on 1 side of the hallway.
- Barriers are used to prevent wandering (Fig. 15-1).
- Hand rails (p. 213) are on both sides of stairs and hallways.
- The person uses hand rails when walking or using stairs.

Furniture
- Furniture is placed for easy movement.
- Furniture is kept in place. It is not re-arranged.
- Chairs have armrests. Armrests give support when standing or sitting.
- A phone, lamp, and personal belongings are within reach.

Beds and Other Equipment
- The bed is at the correct height for the person. Follow the care plan. The bed is raised for bedside care. Then it is lowered to a safe and comfortable level for the person. The distance from the bed to the floor is reduced if the person falls or gets out of bed.
- Bed rails (p. 212) are used according to the care plan.
- A mattress, special mat, or floor cushion is on the floor by the bed (Fig. 15-2). This reduces the chance of injury if the person falls or gets out of bed.
- Wheelchairs, walkers, canes, and crutches fit properly. They are in good repair. Another person's equipment is not used.
- Crutches, canes, and walkers have slip-resistant tips.
- Wheelchair and stretcher safety is followed (Chapter 21).
- Wheel locks (brakes) on beds (p. 214), wheelchairs, stretchers, commodes, and shower chairs are in working order. Wheels are locked (braked) for transfers.
- Linens are checked for sharp objects and for the person's property (dentures, eyeglasses, hearing aids, and so on).

Lighting
- Rooms, hallways, and stairways have good lighting. So do bathrooms and shower/tub rooms.
- Light switches are within reach and easy to find.
- Light switches are at the top and bottom of stairways.
- Night-lights are in bedrooms, hallways, and bathrooms.

Shoes and Clothing
- Slip-resistant footwear is worn. Regular socks (without other footwear), bedroom slippers, and long shoelaces are avoided.
- Shoes fit well. They do not slip up and down on the feet. All shoelaces and straps are fastened.
- Clothing fits properly. Clothing is not loose or dragging on the floor.
- Belts are fastened.
- Padded hip protectors are worn to prevent injury (Fig. 15-3).

Call Lights and Alarms
- The person is taught how to use the call light (Chapter 13).
- The call light is always within the person's reach. This includes when sitting in the chair or on the commode and when in the bathroom and shower/tub room.
- The person is asked to use the call light when help is needed.
  - To get out of bed or a chair or return to bed
  - To walk
  - To get to or from the bathroom
  - To get on or off the toilet, bedpan, or commode
  - To stand to use the urinal
- Call lights are answered promptly. The person may not wait for help.
- Bed, chair, door, floor mat, and belt alarms are used as directed in the care plan. Such devices do not stop the person from falling. They sense when the person tries to get up, get out of bed, or open a door. See "Position Change Alarms."
- Alarms are responded to at once.

Observation
- The person is checked often. This may be every 15 minutes or as required by the care plan. Careful and frequent observation is important.
- Frequent checks are made on persons with poor judgment or memory. This may be every 15 minutes or as required by the care plan.
- Persons at risk for falls are close to the nurses' station.
- Family and friends are asked to visit during busy times. Meal times and shift changes are examples. They are also asked to visit during the evening and night shifts.
- Sitters, companions, or volunteers are provided to stay with the person.

Other
- Color-coded alerts warn of a fall risk. Yellow is common for a fall alert. Besides wristbands (Chapter 14), some agencies also use color-coded blankets, slip-resistant socks, and magnets or stickers on room doors.
- Caution is used when turning corners, entering corridor intersections, and going through doors. You could injure a person coming from the other direction.
- Pull (do not push) wheelchairs, stretchers, carts, and other wheeled equipment through doorways. You lead the way and can see where you are going.
- A safety check is made of the room after visitors leave. (See the inside of the back cover.) They may have lowered a bed rail, moved a call light, or moved a walker out of reach. Or they may have brought an item that could harm the person.

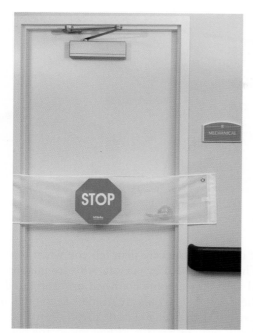

FIGURE 15-1 Barriers are used to prevent wandering.

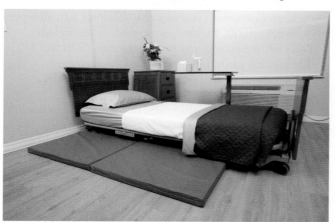

FIGURE 15-2 Floor cushion.

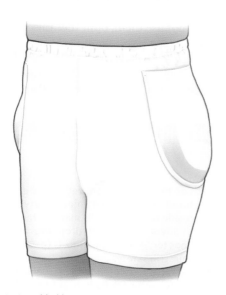

FIGURE 15-3 A padded hip protector. Worn under clothing, the garment helps prevent hip injuries from a fall.

Position Change Alarms

The CMS describes a *position change alarm* as any physical or electronic device that monitors a person's movement and alerts staff of movement. Position change alarms do not include door and elevator alarms that monitor wandering. Types include:

- Chair and bed sensor pads (Fig. 15-4)
- Bedside alarm mats
- Alarms clipped to clothing
- Seat-belt alarms
- Wireless motion sensors

To alert staff, the device makes a sound—alarm, beep, chime, music, and so on. Some play a recorded message. For example: "Please do not get up. Sit down and use your call light for help."

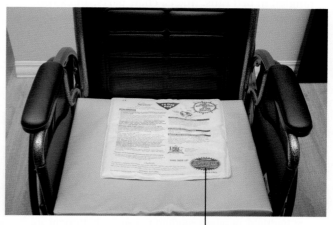

Alarm   Sensor pad

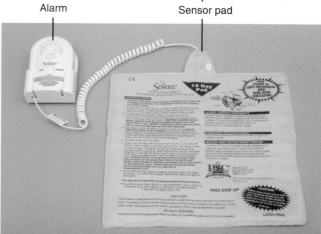

FIGURE 15-4 A position change alarm. This device has a sensor pad connected to an alarm. The alarm sounds when the person moves off of the pad. (NOTE: *Position change alarms do not replace close observation. Careful and frequent observation is needed.*)

Using Position Change Alarms. To use position change alarms safely:

- Follow the manufacturer's instructions.
- Mount the alarm securely out of the person's reach.
- Place the alarm at least 2 feet away from the person's ear. Alarms are loud.
- Test the alarm before leaving the person. If the device does not work, stay with the person. Call for the nurse.
- Respond to alarms at once.
  For an alarm with a cord that attaches (clips) to clothing:
- Attach the clip securely out of the person's reach. The clip is at the back near the shoulder. Check that clothing is not frayed or torn.
- Check the cord. The cord should allow movement for comfort but be short enough to sound if the person moves from the safe area. The cord must not be tangled in bed rails, linens, chair parts, and so on.

Alarms do not replace close observation. Persons at risk for falls are checked often. Careful and frequent observation is important.

See *Promoting Safety and Comfort: Using Position Change Alarms.*

PROMOTING SAFETY AND COMFORT

Using Position Change Alarms

Safety

If position change alarms are used:

- Patterns and routines are monitored. For example, do alarms sound at certain times? Before or after meals, at bedtime, or when needing to use the bathroom are examples.
- Enough supervision is provided for the person's needs.
- Staff must respond to an alarm at once. False alarms are common. As a result, staff do not always respond or do not respond promptly. This increases the risk for falls.

Comfort

Alarms that limit freedom of movement may be considered a restraint (Chapter 16). For example, a person avoids moving because the alarm disrupts staff and other patients or residents. Alarms can cause:

- Embarrassment
- Loss of dignity
- Decreased mobility
- Incontinence
- Sleep problems from the sound of the alarm or fear of moving in bed
- Confusion, fear, agitation, anxiety, or irritation when the alarm sounds

---

Bed Rails

A *bed rail* *(side rail)* is a device that serves as a guard or barrier along the side of the bed. Bed rails are on both sides of the bed. They are raised and lowered (Fig. 15-5). They lock in place with levers, latches, or buttons. Bed rails are quarter (¼), half (½), three quarters (¾), or the full length of the bed. When half-length rails are used, each side has 1 or 2 rails (see Fig. 15-5).

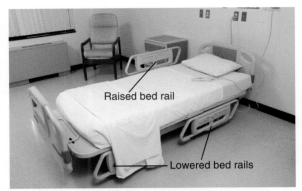

FIGURE 15-5 Bed rails. A far bed rail is raised. The near bed rails are lowered.

The nurse and the care plan tell you when to raise bed rails. They are needed by persons who are unconscious or sedated with drugs. Some confused or disoriented people need them. When bed rails are needed, keep them up at all times except when giving bedside care.

Bed rails present hazards. When raised, the person cannot get out of bed. The person can fall if trying to climb over them. *Entrapment* is also a risk (Chapter 13). The person can get caught, trapped, entangled, or strangled.

Bed rails are considered to be restraints (Chapter 16) if:

- The person cannot get out of bed.
- They cannot or will not be lowered to allow the person to leave the bed.

Bed rails cannot be used unless needed to treat a medical symptom. They must be in the person's best interest. Some people feel safer with bed rails up. Others use them for position changes in bed. The person or legal representative must give written consent for raised bed rails. The need for bed rails is carefully noted in the person's medical record and care plan.

The procedures in this book include bed rails. This helps you learn to use them correctly. The nurse, the care plan, and your assignment sheet tell you who uses bed rails. If a person does not use them, omit the "raise bed rails" and "lower bed rails" steps.

See *Focus on Children and Older Persons: Bed Rails.*
See *Focus on Long-Term Care and Home Care: Bed Rails.*
See *Promoting Safety and Comfort: Bed Rails.*

FOCUS ON CHILDREN AND OLDER PERSONS

Bed Rails

Children

Drop-side cribs do not meet current federal safety standards. Cribs manufactured since June 2011 meet safety standards that ban a drop-side rail. Older cribs may not meet current safety standards. Medical cribs with drop sides are allowed in hospitals. See Chapter 56 and Appendix D (p. 909) for more information about crib safety.

For toddlers and older children, rails placed on beds may cause entrapment (Chapter 13). Rails must fit the child's bed and be installed according to the manufacturer's instructions.

Bed Rails

Long-Term Care

Not all nursing center residents use bed rails. The person's personal choice and condition determine their use. You need to know who does and does not use bed rails. Consult the nurse and the person's care plan.

Home Care

Some home care patients use bed rails. The same risks and safety measures apply. Check the safety of bed rails installed by the family. Look for loose or poor-fitting rails. Tell the nurse if you suspect a problem.

PROMOTING SAFETY AND COMFORT

Bed Rails

Safety

You raise the bed to give care. Follow these safety measures to prevent falling when the bed is raised.

- *For a person who uses bed rails:* Always raise the far bed rail(s) if you are working alone. Raise bed rails on both sides and lower the bed if you need to leave the bedside.
- *For a person who does not use bed rails:* Ask a co-worker to help you. The co-worker stands on the far side of the bed to protect the person from falling.
- Never leave the person alone when the bed is raised.
- Lower the bed to a comfortable and safe level for the person after giving care. Follow the care plan.

If allowed to chart, record your care, safety measures, and any observations. See Figure 15-6 for an example.

Comfort

The person has to reach over raised bed rails for items on the bedside stand and over-bed table (Chapter 13). That is unsafe. Adjust the over-bed table so needed items (water mug, tissues, phone, TV and light controls) are within reach. Ask what other items to place nearby. Always make sure needed items, including the call light, are within reach.

Hand Rails and Grab Bars

Hand rails are in hallways and stairways (Fig. 15-7). They give support to persons who are weak or unsteady when walking.

Grab bars (safety bars) are in bathrooms and in shower/tub rooms (Fig. 15-8). They provide support to sit down or get up from a toilet. They also are used when standing in the shower and to get in and out of the shower or tub.

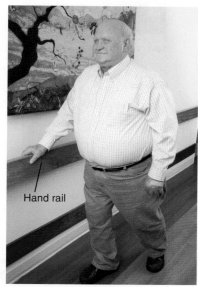

FIGURE 15-7 Hand rails provide support when walking.

DATE: 06/16	TIME: 1415
ACTIVITY AND POSITIONING	

☐ Ambulate	☐ Chair
☐ Self	☒ Bed
☒ Assist of 1	☒ Right side
☐ Assist of 2	☐ Left side
☐ Mechanical lift	☐ Back

Turned Mr. Adams from his back to his right side. Placed pillows under his head, against his back, and under his left leg. He stated he was comfortable with needed items in reach (water mug, phone, tissues, urinal, call light). I told him that I will check on him every 15 minutes and to use the call light if he needs anything.

SAFETY	
☐ Gait belt	☒ Belongings in reach
☐ Slip-resistant shoes	☒ Bed rails raised
☒ Call light in reach	☐ Bed rails lowered
☒ Bed in low position	☐ Bed/chair alarm

FIGURE 15-6 Charting sample.

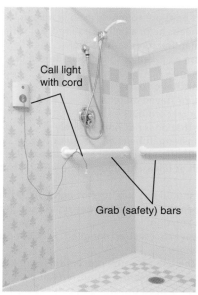

FIGURE 15-8 Grab bars (safety bars) in a shower.

Wheel Locks

Bed wheels let the bed move easily. Wheels have locks (brakes) to prevent the bed from moving (Fig. 15-9). Wheels are locked (braked) at all times except when moving the bed. Make sure bed wheels are locked (braked):

- When giving bedside care
- When you transfer a person to and from bed

Wheelchair and stretcher wheels also are locked (braked) during transfers (Chapter 21). You or the person can be injured if the bed, wheelchair, or stretcher moves.

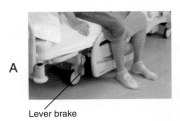

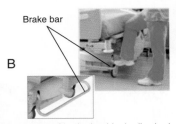

FIGURE 15-9 Examples of bed wheel locks (brakes). **A,** Lever brake. **B,** Brake bar. (Courtesy © Hill-Rom Services, Inc. Reprinted with permission. All rights reserved.)

▊ TRANSFER/GAIT BELTS

A *transfer belt (gait belt)* is a device applied around the waist and used to support a person who is unsteady or disabled (Fig. 15-10). It helps prevent falls and injuries.

- When used to transfer a person (Chapter 21), it is called a *transfer belt.*
- When used to help a person walk (Chapter 35), it is called a *gait belt.*

The belt goes around the waist. Grasp the belt from underneath for support. Use an upward grasp (see Fig. 15-10). A downward grasp at the top of the belt is not secure. If the belt has handles, grasp the belt by the handles (Fig. 15-11).

See *Promoting Safety and Comfort: Transfer/Gait Belts.*
See procedure: *Using a Transfer/Gait Belt.*

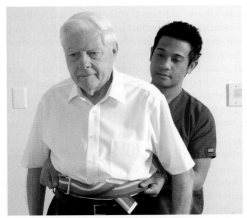

FIGURE 15-10 Transfer/gait belt. The buckle is off-center. Excess strap is tucked into the belt. The nursing assistant grasps the belt from underneath with an upward grasp.

PROMOTING SAFETY AND COMFORT

Transfer/Gait Belts

Safety

Transfer/gait belts are routinely used in nursing centers. If the person needs help, a belt is required. For safe use, always follow the manufacturer's instructions.

Do not use a broken or soiled belt. Before use, check the belt for damage.

- Broken stitches or parts
- Torn, cut, or frayed material
- Broken or cracked buckles
- A buckle that does not hold securely

Some transfer/gait belts have a quick release buckle (Fig. 15-12). Position the buckle at the back where the person cannot reach or release it. Injury could result if the buckle is released.

The belt should be snug but not tight. Slide an open, flat hand between the belt and the person. Adjust the belt if it is too loose or too tight.

Do not leave excess strap dangling. Tuck the excess strap into the belt (see Fig. 15-10).

Remove the belt after the procedure. Do not leave the person alone while wearing a transfer/gait belt.

The standard-sized txansfer/gait belt fits waist sizes up to 51 inches. Bariatric-sized belts fit waist sizes up to 71 inches.

The nurse and care plan tell you what size to use. If the person's waist size is greater than 71 inches, follow the nurse's directions and the care plan.

Using a transfer/gait belt is unsafe for some persons. The belt could cause pressure or rub against care equipment. Check with the nurse and the care plan before using a transfer/gait belt if the person has:

- An ostomy—colostomy, ileostomy, urostomy (Chapters 29 and 52)
- A gastrostomy tube (Chapter 33)
- Chronic obstructive pulmonary disease (Chapter 50)
- An abdominal or chest wound, incision, or drainage tube
- Monitoring equipment
- A hernia (Chapter 51)
- Other conditions or equipment involving the chest or abdomen

Comfort

A transfer/gait belt is always applied over clothing—never over bare skin. Also, it is applied around the waist and under the breasts. Breasts must not be caught under the belt. The belt buckle is never positioned over the person's spine.

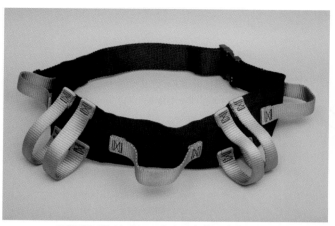

FIGURE 15-11 A transfer/gait belt with handles.

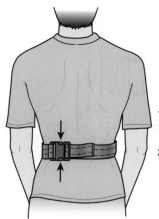

To release the buckle:
1) Press the buttons on both sides of the buckle together.
2) Pull the buckle apart.

FIGURE 15-12 A transfer/gait belt with a quick release buckle. The buckle is positioned off-center at the back.

Using a Transfer/Gait Belt

QUALITY OF LIFE

- Knock before entering the person's room.
- Address the person by name.
- Introduce yourself by name and title.

- Explain the procedure before starting and during the procedure.
- Protect the person's rights during the procedure.
- Handle the person gently during the procedure.

PRE-PROCEDURE

1 See *Promoting Safety and Comfort: Transfer/Gait Belts.*
2 Practice hand hygiene.
3 Obtain a transfer/gait belt of the correct type and size.

4 Identify the person. Check the identification (ID) bracelet against the assignment sheet. Use 2 identifiers (Chapter 14). Also call the person by name.
5 Provide for privacy.

PROCEDURE

6 Assist the person to a sitting position. Apply slip-resistant footwear if not already on.
7 Apply the belt. Hold the belt by the buckle. Wrap the belt around the person's waist over clothing. Do not apply it over bare skin.
  a *For a belt with a metal buckle* (Fig. 15-13, p. 216):
    1) Insert the belt's metal tip into the buckle. Pass the belt through the side with the teeth first (see Fig. 15-13, *A*).
    2) Bring the belt tip across the front of the buckle. Insert the tip through the buckle's smooth side (see Fig. 15-13, *B*).
  b *For a belt with a quick release buckle,* push the belt ends together to secure the buckle.

8 Tighten the belt so it is snug. It should not cause discomfort or impair breathing. You should be able to slide your open, flat hand under the belt. Ask about the person's comfort. If the belt is too loose or too tight, adjust the belt as needed.
9 Make sure that the person's breasts are not caught under the belt.
10 Place the buckle off-center in the front (see Fig. 15-13, *C*) or off-center in the back (see Fig. 15-12) for the person's comfort. A quick release buckle is in the back, out of the person's reach. The buckle is not over the spine.
11 Tuck any excess strap into the belt (see Fig. 15-13, *C*).
12 Complete the transfer (Chapter 21) or ambulation procedure (Chapter 35). Grasp the belt from underneath with 2 hands (see Fig. 15-10). Use an upward grasp. Or grasp the belt by the handles.

POST-PROCEDURE

13 Remove the belt after the procedure in step 12. The person is not left alone wearing the belt.
  a *For a belt with a metal buckle:*
    1) Bring the belt strap back through the buckle's smooth side.
    2) Pull the belt through the side with the teeth.
  b *For a belt with a quick release buckle,* push inward on the quick release buttons (see Fig. 15-12).
  c Remove the belt from the person's waist. Do not drag the belt across the back or waist.
14 Provide for comfort. (See the inside of the back cover.)

15 Place the call light and other needed items within reach.
16 Follow the care plan and the person's preferences for privacy measures to maintain. Leaving the privacy curtain, window coverings, and door open or closed are examples.
17 Complete a safety check of the room. (See the inside of the back cover.)
18 Return the transfer/gait belt to its proper place.
19 Practice hand hygiene.
20 Report and record your care and observations.

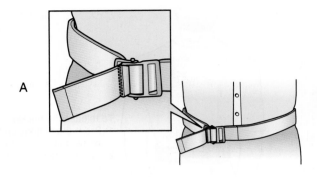

A   The belt is inserted into the buckle.
The belt goes through the side with the teeth first.

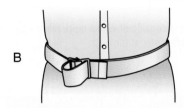

B   The belt is inserted into the buckle's smooth side.

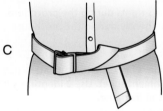

C   The buckle is off-center in the front.
Excess strap is tucked into the belt.

FIGURE 15-13 Applying a transfer/gait belt at the waist. **A** and **B,** The belt is passed through the metal buckle. **C,** Excess strap is tucked in.

THE FALLING PERSON

A person may start to fall when standing or walking. The person may be weak, light-headed, or dizzy. Fainting may occur (Chapter 58). Falling may also be caused by slipping or sliding on spills, waxed floors, throw rugs, or improper shoes. See p. 208 for the causes and risk factors for falls.

Do not try to prevent the fall. You could injure yourself and the person while twisting and straining to prevent the fall. You could lose your balance. You both could fall. Head, wrist, arm, hip, knee, and back injuries could occur.

If a person starts to fall, bring the person close to your body. Ease the person to the floor. This lets you control the direction of the fall. You can also protect the person's head.

Do not let the person move or get up before the nurse checks for injuries. Reassure the person and explain that the nurse will check for injuries before the person is helped up.

If you find a person on the floor, do not move the person. Stay with the person. Call for the nurse.

An incident report is completed after all falls (Chapter 14). The nurse may have you help with the report.

See *Focus on Children and Older Persons: The Falling Person.*
See *Promoting Safety and Comfort: The Falling Person.*
See procedure: *Helping the Falling Person.*

FOCUS ON CHILDREN AND OLDER PERSONS

The Falling Person

Older Persons

Some older persons are confused. Confused persons may not understand why you do not want them to move or get up after a fall. Forcing a person not to move may injure the person and you. You may need to let the person move. Never use force to hold a person down. Stay calm and protect the person from injury. Talk to the person in a quiet, soothing voice. Call for help.

PROMOTING SAFETY AND COMFORT

The Falling Person

Safety

If a bariatric person starts to fall, there is little that you can do. For the person's safety and yours:
- *Do not* use the procedure: *Helping the Falling Person.*
- Move items that could cause injury out of the way. Do so as fast as possible.
- Try to protect the person's head from striking the floor, equipment, or other objects.
- Call for the nurse at once. Stay with the person.
- Assist the health team to move the person from the floor.

Helping the Falling Person

PROCEDURE

1. Stand behind the person with your feet apart. Keep your back straight.
2. Bring the person close to your body as fast as possible (Fig. 15-14, *A*). Use the transfer/gait belt. Or wrap your arms around the person's waist. If necessary, hold the person under the arms.
3. Move your leg so the person's buttocks rest on it (Fig. 15-14, *B*).
4. Lower the person to the floor. The person slides down your leg to the floor (Fig. 15-14, *C*). Bend at your hips and knees as you lower the person.
5. Call for a nurse to check the person. Stay with the person.
6. Follow the nurse's directions to assist with moving the person from the floor (p. 218 and Chapter 19). Get help from other staff if needed. For this procedure, the person is returned to bed.

POST-PROCEDURE

7. Provide for comfort. (See the inside of the back cover.)
8. Place the call light and other needed items within reach.
9. Raise or lower bed rails. Follow the care plan.
10. Complete a safety check of the room. (See the inside of the back cover.)
11. Practice hand hygiene.
12. Report and record the following.
    - How the fall occurred
    - If the person was standing or walking
    - How far the person walked
    - How activity was tolerated before the fall
    - Complaints before the fall
    - How much help the person needed while walking
13. Complete an incident report (Chapter 14).

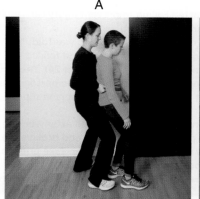
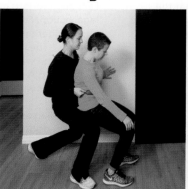
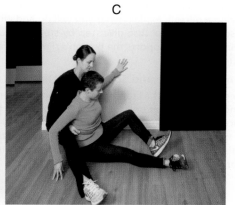

A   B   C

FIGURE 15-14 Helping the falling person. **A,** The falling person is pulled close and supported with the gait belt. **B,** The person's buttocks rest on the nursing assistant's leg. **C,** The person is eased to the floor.

MOVING THE PERSON FROM THE FLOOR

After a fall, the nurse will assess the person for injuries. Special procedures are used to move a person with severe injuries. Assist as the nurse directs.

If there are no injuries or minor injuries, follow the nurse's directions to move the person from the floor.

The Occupational Safety and Health Administration (OSHA) recommends minimal manual lifting or not lifting when possible. If the person can stand alone, the nurse has staff stand by as the person stands up. Or a transfer/gait belt is used to assist the person. A mechanical lift (Chapter 21) may be used (Fig. 15-15). The lift must reach the floor. If a manual lift is required, protect yourself from injury. See Chapter 19.

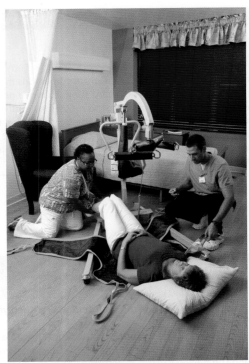

FIGURE 15-15 Moving the person from the floor using a mechanical lift.

FOCUS ON PRIDE

The Person, Family, and Yourself

P ersonal and Professional Responsibility

Safety measures can take time. Resist the urge to take shortcuts. Take the time to:

- Find and use adaptive (assistive) devices.
- Put proper footwear on the person. Footwear is slip-resistant and fits well.
- Raise or lower the bed and bed rails as needed.
- Lock (brake) wheels on beds, stretchers, and wheelchairs.
- Ask for help.
  Take time for safety. Take pride in doing the right thing.

R ights and Respect

Fear of falling does not make a person feel safe. Before moving a person, explain what you will do and what the person needs to do. Also give step-by-step instructions. Good communication supports the person's right to safety and security.

I ndependence and Social Interaction

Some people feel that safety devices limit independence. Using a transfer/gait belt is an example. Listen to the person's concerns. Kindly explain the reason for the safety device. If the person still refuses, tell the nurse. Do not be talked out of a safety measure or using a safety device. Safety is always a priority.

D elegation and Teamwork

Helping co-workers is part of teamwork. A co-worker's patient or resident may ask for your help to move from the chair to the bed, walk to the bathroom, and so on. If you assist the person, you have helped the person and your co-worker.

Being helpful is good, but you must also be safe. You need to know about the person's fall risk and how to move the person safely. You will learn more about transfer and walking procedures in Chapters 21 and 35. You will learn what you need to know before moving a person. Before helping any patient or resident, be sure you have the needed information.

E thics and Laws

Falls are a serious matter. Failing to prevent injury can result in legal action. For example:

- A resident asked repeatedly for help and was told: "I'm busy." The person tried to get up alone and fell.
- A person was using a shower chair (Chapter 24). The floor was wet. A nursing assistant transferred the person from the chair without shoes on the feet. The person slipped and fell.
- A nursing assistant did not lower the bed after working at the bedside. The patient fell out of bed and broke a hip.
  Follow the safety measures in this chapter. Take pride in protecting the person, yourself, and the agency.

FOCUS ON PRIDE: Application

A person is embarrassed about needing a transfer/gait belt and walker. How will you promote safety and dignity? What if the person refuses to use the devices?

REVIEW QUESTIONS

Circle the BEST answer.

1 These statements are about falls. Which is *true?*
   a Most are caused by many risk factors.
   b Serious injuries are unlikely.
   c Falling indoors is not common.
   d Nursing center residents are at decreased risk.

2 Which person has the *lowest* risk of falls?
   a A 75-year-old with confusion
   b A 68-year-old with a history of falls
   c A 60-year-old with a hearing aid
   d An 80-year-old with urinary incontinence

3 A person's care plan includes fall prevention measures. Which should you question?
   a Assist with elimination needs.
   b Keep phone, lamp, and TV controls within reach.
   c Unlock bed wheels when giving bedside care.
   d Complete a safety check after visitors leave the room.

4 You observe the following in the person's room. Which is *unsafe?*
   a The lamp cord is by the chair.
   b The chair has armrests.
   c The night-light is on.
   d The bed is in a low position.

5 You note the following after a person is dressed. Which is *safe?*
   a Pant cuffs are dragging on the floor.
   b The person is wearing slip-resistant shoes.
   c The belt is not fastened.
   d Shoelaces are untied.

6 A resident's care plan includes use of a position change alarm. You hear the alarm sound. What should you do?
   a Find the resident's nursing assistant.
   b Tell the nurse.
   c Assist the person right away.
   d Wait for someone to respond to the alarm.

7 To help prevent falls, you need to report
   a Equipment and supplies being on 1 side of the hallway
   b A floor cushion beside the bed
   c A co-worker pulling a wheelchair through a doorway
   d A loose grab bar (safety bar) in a bathroom

8 Bed rails are used
   a For all persons
   b According to the care plan
   c When you want to use them
   d For persons at high risk for bed entrapment

9 Before transferring a person to bed, you must
   a Raise the bed rails
   b Get a grab bar
   c Lock (brake) the bed wheels
   d Remove the person's shoes

10 A transfer/gait belt is applied
   a To the skin
   b Over clothing at the waist
   c Over the breasts
   d Over a colostomy or ileostomy site

11 To safely use a transfer/gait belt, you must
   a Follow the manufacturer's instructions
   b Be able to slide a closed fist under the belt
   c Leave the belt on if the person is left alone
   d Position the buckle over the person's spine

12 You apply a transfer/gait belt. What should you do with the excess strap?
   a Cut it off.
   b Wrap it around the person's waist.
   c Tuck it into the belt.
   d Let it dangle.

13 A person starts to fall. Your *first* action is to
   a Try to prevent the fall
   b Call for help
   c Bring the person close to your body
   d Lower the person to the floor

14 When a bariatric person falls, you should
   a Try to stop the fall
   b Do nothing
   c Quickly pull the person close to you
   d Try to protect the person's head

15 You found a person lying on the floor. What should you do?
   a Lock the bed wheels.
   b Help the person back to bed.
   c Apply a transfer belt.
   d Call for the nurse.

Answers to Chapter 15 questions are on p. 902.

FOCUS ON PRACTICE

Problem Solving

You are assisting a resident in the bathroom. The resident is not to be left alone while in the bathroom. You hear a position change alarm sound in the hallway right outside the door. What will you do?

Restraint Alternatives and Restraints

OBJECTIVES

- Define the key terms and key abbreviations in this chapter.
- Describe 3 forms of restraint.
- Identify appropriate and inappropriate restraint use.
- Identify restraint alternatives.
- Identify the risk factors related to restraint use.

- Explain the legal aspects of restraint use.
- Describe safety guidelines for restraint use.
- Perform the procedure described in this chapter.
- Explain how to promote PRIDE in the person, the family, and yourself.

KEY TERMS

chemical restraint A drug or drug dosage that:
- Controls behavior or restricts movement and is not standard treatment for the person's condition
- Is used for discipline or convenience and is not required to treat medical symptoms

physical restraint Any manual method or physical or mechanical device, material, or equipment that:
- Is attached to or near a person's body
- Cannot be removed easily by the person
- Restricts freedom of movement or normal access to the body

restraint The restriction of voluntary movement or the control of behavior

restraint alternative Measures used instead of restraint to manage a potentially harmful situation

seclusion Confining a person to a room or area and preventing the person from leaving

KEY ABBREVIATIONS

CMS	Centers for Medicare & Medicaid Services	ROM	Range-of-motion
FDA	Food and Drug Administration	TJC	The Joint Commission
ID	Identification		

Restraints limit a person's freedom of movement and present many dangers. Agency policies and procedures on restraint use must protect the person's rights, ensure safety, and prohibit inappropriate use. A restraint-free setting is the goal.

The Centers for Medicare & Medicaid Services (CMS) has rules for restraint use. While not prohibited, there are limited appropriate uses. Restraints may only be used for a brief time to treat a medical symptom that would require restraint use or for the immediate physical safety of the person or others.

Restraints may be used only when less restrictive measures fail to protect the person or others. Before use, staff must seek to identify and address the condition causing the medical symptom. Restraints must be discontinued as soon as possible.

FORMS OF RESTRAINT

Restraint involves the restriction of voluntary movement or the control of behavior. There are different forms of restraint.
- Physical restraint
- Chemical restraint
- Seclusion

Physical Restraint

The CMS defines *physical restraint* as any manual method or physical or mechanical device, material, or equipment that:
- Is attached to or near a person's body,
- Cannot be removed easily by the person, and
- Restricts freedom of movement or normal access to the body.

BOX 16-1	Physical Restraint Terms and Definitions

- *Manual method*—to hold or limit voluntary movement by using body contact.
- *Remove easily*—the manual method, device, material, or equipment can be removed intentionally by the person in the same manner it was applied by the staff. For example, a person can put bed rails down, untie a knot, or open a buckle. An item that the person *cannot* remove easily may be a restraint.
- *Freedom of movement*—any change in place or position of the body or any part of the body that the person can control. An item that *restricts* freedom of movement or activity may be a restraint.
- *Medical symptom*—an indication or characteristic of a physical or psychological condition. A symptom may be physical, emotional, or behavioral.
- *Discipline*—any action taken by the agency to punish or penalize a patient or resident. *Restraints are not used to discipline a person.*
- *Convenience*—any action taken to control or manage a person's behavior that requires less effort by the staff. The action is not in the person's best interests. *Restraints are not used for staff convenience.*

Modified from Centers for Medicare & Medicaid Services: State operations manual, appendix PP, Baltimore, 2023, Author.

Physical restraint is used only when necessary to treat a medical symptom. *It is never used to discipline a person or for staff convenience.* Box 16-1 explains the terms and definitions used by the CMS regarding physical restraint.

Physical restraint confines a person to an area—bed or chair. Or it prevents movement of a body part. Holding a person down is a form of physical restraint. Some furniture or barriers prevent freedom of movement and may meet the definition of a physical restraint. For example:

- A bed or chair is placed so close to the wall that the person cannot get out of it.
- Bed rails (Chapter 15) are raised to keep the person from getting out of bed. The person cannot lower the rails to get out of bed as desired.
- The design of a chair or mattress prevents a person from getting up.
- A sheet is tucked in so tightly that the person cannot get out of bed.
- Fabric or clothing is fastened in a way that restricts freedom of movement.
- A position change alarm (Chapter 15) is used to monitor movement. The person is afraid to move to avoid setting off the alarm.

The health team must assess the effect that a device (material, equipment) has on the person. They must assess if the person can easily and voluntarily remove the device (material, equipment). For example, a lap-top tray or cushion blocks a person from rising from a chair (Fig. 16-1). The device may be a physical restraint depending on its effect on the person and if the person has freedom of movement from the chair.

Some devices are manufactured as physical restraints for medical use. They are applied to the chest (vest or jacket),

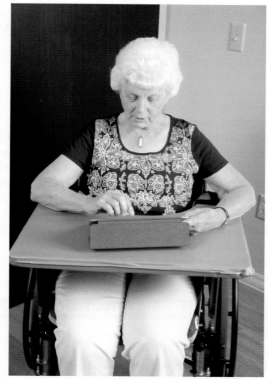

FIGURE 16-1 The health team assesses the effect devices (materials, equipment) have on the person. This lap-top tray may be a restraint for one person but not for another.

waist (belt), wrists or ankles (limb holders), or hands (mitts). See "Laws, Rules, and Guidelines" on p. 224 and "Restraints" on p. 229.

This chapter focuses on physical restraints. The word "restraints" refers to the use of physical restraints for medical use. Restraint is a last resort for protection and treatment. Laws, rules, and guidelines for restraint use must be followed.

See *Focus on Children and Older Persons: Physical Restraint.*

FOCUS ON **CHILDREN AND OLDER PERSONS**

Physical Restraint

Children
Cribs with raised rails are an age-appropriate safety measure for infants and toddlers. Cribs are not considered a restraint.

Older Persons
Dementia can affect behavior, mood, and personality. Symptoms such as aggression, agitation, delusions, and hallucinations can occur. Wandering is common. In Chapter 54 you will learn about causes and care measures for persons with dementia. Care measures include:
- Identifying causes and triggers
- Understanding the person and following his or her routine
- Providing a calm setting
- Using distraction or an activity that is meaningful to the person
  Physical restraint can increase confusion and agitation. The person may try to get free. Serious injury and death are risks (p. 222).

Chemical Restraint

The use of some drugs may be considered restraint. A drug or drug dosage is a *chemical restraint* if it:

- Controls behavior or restricts movement and is not standard treatment for the person's condition.
- Is used for discipline or convenience and is not required to treat medical symptoms.

Treatments should allow the person to function *more* effectively. Reducing the person's ability to function is *not* standard treatment. Using a drug in such a way is considered restraint. For example, a drug makes a person sleepy (sedated) and unable to function at the person's highest level.

Drugs must not be used for discipline or staff convenience. They are used only when required to treat a person's medical symptom.

See *Focus on Children and Older Persons: Chemical Restraint.*

FOCUS ON CHILDREN AND OLDER PERSONS

Chemical Restraint

Older Persons

Drugs used for aggression, agitation, delusions, and hallucinations (antipsychotic drugs) can cause stroke and death in persons with dementia. Such drugs are not approved to treat dementia symptoms. They are very dangerous for persons with dementia.

Practices such as using a drug to quiet a resident or to prevent wandering indicate inappropriate use for staff convenience. *Restraint is never to be used for discipline or convenience.*

Seclusion

Seclusion is another form of restraint. *Seclusion* is confining a person to a room or area and preventing the person from leaving. Seclusion is only used for the immediate safety of the person or others in situations of violence or self-harm.

HISTORY OF RESTRAINT USE

Restraint was once used to prevent falls. However, there is no evidence that restraint use prevents falls. Injuries are more serious from falls in restrained persons than in those not restrained.

Restraint was also used to prevent wandering or interfering with treatment. It was used for confusion, poor judgment, or behavior problems. Older persons were restrained more often than younger persons were. Restraints were viewed as safety measures. However, they can cause serious harm, even death. See "Risks From Restraint Use."

Besides the CMS, the Food and Drug Administration (FDA), state agencies, and The Joint Commission (TJC—an accrediting agency) have restraint guidelines. They do not forbid restraint use. Restraint use is limited to situations in which the person has a medical symptom that warrants the use of a restraint. Also, less restrictive alternatives must be tried and shown to be ineffective first. See "Restraint Alternatives."

Every agency has policies and procedures for restraints. They include identifying persons at risk for harm, harmful behaviors, restraint alternatives, and proper restraint use. Staff training is required.

RESTRAINT ALTERNATIVES

Often there are causes and reasons for harmful behaviors. Knowing and treating the cause can prevent restraint use. The nurse tries to learn what the behavior means.

- Is the person in pain, ill, or injured?
- Is the person short of breath? Do cells have enough oxygen (Chapter 44)?
- Is the person afraid in a new setting?
- Does the person need to use the bathroom?
- Is the person uncomfortable, hot, cold, hungry, or thirsty?
- Is clothing or a wound dressing (Chapter 41) tight or causing discomfort?
- Are body fluids causing skin irritation?
- What are the person's life-long habits?
- Does the person have problems communicating?
- Is the person seeing, hearing, or feeling things that are not real (Chapters 53 and 54)?
- Is the person confused or disoriented (Chapter 54)?
- Are drugs causing the behaviors?

Restraint alternatives are identified in the care plan. *Restraint alternatives* are measures used instead of restraint to manage a potentially harmful situation. The most basic measure is making sure the person's needs are met. See Box 16-2 for examples of restraint alternatives. Individualized interventions are planned, implemented, and evaluated. The person's care plan is changed as needed.

RISKS FROM RESTRAINT USE

Restraints can cause serious injury and death. Box 16-3 lists the risks from restraints. Injuries can occur as the person tries to get free of the restraint. Injuries also occur from using the wrong restraint, applying it wrong, or keeping it on too long. Cuts, bruises, and fractures are common. *The most serious risk is death from strangulation.* See Figures 16-2 and 16-3.

The *Safe Medical Devices Act* applies if a medical device causes illness, injury, or death. Restraints are medical devices. Also, the CMS requires the reporting of any death that occurs:

- While a person is in a restraint.
- Within 24 hours after a restraint was removed.
- Within 1 week after a restraint was removed. This applies if the restraint may have contributed directly or indirectly to the person's death.

See *Promoting Safety and Comfort: Risks From Restraint Use.*

BOX 16-2 Restraint Alternatives

Physical Needs
- Life-long habits and routines are followed.
- Pillows and positioning devices are used.
- Food, fluid, hygiene, and elimination needs are met.
- Needed items are within reach.
- Comfort needs are met. Pain is controlled. See Chapter 36.
- A calm, quiet setting is provided.
- Exercise programs are provided.
- Outdoor time is planned for nice weather.
- Furniture meets the person's needs.
- Observations and visits are made at least every 15 minutes or more often. Follow the care plan.
- The person's room is close to the nurses' station.
- Lighting meets the person's needs and preferences.
- Staff assignments are consistent.
- Sleep is not interrupted.

Safety and Security Needs
- The call light is within reach. The person is reminded to use the call light. Call lights are answered promptly.
- The person wanders in safe areas. Door alarms or knob guards are used to prevent access to unsafe areas.
- All staff are aware of persons who tend to wander.
- Measures are taken to prevent falls and injuries from falls (Chapter 15).
- Walls and furniture corners are padded.
- Procedures and care measures are explained.
- Frequent explanations are given about equipment or devices.
- Confused persons are oriented to person, time, and place. (To *orient* means to remind the person of his or her name and the date, time, and setting.) Calendars and clocks are provided.

Love, Belonging, and Self-Esteem Needs
- Diversion is provided—music, games, relaxation, and so on.
- The person watches videos of family and friends.
- Time is spent in supervised areas (lounge, by the nurses' station).
- Family, friends, and volunteers visit.
- The person has companions or sitters.
- Time is spent with the person.
- Extra time is spent with a person who is restless.
- Reminiscing is done with the person.
- The person does jobs or tasks he or she enjoys and consents to.

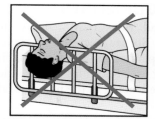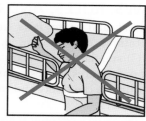

FIGURE 16-2 Restraints can cause injury and death. Incorrect application and trying to get free are causes. Here, the person is caught within and suspended between bed rails while a restraint is used.

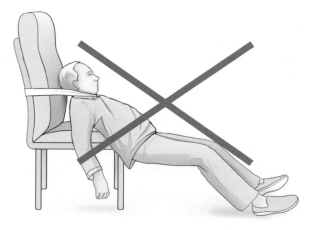

FIGURE 16-3 Death from strangulation is the most serious risk from restraint use.

PROMOTING SAFETY AND COMFORT

Risks From Restraint Use

Safety

If you find a person strangling from a restraint:
- Release the restraint. Or cut the strap if you have scissors in your pocket or within reach.
- Shout for help and for a nurse as you are releasing the restraint.
- Stay with the person. Follow the guidelines for cardiopulmonary resuscitation (CPR) and rescue breathing (Chapter 58). Follow agency policy. Assist the nurse as directed.

BOX 16-3 Risks From Restraint Use

- Constipation
- Contractures
- Cuts and bruises
- Decline in physical function (ability to walk and muscle problems are examples)
- Dehydration
- Falls
- Fractures
- Head trauma

- Incontinence
- Infections: pneumonia and urinary tract
- Nerve injuries
- Pressure injuries
- Social and mental health problems: agitation, aggression, anger, anxiety, delirium, depression, loss of dignity, embarrassment and humiliation, mistrust, loss of self-respect, reduced social contact, withdrawal
- Strangulation

LAWS, RULES, AND GUIDELINES

Federal and state laws and rules (CMS, FDA) for restraint use are followed. So are accrediting agency (TJC) standards. They are part of the agency's policies and procedures for restraint use. The rules are intended to promote the safety and well-being of the person, staff, and others.

- *Unnecessary restraint is prohibited.* Restraints are never used for discipline or convenience. They are only used when necessary to treat medical symptoms warranting restraint use. Unnecessary restraint is false imprisonment (Chapter 5). Legal action may be taken.
- *Restraints are used only after other measures fail to protect the person* (see Box 16-2). The person's care plan lists specific measures to protect the person and others. Many fall prevention measures are restraint alternatives (Chapter 15).
- *Assessment, care planning, and on-going evaluation are required.* The use of a restraint must be individualized. It is based on the person's specific medical symptoms warranting restraint use. There must be on-going evaluation of the continued need for the restraint.
- *A doctor's order is required.* The doctor gives the reason for the restraint, what body part to restrain, what to use, and how long to use it. This information is on the care plan and your assignment sheet. In an "immediate danger" emergency, the order must be obtained during or immediately after a restraint is applied.
- *The least restrictive method is used for the least amount of time.* Some restraints restrict freedom of movement more than others. The method that allows the greatest amount of movement and body access is used. The restraint must be discontinued as soon as possible.
- *Informed consent is required.* The person must understand the reason for the restraint and possible risks. The person is told how the restraint will help medical treatment. If the person cannot give consent, the person's legal representative is given the information. The doctor or nurse provides needed information and obtains consent. The person can refuse the restraint and withdraw consent at any time.
  - The agency has rules for "imminent danger" emergencies. Restraint use must be a last resort for protection. The person's representative is immediately notified. The restraint is discontinued as soon as is safely possible.
- *Careful monitoring and supervision are required when restraints are used.* The restrained person must be properly monitored and supervised. Needs must be met. The person needs to be able to contact staff for help.

See *Focus on Surveys: Laws, Rules, and Guidelines.*

Safety Guidelines

The restrained person must be kept safe (Box 16-4). Also remember these key points.

- *Observe for increased confusion and agitation.* People are aware of restricted movements. They may try to get out of the restraint or struggle to pull at it. Some restrained persons beg others to release them. These behaviors often are viewed as signs of confusion. Confusion can increase because of not understanding what is happening. Provide repeated explanations and reassurance. Report behavior observations.
- *Protect the person's quality of life.* Restraints are used only for a brief time. The care plan must show how to reduce restraint use. You must meet the person's physical, emotional, and social needs.
- *Follow the manufacturer's instructions to safely apply and secure the restraint.* Tight restraints affect circulation and breathing. The person must be comfortable and able to move the restrained part to a limited and safe extent. Restraints must be applied and secured properly.
- *Apply restraints with enough help to protect the person and staff from injury.* In an emergency, restraints may need to be applied quickly. Combative and agitated people can hurt themselves and the staff when restraints are applied. Enough staff members are needed to complete the task safely and quickly.
- *Observe the person at least every 15 minutes or as often as directed by the nurse and the care plan.* Injuries and deaths can result from improper restraint use and poor observation. Prevent complications. Breathing and circulation problems are examples. Constant observation may be required for persons who are:
  - Aggressive, combative, or agitated.
  - At risk for aspiration—breathing food, fluid, vomitus, or an object into the lungs (Chapter 31). Persons who are supine (lying down) and unable to sit up are examples.
  - At risk for suicide (Chapter 53).
- *Remove or release the restraint, re-position the person, and meet basic needs at least every 2 hours.* Or do so as often as noted in the care plan. See Box 16-4.

See *Teamwork and Time Management: Safety Guidelines,* p. 228.

BOX 16-4 | Safety Measures for Using Restraints

Before Applying Restraints

- Do not use sheets, towels, tape, rope, straps, bandages, Velcro, or other items to restrain a person.
- Apply a restraint only after learning about its proper use.
- Demonstrate correct application of the restraint before applying it.
- Use the correct restraint and size. Small restraints are tight. They cause discomfort and agitation and restrict breathing and circulation. Strangulation is a risk from big or loose restraints.
- Use only restraints that have the manufacturer's instructions and warning labels.
  - Read the warning labels. Note the front and back of the restraint.
  - Follow the instructions. Some restraints are safe for bed, chair, and wheelchair use. Others are used only with certain equipment.
- Use intact restraints.
  - Look for broken stitches, tears, cuts, or frayed fabric or straps.
  - Look for missing or loose buckles, locks, hooks, loops, or straps or other damage. The restraint must hold securely.
- Test zippers, buckles, locks, hooks, loops, and other closures. The device must fasten securely.
- Do not alter or repair a restraint.
- Do not use a soiled or damaged restraint. Have the nurse inspect a damaged product.
- Do not use a restraint near a fire, a flame, smoking materials, or other heat sources.

Applying Restraints

- Follow agency policies and procedures and the manufacturer's instructions.
- Do not use a restraint to position a person:
  - On a toilet.
  - On furniture that does not allow for correct application.
  - In a vehicle. The restraint is not a seat belt.
  - In a home setting. Federal law restricts some restraints for use only in health care agencies.
- Position the person in good alignment before applying the restraint (Chapter 19). When in a chair, position the person so the hips are well to the back of the chair.
- Pad bony areas and the skin as directed by the nurse. This prevents pressure and injury from the restraint.
- Follow the manufacturer's application instructions. A restraint applied wrong or backward may cause serious injury or death. Death may occur from suffocation or strangulation.
  - *Vest restraint*—The "V" neck is in front.
  - *Jacket restraint*—The opening is in the back.
  - *Belt restraint when in a chair*—Apply the restraint at a 45-degree angle over the thighs (Fig. 16-4, p. 226).

Applying Restraints—cont'd

- Do not criss-cross straps in the back unless required by the manufacturer's instructions (Fig. 16-5, p. 226). Straps may loosen when the person moves and cause serious injury.
- Secure restraints according to the manufacturer's instructions. Quick release buckles (Fig. 16-6, p. 227) or quick release knots (Fig. 16-7, p. 227) are used. Both are easy to release in an emergency.
- Leave 1 to 2 inches of slack in the straps if directed to do so by the nurse. This allows some movement of the part.
- Secure restraint straps to a safe and secure location out of the person's reach.
  - Bed—Secure the restraint to the movable part of the bed frame (Fig. 16-8, *A*, p. 228). This is the part of the bed frame that moves when raising or lowering the bed. *Never secure restraints to bed rails, head-boards, or foot-boards.*
  - Chair or wheelchair—Secure the straps under the seat (Fig. 16-8, *B*, p. 228).
- Check for snugness after applying the restraint. The restraint should be snug but allow some movement of the restrained part. Follow the manufacturer's instructions. For example:
  - *If applied to the chest or waist*—Make sure the person can breathe easily. A flat hand should slide between the restraint and the person's body (Fig. 16-9, p. 228). Check with the nurse if you have very small or very large hands. Small or large hands could cause a tight or loose restraint.
  - *If applied to a limb*—You should be able to slide 1 finger under the device. Check with the nurse if you have very small or very large fingers. Small or large fingers could cause a tight or loose restraint.
- Make sure that the straps cannot tighten, loosen, slip, slide, or cause too much slack. The straps can change if pulled on by the person. Changing the bed or seat (or cushion) position can also change the straps. Injury or death can result from:
  - Tight straps that can impair breathing and cause suffocation.
  - Loose straps that allow the person to get free of the restraint.
  - Loose straps that allow the person to slip or slide off the bed or chair. The person can become suspended in the restraint (see Figs. 16-2 and 16-3). Chest compression and suffocation can result from strangulation.
- Use bed rail covers or gap protectors as instructed by the nurse (Fig. 16-10, p. 228). The person can become trapped or suspended (see Fig. 16-2) between:
  - The bars of a bed rail
  - The space between half-length (split) bed rails
  - The bed rail and mattress
  - The head-board or foot-board and mattress
- Do not use back cushions when a person is restrained in a chair. If the cushion moves out of place, slack occurs in the straps. Strangulation is a risk if the person slides forward or down from the extra slack.

Continued

BOX 16-4	Safety Measures for Using Restraints—cont'd

After Applying Restraints

- Keep bed rails up when using a vest, jacket, or belt restraint. Also use bed rail covers or gap protectors. Otherwise the person could fall off the bed and strangle on the restraint. Or the person can get caught between half-length bed rails.
- Do not cover the restraint with a sheet, blanket, bedspread, or other covering. The restraint must be within plain view at all times.
- Check the person at least every 15 minutes for safety, comfort, and signs of injury. Or check the person more often as directed by the nurse and the care plan.
- Monitor persons in the supine (back-lying) position constantly. Aspiration is a great risk if vomiting occurs (Chapter 31). Call for the nurse at once.
- Keep scissors in your pocket. In an emergency such as strangulation, cutting the tie may be faster than releasing a knot or buckle. Never leave scissors where the person can reach them. Make sure the person cannot reach the scissors in your pocket.
- Keep the call light and other needed items within the person's reach. Record that this was done.
- Complete a safety check before leaving the room. (See the inside of the back cover.)
- Check the person's circulation at least every 15 minutes or more often as directed by the nurse and the care plan.
  - *For limb holders, mitt restraints, and elbow splints (sleeves)*—You should feel a pulse at a pulse site below the restraint. Fingers or toes should be warm and pink. Tell the nurse at once if:
    - You cannot feel a pulse.
    - Fingers or toes are cold, pale, or blue in color.
    - The person complains of pain, numbness, or tingling in the restrained part.
    - The skin is red or damaged.
  - *For a belt, jacket, or vest restraint*—The person should be able to breathe easily. Also check the position of the restraint, especially in the front and back.

After Applying Restraints—cont'd

- Remove or release the restraint and re-position the person every 2 hours or more often as noted in the care plan. The restraint is removed or released for at least 10 minutes.
- Meet the person's basic needs when the restraint is removed or released.
  - Measure vital signs.
  - Meet elimination needs.
  - Offer food and fluids.
  - Meet hygiene needs.
  - Give skin care.
  - Perform range-of-motion (ROM) exercises or help the person walk. Follow the care plan.
  - Provide for physical and emotional comfort. (See the inside of the back cover.)
- Report to the nurse every time you checked the person and removed or released the restraint. Report your observations and the care given. Follow agency policy for recording. See "Reporting and Recording" on p. 233.

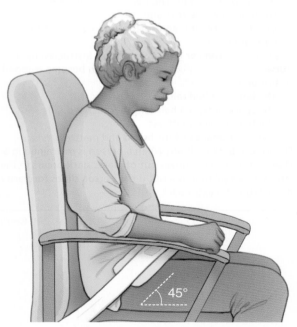

FIGURE 16-4 The belt restraint is at a 45-degree angle over the thighs.

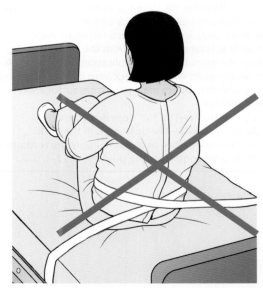

FIGURE 16-5 Never criss-cross vest or jacket straps in the back.

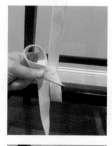

1 Bring the strap down across the front of the bar. Wrap the strap around to the back of the bar.

Cross the loose end over the front of the strap.

Make a loop.

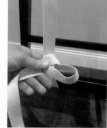

2 Pass the loop through the area where the strap crosses.

Pull to tighten.

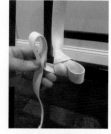

3 Make a second loop with the loose end.

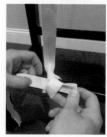

4 Pass the second loop through the first loop.

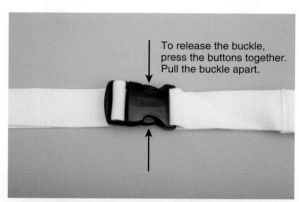

To release the buckle, press the buttons together. Pull the buckle apart.

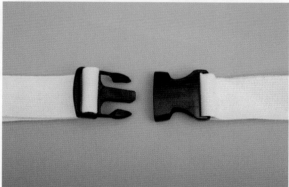

FIGURE 16-6 Quick release buckle.

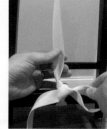

5 Pull to tighten.

Check that the strap is secure.

To untie, pull the loose end.

FIGURE 16-7 Quick release knot. (NOTE: This figure shows only the *method* for tying a quick release knot. The knot should be tied to a secure area out of the person's reach—a movable part of the bed frame or below the chair or wheelchair seat.)

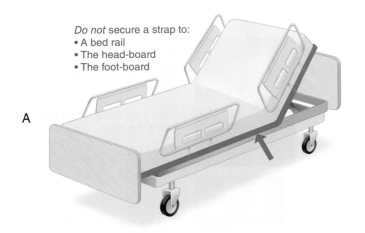

Do not secure a strap to:
• A bed rail
• The head-board
• The foot-board

A

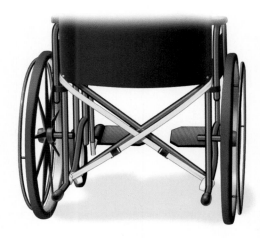

B

FIGURE 16-8 Locations for securing restraint straps. (Note: Straps are secured out of the person's reach.) **A,** On a bed, straps are secured to the movable part of the bed frame. This is the part that moves when raising or lowering the bed. *Do not secure a strap to a bed rail, head-board, or foot-board.* **B,** On a wheelchair, straps are secured to the frame below the seat.

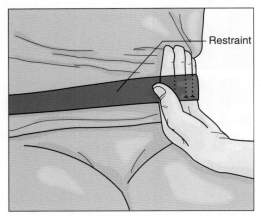

Restraint

FIGURE 16-9 A flat hand slides between the restraint and the person.

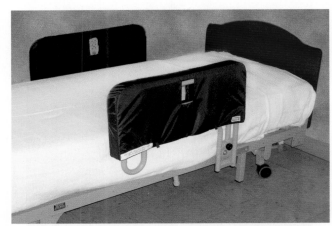

FIGURE 16-10   Bed rail covers. (From Perry AG, Potter PA, Ostendorf WR, et al: *Clinical nursing skills & techniques,* ed 10, St Louis, 2022, Elsevier.)

TEAMWORK AND TIME MANAGEMENT

Safety Guidelines

Make sure you know who is restrained on your unit. When you walk past the person or the person's room, check if the person is safe and comfortable. Answer the person's call light promptly.

RESTRAINTS

Manufactured restraints are made of cloth or other durable materials. Cloth restraints (soft restraints) include limb holders, mitts, splints (sleeves), belts, vests, and jackets.

More restrictive, cuff-style restraints for limbs (arms and legs) are made of more durable materials. These are only used in situations of extreme danger.

Limb Holders

Limb holders applied to the wrists (wrist restraints) limit arm movement (Fig. 16-11). For a brief time, limiting such movement may be necessary if the person:

- Is at risk for pulling out tubes used for life-saving treatment (intravenous [IV] infusion, feeding tube).
- Is at risk for pulling at devices that monitor vital signs.
- Scratches at, pulls at, picks at, or peels the skin, a wound, or a dressing. This can damage the skin or the wound. Limb holders applied to the ankles limit leg movement.

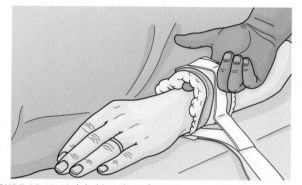

FIGURE 16-11 Limb holder. The soft part is toward the skin. One finger fits between the holder and the wrist.

Mitt Restraints

Hands are placed in mitt restraints. They prevent finger use. They allow hand, wrist, and arm movements. They have the same purpose as wrist restraints. Most mitts are padded (Fig. 16-12).

Some types of mitts are not considered restraints. However, any mitt that is attached to bedding or applied in a way that prevents hand or finger movement is considered a restraint. Also, bulky mitts that significantly reduce the person's ability to use the hands are restraints.

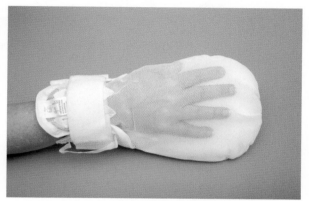

FIGURE 16-12 Mitt restraint.

Elbow Splints

Elbow splints (sleeves) make elbow movement difficult (Fig. 16-13). They prevent scratching and touching incisions or pulling out tubes. When used on 1 arm, such devices may be a restraint alternative. When used on both arms, they are restraints.

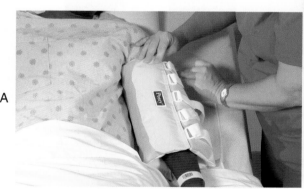
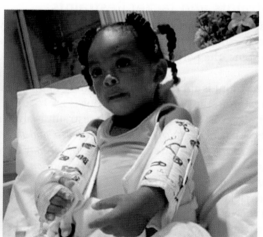

FIGURE 16-13 Elbow splints (sleeves). **A,** Sleeve applied to an adult. **B,** Restraints on a child.
(A, Copyright © Mosby's Clinical Skills: Essentials Collection. B, From Hockenberry MJ, Wilson D, Rodgers CC: *Wong's nursing care of infants and children*, ed 11, St Louis, 2019, Elsevier.)

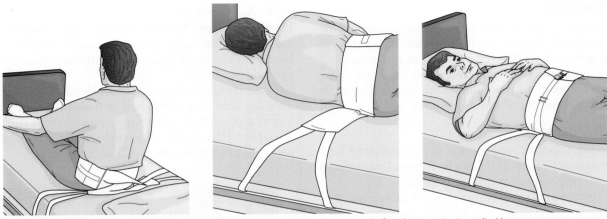

FIGURE 16-14 Belt restraint. (NOTE: The bed rails are raised after the restraint is applied.)

Belt Restraints

Belt restraints prevent the person from getting out of bed or out of a chair. With some types, the person can turn from side to side and sit up in bed (Fig. 16-14).

The belt is applied around the waist and secured to the bed or chair (lap belt). It is applied over a garment. The person can release the quick release type. It is less restrictive than those that only staff can release. Such belts may be considered for persons at risk for falls.

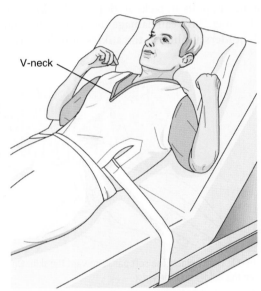

FIGURE 16-15 Vest restraint. The "V" neck is in front. (NOTE: The bed rails are raised after the restraint is applied.)

Vest Restraints and Jacket Restraints

Vest and jacket restraints are applied to the chest. They prevent the person from getting out of bed or out of a chair. With some, the person cannot turn from side to side or sit up.

A jacket restraint is applied with the opening in the back. For a vest restraint, the "V" neck is in front (Fig. 16-15). If needed, the vest crosses in the front. The restraint is always applied over a garment. (*NOTE: The straps of vest and jacket restraints cross in the front. A vest or jacket restraint may have positioning slots in the back* [Fig. 16-16]. *If so, position straps following the manufacturer's instructions.*)

Vest and jacket restraints have life-threatening risks. Death can occur from strangulation. If caught in the restraint, it can become so tight that the person's chest cannot expand to inhale air. The person quickly suffocates and dies. Correct application is critical. *You are advised to only assist the nurse in applying vest and jacket restraints. The nurse should have full responsibility for applying these types of restraints.*

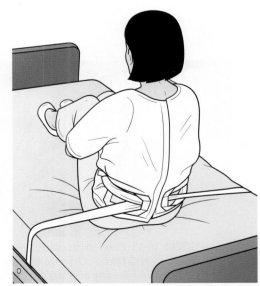

FIGURE 16-16 Jacket restraint with positioning slots in the back. (NOTE: The bed rails are raised after the restraint is applied.)

APPLYING RESTRAINTS

Follow the restraint manufacturer's instructions for application and use. The procedure that follows may be used as a guide to practice applying and using:

- Wrist restraints (limb holders)
- Mitt restraints
- Elbow splints (sleeves)
- A belt restraint
- A vest restraint
- A jacket restraint

See *Focus on Communication: Applying Restraints.*
See *Delegation Guidelines: Applying Restraints.*
See *Promoting Safety and Comfort: Applying Restraints.*
See procedure: *Applying Restraints*, p. 232.

FOCUS ON **COMMUNICATION**

Applying Restraints

If you do not know how to apply a certain restraint, do not do so. Ask the nurse to show you the correct way. You can say: "I've never applied this restraint before. Would you please show me how and then watch me apply it?" Thank the nurse for helping you.

Explain to the person what you will do. Then tell the person what you are doing step-by-step. Always check for safety and comfort.

Place the call light within reach. Make sure the person can use it with the restraint on. Remind the person to call for help if uncomfortable or if anything is needed. Do so as often as needed. For example:

- "How does the restraint feel? Is it too tight? Is it too loose?"
- "Please put your call light on. I want to make sure that you can reach and use it with the restraint on."
- "Please call for help right away if the restraint is too tight."
- "Please call for help right away if you feel pain in your fingers or hands. Also call for me if you feel numbness or tingling."
- "Please call for help right away if you are having problems breathing."
- "Please use your call light if you need anything."

PROMOTING SAFETY AND COMFORT

Applying Restraints

Safety

Restraints can cause serious harm, even death. (See "Risks From Restraint Use" on p. 222.) When needed, restraints must be used correctly and with caution. Application and safety measures vary with the restraint ordered and the manufacturer. *Always read and follow warning labels and follow the manufacturer's instructions for the restraint ordered.* Instructions for 1 restraint may not apply to another. The information, guidelines, and procedure in this chapter do not replace the manufacturer's instructions.

Never use force. Ask a co-worker to help if a person is confused or agitated. The manufacturer may have instructions for applying restraints on such persons. Report problems to the nurse at once.

Check the person at least every 15 minutes or more often as directed by the nurse and the care plan. Make sure the call light is within reach and the person can use it. Ask the person to use the call light at the first sign of problems or discomfort.

Never use a restraint as a seat belt in a car or other vehicle.

Mitt Restraints and Elbow Splints

Mitt restraints and elbow splints are often not secured to the bed or chair. Therefore the person can raise the device to the mouth. Observe the person closely. Watch that the person does not:

- Use the teeth to remove or damage the device.
- Ingest (eat) any material.

The person may be able to walk about. Falls are a risk. Practice safety measures to prevent falls (Chapter 15).

Belt, Vest, and Jacket Restraints

When a belt, vest, or jacket restraint is used, monitor the person's position. Risks include:

- Sliding forward or down in the chair or bed and becoming suspended or entrapped.
- Falling off the chair or mattress and becoming suspended or entrapped.

Comfort

Restraints limit movement. This affects position changes and reaching needed items. Position the person in good alignment before applying a restraint (Chapter 19). Make sure needed items are within reach—call light, water mug, tissues, phone, bed controls, and so on.

DELEGATION GUIDELINES

Applying Restraints

Applying restraints may be considered a delegated nursing task (Chapter 4) in some agencies. You may assist the nurse or the nurse may be allowed to delegate the task to you. Before applying a restraint, you need this information from the nurse and the care plan.

- Why the doctor ordered the restraint.
- What type and size to use.
- Where to apply the restraint.
- How to safely apply the restraint. Have the nurse show you how to apply it. Then show correct application back to the nurse.
- How to correctly position the person.

- What bony areas to pad and how to pad them.
- If bed rails are up or down.
- If bed rail covers or gap protectors are needed.
- What special equipment is needed.
- If the person needs to be checked more often than every 15 minutes. If yes, how often?
- When to apply and release the restraint.
- What observations to report and record. See "Reporting and Recording" on p. 233.
- When to report observations.
- What patient or resident concerns to report at once (see Box 16-4).

Applying Restraints

QUALITY OF LIFE

- Knock before entering the person's room.
- Address the person by name.
- Introduce yourself by name and title.

- Explain the procedure before starting and during the procedure.
- Protect the person's rights during the procedure.
- Handle the person gently during the procedure.

PRE-PROCEDURE

1 Follow *Delegation Guidelines: Applying Restraints*, p. 231. See *Promoting Safety and Comfort: Applying Restraints*, p. 231.
2 Practice hand hygiene and get the following supplies as instructed by the nurse.
   - Correct type and size of restraint
   - Padding for skin and bony areas
   - Bed rail covers or gap protectors (if needed)

3 Arrange items in the person's room.
4 Practice hand hygiene.
5 Identify the person. Check the identification (ID) bracelet against the assignment sheet. Use 2 identifiers (Chapter 14). Also call the person by name.
6 Provide for privacy.

PROCEDURE

7 Position the person for comfort and good alignment.
8 Put the bed rail covers or gap protectors (if needed) on the bed for the person in bed. Follow the manufacturer's instructions.
9 Pad bony areas. Follow the nurse's instructions and the care plan.
10 Read and follow the manufacturer's instructions. Note the front and back of the restraint.
11 *For limb holders to the wrists:*
   a Place the soft or foam part toward the skin.
   b Secure the holder so it is snug but not tight. Make sure you can slide 1 finger under the holder (see Fig. 16-11). Adjust the straps if the holder is too loose or too tight. Check for snugness again.
   c Secure the straps to the movable part of the bed frame out of the person's reach. Use the buckle or a quick release knot.
   d Repeat step 11 (a–c) for the other wrist.
12 *For mitt restraints:*
   a Clean and dry the person's hands.
   b Insert the person's hand into the restraint with the palm down.
   c Wrap the wrist strap around the smallest part of the wrist. Secure the strap with the hook-and-loop or other closure.
   d Secure the restraint to the bed if directed to do so. Secure the straps to the movable part of the bed frame out of the person's reach. Use the buckle or a quick release knot.
   e Check for snugness. Slide 1 finger between the restraint and the wrist. Adjust the straps if the restraint is too loose or too tight. Check for snugness again.
   f Repeat step 12 (b–e) for the other hand.
13 *For elbow splints:*
   a Release or loosen the adjustment straps (hook-and-loop).
   b Position the splint so the buckles are toward the person.
   c Wrap the splint over 1 arm. Or slide the splint up the arm. The splint is centered over the elbow. The opening is toward the inside or top of the arm. Follow the manufacturer's instructions.
   d Secure the splint following the manufacturer's instructions. Use the clips provided by the manufacturer if securing the splint to a sleeve. (This prevents the splint from sliding down the arm.)
   e Check for snugness. Follow the manufacturer's instructions. Adjust the splint if it is too loose or too tight. Check for snugness again.
   f Repeat step 13 (a–e) for the other arm.

14 *For a belt restraint:*
   a Assist the person to a sitting position.
   b Apply the restraint.
   c Remove wrinkles or creases from the front and back.
   d Bring the ties through the slots in the belt if present.
   e Position the straps at a 45-degree angle between the wheelchair seat and sides (see Fig. 16-4). If in bed, help the person lie down.
   f Make sure the person is comfortable and in good alignment.
   g Secure the straps to the movable part of the bed frame. Use the buckle or a quick release knot. The buckle or knot is out of the person's reach. For a wheelchair, criss-cross and secure the straps as in Figure 16-8, *B*.
   h Check for snugness. Slide an open hand between the restraint and the person. Adjust the restraint if it is too loose or too tight. Check for snugness again.
15 *For a vest restraint, assist the nurse as directed.*
   a Assist the person to a sitting position. If in a wheelchair:
      1) The person is as far back in the wheelchair as possible.
      2) The buttocks are against the chair back.
   b Apply the restraint. The "V" neck is in the front.
   c Bring the straps through the slots if the vest criss-crosses (Fig. 16-17).
   d Make sure the side seams are under the arms. Remove wrinkles in the front and back. Close the zipper if the device opens in the back. Or fasten with other closures.
   e Position the straps at a 45-degree angle between the wheelchair seat and sides. If in bed, help the person lie down.
   f Make sure the person is comfortable and in good alignment.
   g Secure the straps to the movable part of the bed frame at waist level. Use the buckle or a quick release knot. The buckle or knot is out of the person's reach. For a wheelchair, criss-cross and secure the straps as in Figure 16-8, *B*.
   h Check for snugness. Slide an open hand between the restraint and the person. Adjust the restraint if it is too loose or too tight. Check for snugness again.

Applying Restraints—cont'd

PROCEDURE—cont'd

16 *For a jacket restraint, assist the nurse as directed.*
  a Assist the person to a sitting position. If in a wheelchair:
     1) The person is as far back in the wheelchair as possible.
     2) The buttocks are against the chair back.
  b Apply the restraint. The jacket opening goes in the back.
  c Make sure the side seams are under the arms. Remove wrinkles in the front and back.
  d Close the back with the zipper or other closures.
  e Position the straps at a 45-degree angle between the wheelchair seat and sides. If in bed, help the person lie down.

  f Make sure the person is comfortable and in good alignment.
  g Secure the straps to the movable part of the bed frame at waist level. Use the buckle or a quick release knot. The buckle or knot is out of the person's reach. For a wheelchair, criss-cross and secure the straps as in Figure 16-8, *B.*
  h Check for snugness. Slide an open hand between the restraint and the person. Adjust the restraint if it is too loose or too tight. Check for snugness again.

POST-PROCEDURE

17 Position the person as the nurse directs.
18 Provide for comfort. (See the inside of the back cover.)
19 Place the call light and other needed items within the person's reach.
20 Raise or lower bed rails. Follow the care plan and the manufacturer's instructions for the restraint.
21 Follow the care plan and the nurse's instructions for privacy measures to maintain.
22 Complete a safety check of the room. (See the inside of the back cover.)
23 Practice hand hygiene.
24 Check the person and the restraint at least every 15 minutes or more often as directed by the nurse and the care plan. Report and record your observations.
  a *For limb holders, mitt restraints, or elbow splints:* Check the pulse, color, and temperature of the restrained parts.
  b *For a belt, vest, or jacket restraint:* Check the person's breathing. Make sure the restraint is properly positioned in the front and back. *Release the restraint and call for the nurse at once if the person is not breathing or is having problems breathing.*

25 Do the following at least every 2 hours for at least 10 minutes.
  a Remove or release the restraint.
  b Measure vital signs.
  c Re-position the person.
  d Meet food, fluid, hygiene, and elimination needs.
  e Give skin care.
  f Perform ROM exercises or help the person walk. Follow the care plan.
  g Provide for physical and emotional comfort. (See the inside of the back cover.)
  h Re-apply the restraint.
26 Complete a safety check of the room. (See the inside of the back cover.)
27 Practice hand hygiene.
28 Report and record your care and observations.

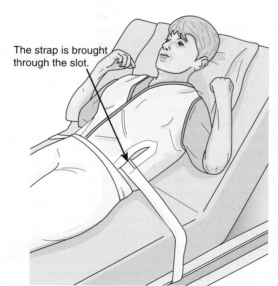

The strap is brought through the slot.

FIGURE 16-17 This vest criss-crosses in front. The straps are brought through the slots. (NOTE: The bed rails are raised after the restraint is applied.)

REPORTING AND RECORDING

Restraint information is recorded in the person's medical record (Fig. 16-18, p. 234). If you apply restraints or care for a restrained person, report and record:

- The restraint type and body part or parts restrained
- Safety measures taken (for example, bed rails padded and up, call light within reach)
- The time you applied the restraint
- The time you removed or released the restraint and for how long
- The person's vital signs
- The care given when the restraint was removed and for how long
- Skin color and condition
- Condition of the extremities
- The pulse felt in the restrained part
- Changes in the person's behavior
  Report the following at once.
- Difficulty breathing
- Pain, numbness, or tingling in the restrained part
- Discomfort
- A tight restraint

RESTRAINT MONITORING

Restraint Type and Location

☐ Limb holder		☒ Mitt		☐ Elbow splint
☐ Right wrist	☐ Right ankle	☒ Right wrist		☐ Right arm
☐ Left wrist	☐ Left ankle	☒ Left wrist		☐ Left arm

☐ Belt	☐ Vest	☐ Jacket	☐ Other:

Care Measures

☒ Restraints released/removed	☒ Food/fluid needs met	☒ Comfort measures
Duration: 20 minutes	☒ ROM/exercise/activity	☒ Skin care and hygiene
☒ Restraints re-applied	☒ Urinary/bowel elimination	☒ Bed rails up and padded
☐ Measures refused	☒ Positioning	☐ Other:
Notified nurse: E. Scott, RN	☒ Call light and needed items in reach	

Vital Signs

Temp 98.4 °F	Pulse 70	R 14	BP 116 / 72 mmHg	Pain 0 /10

Circulation Observations (Normal in blue)

Color: ☒ Pink ☐ Pale ☐ Cyanotic (bluish)

Temperature: ☐ Hot ☒ Warm ☐ Cool ☐ Cold

Sensation: ☒ Good sensation ☐ Numbness/tingling ☐ No sensation

Movement: ☒ Able to move extremities ☐ Unable to move extremities

Pulses: ☒ Pulses present in all extremities ☐ Pulse faint/absent in any extremity

Tell the nurse at once if any observations are abnormal.

Notified nurse: _____

Behavior Observations

☒ Alert	☐ Agitated	☐ Restless	☐ Drowsy
☒ Calm/cooperative	☐ Aggressive	☐ Confused	☐ Sleeping

FIGURE 16-18 Charting sample.

FOCUS ON PRIDE

The Person, Family, and Yourself

Personal and Professional Responsibility

Restraints have many risks. See Box 16-3. Therefore restraint use brings many responsibilities. You must:

- Promote safety and comfort.
- Apply the restraint properly.
- Observe the person closely.
- Meet basic needs.
- Report any concerns to the nurse.

Rights and Respect

You may be asked to assist with restraint alternatives (see Box 16-2). Make a true effort. Be honest. Do not tell the nurse you tried if you did not. Do your best to allow the person the right to freedom from restraint.

Independence and Social Interaction

All restraints limit movement. Independence is restricted. To promote independence:

- Keep the call light within reach at all times. Make sure the person can use it. Tell the person to signal for you if anything is needed. Answer the call light and meet the person's needs promptly.
- Keep needed items within reach. This is most important with restraints that allow hand and arm use. Belt, vest, and jacket restraints and elbow splints are examples.
- Allow choice. For example, let the person choose what to eat and drink when you release the restraint and meet needs.
- Let the person do as much as is safely possible. Personal choice and freedom of movement promote independence, dignity, and self-esteem. Provide care that gives restrained persons the independence they deserve.

Delegation and Teamwork

Care conferences are held to meet the person's safety and care needs. Your input has value. Share your observations and ideas. For example, a person does not try to get out of a chair when looking at photos or reading a book. You share this with the team for the person's care plan.

Ethics and Laws

Imagine the following.

- You need to use the bathroom. Your arms are restrained. You cannot get up or use your call light. You soil yourself with urine.
- You are uncomfortable. You have a vest restraint. You cannot move or turn in bed.
- You are thirsty. Your wrists are restrained. You cannot reach the water mug.
- You hear the fire alarm. You have on a restraint. You cannot get up to move to a safe place. You must wait to be rescued.

What would you do? Would you calmly lie or sit there? Would you try to get free from the restraint? Would you yell for help? Would the staff think that you are uncomfortable? Or would they think that you are agitated and uncooperative? Would you feel angry, embarrassed, or humiliated?

Restraints lessen dignity and freedom. Put yourself in the person's situation. Then you can better understand how the person feels. Treat the person like you would want to be treated—with kindness, caring, respect, and dignity.

FOCUS ON PRIDE: Application

Describe 2 scenarios involving behavior that is dangerous or that interferes with treatment. List ideas for managing the situation without using restraints.

REVIEW QUESTIONS

Circle the BEST answer.

1 Restraints
   a Promote dignity
   b Limit freedom of movement
   c Are a safe fall prevention measure
   d Are calming

2 Restraints may be used
   a For staff convenience
   b For discipline
   c For a person's specific medical symptom
   d When you think they are needed

3 Which is a restraint alternative?
   a Positioning the person's chair close to the wall
   b Using a chair that prevents the person from rising
   c Giving a drug that restricts movement
   d Giving an activity for diversion

4 Which is a restraint?
   a Padding walls and the corners of furniture
   b Bed rails that prevent a person from leaving the bed
   c A supervised lounge area near the nurses' station
   d A crib with raised rails for an infant

5 Physical restraints
   a Can be removed easily by the person
   b Are not allowed by the CMS
   c Require a doctor's order
   d Are safer than other forms of restraint

6 Which statement about restraints is *true?*
   a Restraints are a last resort for protection.
   b A device must be attached to the body to be a restraint.
   c The most restrictive method is best.
   d You can apply a restraint if a restraint alternative fails.

7 An unneeded restraint is applied. Which is *true?*
   a This can lead to charges of false imprisonment.
   b Recording in the medical record is not required.
   c Releasing the restraint every 2 hours is not needed.
   d There is no harm if the restraint was applied properly.

8 The following can occur from restraints. Which is the *most* serious?
   a Fractures
   b Strangulation
   c Pressure injuries
   d Urinary tract infections

9 Which of the following is *safe?*
   a A vest restraint is applied with the "V" neck in the back.
   b Bed rails are left down when a vest restraint is used.
   c A jacket restraint is used to position a person on a toilet.
   d Limb holder straps are secured with quick release knots.

10 A restraint is applied to a person in bed. Where are the straps secured?
   a To the bed rails
   b To the head-board
   c To the movable part of the bed frame
   d To the foot-board

11 A person has a restraint. You check the person and the position of the restraint at least every
   a 15 minutes
   b 30 minutes
   c Hour
   d 3 hours

12 A person has mitt restraints. Which will you report to the nurse at once?
   a The hands are clean, warm, and dry.
   b The person has numbness in the hands.
   c You removed the restraints for 15 minutes.
   d You felt a pulse in both arms.

13 When applying restraints, you should
   a Know when to apply and release them
   b Use force if the person is agitated
   c Allow plenty of slack in the straps
   d Apply a restraint you have not used before

14 A person has a vest restraint. To check for snugness, slide
   a A fist between the vest and the person
   b 1 finger between the vest and the person
   c An open hand between the vest and the person
   d 3 fingers between the vest and the person

15 The correct way to apply any restraint is to follow the
   a Nurse's directions
   b Doctor's orders
   c Care plan
   d Manufacturer's instructions

Answers to Chapter 16 questions are on p. 902.

FOCUS ON **PRACTICE**

Problem Solving

A person uses a wheelchair and often tries to get up without help. The person is at risk for falls. What are some alternatives to restraints that may be tried?

   The health team considers using a lap-top tray with the person's wheelchair. How do you know if a device is a restraint?

OBJECTIVES

- Define the key terms and key abbreviations in this chapter.
- Identify places where microbes live and grow.
- List the signs and symptoms of infection.
- Explain the chain of infection.
- Describe healthcare-associated infections and the persons at risk.
- Explain the difference between medical and surgical asepsis.
- Identify aseptic practices used in the home and in health care settings.

- Explain the rules of hand hygiene.
- Identify 5 moments for hand hygiene during routine care.
- Explain how to care for equipment and supplies.
- Describe disinfection and sterilization methods.
- Explain the Bloodborne Pathogen Standard.
- Describe the principles of surgical asepsis.
- Perform the procedures described in this chapter.
- Explain how to promote PRIDE in the person, the family, and yourself.

KEY TERMS

antibiotic A drug that kills bacteria

antiseptic A substance applied to living tissue that prevents or stops the growth or action of microbes

asepsis The absence *(a)* of disease-producing microbes; *sepsis* means infection

biohazardous waste Items contaminated with blood or other potentially infectious materials (OPIM); regulated medical waste, infectious waste

bloodborne pathogens Microbes that are present in blood and can cause infection

carrier A human (or animal) that is a reservoir for microbes but does not develop the infection

clean technique See "medical asepsis"

communicable disease A disease caused by a pathogen that can spread to others; contagious disease

contagious disease See "communicable disease"

contamination The process of becoming unclean

cross-contamination Passing microbes from 1 person to another by contaminated hands, equipment, or supplies

disinfectant A liquid chemical that can kill many or all pathogens except spores

disinfection The process of killing pathogens

healthcare-associated infection (HAI) An infection that develops in a person cared for in any setting where health care is given; the infection is related to receiving health care

immunity Protection against a certain disease

infection A disease state resulting from the invasion and growth of microbes in the body

infection control Practices and procedures that prevent the spread of infection

medical asepsis Practices used to reduce the number of microbes and prevent their spread from 1 person or place to another person or place; clean technique

microbe See "microorganism"

microorganism A small *(micro)* living thing *(organism)* seen only with a microscope; microbe

non-pathogen A microbe that does not usually cause an infection

normal flora Microbes that live and grow in a certain area

pathogen A microbe that is harmful and can cause an infection

spore A bacterium protected by a hard shell

sterile The absence of *all* microbes

sterile field A work area free of *all* pathogens and non-pathogens (including spores)

sterile technique See "surgical asepsis"

sterilization The process of destroying *all* microbes

surgical asepsis Practices used to remove *all* microbes; sterile technique

vaccination Giving a vaccine to produce immunity against an infectious disease

vaccine A preparation containing dead or weakened microbes

vector An animal or insect that transmits disease

vehicle Any substance that transmits microbes

KEY ABBREVIATIONS

AIDS	Acquired immunodeficiency syndrome	**HIV**	Human immunodeficiency virus
CDC	Centers for Disease Control and Prevention	**MDRO**	Multidrug-resistant organism
C. diff	*Clostridioides difficile; Clostridium difficile*	**MRSA**	Methicillin-resistant *Staphylococcus aureus*
cm	Centimeter	**OPIM**	Other potentially infectious materials
E. coli	*Escherichia coli*	**OSHA**	Occupational Safety and Health Administration
EPA	Environmental Protection Agency	**PPE**	Personal protective equipment
GI	Gastro-intestinal	**VRE**	Vancomycin-resistant *Enterococcus*
HAI	Healthcare-associated infection	**WHO**	World Health Organization
HBV	Hepatitis B virus		

An *infection* is a disease state resulting from the invasion and growth of microbes in the body. Infection is a major safety and health hazard. Minor infections are short-term. However, some infections are serious and can cause death. Infants, older persons, and disabled persons are at risk. Certain practices and procedures prevent the spread of infection *(infection control)*. The goal is to protect patients, residents, visitors, and staff from infection.

MICROORGANISMS

A *microorganism (microbe)* is a small *(micro)* living thing *(organism)* seen only with a microscope. Commonly called *germs*, microbes are everywhere—mouth, nose, respiratory tract, stomach, and intestines. They are on the skin and in the air, soil, water, and food. They are on animals, clothing, and furniture. Some microbes are helpful. Others are harmful.

Non-Pathogens and Pathogens

Non-pathogens are microbes that do not usually cause an infection. Microbes that are harmful and can cause infections are called *pathogens*. There are different types of pathogens.

- *Bacteria*—small, 1-celled organisms. Bacteria have a variety of sizes, shapes, and arrangements (Fig. 17-1). Some produce resistant forms called spores. *Spores* are bacteria protected by a hard shell. They are hard to destroy. Bacteria can infect any body system. However, not all bacteria cause infection.
- *Viruses*—particles that multiply inside living cells. Viruses use the host cell to replicate (produce more viruses). New viruses exit the cell. The host cell is damaged or destroyed. Viruses cause many diseases including the common cold, influenza, herpes, acquired immunodeficiency syndrome (AIDS), and hepatitis.
- *Fungi*—plant-like organisms. They cannot produce their own food. They rely on other organisms for food. Yeast and mold are fungi. The skin, nails, and mucous membranes are common infection sites. Infections of the lungs, blood, and brain tissue can occur. *Candida* infections occur from the overgrowth of yeast. Infections can occur in the mouth and throat (thrush), esophagus, vagina, skin, and other body parts.
- *Protozoa*—1-celled organisms that are larger than bacteria. They can infect the blood, brain, intestines, and other body areas.

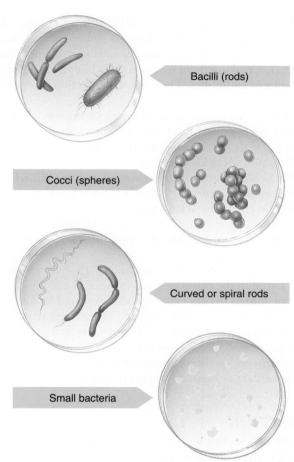

FIGURE 17-1 Bacteria vary in size and shape. They may be arranged as a single bacterium or in pairs, strings, or clusters. (Modified from Thibodeau G, Patton K: *The human body in health and disease*, ed 4, St Louis, 2005, Elsevier.)

Requirements of Microbes

Microbes need a reservoir. The *reservoir* is the place where the microbe lives and grows. People, plants, animals, the soil, food, and water are common reservoirs. Microbes can also live on wet or dry items and surfaces in the person's setting.

Microbes need *water* and *nourishment* from the reservoir. Most need *oxygen* to live (aerobic). Others do not (anaerobic). A *warm* and *dark* environment is needed. Most grow best at body temperature. They are destroyed by heat and light.

Normal Flora

Microbes that live and grow in a certain area are called *normal flora*. They are non-pathogens where they normally live and grow. When transmitted to another site or host, they become pathogens. For example, *Escherichia coli* (*E. coli*) is normally present in the colon. If it enters the urinary system, it can cause an infection.

Multidrug-Resistant Organisms

Multidrug-resistant organisms (MDROs) are microbes that can resist the effects of antibiotics. *Antibiotics* are drugs that kill bacteria. Sometimes bacteria can change their structures, making them harder to kill. They can live in the presence of antibiotics. Therefore the infections they cause are hard to treat.

MDROs are caused by prescribing antibiotics when not needed (over-prescribing). Not taking antibiotics for the length of time prescribed is another cause.

Common MDROs are:
- *Methicillin-resistant Staphylococcus aureus (MRSA)*. *Staphylococcus aureus* ("staph") is found in the nose and on the skin. MRSA is resistant to antibiotics often used for "staph" infections. MRSA can cause serious wound and bloodstream infections and pneumonia.
- *Vancomycin-resistant Enterococcus (VRE)*. *Enterococcus* is found in the intestines and in feces. It can be transmitted to other sites by contaminated hands, toilet seats, care equipment, and other items that the hands touch. Enterococci can cause urinary tract, wound, pelvic, and other infections. Enterococci resistant to vancomycin (an antibiotic) are called *vancomycin-resistant Enterococcus (VRE)*.

INFECTION

People can be sick with signs and symptoms of an infection. Or they can have a pathogen present but not have signs or symptoms. This is called *colonization*. A colonized person can still pass the microbe on to others.

For an infection to occur, microbes must enter the body, invade tissues, multiply, and cause the body to respond. A *localized infection* is in a body part. A *systemic infection* involves the whole body. (*Systemic* means entire.) The person has some or all of the signs and symptoms listed in Box 17-1.

See *Focus on Children and Older Persons: Infection*.
See *Focus on Surveys: Infection*.

BOX 17-1	Infection—Signs and Symptoms

- *Fever* (elevated body temperature)
- Pulse and respirations: increased
- Chills
- Pain, tenderness, or limited use of a body part
- Fatigue and loss of energy
- Appetite: loss of (*anorexia*)
- Nausea and vomiting
- Diarrhea
- Rash
- Sores on mucous membranes
- Redness and swelling of a body part
- Discharge or drainage from the infected area
- Heat or warmth in a body part
- Headache
- Muscle aches
- Joint pain
- Confusion

FOCUS ON CHILDREN AND OLDER PERSONS
Infection

Older Persons
The immune system protects the body from disease and infection (Chapter 10). Changes occur in this system with aging, making older persons at risk for infection.

An older person may not show the signs and symptoms in Box 17-1. The person may have a slight fever or no fever at all. Redness and swelling may be very slight. The person may not complain of pain. Confusion and delirium may occur (Chapter 54).

An infection can be life-threatening before the older person shows signs and symptoms. Report minor behavior or condition changes at once.

Healing takes longer in older persons. Therefore an infection can prolong rehabilitation. Independence and quality of life are affected.

FOCUS ON SURVEYS
Infection

Infection control practices are a focus of surveys. You may be asked about the signs and symptoms of infection.
- What you do when you observe them
- Who you tell

The Chain of Infection

Communicable diseases (contagious diseases) are diseases caused by pathogens that can spread to others. Understanding how infections occur can help prevent the spread of the pathogens that cause them.

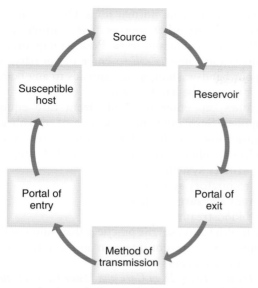

FIGURE 17-2 The chain of infection. (Redrawn and modified from Potter PA, Perry AG, Stockert PA, Hall AM: *Fundamentals of nursing*, ed 10, St Louis, 2021, Elsevier.)

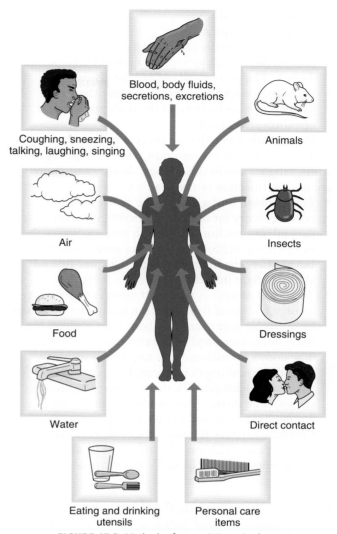

FIGURE 17-3 Methods of transmitting microbes.

The chain of infection explains how infections occur. See Figure 17-2. The chain of infection involves a:

- Source—A pathogen.
- Reservoir—The pathogen needs a place to grow and multiply. See "Requirements of Microbes." Human reservoirs (hosts) may or may not show signs of illness. A *carrier* is a human (or animal) that is a reservoir for microbes but does not develop the infection. A carrier is colonized with the microbe. Carriers can pass pathogens to others.
- Portal of exit—The pathogen needs a way to leave the reservoir. Pathogens can exit the body through blood and body fluids. The respiratory, gastro-intestinal (GI), urinary, and reproductive tracts and breaks in the skin are exit sites.
- Method of transmission—The pathogen is *transmitted* (moved) to another host (Fig. 17-3). See "Transmission."
- Portal of entry—The pathogen enters the body. Portals of entry and exit are the same—the respiratory, GI, urinary, and reproductive tracts; breaks in the skin; and blood. Mucous membranes at body openings are important natural entry sites.
- Susceptible host—The transmitted microbe needs a host where it can grow and multiply. Susceptible hosts are at risk for infection. See "Susceptible Hosts."

Transmission. A pathogen can be transmitted (moved) to a susceptible person in different ways. A person can have *direct contact* with the source through person-to-person contact. Or there can be *indirect contact* through another means.

- A *vehicle* is any substance that transmits microbes. Food, water, and objects and surfaces (fomites) are examples.
- A *vector* is an animal or insect that transmits disease. Mosquitos, ticks, and fleas are common vectors.

In health care settings, the major transmission methods are:

- *Contact (touch).* For example, staff touch an item or surface containing a pathogen and then give care without cleaning the hands.
- *Droplets (splashes or sprays).* This occurs through coughing and sneezing. Droplets carry microbes short distances. Microbes can transfer to another person's eyes, nose, or mouth.
- *Airborne (inhalation).* Some microbes can spread over longer distances through the air.
- *Sharps injuries.* The skin barrier is broken by a used needle or other used sharp instrument. Pathogens present in blood can transmit infections (p. 249).

Susceptible Hosts. Susceptible hosts include persons who:

- Were exposed to the pathogen.
- Are very young or who are older.
- Have other health problems.
- Have weakened immune systems.

So are persons who:
- Have poor nutrition.
- Are not immune (by vaccination or naturally). An *immune* person has protection against a certain disease. The person will not get the disease.
- Have extra ways for microbes to enter the body. Medical devices inserted in the body and surgical openings are examples.
- Do not follow practices to prevent infection.

The ability to resist infection relates to age, nutrition, stress, fatigue, and health. Drugs, disease, and injury also are factors. Infection can be deadly for:
- *Burn patients.* Burns destroy the skin, providing a portal of entry for microbes. Microbes are from the person's normal flora, the health care setting, or the health team. MRSA and VRE are great concerns. Burns affect the immune system (Chapter 10) and the ability to fight infection.
- *Transplant patients.* A *transplant* involves transferring an organ or tissue from 1 person to another person or from 1 body part to another body part. Kidney, liver, heart, lung, bone, and skin transplants are examples. The body's normal immune response is to attack (reject) the new organ or tissue. Drugs are given to prevent rejection. The drugs suppress (prevent) the immune system from producing antibodies. Antibodies are needed to fight infection.
- *Chemotherapy patients.* Some chemotherapy drugs given to treat cancer (Chapter 48) affect the production of white blood cells (WBCs). WBCs are needed to fight infection.

Healthcare-Associated Infections

A *healthcare-associated infection (HAI)* is an infection that develops in a person cared for in any setting where health care is given. The infection is related to receiving health care. (See Box 17-2 for examples.) HAIs also are called nosocomial infections. (*Nosocomial* comes from the Greek word for hospital.) HAIs can occur in any health care setting including hospitals, nursing centers, clinics, and home care settings.

BOX 17-2	Healthcare-Associated Infections: Examples

- *Clostridioides difficile* (also known as *Clostridium difficile* or *C. diff*)—Chapter 29
- Gastro-intestinal infections (norovirus)—Chapter 29
- Hepatitis A, B, and C—Chapter 51
- Human immunodeficiency virus (HIV)—Chapter 48
- Influenza—Chapter 50
- Methicillin-resistant *Staphylococcus aureus* (MRSA)—p. 238
- Tuberculosis (TB)—Chapter 50
- Vancomycin-resistant *Enterococcus* (VRE)—p. 238

Modified from Centers for Disease Control and Prevention: Healthcare-associated infections (HAI): diseases and organisms in healthcare settings, Atlanta, page reviewed October 7, 2019.

HAIs are caused by normal flora. Or they are caused by microbes from other sources. For example, *E. coli* is normally in the colon and feces. Poor wiping after bowel movements can cause *E. coli* to enter the urinary system. With poor hand-washing, *E. coli* spreads to any body part, thing, or person the hands touch.

Microbes can enter the body from care equipment and supplies. Such items must be free of microbes. Staff can transfer microbes from 1 person to another and from themselves to others. Common sites for HAIs are:
- The urinary system
- The respiratory system
- Wounds and surgical sites
- The bloodstream

The health team uses the practices that follow and those in Chapter 18 to prevent infection and stop the spread of infection once it occurs.

See *Focus on Long-Term Care and Home Care: Healthcare-Associated Infections.*

FOCUS ON LONG-TERM CARE AND HOME CARE

Healthcare-Associated Infections

Home Care

An HAI does not apply to every infection acquired by a home care patient. Rather, it applies to any infection associated with a medical, surgical, or nursing measure. It results from receiving care.

ASEPSIS

Microbes are everywhere. Measures are needed to prevent microbes from causing infection. *Asepsis* is the absence *(a)* of disease-producing microbes. (*Sepsis* means infection.) The health team practices measures to achieve asepsis.

Medical asepsis (clean technique) involves the practices used to:
- Reduce the number of microbes.
- Prevent microbes from spreading from 1 person or place to another person or place.

Extra precaution must be taken any time the skin or tissues are entered. During surgery is an example. *All* microbes must be removed, not just pathogens. *Surgical asepsis (sterile technique)* involves the practices used to remove *all* microbes. *Sterile* means the absence of *all* microbes. Pathogens and non-pathogens are removed.

Contamination is the process of becoming unclean.
- In medical asepsis, an item or area is *clean* when it is free of pathogens. The item or area is *contaminated* when pathogens are present.
- A sterile item or area is *contaminated* when pathogens or non-pathogens are present.

Cross-contamination is passing microbes from 1 person to another by contaminated hands, equipment, or supplies (Fig. 17-4). Medical asepsis and surgical asepsis (p. 252) prevent cross-contamination.

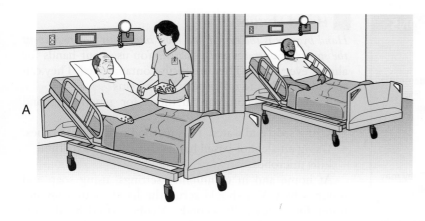

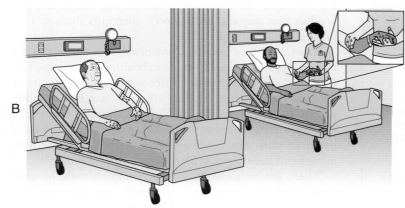

FIGURE 17-4 Cross-contamination. **A,** Microbes on the person's skin are transmitted to the nursing assistant's hands. **B,** The nursing assistant's contaminated hands transmit microbes from 1 person to another.

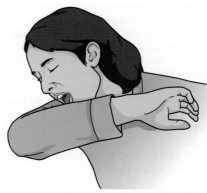

FIGURE 17-5 Sneezing into the upper arm.

Common Aseptic Practices

Aseptic practices break the chain of infection. You practice them in your daily life. You will learn how aseptic practices apply to your work. For example, to prevent the spread of microbes, you wash your hands:

* After elimination.
* After changing tampons or sanitary pads.
* After contact with your own or another person's blood or body fluids—saliva, vomit, urine, feces (stools), vaginal discharge, mucus, semen, wound drainage, pus, or respiratory secretions.
* After coughing, sneezing, or blowing your nose.
* Before and after handling, preparing, or eating food.
* After smoking.

These measures also protect yourself and others.

* Provide all persons with their own linens and personal care items.
* Cover your nose and mouth when coughing, sneezing, or blowing your nose. If without tissues, cough or sneeze into your upper arm (Fig. 17-5). Do not cough or sneeze into your hands.
* Bathe, wash hair, and brush your teeth regularly.
* Wash fruit and raw vegetables before eating or serving them.
* Wash cooking and eating utensils with soap and water after use.

See *Focus on Children and Older Persons: Common Aseptic Practices*, p. 242.

See *Focus on Long-Term Care and Home Care: Common Aseptic Practices*, p. 242.

FOCUS ON CHILDREN AND OLDER PERSONS
Common Aseptic Practices

Older Persons
Dementia can affect a person's judgment. Persons with dementia may no longer practice their own aseptic measures well. They need reminders and help. Assist them with hand-washing:
- After elimination
- After coughing, sneezing, or blowing the nose
- Before and after they eat or handle food
- Any time their hands are soiled
  Check and clean their hands and fingernails often. They may not tell you when soiling occurs. Some are unable to tell you.

FOCUS ON LONG-TERM CARE AND HOME CARE
Common Aseptic Practices

Home Care
You must prevent the spread of microbes in home settings. Also, protect the person from microbes brought into the home. Common aseptic measures are needed. See "Supplies and Equipment" on p. 247 and "Other Aseptic Measures" on p. 248. Also protect the person from foodborne illnesses (Chapter 31).

Microbes easily grow and spread in bathrooms. The entire family must help keep the bathroom clean. Aseptic measures are needed when the bathroom is used.
- Flush the toilet after each use.
- Rinse the sink after washing, shaving, or oral hygiene.
- Wipe out the tub or shower after each use.
- Remove and dispose of hair from the sink, tub, or shower.
- Hang towels to dry. Or place them in a hamper.
- Wipe up spills—water, personal care products, and so on.
  Wear utility gloves to clean bathrooms. Use a disinfectant or water and detergent to clean all surfaces.
- Toilet surfaces—bowl, seat, and all outside areas
- The floor
- The shower or tub
- Towel racks
- Toilet paper holder, toothbrush holder, and soap holders
- The mirror (use a glass cleaner)
- The sink
- Window sills
  To clean bathrooms, you also need to:
- Mop uncarpeted floors. Vacuum carpeted floors.
- Empty wastebaskets.
- Put out clean towels and washcloths.
- Open bathroom windows for a short time and use air fresheners. These actions reduce odors and provide a fresh smell.
- Wash bath mats, the wastebasket, and the laundry hamper weekly.
- Replace toilet paper and facial tissue as needed.
  The care plan and assignment sheet tell you when to clean other areas of the home. For general housekeeping:
- Wipe up spills right away.
- Dust furniture and blinds.
- Vacuum or mop floors. Damp-mop uncarpeted floors at least weekly.
- Sweep daily or more often if needed. Use a dustpan to collect dust, crumbs, and other things swept up.
- Wash clothes and linens.

Hand Hygiene

Hand hygiene is the easiest and most important way to prevent the spread of microbes and infection. You use your hands for almost everything. They are easily contaminated. They can spread microbes to other persons or items (see Fig. 17-4).

There are 2 common methods for practicing hand hygiene.
- Using soap and water. This method removes microbes.
- Using an alcohol-based hand sanitizer. This method kills microbes.

At home and in community settings, using soap and water is best. You should scrub the hands with soap and water for at least 20 seconds. Alcohol-based hand sanitizer is useful when soap and water are not available. Use a product that contains at least 60% (percent) alcohol. This is listed on the product's label.

The Centers for Disease Control and Prevention (CDC) has guidelines for hand hygiene in health care settings. The CDC recommends the use of alcohol-based hand sanitizer for most health care situations (unless hands are visibly soiled). According to the CDC, hand sanitizer is effective at reducing the number of microbes that may be on the hands of staff. Also, staff are often more compliant with using hand sanitizer compared to soap and water.

There are times when soap and water should be used instead of hand sanitizer in health care settings. See Box 17-3 for the rules of hand hygiene.

See *Focus on Surveys: Hand Hygiene.*
See *Promoting Safety and Comfort: Hand Hygiene.*
See procedure: *Hand-Washing,* p. 245.
See procedure: *Using an Alcohol-Based Hand Sanitizer,* p. 245.

FOCUS ON SURVEYS
Hand Hygiene

Hand hygiene is a focus of surveys. A surveyor may:
- Observe how you wash your hands or use an alcohol-based hand sanitizer.
- Observe when you practice hand hygiene.
- Ask you questions about:
  - When to wash your hands with soap and water
  - When to use an alcohol-based hand sanitizer

PROMOTING SAFETY AND COMFORT
Hand Hygiene

Safety
Hand hygiene is very important. Your hands can pick up microbes from a person, place, or thing and transfer them to other people, places, or things. Know when to practice hand hygiene (see Box 17-3 and p. 246). Be careful and thorough.

Comfort
You will practice hand hygiene frequently during your shift. Hand lotions and hand creams help prevent chapping and dry skin. Use an agency-approved lotion or cream.

BOX 17-3	**Rules for Hand Hygiene in Health Care Settings**

When to Use Soap and Water

Wash your hands (with soap and water):

- When they are visibly dirty or soiled. Soiling may be from blood or a body fluid. Body fluids include secretions such as saliva or nasal secretions and excretions such as urine, feces (stools), or vomit.
- Before eating.
- After using the restroom.
- After caring for a person with known or suspected infectious diarrhea. *Clostridioides difficile (C. diff)* and norovirus are discussed in Chapter 29.
- After known or suspected exposure to spores. *C. diff* and anthrax spores are examples.
- If an alcohol-based hand sanitizer is not available.

When to Use Alcohol-Based Hand Sanitizer

Use an alcohol-based hand sanitizer for hand hygiene if your hands are not visibly soiled:

- Before touching a patient or resident.
- Before performing a clean or aseptic task. Such tasks involve contact with mucous membranes, non-intact skin, or an invasive medical device. (*Invasive* means entering the body.)
- Before moving from a soiled body site to a clean body site on the same person.
- After contact with blood, body fluids, or contaminated items or surfaces.
- After touching a patient or resident.
- After touching items close to a patient or resident. This includes equipment.
- After removing gloves.

How to Use Soap and Water

Follow these rules for washing your hands with soap and water. See procedure: *Hand-Washing*, p. 245.

- Wash your hands under warm running water. Do not use hot water.
- Stand away from the sink. Do not let your hands, body, or uniform touch the sink. The sink is contaminated. See Figure 17-6.
- Do not touch the inside of the sink at any time.
- Keep your hands and forearms lower than your elbows. If you hold your hands and forearms up, dirty water runs from your hands to your forearms and elbows. Those areas become contaminated.

How to Use Soap and Water—cont'd

- Wet your hands with water first. Then apply the amount of soap recommended by the manufacturer.
- Rub your palms together (Fig. 17-7, p. 244) and interlace your fingers (Fig. 17-8, p. 244) to work up a good lather. The rubbing action helps remove microbes and dirt.
- Pay attention to areas often missed during hand-washing—thumbs, knuckles, sides of the hands, little fingers, and under the nails.
- Clean fingernails by rubbing the fingertips against your palms (Fig. 17-9, p. 244).
- Use a nail file or orangewood stick to clean under fingernails (Fig. 17-10, p. 244). Microbes grow easily under the fingernails.
- Wash your hands for at least 20 seconds. Wash longer if they are dirty or soiled. Use your judgment and follow agency policy.
- Use clean, dry paper towels to dry your hands.
- Dry your hands starting at the fingertips. Work up to your forearms (Fig. 17-11, p. 244). You will dry the cleanest area first.
- Use a clean, dry paper towel to turn the water off (Fig. 17-12, p. 244). Faucets are contaminated. The paper towel prevents you from contaminating your clean hands.

How to Use Alcohol-Based Hand Sanitizer

Follow these rules when decontaminating your hands with an alcohol-based hand sanitizer. See procedure: *Using an Alcohol-Based Hand Sanitizer*, p. 245.

- Apply the product to the palm of 1 hand. Follow the manufacturer's instructions for the amount to use.
- Rub your hands together.
- Cover all surfaces of your hands and fingers.
- Continue rubbing your hands together until your hands are dry. It should take about 20 seconds.

Lotions and Creams

- Use hand lotion or cream to prevent the skin from chapping and drying. Skin breaks can occur in chapped and dry skin. Skin breaks are portals of entry for microbes.
- Use an agency-approved lotion. Other lotions can interfere with hand sanitizing products.

Modified from Centers for Disease Control and Prevention: Guidelines for hand hygiene in health-care settings, *Morbidity and Mortality Weekly, Report 51 (RR-16), October 2002. (*NOTE: *Updated from Centers for Disease Control and Prevention:* Frequent questions about hand hygiene, *last reviewed November 4, 2022, and* Hand hygiene in healthcare settings: healthcare providers, *last reviewed January 8, 2021.)*

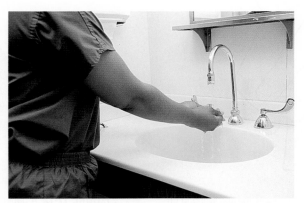

FIGURE 17-6 The uniform does not touch the sink. Hands are lower than the elbows. Hands do not touch the inside of the sink.

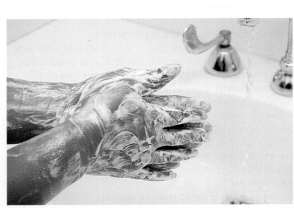

FIGURE 17-7 The palms are rubbed together to work up a good lather.

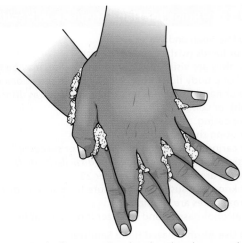

FIGURE 17-8 The fingers are interlaced to clean between the fingers.

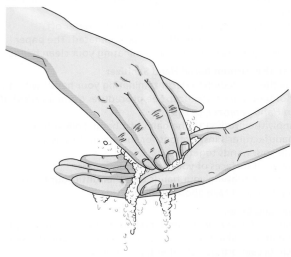

FIGURE 17-9 The fingertips are rubbed against the palms to clean under the fingernails.

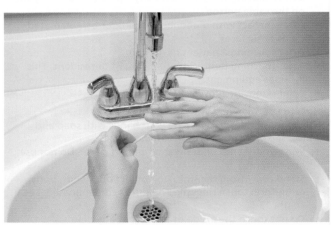

FIGURE 17-10 An orangewood stick is used to clean under the fingernails.

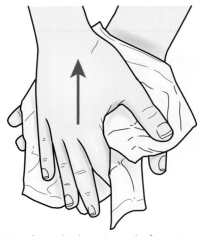

FIGURE 17-11 Hands are dried starting at the fingertips and working up to the forearms.

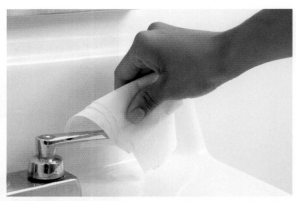

FIGURE 17-12 A paper towel is used to turn off the faucet.

Hand-Washing

PROCEDURE

1 See *Promoting Safety and Comfort: Hand Hygiene*, p. 242.
2 Make sure you have soap, paper towels, an orangewood stick or nail file, and a wastebasket. Get any missing items.
3 Push your watch up your arm 4 to 5 inches. Push long uniform sleeves up too.
4 Stand away from the sink so your clothes do not touch the sink (see Fig. 17-6). Stand so the soap and faucet are easy to reach. Do not touch the inside of the sink at any time.
5 Turn on and adjust the water until it feels warm.
6 Wet your wrists and hands. Keep your hands lower than your elbows. Be sure to wet the area 3 to 4 inches above your wrists.
7 Apply about 1 teaspoon of soap to your hands. Follow the manufacturer's instructions for the amount to use.
8 Rub your palms together and interlace your fingers to work up a good lather (see Fig. 17-7). Lather your wrists, hands, and fingers. Keep your hands lower than your elbows. Steps 8 through 10 should last at least 20 seconds.

9 Wash each hand and wrist thoroughly. Clean the back of your fingers and between your fingers (see Fig. 17-8).
10 Clean under the fingernails. Rub your fingertips against your palms (see Fig. 17-9).
11 Clean under the fingernails with a nail file or orangewood stick (see Fig. 17-10). Do this for the first hand-washing of the day and when your hands are visibly soiled.
12 Rinse your wrists, hands, and fingers well. Water flows from above the wrists to your fingertips.
13 Repeat steps 7 through 12, if needed.
14 Dry your fingers, hands, and wrists with clean, dry paper towels. Pat dry starting at your fingertips (see Fig. 17-11).
15 Discard used paper towels into the wastebasket.
16 Use a clean, dry paper towel to turn off the water. This prevents you from contaminating your clean hands (see Fig. 17-12). Or use knee or foot controls to turn off the faucet.
17 Discard the paper towel into the wastebasket.

Using an Alcohol-Based Hand Sanitizer

PROCEDURE

1 See *Promoting Safety and Comfort: Hand Hygiene*, p. 242.
2 Apply a palmful of an alcohol-based hand sanitizer into a cupped hand (Fig. 17-13). Follow the manufacturer's instructions for the amount to use.
3 Rub your hands together. Cover all surfaces of the hands and fingers (see Fig. 17-13).
  a Rub your palms together.
  b Rub the palm of 1 hand over the back of the other. Do the same for the other hand.

  c Rub your palms together with your fingers interlaced.
  d Interlock your fingers. Rub your fingers back and forth.
  e Rub the thumb of 1 hand in the palm of the other. Do the same for the other thumb.
  f Rub the fingers of 1 hand into the palm of the other hand. Use a circular motion. Do the same for the fingers of the other hand.
4 Continue rubbing your hands until they are dry.

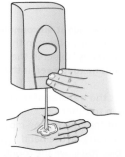
Apply a palmful of an alcohol-based hand sanitizer into a cupped hand.

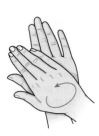
Rub the palms together.

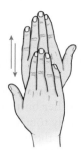
Rub the palm of 1 hand over the back of the other hand. Repeat for the other hand.

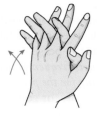
Rub the palms together with the fingers interlaced.

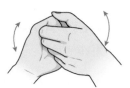
Interlock the fingers and rub back and forth.

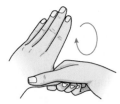
Rub the thumb of 1 hand in the palm of the other hand. Repeat for the other thumb.

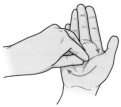
Rub the fingers of 1 hand into the palm of the other hand with circular motions. Repeat for the fingers on the other hand.

FIGURE 17-13 Using an alcohol-based hand sanitizer.

Your 5 Moments for Hand Hygiene

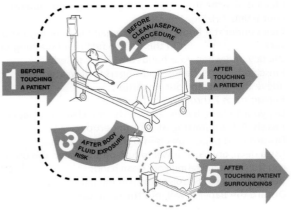

FIGURE 17-14 WHO's 5 Moments for Hand Hygiene. (NOTE: Dashed lines mark the separation of the zones. The "patient zone" is within the dashed lines. The "health-care area" is outside the dashed lines.) (From World Health Organization, *SAVE LIVES: Clean your hands, 2024.*)

Moments for Hand Hygiene. The World Health Organization (WHO) has promoted "5 Moments for Hand Hygiene" in an effort to improve health care worker hand hygiene (Fig. 17-14). The WHO's model describes 2 "zones"—the "patient zone" and the "health-care area."

The "patient zone" includes the patient or resident and the person's close surroundings. This zone typically involves a bed. However, it also applies to other situations. A patient or resident seated in a chair is an example. The "patient zone" involves:

- *The person*
- *Items the person touches or has direct contact with*—bed rails, the bedside table, bed linens, medical equipment near the person
- *Objects frequently touched by health care workers while caring for the person*—bed controls; other buttons, monitors, or controls; other frequently touched objects

In the "patient zone," it is assumed that the person's normal flora quickly contaminate the area. Also, that area is cleaned before another patient or resident uses it.

The "health-care area" includes all objects outside of the "patient zone." The health care facility and other patients or residents within their "patient zones" are part of the "health-care area." The "health-care area" is considered to be contaminated with microbes that may be harmful if brought into a "patient zone."

The WHO has identified 5 moments when hand hygiene is essential. See Box 17-4 and Figure 17-14. During routine care, always practice hand hygiene at these times. If 2 moments occur together, a single act of hand hygiene covers both moments.

See *Promoting Safety and Comfort: Moments for Hand Hygiene.*

BOX 17-4	WHO's 5 Moments for Hand Hygiene

Moment 1: Before Touching a Patient or Resident
- This moment occurs between the last contact with an object in the health care area and the first contact with the person.
- This protects the person. It prevents the transfer of microbes from the health care setting to the person.
- For example, you touch the door handle to enter the room. You practice hand hygiene before touching the arm to check the person's identification (ID) bracelet.

Moment 2: Before a Clean/Aseptic Procedure
- This moment occurs between the last contact with any object (even within the patient zone) and before a task involving contact with mucous membranes, non-intact skin, or invasive medical devices.
- This protects the person. It prevents the transfer of microbes to a site that can cause an infection.
- For example, you had contact with items near the person. You practice hand hygiene immediately before performing oral care.

Moment 3: After Body Fluid Exposure Risk
- This moment occurs after a task that exposes the hands to body fluids. Hand hygiene must occur before contact with any other object (even within the patient zone).
- This protects the person and others. It prevents transmission of microbes between a soiled and a clean body site on the same person. It also prevents the transfer of microbes to the health care worker and then to others.
- For example, you had contact with urine during bathing. You practice hand hygiene before touching clean clothes to dress the person.

Moment 4: After Touching a Patient or Resident
- This moment occurs after contact with the person and before touching an object in the health care area.
- This protects others. It prevents the transfer of microbes to the health care area and then to others.
- For example, you turn and re-position a patient. You practice hand hygiene after touching the person. You leave the room.

Moment 5: After Touching Patient or Resident Surroundings
- This moment occurs after touching any object in the patient zone and before touching any object in the health care area. Hand hygiene is needed even if the person is not touched.
- This protects others. It prevents the transfer of microbes to the health care area and then to others.
- For example, you bring a resident fresh water and move the over-bed table closer to the bed. You practice hand hygiene after touching the over-bed table. You leave the room.

Modified from World Health Organization: WHO guidelines on hand hygiene in health care, *2009.*

PROMOTING SAFETY AND COMFORT
Moments for Hand Hygiene

Safety
Depending on the procedure and care setting, some supplies and equipment are gathered in the "health care area" before entering the "patient zone." For the procedures in this book, hand hygiene is indicated at the following times when supplies are likely to be gathered in the "health care area":
- Before gathering supplies and equipment
- Before touching the person

Supplies and Equipment

Disposable supplies and equipment help prevent the spread of infection. Discard single-use items after use. A person uses multi-use items many times. They include plastic bed-pans, urinals, wash basins, and water mugs. Label multi-use items with the person's name and room and bed number. Do not "borrow" them for another person.

Non-disposable items are cleaned and then disinfected. Items requiring sterilization are sterilized, usually by the supply department.

Cleaning.

Cleaning reduces the number of microbes present. It also removes organic matter such as food, blood, and body fluids. *Organic matter* comes from living plants and animals and will decay.

To clean equipment:

- Wear personal protective equipment (PPE) to clean items contaminated with blood or body fluids. PPE includes gloves, a mask, a gown, and goggles or a face shield. See Chapter 18.
- Work from *clean* to *dirty* areas. If you work from a *dirty* to *clean* area, the *clean* area becomes contaminated (*dirty*).
- Rinse the item in cold water to remove organic matter. Heat makes organic matter thick, sticky, and hard to remove.
- Wash the item with soap and hot water.
- Scrub thoroughly. Use a brush if necessary.
- Rinse the item in warm water.
- Follow agency procedures for drying, disinfection, or sterilization as needed.
- Follow agency procedures to clean and disinfect equipment and the sink used for cleaning.
- Discard PPE.
- Practice hand hygiene.

Disinfection.

Disinfection is the process of killing pathogens. Spores (p. 237) are not destroyed. Spores are killed by very high temperatures.

Disinfectants are used for objects and surfaces. A *disinfectant* is a liquid chemical that can kill many or all pathogens except spores. Disinfectants are used to clean counters, tubs, showers, and re-usable items. Such items include:

- Blood pressure cuffs
- Commodes and bedpans
- Shower chairs
- Wheelchairs and stretchers
- Furniture

Federal laws require that all disinfectants be registered with the United States Environmental Protection Agency (EPA). See Figure 17-15 for how to read a disinfectant label.

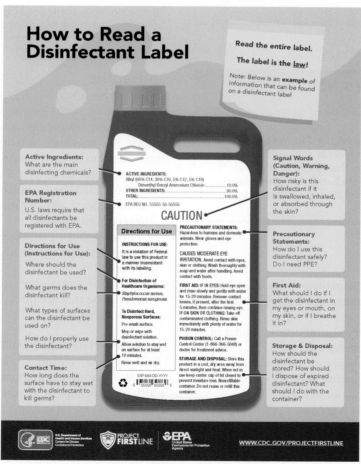

FIGURE 17-15 How to read a disinfectant label. (From United States Environmental Protection Agency and Centers for Disease Control and Prevention, Department of Health and Human Services.)

Agencies have policies and procedures for cleaning and disinfection. A disinfectant needs to remain wet on the object or surface for a certain length of time *(contact time)* to kill microbes. Follow agency practices and the product manufacturer's instructions for disinfectant use.

See *Focus on Long-Term Care and Home Care: Disinfection.*
See *Promoting Safety and Comfort: Disinfection.*

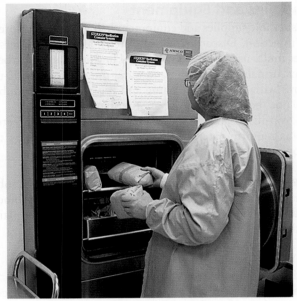

FIGURE 17-16 An autoclave.

FOCUS ON LONG-TERM CARE AND HOME CARE

Disinfection

Home Care
Detergent and hot water are used for cooking, eating, and drinking utensils and linens. Household disinfectants are used for surfaces—floors, toilets, tubs, and showers. Use the products the family prefers or as the nurse instructs.

A bleach solution may be used in home settings. Follow the directions on the product label to make a bleach solution. The CDC recommends the following measurements if the product does not have directions. Use 5 tablespoons (⅓ cup) of bleach to 1 gallon of water. Or use 4 teaspoons of bleach to 1 quart of water. Use room temperature water. Follow the manufacturer's instructions for applying the solution to surfaces. Bleach solutions are less effective after 24 hours. A new solution must be made daily. Do not mix bleach (or any disinfectant) with other cleaners or disinfectants.

FOCUS ON LONG-TERM CARE AND HOME CARE

Sterilization

Home Care
Sterilizing requires the use of special equipment. Sterile items needed in the home are purchased as sterile.

PROMOTING SAFETY AND COMFORT

Disinfection

Safety
Disinfectants can burn and irritate the skin. Wear gloves to prevent skin irritation. Utility gloves or rubber household gloves provide more protection than disposable gloves.

Read the product label before handling a disinfectant. Follow the directions for use and storage. Store products safely (Chapter 14).

Sterilization. *Sterilization* is the process of destroying *all* microbes. Non-pathogens, pathogens, and spores are destroyed. Very high temperatures are used. Heat destroys microbes.

Liquid or gas chemicals, dry heat, and steam under pressure are sterilization methods. An *autoclave* (Fig. 17-16) is a pressure steam sterilizer. Glass, surgical items, and metal items are autoclaved. High temperatures destroy plastic and rubber items. They are not autoclaved.

See *Focus on Long-Term Care and Home Care: Sterilization.*

Antiseptics

An *antiseptic* is a substance applied to living tissue that prevents or stops the growth or action of microbes. (*Anti* means against. *Sepsis* means infection.) The substance either inhibits the microbe's activity or destroys the microbe. Antiseptics can be used on the skin or mucous membranes.

Antiseptic products have a variety of uses. For example:
- Alcohol-based hand sanitizer is used during routine care.
- An antiseptic is applied to a patient's skin before surgery (Chapter 40).
- A nurse applies an antiseptic to the area around a patient's urethra before inserting a urinary catheter (Chapter 28).
- You use antiseptic wipes to clean the parts of your stethoscope that are placed in your ears and on the person (Chapter 34).

Other Aseptic Measures

Hand hygiene, cleaning, disinfection, sterilization, and antiseptic use are important aseptic measures used in health care settings. So are the measures listed in Box 17-5. They are also useful in home settings and in every-day life.

BOX 17-5 Aseptic Measures

Controlling Reservoirs (You, the Person, and the Person's Setting)
- Provide for hygiene needs (Chapters 23 and 24).
- Wash contaminated areas with soap and water. Feces (stools), urine, blood and other body fluids (including secretions and excretions) can contain microbes.
- Use leak-proof plastic bags for soiled tissues, linens, and other items.
- Keep tables, counters, wheelchair trays, and other surfaces clean and dry.
- Keep linens clean and dry.
- Label bottles with the person's name and the date the bottle was opened.
- Keep bottles and fluid containers tightly capped or covered.
- Keep drainage containers below the drainage site (Chapters 28 and 41).
- Empty drainage containers and dispose of drainage following agency policy. Usually drainage containers are emptied every shift. The nurse may have you empty them more often.
- Follow agency practices to clean and disinfect objects and surfaces in the health care setting.

Controlling Transmission
- Provide all persons with their own personal care equipment. This includes wash basins, bedpans, urinals, commodes, and eating and drinking utensils.
- Do not take equipment from 1 person's room to use for another person. Even if un-used, do not take the item from 1 room to another.
- Hold equipment and linens away from your uniform (Fig. 17-17).
- Practice hand hygiene. See Box 17-3.
- Assist the person with hand-washing.
  - Before and after eating
  - After elimination
  - After changing tampons, sanitary napkins, or other personal hygiene products
  - After contact with blood or body fluids (including secretions or excretions)
- Prevent dust movement. Do not shake linens or equipment. Use a damp cloth for dusting.
- Clean from *clean* to *dirty* areas to prevent soiling a clean area.

Controlling Transmission—cont'd
- Clean away from your body. Do not dust, brush, or wipe toward yourself. Otherwise you transmit microbes to your skin, hair, and clothing.
- Flush urine and feces (stools) down the toilet. Avoid splatters and splashes.
- Pour contaminated liquids directly into sinks or toilets as appropriate. Avoid splashing onto other areas.
- Do not sit on the person's bed or chair. You will pick up microbes and transfer them to other surfaces that you sit on.
- Do not use items on the floor. The floor is contaminated.
- Follow agency cleaning and disinfection procedures for:
  - Items used for more than 1 person. Tubs, showers, and shower chairs are examples.
  - Items soiled with body fluids. Bedpans, urinals, and commodes are examples.
  - Items and surfaces that are touched often.
- Report pests—ants, spiders, mice, and so on.

Controlling Portals of Exit and Entry
- Provide good oral hygiene and skin care (Chapters 23 and 24). This promotes intact skin and mucous membranes.
- Protect the skin from injury.
  - Do not let the person lie on tubes or other items.
  - Make sure linens are dry and wrinkle-free (Chapter 22).
  - Turn and re-position the person as directed by the nurse and care plan (Chapters 19 and 20).
- Assist with or clean the genital area after elimination. (See "Perineal Care" in Chapter 24.) Wipe and clean from the urethra (cleanest area) to the rectum (dirtiest area). This helps prevent urinary tract infections.
- Cover the nose and mouth to cough or sneeze. Provide tissues. Discard tissues after use.
- Make sure drainage tubes are properly connected. This prevents microbes from entering the drainage system.
- Wear PPE as needed (Chapter 18).

Protecting the Susceptible Host
- Follow the care plan to meet nutrition and fluid needs (Chapters 30, 31, 32, and 33). This helps prevent infection.
- Assist with deep-breathing and coughing exercises as directed (Chapter 44). This helps prevent respiratory infections.

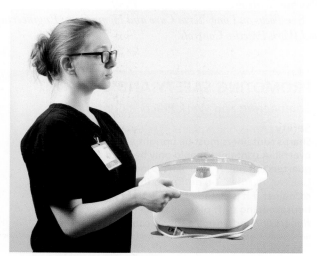

FIGURE 17-17 Hold equipment away from your uniform.

BLOODBORNE PATHOGEN STANDARD

Bloodborne pathogens are microbes that are present in blood and can cause infection. The human immunodeficiency virus (HIV) and the hepatitis B virus (HBV) are examples (Chapters 48 and 51). Persons who come into contact with bloodborne pathogens are at risk for infection and illness.

The goal of the Occupational Safety and Health Administration (OSHA) is to ensure safe working conditions. The *Bloodborne Pathogen Standard* is a regulation of OSHA. It protects the health team from exposure to bloodborne pathogens.

The standard has requirements for employers to follow in order to protect workers who may be exposed to blood or other potentially infectious materials (OPIM) in their work. OPIM may contain blood. Body fluids such as semen, vaginal secretions, saliva in dental procedures, and any body fluid visibly contaminated with blood are some OPIM.

The following body fluids are generally *not* considered OPIM—urine, feces (stools), nasal secretions, sputum, vomit, breast-milk, and saliva (other than in dental procedures). Standard Precautions (Chapter 18) are used for contact with such body fluids. Standard Precautions assume that every person is infected or colonized with a pathogen that can be transmitted in the health care setting. Precautions are used when handling such body fluids. However, they are generally not considered a source of bloodborne pathogens unless blood is visible. See "Standard Precautions" in Chapter 18.

Staff at risk for exposure to blood or OPIM receive free training. It occurs upon employment and yearly. Training is also done for new or changed tasks involving exposure to bloodborne pathogens.

Infection prevention and follow-up measures in the Bloodborne Pathogen Standard include:

* Vaccination against hepatitis B
* Engineering and work practice controls to reduce exposure
* The use of personal protective equipment (PPE)
* Regulations for equipment, work surfaces, biohazardous waste, and laundry
* Requirements for exposure incidents

See *Promoting Safety and Comfort: Bloodborne Pathogen Standard*.

PROMOTING SAFETY AND COMFORT
Bloodborne Pathogen Standard

Safety
The agency identifies staff at risk for exposure to blood or OPIM. All caregivers and laundry, supply, and housekeeping staffs are at risk. Training includes:
* The causes, signs, and symptoms of bloodborne diseases
* How bloodborne pathogens are spread
* The tasks that might cause exposure
* The use and limits of safe work practices and PPE
* Information about the hepatitis B vaccination
* Who to contact and what to do in an emergency
* Information on reporting an exposure incident, post-exposure evaluation, and follow-up

Hepatitis B Vaccination

A *vaccination* involves giving a vaccine to produce immunity against an infectious disease. *Immunity* means that a person has protection against a certain disease. A *vaccine* is a preparation containing dead or weakened microbes. The hepatitis B vaccine produces immunity against hepatitis B.

The hepatitis B vaccination involves 3 injections (shots). Injection 2 is given 1 month after the first. Injection 3 is given 6 months after the first. The vaccination can be given before or after HBV exposure.

The agency must offer the hepatitis B vaccination after you are trained about the vaccine and within 10 days of your first working day. The agency pays for it. You can refuse the vaccination. If so, you must sign a statement refusing the vaccine. You can have the vaccination at a later date if you want.

Engineering and Work Practice Controls

Engineering controls isolate or remove bloodborne pathogen hazards from the workplace. For example, broken glass is safely cleaned up and discarded using a brush and dust pan. Pieces are placed in a puncture-resistant container. The hands (even gloved hands) are not used to pick up broken glass.

Work practice controls reduce the likelihood of exposure. All tasks involving blood or OPIM are done in ways to limit splatters, splashes, and sprays. Producing droplets also is avoided.

Health care workers:
* Do not eat, drink, smoke, apply cosmetics or lip balm, or handle contact lenses in areas of exposure.
* Do not store food or drinks where blood or OPIM are kept.
* Practice hand hygiene after removing gloves.
* Wash hands as soon as possible after skin contact with blood or OPIM.
* Never re-cap, bend, or remove needles by hand. A mechanical means (forceps) or a 1-handed method is used.
* Never shear or break needles.
* Discard needles and sharp instruments (such as razors) in containers that are closable, puncture-resistant, and leak-proof. Containers have the *BIOHAZARD* symbol. The color red is used to designate a hazard. See Figure 17-18.

See *Promoting Safety and Comfort: Engineering and Work Practice Controls*.

See *Focus on Long-Term Care and Home Care: Engineering and Work Practice Controls*.

PROMOTING SAFETY AND COMFORT
Engineering and Work Practice Controls

Safety
Sharps containers must be upright and not allowed to overfill. A container should only be filled about three quarters (¾) full. A "full" line is indicated on the label (see Fig. 17-18, *B*). Do not try to fit 1 more item in the container if it is already too full. Notify the nurse or housekeeping staff of a full container. *Never stick your fingers or hands inside a sharps container.*

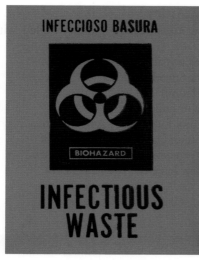 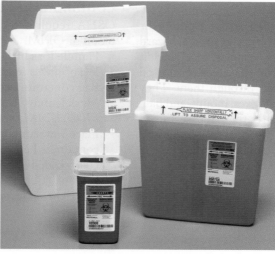 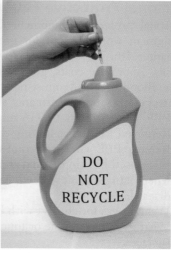

A B C

FIGURE 17-18 **A,** *BIOHAZARD* symbol. **B,** FDA-cleared sharps containers. **C,** Household disposable sharps container labeled with "Do Not Recycle." The needle with syringe is inserted "point first." (NOTE: "FDA" stands for Food and Drug Administration.) (B, From Warekois RS, Robinson R, Primrose PB: *Phlebotomy worktext and procedures manual*, ed 5, St Louis, 2020, Elsevier.)

FOCUS ON LONG-TERM CARE AND HOME CARE

Engineering and Work Practice Controls

Home Care

Sharp instruments are used in home care. The patient or family may use syringes and needles. You may use safety razors for shaving (Chapter 25) and lancets for blood glucose testing (Chapter 39). Proper disposal:

- Protects neighbors, children, pets, janitors, housekeepers, sanitation workers, and sewage treatment workers from injury and infection.
- Prevents needle sharing and re-using sharps.
- Protects the environment.

According to the EPA and the Food and Drug Administration (FDA):

- Do not throw loose needles, syringes, or sharps into the trash.
- Do not flush needles, syringes, or sharps down the toilet.
- Do not put needles, syringes, or sharps in recycling containers.
- Properly store used needles, syringes, and sharps. Put them in an FDA-cleared sharps container right after use. If not available, a hard plastic household container is an alternative (see Fig. 17-18, C). The container must be puncture-resistant and leak-proof with a secure, puncture-resistant lid. The container must remain upright during use. Detergent bottles with screw-on lids may be used.
  - Label the container with a "Do Not Recycle" or "SHARPS" label.
  - Put sharps in the container point-first.
  - Do not use containers that break or puncture easily—milk cartons, water bottles, soda cans, and glass containers.
  - Keep storage containers where children cannot reach them.
  - When the container is three quarters (¾) full, secure the lid in place with heavy tape for added protection.

For sharps container disposal, the nurse and care plan tell you what to use at the person's address. The EPA describes these disposal options.

- *Drop-off collection sites.* Sharps containers are taken to a collection site. Hospitals, doctors' offices, clinics, pharmacies, health departments, and police and fire stations are examples. So are medical waste facilities.
- *Household hazardous waste collection sites.* Sharps containers are taken to a collection site that accepts other household hazardous waste.
- *Residential special waste pick-up services.* Some communities offer pick-up services. There may be regular pick-up times or the person calls for pick-up.
- *Syringe-exchange programs.* Used needles and syringes are exchanged for new ones. The agency operating the program disposes of used ones.
- *Mail-back programs.* Used sharps are placed in special containers and mailed to a collection site. U.S. Postal Service procedures are followed. The program works well for rural areas.
- *Home needle destruction devices.* Such devices clip, melt, or burn the needle. The syringe and destroyed needle are placed in the trash.

Some states allow household sharps containers to be discarded in regular trash. In some areas, this is not legal. Follow community guidelines. Do not recycle a household sharps container.

Personal Protective Equipment

Personal protective equipment (PPE) is the clothing or equipment worn by staff for protection against a hazard (Chapter 18). This includes gloves, goggles, face shields, masks, laboratory coats, gowns, shoe covers, and surgical caps. Blood or OPIM must not pass through them. They protect clothes, under-garments, skin, eyes, mouth, and hair.

PPE is free to staff. OSHA requires these measures.
- Remove PPE before leaving the work area.
- Remove PPE when it becomes contaminated.
- Place used PPE in marked areas or containers when being stored, washed, decontaminated, or discarded.
- Wear gloves for contact with blood or OPIM.
- Wear gloves to handle or touch contaminated items or surfaces.
- Replace worn, punctured, or contaminated gloves.
- Never wash or decontaminate disposable gloves for re-use.
- Discard utility gloves that show signs of cracking, peeling, tearing, or puncturing. Utility gloves are decontaminated for re-use if the process will not ruin them.

Equipment and Work Surfaces

Contaminated equipment and work surfaces are cleaned and decontaminated with a proper disinfectant.
- Upon completing tasks
- At once for obvious contamination
- At the end of your work shift when surfaces became contaminated since the last cleaning

Biohazardous Waste

Some waste is hazardous. Also known as *regulated medical waste* or *infectious waste*, **biohazardous waste** involves items contaminated with blood or other potentially infectious materials (OPIM). (*Bio* means life. *Hazardous* means dangerous or harmful.) Such waste requires special handling.

Closable, leak-proof containers that are color-coded in red with the *BIOHAZARD* symbol (see Fig. 17-18, *A*) are used to collect:
- Liquid or semi-liquid blood or OPIM
- Items contaminated with blood or OPIM
- Items caked with dried blood or OPIM
- Contaminated sharps—needles, syringes, razors, and other sharp items. (Containers for contaminated sharps must be puncture-resistant.)

State and local guidelines and regulations determine what is considered biohazardous waste. The amount of soiling is a factor. Follow agency policies and procedures for handling contaminated trash, equipment, and supplies.

Contaminated Laundry

OSHA requires these measures for laundry soiled with blood or OPIM.
- Handle it as little as possible.
- Wear gloves or other needed PPE.
- Bag contaminated laundry where it is used.
- Mark laundry bags or containers with the *BIOHAZARD* symbol for laundry sent off-site.
- Place wet, contaminated laundry in leak-proof containers before transport. The containers are color-coded in red or have the *BIOHAZARD* symbol.

See *Focus on Surveys: Contaminated Laundry.*

Exposure Incidents

An *exposure incident* is any eye, mouth, other mucous membrane, non-intact skin, or parenteral contact with blood or OPIM. *Parenteral* means piercing the mucous membranes or the skin. Causes include needle-sticks, human bites, cuts, and abrasions.

Report an exposure incident at once. Medical evaluation, follow-up, and testing are free. Your blood is tested for HIV and HBV. If you refuse testing, the blood sample is kept for at least 90 days. Testing is done later if you desire.

You are told about medical conditions related to the exposure that may need treatment. You receive a written opinion within 15 days after the evaluation is complete.

The *source individual* is the person whose blood or body fluids are the source of an exposure incident. The source's blood is tested for HIV and HBV. The agency informs you about laws affecting the source's identity and test results.

SURGICAL ASEPSIS

Surgical asepsis (sterile technique) is required any time the skin or sterile tissues are entered. The items used and the work area must be sterile—absent of *all* microbes (p. 240).

Surgery and labor and delivery areas require surgical asepsis. So do many tests and nursing procedures. If a break occurs in sterile technique, microbes can enter the body. Infection is a risk.

Assisting With Sterile Procedures

You may assist with sterile procedures. If so, you need to understand the principles and practices of sterile technique. See Box 17-6.

Items used for the procedure are kept sterile. If an item is contaminated, infection is a risk.

A sterile field is needed. A *sterile field* is a work area free of *all* pathogens and non-pathogens (including spores). See Figure 17-19.

See *Delegation Guidelines: Assisting With Sterile Procedures*, p. 254.

BOX 17-6	Surgical Asepsis: Principles and Practices

- The edges of a sterile field are contaminated.
  - A 1-inch (2.5-centimeter [cm]) margin around the sterile field is considered contaminated (see Fig. 17-19).
  - Place all sterile items inside the sterile area.
  - Items within and outside the 1-inch (2.5-cm) margin are contaminated.
- A sterile item can touch only another sterile item.
  - If a sterile item touches a clean item, the sterile item is contaminated.
  - If a clean item touches a sterile item, the sterile item is contaminated.
  - A sterile package is contaminated if open, torn, punctured, wet, or moist.
  - A sterile package is contaminated when the expiration date has passed.
  - Place only sterile items on a sterile field.
  - Sterile gloves or sterile forceps are used to handle other sterile items (Fig. 17-20).
  - Consider any item to be contaminated if not sure of its sterility.
  - Do not use contaminated items. They are discarded or re-sterilized.
- A sterile field or sterile items are always kept within your vision and above the waist.
  - If you cannot see an item, it is contaminated.
  - If the item is below your waist, it is contaminated.
  - Keep sterile-gloved hands above your waist and in your sight.
  - Do not leave a sterile field unattended.
  - Do not turn your back on a sterile field.
- Airborne microbes can contaminate sterile items or a sterile field.
  - Prevent drafts. Close the door and avoid extra movements. Ask other staff in the room to avoid extra movements.
  - Avoid coughing, sneezing, talking, or laughing over a sterile field. Turn your head away from the sterile field if you must talk.
  - Wear a mask if you need to talk during the procedure.
  - Do not assist with sterile procedures if you have a respiratory infection.
  - Do not reach over a sterile field.
- Fluid flows downward, in the direction of gravity.
  - Hold wet items down (see Fig. 17-20). If held up, fluid flows down into a contaminated area.
- The sterile field is kept dry unless the area below it is sterile.
  - The sterile field is contaminated if it gets wet and the area below it is not sterile.
  - Avoid spilling and splashing when pouring sterile fluids into sterile containers.
- Honesty is essential to sterile technique.
  - Be honest if you contaminate an item or sterile field, even if other staff do not notice.
  - Report contamination or suspected contamination to the nurse.
  - Remove the contaminated item and correct the matter. The procedure may need to start over with new sterile supplies. Follow the nurse's directions.

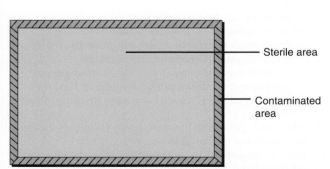

FIGURE 17-19 A sterile field. A 1-inch (2.5 cm) margin around the sterile field is considered contaminated. The shading and slash marks show that the 1-inch (2.5 cm) margin is contaminated.

Sterile area

Contaminated area

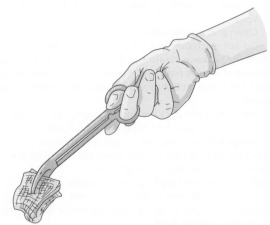

FIGURE 17-20 Sterile forceps are used to handle sterile items.

DELEGATION GUIDELINES

Assisting With Sterile Procedures

Sterile procedures are usually not delegated to nursing assistants. If a procedure requires sterile gloves, the nurse instructs about the reason for using sterile gloves. See "Sterile Gloving." You may assist with sterile procedures. Before doing so, make sure that:

- Your state allows you to perform the task.
- The task is in your job description.
- You have the necessary education and training.
- You know how to use the agency's equipment and supplies.
- You and the nurse review what is expected.
- The nurse is present to provide direction.
  Before assisting with a sterile procedure, you need this information from the nurse.
- The procedure to be done
- What gloves to wear—sterile or non-sterile
- What you are expected to do
- What you can and cannot touch
- What concerns to report at once

Sterile Gloving

Before donning (putting on) sterile gloves, the sterile field is set up. After sterile gloves are on, you can handle sterile items within the sterile field. Do not touch anything outside the sterile field.

Sterile gloves are single-use. They come in many sizes to fit snugly. The insides are powdered for ease in donning gloves. The right and left gloves are marked on the package.

See *Promoting Safety and Comfort: Sterile Gloving.*
See procedure: *Sterile Gloving.*

PROMOTING SAFETY AND COMFORT

Sterile Gloving

Safety

Always keep sterile gloved hands above your waist and within your vision. Touch only items within the sterile field. If you contaminate the gloves, remove them. Tell the nurse what happened. Practice hand hygiene and put on a new pair. Replace gloves that are torn, cut, or punctured.

Comfort

If you, the nurse, or the person contaminates your gloves, they must be removed. When collecting supplies, get an extra pair of gloves. The gloves are in the room if the first pair is contaminated. Care can continue with little delay.

Sterile Gloving

PROCEDURE

1 Follow *Delegation Guidelines: Assisting With Sterile Procedures.* See *Promoting Safety and Comfort: Sterile Gloving.*
2 Practice hand hygiene.
3 Inspect the package of sterile gloves for sterility.
 a Check the expiration date.
 b See if the package is dry.
 c Check for tears, holes, punctures, and water marks.
4 Create a work surface with enough room.
 a Arrange the work surface at waist level and within your vision.
 b Clean and dry the work surface.
 c Do not reach over or turn your back on the work surface.
5 Open the package. Grasp the flaps. Gently peel them back.
6 Remove the inner package. Place it on your work surface.
7 Note the labels on the inner package—*left, right, up,* and *down.*
8 Arrange the inner package for left, right, up, and down. Left glove is on your left; right glove is on your right. Glove openings are near you; fingers point away from you.
9 Grasp the folded edges of the inner package. Use the thumb and index finger of each hand.
10 Fold back the inner package to expose the gloves (Fig. 17-21, *A*). Do not touch or otherwise contaminate the inside package or the gloves. The inside of the inner package is a sterile field.
11 Note that about 2 to 3 inches of each glove is folded so the inside of the glove is to the outside. This is called the *cuff.* The insides of the gloves (including the cuff portion facing out) are considered *not sterile.* These are the only parts that you can touch with bare hands.

12 Put on the right glove if you are right-handed. Put on the left glove if you are left-handed.
 a Pick up the glove with your other hand. Use your thumb and index and middle fingers. Touch only the cuff and inside of the glove (Fig. 17-21, *B*).
 b Turn the hand to be gloved palm side up.
 c Slide your fingers and hand into the glove (Fig. 17-21, *C*).
 d Pull the glove up over your hand. If some fingers get stuck, leave them that way until the other glove is on. *Do not use your ungloved hand to straighten the glove. Do not let the outside of the glove touch any non-sterile surface.*
 e Leave the cuff folded at the wrist.
13 Put on the other glove. Use your gloved hand.
 a Reach under the cuff of the second glove. Use the 4 fingers of your gloved hand (Fig. 17-21, *D*).
 b Put on the second glove (Fig. 17-21, *E*). Your gloved hand cannot touch the cuff or any surface. Hold the thumb of your first gloved hand away from the other hand.
14 Adjust each glove with the other hand. The gloves should be smooth and comfortable (Fig. 17-21, *F*).
15 Slide the fingers of 1 hand under the cuff of the glove on the other hand. Touch only the outer surface of the glove. Pull upward to unfold the cuff (Fig. 17-21, *G*). Repeat for the other hand.
16 Touch only sterile items.
17 Remove and discard the gloves. See Chapter 18.
18 Practice hand hygiene.

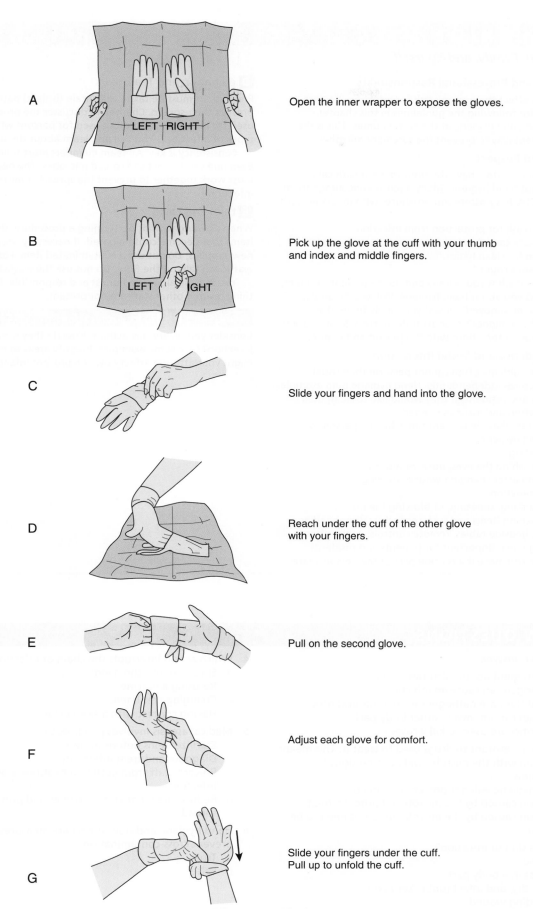

A   Open the inner wrapper to expose the gloves.

B   Pick up the glove at the cuff with your thumb and index and middle fingers.

C   Slide your fingers and hand into the glove.

D   Reach under the cuff of the other glove with your fingers.

E   Pull on the second glove.

F   Adjust each glove for comfort.

G   Slide your fingers under the cuff. Pull up to unfold the cuff.

FIGURE 17-21 Sterile gloving.

FOCUS ON PRIDE

The Person, Family, and Yourself

Personal and Professional Responsibility

Your actions affect the person's risk for infection. You are responsible for following the guidelines in this chapter. Practice good hand hygiene at the correct times. This is the most important way to prevent the spread of microbes.

Rights and Respect

The person and visitors have the right to ask health care workers about hand hygiene. Many agencies encourage them to ask. The CDC has posters and brochures with messages such as:

* "It's OK to ask for protection from infection."
* "Ask for safe care. Ask for clean hands."
* "Speak up for clean hands."
* "Clean hands count."

Think about what you will say and do if a patient, resident, or visitor asks you about hand hygiene. Will you be angry, embarrassed, or annoyed? Or will you kindly thank the person for the reminder? Your attitude matters. Show a good attitude in your interactions with the person and visitors.

Independence and Social Interaction

Patients and residents often cannot perform their usual hygiene measures independently. Hand hygiene is an example. Ask patients and residents if they would like to clean their hands. Ask often and assist as needed.

The CDC lists these important times for the person to perform hand hygiene.

* Before eating
* Before touching the eyes, nose, or mouth
* Before and after changing wound dressings
* After elimination
* After coughing, sneezing, or blowing the nose
* After touching items and surfaces such as door handles, bed rails, bedside tables, remote controls, or the phone Hand hygiene is important for patients and residents.

Encourage it and make it a routine part of the person's care.

Delegation and Teamwork

Precautions must be taken to contain (isolate) pathogens and prevent their spread. Chapter 18 discusses the precautions used for all persons and those used for persons with certain types of infections. You will also learn about the use of PPE.

Consistency is key. All team members must follow the rules. Even one careless act can spread microbes. The health team must work together to prevent the spread of microbes and infection.

Ethics and Laws

When assisting with or performing a procedure, do not use items that become contaminated. If necessary, stop and get new supplies. Do not use a contaminated item. For example, a washcloth falls on the floor. Do not use the washcloth.

You may be alone. Be honest and responsible. Do the right thing, even if other staff are not present.

FOCUS ON PRIDE: Application

Consider your every-day actions. How do they prevent infection? Give some examples. Identify areas to improve. How might your attitude affect how you prevent infection at work?

REVIEW QUESTIONS

Circle the BEST answer.

1 Which statement about microbes is true?
   a A pathogen can cause an infection.
   b Normal flora are pathogens in their natural sites.
   c Microbes cannot invade other body parts.
   d Antibiotics are used to kill viruses.

2 A microbe is resistant to drugs used to treat it. This means
   a Infection with the microbe will have no signs or symptoms
   b Hand hygiene will not prevent its spread
   c Infection caused by the microbe is harder to treat
   d Infection caused by the microbe does not need to be treated

3 Which is a sign of infection?
   a A bruise
   b Redness in a body part
   c Warm, dry, and intact (unbroken) skin
   d A bleeding wound

4 Which action interrupts the chain of infection?
   a Sneezing into the hands
   b Refusing a vaccine
   c Changing wet linens
   d Having contact with a sick person

5 Medical asepsis involves practices to
   a Sterilize items before surgery
   b Diagnose and treat infections
   c Prevent staff from getting a healthcare-associated infection
   d Reduce the number of microbes and prevent microbe spread

6 Hand hygiene and disinfection are measures used to prevent cross-contamination.
   a True
   b False

7 If an item is "sterile," this means that
 a There are only non-pathogens on the item
 b The item has been cleaned with soap and hot water
 c There are no microbes on the item
 d The item has been cleaned with an antiseptic

8 Unless hands are visibly soiled, which is used for hand hygiene in *most* health care situations?
 a Soap and water
 b Alcohol-based hand sanitizer
 c Disinfectant spray
 d Hot water

9 You have blood on your hand. What should you do?
 a Wash your hands with soap and water.
 b Use an alcohol-based hand sanitizer.
 c Rinse your hands.
 d Wash your hands with a disinfectant.

10 You move from a soiled body site to a clean body site. Your hands are not visibly soiled. What should you do?
 a Wash your hands after the next task.
 b Use an alcohol-based hand sanitizer.
 c Rinse your hands with water.
 d Continue care without hand hygiene.

11 When washing your hands with soap and water, you should
 a Stand with your body against the sink
 b Hold your hands and forearms up
 c Scrub the hands for 10 seconds
 d Dry from the fingertips toward the forearms

12 To use an alcohol-based hand sanitizer correctly
 a Wash your hands before applying the hand sanitizer
 b Rinse your hands after applying the hand sanitizer
 c Rub the product only on the palms of your hands
 d Rub your hands together until they are dry

13 Hand hygiene is performed before touching a person. This prevents the transfer of microbes from the health care setting to the person.
 a True
 b False

14 Why do you practice hand hygiene immediately before a procedure that involves mucous membranes?
 a To protect yourself
 b To protect the person
 c To protect other staff
 d To protect other patients or residents

15 You touch items in the person's room but do not touch the person. You are going to leave the room. Hand hygiene
 a Is optional
 b Is not needed if the person was not touched
 c Is not needed if there was no contact with body fluids
 d Is needed after touching items in the person's room

16 When cleaning equipment
 a Rinse the item in hot water before cleaning
 b Wash the item with soap and cold water
 c Use a brush if necessary
 d Work from dirty to clean areas

17 Which shows that you know how to use a disinfectant safely?
 a You use the product on intact skin.
 b You dry an item immediately after applying the disinfectant.
 c You mix it with another disinfectant to kill more microbes.
 d You read and follow the directions on the product label.

18 To control a portal of exit
 a Cover the mouth and nose with tissues when coughing
 b Position a drainage container above the drainage site
 c Clean the genital area from the rectum to the urethra
 d Leave an open wound uncovered

19 Which measure prevents the transmission of microbes
 a Sharing personal care equipment
 b Holding linens against your uniform
 c Disinfecting a shower chair after use
 d Sitting on the person's bed

20 The Bloodborne Pathogen Standard is a regulation of OSHA to protect workers from exposure to pathogens present in blood.
 a True
 b False

21 Bloodborne pathogens are spread through
 a Only blood
 b Blood and other potentially infectious materials
 c Close contact
 d Coughing and sneezing

22 According to the Bloodborne Pathogen Standard, you should
 a Wear PPE home so you can clean it
 b Discard a used razor in a wastebasket
 c Wear a torn glove
 d Be offered a hepatitis B vaccine

23 Blood splashed in your eye at work. Which is *true?*
 a You do not have to report the exposure.
 b You pay for required tests after the exposure.
 c You can refuse HIV and HBV testing.
 d The source individual is not tested for HIV or HBV.

24 Which statement about surgical asepsis is *true?*
 a The outside margin of a sterile field is considered sterile.
 b Wet sterile items are held up.
 c A torn sterile package is still sterile.
 d If you are not sure if an item is sterile, it is considered contaminated.

25 You have on sterile gloves. You can touch
 a Clean items
 b Items on the sterile field
 c Items below your waist
 d Your face and uniform

Answers to Chapter 17 questions are on p. 902.

FOCUS ON **PRACTICE**

Problem Solving

Two residents share a room. You make both beds without practicing hand hygiene between beds. Why is this a problem? When should you practice hand hygiene? Can you use an alcohol-based hand sanitizer? When must you use soap and water?

Isolation Precautions

- Define the key terms and key abbreviations in this chapter.
- Identify when Standard Precautions and Transmission-Based Precautions are used.
- Explain the purpose of Standard Precautions.
- Describe how to follow Standard Precautions.
- Explain the purpose of Enhanced Barrier Precautions in nursing centers.
- Explain the purpose of Transmission-Based Precautions.
- Identify 3 types of Transmission-Based Precautions.

- Describe the rules for Transmission-Based Precautions.
- Explain how to use personal protective equipment.
- Describe infection control measures for handling used laundry, supplies, and equipment.
- Describe infection control measures when collecting specimens and transporting persons.
- Perform the procedures described in this chapter.
- Explain how to promote PRIDE in the person, the family, and yourself.

KEY TERMS

infection control Practices and procedures that prevent the spread of infection

personal protective equipment (PPE) The clothing or equipment worn by staff for protection against a hazard

KEY ABBREVIATIONS

CDC	Centers for Disease Control and Prevention
EBP	Enhanced Barrier Precautions
MDRO	Multidrug-resistant organism

PPE	Personal protective equipment
TB	Tuberculosis

Infection control is the practices and procedures that prevent the spread of infection. A goal is to isolate (contain) and prevent the spread of pathogens. In health care settings, the *Guideline for Isolation Precautions: Preventing Transmission of Infectious Agents in Healthcare Settings 2007* is followed. It is a guideline of the Centers for Disease Control and Prevention (CDC).

The CDC guideline has 2 main tiers of precautions.
- *Standard Precautions*—used in all situations for all persons.
- *Transmission-Based Precautions*—used when persons have or may have certain infections. More precautions are needed.

STANDARD PRECAUTIONS

Standard Precautions are basic precautions used in health care settings (Box 18-1). They:
- Reduce the risk of spreading pathogens.
- Reduce the risk of spreading known and unknown infections.

Standard Precautions are used for all persons whenever care is given. Standard Precautions prevent the spread of infection from:
- Blood.
- All body fluids (except sweat). This includes secretions and excretions even if blood is not visible. Nasal secretions, saliva, sputum, urine, feces (stools), vomit, and breast-milk are examples. Sweat is not known to spread infection.
- Non-intact skin (skin with open breaks).
- Mucous membranes.

See *Focus on Long-Term Care and Home Care: Standard Precautions*, p. 260.

BOX 18-1	Standard Precautions

Hand Hygiene
- Follow the rules of hand hygiene. See Chapter 17.
- Touch surfaces close to the person only when necessary. This prevents contaminating clean hands from room or care setting surfaces. It also prevents transmitting pathogens from contaminated hands to other surfaces.
- Do not wear fake nails or nail extenders for contact with persons at risk for infection or other adverse outcomes. Microbes can live under fake nails even after hand hygiene. (NOTE: Non-natural nails are not allowed in some agencies.)

Personal Protective Equipment (PPE) (p. 264)
- Wear personal protective equipment (PPE) when contact with blood or body fluids is likely.
- Do not contaminate your clothing or skin when removing PPE.
- Remove and discard PPE before leaving the person's room or care setting.

Gloves
- Wear gloves when contact with the following is likely.
  - Blood or other potentially infectious materials (Chapter 17)
  - Body fluids (including secretions and excretions)
  - Mucous membranes
  - Non-intact skin
  - Skin or equipment that may be contaminated (for example, from urine or feces [stools])
- Wear gloves that fit and are needed for the task.
  - Wear disposable gloves for direct care.
  - Wear disposable gloves or utility gloves to clean equipment or care settings.
- Remove gloves before going to another person. Do not wear the same pair of gloves for the care of more than 1 person.
- Change gloves during care if your hands will move from a soiled body site to a clean body site. Moving from perineal care (Chapter 24) to oral care (Chapter 23) is an example.
- Remove gloves carefully to prevent hand contamination. See "Donning and Removing PPE" on p. 266.
- Do not wash gloves for re-use.

Gowns
- Wear a gown to protect your skin and clothing when contact with blood or body fluids is likely.
- Wear a gown for direct contact with a person who has uncontained secretions or excretions. Diarrhea is an example.
- Remove the gown and perform hand hygiene before leaving the person's room.
- Do not re-use gowns, even for repeat contact with the same person.

Mouth, Nose, and Eye Protection
- Wear PPE—masks, goggles, face shields, or a combination of each—for procedures and tasks that are likely to cause splashes and sprays of blood or body fluids.
- Wear the correct PPE for the procedure or task.
- Wear gloves, a gown, and 1 of the following for procedures or tasks likely to cause sprays of respiratory secretions.
  - A face shield that fully covers the front and sides of the face
  - A mask with attached shield
  - A mask and goggles

Respiratory Hygiene/Cough Etiquette
- Instruct persons with respiratory symptoms to:
  - Cover the nose and mouth to cough or sneeze.
  - Use tissues to contain respiratory secretions.
  - Dispose of tissues in the nearest no-touch waste container.
  - Perform hand hygiene after contact with respiratory secretions.
- Provide visitors with masks according to agency policy.

Care Equipment
- Wear the correct PPE to handle:
  - Care equipment that is visibly soiled with blood or body fluids
  - Care equipment that may have been in contact with blood or body fluids
- Remove organic material before disinfection and sterilization procedures (Chapter 17). Follow agency policy for using cleaning agents.

Care of the Environment
- Follow agency procedures to clean and maintain surfaces. Care setting surfaces and care equipment are examples. Surfaces near the person may need frequent cleaning and maintenance—door knobs, bed rails, over-bed tables, walker and cane handles, toilet surfaces and areas, and so on.
- Follow agency procedures to clean and disinfect multi-use electronic equipment. This includes:
  - Items used by patients and residents
  - Items used to give care
  - Mobile devices that are moved in and out of patient or resident rooms
- Follow these rules for children's toys. This includes toys in waiting areas.
  - Select toys that are easy to clean and disinfect.
  - Do not allow stuffed, furry toys if they will be shared.
  - Clean and disinfect large stationary toys (for example, climbing equipment) at least weekly and when visibly soiled.
  - Rinse toys with water after disinfection if they are likely to be mouthed by children. Or wash them in a dishwasher.
  - Clean and disinfect a toy at once when it needs cleaning. Or store the toy in a labeled container away from toys that are clean and ready for use.

Textiles and Laundry
- Handle used textiles and fabrics (linens) with minimal (the least amount of) agitation. This prevents contamination of air, surfaces, and other persons.

Worker Safety
- Protect yourself and others from exposure to bloodborne pathogens. This includes handling needles and other sharps. See "Bloodborne Pathogen Standard" in Chapter 17.
- Use a mouthpiece, resuscitation bag, or other ventilation device for resuscitation to prevent contact with the person's mouth and oral secretions. See Chapter 58.

Patient or Resident Placement
- A private room is preferred if the person is at risk for transmitting infection to others.
- Follow the nurse's directions if a private room is not available.

Modified from Siegel JD, Rhinehart E, Jackson M, Chiarello L, and the Healthcare Infection Control Practices Advisory Committee: Guideline for isolation precautions: preventing transmission of infectious agents in healthcare settings 2007, *Atlanta, last update July 2023, Centers for Disease Control and Prevention.*

TRANSMISSION-BASED PRECAUTIONS

With some infections, transmission is not prevented with Standard Precautions alone. When a person is known or suspected to have such an infection, Transmission-Based Precautions are needed along with Standard Precautions. Transmission-Based Precautions are commonly called "isolation precautions."

There are 3 types of Transmission-Based Precautions. Some infections require more than 1 type of precaution.

- *Contact*—involves touch. The pathogen spreads through touching the person or items and surfaces near the person.
- *Droplet*—involves respiratory droplets. The pathogen spreads through close contact with respiratory secretions.
- *Airborne*—involves air. The pathogen is able to suspend in the air. It can be transmitted over long distances.

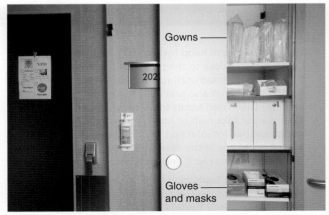

FIGURE 18-1 Personal protective equipment is in a cabinet outside the person's room.

Personal protective equipment (PPE) is required. Needed PPE depends on how the pathogen is spread. Gloves, a gown, a mask or respirator, and goggles or a face shield may be needed. The CDC provides guidelines on what PPE to wear and how to safely apply and remove it. See "Personal Protective Equipment" on p. 264.

Disposable (single-use) equipment is used when possible. Or dedicated equipment is kept in the room. *Dedicated equipment* is only used for 1 person. For example, a thermometer and blood pressure equipment are kept in the room. The equipment is not removed for use on another person. Equipment that must be shared is disinfected after use. A mechanical lift (Chapter 21) is an example.

In this chapter, "isolation room" refers to the room of a person who needs Transmission-Based Precautions. The nurse may have you help set up an isolation room. Follow agency procedures. The following are common.

- PPE is in a cart or cabinet outside the room (Fig. 18-1). Or supplies are in an adjoining room (*anteroom*) with items for hand hygiene. Re-stock supplies as needed.
- A sign is posted outside the room to alert staff and visitors of needed precautions (Fig. 18-2).
- A wastebasket and linen cart are inside the room. Color-coded or red bags with the *BIOHAZARD* label (Chapter 17) are not required. However, follow agency policies and procedures.
- Dedicated equipment, leak-proof plastic bags, and a disinfectant are supplied.

The rules in Box 18-2 are a guide for giving safe care when using Transmission-Based Precautions. See Box 18-3 (p. 262) for the CDC's guidelines for the 3 types of Transmission-Based Precautions. Agency policies may differ from those in this text.

See *Focus on Communication: Transmission-Based Precautions*, p. 263.

See *Focus on Surveys: Transmission-Based Precautions*, p. 263.

See *Delegation Guidelines: Transmission-Based Precautions*, p. 263.

See *Promoting Safety and Comfort: Transmission-Based Precautions*, p. 263.

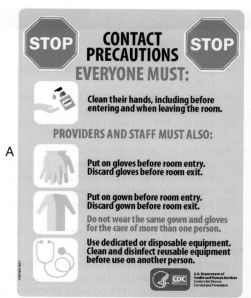

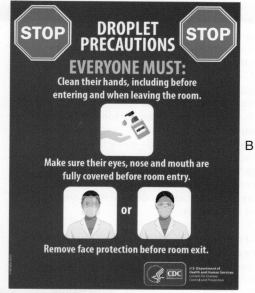

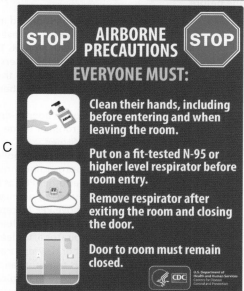

FIGURE 18-2 Sample signs for Transmission-Based Precautions. The sign is posted outside the room to alert staff and visitors of needed precautions. **A,** Contact Precautions. **B,** Droplet Precautions. **C,** Airborne Precautions. (From Centers for Disease Control and Prevention, Department of Health and Human Services.)

BOX 18-2	Rules for Transmission-Based Precautions

- Tell the nurse if you have any cuts, open skin areas, a sore throat, vomiting, or diarrhea.
- Collect all needed items before entering the room.
- Wear required PPE (see Box 18-3).
- Do not touch your hair, nose, mouth, eyes, or other body parts.
- Do not touch any clean area or object if your hands are contaminated.
- Wash your hands with soap and water if they are visibly dirty or contaminated with blood or body fluids (including secretions and excretions). Follow the rules for hand hygiene (Chapter 17).
- Place clean items on paper towels.
- Do not shake linens.
- Use paper towels to handle contaminated items.
- Use paper towels to turn faucets on and off.

- Use a paper towel to open the door to the person's room. Discard it after use.
- Do not contaminate equipment and supplies. Floors are contaminated. So is any object on the floor or that falls to the floor.
- Clean floors with mops wetted with a disinfectant solution.
- Prevent drafts. Drafts can carry some microbes in the air.
- Remove items from the room in leak-proof plastic bags.
- Follow agency procedures to remove and transport re-usable and disposable items. For meal trays:
    - Place re-usable dishes, drinking vessels, eating utensils, and trays in a leak-proof plastic bag (p. 272).
    - Discard disposable dishes, drinking vessels, eating utensils, and trays in the waste container in the person's room.

| BOX 18-3 | Transmission-Based Precautions |

Contact Precautions
- Used for persons with known or suspected infections or conditions that increase the risk of contact (touch) transmission.
- Patient or resident placement:
  - A single room is preferred.
  - If a room is shared with another person not infected with the same agent:
    - Keep the persons separated—more than 3 feet apart.
    - Keep the privacy curtain between the beds closed.
    - Change PPE and practice hand hygiene between contact with persons in the same room. Do so regardless of whether 1 or both persons are on Contact Precautions.
- Gloves:
  - Wear gloves to touch the person's intact skin or surfaces or items near the person.
  - Don (put on) gloves upon entry into the person's room or care setting.
  - Remove gloves and practice hand hygiene before leaving the person's room.
- Gown:
  - Wear a gown when clothing may have direct contact with the person.
  - Wear a gown when contact is likely with surfaces or equipment near the person.
  - Don the gown upon entry into the person's room or care setting.
  - Remove the gown and practice hand hygiene before leaving the person's room.
  - Make sure your clothing and skin do not touch potentially contaminated surfaces after removing the gown.
- Patient or resident transport:
  - Limit transport and movement of the person outside of the room to medically necessary purposes.
  - Cover the infected area of the person's body.
  - Remove and discard contaminated PPE and practice hand hygiene before transporting the person.
  - Don clean PPE to handle the person at the transport destination.
- Care equipment:
  - Follow Standard Precautions.
  - Use disposable equipment when possible. If possible, leave non-disposable equipment in the person's room.
  - Clean and disinfect non-disposable and multiple-use equipment before use on another person.

Droplet Precautions
- Used for persons known or suspected to be infected with pathogens transmitted by respiratory droplets. Such droplets come from coughing, sneezing, or talking.
- Patient or resident placement:
  - A single room is preferred.
  - If a room is shared with another person who is not infected with the same agent:
    - Keep the persons separated—more than 3 feet apart. Some infections require at least 6 feet of separation.
    - Keep the privacy curtain between the beds closed.
    - Change PPE and practice hand hygiene between contact with persons in the same room. Do so regardless of whether 1 or both persons are on Droplet Precautions.

Droplet Precautions—cont'd
- PPE:
  - Don a mask upon entry into the person's room or care setting.
  - Wear other PPE as required for the pathogen or as required by agency policy.
  - Remove PPE and practice hand hygiene before leaving the person's room.
- Patient or resident transport:
  - Limit transport and movement of the person outside of the room to medically necessary purposes.
  - Have the person wear a mask.
  - Instruct the person to follow Respiratory Hygiene/Cough Etiquette (see Box 18-1).
  - No mask is required for staff transporting the person.

Airborne Precautions
- Used for persons known or suspected to be infected with pathogens transmitted person-to-person by the airborne route. Tuberculosis (TB), measles, chicken pox, and smallpox are examples.
- The person is placed in an airborne infection isolation room (AIIR). If not available, the person is transferred to an agency with an AIIR. The room door is kept closed except when someone enters or leaves the room.
- Staff susceptible to the infection do not enter the room (if immune staff members are available to give care).
- PPE:
  - Wear an agency-approved respirator when entering the room or home when TB or smallpox is suspected or confirmed.
  - Follow agency policy for respiratory protection for other airborne infections.
  - Wear other PPE as required for the pathogen or as required by agency policy.
  - Remove PPE (except for a respirator) and practice hand hygiene before leaving the person's room. Remove a respirator after leaving and closing the door.
- Patient or resident transport:
  - Limit transport and movement of the person outside of the room to medically necessary purposes.
  - Have the person wear a surgical mask.
  - Instruct the person to follow Respiratory Hygiene/Cough Etiquette (see Box 18-1).
  - Cover skin lesions infected with the microbe.
  - No mask or respirator is required for staff transporting the person if the person is wearing a mask and skin lesions are covered.

Modified from Siegel JD, Rhinehart E, Jackson M, Chiarello L, and the Healthcare Infection Control Practices Advisory Committee: Guideline for isolation precautions: preventing transmission of infectious agents in healthcare settings 2007, *Atlanta, last update July 2023, Centers for Disease Control and Prevention.*

Transmission-Based Precautions

The health team and visitors must know what PPE to use. Signs are a common way to communicate the type of precaution and the needed PPE (see Fig. 18-2). Signs are posted at the person's doorway. In long-term care settings, signs may instruct visitors to see the nurse before entering the person's room.

Visitors may ask why PPE is needed. Some visitors ignore signs or requests to wear PPE. Politely communicate with the person and visitors about PPE. For example, you can say: "Please wear this mask. It is our policy to protect you, your family member, and others." Tell the nurse if the person or visitors have more questions. Also tell the nurse if someone refuses to wear PPE.

If you see a staff member not wearing needed PPE, remind the person. You can also offer to get the person PPE. For example, you can say:
- "I'll get you the mask that you need."
- "Here are gloves and a gown you need."
Be polite. Tell the nurse if the person refuses.

Transmission-Based Precautions

When a person requires Transmission-Based Precautions, surveyors will observe if staff:
- Wash their hands correctly and at the correct times.
- Change gloves after providing personal care.
- Don, wear, and dispose of PPE correctly.

DELEGATION GUIDELINES

Transmission-Based Precautions

If a person needs Transmission-Based Precautions, review the type with the nurse. Also check with the nurse and care plan about:
- What PPE to use
- What special measures are needed
- What equipment to use—disposable or dedicated

PROMOTING SAFETY AND COMFORT

Transmission-Based Precautions

Safety
Preventing the spread of infection is important. Transmission-Based Precautions protect everyone—patients, residents, visitors, staff, and you. If you are careless, everyone's safety is at risk.

Social and Emotional Needs

With Transmission-Based Precautions, the person is more isolated and knows the disease can spread to others. Visitor restrictions may be required. Or visitors might avoid the person. Staff may not enter as often because of needed PPE. The person may feel ashamed, guilty, or dirty. Sadness and loneliness are common.

Do not avoid the person. Do not complain about the need for PPE or other precautions. When giving care, talk to the person. Show kindness and respect. Listen with interest. You can also suggest that the person call family and friends. Assist the person if needed. These actions can help meet social and emotional needs.

See *Focus on Communication: Social and Emotional Needs*.

See *Focus on Children and Older Persons: Social and Emotional Needs*.

Social and Emotional Needs

Some questions or statements can make the person feel dirty or ashamed. Be careful what you say. For example, do not say:
- "How did you get that?"
- "I'm afraid to touch you."
- "Don't breathe on me."

Social and Emotional Needs

Children
Goggles, face shields, masks, and gowns may scare infants and children. Parents and staff look different. Gloves and gowns prevent skin-to-skin contact with parents. Because of likely contamination, toys and comfort items (blankets, stuffed animals) may be kept from the child. This increases the child's distress.

The nurse teaches the child and family about needed precautions. Simple explanations are given to the child. Depending on age, the nurse may give the child a mask and goggles or face shield to touch and play with.

Older Persons
Some older persons have dementia. PPE may increase confusion and cause fear and agitation. These measures can help.
- Tell the person who you are and what you need to do.
- Use a calm, soothing voice.
- Do not rush the person.
- Use touch to reassure the person.
- Follow the care plan and the nurse's instructions for other measures to help the person.
- Report signs of increased confusion or behavior changes.

PERSONAL PROTECTIVE EQUIPMENT

Personal protective equipment (PPE) is the clothing or equipment worn by staff for protection against a hazard. PPE protects you and prevents the spread of microbes.

- For Standard Precautions, PPE is worn when contact with blood or body fluids is likely. The *task* determines what is needed.
- For Transmission-Based Precautions, PPE is worn regularly when giving care. The *infection* determines what is needed.

PPE includes gowns, masks and respirators, goggles and face shields, and gloves. If you are unsure of what PPE to wear, ask the nurse.

See *Teamwork and Time Management: Personal Protective Equipment.*

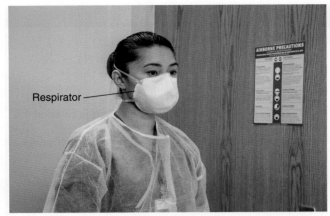

FIGURE 18-3 A respirator. (Modified from Stein L, Hollen C: *Concept-based clinical nursing skills,* ed 2, St Louis, 2023, Elsevier.)

TEAMWORK AND TIME MANAGEMENT

Personal Protective Equipment

Putting on (donning) and removing PPE take time and effort. Once on, you must remove PPE before leaving the room. Therefore you need to plan your time and work to stay in the room.

- Meet the needs of other patients or residents first.
- Ask a co-worker to answer call lights for you. Ask politely.
- Gather needed care items for the room.
- Make sure the person's needs are met before leaving.
- Complete a safety check of the room. (See the inside of the back cover.)
- Tell the person when you will return to the room.

Gowns

Gowns protect your clothes and body from contact with blood and body fluids. They also protect against splashes and sprays. Gowns are worn with gloves and with other PPE as needed.

A gown must completely cover your body front from the neck to the knees. The long sleeves have tight cuffs. The gown opens at the back and wraps around your back to cover your uniform. It is tied in the back at the neck and waist. *The gown front and sleeves are considered contaminated.*

Gowns are used once. A wet gown is contaminated. Hold water basins and wet items out away from the gown. Avoid contact with wet surfaces. Remove a wet gown and put on a dry one. Discard disposable gowns after use.

Masks and Respirators

You wear disposable masks:

- To prevent contact with infectious materials from the person. Respiratory secretions and splashes or sprays of blood or body fluids are examples.
- To protect the person from infectious agents carried in your mouth or nose during sterile procedures.

A wet or moist mask is contaminated. Breathing can cause masks to become wet or moist. Apply a new mask when contamination occurs.

A mask fits snugly over your nose and mouth. Practice hand hygiene before putting on a mask. To remove a mask, touch only the ties or the elastic bands. *The front of the mask is contaminated.*

Agency-approved respirators (Fig. 18-3) are worn when caring for persons with infections spread by the airborne route. TB is an example (Chapter 50).

Respirator Fit. There are different types and sizes of respirators. A respirator must fit the user securely. Employers provide fit testing and training on how to check for a proper seal.

Fit testing is done to check that a respirator fits the user and is comfortable. An improper fit lessens the respirator's protection. Fit testing is required before a respirator is worn on the job, yearly, and if there are physical changes that may affect fit. Significant weight change, facial scarring, or dental work are examples.

With a proper fit and proper application, there is minimal leakage around the edges of the respirator. A *user seal check* is to be done *every time* a respirator is worn. The check ensures that the respirator fits and has been donned (put on) properly. Follow the manufacturer's instructions to check for a proper seal.

Goggles and Face Shields

Splashes and sprays can occur when you give care, clean items, or dispose of fluids. Goggles protect your eyes from splashing or spraying of blood and body fluids. Face shields protect your eyes and other areas of your face.

The front (outside) of goggles or a face shield is contaminated. The headband, ties, or ear-pieces used to secure the device are clean. Use them to remove the device after hand hygiene when they are safe to touch with bare hands. Lift the ties or ear-pieces from the back when removing the device.

Discard disposable goggles or face shields after use. Reusable eyewear is cleaned and disinfected before re-use. It is washed with soap and water. Then a disinfectant is used.

See *Promoting Safety and Comfort: Goggles and Face Shields.*

PROMOTING SAFETY AND COMFORT

Goggles and Face Shields

Safety

Eyeglasses and contact lenses do not provide eye protection. The face shield must fit over eyeglasses with minimal gaps.

Goggles do not provide splash or spray protection to other parts of your face.

Gloves

A natural barrier, the skin prevents microbes from entering the body. Small skin breaks on the hands and fingers are common and may be hard to see. Disposable gloves provide a barrier. They protect:

- You from the person's pathogens
- The person from microbes on your hands

Wear gloves when contact with blood, body fluids (including secretions and excretions), mucous membranes, or non-intact skin is likely. Contact may be directly with blood or body fluids. Or contact may be with contaminated items or surfaces.

Wearing gloves is the most common measure for Standard Precautions and Transmission-Based Precautions. See Box 18-4 for guidelines to follow when using gloves.

See *Promoting Safety and Comfort: Gloves.*

PROMOTING SAFETY AND COMFORT

Gloves

Safety

Some gloves are made of latex (a rubber product). Latex allergies can cause skin rashes. Difficulty breathing and shock are more serious problems. Report skin rashes, breathing problems, or symptoms of shock (Chapter 58) to the nurse at once.

You may have a latex allergy. Some patients and residents are allergic to latex. This is noted on the care plan and your assignment sheet. Latex-free gloves are worn for latex allergies.

Comfort

Gloves are needed when contact with blood, body fluids, mucous membranes, or non-intact skin is likely. Gloves are not needed when such contact is not likely. Back massages and brushing and combing hair are examples if the skin is intact. To reduce exposure to latex, wear gloves only when needed.

BOX 18-4	Rules for Glove Use

When to Wear Gloves
- Wear gloves when contact with blood, body fluids (including secretions and excretions), mucous membranes, or non-intact skin is likely. This includes items that are or may be soiled with blood or body fluids.
- Wear gloves as required by Transmission-Based Precautions.

Applying Gloves
- Apply to dry hands. Gloves are easier to put on dry hands.
- Do not tear gloves when putting them on. Carelessness, long fingernails, and rings can tear gloves. Blood and body fluids can enter the glove through a tear. This contaminates your hand.
- Put on gloves last when worn with other PPE.
- Make sure gloves cover your wrists. If you wear a gown, gloves cover the cuffs (Fig. 18-4).

When to Remove or Change Gloves
- Remove damaged gloves at once. Torn, cut, or punctured gloves need to be removed. Practice hand hygiene and apply a new pair.
- Remove gloves when hand hygiene is needed during care (Chapter 17). Practice hand hygiene. Apply clean gloves if they are needed for the next task. During care, hand hygiene is needed:
  - Before clean or aseptic tasks
  - Before moving from a soiled body site to a clean body site on the same person
  - After tasks involving contact with blood or body fluids
- Remove gloves and practice hand hygiene before touching portable computer keyboards or other equipment that is moved from room to room.
- Remove gloves and practice hand hygiene before contact with another person. Never wear the same pair of gloves for the care of more than 1 person.

Removing Gloves
- *Consider the outside of gloves to be contaminated.* Remove gloves so the inside part is on the outside. The inside is clean.
- Discard gloves after use. Gloves are only worn once.
- Practice hand hygiene after removing gloves.

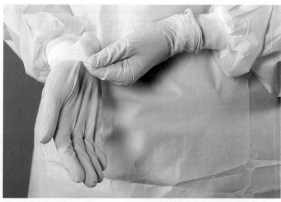

FIGURE 18-4 The gloves cover the gown cuffs.

Donning and Removing PPE

The PPE worn depends on the task to be done or the type of Transmission-Based Precautions needed. Non-sterile gloves are the most common PPE used. See Figure 18-5 for how to apply gloves. Any time a gown is worn, gloves are also needed. Gloves cover the gown cuffs (see Fig. 18-4).

According to the CDC, PPE may safely be donned (put on) using more than 1 method. You need training and practice using your agency's equipment and procedures.

Practice hand hygiene before donning PPE. The CDC lists the following order for donning as an example. See Figure 18-6.

1 Gown
2 Mask or respirator
3 Eyewear (goggles or face shield)
4 Gloves

PPE should not be adjusted while giving care. For example, do not retie a gown or adjust a mask or respirator. Be sure PPE is applied correctly before giving care.

See *Promoting Safety and Comfort: Donning and Removing PPE.*

See procedure: *Donning Personal Protective Equipment.*

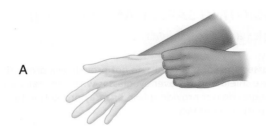
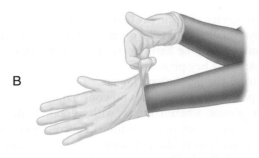

FIGURE 18-5 Applying (donning) gloves. **A**, Grasp the first glove at the wrist area. Carefully pull on the glove. **B**, Grasp the second glove at the wrist area. Carefully pull on the glove. Avoid touching your wrist and forearm with the gloved hand. Do not tear the gloves.

SEQUENCE FOR PUTTING ON PERSONAL PROTECTIVE EQUIPMENT (PPE)

The type of PPE used will vary based on the level of precautions required, such as standard and contact, droplet or airborne infection isolation precautions. The procedure for putting on and removing PPE should be tailored to the specific type of PPE.

1. GOWN
- Fully cover torso from neck to knees, arms to end of wrists, and wrap around the back
- Fasten in back of neck and waist

2. MASK OR RESPIRATOR
- Secure ties or elastic bands at middle of head and neck
- Fit flexible band to nose bridge
- Fit snug to face and below chin
- Fit-check respirator

3. GOGGLES OR FACE SHIELD
- Place over face and eyes and adjust to fit

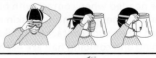

4. GLOVES
- Extend to cover wrist of isolation gown

USE SAFE WORK PRACTICES TO PROTECT YOURSELF AND LIMIT THE SPREAD OF CONTAMINATION

- Keep hands away from face
- Limit surfaces touched
- Change gloves when torn or heavily contaminated
- Perform hand hygiene

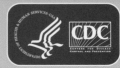

CS250672-E

FIGURE 18-6 Donning PPE. (From Centers for Disease Control and Prevention, Department of Health and Human Services.)

PROMOTING SAFETY AND COMFORT
Donning and Removing PPE

Safety

Some severe and deadly infections require additional PPE—full face shield, helmet, or headpiece; coveralls with socks or special gowns; double gloving; boot or shoe covers; and aprons. Special training is needed to care for such patients and for donning and removing the PPE.

Some states and agencies have different procedures for donning or removing PPE. Follow your state's procedures for your state competency exam. Follow your agency's procedures when working.

Donning Personal Protective Equipment

PROCEDURE

1 Follow *Delegation Guidelines: Transmission-Based Precautions*, p. 263. See *Promoting Safety and Comfort*:
   a *Transmission-Based Precautions*, p. 263
   b *Goggles and Face Shields*, p. 265
   c *Gloves*, p. 265
   d *Donning and Removing PPE*
2 Remove your watch and all jewelry.
3 Roll up long uniform sleeves.
4 Practice hand hygiene.
5 Put on a gown (see Fig. 18-6).
   a Hold a clean gown out in front of you.
   b Unfold the gown. Face the back (opening) of the gown. Do not shake it.
   c Put your hands and arms through the sleeves.
   d Make sure the gown covers you from your neck to your knees. It must cover your arms to the end of your wrists.
   e Tie the strings at the back of the neck.
   f Over-lap the back of the gown. Make sure it covers your uniform. The gown should be snug, not loose.
   g Tie the waist strings. Tie them at the back or the side. Do not tie them in front.

6 Put on a mask or respirator (see Fig. 18-6 and Fig. 18-7).
   a Pick up a mask by its upper ties. Do not touch the part that will cover your face.
   b Place the mask over your nose and mouth (Fig. 18-7, *A*).
   c Place the upper strings above your ears. Tie them at the back in the middle of your head (Fig. 18-7, *B*).
   d Tie the lower strings at the back of your neck (Fig. 18-7, *C*). The lower part of the mask is under your chin.
   e Pinch the metal band around your nose. The top of the mask must be snug over your nose. If you wear eyeglasses, the mask must be snug under the bottom of the eyeglasses.
   f Make sure the mask is snug over your face and under your chin.
7 Put on goggles or a face shield (if needed and if not part of the mask) (see Fig. 18-6).
   a Place the device over your face and eyes.
   b Adjust the device to fit.
8 Put on gloves (see Fig. 18-5). Make sure the gloves cover the wrists of the gown (see Fig. 18-4).

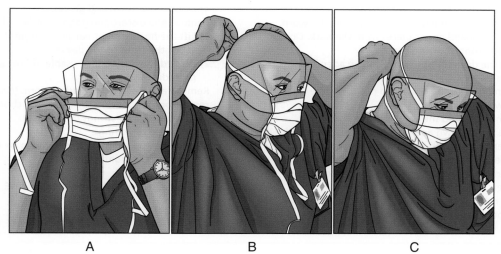

A   B   C

FIGURE 18-7 Donning a mask. (NOTE: The mask has a face shield.) **A,** The mask covers the nose and mouth. **B,** Upper strings are tied at the back of the head. **C,** Lower strings are tied at the back of the neck.

PPE is removed at the doorway before leaving the person's room. If a respirator is worn, it is removed after leaving the person's room and closing the door. Sometimes goggles or a face shield is also removed at this time after hand hygiene. Follow your agency's procedures.

PPE is removed slowly and carefully to avoid contaminating your body and uniform. More than 1 method may be used to safely remove PPE. The CDC gives 2 examples.

Method 1:

1 Gloves
2 Eyewear (goggles or face shield)
3 Gown
4 Mask or respirator

Method 2:

1 Gown and gloves
2 Eyewear (goggles or face shield)
3 Mask or respirator

Practice hand hygiene after removing PPE. Practice hand hygiene between steps if your hands become contaminated. Then practice hand hygiene again after removing all PPE.

See procedure: *Removing Personal Protective Equipment*.

Removing Personal Protective Equipment

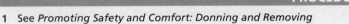

PROCEDURE

1 See *Promoting Safety and Comfort: Donning and Removing PPE*, p. 267.
2 Remove and discard PPE using a method that prevents contamination of your body and uniform (Fig. 18-8). Practice hand hygiene between each step if your hands become contaminated.
3 *Method 1:* Remove gloves, goggles or face shield, gown, mask or respirator (see Fig. 18-8, *A*).
   a Remove and discard the gloves (Fig. 18-9, p. 271).
     1) Make sure that glove touches only glove.
     2) Grasp a glove at the palm (Fig. 18-9, *A*). Grasp it on the outside.
     3) Pull the glove down over your hand so it is inside-out (Fig. 18-9, *B*).
     4) Hold the removed glove with your other gloved hand.
     5) Reach inside the other glove. Use the first 2 fingers of the ungloved hand (Fig. 18-9, *C*).
     6) Pull the glove down (inside-out) over your hand and the other glove (Fig. 18-9, *D*).
     7) Discard the gloves.
   b Remove and discard the goggles or face shield if worn.
     1) Lift the headband or ear-pieces from the back. Do not touch the front of the device.
     2) Discard the device. If re-usable, follow agency procedures.
   c Remove and discard the gown. Do not touch the outside of the gown.
     1) Untie the neck and the waist strings.
     2) Pull the gown down and away from your neck and shoulders. Only touch the inside of the gown.
     3) Turn the gown inside-out as it is removed. Hold it at the inside shoulder seams and bring your hands together.
     4) Fold or roll up the gown away from you. Keep it inside-out. Do not let the gown touch the floor.
     5) Discard the gown.

   d Remove and discard the mask if worn. (NOTE: Remove a respirator after leaving the room and closing the door.)
     1) Untie the lower strings of the mask.
     2) Untie the top strings.
     3) Hold the top strings. Remove the mask without touching the front of the mask.
     4) Discard the mask.
4 *Method 2:* Remove gown and gloves, goggles or face shield, mask or respirator (see Fig. 18-8, *B*, p. 270).
   a Remove and discard the gown and gloves.
     1) Grasp the gown in front with your gloved hands. Pull away from your body so the ties break. Only touch the outside of the gown.
     2) Fold or roll the gown inside-out into a bundle while removing the gown. Keep it inside-out. Do not let the gown touch the floor.
     3) Peel off your gloves as you remove the gown. Only touch the inside of the gloves and gown with your bare hands.
     4) Discard the gown and gloves.
   b Remove and discard the goggles or face shield.
     1) Lift the headband or ear-pieces from the back. Do not touch the front of the device.
     2) Discard the device. If re-usable, follow agency procedures.
   c Remove and discard the mask if worn. (NOTE: Remove a respirator after leaving the room and closing the door.)
     1) Untie the lower strings of the mask.
     2) Untie the top strings.
     3) Hold the top strings. Remove the mask without touching the front of the mask.
     4) Discard the mask.
5 Practice hand hygiene after removing all PPE.

HOW TO SAFELY REMOVE PERSONAL PROTECTIVE EQUIPMENT (PPE) EXAMPLE 1

There are a variety of ways to safely remove PPE without contaminating your clothing, skin, or mucous membranes with potentially infectious materials. Here is one example. **Remove all PPE before exiting the patient room** except a respirator, if worn. Remove the respirator **after** leaving the patient room and closing the door. Remove PPE in the following sequence:

1. GLOVES

- Outside of gloves are contaminated!
- If your hands get contaminated during glove removal, immediately wash your hands or use an alcohol-based hand sanitizer
- Using a gloved hand, grasp the palm area of the other gloved hand and peel off first glove
- Hold removed glove in gloved hand
- Slide fingers of ungloved hand under remaining glove at wrist and peel off second glove over first glove
- Discard gloves in a waste container

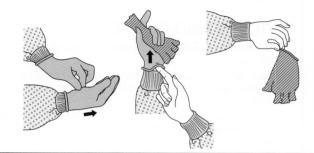

2. GOGGLES OR FACE SHIELD

- Outside of goggles or face shield are contaminated!
- If your hands get contaminated during goggle or face shield removal, immediately wash your hands or use an alcohol-based hand sanitizer
- Remove goggles or face shield from the back by lifting head band or ear pieces
- If the item is reusable, place in designated receptacle for reprocessing. Otherwise, discard in a waste container

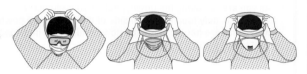

3. GOWN

- Gown front and sleeves are contaminated!
- If your hands get contaminated during gown removal, immediately wash your hands or use an alcohol-based hand sanitizer
- Unfasten gown ties, taking care that sleeves don't contact your body when reaching for ties
- Pull gown away from neck and shoulders, touching inside of gown only
- Turn gown inside out
- Fold or roll into a bundle and discard in a waste container

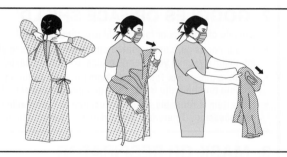

4. MASK OR RESPIRATOR

- Front of mask/respirator is contaminated — DO NOT TOUCH!
- If your hands get contaminated during mask/respirator removal, immediately wash your hands or use an alcohol-based hand sanitizer
- Grasp bottom ties or elastics of the mask/respirator, then the ones at the top, and remove without touching the front
- Discard in a waste container

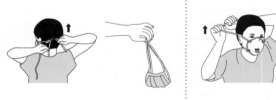

5. WASH HANDS OR USE AN ALCOHOL-BASED HAND SANITIZER IMMEDIATELY AFTER REMOVING ALL PPE

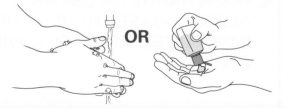

PERFORM HAND HYGIENE BETWEEN STEPS IF HANDS BECOME CONTAMINATED AND IMMEDIATELY AFTER REMOVING ALL PPE

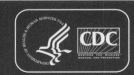

CS250672-E

FIGURE 18-8 A, Removing PPE: Method 1.

Continued

HOW TO SAFELY REMOVE PERSONAL PROTECTIVE EQUIPMENT (PPE) EXAMPLE 2

Here is another way to safely remove PPE without contaminating your clothing, skin, or mucous membranes with potentially infectious materials. **Remove all PPE before exiting the patient room** except a respirator, if worn. Remove the respirator **after** leaving the patient room and closing the door. Remove PPE in the following sequence:

1. GOWN AND GLOVES

- Gown front and sleeves and the outside of gloves are contaminated!
- If your hands get contaminated during gown or glove removal, immediately wash your hands or use an alcohol-based hand sanitizer
- Grasp the gown in the front and pull away from your body so that the ties break, touching outside of gown only with gloved hands
- While removing the gown, fold or roll the gown inside-out into a bundle
- As you are removing the gown, peel off your gloves at the same time, only touching the inside of the gloves and gown with your bare hands. Place the gown and gloves into a waste container

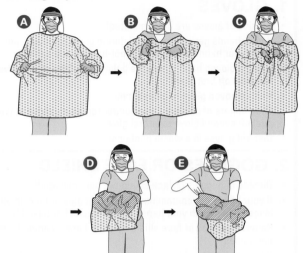

2. GOGGLES OR FACE SHIELD

- Outside of goggles or face shield are contaminated!
- If your hands get contaminated during goggle or face shield removal, immediately wash your hands or use an alcohol-based hand sanitizer
- Remove goggles or face shield from the back by lifting head band and without touching the front of the goggles or face shield
- If the item is reusable, place in designated receptacle for reprocessing. Otherwise, discard in a waste container

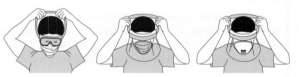

3. MASK OR RESPIRATOR

- Front of mask/respirator is contaminated — DO NOT TOUCH!
- If your hands get contaminated during mask/respirator removal, immediately wash your hands or use an alcohol-based hand sanitizer
- Grasp bottom ties or elastics of the mask/respirator, then the ones at the top, and remove without touching the front
- Discard in a waste container

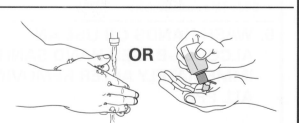

4. WASH HANDS OR USE AN ALCOHOL-BASED HAND SANITIZER IMMEDIATELY AFTER REMOVING ALL PPE

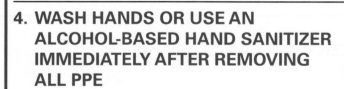

PERFORM HAND HYGIENE BETWEEN STEPS IF HANDS BECOME CONTAMINATED AND IMMEDIATELY AFTER REMOVING ALL PPE

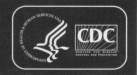

CS250672-E

FIGURE 18-8, cont'd B, Removing PPE: Method 2. (From Centers for Disease Control and Prevention, Department of Health and Human Services.)

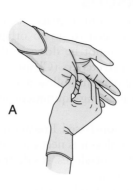
A
Grasp the glove
at the palm.

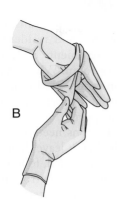
B
Pull the glove down
over the hand.
The glove is inside-out.

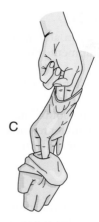
C
Insert the fingers of the
ungloved hand inside
the other glove.

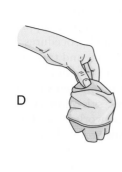
D
Pull the glove down and over
the other hand and glove.
The glove is inside-out.

FIGURE 18-9 Removing gloves.

USED LAUNDRY

Laundry commonly includes bed linens, towels and wash-cloths, and personal clothing or patient gowns. Standard Precautions are used to prevent the transmission of microbes when handling used laundry. Wear gloves if contact with blood or body fluids is likely. Hold laundry away from your body and uniform. Do not shake items or place them on the floor. Do not place used items on a clean item or surface. Place used laundry in leak-proof containers or bags where it was used. Close containers or tie bags securely before transport to the agency's collection or laundering area.

Follow agency policies and procedures for collecting and transporting used laundry from an isolation room. The CDC's guidance is to follow Standard Precautions without special practices. According to the CDC, use of a second bag (double-bagging) is not routinely needed. See "Double-Bagging."

▌ DOUBLE-BAGGING

Using a second bag (double-bagging) is only done if the outside of a bag is visibly soiled or if the contents have leaked through and the bag is wet (Fig. 18-10). If double-bagging is needed, follow your agency's procedures. The following procedure describes how to double-bag items from an isolation room.

See procedure: *Double-Bagging*.

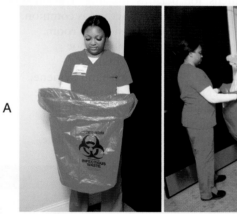

A
B

FIGURE 18-10 Double-bagging. A soiled (dirty) bag is placed in a clean bag. **A,** A cuff is made on the clean bag. **B,** One nursing assistant is in the room by the doorway. The other is outside the doorway. The dirty bag is placed inside the clean bag. (NOTE: A *BIOHAZARD* bag is only used when soiling involves blood or other potentially infectious materials [Chapter 17] or as required by agency policy.)

▌▌ Double-Bagging

PROCEDURE

1 Ask a co-worker to help you. Have your co-worker stand outside the doorway. You remain in the room.
2 Seal the *dirty* bag securely.
3 Ask your co-worker to make a wide cuff on a *clean* bag. It is held wide open. The cuff protects the hands from contamination (see Fig. 18-10, *A*).
4 Place the *dirty* bag into the *clean* bag (see Fig. 18-10, *B*). Do not touch the outside of the *clean* bag.

5 Have your co-worker seal the *clean* bag. Follow agency procedures for use of color-coded or *BIOHAZARD* bags (Chapter 17).
6 Have your co-worker take the bag to the appropriate department for laundering, disinfection, sterilization, or disposal.

USED SUPPLIES AND EQUIPMENT

See Chapter 17 for the measures used to clean and disinfect or sterilize re-usable supplies and equipment. Follow agency policies and procedures to:

- Handle, contain, and transport items contaminated with blood or body fluids.
- Remove re-usable items from an isolation room. The following process is commonly used to bag items for removal.
  - Have a co-worker stand outside the door with an open, leak-proof, clean plastic bag.
  - Place the item inside the bag without contaminating the outside of the bag.
  - Have your co-worker seal the bag and take the item to the appropriate area for cleaning and disinfection.

COLLECTING SPECIMENS

Blood and body fluids often require laboratory testing (Chapter 39). Wear PPE as required for the task to collect the specimen. Place the specimen container in a plastic specimen bag labeled with the *BIOHAZARD* symbol (Chapter 17) for transport to the laboratory. Do not let the specimen container touch the outside of the bag.

Follow agency policies and procedures to collect and transport specimens for persons needing Transmission-Based Precautions. The following method is common.

- Leave the *BIOHAZARD* bag outside the room.
- Collect the specimen (Chapter 39). Do not contaminate the outside of the container.
- Remove and discard PPE. Practice hand hygiene.
- Use a paper towel to pick up the container. Place the specimen in the *BIOHAZARD* bag. Do not contaminate the outside of the bag.
- Discard the paper towel. Practice hand hygiene.

TRANSPORTING PERSONS

To *transport* means to move from 1 place to another. Patients and residents often need to go to other areas for treatments or tests that cannot be done in the person's room. Wheelchairs and stretchers (Chapter 21) are commonly used to move the person. Follow agency policies and procedures for disinfecting equipment used for transport.

Persons needing Transmission-Based Precautions usually do not leave their rooms unless it is necessary. If transport is needed, follow agency procedures. A safe transport protects others from the infection.

- Staff in the receiving area need to know that the person requires isolation precautions. They need to know the type of precaution and the PPE needed.
- The person wears a clean gown or pajamas.
- Barriers are used as needed (see Box 18-3). For example:
  - Tissues and a leak-proof bag are provided for respiratory secretions. Used tissues are placed in the bag.
  - Skin lesions or infected or draining areas are covered.
  - The person wears a mask as required.
- Staff do not wear contaminated PPE during the transport.
- Only the person and transport staff enter an elevator when one is needed. This prevents others from having exposure to infection.
- Staff don clean PPE to handle the person at the transport destination.
- Transport equipment is disinfected after use.

FOCUS ON **PRIDE**

The Person, Family, and Yourself

Personal and Professional Responsibility

Be sure you understand this information and the rules of hand hygiene in Chapter 17 well. Ask your instructor if you have questions. At work, ask the nurse if you have questions about needed PPE or other infection control measures.

Rights and Respect

Transmission-Based Precautions require extra time and effort. The person must not feel like a burden. Watch your verbal and nonverbal communication (Chapter 7).

Independence and Social Interaction

The person on Transmission-Based Precautions may feel isolated and lonely. Visiting with the person and providing hobby or reading materials can help. Remember, items brought into the room become contaminated. Disinfect or discard the items according to agency policy.

Delegation and Teamwork

Good teamwork is helpful when patients or residents need Transmission-Based Precautions. You can tie a gown for a co-worker. You can answer call lights while co-workers provide care in an isolation room. And you can bring any needed supplies to the doorway of the room.

Communicate with co-workers when you will be in a room for a long period of time. Politely ask if they can answer call lights for you. Thank them for their help.

Ethics and Laws

When a person has an infectious disease, remember that the pathogen is undesirable, not the person. Show kindness and respect. Treat the person with dignity.

FOCUS ON **PRIDE**: *Application*

Explain the emotional and social effects of Transmission-Based Precautions. How can you help meet these needs?

REVIEW QUESTIONS

Circle the BEST answer.

1 Which statement about Standard Precautions is *true?*
   a They are used for all persons.
   b The 3 types are contact, droplet, and airborne.
   c They are used only in hospitals.
   d They require a doctor's order.

2 Transmission-Based Precautions are used for
   a All persons
   b Persons who have or may have certain infections
   c Persons recovering from surgery
   d Staff who are at risk for infection

3 What PPE is needed to move and position a patient requiring Contact Precautions?
   a A gown and gloves
   b A gown, mask, and gloves
   c A gown, mask, goggles, and gloves
   d None

4 A patient requires Droplet Precautions. There is 1 mask left outside the room. You should
   a Not use the mask
   b Use the mask and return it for re-use
   c Use the mask and re-stock the masks
   d Wait until a co-worker re-stocks the masks to give care

5 A resident requires Transmission-Based Precautions. You can
   a Use linens that fall on the floor
   b Touch your hair and face in the person's room
   c Use a leak-proof plastic bag to remove a meal tray from the room
   d Keep PPE on when leaving the room to get supplies

6 To remove a gown safely
   a Roll the gown so the outside of the gown is on the outside of the roll
   b Touch the inside with gloved hands
   c Touch the ties with gloved hands
   d Do not touch the front and sleeves with ungloved hands

7 A mask
   a Is removed before other PPE is removed
   b Is contaminated when moist
   c Is the same as a respirator
   d Should fit loosely for breathing

8 To use PPE correctly
   a Never change gloves in the person's room
   b Tie a gown's waist strings in front
   c Don gloves first when applying PPE
   d Apply new PPE for each person

9 Which task requires gloves?
   a Measuring blood pressure
   b Giving a back massage
   c Collecting a urine specimen
   d Moving the person up in bed

10 A glove tears while giving care. You should
   a Continue giving care with the glove
   b Apply a second glove over the torn glove
   c Remove gloves and finish the task without gloves
   d Remove gloves, practice hand hygiene, and apply new gloves

11 You assist a person with wiping after a bowel movement. Then you provide oral care. Which is *correct?*
   a Hand hygiene and clean gloves are needed for oral care.
   b Gloves are not needed for either task.
   c You can wear the same pair of gloves for both tasks.
   d You can change gloves without practicing hand hygiene.

12 Which can contaminate your skin when removing gloves?
   a You touch the inner part of a glove with an ungloved finger.
   b You touch the outer part of a glove with an ungloved hand.
   c You touch the outer part of a glove with a gloved hand.
   d You roll a glove inside-out as it is removed.

13 A face shield is worn
   a For Contact Precautions
   b When splashing of body fluids may occur
   c If you have an eye infection
   d As a substitute for a mask or respirator

14 Which shows you understand how to handle laundry safely?
   a You shake a blanket to remove crumbs from it.
   b You hold linens against your uniform.
   c You place used linens on the floor.
   d You wear gloves to handle a sheet soiled with urine.

15 A person on Droplet Precautions needs a specimen collected. You need to
   a Avoid contaminating the outside of the *BIOHAZARD* bag
   b Wear PPE to deliver the specimen to the laboratory for testing
   c Transport the person to the laboratory to collect the specimen
   d Have the person wear a mask while collecting the specimen

Answers to Chapter 18 questions are on p. 902.

FOCUS ON **PRACTICE**

Problem Solving

You plan to do the following for 1 patient. Identify when to practice hand hygiene and apply gloves. Do you need to change gloves before any tasks?
- Help the person move from the bed to a chair.
- Empty urine from the person's urinal (a container that holds urine).
- Brush and floss the person's teeth.

Safe Handling and Positioning

OBJECTIVES

- Define the key terms and key abbreviations in this chapter.
- Explain the purpose of safe handling and positioning.
- Identify the risk factors for work-related injuries.
- Identify the activities at high risk for work-related injuries, including back injuries.
- Identify the causes, signs, and symptoms of back injuries.
- Explain how to prevent work-related injuries.

- Describe the principles and rules of body mechanics.
- Identify the elements of an effective safe handling program.
- Explain the safety and comfort measures needed when positioning persons.
- Position persons in the basic bed positions and in a chair.
- Explain how to promote PRIDE in the person, the family, and yourself.

KEY TERMS

base of support The area on which an object rests
body alignment The way the head, trunk, arms, and legs align with one another; posture
body mechanics Using the body in an efficient and careful way
dorsal recumbent position The back-lying or supine position
ergonomics The science of designing a job to fit the worker; *ergo* means work, *nomos* means law
Fowler's position A semi-sitting position; the head of the bed is raised between 45 and 60 degrees
high-Fowler's position A variation of Fowler's position; the head of the bed is raised 60 to 90 degrees
lateral position The person lies on 1 side or the other; side-lying position

musculo-skeletal disorders (MSDs) Injuries and disorders of the muscles, tendons, ligaments, joints, and cartilage
posture See "body alignment"
prone position The person lies on the abdomen with the head turned to 1 side
semi-Fowler's position A variation of Fowler's position; the head of the bed is raised 30 degrees
semi-prone position The person lies on the side of the abdomen
side-lying position See "lateral position"
supine position The back-lying or dorsal recumbent position

KEY ABBREVIATIONS

MSD   Musculo-skeletal disorder

OSHA   Occupational Safety and Health Administration

Injuries can occur from activities done on the job. Handling and positioning refer to procedures that involve the movement and alignment of another person's body. Such procedures are a frequent part of the nursing assistant role. Handling and positioning activities place nursing assistants at high risk for injury. The principles of body mechanics, safe handling, and proper positioning help protect you and the person from injury.

See *Body Structure and Function Review: The Musculo-Skeletal System*. For greater detail, see Chapter 10.

BODY STRUCTURE AND FUNCTION REVIEW

The Musculo-Skeletal System

 Bones are hard, rigid structures that provide structure and bear the body's weight. A *joint* is the point at which 2 or more bones meet. *Cartilage* is connective tissue at the end of bones. It cushions the joint so that the bone ends do not rub together. *Ligaments* are strong bands of connective tissue that connect bones at a joint. *Skeletal muscles* are attached to bones. *Tendons* are strong bands of connective tissue that connect muscles to bones. Working together, these structures provide the framework for the body, maintain posture, and allow the body to move. Injuries can occur in any structure in the musculo-skeletal system.

WORK-RELATED INJURIES

Musculo-skeletal disorders (MSDs) are injuries and disorders of the muscles, tendons, ligaments, joints, and cartilage. They can be caused or made worse by the work setting. The lower back and shoulders are often affected. Injuries can involve the nervous system.

Sprains and strains are common.
* *Sprain*—Ligaments are stretched or torn. Symptoms include pain, bruising, swelling, and not being able to use the joint.
* *Strain*—Muscles or tendons are stretched or torn. Symptoms include pain, muscle spasms, swelling, cramping, and problems moving.

MSDs can develop slowly over weeks, months, and years. Or they can occur from 1 event. Early signs and symptoms include pain, difficulty moving, or swelling. Numbness, tingling, stiff joints, and muscle weakness can occur. Disabilities can result. Time off work is often needed.

MSD Risk Factors

The Occupational Safety and Health Administration (OSHA) has identified MSD risk factors. An MSD is more likely if risk factors are combined. For example, a task involves both force and repeating actions.
* *Force*—the amount of physical effort needed for a task. Lifting or transferring heavy persons, preventing falls, and sudden motions are examples.
* *Repeating action*—doing the same motion or series of motions often or continually. Re-positioning persons and transfers to and from beds, chairs, and commodes without adequate rest breaks are examples.
* *Awkward postures*—assuming positions that place stress on the body. Examples are reaching above shoulder height, kneeling, squatting, leaning over a bed, bending, or twisting the torso while lifting. (The torso [trunk] is the chest and abdomen.)
* *Heavy lifting*—manually lifting people who cannot move themselves.

According to the U.S. Department of Labor, nursing assistants are at great risk. The tasks listed in Box 19-1 are high risk for MSDs.

BOX 19-1	Musculo-Skeletal Disorders: Risk Factors for Nursing Assistants

* Transfers—to and from beds, chairs, wheelchairs, toilets, stretchers, and bathtubs
* Trying to stop a person from falling
* Picking up a person from the floor to the bed
* Lifting alone
* Lifting persons who are confused or uncooperative
* Lifting persons who cannot support their own weight
* Lifting heavy persons
* Weighing a person
* Moving a person up in bed
* Re-positioning a person in a bed or in a chair
* Changing an incontinence product
* Making beds
* Dressing and undressing a person
* Feeding a person in bed
* Giving a bed bath
* Applying anti-embolism stockings
* Prolonged holding of a body part for care measures—arm, leg, abdomen, skin fold

Back Injuries. Back injuries are major threats. These and other factors can lead to back disorders.
* Reaching while lifting
* Poor posture when sitting or standing
* Staying in 1 position too long
* Poor body mechanics (p. 276) when lifting, pushing, pulling, or carrying objects
* Poor physical condition—not having the strength or endurance to perform tasks without strain
* Repeated lifting of items, equipment, or persons
* Shifting weight when a person loses balance or strength while moving
* Twisting or bending while lifting or during a task
* Maintaining a bent posture such as leaning over a bed
* Reaching over raised bed rails
* Working in confined, crowded, or cluttered areas (rooms, bathrooms, hallways)
* Fatigue
* Poor footing, such as on slippery floors
* Lifting with forceful movement

Injuries can occur from repeated activities or from 1 event. Signs and symptoms include:
* Pain when trying to assume a normal posture
* Decreased mobility
* Pain when standing or rising from a seated position

See *Promoting Safety and Comfort: Back Injuries.*

PROMOTING SAFETY AND COMFORT
Back Injuries

Safety
The activities listed in Box 19-1 are related to back injuries. Follow the rules and safety measures in this chapter to prevent back injuries. Be very careful during tasks associated with back injuries. Get help and avoid lifting and bending the back when possible. Protect yourself from injury.

Preventing MSDs

A safe work setting is free of hazards that cause or may cause death or serious physical harm to staff. Employers must make reasonable attempts to prevent or reduce hazards.

Ergonomics is the science of designing a job to fit the worker. (*Ergo* means work. *Nomos* means law.) It involves changing the task, work station, equipment, and tools to help reduce stress on the worker's body. The goal is to eliminate a serious work-related MSD.

Your employer has a role in preventing MSDs. So do you. Moving and transfer procedures are major risk factors for injury. The principles of body mechanics and safe handling programs are intended to prevent injury.

Always report a work-related injury as soon as possible. Early attention can prevent the problem from becoming worse. Also, injuries are often less serious and less costly to treat with early attention.

PRINCIPLES OF BODY MECHANICS

Body mechanics means using the body in an efficient and careful way. It involves good posture, balance, and using your strongest and largest muscles for work. Fatigue and injury can result from the incorrect use and positioning of the body during activity or rest.

Body alignment (posture) is the way the head, trunk, arms, and legs align with one another. Good alignment lets the body move and function with strength and efficiency. Standing, sitting, and lying down require good alignment.

Base of support is the area on which an object rests. A good base of support is needed for balance (Fig. 19-1). When standing, your feet are your base of support. Stand with your feet apart for a wider base of support and more balance.

Your strongest and largest muscles are in the shoulders, upper arms, hips, and thighs. Use these muscles to handle and move persons and heavy objects. Otherwise, you place strain and exertion on the smaller and weaker muscles. This causes fatigue and injury. *Back injuries are a major risk.* For good body mechanics:

- Bend your knees and squat to lift a heavy object (Fig. 19-2). Do not bend from your waist. Bending from the waist places strain on small back muscles.
- Hold items close to your body and base of support (see Fig. 19-2). This involves upper arm and shoulder muscles. Holding objects away from the body places strain on small muscles in the lower arms.

All activities require good body mechanics. The principles of body mechanics apply in the work setting and at home. They apply whether you are moving an item or a person. Follow the rules in Box 19-2.

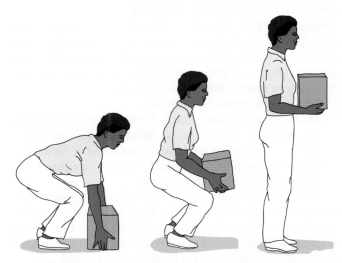

FIGURE 19-2 Picking up a box using good body mechanics.

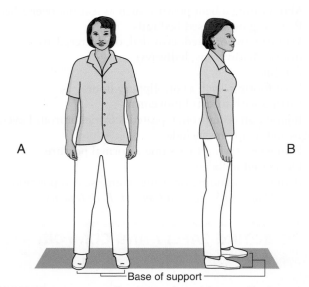

FIGURE 19-1 A, Anterior (front) view of an adult in good body alignment. The feet are apart for a wide base of support. **B,** Lateral (side) view of an adult with good posture and alignment.

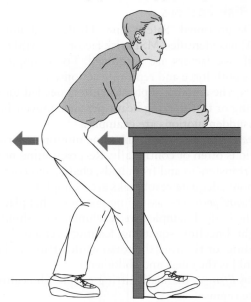

FIGURE 19-3 Move your rear leg back when pulling.

BOX 19-2	Rules of Body Mechanics

- Keep your body in good alignment with a wide base of support. Your feet are at least 12 inches apart or shoulder-width apart.
- Use an upright working posture. Bend your legs. Do not bend your back.
- Use the stronger and larger muscles in your shoulders, upper arms, thighs, and hips.
- Keep objects close to your body to lift, move, or carry them (see Fig. 19-2).
- Avoid bending and reaching. Raise the bed and over-bed table to waist level or to a comfortable working height.
- Face your work area. This prevents twisting.
- Push, slide, or pull heavy objects when you can rather than lifting them. Pushing is easier than pulling.
- Widen your base of support to push or pull. Move your front leg forward when pushing. Move your rear leg back when pulling (Fig. 19-3).
- Use both hands and arms to lift, move, or carry objects.
- Turn your whole body to change direction. Do not twist.
- Work with smooth and even movements. Avoid sudden or jerky motions.
- Do not lean over a person to give care.
- *Get help from a co-worker to move persons or heavy objects. Do not lift or move them by yourself.*
- Bend your hips and knees to lift heavy objects from the floor (see Fig. 19-2). Straighten your back as the object reaches thigh level. Your leg and thigh muscles work to raise the item off the floor and to waist level.
- Do not lift objects higher than chest level. Do not lift above your shoulders. Use a step stool or ladder to reach an object higher than chest level.

SAFE HANDLING PROGRAMS

Proper body mechanics alone do not prevent injury. Health care agencies must plan other ways to protect workers. *Safe handling programs* help reduce the risk of injury to staff and patients or residents from transferring, lifting, re-positioning, and other moving activities.

A safe handling program begins at the management level. OSHA identifies the following elements of an effective program.

- Management is committed to implementing a safe handling program. Policies are in place. Management and departments support the program.
- Staff are involved in the process of planning and implementing the program.
- Hazards are identified and addressed with safety measures.
- Transfer and lifting devices are part of the plan. Staff are involved in the selection of patient or resident handling devices.
- Staff have the needed equipment to avoid manual lifting. Assist devices and mechanical lifts are examples (Chapters 20 and 21).
- Care planning includes safe moving and transfer procedures.
- Staff are trained. Training includes hazard awareness, safe use of transfer and lift equipment and other devices, and safe practices for patient or resident handling.
- The program is reviewed and evaluated.

The guidelines in Box 19-3 outline the safety measures to follow during moving and transfer procedures. You will learn about the specific moving and transfer procedures in Chapters 20 and 21.

See *Promoting Safety and Comfort: Safe Handling Programs*, p. 278.

BOX 19-3	Guidelines for Safe Handling

General Guidelines

- Wear shoes with good traction. Avoid shoes with worn-down soles or sides. Good traction helps prevent slips or falls.
- Use assist equipment and devices (Chapters 20 and 21) when possible instead of lifting and moving the person manually. Follow the care plan.
- Get help from other staff. The nurse and care plan tell you the number of staff needed for a task.
- Plan and prepare for the task. For example, know what equipment is needed, where to place chairs or wheelchairs, and what side of the bed to work on.
- Schedule harder tasks early in your shift.
- Balance lighter and harder tasks. Plan to complete a lighter task after a harder one.
- Lock (brake) bed wheels and wheelchair or stretcher wheels.
- Tell the person how to help. Give clear, simple instructions. Give the person time to respond.
- Do not hold or grab the person under the underarms.
- Do not let the person hold or grasp you around your neck.
- Follow the person's care plan for specific measures.

Manual Lifting

- Minimize or eliminate manual lifting when possible.
- Stand with good posture. Keep your back straight.

Manual Lifting—cont'd

- Bend your legs, not your back.
- Use the large muscles in your legs to do the work.
- Face the person.
- Do not twist or turn. Pick up your feet and pivot (turn) your whole body in the direction of the move.
- Keep what you are moving close to you.
- Move the person toward you, not away from you.
- Use a wide, balanced base of support. Stand with 1 foot slightly ahead of the other.
- Use smooth, even movements. Avoid jerking movements.
- Lift on the "count of 3" when lifting with others. Everyone lifts at the same time.

Transfer/Gait Belts (Chapter 15)

- Keep the person as close to you as possible.
- Avoid bending your back, reaching, or twisting for these and other nursing tasks:
  - Applying or removing a transfer/gait belt
  - Lowering the person to the chair, bed, toilet, or floor
  - Helping the person walk
- Use a gentle rocking motion to help the person stand. The rocking motion gives strength and force as you help the person stand.

Continued

BOX 19-3	Guidelines for Safe Handling—cont'd

Moving the Person in Bed (Chapter 20)
- Adjust the bed height to a safe and comfortable working height.
- Lower the bed rail.
- Work on the side where the person will be closest to you.
- Place equipment or other items close to you at waist level or at a comfortable working height.
- Use friction-reducing devices (Chapters 20 and 21).

Stand and Pivot Transfers (Chapter 21)
- Use assist devices as directed. Follow the care plan.
- Use a transfer belt as directed. The nurse may have you use a transfer belt with handles. See Chapter 15.
- Plan the transfer so the person's strong side moves first.
- Lower the bed so the person can place the feet on the floor.
- Get the person close to the edge of the bed or the chair.
- Block the person's weak leg with your legs or knees. If the position is awkward:
  - Use a transfer belt with handles.
  - Straddle your legs around the person's weak leg.
- Keep your feet at least shoulder-width apart.
- Bend your legs. Do not bend your back.
- Have the person lean forward slightly. Use a gentle rocking motion to help the person stand. The rocking motion gives strength and force as you help the person stand.
- Pivot (turn) with your feet. Do not twist.

Lateral Transfers (Chapter 21)
- Position surfaces close to each other. (A lateral transfer involves 2 horizontal surfaces. For example, a person is moved from a bed to a stretcher.)
- Adjust surfaces to about waist height or to a comfortable working height. Do 1 of the following as directed by the nurse and care plan.
  - Adjust the surfaces to the same level.
  - Adjust the receiving surface so it is slightly lower (about ½ inch) than the surface the person is on. This allows the use of gravity. For example, the stretcher surface (receiving surface) is slightly lower than the bed for a bed to stretcher transfer.

Lateral Transfers (Chapter 21)—cont'd
- Have staff on both sides—staff on the receiving side and staff at the side of the surface the person is on.
- Lower bed rails and stretcher side rails.
- Use friction-reducing devices. Get a good hand-hold. Roll up the sides of the device. Or use a device with handles.
- Kneel on the bed or stretcher if needed to prevent extended reaching and bending your back.
- Move the person on the "count of 3." Use a smooth, push-pull motion. Do not reach across the person.

Transporting the Person and Equipment
- Push, do not pull.
- Keep the load close to your body.
- Use an upright posture.
- Push with your whole body, not just your arms.
- Move down the center of the hallway. This helps avoid collisions.
- Watch out for door handles and high thresholds on floors. These can cause abrupt stops.

Transferring the Person From the Floor
- Avoid manual lifting when possible. Assist as the nurse directs. See Chapter 15.
- See "Manual Lifting" if a manual lift is required and there are no injuries or minor injuries.
  - Roll the person onto the side.
  - Position an assist device. A blanket or drawsheet (Chapter 22) are examples. Avoid reaching across the person.
  - Have at least 2 staff members on each side. The larger the person, the more staff are needed.
  - Bend your knees, not your back. Do not twist.
  - For the lift:
    - Kneel on 1 knee.
    - Grasp the drawsheet, blanket, or other device.
    - Lift smoothly with your legs as you stand. Stand together on the "count of 3." Do not bend your back.

Modified from Cal/OSHA: A back injury prevention guide for health care providers, Sacramento, Calif., 1997, Author; Occupational Safety and Health Administration: Guidelines for nursing homes: ergonomics for the prevention of musculoskeletal disorders, Washington, DC, revised March 2009, Author.

PROMOTING SAFETY AND COMFORT

Safe Handling Programs

Safety
Transfer and lifting devices do not only benefit staff. Such devices can help protect patients and residents from falls, bruising, and skin tears (Chapter 41).

Comfort
Patients, residents, and their families are more at ease when taught about how transfer and lifting devices can prevent injury. The nurse provides this teaching. You must explain a move or transfer before you perform the procedure. See Chapters 20 and 21.

POSITIONING THE PERSON

The person must be positioned correctly at all times. Regular position changes and good alignment promote comfort and well-being. Breathing is easier. Circulation is promoted. Pressure injuries and contractures are prevented. A *contracture* is the lack of joint mobility caused by the abnormal shortening of a muscle (Chapter 35).

Many patients and residents are able to move and turn when in bed or a chair. Some need reminding or help to adjust their positions. Others depend entirely on the nursing team for position changes.

Whether in bed or a chair, the person is re-positioned at least every 2 hours or more often. Follow the nurse's instructions and the care plan. To safely position a person:

- Use good body mechanics.
- Follow the care plan for use of assist devices (Chapters 20 and 21).
- Ask a co-worker to help you if needed.
- Explain the procedure to the person.
- Provide for privacy.
- Be gentle when moving the person.
- Use pillows as directed by the nurse for support and alignment.
- Provide for comfort after positioning. (See the inside of the back cover.)
- Place the call light and other needed items within reach after positioning.
- Complete a safety check before leaving the room. (See the inside of the back cover.)

See *Focus on Communication: Positioning the Person.*
See *Delegation Guidelines: Positioning the Person.*
See *Promoting Safety and Comfort: Positioning the Person.*

FOCUS ON **COMMUNICATION**

Positioning the Person

Moving can be painful. Some older persons have painful joints. Pain is common after surgery or an injury. Avoid causing pain when positioning the person. Explain what you will do before and during the procedure. Move the person slowly and gently. Give the person time to tell you if a movement is painful. Make sure the person is comfortable. You can say:
- "Am I hurting you?"
- "Please tell me if I'm moving you too fast."
- "Please tell me if you feel pain or discomfort."
- "Do you need a pillow adjusted?"
- "Are you comfortable?"
- "How can I help make you more comfortable?"

DELEGATION GUIDELINES

Positioning the Person

Many routine nursing tasks involve positioning and re-positioning. You need this information from the nurse and the care plan.
- Position or positioning limits ordered by the doctor
- How often to turn and re-position the person
- How many staff members need to help you
- What assist devices to use (Chapters 20 and 21)
- What skin care measures to perform (Chapter 24)
- What range-of-motion exercises to perform (Chapter 35)
- Where to place pillows
- What positioning devices and protective devices are needed and how to use them (Chapters 35 and 42)
- What observations to report and record
- When to report observations
- What patient and resident concerns to report at once

PROMOTING SAFETY AND COMFORT

Positioning the Person

Safety
Pressure injuries are serious threats from lying or sitting too long in 1 place. Wet, soiled, and wrinkled linens are other causes. When you re-position a person, make sure linens are clean, dry, and wrinkle-free. Change or straighten linens as needed. Follow the care plan for prevention measures and protective devices to use. See Chapter 42.

Contractures can develop from staying in 1 position too long (Chapter 35). Re-positioning, exercise, and activity help prevent contractures.

Comfort
Pillows and positioning devices (Chapter 42) support body parts and provide good alignment. This promotes comfort. Place pillows and positioning devices as directed by the nurse and the care plan.

Older persons may have limited range of motion in their necks and other joints. (*Range of motion* is the movement of a joint to the extent possible without causing pain. See Chapter 35.) Some positions may not be comfortable for them. Ask about comfort. Do not leave the person in an uncomfortable position.

Fowler's Positions

Fowler's position is a semi-sitting position. The head of the bed is raised between 45 and 60 degrees (Fig. 19-4). The knees may be slightly elevated. Variations of Fowler's position include:

- *Semi-Fowler's position*—the head of the bed is raised 30 degrees. In some agencies, semi-Fowler's position includes raising the knee portion of the bed 15 degrees.
- *High-Fowler's position*—the head of the bed is raised 60 to 90 degrees.

For good alignment:
- The spine is straight.
- The head is supported with a small pillow.
- The arms are supported with pillows.

The nurse may have you place small pillows under the lower back, thighs, and ankles. Persons with heart and respiratory disorders usually breathe easier in Fowler's position.

See *Focus on Math: Fowler's Positions*, p. 280.

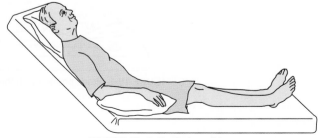

FIGURE 19-4 Fowler's position.

FOCUS ON MATH

Fowler's Positions

+− When 2 lines meet, an angle is formed. Angles are
×÷ measured in degrees (°). Degrees range from 0 to 360.
With bed positions, you need a basic understanding of
angle measurements between 0° and 90°.
To estimate the angle:

1 Use the bed frame and the head of the bed as the 2 lines.
2 Estimate the angle from the bed frame to the head of the
bed. See Figure 19-5.

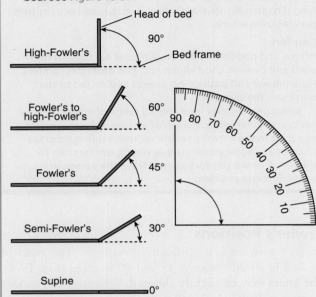

FIGURE 19-5 Measuring bed angles. The angle is measured from
the bed frame to the back of the head of the bed. As the head of the
bed rises, the angle increases.

Supine Position

The *supine position (dorsal recumbent position)* is the
back-lying position (Fig. 19-6).
• The bed is flat.
• The head and shoulders are supported on a pillow.
• Arms and hands are at the sides. You can support the
arms with regular pillows. Or you can support the
hands on small pillows with the palms down.
The nurse may have you place a small pillow under the
lower back and thighs. A pillow under the lower legs lifts
the heels off of the bed. This prevents the heels from rubbing on the sheets.

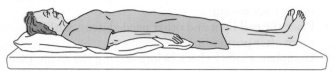

FIGURE 19-6 Supine position.

Prone Position

In the *prone position*, the person lies on the abdomen with
the head turned to 1 side.
• The bed is flat.
• Small pillows are under the head, abdomen, and lower
legs (Fig. 19-7).
• Arms are flexed at the elbows with the hands near the
head.
You also can position a person with the feet hanging
over the end of the mattress (Fig. 19-8). A pillow is not
needed under the feet.

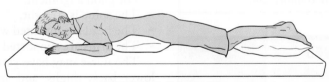

FIGURE 19-7 Prone position.

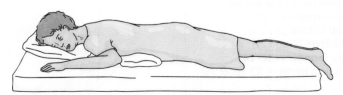

FIGURE 19-8 Prone position with the feet hanging over the edge of the mattress.

Semi-Prone Position

In the *semi-prone position*, the person lies on the side of the abdomen.

- The bed is flat.
- A pillow is under the person's head and shoulder.
- The top leg is sharply flexed (bent). The top leg does not rest on the bottom leg. The top leg and ankle are supported with a pillow.
- The bottom arm is behind the person.
- The top arm is flexed. The arm and hand are supported with a pillow.

The left semi-prone position is used for certain procedures involving the bowel (Chapter 29). In the *left semi-prone position*, the person lies on the left side of the abdomen. The right leg is flexed and supported. The left arm is behind the person. The right arm and hand are supported. See Figure 19-9.

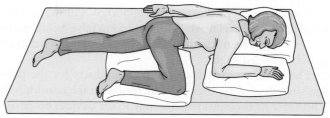

FIGURE 19-9 Left semi-prone position.

Lateral Position

In the *lateral position (side-lying position)*, the person lies on 1 side or the other (Fig. 19-10).

- The bed is flat.
- A pillow is under the head and neck.
- The top leg is flexed. The top leg does not rest on the bottom leg. The top leg and ankle are supported with a pillow. The bottom leg may be flexed for comfort.
- A pillow is against the person's back. The person rolls back against the pillow so that the back is at a 45-degree angle with the mattress.
- Both arms are in front of the body. The top arm is flexed (bent). The arm and hand are supported with a pillow.

A variation of this position is the *30-degree lateral position*. The back is at a 30-degree angle with the mattress. This prevents pressure on the hip that can lead to pressure injuries (Chapter 42).

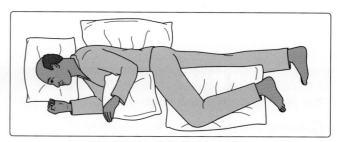

FIGURE 19-10 Lateral position.

Chair Position

A person in a chair must hold the upper body and head upright. If not, poor alignment results. For good alignment:

- The person's back and buttocks are against the back of the chair.
- Feet are flat on the floor or wheelchair footplates. Never leave feet unsupported.
- Backs of the knees and calves are slightly away from the edge of the seat (Fig. 19-11).

The nurse may have you put a small pillow between the person's lower back and the chair. This supports the lower back. *Remember, a pillow is not used behind the back if restraints are used* (Chapter 16).

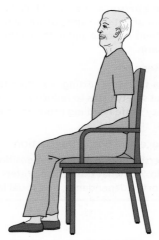

FIGURE 19-11 Chair position.

Support Devices. Sliding down in the seat, leaning forward, and leaning to the side cause poor alignment. Some persons need postural support devices. Special cushions, back supports, side (lateral) supports, and padded footrests are examples.

Weak or paralyzed arms are supported. Pillows or elevated armrests are used. Some persons have positioners (Fig. 19-12). The nurse may have you position the wrists at a slight upward angle.

The health team selects the best products for the person's needs. Safety, dignity, and function are considered. The nurse or therapist teaches how to use devices properly.

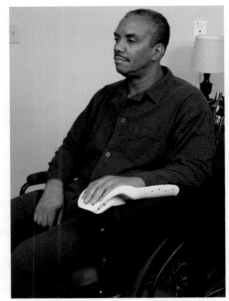

FIGURE 19-12 Elevated armrest and positioner.

FOCUS ON PRIDE

The Person, Family, and Yourself

Personal and Professional Responsibility

You make decisions daily about protecting yourself.

- Do you bend at the waist or the hips and knees to lift objects?
- Do you reach or use a step stool to get high objects?
- Do you exercise for strength and endurance?
- Do you raise the bed when giving bedside care?
- Do you move a person alone or get help?

Your decisions affect the safety of yourself and others. Use good judgment at home and in the workplace. Protect yourself from harm.

Rights and Respect

OSHA requires a safe work setting. You have the right to ask employers about safety plans to reduce your risk of injury. Ask about the agency's safe handling program, staff training, and safety practices.

Independence and Social Interaction

Talk with the person before and during positioning. Explain what you will do. Ask what the person prefers. Doing so promotes comfort, independence, and social interaction.

Delegation and Teamwork

Know which tasks increase your risk for injury. Use caution when doing them. Get help when needed.

Thinking that injuries happen only to others is dangerous. Anyone can be injured. Your safety is important. Take pride in working carefully.

Ethics and Laws

Failure to move and position the person correctly places the person at risk. For example, a person develops a pressure injury after being slumped in a chair for 3 hours. Or a person is injured from being moved without enough help. You must give care in a way that maintains or improves quality of life, health, and safety.

FOCUS ON PRIDE: Application

What changes will you make in your daily life to protect yourself from injury? How do you plan to protect yourself in the workplace?

REVIEW QUESTIONS

Circle the BEST answer.

1 Handling and positioning
   a Are not a common part of the nursing assistant role
   b Are tasks that have a low risk of injury for you
   c Can injure you but not the person
   d Must be practiced safely to protect you and the person

2 Risk of MSDs decreases with
   a Repeating actions
   b Awkward postures
   c Avoiding manual lifting when possible
   d Greater force

3 Regular work tasks include moving persons in bed, transfers to and from bed, dressing, and giving bed baths. These activities
   a Place you at risk for injury
   b Are safe if you usually use good body mechanics
   c Cannot be included in safe handling program planning
   d Cannot be done safely

4 Which statement about back injuries is *true?*
   a Back injuries cannot be prevented.
   b Pain when assuming a normal posture is a symptom.
   c Back injuries are a minor problem.
   d Bending when making beds does not cause back injuries.

5 The purpose of ergonomics is to
   a Reduce stress on the worker's body
   b Discourage time off work due to injury
   c Hold employees responsible for injuries on the job
   d Manage the cost of treating work-related injuries

6 Good body mechanics involve
   a Lifting a heavy object alone
   b Twisting to change direction
   c Reaching to give care
   d Having a wide base of support

7 Proper body mechanics alone prevent injury during handling and positioning procedures.
   a True
   b False

8 Which is an example of good alignment?
   a Being slumped in a bed
   b Sitting upright in a chair
   c Leaning to the side in a wheelchair
   d Walking with the head down and the back bent forward

9 Which action shows poor body mechanics?
   a Holding a meal tray close to your body
   b Raising the over-bed table to prevent bending
   c Leaning over a raised bed rail to give care
   d Using both hands and arms to lift an object

10 You need to move a large chair in a resident's room. You should
   a Push or slide the chair
   b Lift and carry the chair
   c Ask the nurse to move the chair for you
   d Pull the chair using quick, jerking motions

11 You ask about safe handling practices during a job interview. Which reply communicates a commitment to safe handling?
   a "You will not get hurt if you use good body mechanics."
   b "Why do you ask? Do you have back problems?"
   c "You look healthy. I am sure you will be fine."
   d "Staff are trained on hazards and how to safely use equipment to prevent injury."

12 Which statement about positioning is *true?*
   a Re-positioning helps prevent pressure injuries and contractures.
   b Circulation is not affected by positioning.
   c Position changes are avoided if moving causes pain.
   d Persons in chairs do not need to be re-positioned.

13 A resident is to be re-positioned at least every 2 hours. You last re-positioned the person at 0800. At 0900 the person is slumped in bed. You should
   a Wait until 1000 to re-position the person
   b Re-position the person when it is convenient
   c Re-position the person at 0900
   d Wait until the person asks to be re-positioned

14 You position a resident in the lateral position. Where do you place the call light?
   a At the foot of the bed
   b At the head of the bed
   c Behind the person
   d Within the person's reach

15 For Fowler's position
   a The bed is flat
   b The head of the bed is raised 45 to 60 degrees
   c The person's head is turned to 1 side
   d The feet hang over the edge of the mattress

16 The back-lying position is called
   a The prone position
   b The supine position
   c The lateral position
   d High-Fowler's position

17 A pillow is placed against the person's back in
   a A chair while restraints are used
   b The prone position
   c The lateral position
   d The semi-prone position

18 For proper alignment in a chair, the person's feet
   a Are flat on the floor
   b Are able to touch the floor with the toes
   c Are dangling
   d Are positioned on pillows

Answers to Chapter 19 questions are on p. 902.

FOCUS ON **PRACTICE**

Problem Solving

To complete tasks quickly, you do not raise the bed to a comfortable working height. You move persons alone instead of getting help. You lean over the bed instead of moving to the other side. Why do these actions put you at increased risk for injury?

You now have back pain. Your walking is affected. How does this affect your work and daily life? How could you have avoided this problem?

Moving the Person

- Define the key terms and key abbreviation in this chapter.
- Explain how to prevent work-related injuries during moving procedures.
- Identify the delegation information needed before moving the person.
- Identify comfort and safety measures for moving the person.

- Explain how to plan and prepare for a safe move.
- Explain the purpose of friction-reducing devices.
- Perform the procedures described in this chapter.
- Explain how to promote PRIDE in the person, the family, and yourself.

KEY TERMS

bed mobility How a person moves to and from a lying position, turns from side to side, and re-positions in a bed or other sleeping furniture
friction The rubbing of 1 surface against another

logrolling Turning the person as a unit, in alignment, with 1 motion
shearing When the skin sticks to a surface while muscles slide in the direction the body is moving

KEY ABBREVIATION

ID   Identification

You will move persons often. You will assist with bed mobility. *Bed mobility* is how a person moves to and from a lying position, turns from side to side, and re-positions in a bed or other sleeping furniture. You also position the person in chairs and wheelchairs.

Moving procedures involve lifting, awkward postures, and repeated motions. These increase your risk for injury. You must prevent work-related injuries during moving procedures. See Chapter 19.

Good body mechanics alone will not prevent injury. The Occupational Safety and Health Administration (OSHA) recommends:

- Minimizing manual lifting in all cases
- Eliminating manual lifting when possible

You must work carefully to protect yourself and the person from injury.

See *Focus on Communication: Moving the Person.*
See *Delegation Guidelines: Moving the Person.*
See *Promoting Safety and Comfort: Moving the Person.*

FOCUS ON **COMMUNICATION**

Moving the Person

Moving can be painful after an injury or surgery. Many older persons have painful joints. Provide for comfort and avoid causing pain. You can say:

- "Please tell me when you feel pain or discomfort."
- "Do you need a pillow adjusted?"
- "Are you comfortable?"
- "How can I make you more comfortable?"

DELEGATION GUIDELINES

Moving the Person

Moving procedures are routine nursing tasks. Many tasks involve moving persons. Before moving a person, you need this information from the nurse and the care plan.

- The person's height and weight.
- How much help the person needs. These terms may be used.
  - *Independent*—moves without help from another person.
  - *Set-up or clean-up assistance*—requires help to get or put away items before or after the move. The person performs the move without help.
  - *Supervision or touching assistance*—moves without help but needs supervision or cues. To *cue* means to remind the person what to do. Touching or steadying may occur.
  - *Partial (moderate) assistance*—staff lift, hold, or support the body. *Less than half* of the effort is done by staff.
  - *Substantial (maximal) assistance*—staff lift, hold, or support the body. *More than half* of the effort is done by staff.
  - *Dependent*—staff move the person. *All* of the effort is done by staff. (Or 2 or more staff are required to complete the move.)
- The person's physical abilities. Does the person have strength in the arms and legs?
- If the person has a weak side. If yes, which side?
- If the person has problems that increase the risk of injury. Weakness, dizziness, confusion, hearing or vision problems, recent surgery, and fragile skin are examples.
- The person's ability to follow directions.
- Possible behavior problems. Combative, agitated, uncooperative, and unpredictable behaviors are examples.
- The number of staff needed to complete the task safely.
- Any doctor's orders for moving the person.
- What procedure to use.
- What equipment or devices to use.
- What observations to report and record:
  - Who helped you with the move
  - How much help the person needed
  - How the person tolerated the move
  - How you positioned the person
  - Complaints of pain or discomfort
  - Signs of skin breakdown or pressure injury (Chapter 42)
- When to report observations.
- What patient or resident concerns to report at once.

PROMOTING SAFETY AND COMFORT

Moving the Person

Safety

For all moving procedures, you need to move the person carefully. Keep the person in good alignment during and after the move. Make sure the face, nose, and mouth are not obstructed (blocked) by a pillow or other device.

In nursing centers, follow agency policies and procedures for using Enhanced Barrier Precautions for high-contact tasks. See Chapter 18.

Comfort

Explain what you will do and how the person can help. Be courteous. Treat the person with dignity. Screen and cover the person for privacy. These measures promote mental comfort.

Use pillows and other positioning and protective devices as directed by the nurse and the care plan (Chapters 35 and 42). If a pillow is allowed under the person's head, position it so it supports the head and neck.

PLANNING A SAFE MOVE

Each person is different. Careful planning is needed to move the person safely. You must know about the person's physical abilities and the number of staff needed. The number of staff depends on the person's height, weight, cognitive function, and physical abilities.

The nurse and care plan tell you what procedure to use and the equipment or devices needed. Always follow the manufacturer's instructions. You should be trained to use your agency's equipment and devices safely. Ask for any needed training. Use equipment and devices correctly.

See *Focus on Communication: Planning a Safe Move.*

See *Teamwork and Time Management: Planning a Safe Move.*

See *Promoting Safety and Comfort: Planning a Safe Move,* p. 286.

FOCUS ON **COMMUNICATION**

Planning a Safe Move

Before beginning a procedure, tell the person what you and your co-workers will do. Also explain what the person needs to do. Just before the move, remind the person what will happen.

The procedures in this chapter have you move the person on the "count of 3." Staff smoothly move the person at the same time. One co-worker leads by counting. Decide who will count before the move. Be sure the person and staff know who is leading and what to do. You can say:

We will help you move up in bed. I will count "1, 2, 3." When I say "3," push against the bed with your feet. We will help you move when I say "3."

TEAMWORK AND TIME MANAGEMENT

Planning a Safe Move

Patients and residents are moved, turned, and re-positioned often. Some procedures are best done by at least 2 staff members.

Friendships are common among co-workers. And some working relationships are better than others. Do not just ask for help from or give help to friends or those with whom you work well. Include all co-workers. This includes new staff and those from other units.

PROMOTING SAFETY AND COMFORT

Planning a Safe Move

Safety

Decide how to move the person before the procedure. Ask needed staff to help before you begin. To prevent injury:

- Follow the rules of body mechanics (Chapter 19). Stand with a wide base of support and good posture. Bend your hips and knees, not your back.
- Have help to move persons who cannot move alone. Use friction-reducing devices as instructed by the nurse and the care plan.

  Beds are raised to move persons in bed. This reduces bending and reaching. You must:
- Use the bed correctly. Be sure bed wheels are locked (braked) before a move.
- Protect the person from falling when the bed is raised (Chapter 15). Follow the care plan for bed rail use. Ask a co-worker to help you if needed. Never leave the person alone when the bed is raised.
- Lower the bed to a comfortable and safe level for the person after giving care. Follow the care plan.

  You need to plan how to protect tubes and devices connected to the person. Intravenous (IV) tubing (Chapter 33), urine drainage systems (Chapter 28), and wound drains (Chapter 41) are examples.

  If needed, move furniture to provide moving space. Return the furniture to its proper place after the move.

PROTECTING THE SKIN

Friction and shearing injure the skin (Fig. 20-1). Both cause infection and pressure injuries (Chapter 42).

- *Friction* is the rubbing of 1 surface against another. When moved in bed, the person's skin rubs against the sheet.
- *Shearing* is when the skin sticks to a surface while muscles slide in the direction the body is moving. It occurs when the person slides down in bed or is moved in bed.

Older persons are at great risk for skin damage from shearing. Their fragile skin is easily torn. Protect the skin during moving procedures. Ask a co-worker to help you. Move the person carefully and gently. Use a friction-reducing device.

See *Focus on Surveys: Protecting the Skin.*

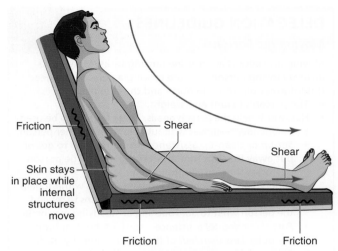

FIGURE 20-1 Friction and shearing injure the skin and underlying tissues and blood vessels. (Modified from Gosnell K, Cooper K: *Foundations of nursing*, ed 9, St Louis, 2023, Elsevier.)

Friction-Reducing Devices

Friction-reducing devices (assist devices) protect the person's skin from injury. They also help prevent work-related injuries. Examples of devices placed under the person include:

- Turning pads or turning sheets (Fig. 20-2)
- Slide sheets (Fig. 20-3)
- Drawsheets (Chapter 22) or flat sheets folded in half
- Large re-usable waterproof under-pads (Chapter 22)

  With these devices, the person is moved evenly. Shearing and friction are reduced. At least 2 staff members are needed to move the person. See "Moving Persons in Bed" on p. 288.

  When able, the person moves alone or helps with the move. The person may use a trapeze (Fig. 20-4). A *trapeze* is a bar that hangs from an over-bed frame. The person grasps the bar with both hands to lift the trunk (torso) off of the bed. The person uses it to move in bed alone or with the help of staff (p. 290).

  See *Promoting Safety and Comfort: Friction-Reducing Devices.*

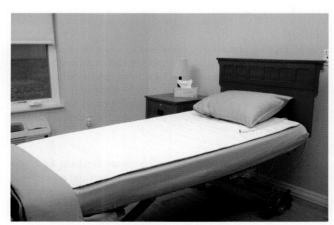

FIGURE 20-2 Turning pad.

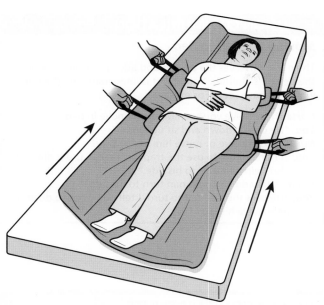

FIGURE 20-3 A slide sheet.

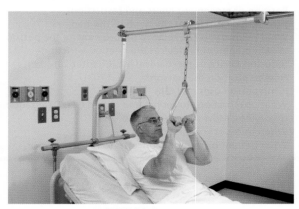

FIGURE 20-4 A trapeze.

PROMOTING SAFETY AND COMFORT

Friction-Reducing Devices

Safety

Disposable, single-use under-pads are not strong enough to hold the person's weight during a move. Re-usable under-pads are stronger. Ask the nurse if the person's under-pad is safe to use for moving. For safety, the under-pad must:

• Be strong enough to support the person's weight.
• Be long enough. It should extend from the person's head or shoulders (depending on the person's ability to lift the head and neck) to above the knees or lower.
• Be wide enough for staff to get a firm grip.

Slide sheets are made of slick material. After using a slide sheet, remove it. If left in place, the person can slide down in bed or off of the bed.

Positioning Friction-Reducing Devices. For a device manufactured as a friction-reducing device, use it following the manufacturer's instructions.

Some slide sheets can be positioned with the person lying flat. The device is folded, placed under the person beginning at the head or foot, and unfolded beneath the person. Follow the manufacturer's instructions to position the device.

Turning (rolling) to position a device is common (Fig. 20-5). You and at least 1 co-worker:

1 Turn the person to 1 side. See "Turning Persons" on p. 293.
2 Place the device on the bed. Open and fan-fold it toward the person. The device is positioned from the head to above the knees or lower.
3 Tell the person that there will be a "bump" to roll over. Assure the person that he or she will not fall.
4 Turn the person to the other side. The person rolls over the device.
5 Pull the device tightly. Smooth any wrinkles.
6 Roll the person onto the back. The person is lying on the device.

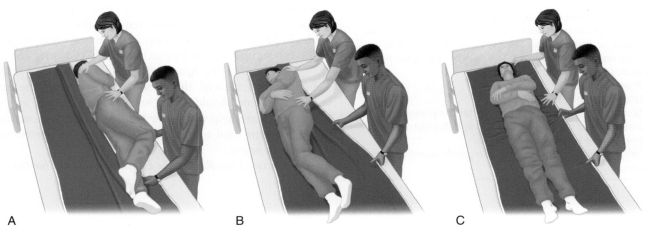

A   B   C

FIGURE 20-5 Turning the person to position a friction-reducing device. **A,** The person is turned to the side. The device is placed on the bed and fan-folded toward the person. **B,** The person is rolled to the other side. The device is pulled tightly. **C,** The person is rolled onto the back. The person is lying on the device.

MOVING PERSONS IN BED

Some persons can move and turn in bed without help. Others need help from 2 or more people. Those who are weak, unconscious, paralyzed, or in casts need help. Sometimes a mechanical lift (Chapter 21) is needed. Follow the guidelines in Box 20-1 to move persons in bed.

See *Focus on Children and Older Persons: Moving Persons in Bed.*

See *Focus on Communication: Moving Persons in Bed.*

See *Delegation Guidelines: Moving Persons in Bed.*

BOX 20-1	Guidelines for Moving Persons in Bed

- Follow the guidelines to prevent work-related injuries (Chapter 19).
- Know how much help and what equipment or friction-reducing devices you need. Follow the nurse's directions and the care plan. The nurse uses the person's weight to plan a safe move.
  - *Persons fully able to assist*—staff assistance is not needed. Staff stand by for safety and provide cues as needed.
  - *Persons partially able to assist:*
    - *The person weighs less than 200 pounds*—2 to 3 staff members and a friction-reducing device are used.
    - *The person weighs more than 200 pounds*—at least 3 staff members and a friction-reducing device are used.
  - *Persons unable to assist*—a mechanical lift and at least 2 staff members are needed. See "Using a Mechanical Lift" in Chapter 21.

Modified from Occupational Safety and Health Administration: Guidelines for nursing homes: ergonomics for the prevention of musculoskeletal disorders, Washington, DC, revised March 2009, Author.

FOCUS ON CHILDREN AND OLDER PERSONS

Moving Persons in Bed

Older Persons

Persons with dementia may not understand what you are doing. They may resist your efforts. The person may shout, grab you, or try to hit you. Always have a co-worker help you. Do not force the person. The person's care plan has measures for safe care. For example:

- Proceed slowly.
- Use a calm, pleasant voice.
- Distract the person. For example, let the person hold a washcloth or other soft object. This helps distract the person and keeps the hands busy.

Tell the nurse at once if you have problems moving the person.

FOCUS ON COMMUNICATION

Moving Persons in Bed

The nurse observes the person and asks questions to assess the person's abilities. Your input is important. Tell the nurse what you have seen. For example:

Nurse: "How have you seen Mr. Boyd move in bed?"
You: "He can lie down and sit up alone."
Nurse: "Do you cue or move him in any way?"
You: "I remind him to use the trapeze. He can use it alone. I also help him turn to his side."
Nurse: "How do you help him turn to his side?"
You: "He uses the bed rail to turn. I tell him what to do and help move his legs."

DELEGATION GUIDELINES

Moving Persons in Bed

Before moving a person in bed, you need this information from the nurse and the care plan.

- The number of staff needed to safely move the person
- Position or movement limits and restrictions
- How far you can lower the head of the bed
- What pillows you can remove before moving the person
- What equipment or devices are needed—friction-reducing device or mechanical lift (Chapter 21)
- How to position the person
- If the person uses bed rails
- What observations to report and record (see *Delegation Guidelines: Moving the Person*, p. 285)
- When to report observations
- What patient or resident concerns to report at once

Raising the Person's Head and Shoulders

Sometimes you raise the person's head and shoulders to give care. Moving the pillow requires this procedure. It also is done when changing garments in bed when the person can sit up and lean forward with help (Chapter 26).

You can raise the head and shoulders easily and safely by locking arms with the person and supporting the person's neck and shoulders. *Do not pull on the person's arm or shoulder.* Have help with older persons and with those who are heavy or hard to move. This protects the person and you from injury.

See procedure: *Raising the Person's Head and Shoulders.*

Raising the Person's Head and Shoulders

QUALITY OF LIFE

- Knock before entering the person's room.
- Address the person by name.
- Introduce yourself by name and title.

- Explain the procedure before starting and during the procedure.
- Protect the person's rights during the procedure.
- Handle the person gently during the procedure.

PRE-PROCEDURE

1 Follow *Delegation Guidelines:*
   a *Moving the Person*, p. 285
   b *Moving Persons in Bed*
   See *Promoting Safety and Comfort*:
   a *Moving the Person*, p. 285
   b *Planning a Safe Move*, p. 286
2 Ask a co-worker to help you if needed.

3 Practice hand hygiene.
4 Identify the person. Check the identification (ID) bracelet against the assignment sheet. Use 2 identifiers (Chapter 14). Also call the person by name.
5 Provide for privacy.
6 Lock (brake) the bed wheels.
7 Raise the bed for body mechanics. Bed rails are up if used.

PROCEDURE

8 If you are working alone and the person has a weaker side, stand on the weak side. Have your co-worker stand on the other side of the bed (if needed).
9 Lower 1 or both bed rails if up. Raise the head of the bed.
10 Lock arms and support the person's neck and shoulders.
   a Place your near arm behind the person's near arm and shoulder. Have the person do the same to your arm. The person's hand rests on your shoulder. See Figure 20-6, *A*. If working with a co-worker, your co-worker does the same on the other side (Fig. 20-7, *A*, p. 290).
   b Bring your other arm around the person's back. Grasp the person's far shoulder. Your arm supports the neck and shoulder (Fig. 20-6, *B*). If working with a co-worker, your co-worker also places a hand behind the back to support the person (Fig. 20-7, *B*, p. 290).

11 Help the person lean forward on the "count of 3" (Fig. 20-6, *C*).
12 Continue to support the person with your near arm if needed. Give care with your far arm. If working with a co-worker, one of you supports the person. The other gives care (Fig. 20-7, *C*, p. 290).
13 Help the person lie down. Provide support with your locked arm. Support the person's neck and shoulders with your other arm. Your co-worker does the same.

POST-PROCEDURE

14 Position the person in good alignment. Lower the head of the bed to a position of comfort.
15 Provide for comfort. (See the inside of the back cover.)
16 Place the call light and other needed items within reach.
17 Lower the bed to a safe and comfortable level. Follow the care plan.
18 Raise or lower bed rails. Follow the care plan.

19 Follow the care plan and the person's preferences for privacy measures to maintain. Leaving the privacy curtain, window coverings, and door open or closed are examples.
20 Complete a safety check of the room. (See the inside of the back cover.)
21 Practice hand hygiene.
22 Report and record your care and observations.

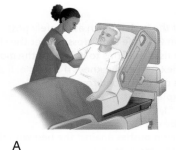 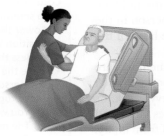 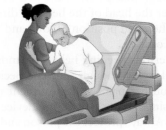

A   B   C

FIGURE 20-6 Raising the person's head and shoulders. **A,** You and the person lock arms. Place your near arm behind the person's near arm and shoulder. The person does the same to your arm. **B,** Bring your other arm around the person's back. Grasp the person's far shoulder. Your arm supports the neck and shoulder. **C,** Help the person lean forward.

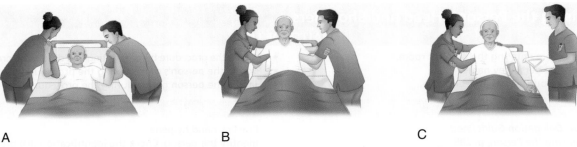

A   **B**   **C**

FIGURE 20-7 Raising the person's head and shoulders with a co-worker. **A,** You and your co-worker lock arms with the person. **B,** You both place an arm behind the person's back, supporting the neck and shoulders. You both help the person lean forward. **C,** One of you supports the person. The other gives care.

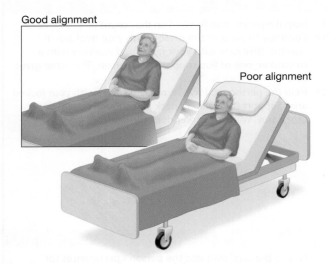

Good alignment

Poor alignment

FIGURE 20-8 A person in poor alignment after sliding down in bed.

Moving the Person Up in Bed

When the head of the bed is raised, it is easy to slide down toward the middle and foot of the bed (Fig. 20-8). Moving the person up in bed promotes good alignment and comfort.

Persons who are fully able to assist can move up in bed alone. Some need cues (direction) from staff. For example, a person pushes off of the bed with the arms and feet. You lower the head of the bed and direct the person in the move. Then you position pillows and raise the head of the bed for comfort.

For persons needing help, 2 or more staff members are needed. Having enough staff is especially important when the person has pain with movement or is heavy, weak, or older. Using a friction-reducing device promotes safety and comfort. Always protect the person and yourself from injury.

See *Promoting Safety and Comfort: Moving the Person Up in Bed*.

See procedure: *Moving the Person Up in Bed With a Friction-Reducing Device*.

PROMOTING SAFETY AND COMFORT
Moving the Person Up in Bed

Safety

The procedure that follows is a general procedure for use with a trapeze or a drawsheet, waterproof under-pad, or slide sheet. For other manufactured friction-reducing devices, follow the manufacturer's instructions.

This procedure is done with at least 2 staff members. More may be needed. Use the guidelines in Box 20-1. Follow the care plan and the nurse's directions. Work from the side of the bed. Do not pull the person from the head of the bed.

For persons with bariatric needs, the care plan may include:

- Positioning the bed in Trendelenburg's position with the head of the bed lowered and the foot of the bed raised (Chapter 13). Gravity helps with the move. (*Gravity* is a natural force that pulls things downward.) The position is used only if tolerated by the person and allowed by the doctor.
- Leaving a friction-reducing device under the person. The device is covered with a drawsheet. Leaving the device in place reduces the risk of injuries from placing and removing the device.
- Using a bariatric lift.

Do not let the person's head hit the head-board when moving up in bed. If the person can be without a pillow, place it upright against the head-board.

Comfort

For a smoother move:
- Lower the head of the bed as much as is safely possible.
- Position the person with the arms crossed over the chest (unless the person uses the arms to help with the move).
- Have the person flex (bend) the knees if possible. If able, the person pushes off of the bed to assist.
- Move together. Explain that:
  - You will count "1, 2, 3."
  - The move will be on "3."
  - On "3," the person pushes against the bed with the feet (if able). Staff move together.
- Use a smooth, even movement. Repeat the move if needed.

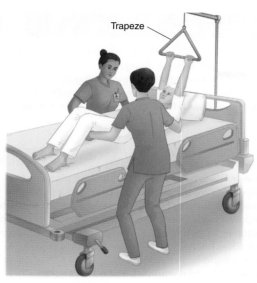

FIGURE 20-9 Moving a person up in bed with a trapeze.

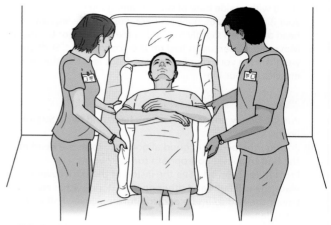

FIGURE 20-10 Moving a person up in bed with a drawsheet. Rolled close to the person, the drawsheet is held near the shoulders and hips.

Moving the Person Up in Bed With a Friction-Reducing Device

QUALITY OF LIFE

- Knock before entering the person's room.
- Address the person by name.
- Introduce yourself by name and title.

- Explain the procedure before starting and during the procedure.
- Protect the person's rights during the procedure.
- Handle the person gently during the procedure.

PRE-PROCEDURE

1 Follow *Delegation Guidelines*:
  a *Moving the Person*, p. 285
  b *Moving Persons in Bed*, p. 288
  See *Promoting Safety and Comfort*:
  a *Moving the Person*, p. 285
  b *Planning a Safe Move*, p. 286
  c *Friction-Reducing Devices*, p. 287
  d *Moving the Person Up in Bed*
2 Ask at least 1 co-worker to help you.

3 Practice hand hygiene and get the needed friction-reducing device if it is not already in place. (This procedure instructs on a move with a trapeze and a move with a friction-reducing device under the person.)
4 Identify the person. Check the ID bracelet against the assignment sheet. Use 2 identifiers (Chapter 14). Also call the person by name.
5 Provide for privacy.
6 Lock (brake) the bed wheels.
7 Raise the bed for body mechanics. Bed rails are up if used.

PROCEDURE

8 Stand on 1 side of the bed. Your co-worker stands on the other side.
9 Lower the head of the bed to a level appropriate for the person. It is as flat as possible.
10 Lower the bed rails if up.
11 Remove pillows as directed by the nurse. Place a pillow upright against the head-board if the person can be without it.
12 *If using a trapeze:*
  a Have the person grasp the trapeze and flex both knees.
  b Place 1 arm under the person's shoulder and 1 arm under the thighs. Your co-worker does the same. Grasp each other's forearms (Fig. 20-9). Or use a friction-reducing device under the person (step 13).

13 *If using a friction-reducing device under the person:*
  a Position the device. (See "Positioning Friction-Reducing Devices" on p. 287.)
  b Have the person cross the arms over the chest (unless the person uses the arms to assist with the move).
  c Roll the sides of the device up close to the person. (Note: Omit this step if the device has handles.)
  d Grasp the device firmly near the person's shoulders and hips (Fig. 20-10). Or grasp it by the handles. Be sure the person's head is supported.
14 Explain that:
  a You will count "1, 2, 3."
  b The move will be on "3."
  c On "3," the person needs to push against the bed with the feet if able. If using a trapeze, the person will pull up with the trapeze.

Continued

Moving the Person Up in Bed With a Friction-Reducing Device—cont'd

PROCEDURE—cont'd

15 Stand with a wide base of support and good posture. Bend your hips and knees, not your back. Position the leg near the head of the bed slightly forward in the direction of the move.

16 Move the person up in bed on the "count of 3." Shift your weight from your rear leg to your front leg. Use the strong muscles in your legs.

17 Repeat steps 15 and 16 if necessary.

18 Unroll the sides of the friction-reducing device if used. (NOTE: Omit this step if the device has handles.) Remove a slide sheet if used. Have the person release the trapeze.

POST-PROCEDURE

19 Put the pillow under the person's head and neck. Straighten linens.

20 Position the person in good alignment. Raise the head of the bed to a level appropriate for the person.

21 Provide for comfort. (See the inside of the back cover.)

22 Place the call light and other needed items within reach.

23 Lower the bed to a safe and comfortable level. Follow the care plan.

24 Raise or lower bed rails. Follow the care plan.

25 Follow the care plan and the person's preferences for privacy measures to maintain. Leaving the privacy curtain, window coverings, and door open or closed are examples.

26 Complete a safety check of the room. (See the inside of the back cover.)

27 Practice hand hygiene.

28 Report and record your care and observations.

Moving the Person to the Side of the Bed

Re-positioning and care procedures require moving the person to the side of the bed. For example:

- Bathing in a bed may require reaching over the person. You reach less if the person is near you.
- Before turning the person into the lateral (side-lying) position, you move the person to the side of the bed. Otherwise, after turning, the person lies on the side of the bed—not in the middle.

In 1 method, the person is moved in segments (Fig. 20-11). Sometimes you can do this alone if the person is small in size. Using a friction-reducing device helps prevent pain, skin damage, and injury to the bones, joints, and spinal cord. Follow the guidelines for moving persons in bed (Box 20-1). A mechanical lift (Chapter 21) may be needed.

See *Promoting Safety and Comfort: Moving the Person to the Side of the Bed.*

See procedure: *Moving the Person to the Side of the Bed.*

PROMOTING SAFETY AND COMFORT

Moving the Person to the Side of the Bed

Safety

Use the method and equipment that are best for the person. The nurse and the care plan tell you which method to use. The wrong method could cause serious injury. This is very important for person who are older, have arthritis and painful joints, or are recovering from spinal cord injury or surgery.

Only move the person alone in segments if the person is small in size and you are comfortable doing so. To move the person in segments, move the person toward you, not away from you. Stand with a wide base of support and good posture. Bend your hips and knees, not your back. Position 1 leg in front of the other. When moving, shift your weight to your rear leg.

To use a friction-reducing device, you need at least 1 co-worker to help you. More staff members may be needed. Remove a slide sheet after use.

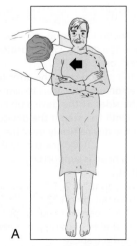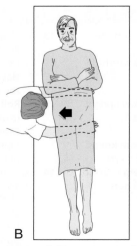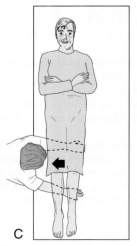

FIGURE 20-11 Moving the person to the side of the bed in segments. **A,** The upper part of the body is moved. **B,** The lower part of the body is moved. **C,** The legs and feet are moved. (CAUTION: Only perform this method alone if the person is small in size and you are comfortable doing so.)

Moving the Person to the Side of the Bed

QUALITY OF LIFE

- Knock before entering the person's room.
- Address the person by name.
- Introduce yourself by name and title.

- Explain the procedure before starting and during the procedure.
- Protect the person's rights during the procedure.
- Handle the person gently during the procedure.

PRE-PROCEDURE

1 Follow *Delegation Guidelines:*
   a *Moving the Person,* p. 285
   b *Moving Persons in Bed,* p. 288
   See *Promoting Safety and Comfort:*
   a *Moving the Person,* p. 285
   b *Planning a Safe Move,* p. 286
   c *Friction-Reducing Devices,* p. 287
   d *Moving the Person to the Side of the Bed*
2 Ask at least 1 co-worker to help you as needed.

3 Practice hand hygiene and get the needed friction-reducing device if it is not already in place. (This procedure uses a drawsheet.)
4 Identify the person. Check the ID bracelet against the assignment sheet. Use 2 identifiers (Chapter 14). Also call the person by name.
5 Provide for privacy.
6 Lock (brake) the bed wheels.
7 Raise the bed for body mechanics. Bed rails are up if used.

PROCEDURE

8 Stand on the side of the bed to which you will move the person.
9 Lower the head of the bed to a level appropriate for the person. It is as flat as possible.
10 Lower the bed rail near you if bed rails are used. (Both bed rails are lowered for Method 2.)
11 Remove pillows as directed by the nurse.
12 Cross the person's arms over the chest.
13 Stand with a wide base of support and good posture. Bend your hips and knees, not your back. One foot is in front of the other.
14 *Method 1—moving the person in segments:*
   a Place your arm under the person's neck and shoulders. Grasp the far shoulder.
   b Place your other arm under the mid-back.
   c Move the upper part of the person's body toward you. Rock backward. Shift your weight to your rear leg (see Fig. 20-11, *A*).

   d Place 1 arm under the person's waist and 1 under the thighs.
   e Rock backward to move the lower part of the person toward you (see Fig. 20-11, *B*).
   f Place your arms under the person's thighs and calves. Repeat the procedure for the legs and feet (see Fig. 20-11, *C*).
15 *Method 2—moving the person with a drawsheet:*
   a Position the drawsheet if it is not already under the person.
   b Roll up the drawsheet close to the person (see Fig. 20-10).
   c Grasp the rolled-up drawsheet near the person's shoulders and hips. Your co-worker does the same. Be sure the person's head is supported.
   d Rock backward on the "count of 3," moving the person toward you. Your co-worker rocks backward slightly and then forward toward you while keeping the arms straight.
   e Unroll the drawsheet. Remove any wrinkles.

POST-PROCEDURE

16 Put the pillow under the person's head and neck. Straighten linens.
17 Turn and position the person on the side. See "Turning Persons." Or return the person to the center of the bed after completing care at the side of the bed.
18 Position the person in good alignment.
19 Provide for comfort. (See the inside of the back cover.)
20 Place the call light and other needed items within reach.
21 Lower the bed to a safe and comfortable level. Follow the care plan.

22 Raise or lower bed rails. Follow the care plan.
23 Follow the care plan and the person's preferences for privacy measures to maintain. Leaving the privacy curtain, window coverings, and door open or closed are examples.
24 Complete a safety check of the room. (See the inside of the back cover.)
25 Practice hand hygiene.
26 Report and record your care and observations.

TURNING PERSONS

Turning persons onto their sides helps prevent complications from immobility and bed rest (Chapter 35). Procedures and care measures often require the side-lying position. You also may turn the person to position and remove friction-reducing devices.

You turn the person toward you or away from you (Fig. 20-12, p. 294). The direction depends on the person's condition and the situation.

Many older persons have painful joints and arthritis in their spines, hips, and knees. Less painful, logrolling (p. 295) is preferred for turning these persons.

See *Delegation Guidelines: Turning Persons,* p. 294.
See *Promoting Safety and Comfort: Turning Persons,* p. 294.
See procedure: *Turning and Positioning the Person on the Side,* p. 295.

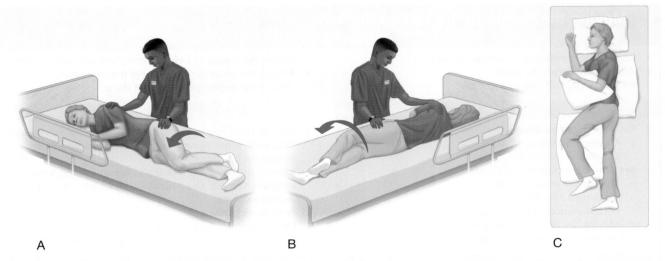

FIGURE 20-12 Turning and positioning the person on the side (lateral position). **A,** Turning the person away from you. **B,** Turning the person toward you. **C,** Positioning on the side with pillows for support.

DELEGATION GUIDELINES

Turning Persons

Before turning and positioning a person, you need this information from the nurse and the care plan.
- How much help the person needs
- The number of staff needed for safety
- The person's comfort level and painful body parts
- If logrolling is needed
- What friction-reducing device to use (if needed)
- What positioning and protective devices to use (Chapters 35 and 42)
- Where to place pillows
- What observations to report and record (See *Delegation Guidelines: Moving the Person*, p. 285)
- When to report observations
- What patient or resident concerns to report at once

PROMOTING SAFETY AND COMFORT

Turning Persons

Safety

Do not turn a person away from you with the far bed rail down. You can do 1 of the following instead.
- Turn the person toward a co-worker positioned on the other side of the bed.
- Raise the bed rail on the side near you. Go to the other side of the bed. Turn the person toward you.

When positioned on the side, the person does not lie on the bottom arm. The top leg is flexed (bent) in front of the bottom leg and supported. This prevents contact between the knees and ankles that can cause pressure injuries (Chapter 42). Make sure the person's face, nose, and mouth are not obstructed (blocked) by a pillow or other device.

Comfort

Move the person to the side of the bed (p. 292) before turning and positioning the person on the side. Move the person to the side of the bed opposite to where you will turn. The person is in the center of the bed after the turn.

After turning, position the person in good alignment. Use pillows as directed to support the person in the lateral (side-lying) position. Placing a pillow in the following places is common for comfort and alignment.
- Under the head and neck
- Against the back
- Supporting the top arm and hand
- Supporting the top leg and ankle

Turning and Positioning the Person on the Side

QUALITY OF LIFE

- Knock before entering the person's room.
- Address the person by name.
- Introduce yourself by name and title.

- Explain the procedure before starting and during the procedure.
- Protect the person's rights during the procedure.
- Handle the person gently during the procedure.

PRE-PROCEDURE

1 Follow *Delegation Guidelines:*
  a *Moving the Person*, p. 285
  b *Moving Persons in Bed*, p. 288
  c *Turning Persons*
  See *Promoting Safety and Comfort:*
  a *Moving the Person*, p. 285
  b *Planning a Safe Move*, p. 286
  c *Moving the Person to the Side of the Bed*, p. 292
  d *Turning Persons*

2 Practice hand hygiene.
3 Identify the person. Check the ID bracelet against the assignment sheet. Use 2 identifiers (Chapter 14). Also call the person by name.
4 Provide for privacy.
5 Lock (brake) the bed wheels.
6 Raise the bed for body mechanics. Bed rails are up if used.

PROCEDURE

7 Stand on the side of the bed opposite to where you will turn the person.
8 Lower the head of the bed to a level appropriate for the person. It is as flat as possible.
9 Lower the bed rail.
10 Move the person to the side near you. See procedure: *Moving the Person to the Side of the Bed*, p. 293.
11 Cross the person's arms over the chest. Cross the leg near you over the far leg.
12 *Turning the person away from you:*
  a Stand with a wide base of support and good posture. Bend your hips and knees, not your back. One foot is in front of the other.
  b Place 1 hand on the person's shoulder. Place the other on the hip near you.
  c Roll the person gently away from you toward the raised bed rail (see Fig. 20-12, *A*).
  d Shift your weight from your rear leg to your front leg. If the person can assist with the turn, have the person grasp the far bed rail when able.

13 *Turning the person toward you:*
  a Raise the bed rail.
  b Go to the other side of the bed. Lower the bed rail.
  c Stand with a wide base of support and good posture. Bend your hips and knees, not your back. One foot is in front of the other.
  d Place 1 hand on the person's shoulder. Place the other on the far hip.
  e Roll the person gently toward you (see Fig. 20-12, *B*). Shift your weight from your front leg to your rear leg.
14 Position the person (see Fig. 20-12, *C*). Follow the nurse's directions and the care plan. For a lateral (side-lying) position:
  a Place a pillow under the head and neck.
  b Adjust the shoulder. The person should not be on an arm.
  c Position a pillow against the back.
  d Place a small pillow under the top arm and hand.
  e Flex (bend) the top hip and knee. Support the top leg and ankle on a pillow. The top leg does not rest on the bottom leg.

POST-PROCEDURE

15 Provide for comfort. (See the inside of the back cover.)
16 Place the call light and other needed items within reach.
17 Lower the bed to a safe and comfortable level. Follow the care plan.
18 Raise or lower bed rails. Follow the care plan.
19 Follow the care plan and the person's preferences for privacy measures to maintain. Leaving the privacy curtain, window coverings, and door open or closed are examples.

20 Complete a safety check of the room. (See the inside of the back cover.)
21 Practice hand hygiene.
22 Report and record your care and observations.

Logrolling

Logrolling is turning the person as a unit, in alignment, with 1 motion. The head, neck, and spine are kept straight. The procedure is used to turn:

- Older persons with painful joints or arthritis of the spine, hip, or knee.
- Persons recovering from hip fractures.
- Persons with spinal cord injuries or after spinal cord surgery.
  See *Promoting Safety and Comfort: Logrolling.*
  See procedure: *Logrolling the Person*, p. 296.

PROMOTING SAFETY AND COMFORT

Logrolling

Safety
For logrolling, 2 or 3 staff members are needed. If the person is tall or heavy, at least 3 are needed. You may use a friction-reducing device (p. 286).

After spinal cord injury or surgery, the head, neck, and spine are kept straight. A device on the neck (cervical collar) helps maintain alignment. The doctor or nurse stands at the head of the bed and holds the head, neck, and spine straight during the move. The doctor (nurse) directs the move step-by-step. Assist as directed. Position the person and use pillows as directed.

Logrolling the Person

QUALITY OF LIFE

- Knock before entering the person's room.
- Address the person by name.
- Introduce yourself by name and title.

- Explain the procedure before starting and during the procedure.
- Protect the person's rights during the procedure.
- Handle the person gently during the procedure.

PRE-PROCEDURE

1 Follow *Delegation Guidelines:*
   a *Moving the Person*, p. 285
   b *Moving Persons in Bed*, p. 288
   c *Turning Persons*, p. 294
   See *Promoting Safety and Comfort:*
   a *Moving the Person*, p. 285
   b *Planning a Safe Move*, p. 286
   c *Friction-Reducing Devices*, p. 287
   d *Turning Persons*, p. 294
   e *Logrolling*, p. 295

2 Ask a co-worker to help you.
3 Practice hand hygiene and get the needed friction-reducing device if it is not already in place. (This procedure uses a turning pad.)
4 Identify the person. Check the ID bracelet against the assignment sheet. Use 2 identifiers (Chapter 14). Also call the person by name.
5 Provide for privacy.
6 Lock (brake) the bed wheels.
7 Raise the bed for body mechanics. Bed rails are up if used.

PROCEDURE

8 Stand on the side opposite to which you will turn the person. Your co-worker stands on the other side.
9 Make sure the bed is flat.
10 Lower the bed rails if used.
11 Position the turning pad or other friction-reducing device if needed.
12 Move the person as a unit to the side of the bed near you. Use the turning pad. (If the person has a spinal cord injury or had spinal cord surgery, assist the nurse as directed.)
13 Place the person's arms across the chest. Place a pillow between the knees.
14 Raise the bed rail if used.
15 Go to the other side.

16 Stand near the shoulders and chest. Your co-worker stands near the hips and thighs.
17 Stand with a wide base of support and good posture. Bend your hips and knees, not your back. One foot is in front of the other.
18 Ask the person to hold the body rigid.
19 Grasp the turning pad as show in Figure 20-13, *A.* Or position your hands as shown in Figure 20-13, *B* if a friction-reducing device is not used.
20 Roll the person toward you. Turn the person as a unit.
21 Position the person in good alignment. Use pillows as directed by the nurse and care plan.

POST-PROCEDURE

22 Provide for comfort. (See the inside of the back cover.)
23 Place the call light and other needed items within reach.
24 Lower the bed to a safe and comfortable level. Follow the care plan.
25 Raise or lower bed rails. Follow the care plan.

26 Follow the care plan and the person's preferences for privacy measures to maintain. Leaving the privacy curtain, window coverings, and door open or closed are examples.
27 Complete a safety check of the room. (See the inside of the back cover.)
28 Practice hand hygiene.
29 Report and record your care and observations.

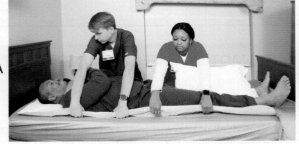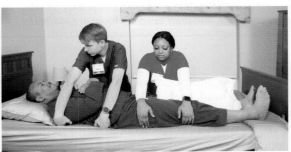

FIGURE 20-13 Logrolling. A pillow is between the person's legs. The arms are crossed on the chest. The person is on the far side of the bed. The person is turned as a unit. **A,** With a turning pad. **B,** Without a turning pad.

SITTING ON THE SIDE OF THE BED (DANGLING)

You will assist patients and residents to sit on the side of the bed *(dangle)*. The procedure is part of some tasks—assisting the person to stand, transferring from bed to chair, partial bath, and others. While dangling the legs, the person coughs and deep breathes. Moving the legs back and forth in circles stimulates circulation.

Patients and residents may become dizzy or faint when getting out of bed too fast. Activity may increase in stages—lying flat, to lying with the head of the bed raised, to dangling, to sitting in a chair, and then to walking. This is common after surgery. The person may need to sit on the side of the bed for 1 to 5 minutes before transferring or walking.

Persons with weakness or balance problems need support. If dizziness or fainting occurs while in bed, lay the person down. If standing, have the person sit or lie down. Tell the nurse at once. See "The Falling Person" in Chapter 15 for safety measures for falling. See Chapter 58 for fainting.

See *Focus on Children and Older Persons: Dangling.*
See *Delegation Guidelines: Dangling.*
See *Promoting Safety and Comfort: Dangling*, p. 298.
See procedure: *Sitting on the Side of the Bed (Dangling)*, p. 298.

FOCUS ON CHILDREN AND OLDER PERSONS

Dangling

Older Persons
Older persons may have circulatory changes. They may become dizzy or faint when getting up too fast. Let them sit on the side of the bed for a few minutes before standing.

DELEGATION GUIDELINES

Dangling

The nurse may ask you to help a person sit on the side of the bed. Before the dangling procedure, you need this information from the nurse and the care plan.

* Areas of weakness. For example, if the arms are weak, the person cannot hold on to the mattress for support. If the left side is weak, turn the person onto the stronger right side. The person uses the right arm to help move from the lying to sitting position.
* The amount of help the person needs.
* If you need a co-worker to help you.
* If the bed is raised or in a low position. If the person will walk or transfer to a chair, the bed is in a low position safe for a transfer (Chapter 21).
* How long the person needs to sit on the side of the bed.
* What exercises are to be done while dangling.
  * Range-of-motion exercises (Chapter 35)
  * Deep-breathing and coughing exercises (Chapter 44)
* What observations to report and record (Fig. 20-14):
  * Pulse and respiratory rates (Chapter 34)
  * Pale or bluish skin color *(cyanosis)*
  * Complaints of dizziness, light-headedness, or difficulty breathing
  * How long the person dangled
  * The observations listed in *Delegation Guidelines: Moving the Person*, p. 285
* When to report observations.
* What patient or resident concerns to report at once.

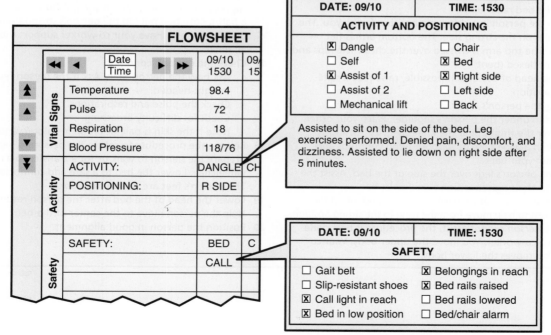

FIGURE 20-14 Charting sample—sitting on the side of the bed (dangling).

PROMOTING SAFETY AND COMFORT

Dangling

Safety

Weakness and balance problems can occur after illness, injury, surgery, and bed rest. Some disabilities affect sitting and balance. Support the person who is sitting on the side of the bed. Have a co-worker help you. This protects the person from falling and other injuries.

As the person sits on the side of the bed, you observe the person. Lay the person down and tell the nurse at once if the person:

- Is dizzy or light-headed.
- Has an abnormal pulse or respirations.
- Has difficulty breathing.
- Has pale or bluish skin.

Comfort

Do not leave the person alone. Provide support at all times.

Provide for warmth during the procedure. Help the person put on a robe. Or cover the shoulders and back with a bath blanket (Chapter 22).

The person may want to perform hygiene measures while sitting on the side of the bed. Oral hygiene and washing the face and hands are examples. These measures are refreshing and stimulate circulation. Follow the nurse's directions and the care plan.

Sitting on the Side of the Bed (Dangling)

QUALITY OF LIFE

- Knock before entering the person's room.
- Address the person by name.
- Introduce yourself by name and title.

- Explain the procedure before starting and during the procedure.
- Protect the person's rights during the procedure.
- Handle the person gently during the procedure.

PRE-PROCEDURE

1 Follow *Delegation Guidelines*:
  a *Moving the Person*, p. 285
  b *Dangling*, p. 297
  See *Promoting Safety and Comfort*:
  a *Moving the Person*, p. 285
  b *Planning a Safe Move*, p. 286
  c *Dangling*
2 Ask a co-worker to help you if needed.

3 Practice hand hygiene.
4 Identify the person. Check the ID bracelet against the assignment sheet. Use 2 identifiers (Chapter 14). Also call the person by name.
5 Provide for privacy.
6 Lock (brake) the bed wheels.
7 Raise the bed for body mechanics. Bed rails are up if used.

PROCEDURE

8 Decide which side of the bed to use. Stand on that side.
9 Lower the bed rail if up.
10 Position the person in a side-lying position facing you. The person lies on the strong side. The bottom arm is flat on the bed. The top arm is crossed over the chest. The hips and knees are flexed (bent).
11 Raise the head of the bed. If possible, raise it to a semi-sitting position.
12 Stand by the person's hips.
13 Slide 1 arm under the person's shoulder. Place your other hand over the thighs near the knees (Fig. 20-15, *A*).
14 Stand with a wide base of support. Bend your hips and knees, not your back.
15 Move the person's legs over the side of the bed. Assist the person to an upright position (Fig. 20-15, *B*).
  a *If the person can assist*, have the person push off of the mattress to help move from the lying to the sitting position.
  b *If the person cannot assist*, the procedure is best done with a co-worker. You move the upper body. Your co-worker moves the lower body.

16 Have the person hold on to the edge of the mattress. This supports the person in the sitting position. If possible, raise a half-length bed rail (on the person's strong side) for the person to grasp. Have your co-worker support the person at all times.
17 Check the person's condition.
  - Ask how the person feels. Ask if the person feels dizzy or light-headed.
  - Check the pulse and respirations.
  - Check for difficulty breathing.
  - Note if the skin is pale or bluish in color *(cyanosis)*.
18 Reverse the procedure to return the person to bed. (Or prepare the person to walk or for a transfer to a chair or wheelchair. Lower the bed to a safe and comfortable level. The person's feet are flat on the floor.)
19 Lower the head of the bed after the person returns to bed. Help the person move to the center of the bed.
20 Position the person in good alignment.

Sitting on the Side of the Bed (Dangling)—cont'd
POST-PROCEDURE

21 Provide for comfort. (See the inside of the back cover.)
22 Place the call light and other needed items within reach.
23 Lower the bed to a safe and comfortable level. Follow the care plan.
24 Raise or lower bed rails. Follow the care plan.
25 Follow the care plan and the person's preferences for privacy measures to maintain. Leaving the privacy curtain, window coverings, and door open or closed are examples.

26 Complete a safety check of the room. (See the inside of the back cover.)
27 Practice hand hygiene.
28 Report and record your observations.

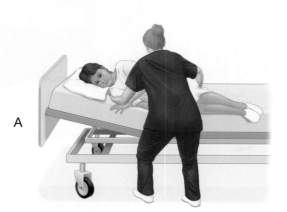 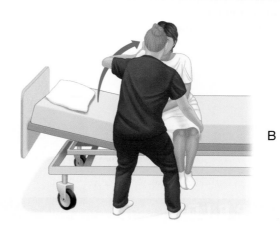

FIGURE 20-15 Helping the person sit on the side of the bed. **A,** The person is in a side-lying position. One arm is under the person's shoulder. The other is over the thighs near the knees. **B,** The person sits upright as the legs are moved over the edge of the bed.

RE-POSITIONING IN A CHAIR OR WHEELCHAIR

The person can slide down in a chair or wheelchair. For good alignment and safety, the person's back and buttocks must be against the back of the chair.

Follow the nurse's directions and the care plan for the best way to re-position a person in a chair or wheelchair. *Do not pull the person from behind the chair or wheelchair.*

Use the following method if the person is alert, cooperative, and able to assist. The person must be able to follow directions. And the person must have the strength to help.

1 Lock (brake) the wheelchair wheels. Remove or swing front rigging out of the way. See Chapter 21 for wheelchair safety.
2 Position the person's feet flat on the floor.
3 Apply a transfer belt (Chapter 15).
4 Position the person's arms on the armrests.
5 Stand in front of the person. Block the person's knees and feet with your knees and feet.
6 Grasp the transfer belt on each side while the person leans forward.
7 Ask the person to push with the feet and arms on the "count of 3."
8 Move the person back into the chair on the "count of 3" as the person pushes with the feet and arms (Fig. 20-16).
9 Remove the transfer belt.

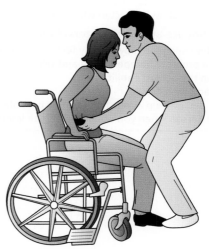

FIGURE 20-16 Re-positioning the person in a wheelchair. A transfer belt is used to move the person to the back of the chair.

The following method may be used if the person cannot assist and the chair reclines.

1 Ask at least 1 co-worker to help you.
2 Lock (brake) the wheels.
3 Recline the chair.
4 Position a friction-reducing device under the person.
5 Grasp the device (Fig. 20-17).
6 Use the device to move the person up. See procedure: *Moving the Person Up in Bed With a Friction-Reducing Device*, p. 291. Remove a slide sheet if used.

A mechanical lift (Chapter 21) is used if:

• The person cannot assist.
• The chair does not recline.

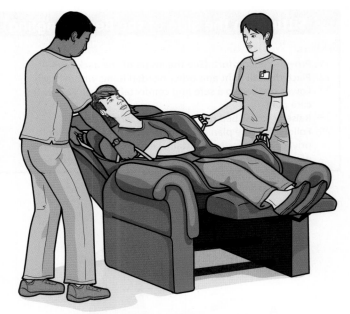

FIGURE 20-17 Re-positioning in a reclining chair.

FOCUS ON PRIDE

The Person, Family, and Yourself

Personal and Professional Responsibility

You will practice moving and positioning procedures in your training program. Practice with other students. Be willing to act as the patient or resident to help other students practice. Use your practice time wisely.

Rights and Respect

How would you feel if these statements were made to you?
• "You're too heavy. I need to get help to move you."
• "I'll get hurt if I try to move you."
   What you say affects the person's self-esteem. Choose your words carefully. Show respect in what you say.

Independence and Social Interaction

Persons who need help moving may feel embarrassed or helpless. To promote independence and self-esteem:
• Focus on the person's abilities.
• Encourage the person.
• Let the person help as much as is safely possible.
• Tell the person when you notice even small improvements.

Delegation and Teamwork

Many moving procedures are safer when done by 2 or more workers. This is very important when caring for bariatric persons. Moving a person without enough help can harm you, your co-workers, and the person. Work as a team to protect yourself and others from injury.

Ethics and Laws

Before a move, explain what you will do and what the person needs to do. Ask if the person has any questions or preferences. The person may suggest an easier or more comfortable method. Always listen. Ignoring the person is wrong. If the method is not safe, explain why. Ask the nurse if you do not know how to answer or if you are unsure how to safely move the person.

FOCUS ON PRIDE: Application

Most moving procedures require a team effort. How well do you work with others? What can you improve?

REVIEW QUESTIONS

Circle the BEST answer.

1 You move the person on the "count of 3" to
 a Save time
 b Distract the person from the move
 c Move the person smoothly
 d Move the person slowly

2 Which term describes needing the *most* assistance with a move?
 a Independent
 b Supervision assistance
 c Partial (moderate) assistance
 d Dependent

3 Before moving a person, you must know what the person is able to do.
 a True
 b False

4 A resident with dementia needs to be moved up in bed. You should
 a Avoid rushing
 b Wait until the person is asleep
 c Move the person alone
 d Continue if the person resists the move

5 Drawsheets and slide sheets are used to
 a Promote privacy
 b Reduce friction
 c Promote independence
 d Improve posture

6 A waterproof under-pad can be used to move a person in bed if it
 a Is disposable
 b Is dry
 c Is strong enough, long enough, and wide enough
 d Can be left in place

7 You need to turn a person to position a friction-reducing device. The person has painful joints and cannot assist. You should
 a Move the person without the device
 b Position the device by yourself
 c Get help and logroll the person to position the device
 d Refuse to move the person

8 A person is fully able to assist with moving up in bed. You should
 a Stand by and provide cues as needed
 b Pull the person up in bed by yourself
 c Ask 1 co-worker to help move the person
 d Ask 2 co-workers to help move the person

9 A person is partially able to assist with moving up in bed. You should
 a Stand by for safety but not assist
 b Move the person up in bed by yourself
 c Tell the person not to assist to avoid injury
 d Ask for help and get a friction-reducing device

10 Before turning a person onto the side, you
 a Move the person to the middle of the bed
 b Move the person to the side of the bed
 c Raise the head of the bed 30 degrees
 d Position a pillow against the back

11 A patient with a spinal cord injury is turned with
 a The logrolling procedure
 b A transfer belt
 c A mechanical lift
 d A pillow under the head and neck

12 You turn and position a person on the side. Which is *safe?*
 a The pillow under the top arm is covering the face.
 b The person is lying on the bottom arm.
 c The top leg is flexed and supported so the knees and ankles do not touch.
 d The person's face is up against the bed rail.

13 You are helping an older person sit on the side of the bed before standing. Which is *true?*
 a The person should sit only for a few seconds before standing.
 b Circulatory changes can cause dizziness.
 c Difficulty breathing during the procedure is normal.
 d Moving the person quickly promotes comfort.

14 To protect the person's rights during dangling
 a Leave the room as the person dangles
 b Perform the procedure alone
 c Do not ask how the person feels
 d Close the privacy curtain

15 A person is able to help move. To re-position the person in a wheelchair
 a Pull the person from behind
 b Unlock the wheelchair wheels
 c Position the person's feet flat on the floor
 d Position the person's arms across the chest

Answers to Chapter 20 questions are on p. 902.

FOCUS ON **PRACTICE**

Problem Solving

A person with right-sided weakness needs to sit on the side of the bed (dangle). Which side of the bed is best—right, left, or either? Why? The person becomes pale and dizzy while dangling. What will you do?

OBJECTIVES

- Define the key terms and key abbreviation in this chapter.
- Explain how to prevent work-related injuries during transfers.
- Identify the delegation information needed to transfer a person.
- Identify comfort and safety measures for transferring the person.

- Explain wheelchair and stretcher safety.
- Perform the procedures described in this chapter.
- Explain how to promote PRIDE in the person, the family, and yourself.

KEY TERMS

lateral transfer When a person moves between 2 horizontal surfaces

pivot To turn one's body from a set standing position
transfer How a person moves to and from a surface

KEY ABBREVIATION

ID   Identification

Patients and residents are moved to and from surfaces such as beds, chairs, wheelchairs, shower chairs, commodes, toilets, and stretchers. A *transfer* is how a person moves to and from a surface. The amount of help needed and the method used vary with the person's abilities. You will assist with transfers often.

Rules for body mechanics and the safety measures for preventing work-related injuries apply to transfers (Chapter 19). So do the rules for moving persons (Chapter 20). Protect yourself and the person from injury. Use your body and transfer devices and equipment correctly.

See *Focus on Communication: Transferring the Person.*

See *Teamwork and Time Management: Transferring the Person.*

See *Delegation Guidelines: Transferring the Person.*

See *Promoting Safety and Comfort: Transferring the Person.*

FOCUS ON **COMMUNICATION**

Transferring the Person

Transfers can be painful for older persons and after an injury or surgery. Ask about comfort. Remind the person to tell you about discomfort.

- "Please tell me if you feel pain or discomfort."
- "Tell me to stop if you feel pain."

Before any transfer, tell the person what you and your co-workers will do. Also explain what the person needs to do. Give step-by-step instructions during the procedure.

The procedures in this chapter explain how to transfer on the "count of 3." You and the person or you and your co-workers move at the same time. For example:

I will help you transfer to the chair. I will count "1, 2, 3." When I say "3," push on the mattress with your hands and stand. I will steady you with the transfer belt as you stand. You will turn so your legs touch the seat's edge. Grab the chair's armrests. I will help you sit.

TEAMWORK AND TIME MANAGEMENT
Transferring the Person

Some agencies have "lift teams" that perform most transfer procedures. They use assist equipment and do not manually lift a person unless necessary. The nurse coordinates with the lift team before scheduled procedures. The team can also be contacted for unscheduled transfers.

Follow agency procedures to check or add to the lift team's schedule. If the person is on the schedule, check to make sure that the procedure was done. Unscheduled or unexpected events can cause delays. Thank the team for the work they do. Their work protects patients, residents, and you from injury.

Some transfer devices are used by other staff members. Mechanical lifts (p. 317) are examples. After using a shared device, return it to the storage area. Do not leave the device in a person's room or other area. Co-workers should not have to search for a device.

DELEGATION GUIDELINES
Transferring the Person

Transfer procedures are routine nursing tasks. They include stand and pivot transfers (p. 306), lateral transfers (p. 313), and transfers using a mechanical lift (p. 317). Before transferring a person, you need information from the nurse and care plan.
- What procedure to use.
- The person's weight and height.
- How much help the person needs. These terms may be used.
  - *Independent*—transfers without help from another person.
  - *Set-up or clean-up assistance*—requires help to get or put away items before or after the transfer. The person transfers without help.
  - *Supervision or touching assistance*—the person transfers without help but needs supervision or cues. Touching or steadying may occur.
  - *Partial (moderate) assistance*—staff lift, hold, or support the body. *Less than half* of the effort is done by staff.
  - *Substantial (maximal) assistance*—staff lift, hold, or support the body. *More than half* of the effort is done by staff.
  - *Dependent*—staff transfer the person. *All* of the effort is done by staff. (Two or more staff and a mechanical lift are required to complete the transfer.)
- The person's physical abilities.
  - Can the person sit up, stand up, or walk without help?
  - Does the person have strength in the arms and legs?
  - Does the person have a weak side. If yes, which side?
- If the person has problems that increase the risk of injury. Dizziness, confusion, hearing or vision problems, recent surgery, and fragile skin are examples.
- The person's ability to follow directions.
- If behavior problems are likely. Combative, agitated, uncooperative, and unpredictable behaviors are examples.
- The number of staff needed for a safe transfer.
- What equipment or devices to use.
  - *Stand and pivot transfer*—transfer belt, wheelchair, stand-assist device (p. 306), positioning devices, wheelchair cushion, position change alarm, and so on
  - *Lateral transfer*—friction-reducing device (Chapter 20) or other lateral transfer device (p. 313)
  - *Mechanical lift transfer*— stand-assist mechanical lift or full-sling mechanical lift (p. 317)
- What observations to report and record:
  - The amount of help needed to transfer the person
  - How the person helped with the procedure
  - How the person tolerated the transfer
  - How you positioned the person
  - The person's pulse, respirations, and blood pressure if asked to measure them before, during, or after the procedure
  - Complaints of dizziness, pain, discomfort, difficulty breathing, weakness, or fatigue
  - Who helped you with the transfer
- When to report observations.
- What patient or resident concerns to report at once.

PROMOTING SAFETY AND COMFORT
Transferring the Person

Safety

To prevent injury to fragile bones and joints:
- Follow the rules of body mechanics and the safety measures for preventing work-related injuries (Chapter 19).
- Have help to transfer the person.
- Use assist devices as directed by the nurse and the care plan. Wheelchair, walker or cane (Chapter 35), and transfer belt (Chapter 15) are examples.
- Transfer the person carefully and in good alignment.

Decide how to transfer the person before beginning. Ask needed staff to help. Arrange the room to allow enough space for a safe transfer. Correctly place the chair, wheelchair, or other device. Also plan to protect tubes or devices connected to the person.

Raise or lower the bed to a safe and comfortable level for the transfer. If the person will stand, the feet must be flat on the floor. For a lateral transfer, the bed is at a safe working height for staff.

In nursing centers, follow agency policies and procedures for using Enhanced Barrier Precautions for high-contact tasks. See Chapter 18.

Comfort

To promote mental comfort:
- Explain what you will do and how the person can help.
- Screen and cover the person for privacy.
- Reassure the person that mechanical lifts (p. 317) are safe.
To promote physical comfort:
- Keep the person in good alignment.
- Do not pull on any part of the person's body.
- Raise the head of the bed as soon as possible. Lying flat for too long can cause discomfort and trouble breathing.
- Use pillows and other positioning devices as directed by the nurse and the care plan.

WHEELCHAIR AND STRETCHER SAFETY

Wheelchairs are useful for people who cannot walk or who have severe problems walking (Fig. 21-1). You use the hand grips/push handles to move the wheelchair. Or the person moves it using the hand rims or with the feet. Motorized wheelchairs have controls operated by the hand, chin, mouth, or other means.

Stretchers (Fig. 21-2) are used to transport persons who cannot sit up or who are very ill. The stretcher is covered with a fitted stretcher sheet or a folded flat sheet. A pillow and extra blankets are on hand. If the nurse allows, raise the head of the stretcher to a Fowler's or semi-Fowler's position (Chapter 19) for comfort.

Follow the safety measures in Box 21-1 to use wheelchairs and stretchers. The person can fall from the wheelchair or stretcher. Or the person can fall during transfers to and from the wheelchair or stretcher.

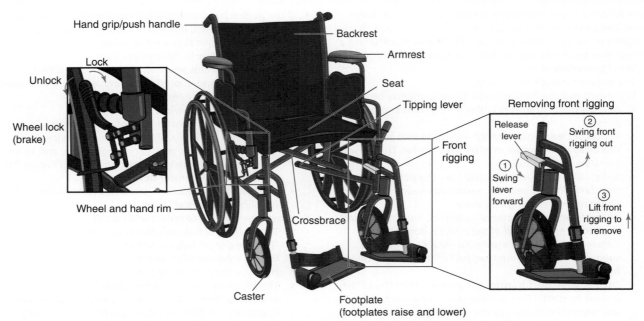

FIGURE 21-1 Parts of a wheelchair. (NOTE: Insets show how to lock [brake] the wheels and remove front rigging.)

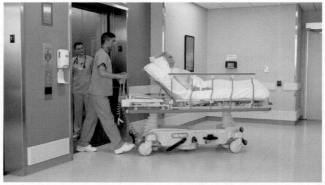

FIGURE 21-2 A stretcher. The stretcher is moved feet first. (Courtesy © Hill-Rom Services, Inc. Reprinted with permission. All rights reserved.)

| BOX 21-1 | **Wheelchair and Stretcher Safety** |

Wheelchair Safety
Maintenance

- Check that you can lock and unlock the wheel locks (brakes).
- Check for flat or loose tires. A wheel lock (brake) will not work on a flat or loose tire.
- Make sure wheel spokes are intact. Damaged, broken, or loose spokes can interfere with moving the wheelchair or locking (braking) the wheels.
- Make sure the casters point forward. This keeps the wheelchair balanced and stable.
- Clean the wheelchair according to agency policy.
- Follow the safety measures to prevent equipment accidents (Chapter 14).

Transfers

- Lock (brake) both wheels before you transfer a person to or from the wheelchair (see Fig. 21-1). Make sure bed wheels are locked.
- Remove the near armrest (if removable) for lateral transfers (p. 313) to and from the bed, toilet, commode, tub, or car. Leave the armrests in place if the person will push off of them to stand.
- Raise the footplates and remove or swing front rigging out of the way for transfers to and from the wheelchair. Figure 21-1 shows how to remove front rigging.
- Do not let the person stand on the footplates.
- Do not let the footplates fall back onto the person's legs.
- Position the person's feet on the footplates after the transfer. The feet must not touch or drag on the floor when the chair is moving.
- Provide needed wheelchair accessories—safety belt, pouch, tray, lap-board, cushion.

Transport

- Follow the care plan for the number of staff needed for a safe transport. This depends on:
  - The person's weight
  - If the person is cooperative
  - If the wheelchair is motorized
- Push the chair forward to transport the person. Do not pull the chair backward unless going through a doorway or down a steep ramp or incline.
- Follow the nurse's or physical therapist's instructions on how to move a wheelchair up and down a ramp.
  - *Going up a ramp*—Push the wheelchair forward (Fig. 21-3, *A*, p. 306).
  - *Going down a ramp*—Pull the wheelchair backward. Look behind as needed to go down safely (Fig. 21-3, *B*, p. 306).

Wheelchair Safety—cont'd
Transport—cont'd

- Follow the nurse's or physical therapist's instructions on how to move a wheelchair over a curb.
- *Going up a curb*—Push the wheelchair forward (Fig. 21-4, *A*, p. 306).
  - Position the wheelchair so the front casters are at the curb.
  - Tilt the wheelchair back so the front casters are above the curb.
  - Push the wheelchair forward until you can set the wheelchair down over the curb. Lower the front casters once past the curb.
  - Push the rear wheels up over the curb.
- *Going down a curb*—Pull the wheelchair backward (Fig. 21-4, *B*, p. 306).
  - Position the wheelchair so the rear wheels are at the curb.
  - Lower the rear wheels down and away from the curb.
  - Tilt the wheelchair back. Pull the wheelchair backward to bring the front casters over the curb. Lower the front casters once past the curb.
- Follow the care plan for keeping the wheels locked (braked) when not moving the wheelchair. Locking (braking) the wheels prevents the chair from moving when the person moves to or from the chair. Leaving the wheels locked may be viewed as a restraint (Chapter 16).

Stretcher Safety

- Have 2 or more co-workers help you transfer the person to or from the stretcher.
- Lock (brake) the stretcher wheels before the transfer.
- Follow the care plan for the number of staff needed for a safe transport. As many as 4 staff members may be needed. This depends on:
  - The person's weight
  - If the person is cooperative
- Use the safety straps if the stretcher has them. Fasten the safety straps when the person is properly positioned on the stretcher.
- Raise the side rails. Keep them up during the transport.
- Make sure the person's arms, hands, legs, and feet do not dangle through the side rail bars.
- Stand at the head of the stretcher. Another staff member may be positioned near the foot to help guide the stretcher.
- Move the stretcher feet first (see Fig. 21-2). The staff member at the head of the stretcher watches the person's breathing and color during the transport.
- Do not leave the person alone.
- Follow the safety measures to prevent equipment accidents (Chapter 14).

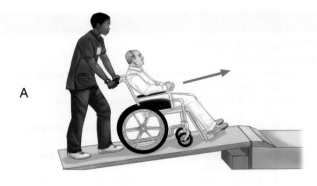

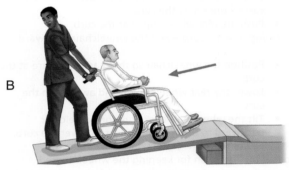

FIGURE 21-3 A, Moving a wheelchair up a ramp. **B,** Moving a wheelchair down a ramp.

STAND AND PIVOT TRANSFERS

Some persons can stand and pivot. *Pivot* means to turn one's body from a set standing position. A stand and pivot transfer is used if:

- The legs are strong enough to bear (support) some or all of the person's weight.
- The person can cooperate and follow directions.
- The person can assist with the transfer.
  See *Promoting Safety and Comfort: Stand and Pivot Transfers.*

PROMOTING SAFETY AND COMFORT

Stand and Pivot Transfers

Safety

You need to know about any areas of weakness. For example, if the arms are weak, the person cannot hold on to the mattress for support. If the left side is weak, the person should get out of bed on the stronger right side. The person uses the right arm to help move.

The person wears slip-resistant footwear for stand and pivot transfers. Such footwear helps prevent slipping, sliding, and falls. Tie shoelaces securely. Otherwise the person can trip and fall.

Long gowns and robes can cause the person to trip and fall. Also avoid robes with long ties.

Lock (brake) bed and wheelchair wheels and wheels on other devices. This prevents the bed and the device from moving during the transfer. Otherwise the person can fall. You also are at risk for injury.

The person must not put his or her arms around your neck. Otherwise the person can pull you forward or cause you to lose balance. Neck, back, and other injuries are possible. To stand, the person pushes off the mattress or the chair or wheelchair armrests. Or the person uses a bed rail or stand-assist device (Fig. 21-5). Follow the care plan and the nurse's directions.

Comfort

After the transfer, position the person in good alignment. Place the call light and other needed items within reach.

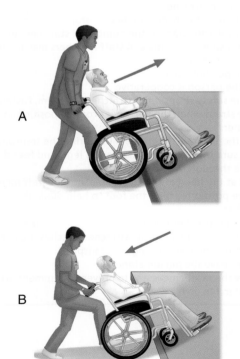

FIGURE 21-4 A, Moving a wheelchair up a curb. **B,** Moving a wheelchair down a curb.

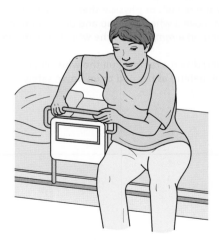

FIGURE 21-5 Stand-assist bed attachment.

Transfer Belts

Transfer belts (gait belts) are discussed in Chapter 15. They are used to:

- Support patients and residents during transfers.
- Re-position persons in chairs and wheelchairs (Chapter 20).
- Assist with ambulation (Chapter 35).

Wider belts have padded handles. They are easier to grip and allow better control should the person fall.

Bed to Chair or Wheelchair Transfers

Safety is important for chair and wheelchair transfers. Help the person out of bed on the person's strong side. If the left side is weak and the right side is strong, get the person out of bed on the right side. The strong side moves first. It pulls the weaker side along. Transfers from the weak side are awkward and unsafe.

See *Focus on Surveys: Bed to Chair or Wheelchair Transfers.*

See *Promoting Safety and Comfort: Bed to Chair or Wheelchair Transfers.*

See procedure: *Transferring the Person to a Chair or Wheelchair.*

FOCUS ON SURVEYS

Bed to Chair or Wheelchair Transfers

Agencies must ensure that nursing assistants can safely perform the skills needed for safe care. Surveyors will observe how nursing assistants function. One skill of focus is transferring a person from the bed to a wheelchair.

PROMOTING SAFETY AND COMFORT

Bed to Chair or Wheelchair Transfers

Safety

The chair or wheelchair must support the person's weight. The number of staff needed depends on the person's abilities, condition, and size (weight and height). Sometimes you need a mechanical lift (p. 317).

If not using a mechanical lift, use a transfer belt. It is safer for the person and you. Putting your arms around the person and grasping the shoulder blades is another method. This can cause the person discomfort and be stressful for you. Use this method only if the nurse and care plan direct and you are comfortable doing so.

Bed and wheelchair wheels are locked (braked) for a safe transfer. After the transfer, unlock the wheelchair wheels (release the brakes) to position the wheelchair as the person prefers. Then lock (brake) the wheels or keep them unlocked according to the care plan. Locked wheels may be viewed as restraints if the person cannot unlock them to move the wheelchair (Chapter 16). However, falls and other injuries are risks if the person tries to stand when the wheels are unlocked.

Comfort

Many wheelchairs and bedside chairs have vinyl seats and backs. Vinyl holds body heat. The person becomes warm and perspires (sweats) more. If needed, cover the back and seat with a folded bath blanket. This increases comfort.

Some people have wheelchair cushions or positioning devices. Follow the manufacturer's instructions for how to use and place a device. Ask the nurse if you need help.

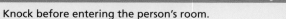

Transferring the Person to a Chair or Wheelchair

QUALITY OF LIFE

- Knock before entering the person's room.
- Address the person by name.
- Introduce yourself by name and title.

- Explain the procedure before starting and during the procedure.
- Protect the person's rights during the procedure.
- Handle the person gently during the procedure.

PRE-PROCEDURE

1 Follow *Delegation Guidelines: Transferring the Person*, p. 303. See *Promoting Safety and Comfort:*
   a *Transfer/Gait Belts*, Chapter 15
   b *Transferring the Person*, p. 303
   c *Stand and Pivot Transfers*
   d *Bed to Chair or Wheelchair Transfers*
2 Practice hand hygiene and get the following supplies.
   - Wheelchair or arm chair
   - Bath blanket or cushion (if needed)
   - Lap blanket (if used)
   - Robe (if needed) and slip-resistant footwear
   - Paper towel or towel (if needed)
   - Transfer belt (if needed)

3 Arrange items in the person's room.
4 Practice hand hygiene.
5 Identify the person. Check the identification (ID) bracelet against the assignment sheet. Use 2 identifiers (Chapter 14). Also call the person by name.
6 Provide for privacy.
7 Decide which side of the bed to use. Move furniture as needed for a safe transfer.

Continued

Transferring the Person to a Chair or Wheelchair—cont'd

PROCEDURE

8 Raise the wheelchair footplates for a wheelchair transfer. Remove or swing front rigging out of the way if possible. Position the chair or wheelchair beside the bed on the person's strong side.
  a If at the head of the bed, it faces the foot of the bed.
  b If at the foot of the bed, it faces the head of the bed.
  c The armrest almost touches the bed.

9 Place a folded bath blanket or cushion on the seat (if needed).

10 Lock (brake) wheelchair wheels. Make sure bed wheels are locked.

11 Fan-fold top linens to the foot of the bed.

12 Place the paper towel or towel under the person's feet. (This protects linens from footwear.) Put footwear on the person. Or apply footwear when the person is seated on the side of the bed (step 14).

13 Lower the bed to a safe and comfortable level for the person. Follow the care plan.

14 Help the person sit on the side of the bed (Chapter 20). Feet must be flat on the floor.

15 Be sure the person's clothing will properly cover the person during the transfer. Help the person put on a robe if needed.

16 Apply the transfer belt if needed (Chapter 15). It is applied at the waist over clothing.

17 *Method 1—using a transfer belt:*
  a Stand in front of the person.
  b Have the person hold on to the mattress.
  c Make sure the feet are flat on the floor.
  d Have the person lean slightly forward.
  e Grasp the transfer belt at each side. Grasp the handles or grasp the belt from underneath. Hands are in an upward position (upward grasp). See Chapter 15.
  f Prevent the person from sliding or falling. Do 1 of the following.
    1) Brace your knees against the person's knees. Block the feet with your feet (Fig. 21-6).
    2) Use the knee and foot of 1 leg to block the person's weak leg or foot. Place your other foot slightly behind you for balance.
    3) Straddle your legs around the weak leg.
  g Explain the following.
    1) You will count "1, 2, 3."
    2) The move will be on "3."
    3) On "3," the person pushes down on the mattress and stands.
  h Ask the person to push down on the mattress and stand on the "count of 3." Assist the person to a standing position as you straighten your knees (Fig. 21-7, *A*).

18 *Method 2—no transfer belt:* (NOTE: Use this method only if directed by the nurse and the care plan and you are comfortable doing so.)
  a Follow steps 17 (a–c).
  b Place your hands under the person's arms. Your hands are around the person's shoulder blades (Fig. 21-7, *B*).
  c Have the person lean slightly forward.
  d Prevent the person from sliding or falling using 1 of the methods in step 17 (f).
  e Explain the "count of 3." See step 17 (g).
  f Ask the person to push down on the mattress and to stand on the "count of 3." Assist the person to a standing position as you straighten your knees.

19 Support the person in the standing position. Hold the transfer belt or keep your hands around the shoulder blades. Steady the person to prevent sliding or falling.

20 Help the person pivot (turn). Have the person grasp the far arm of the chair or wheelchair (Fig. 21-8). The legs will touch the edge of the seat.

21 Continue to help the person pivot (turn) until the other armrest is grasped.

22 Lower the person into the chair or wheelchair as you bend your hips and knees (Fig. 21-9). The person leans slightly forward and bends the elbows and knees.

23 Make sure the hips are to the back of the seat. Position the person in good alignment.

24 Remove the transfer belt if used.

25 Attach wheelchair front rigging for a wheelchair transfer. Position the person's feet on the footplates.

26 Cover the person's lap and legs with a lap blanket (if used). Keep the blanket off the floor and the wheels.

27 Position the chair as the person prefers. Lock (brake) wheelchair wheels according to the care plan.

POST-PROCEDURE

28 Provide for comfort. (See the inside of the back cover.)

29 Place the call light and other needed items within reach.

30 Follow the care plan and the person's preferences for privacy measures to maintain. Leaving the privacy curtain, window coverings, and door open or closed are examples.

31 Complete a safety check of the room. (See the inside of the back cover.)

32 Practice hand hygiene.

33 Report and record your care and observations.

34 See procedure: *Transferring the Person From a Chair or Wheelchair to Bed* (p. 310) to return the person to bed.

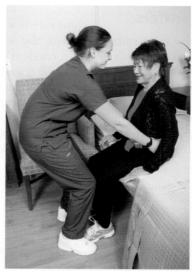

FIGURE 21-6 The person's knees and feet are blocked by the nursing assistant's knees and feet.

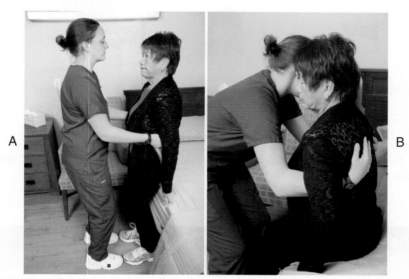

FIGURE 21-7 The person is assisted to a standing position. **A,** *Method 1*—with a transfer belt. The person is supported with the transfer belt. **B,** *Method 2*—without a transfer belt. The hands are under the person's arms and around the shoulder blades.

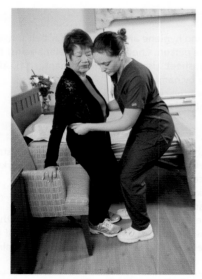

FIGURE 21-8 The person pivots (turns) and grasps the far arm of the chair.

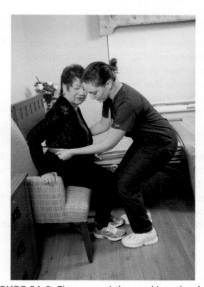

FIGURE 21-9 The person is lowered into the chair.

Chair or Wheelchair to Bed Transfers

Chair or wheelchair to bed transfers have the same rules as bed to chair transfers. If the person is weak on 1 side, transfer the person so that the strong side moves first. Position the person so the strong side is near the bed. See Figure 21-10. The strong side moves first.

You may have to move the chair or wheelchair. If you cannot safely move a chair alone, have help to move the chair or to transfer the person. For example, a resident's right side is weak. The left side is strong. To transfer out of bed, the wheelchair was on the left side of the bed. The resident's left side (strong side) moved first. Now you will transfer the resident back to bed. Position the wheelchair on the other side of the bed (right side). The resident's stronger left side will be near the bed for a safer transfer.

See procedure: *Transferring the Person From a Chair or Wheelchair to Bed.*

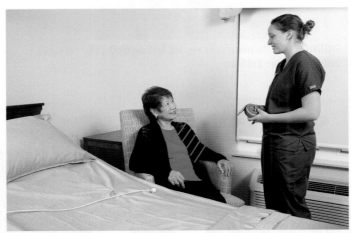

FIGURE 21-10 The person's strong side is near the bed for a transfer to bed. (Note: The "weak" side is indicated by slash marks.)

Transferring the Person From a Chair or Wheelchair to Bed

QUALITY OF LIFE

- Knock before entering the person's room.
- Address the person by name.
- Introduce yourself by name and title.

- Explain the procedure before starting and during the procedure.
- Protect the person's rights during the procedure.
- Handle the person gently during the procedure.

PRE-PROCEDURE

1 Follow *Delegation Guidelines: Transferring the Person,* p. 303. See *Promoting Safety and Comfort:*
  a *Transfer/Gait Belts* (Chapter 15)
  b *Transferring the Person,* p. 303
  c *Stand and Pivot Transfers,* p. 306
  d *Bed to Chair or Wheelchair Transfers,* p. 307

2 Practice hand hygiene and get a transfer belt if needed.
3 Identify the person. Check the ID bracelet against the assignment sheet. Use 2 identifiers (Chapter 14). Also call the person by name.
4 Provide for privacy.
5 Move furniture as needed for a safe transfer.

PROCEDURE

6 Raise the head of the bed to a sitting position. Be sure the bed is at a safe and comfortable level for the person. Follow the care plan. When the person transfers to the bed, the feet must be flat on the floor when sitting on the side of the bed.
7 Move the call light so it is on the strong side when the person is in bed.

8 Position the chair or wheelchair so the person's strong side is next to the bed (see Fig. 21-10). Have a co-worker help you if necessary.
9 Lock (brake) the wheelchair and bed wheels.
10 Remove and fold the lap blanket.
11 Lift the person's feet from the footplates. Raise the footplates. Remove or swing front rigging out of the way. Put slip-resistant footwear on the person if not already done.

Transferring the Person From a Chair or Wheelchair to Bed—cont'd

PROCEDURE—cont'd

12 Apply the transfer belt if needed.

13 Make sure the person's feet are flat on the floor.

14 Stand in front of the person.

15 Have the person hold on to the armrests. (If the nurse directs you to do so, place your arms under the person's arms. Your hands are around the shoulder blades.)

16 Have the person lean slightly forward.

17 Grasp the transfer belt on each side if using it. Grasp underneath the belt. Hands are in an upward position (upward grasp).

18 Prevent the person from sliding or falling. Do 1 of the following.
  a Brace your knees against the person's knees. Block the feet with your feet.
  b Use the knee and foot of 1 leg to block the person's weak leg or foot. Place your other foot slightly behind you for balance.
  c Straddle your legs around the person's weak leg.

19 Explain the "count of 3." See procedure: *Transferring the Person to a Chair or Wheelchair*, p. 307.

20 Ask the person to push down on the armrests on the "count of 3." Assist the person into a standing position as you straighten your knees.

21 Support the person in the standing position. Hold the transfer belt or keep your hands around the shoulder blades. Steady the person to prevent sliding or falling.

22 Help the person pivot (turn) to reach the edge of the mattress. The legs will touch the mattress. The person can reach the mattress with both hands.

23 Lower the person onto the bed as you bend your hips and knees. The person leans slightly forward and bends the elbows and knees.

24 Remove the transfer belt.

25 Remove the robe (if worn) and footwear.

26 Help the person lie down.

POST-PROCEDURE

27 Provide for comfort. (See the inside of the back cover.)

28 Place the call light and other needed items within reach.

29 Be sure the bed is at a safe and comfortable level. Raise or lower bed rails. Follow the care plan.

30 Arrange furniture to meet the person's needs.

31 Follow the care plan and the person's preferences for privacy measures to maintain. Leaving the privacy curtain, window coverings, and door open or closed are examples.

32 Complete a safety check of the room. (See the inside of the back cover.)

33 Practice hand hygiene.

34 Report and record your care and observations.

Transferring the Person To and From the Toilet

Using the bathroom for elimination promotes privacy, dignity, self-esteem, and independence. However, bathrooms are often small with little room for you or a wheelchair. Therefore transfers with wheelchairs and toilets are often hard. Falls and work-related injuries are risks.

Sometimes mechanical lifts (p. 317) are used for toilet transfers. The following procedure can be used if the person can stand and pivot from the wheelchair to the toilet.

See *Promoting Safety and Comfort: Transferring the Person To and From the Toilet.*

See procedure: *Transferring the Person To and From the Toilet*, p. 312.

PROMOTING SAFETY AND COMFORT
Transferring the Person To and From the Toilet

Safety

Make sure the person has an elevated (raised) toilet seat. The toilet seat and wheelchair are at the same level.

A standard toilet has a weight limit of 350 pounds. For persons with bariatric needs:

• A steel, floor-mounted toilet is best. Wall-mounted toilets should not be used.

• A bariatric commode (Chapter 27) is used if the bathroom does not have a floor-mounted toilet.

Have the person use grab bars (Chapter 15). They are used to get on and off the toilet. Check that they are secure. If loose, tell the nurse. Do not use grab bars that are not secure.

Follow Standard Precautions. Wear gloves and practice hand hygiene as needed.

Transferring the Person To and From the Toilet

QUALITY OF LIFE

- Knock before entering the person's room.
- Address the person by name.
- Introduce yourself by name and title.

- Explain the procedure before starting and during the procedure.
- Protect the person's rights during the procedure.
- Handle the person gently during the procedure.

PRE-PROCEDURE

1 Follow *Delegation Guidelines: Transferring the Person*, p. 303. See *Promoting Safety and Comfort*:
   a *Transfer/Gait Belts* (Chapter 15)
   b *Transferring the Person*, p. 303
   c *Stand and Pivot Transfers*, p. 306
   d *Bed to Chair or Wheelchair Transfers*, p. 307
   e *Transferring the Person To and From the Toilet*, p. 311

2 Practice hand hygiene and get the following supplies.
   - Transfer belt
   - Slip-resistant footwear (if not already on)
3 Provide for privacy.

PROCEDURE

4 Put slip-resistant footwear on the person (if not already on).
5 Wheel the wheelchair into the bathroom near the toilet. Close the bathroom door for privacy.
6 Lift the person's feet from the footplates. Raise the footplates. Remove or swing front rigging out of the way.
7 Position the wheelchair close to the toilet. It is best to have the person's strong side near the toilet. Grab bars are within reach.
   a *Method 1*—at the front of the toilet (Fig. 21-11, *A*).
   b *Method 2*—next to the toilet (Fig. 21-11, *B*).
8 Lock (brake) the wheelchair wheels.
9 Apply the transfer belt.
10 Help the person unfasten clothing.
11 Use the transfer belt to help the person stand and pivot (turn) or step to the toilet. See procedure: *Transferring the Person From a Chair or Wheelchair to Bed*, p. 310. The person uses the grab bars for support.
12 Support the person with the transfer belt while the person lowers clothing. Or have the person hold on to the grab bars as you lower clothing.
13 Use the transfer belt to lower the person onto the toilet seat. Check for proper positioning on the toilet.
14 Remove the transfer belt.
15 Tell the person you will stay nearby. Remind the person to use the call light or call for you when help is needed. Stay with the person if required by the care plan.

16 Close the bathroom door for privacy.
17 Stay near the bathroom. Complete other tasks in the person's room. Check on the person every 5 minutes.
18 Knock on the bathroom door when the person calls for you.
19 Help with wiping, perineal care (Chapter 24), flushing, and hand-washing as needed. Wear gloves and practice hand hygiene after removing the gloves.
20 Apply the transfer belt.
21 Use the transfer belt to help the person stand.
22 Help the person raise and secure clothing as needed.
23 Use the transfer belt to transfer the person to the wheelchair. See procedure: *Transferring the Person to a Chair or Wheelchair*, p. 307.
24 Make sure the person's buttocks are to the back of the seat. Position the person in good alignment.
25 Remove the transfer belt.
26 Roll the wheelchair back away from the toilet. Re-attach front rigging. Lower the footplates. Position the feet on the footplates.
27 Cover the lap and legs with a lap blanket. Keep the blanket off the floor and wheels.
28 Position the chair as the person prefers. Lock (brake) the wheelchair wheels according to the care plan.

POST-PROCEDURE

29 Provide for comfort. (See the inside of the back cover.)
30 Place the call light and other needed items within reach.
31 Follow the care plan and the person's preferences for privacy measures to maintain. Leaving the privacy curtain, window coverings, and door open or closed are examples.

32 Complete a safety check of the room. (See the inside of the back cover.)
33 Practice hand hygiene.
34 Report and record your care and observations.

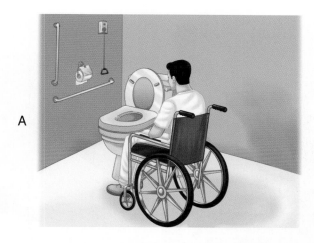

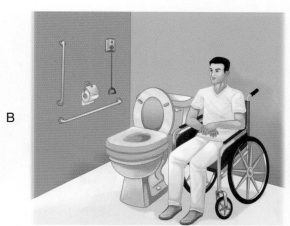

FIGURE 21-11 Wheelchair positions for a transfer to the toilet. **A,** The wheelchair is at the front of the toilet. **B,** The wheelchair is next to the toilet.

LATERAL TRANSFERS

A *lateral transfer* moves a person between 2 horizontal surfaces. The person slides from 1 surface to the other. A transfer from a bed to a stretcher is an example.

Lateral Transfer Devices

Friction and shearing injure the skin (Chapter 20). Infection and pressure injuries can result (Chapter 42). Friction-reducing devices (Chapter 20) protect the skin during lateral transfers. They also protect staff from injury.

Lateral transfer devices to reduce friction include:

- Turning pads or turning sheets (Chapter 20)
- Drawsheets (Chapter 22)
- Large re-usable waterproof under-pads (Chapter 22)
- Slide sheets, slide boards, air-assisted (inflatable) devices, or other lateral sliding aids (lateral transfer devices) (Fig. 21-12, p. 314)

A transfer board (sliding board) (Fig. 21-13, p. 314) may be used for seated lateral transfers if:

- The person has upper body strength.
- The person has good sitting balance.
- There is enough room to position the 2 surfaces close together.

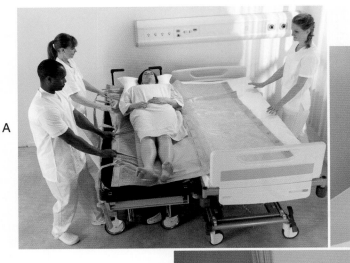
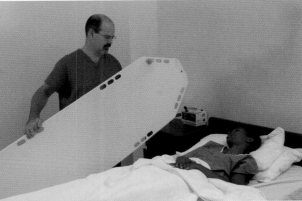
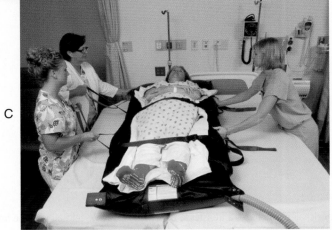

FIGURE 21-12 Lateral sliding aids (lateral transfer devices). **A,** Slide sheet. **B,** Slide board. **C,** Air-assisted transfer device. (A, Used with permission of Arjo Inc. B, Modified from and C, From Perry AG, Potter PA, Laplante N, Ostendorf WR: *Clinical nursing skills & techniques,* ed 10, St Louis, 2022, Elsevier.)

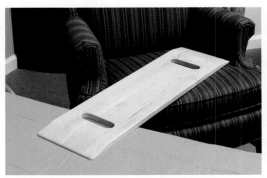

FIGURE 21-13 Transfer board (sliding board) for seated transfers to and from surfaces.

Moving the Person to a Stretcher

A friction-reducing device is used for transfers to and from stretchers. At least 2 or 3 staff are needed for a safe transfer.

- *If the person weighs less than 200 pounds*—a friction-reducing device or lateral sliding aid (lateral transfer device) is used.
- *If the person weighs more than 200 pounds*—a lateral sliding aid (lateral transfer device) or other device is used as directed. At least 3 staff members are needed. Or a mechanical ceiling lift (p. 318) is used.

The person's weight must not exceed the stretcher's weight limit. For persons with bariatric needs, use a bariatric stretcher. Check for an "EC" (expanded capacity) or "Bariatric" label and the weight limit. The nurse and care plan may also direct staff to:

- Position the stretcher so it is ½ inch lower than the bed.
- Use a lateral transfer device, bariatric ceiling lift (p. 318), or other device as directed.
- Transfer the person from his or her strong side.
- Apply an abdominal binder if the person's abdomen is in the way. See Chapter 41.

See *Promoting Safety and Comfort: Moving the Person to a Stretcher*.

See procedure: *Moving the Person to a Stretcher*.

PROMOTING SAFETY AND COMFORT
Moving the Person to a Stretcher

Safety

Protect yourself and the person from injury. Make sure you have enough help. At least 2 or 3 staff are needed. Practice good body mechanics and follow the guidelines for preventing work-related injuries (Chapter 19). Avoid extended reaches and bending your back.

Position the stretcher and bed surfaces as close as possible to each other. Follow the rules for stretcher safety (see Box 21-1). Make sure the bed and stretcher wheels are locked (braked).

Follow the manufacturer's instructions for placing and using a lateral transfer device. Ask for help if you are unsure how to use the device properly.

Moving the Person to a Stretcher

QUALITY OF LIFE

- Knock before entering the person's room.
- Address the person by name.
- Introduce yourself by name and title.
- Explain the procedure before starting and during the procedure.
- Protect the person's rights during the procedure.
- Handle the person gently during the procedure.

PRE-PROCEDURE

1. Follow *Delegation Guidelines: Transferring the Person,* p. 303. See *Promoting Safety and Comfort:*
   a *Transferring the Person,* p. 303
   b *Moving the Person to a Stretcher*
2. Ask at least 1 or 2 staff members to help you.
3. Practice hand hygiene and get the following supplies.
   - Stretcher covered with a sheet
   - Bath blanket or sheet
   - Pillow(s) if needed
   - Lateral transfer device (this procedure uses a slide board)
4. Arrange items in the person's room.
5. Practice hand hygiene.
6. Identify the person. Check the ID bracelet against the assignment sheet. Use 2 identifiers (Chapter 14). Also call the person by name.
7. Provide for privacy.
8. Move furniture as needed for space.

PROCEDURE

9. Raise the bed for body mechanics. Lower the head of the bed. It is as flat as possible. Lower the bed rails if used. Bed wheels are locked (braked).
10. Fan-fold top linens to the foot of the bed.
11. Position the lateral transfer device. (See Chapter 20 for how to position friction-reducing devices.) Follow the manufacturer's instructions and the nurse's directions. To position a slide board:
    a Loosen the drawsheet if it is tucked in. Use the drawsheet to assist with turning.
    b Turn the person to the side. Turn the person toward you.
    c Have a co-worker place the slide board on the bed.
    d Turn the person onto the back. The person is lying on the board. The drawsheet is between the board and the person.

Continued

Moving the Person to a Stretcher—cont'd

PROCEDURE—cont'd

12 Have a co-worker position the stretcher next to the bed. Hold the far side of the drawsheet to protect the person from falling.

13 Raise the stretcher as directed by the nurse. It is either at the same level as the bed or slightly lower (about ½ inch).

14 Lock (brake) the stretcher wheels.

15 Position yourself and co-workers.
   a 1 or 2 workers stand at the side of the stretcher.
   b 1 worker remains at the side of the bed.

16 Grasp the handles on the slide board.

17 Slide the person to the stretcher on the "count of 3." See Figure 21-14. Be sure the person is fully on the stretcher.

18 Have the worker(s) on the stretcher side hold the far side of the drawsheet to protect the person from falling. Unlock the stretcher wheels (release the brakes). Move the stretcher away from the side of the bed.

19 Remove the slide board.
   a Lock (brake) the stretcher wheels.
   b Have the worker(s) use the drawsheet to turn the person. Turn toward the worker(s).
   c Remove the slide board.
   d Turn the person onto the back. The person is centered on the stretcher.

20 Place a pillow under the person's head and neck if allowed. Raise the head of the stretcher if allowed.

21 Cover the person. Provide for comfort.

22 Fasten the safety straps if present. Raise the side rails.

23 Unlock the stretcher wheels (release the brakes). Transport the person.

POST-PROCEDURE

24 Practice hand hygiene.

25 Report and record:
   • The time of the transport
   • Where the person was transported to
   • Who went with the person
   • How the transfer was tolerated

26 Reverse the procedure to return the person to bed.

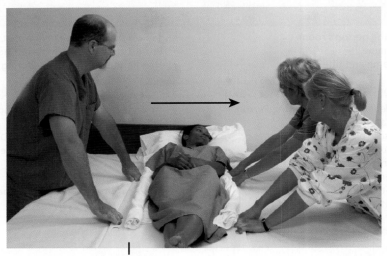

Slide board

FIGURE 21-14 Using a slide board to transfer from a bed to a stretcher. (Modified from Perry AG, Potter PA, Laplante N, Ostendorf WR: *Clinical nursing skills & techniques*, ed 10, St Louis, 2022, Elsevier.)

MECHANICAL LIFTS

Mechanical lifts are used for transfers to and from beds, chairs, wheelchairs, stretchers, tubs (whirlpool tubs), shower chairs, toilets, commodes, or vehicles. They are used for persons who:

- Need weight-bearing support to transfer
- Cannot assist with transfers
- Are too heavy for staff to move

There are manual, battery-operated, and electric lifts. Two types are common.

- *Stand-assist mechanical lifts* (Fig. 21-15, *A* and Fig. 21-16, *A*) are for persons who require some help with transfers and can:
  - Bear (support) some weight.
  - Follow directions.
  - Sit on the side of the bed with or without help.
  - Bend the hips, knees, and ankles.
- *Full-sling mechanical lifts* (Fig. 21-15, *B* and Fig. 21-16, *B*) are for persons who:
  - Cannot assist with transfers.
  - Are partially able or unable to bear (support) weight.
  - Are heavy.
  - Have physical limits preventing other types of transfers.

Some lifts are mounted on the ceiling. Your agency may have floor or ceiling-mounted bariatric lifts (Fig. 21-17, p. 318).

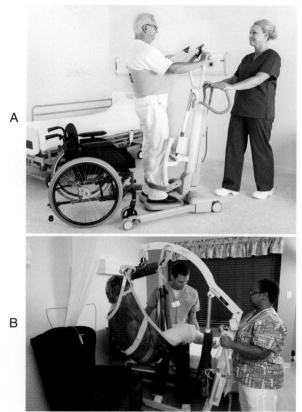

FIGURE 21-15 A, A stand-assist mechanical lift supports the upper body. **B,** A full-sling mechanical lift supports the entire body. (A, Used with permission of Arjo Inc.)

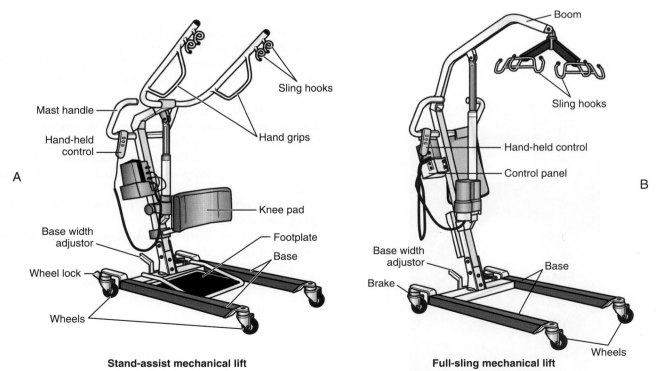

Stand-assist mechanical lift   **Full-sling mechanical lift**

FIGURE 21-16 Mechanical lift parts. **A,** Parts of a stand-assist mechanical lift. **B,** Parts of a full-sling mechanical lift.

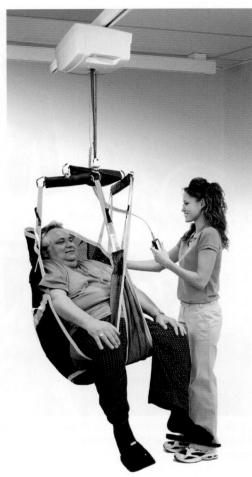

FIGURE 21-17 Bariatric ceiling lift. (Courtesy MedCare Products, Burnsville, Minn.)

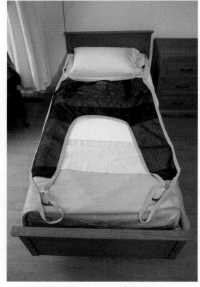

FIGURE 21-18 A full-sling.

Slings

The sling used depends on the lift type and the person's size, condition, and care needs. Slings are padded, unpadded, or made of mesh. Stand-assist slings support the upper body (see Fig. 21-15, *A*). Full-slings support the entire body (see Fig. 21-15, *B*). There are many types of full-slings.

- *Standard full-sling*—for normal transfers (Fig. 21-18).
- *Bathing sling*—for transfers from the bed or chair into a bathtub. Depending on the manufacturer's instructions, the sling may be left in place and attached to the lift during the bath.
- *Toileting sling*—the sling bottom is open.
- *Amputee sling*—for the person who has had both legs amputated.
- *Bariatric sling*—for use with a bariatric lift. There are also bariatric bathing and toileting slings. The nurse may have you leave the sling under the person when seated for short periods or at all times. If left in place, the person is not turned from side-to-side to place and remove the sling for each transfer. This reduces the risk of injury to the person and staff.

The nurse and care plan tell you what type and size sling to use. You must use a sling designed for use with the mechanical lift. Follow agency policy and the manufacturer's instructions for using slings and washing contaminated slings. A sling is contaminated if it:

- Has any visible sign of blood or body fluids.
- Is used on a person's bare skin.
- Is used to bathe a person.

▨ Using a Mechanical Lift

When used properly, mechanical lifts can reduce the risk of injury to patients or residents and staff. There are risks from improper use. Falls from mechanical lifts can cause head trauma, fractures, and death. You must use lifts safely. See Box 21-2 for the guidelines for safe use of mechanical lifts.

There are different types of mechanical lifts. Always follow the manufacturer's instructions. The procedures that follow are used as a guide.

See *Delegation Guidelines: Using a Mechanical Lift.*

See *Promoting Safety and Comfort: Using a Mechanical Lift.*

See procedure: *Transferring the Person Using a Stand-Assist Mechanical Lift*, p. 320.

See procedure: *Transferring the Person Using a Full-Sling Mechanical Lift*, p. 321.

BOX 21-2	Guidelines for Using Mechanical Lifts

Training
- Receive training before using a lift on a patient or resident. You must know how to operate the lift.
- Follow the manufacturer's instructions for the lift. Knowing how to use 1 lift does not mean you know how to use others. If you have not used a certain lift before, ask for training. Ask the nurse to help you until you are comfortable using a lift.

Operation
- Use the correct sling for the lift. Use a sling approved for use by the lift's manufacturer.
- Use the correct sling size. The person's weight and size determine sling size. Follow the person's care plan.
- Do not exceed the weight limit of the sling or the lift.
- Follow the manufacturer's instructions for proper sling positioning.
- Position the person's arms correctly. For a stand-assist mechanical lift, the sling straps are under the arms. The person grasps the lift's hand grips. Arms are inside the sling straps when using a full-sling mechanical lift.
- Make sure the person is not restless or agitated. If the person is, do not attempt the transfer. Tell the nurse.
- Have enough help. One or 2 staff members are needed for a stand-assist mechanical lift. Follow the manufacturer's instructions and agency policy. Two staff members are needed to safely use a full-sling mechanical lift. Current federal regulations require that at least 1 staff member be 18 years of age or older.
- Ensure that the straps are securely fastened during operation.

Operation—cont'd
- Position the base in the wide (open) position when lifting, lowering, and moving. The lift's base widens (opens) and narrows (closes). The lift is most stable with the base in the wide (open) position. Narrowing may be needed briefly to move through a narrow area. Return the base to the wide (open) position as soon as possible.
- Lock (brake) the wheels on the receiving surface—bed, chair, wheelchair, stretcher, shower chair, and so on.
- Follow the manufacturer's instructions for locking (braking) the lift's wheels. For many lifts, the wheels are unlocked during lifting and lowering. This allows the lift to stabilize (become steady). For some stand-assist lifts, the wheels are locked (braked) when lifting and lowering.
- Use the handles to move the lift. Do not push on other parts of the lift. This may cause the lift to tilt.
- Stay with the person when using a lift. Never leave the person unattended (alone) in the lift.

Maintenance
- Inspect the sling for damage. Sling fabric and straps must not be frayed or torn. If a sling has signs of wear, do not use it.
- Follow the manufacturer's instructions for washing and maintaining slings.
- Be sure a battery-powered lift has well-charged batteries.
- Tell the nurse when a lift needs repair or does not work properly. Do not use a lift that is not working properly.
- Follow the agency's safety practices for inspecting and reporting worn or damaged items.

DELEGATION GUIDELINES

Using a Mechanical Lift

Before using a mechanical lift, you need the information in *Delegation Guidelines: Transferring the Person* on p. 303. You also need the following information from the nurse and the care plan.
- What lift to use—stand-assist mechanical lift or full-sling mechanical lift.
- The lift's weight limit. Do not exceed the lift's weight limit.
- What type of sling to use.
- What size sling to use.
- If you need to apply an abdominal binder (Chapter 41). For the person with bariatric needs, an abdominal binder may be needed.

PROMOTING SAFETY AND COMFORT

Using a Mechanical Lift

Safety
Follow the guidelines in Box 21-2 for using a mechanical lift properly. Ask the nurse if you have questions.
   For persons with bariatric needs:
- Make sure the receiving surface (bed, chair, wheelchair, stretcher, and so on) has expanded capacity for the person's weight.
- Use a chair or wheelchair with arms that you can remove or lower.
- Use an abdominal binder (Chapter 41) as directed by the nurse and the care plan.
   Use caution when moving the lift. Floor thresholds, uneven floor surfaces, and thick carpets can cause:
- Difficulty rolling the lift
- Imbalance of the lift
- More exertion (work) for staff

Comfort
The person is lifted up and off the bed or chair. Falling is a common fear. For mental comfort, always explain the procedure before you begin. Also show the person how the lift works.

Transferring the Person Using a Stand-Assist Mechanical Lift

QUALITY OF LIFE

- Knock before entering the person's room.
- Address the person by name.
- Introduce yourself by name and title.

- Explain the procedure before starting and during the procedure.
- Protect the person's rights during the procedure.
- Handle the person gently during the procedure.

PRE-PROCEDURE

1 Follow *Delegation Guidelines:*
   a *Transferring the Person*, p. 303
   b *Using a Mechanical Lift*, p. 319
   See *Promoting Safety and Comfort:*
   a *Transferring the Person*, p. 303
   b *Using a Mechanical Lift*, p. 319
2 Ask a co-worker to help you (if needed).
3 Practice hand hygiene and get the following supplies.
   • Stand-assist mechanical lift and sling
   • Arm chair or wheelchair

   • Slip-resistant footwear
   • Bath blanket or cushion (if needed)
   • Lap blanket (if used)
4 Arrange items in the person's room.
5 Practice hand hygiene.
6 Identify the person. Check the ID bracelet against the assignment sheet. Use 2 identifiers (Chapter 14). Also call the person by name.
7 Provide for privacy.

PROCEDURE

8 Place the chair (wheelchair) at the head of the bed. It is even with the head-board and about 1 foot away from the bed. Lock (brake) the wheelchair wheels. Place a folded bath blanket or cushion in the seat if needed.
9 Assist the person to a seated position on the side of the bed. See procedure: *Sitting on the Side of the Bed (Dangling)* in Chapter 20. The person's feet are flat on the floor. Bed wheels are locked (braked).
10 Put footwear on the person.
11 Apply the sling.
   a Position the sling at the lower back.
   b Bring the straps around to the front of the chest. The straps are positioned under the arms.
   c Secure the waist belt around the person's waist. Adjust the belt so it is snug but not tight.
12 Position the lift in front of the person.
13 Widen the lift's base.
14 Lock (brake) the lift's wheels.
15 Have the person place the feet on the footplate and the knees against the knee pad. Assist as needed. If the lift has a knee strap, secure the strap around the legs. Adjust the strap so it is snug but not tight.
16 Attach the sling to the sling hooks.
17 Have the person grasp the lift's hand grips.
18 Unlock the lift's wheels (release the brakes) following the manufacturer's instructions.

19 Raise the person slightly off the bed. Check that the sling is secure, the feet are on the footplate, and the knees are against the knee pad (Fig. 21-19, *A*). If not, lower the person and correct the problem.
20 Raise the lift until the person is clear of the bed (Fig. 21-19, *B*). Or raise the person to a standing position (Fig. 21-19, *C*). Follow the care plan.
21 Adjust the base's width to move from the bed to the chair (wheelchair) only if needed. Keep the base in the wide (open) position as much as possible.
22 Move the lift to the chair (wheelchair). The person's back is toward the seat.
23 Lower the person into the chair (wheelchair). Guide the person into the seat. See Figure 21-19, *D* and *E*.
24 Lock (brake) the lift's wheels following the manufacturer's instructions.
25 Unhook the sling from the sling hooks.
26 Unbuckle the waist belt. Remove the sling.
27 Unlock the lift's wheels (release the brakes).
28 Have the person lift the feet off of the footplate. Assist as needed. Move the lift. Position the feet flat on the floor or on the wheelchair footplates.
29 Cover the lap and legs with a lap blanket (if used). Keep it off the floor.

POST-PROCEDURE

30 Provide for comfort. (See the inside of the back cover.)
31 Place the call light and other needed items within reach.
32 Follow the care plan and the person's preferences for privacy measures to maintain. Leaving the privacy curtain, window coverings, and door open or closed are examples.

33 Complete a safety check of the room. (See the inside of the back cover.)
34 Practice hand hygiene.
35 Report and record your care and observations.
36 Reverse the procedure to return the person to bed.

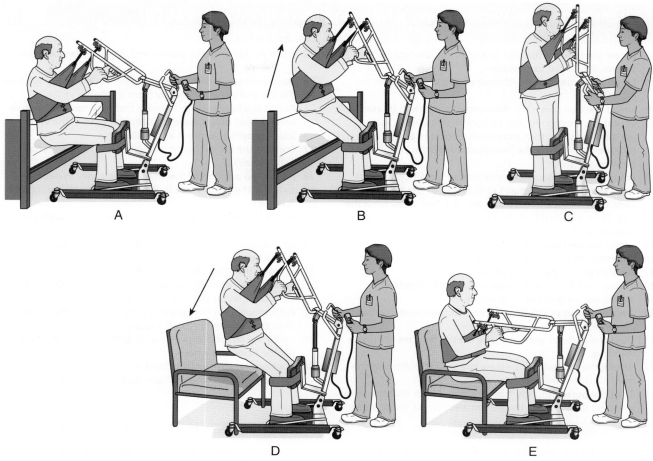

FIGURE 21-19 Using a stand-assist mechanical lift. **A,** The sling is around the person's lower back. The straps are under the arms. The waist belt is secure. Feet are on the footplate. The person holds the hand grips. **B,** The lift is raised. **C,** The person is in a standing position. **D,** The person is lowered into the chair. **E,** The person is seated. The back is against the back of the chair.

Transferring the Person Using a Full-Sling Mechanical Lift

QUALITY OF LIFE

- Knock before entering the person's room.
- Address the person by name.
- Introduce yourself by name and title.

- Explain the procedure before starting and during the procedure.
- Protect the person's rights during the procedure.
- Handle the person gently during the procedure.

PRE-PROCEDURE

1 Follow *Delegation Guidelines:*
   a *Transferring the Person*, p. 303
   b *Using a Mechanical Lift*, p. 319
   See *Promoting Safety and Comfort:*
   a *Transferring the Person*, p. 303
   b *Using a Mechanical Lift*, p. 319
2 Ask a co-worker to help you.
3 Practice hand hygiene and get the following supplies.
   - Full-sling mechanical lift and sling
   - Arm chair or wheelchair
   - Footwear
   - Bath blanket or cushion (if needed)
   - Lap blanket (if used)

4 Arrange items in the person's room.
5 Practice hand hygiene.
6 Identify the person. Check the ID bracelet against the assignment sheet. Use 2 identifiers (Chapter 14). Also call the person by name.
7 Provide for privacy.
8 Raise the bed for body mechanics. Bed rails are up if used.

Continued

Transferring the Person Using a Full-Sling Mechanical Lift—cont'd

PROCEDURE

9 Lower the head of the bed to a level appropriate for the person. It is as flat as possible.

10 Stand on 1 side of the bed. Your co-worker stands on the other side.

11 Lower the bed rails if up. Bed wheels are locked (braked).

12 Center the sling under the person (Fig. 21-20, A). To position the sling, turn the person from side to side (Chapter 20). Follow the manufacturer's instructions to position the sling.

13 Position the person in the semi-Fowler's position.

14 Place the chair (wheelchair) at the head of the bed. It is even with the head-board and about 1 foot away from the bed. Place a folded bath blanket or cushion in the seat if needed. Lock (brake) the wheelchair wheels.

15 Lower the bed so it is level with the chair.

16 Raise the lift to position it over the person.

17 Position the lift over the person (Fig. 21-20, B).

18 Widen the lift's base. Lock (brake) the lift wheels.

19 Attach the sling to the sling hooks (Fig. 21-20, C).

20 Raise the head of the bed to a comfortable level for the person.

21 Cross the person's arms over the chest. The arms are inside the sling.

22 Unlock the lift's wheels (release the brakes) following the manufacturer's instructions.

23 Raise the person slightly from the bed. Check that the sling is secure. If not, lower the person and correct the problem.

24 Raise the lift until the person and sling are free of the bed (Fig. 21-20, D).

25 Have your co-worker support the person's legs as you move the lift and the person away from the bed (Fig. 21-20, E).

26 Adjust the base's width to move from the bed to the chair (wheelchair) only if needed. Keep the base in the wide (open) position as much as possible.

27 Position the lift so the person's back is toward the chair (wheelchair).

28 Adjust the position of the chair (wheelchair) as needed to lower the person into it. Wheelchair wheels are locked (braked).

29 Lower the person into the chair (wheelchair). Guide the person into the seat (Fig. 21-20, F).

30 Lock (brake) the lift wheels following the manufacturer's instructions.

31 Unhook the sling. Unlock the lift's wheels (release the brakes). Move the lift away from the person. Remove the sling from under the person unless otherwise indicated.

32 Put footwear on the person. Position the feet flat on the floor or on the wheelchair footplates.

33 Cover the lap and legs with a lap blanket (if used). Keep it off the floor and wheels.

34 Position the chair (wheelchair) as the person prefers. Lock (brake) the wheelchair wheels according to the care plan.

POST-PROCEDURE

35 Provide for comfort. (See the inside of the back cover.)

36 Place the call light and other needed items within reach.

37 Follow the care plan and the person's preferences for privacy measures to maintain. Leaving the privacy curtain, window coverings, and door open or closed are examples.

38 Complete a safety check of the room. (See the inside of the back cover.)

39 Practice hand hygiene.

40 Report and record your care and observations.

41 Reverse the procedure to return the person to bed. Follow the manufacturer's instructions to position a sling on a person seated in a chair or wheelchair. The following method is common.

  a Have the person lean forward. Have your co-worker help the person if needed.

  b Slide the sling behind the person's back. Tuck the sling down along the back to the seat of the chair or wheelchair.

  c Bring the leg straps around the sides of the person. The straps are at the sides of the legs.

  d Pass the leg straps under the legs.

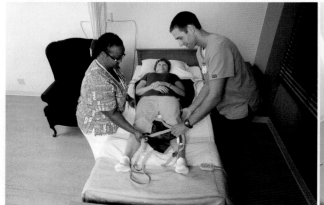
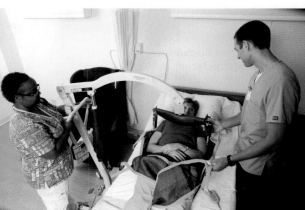

A   B

FIGURE 21-20 Using a full-sling mechanical lift. **A,** The sling is positioned under the person. **B,** The lift is over the person.

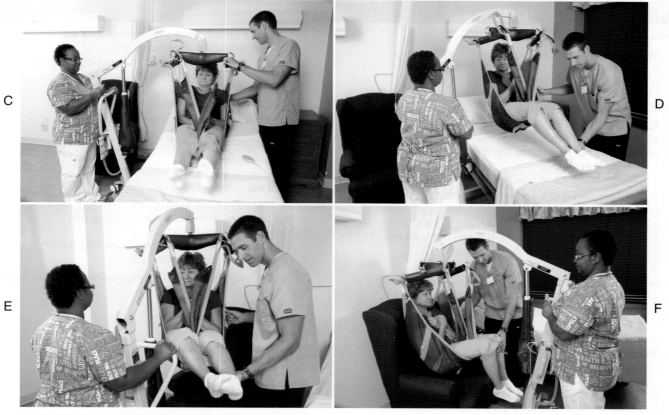

FIGURE 21-20, cont'd **C,** The sling is attached to the lift. **D,** The lift is raised until the sling and person are off the bed. **E,** The legs are supported. The person and lift are moved away from the bed. **F,** The person is guided into a chair.

FOCUS ON **PRIDE**

The Person, Family, and Yourself

Personal and Professional Responsibility

Take time to plan and prepare for a transfer. Gather needed items. Organize the room and equipment. Remember to:
- Position the chair, wheelchair, stretcher, and so on for a safe transfer. Lock (brake) wheels.
- Raise footplates and remove wheelchair front rigging or swing it out of the way.
- Adjust the bed to a safe and comfortable height.
- Make sure a mechanical lift is charged.
- Move furniture or clutter out of the way.

Rights and Respect

Respect privacy during transfers. Close privacy curtains, doors, and window coverings. Properly cover the person. For example, a patient gown opens in the back. Apply a robe or another gown to cover the person's backside. Use a covering that is safe for transfers.

Independence and Social Interaction

How you speak to the person makes a difference. To give directions:
- Speak slowly and clearly.
- Talk loudly enough for the person to hear you.
- Speak calmly and kindly. Never yell at or insult the person.
- Face the person and use eye contact when possible.
- Give 1 direction at a time.
- Repeat directions as needed. Be patient.
- Ask if the person has questions before proceeding.

Your speech and tone must convey dignity. Show you value the person through respectful interactions.

Delegation and Teamwork

You need help to transfer a person. Your co-workers are busy. Do you ask for help? Or do you try to move the person alone? Never be afraid to ask for help. Ask politely and say thank you. Work as a team for the person's safety and to protect yourself and others from injury.

Ethics and Laws

The right way to transfer is not always the quickest way. Do not pull on the person's clothing or arm, underarm, or other body part. Choose to give care correctly. Take pride in giving care in a way that prevents harm and promotes comfort and safety.

FOCUS ON **PRIDE**: *Application*

Explaining procedures improves with practice. Practice explaining a transfer from the bed to a chair using:
- A stand and pivot transfer
- A stand-assist mechanical lift
- A full-sling mechanical lift

REVIEW QUESTIONS

Circle the BEST answer.

1 To promote comfort during a transfer
 a Pull the person to a standing position
 b Explain the procedure
 c Let the person choose the procedure
 d Open the privacy curtain

2 For a safe transfer to a chair
 a Tell the person to grasp you around your neck
 b Pull the person's arms to stand
 c Manually lift the person
 d Move furniture and equipment as needed

3 You are preparing to transfer a person. Which statement promotes comfort?
 a "I'll move you quickly. The pain will be brief."
 b "I can leave the door open. This will not take long."
 c "Please tell me to stop if you feel pain."
 d "I'm nervous. I don't want to drop you."

4 A person uses a wheelchair. Which measure is *unsafe?*
 a The wheels are locked (braked) for transfers
 b The chair is pulled backward for transport.
 c The feet are positioned on the footplates.
 d The casters point forward.

5 To use a stretcher safely
 a Lock (brake) the wheels for transfers to and from the stretcher
 b Transfer a person to a stretcher without help
 c Lower the side rails during a transport
 d Move the stretcher head first

6 A stand and pivot transfer is *unsafe* for a person who
 a Is hard of hearing but can follow directions
 b Can bear (support) some weight with the legs
 c Is confused and combative
 d Uses a transfer belt

7 A person has a weak side. For transfers,
 a The strong side moves first
 b The weak side moves first
 c Pillows are used for support
 d The transfer belt is not used

8 Which is *unsafe* for a stand and pivot transfer to a wheelchair?
 a The wheelchair's front rigging is removed.
 b The person's feet are flat on the floor.
 c The person is wearing slip-resistant footwear.
 d The wheelchair is behind you as you face the person.

9 To transfer a person from a wheelchair to a toilet
 a Position the wheelchair facing the toilet
 b Remove the transfer belt when lowering clothing
 c Have the person hold on to the grab bar for support
 d Keep the bathroom door open

10 Which is used for a lateral transfer from a bed to a stretcher?
 a Slide sheet
 b Transfer belt
 c Stand-assist mechanical lift
 d Grab bar

11 When using a mechanical lift
 a Position the lift on the person's strong side
 b Collect a battery and a transfer belt
 c Compare the person's weight to the lift's weight limit
 d Allow the person to control the lift

12 For a safe transfer with a full-sling mechanical lift, at least
 a 1 worker is needed
 b 2 workers are needed
 c 3 workers are needed
 d 4 workers are needed

13 You are using a stand-assist mechanical lift. Which is *unsafe?*
 a The person is holding the lift's hand grips.
 b The person's feet are on the footplate.
 c The lift's base is narrow when lifting.
 d The person's knees are against the knee pad.

14 After a transfer, which should you do *first?*
 a Report to the nurse.
 b Return the mechanical lift to the storage area.
 c Record the procedure.
 d Place the call light within reach.

Answers to Chapter 21 questions are on p. 902.

FOCUS ON PRACTICE

Problem Solving

You are preparing to transfer a resident using a stand and pivot transfer. Today the person is weaker than usual and unsteady. The person cannot bear (support) weight with the legs. What will you do?

Bedmaking

OBJECTIVES

- Define the key terms and key abbreviation in this chapter.
- Describe closed, open, occupied, and surgical beds.
- Explain when to change bed linens.
- Identify the linens used for bedmaking.
- Explain the purposes of drawsheets and waterproof under-pads and how to use them.

- Handle linens following the rules of medical asepsis.
- Perform the procedures described in this chapter.
- Explain how to promote PRIDE in the person, the family, and yourself.

KEY TERMS

bath blanket A covering used for privacy and warmth during bathing, hygiene, and other care measures
drawsheet A small sheet placed over the middle of the bottom sheet to keep the mattress and bottom linens clean

occupied In use
waterproof under-pad An absorbent pad with a quilted top layer and a waterproof bottom layer

KEY ABBREVIATION

ID	Identification

Beds are made every day. Clean, dry, and wrinkle-free beds:
- Promote comfort.
- Prevent skin breakdown.
- Prevent pressure injuries (Chapter 42).

Beds are usually made in the morning after baths. Or they are made while the person is in the shower, up in the chair, or out of the room. To keep beds neat and clean:
- Change linens when they are wet, soiled, or damp.
- Straighten linens when loose or wrinkled and at bedtime.
- Check for and remove food and crumbs after meals and snacks.
- Check linens for dentures, eyeglasses, hearing aids, sharp objects, and other items.

TYPES OF BEDS

Beds are made in these ways.
- A *closed bed* is not in use (Fig. 22-1, p. 326). The bed is ready for a new patient or resident. In nursing centers, closed beds are made for residents who are up during the day.
- An *open bed* is ready for use (Fig. 22-2, p. 326). Top linens are fan-folded to the foot (end) of the bed so the person can get into bed.
- An *occupied bed* is made with the person in it (Fig. 22-3, p. 326). *Occupied* means in use.
- A *surgical bed* is made to transfer a person from a stretcher to a bed (Fig. 22-4, p. 326). This includes an ambulance stretcher.

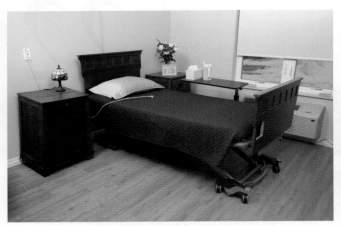

FIGURE 22-1 Closed bed.

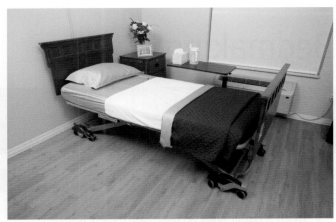

FIGURE 22-2 Open bed. Top linens are fan-folded to the foot of the bed.

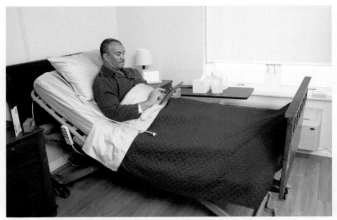

FIGURE 22-3 Occupied bed.

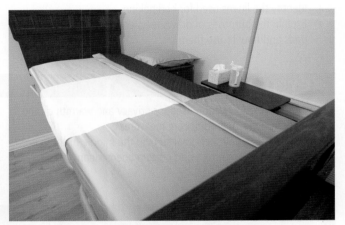

FIGURE 22-4 Surgical bed.

LINENS

Beds in health care settings are at least made with a bottom sheet, top sheet, bedspread, and a pillow with a pillowcase. Bottom sheets are flat (without elastic) or fitted. A fitted sheet has elastic in the sides of the sheet. The sheet is made to fit securely around the mattress. Fitted bottom sheets are common.

A mattress pad may be placed on top of the mattress for comfort and mattress protection. Drawsheets and waterproof under-pads are common. See "Drawsheets and Waterproof Under-Pads." An extra blanket may be applied for warmth. Personal items such as throw blankets, quilts, and decorative pillows are common in nursing centers.

Patient and resident rooms also need linens for personal hygiene. These include bath towels, hand towels, washcloths, gowns or pajamas, and bath blankets. A *bath blanket* is a covering used for privacy and warmth during bathing, hygiene, and other care measures. A bath blanket is used to cover the person when making an occupied bed (p. 335).

Drawsheets and Waterproof Under-Pads

A *drawsheet* is a small sheet placed over the middle of the bottom sheet to keep the mattress and bottom linens clean (Fig. 22-5). The drawsheet absorbs moisture and reduces heat retention. A flat sheet folded in half can serve as a drawsheet. Drawsheets are often used as assist devices to move and transfer persons in bed (Chapters 20 and 21).

A *waterproof under-pad* is an absorbent pad with a quilted top layer and a waterproof bottom layer (Fig. 22-6). Waterproof under-pads come in different sizes. They are commonly used for incontinence (Chapter 27) to protect the bottom linens and mattress from being soiled. Disposable bed protectors may also be used (Fig. 22-7). "Soaker pad" and "chux pad" are other names.

A waterproof under-pad may be used for moving and transfers if the device is strong enough and large enough. Disposable bed protectors are not strong enough to be used for these purposes. See Chapter 20.

Drawsheets and waterproof under-pads are cleaned for re-use. They are placed in linen bags when wet, when soiled, or when it is time for a linen change. Disposable bed protectors are discarded in the trash.

See *Focus on Long-Term Care and Home Care: Drawsheets and Waterproof Under-Pads.*

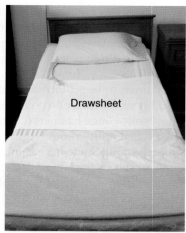

FIGURE 22-5 A drawsheet is placed across the middle of the bed on top of the bottom sheet.

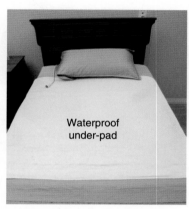

FIGURE 22-6 A waterproof under-pad is padded on top. It has an absorbent middle layer and a waterproof bottom layer.

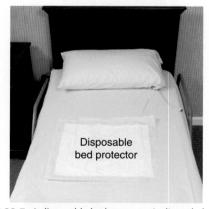

FIGURE 22-7 A disposable bed protector is discarded after use.

> ### FOCUS ON **LONG-TERM CARE AND HOME CARE**
>
> *Drawsheets and Waterproof Under-Pads*
>
> #### Home Care
> A flat sheet folded in half can serve as a drawsheet. A twin-sized sheet is easier to use for this purpose. The nurse tells you what to use.
>
> Medical supply stores and many drugstores sell waterproof under-pads. The nurse discusses the need for these items with the person and family.
>
> Some home care patients and families use plastic mattress protectors. If so, tell the nurse. The nurse can assess what is safe for the person. Plastic mattress protectors only protect the mattress. They do not prevent the soiling of other linens.
>
> Do not use plastic trash bags or dry-cleaning bags. They are not strong enough to protect the linens and mattress. They slide easily and move out of place. Suffocation is a risk if the bag covers the person's nose and mouth.

Collecting Linens

Do not collect unneeded linens. Once in the person's room, extra linens are considered contaminated. You cannot use them for another person.

Collect linens in the order of use. That way you avoid fumbling with linens for the piece you need. Linens stay neat and clean in your stack. Bed linens are used in the following order.

- Mattress pad (if needed)
- Bottom sheet (flat or fitted)
- Drawsheet (if needed)
- Waterproof under-pad (if needed)
- Top sheet
- Blanket (if needed)
- Bedspread
- Pillowcase(s)

When collecting linens for bedmaking, it is common to collect linens for personal hygiene. You may need to collect towels (bath and hand), washcloths, a gown or pajamas, and a bath blanket.

Use 1 hand to hold the linens. Use your other hand to pick them up. The first item to use is at the bottom of the stack. To get it on top, place your hand over the stack. Then turn the stack over onto the other hand (Fig. 22-8, p. 328). The first item to use is now on top.

Handling Linens

When handling linens and making beds, practice medical asepsis. Your uniform is considered *dirty*. Always hold linens away from your body and uniform (see Fig. 22-8). Never shake linens. Shaking them spreads microbes. Place clean linens on a clean surface. Never put clean or used linens on the floor.

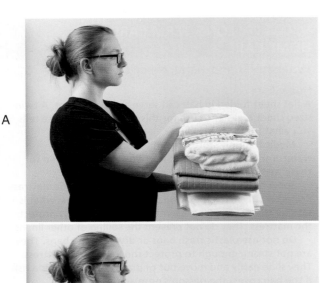

A

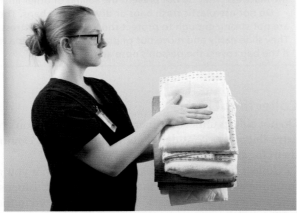

B

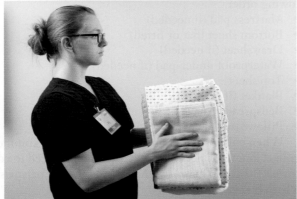

C

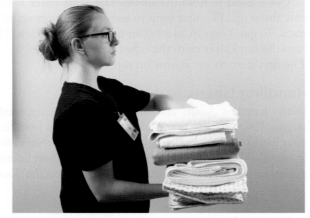

D

FIGURE 22-8 Collecting linens. Linens are held away from the body and uniform. **A,** One hand is placed over the top of the stack of linens. **B, C,** and **D,** The stack of linens is turned onto the other hand.

Used Linens. Used linens are handled carefully to prevent the spread of microbes. Remove used linens 1 piece at a time. Roll each piece away from you (Fig. 22-9). Roll soiled linens so the soiled side is inside the roll and away from you.

Leak-proof containers or bags (linen bags, laundry bags) are used to collect linens for transport to laundering areas. Some agencies have soiled linen hampers (containers, carts) in hallways or in a soiled utility room (Fig. 22-10). Others have hampers in each room. Some have laundry chutes.

The procedures in this chapter use a laundry bag. Follow agency policies and procedures for collecting and transporting used linens for laundering. See Box 22-1 for guidelines for handling used linens.

See *Focus on Surveys: Used Linens.*

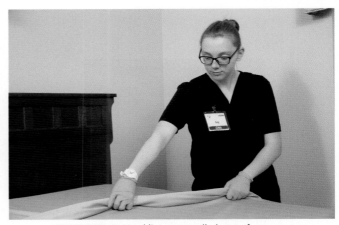

FIGURE 22-9 Used linens are rolled away from you.

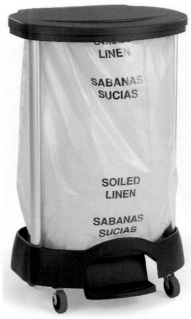

FIGURE 22-10 A hamper for used linens.

BOX 22-1	Guidelines for Handling Used Linens

- Follow Standard Precautions (Chapter 18) and the Bloodborne Pathogen Standard (Chapter 17). Wear gloves and any other needed personal protective equipment when handling soiled linens.
- Hold linens away from your body and uniform.
- Handle linens carefully with minimal agitation. Never shake them. Shaking spreads microbes.
- Do not place linens on the floor.
- Do not place used linens on clean linens or on a clean surface. The over-bed table is an example.
- Do not rinse or sort linens in the areas where they were used. For example, do not rinse a soiled waterproof under-pad in the person's bathroom.
- Bag used linens in the room where they were used.
  - Use a *BIOHAZARD* label (*BIOHAZARD* bag) for linens contaminated with blood or other potentially infectious materials (Chapter 17) as required by agency policy.
  - Follow agency policies and procedures for collecting and transporting used linens when Transmission-Based Precautions are needed (Chapter 18).
  - Tie the bag securely.
  - Do not carry used linens un-bagged outside of the person's room.
- Place used linens in the correct container. Other containers in the same location may be for trash.
- Do not over-fill a hamper or laundry bag. The hamper's lid will not close. The person emptying the hamper or lifting the bag may be injured.
- Empty containers as needed. Some units assign a person to empty linen containers. Be helpful. Show good teamwork. If you see a full hamper, empty it. The person assigned the task may be busy.
- Clean up after yourself. If you fill a hamper, empty it. If you place an item inside that will cause an odor, empty the hamper.
- Do not place un-bagged linens in a laundry chute. Bag the items and tie the bag securely to prevent linens from falling out in the chute.

FOCUS ON SURVEYS

Used Linens

Used linens may contain microbes and blood or body fluids. You must help prevent the spread of infection. Surveyors will observe:

- How you transport linens.
- If you practice hand hygiene after handling used linens.
- If you use a second bag (double-bagging) when:
  - The outside of the laundry bag is visibly contaminated.
  - The contents have wet through to the outside of the bag.
- If you bag contaminated linens where they were used. The person's room and the shower room are examples.

MAKING BEDS

In hospitals, bottom and top sheets, the drawsheet, the waterproof under-pad (if used), and pillowcases are usually changed daily. If still clean, the bedspread can be re-used for the same person. If needed, mattress pads and blankets can also be re-used if still clean.

In nursing centers, linens are not changed every day. A complete linen change is usually done on the person's bath or shower day. This may be 1 or 2 times a week. On other days, the bed is made with the same linens.

Linens are not re-used if soiled, wet, or wrinkled. Change wet, damp, or soiled linens right away. Safety and medical asepsis are important for bedmaking. Follow the guidelines in Box 22-2.

Sometimes a special mattress is used to prevent or treat pressure injuries (Chapter 42). Air flows through the mattress for pressure relief. Follow the manufacturer's instructions and agency procedures for linens used with special mattresses.

See *Focus on Long-Term Care and Home Care: Making Beds*, p. 330.

See *Delegation Guidelines: Making Beds*, p. 330.

See *Promoting Safety and Comfort: Making Beds*, p. 330.

BOX 22-2	Bedmaking Guidelines

- Follow the guidelines for handling used linens in Box 22-1.
- Use good body mechanics at all times (Chapter 19).
- Follow the rules in Chapters 20 and 21 to safely move and transfer the person. You move the person when you make an occupied bed. You may transfer the person out of bed to make a closed or open bed.
- Practice hand hygiene before handling clean linens.
- Remove gloves and practice hand hygiene after removing soiled linens and before touching clean linens.
- Bring only needed linens to the person's room. Extra linens are considered contaminated. You cannot use extra linens for another person.
- Place clean linens on a clean surface. Use the bedside chair, over-bed table, or bedside stand. Place a barrier (towel, paper towel, disposable bed protector) between the clean surface and the linens if required by agency policy.
- Do not use torn or frayed linens.
- Never shake any linens—used or clean.
- Hold all linens away from your body and uniform. Do not let used or clean linens touch your uniform.
- Keep bottom linens tucked in and wrinkle-free.
- Straighten and tighten loose linens as needed.
- Move the bed and furniture as needed to allow room to move around the bed.
- Change wet, damp, or soiled linens right away.

FOCUS ON LONG-TERM CARE AND HOME CARE

Making Beds

Long-Term Care

Some residents bring linens from home. Use them to make the bed. They are the person's property, and they need to be protected from loss and damage. Follow agency practices to prevent confusion with another person's property.

Promote personal choice. Some centers have colored or printed linens. The person can choose what color to use. Ask how many pillows or blankets the person wants. If possible, the person chooses the time when you make the bed.

Home Care

Linen changes in the home are usually done 1 or 2 times a week. Follow the person's routine. Change linens more often if the person asks you to do so. Always change linens that are wet, damp, soiled, or very wrinkled. Contact the nurse if the person refuses a linen change.

Some home care patients have hospital beds. Others have twin-, full-, queen-, or king-sized beds. Sofa sleepers, cots, or recliners may be used for sleep. Make the bed (or sleeping surface) as the person wishes. Follow the rules in Box 22-2. If the person's wishes are not safe, tell the nurse.

You may have laundry responsibilities. Wash linens when soiling is fresh to help prevent staining. Urine, feces (stools), vomit, and blood can stain linens. Follow these guidelines.
- Wear gloves if contact with blood or body fluids is likely.
- Rinse the item in cold water to remove the substance.
- Treat the stain. The person may use a stain-removing agent. Read and follow the manufacturer's instructions. Or follow the nurse's directions.
- Wash and dry linens as the person prefers.

DELEGATION GUIDELINES

Making Beds

Bedmaking is a routine nursing task. Before making a bed, you need this information from the nurse and the care plan.
- What bed to make—closed, open, occupied, or surgical.
- If a drawsheet, waterproof under-pad, or disposable bed protector is needed.
- If the person uses bed rails.
- The person's treatment, therapy, and activity schedules. For example, change a patient's linens after a treatment. Or make a resident's bed while the person is in physical therapy.
- Position restrictions or the person's movement or activity limits.
- How to position the person and the positioning devices needed.
- If the bed needs to be locked into a certain position (Chapter 13).
- When to report observations.
- What patient or resident concerns to report at once.

PROMOTING SAFETY AND COMFORT

Making Beds

Safety

You need to raise the bed for body mechanics. The bed also is as flat as possible. Return the bed to the correct position when you are done. Lock the bed in position if ordered.

Bed wheels are locked (braked) during bedmaking. You may need to move the bed to avoid reaching. Unlock the wheels (release the brakes) to move the bed. Then lock (brake) the wheels.

Linens may contain blood or body fluids. Wear gloves to remove soiled linens from the bed. Follow Standard Precautions and the Bloodborne Pathogen Standard. The procedures in this chapter include glove use. (For skills tested in your state, wear gloves as required by your state's competency exam.) Practice hand hygiene after removing and discarding soiled gloves and before touching clean items or surfaces.

In nursing centers, follow agency policies and procedures for using Enhanced Barrier Precautions for high-contact tasks. See Chapter 18.

After making a bed, lower the bed to the correct level for the person. Follow the care plan. Raise or lower bed rails according to the care plan.

The Closed Bed

Closed beds are made for:
- Nursing center residents and home care patients who are up for most or all of the day. Top linens are folded back at bedtime. New linens are used as needed.
- New patients and residents. The bed is made after the bed system (Chapter 13) is cleaned and disinfected. New linens are needed for the entire bed.

The procedure that follows explains how to make as much of 1 side of the bed as possible before moving to the other side. This saves time and energy. It also prepares you for what to do when the bed is occupied.

Another method is to place each item fully on the bed before moving to the next item. The bottom sheet is applied and fully tucked in on both sides, then the drawsheet is applied, and so on. This requires more trips from side to side. But, for some, it is easier to get linens tight and wrinkle-free.

See procedure: *Making a Closed Bed.*

Making a Closed Bed

QUALITY OF LIFE

- Knock before entering the person's room.
- Address the person by name.
- Introduce yourself by name and title.

- Explain the procedure before starting and during the procedure.
- Protect the person's rights during the procedure.
- Handle the person gently during the procedure.

PRE-PROCEDURE

1 Follow *Delegation Guidelines: Making Beds.* See *Promoting Safety and Comfort: Making Beds.*
2 Practice hand hygiene and get the following clean linens and supplies.
   - Mattress pad (if needed)
   - Bottom sheet (flat sheet or fitted sheet)
   - Drawsheet (if needed)
   - Waterproof under-pad (if needed)
   - Top sheet
   - Blanket (if needed)
   - Bedspread

   - A pillowcase for each pillow
   - Personal hygiene linens (as needed)—bath towel, hand towel, washcloth, gown or pajamas, bath blanket
   - Gloves
   - Laundry bag
   - Towel, paper towels, or disposable bed protector (as a barrier for clean linens)

3 Arrange items in the person's room. Place linens on a clean surface. First place the barrier between the clean surface and clean linens if required by agency policy.
4 Raise the bed for body mechanics. Bed rails are down.

PROCEDURE

5 Put on gloves if contact with blood or body fluids may occur.
6 Remove linens. Roll each piece away from you. Place each piece in a laundry bag. (NOTE: If a disposable bed protector is used, discard it in the trash. Do not put it in the laundry bag.)
7 Clean the bed frame and mattress (if this is your job).
8 Remove and discard the gloves. Practice hand hygiene.
9 Move the mattress to the head of the bed.
10 Put the mattress pad on the mattress (if used). It is even with the head of the mattress.
11 Apply the bottom sheet to 1 side of the bed. Unfold the sheet length-wise. Place the center crease in the middle of the bed.
   a *For a flat sheet:*
      1) Place the lower edge even with the foot of the mattress (Fig. 22-11, *A*, p. 332).
         a) If there is a large and small hem, the large hem is at the head. The small hem is at the foot.
         b) Place the stitched side of the hem downward, away from the person. Hem-stitching can be rough. The smooth side is up, against the skin.
      2) Open and fan-fold the sheet to the other side of the bed (Fig. 22-11, *B*, p. 332).
      3) Tuck the top of the sheet under the mattress. Smooth the sheet from the head to the foot.
      4) Make a mitered corner at the top. Tuck in the sheet along the side of the mattress. See Figure 22-12, p. 333.
   b *For a fitted sheet* (Fig. 22-13, p. 333):
      1) Open and fan-fold the sheet to the other side of the bed.
      2) Tuck the corners over the mattress at the head and the foot of the bed on 1 side.
12 Place the drawsheet (if used) on the bed. It is in the middle of the mattress. Open and fan-fold the drawsheet to the other side of the bed. Tuck the drawsheet under the mattress.

13 Go to the other side of the bed.
14 Tuck in the bottom sheet on the other side of the bed. Make sure the sheet is smooth and tight without wrinkles.
   a *For a flat sheet*, miter the top corner. Tuck in the sheet along the side of the mattress.
   b *For a fitted sheet*, tuck the corners over the mattress at the head and the foot of the bed.
15 Pull the drawsheet tight so there are no wrinkles (Fig. 22-14, p. 333). Tuck in the drawsheet.
16 *If using a waterproof under-pad*, place the waterproof under-pad on the bed. It is in the middle of the mattress.
17 Put the top sheet on the bed.
   a Unfold it length-wise with the center crease in the middle.
   b Place the top edge even with the head of the mattress.
      1) If there is a large hem and small hem, the large hem is at the head. The small hem is at the foot.
      2) Place the stitched side of the hem outward, away from the person. The smooth side is down, against the skin.
   c Open and fan-fold the sheet to the other side of the bed. Do not tuck the sheet in yet. Never tuck top linens in on the sides.
18 Place the blanket on the bed (if used).
   a Unfold it with the center crease in the middle.
   b Put the top edge about 6 to 8 inches from the head of the mattress.
   c Open and fan-fold the blanket to the other side.
19 Place the bedspread on the bed (Fig. 22-15, p. 334).
   a Unfold it with the center crease in the middle.
   b Place the top edge even with the head of the mattress.
   c Open and fan-fold the bedspread to the other side.

Continued

Making a Closed Bed—cont'd

PROCEDURE—cont'd

20 Go to the other side.

21 Bring the top linens down over the side of the bed. Straighten all top linens. Make sure the bedspread facing the door is even. It covers all top linens.

22 Tuck in top linens together at the foot of the bed so they are smooth and tight. Miter the corners at the foot of the bed (see Fig. 22-12, *A, B,* and *C*). Leave the top linens untucked at the sides.

23 Put the pillowcase on the pillow. The zipper, tag, or seam end of the pillow is inserted first. Keep the pillow and pillowcase away from your body and uniform. Figures 22-16 and 22-17 (p. 334) show 2 ways to insert the pillow into the pillowcase. Fold extra material under the pillow at the open end of the pillowcase.

24 Follow the person's preference and agency practices for finishing the bed. The bed should look neat and wrinkle-free. Linens are not touching the floor. For a neat appearance, the open end of the pillowcase does not face the door. The following methods are common.

  a *Method 1*—Turn the top hem of the bedspread under the blanket to form a cuff. Turn the top sheet over the bedspread. Hem-stitching is down. The smooth side is up. Place the pillow on the bed. See Figure 22-18 (p. 335).

  b *Method 2*—Fold the top of the bedspread back (enough to fit the pillow in the area). Place the pillow on the bed. Bring the bedspread up over the pillow. Tuck the bedspread under the pillow as in Figure 22-19 (p. 335).

  c *Method 3*—Pull the bedspread up to the head of the mattress. Place the pillow on top. See Figure 22-1.

POST-PROCEDURE

25 Provide for comfort. (See the inside of the back cover.) NOTE: Omit this step if the bed is prepared for a new patient or resident.

26 Attach the call light to the bed. Or place it within the person's reach.

27 Lower the bed to a safe level. Follow the care plan. The bed wheels are locked (braked).

28 Raise or lower bed rails. Follow the care plan or the nurse's directions.

29 Put the towels, washcloth, gown or pajamas, and bath blanket in the bedside stand.

30 Complete a safety check of the room. (See the inside of the back cover.)

31 Follow agency policy for used linens.

32 Practice hand hygiene.

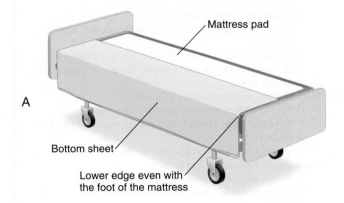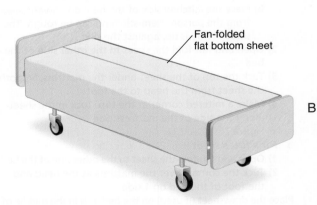

FIGURE 22-11 Applying a flat bottom sheet. **A,** The bottom sheet is on the bed with the center crease in the middle. The lower edge of the sheet is even with the foot of the mattress. **B,** The sheet is fan-folded to the other side of the bed.

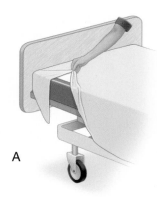

Tuck the sheet under the mattress at the head of the bed.

Raise the side of the sheet up onto the mattress to make a triangle.

A

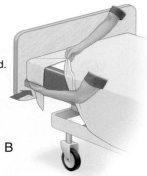

Tuck the remaining portion of the sheet under the mattress.

B

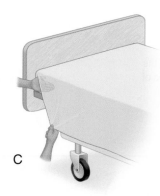

Bring the raised portion of the sheet down off of the mattress.

C

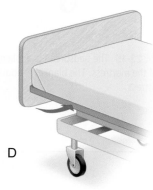

Tuck in the entire side of the sheet along the mattress.

The sheet should be tight and wrinkle-free.

D

FIGURE 22-12 Making a mitered corner.

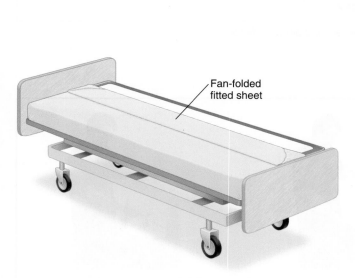

Fan-folded fitted sheet

FIGURE 22-13 Applying a fitted bottom sheet.

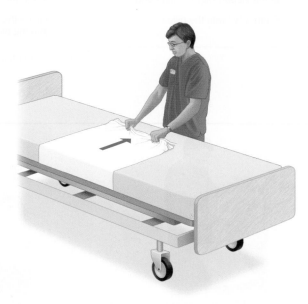

FIGURE 22-14 The drawsheet is pulled tight to remove wrinkles. The drawsheet is tucked in under the sides of the mattress.

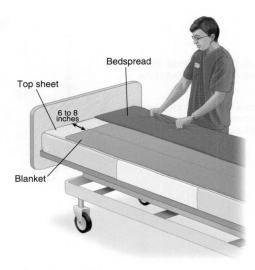

FIGURE 22-15 The bedspread is applied. The top sheet is even with the head of the mattress. The blanket is about 6 to 8 inches from the head of the mattress.

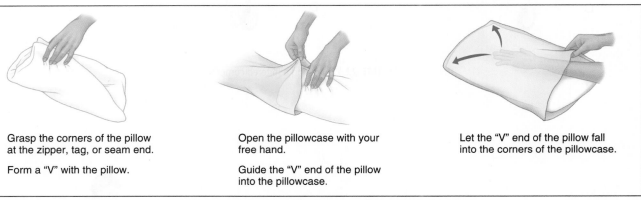

Grasp the corners of the pillow at the zipper, tag, or seam end.

Form a "V" with the pillow.

Open the pillowcase with your free hand.

Guide the "V" end of the pillow into the pillowcase.

Let the "V" end of the pillow fall into the corners of the pillowcase.

FIGURE 22-16 Putting a pillowcase on a pillow—*Method 1.*

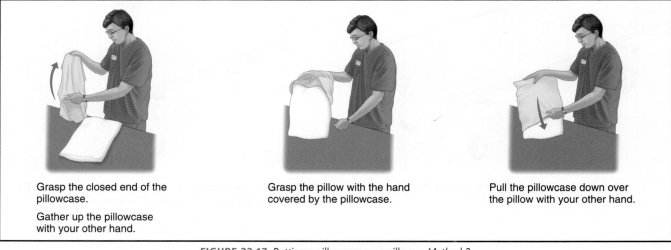

Grasp the closed end of the pillowcase.

Gather up the pillowcase with your other hand.

Grasp the pillow with the hand covered by the pillowcase.

Pull the pillowcase down over the pillow with your other hand.

FIGURE 22-17 Putting a pillowcase on a pillow—*Method 2.*

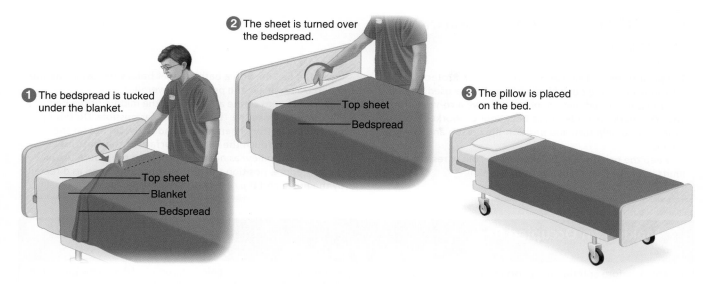

① The bedspread is tucked under the blanket.

Top sheet
Blanket
Bedspread

② The sheet is turned over the bedspread.

Top sheet
Bedspread

③ The pillow is placed on the bed.

FIGURE 22-18 Finishing a closed bed by making a cuff with the top linens.

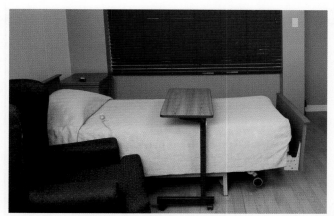

FIGURE 22-19 A closed bed with the pillow under the bedspread. The bedspread is tucked under the pillow.

The Open Bed

A closed bed becomes an open bed by fan-folding the top linens to the foot of the bed. The person can get into bed with ease. An open bed is commonly made for:

- Newly admitted persons arriving by wheelchair
- Persons who are getting ready for bed
- Persons who are out of bed for a short time

For a newly admitted person, make a closed bed with new linens. See procedure: *Making a Closed Bed* on p. 331. When finishing the bed, fan-fold top linens neatly to the foot of the bed (see Fig. 22-2). See "Making Beds" on p. 329 for other times new linens are needed. Otherwise, use the linens already on the bed. Fan-fold the top linens and check that the bed is neat and wrinkle-free. Neaten the bed as needed.

Before leaving, complete a safety check of the room. (See the inside of the back cover.) Make sure the call light and other needed items will be within reach. The bed is at a safe level.

The Occupied Bed

You make an occupied bed when the person stays in bed. The person is rolled to the side and used bottom linens are tucked under the person. Clean bottom linens are put on that side of the bed. Then the person is rolled back onto the clean bottom linens to finish the other side of the bed.

Explain each step to the person before it is done. This is important even if the person cannot respond.

See *Focus on Communication: The Occupied Bed*.
See *Promoting Safety and Comfort: The Occupied Bed*, p. 336.
See procedure: *Making an Occupied Bed*, p. 336.

FOCUS ON **COMMUNICATION**

The Occupied Bed

After making an occupied bed, ask about the person's comfort.

- "Are you comfortable?"
- "How can I make you more comfortable?"
- "Are you warm enough?"
- "Do you feel any creases or wrinkles?"
- "Can I adjust your pillow?"

After making the bed, thank the person for cooperating.

PROMOTING SAFETY AND COMFORT

The Occupied Bed

Safety

The person lies on 1 side and then the other. Protect the person from falling out of bed. If bed rails are used, the far bed rail is up. If bed rails are not used, have a co-worker help you. You work on 1 side of the bed. Your co-worker is on the other side to help turn and position the person and prevent falling.

Keep the person in good alignment. Follow restrictions or limits in the person's movement or position.

Comfort

Cover the person with a bath blanket before removing the top sheet. Do not leave the person uncovered.

Tucked linens create a "bump" in the middle of the bed. For comfort, make the "bump" as low as possible. Do this by fan-folding bottom linens neatly and flatly. Do not let the person's body touch the exposed surface of the mattress.

Adjust the pillow as needed during the procedure. After the procedure, position the person for comfort and as directed by the nurse and the care plan.

Making an Occupied Bed

QUALITY OF LIFE

- Knock before entering the person's room.
- Address the person by name.
- Introduce yourself by name and title.

- Explain the procedure before starting and during the procedure.
- Protect the person's rights during the procedure.
- Handle the person gently during the procedure.

PRE-PROCEDURE

1. Follow *Delegation Guidelines: Making Beds*, p. 330. See *Promoting Safety and Comfort*:
   a. *Making Beds*, p. 330
   b. *The Occupied Bed*
2. Ask a co-worker to help you if needed.
3. Practice hand hygiene and get the following supplies.
   - Clean linens (see procedure: *Making a Closed Bed*, p. 331)
   - Bath blanket
   - Gloves
   - Laundry bag
   - Towel, paper towels, or disposable bed protector (as a barrier for clean linens)

4. Arrange items in the person's room. Place linens on a clean surface. First place the barrier between the clean surface and clean linens if required by agency policy.
5. Practice hand hygiene.
6. Identify the person. Check the identification (ID) bracelet against the assignment sheet. Use 2 identifiers (Chapter 14). Also call the person by name.
7. Provide for privacy.
8. Move the call light off of the bed.
9. Raise the bed for body mechanics. Bed rails are up if used. Bed wheels are locked (braked).
10. Lower the head of the bed. It is as flat as possible.

PROCEDURE

11. Put on gloves if contact with blood or body fluids may occur.
12. Loosen top linens at the foot of the bed.
13. Lower the bed rail near you if up.
14. Fold and remove the bedspread (Fig. 22-20). Do the same for the blanket (if used). Place each over the chair or on a clean surface.
15. Cover the person with a bath blanket.
    a. Unfold the bath blanket over the top sheet.
    b. Have the person hold the bath blanket. If the person is unable, tuck the top part under the person's shoulders.
    c. Grasp the top sheet under the bath blanket at the shoulders. Bring the sheet down toward the foot of the bed. Remove the sheet from under the blanket (Fig. 22-21, p. 338). Place it in the laundry bag.
16. Explain the safety measures you have taken to prevent falling from the bed. Help the person turn onto the side facing away from you. Adjust the pillow for comfort.
17. Loosen bottom linens on the side of the bed near you.
18. Fan-fold bottom linens 1 at a time toward the person (Fig. 22-22, p. 338). If re-using a mattress pad, do not fan-fold it.
19. Remove and discard the gloves. Practice hand hygiene. Put on clean gloves if you will handle soiled linens again on the other side of the bed.

20. Place a clean mattress pad on the bed if needed. Unfold it length-wise with the center crease in the middle. Fan-fold the top part toward the person. If re-using a mattress pad, straighten and smooth any wrinkles.
21. Place the bottom sheet on the side of the bed near you. For a flat sheet, see step 11 (a) in the procedure: *Making a Closed Bed* on p. 331. For a fitted sheet, tuck the corners over the mattress at the head and the foot of the bed on the side near you. Fan-fold the sheet toward the person.
22. *If using a drawsheet* (Fig. 22-23, p. 338):
    a. Place the drawsheet on the bed. It is in the middle of the mattress.
    b. Open the drawsheet.
    c. Fan-fold it toward the person.
    d. Tuck in excess fabric at the side of the bed.
23. *If using a waterproof under-pad:*
    a. Place the waterproof under-pad on the bed. It is in the middle of the mattress.
    b. Fan-fold it toward the person.
24. Explain to the person that there is a "bump" to roll back over. Help the person turn toward you. Adjust the pillow for comfort.
25. Raise the bed rail. Go to the other side and lower the bed rail. (Note: Omit this step if you are working with a co-worker. Your co-worker removes used linens and places clean linens on the other side of the bed.)

Making an Occupied Bed—cont'd

PROCEDURE—cont'd

26 Loosen and remove the bottom linens (Fig. 22-24, *A*, p. 338). Remove 1 piece at a time. Place each piece in the laundry bag. (NOTE: If a disposable bed protector is used, discard it in the trash. Do not put it in the laundry bag.)
27 Remove and discard gloves. Practice hand hygiene.
28 Straighten and smooth the mattress pad if used.
29 Pull the clean bottom sheet toward you and tuck it in. For a flat sheet, make a mitered corner at the top. Tuck the sheet under the mattress from the head to the foot of the bed. For a fitted sheet, tuck the corners over the mattress at the head and the foot of the bed.
30 Pull the drawsheet tightly toward you and tuck it in (Fig. 22-24, *B*, p. 338).
31 Position the person supine in the center of the bed. Adjust the pillow for comfort.
32 Put the top sheet on the bed. Unfold it length-wise with the center crease in the middle. The large hem is even with the head of the mattress. Hem-stitching is on the outside.
33 Have the person hold the top sheet so you can remove the bath blanket. Or tuck the top sheet under the person's shoulders. Remove the bath blanket. Place it in the laundry bag.
34 Unfold the blanket on the bed if used. The center crease is in the middle and it covers the person. The upper hem is 6 to 8 inches from the head of the mattress.
35 Unfold the bedspread on the bed. The center crease is in the middle and it covers the person. The top hem is even with the head of the mattress.
36 Straighten and smooth top linens.
37 Raise the bed rail. Go to the foot of the bed.
38 Make a 2-inch toe pleat across the foot of the bed (Fig. 22-25, p. 339). The pleat (fold) is about 6 to 8 inches from the foot of the bed. The pleat prevents pressure on the toes from top linens.
39 Tuck in all top linens together at the foot of the bed. Avoid removing the toe pleat. Miter the corners at the foot of the bed. Leave the top linens untucked at the sides.
40 Follow the person's preference and agency practices for finishing the bed. If a blanket is used, turn the top hem of the bedspread under the blanket to make a cuff. Bring the top sheet down over the bedspread to form a cuff.
41 Change the pillowcase(s).

POST-PROCEDURE

42 Provide for comfort. (See the inside of the back cover.)
43 Place the call light and other needed items within reach.
44 Lower the bed to a safe and comfortable level. Follow the care plan. The bed wheels are locked (braked).
45 Raise or lower bed rails. Follow the care plan.
46 Put the clean towels, washcloth, gown or pajamas, and bath blanket in the bedside stand.
47 Follow the care plan and the person's preferences for privacy measures to maintain. Leaving the privacy curtain, window coverings, and door open or closed are examples.
48 Complete a safety check of the room. (See the inside of the back cover.)
49 Follow agency policy for used linens.
50 Practice hand hygiene.
51 Report and record your care and observations.

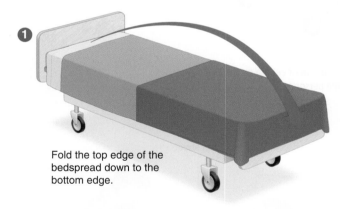
Fold the top edge of the bedspread down to the bottom edge.

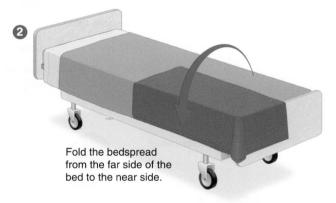
Fold the bedspread from the far side of the bed to the near side.

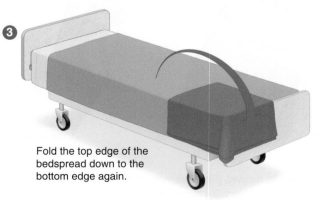
Fold the top edge of the bedspread down to the bottom edge again.

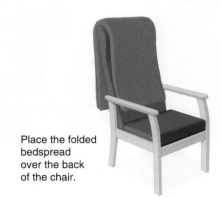
Place the folded bedspread over the back of the chair.

FIGURE 22-20 Folding linens for re-use.

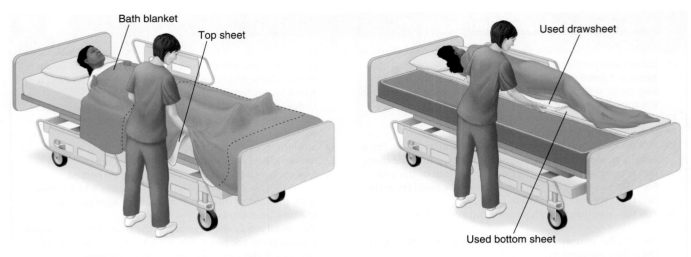

FIGURE 22-21 The person holds on to the bath blanket. The top sheet is removed from under the bath blanket.

FIGURE 22-22 Used bottom linens are tucked under the person.

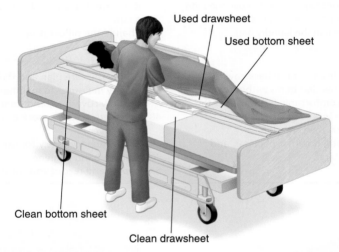

FIGURE 22-23 A clean bottom sheet and drawsheet are on the bed. Both are fan-folded and tucked under the person.

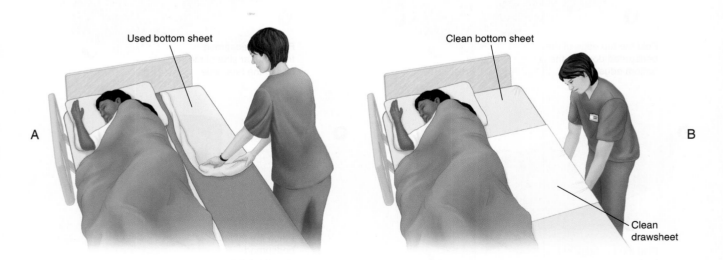

FIGURE 22-24 **A,** The person is turned to the other side. Used linens are removed. (Gloves are removed and hand hygiene is performed before touching clean linens.) **B,** The clean bottom linens are pulled through and tucked in.

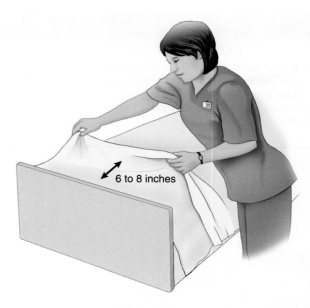

FIGURE 22-25 Making a toe pleat. Pull up on the top linens. Make a 2-inch pleat (fold) across the foot of the bed. The pleat is 6 to 8 inches from the foot of the bed.

6 to 8 inches

The Surgical Bed

The surgical bed also is called a *recovery bed* or *post-operative bed*. Top linens are folded to the side to transfer the person from a stretcher to the bed. These beds are made for persons:

- Returning to their rooms from surgery. A complete linen change is needed.
- Arriving at the agency by ambulance. A complete linen change is needed if the person:
  - Is a new patient or resident.
  - Is returning to the agency from the hospital.
- Going by stretcher to treatment or therapy areas. A complete linen change is not needed.
- Using portable tubs (Chapter 24). Because of bathing, a complete linen change is needed.

See *Promoting Safety and Comfort: The Surgical Bed*.
See procedure: *Making a Surgical Bed*.

PROMOTING SAFETY AND COMFORT

The Surgical Bed

Safety
Chapter 21 explains stretcher safety and transfers involving a stretcher. Leave the bed raised to prepare for the arrival of the stretcher. After the transfer, lower the bed to a safe and comfortable level for the person. Bed wheels are locked (braked). Raise or lower bed rails according to the care plan.

Making a Surgical Bed

PRE-PROCEDURE

1. Follow *Delegation Guidelines: Making Beds*, p. 330. See *Promoting Safety and Comfort*:
   a. *Making Beds*, p. 330
   b. *The Surgical Bed*
2. Practice hand hygiene and get the following supplies.
   - Clean linens (see procedure: *Making a Closed Bed*, p. 331)
   - Gloves
   - Laundry bag
   - Equipment requested by the nurse
   - Towel, paper towels, or disposable bed protector (as a barrier for clean linens)
3. Arrange items in the person's room. Place linens on a clean surface. First place the barrier between the clean surface and clean linens if required by agency policy.
4. Move the call light off of the bed.
5. Raise the bed for body mechanics. Bed rails are down.

PROCEDURE

6. Put on gloves if contact with blood or body fluids may occur.
7. Remove and place the used linens in the laundry bag. Remove gloves. Practice hand hygiene after removing and discarding them.
8. Make a closed bed (see procedure: *Making a Closed Bed*, p. 331). Do not tuck top linens under the mattress.
9. Fold all top linens at the foot of the bed back onto the bed. The fold is even with the edge of the mattress (Fig. 22-26, *A*, p. 340).
10. Know on which side of the bed the stretcher will be placed. Fan-fold linens length-wise to the other side of the bed (Fig. 22-26, *B*, p. 340).
11. Put a pillowcase on each pillow.
12. Place the pillow(s) on a clean surface.

Continued

Making a Surgical Bed—cont'd

POST-PROCEDURE

13 Leave the bed in the high position.
14 Leave both bed rails down.
15 Put the clean towels, washcloth, gown or pajamas, and bath blanket in the bedside stand.
16 Move furniture away from the bed. Allow room for the stretcher and the staff.

17 Do not attach the call light to the bed.
18 Complete a safety check of the room. (See the inside of the back cover.)
19 Follow agency policy for used linens.
20 Practice hand hygiene.

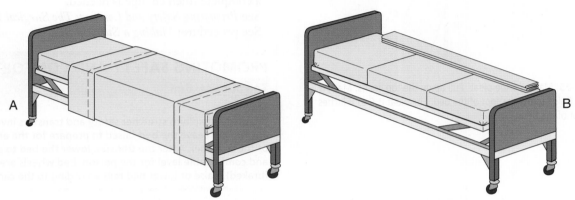

FIGURE 22-26 Surgical bed. **A,** The bottom of the top linens is folded back onto the bed. The fold is even with the edge of the mattress. **B,** Top linens are fan-folded length-wise to the side of the bed.

FOCUS ON PRIDE

The Person, Family, and Yourself

Personal and Professional Responsibility

You are responsible for providing a neat and orderly setting. The bed must be clean and well made. If the person stays in bed, straighten and tighten linens as needed. These actions promote comfort and quality of life.

Rights and Respect

Nursing center residents often bring bedspreads, blankets, and so on from home. The items have meaning and value. For example, a resident uses a quilt at night. Made by a family member, the sight and smell of the quilt remind the person of home.

Protect personal items from loss and damage. Handle the person's belongings with care and respect.

Independence and Social Interaction

Allow personal choice when possible. For example, the person chooses what time you make the bed. What is best for you may not be best for the person. Consider the person's preferences when planning your day and managing time. The more choices are allowed, the greater the person's sense of control and independence.

Delegation and Teamwork

Making beds with a co-worker is faster, easier, and safer. Make 1 side of the bed while your co-worker makes the other. Always thank your co-worker for helping you. Also, be willing to help others.

Ethics and Laws

Leaving a person to lie on wet or soiled linens is neglect. Check persons at risk for wetting or soiling often. This may be from perspiration (sweat), urine, or feces (stools). Change wet or soiled linens as often as needed.

FOCUS ON PRIDE: Application

Do you make your bed at home every day? If yes, why? If no, why? Explain why the look and feel of the bed can affect the person's comfort and safety.

REVIEW QUESTIONS

Circle the BEST answer.

1 A resident is showering and will be out of bed for the day. You will
   a Make an occupied bed
   b Re-use the linens and make a closed bed
   c Make a closed bed with clean linens
   d Make an open bed with clean linens

2 To transfer a person from a stretcher to the bed, you make
   a A closed bed
   b An open bed
   c An occupied bed
   d A surgical bed

3 When making beds
   a Leave wrinkles in the bottom sheet
   b Check the bed for eyeglasses and other items
   c Shake clean linens to unfold them
   d Take extra linens to another person's room

4 When removing used linens
   a Remove 1 piece at a time
   b Roll all linens together for removal
   c Roll linens toward your body
   d Shake linens to remove crumbs

5 When handling used linens
   a Place them on the floor until you finish making the bed
   b Hold them against your uniform
   c Carry them outside of the room un-bagged
   d Wear gloves to remove linens soiled with urine

6 You have applied a waterproof under-pad correctly if
   a It is in the middle of the mattress
   b The quilted side is down
   c It is under the bottom sheet
   d The corners are mitered

7 A complete linen change is done when
   a The waterproof under-pad is wet
   b The bed is made for a new person
   c The person returns from therapy
   d Linens are loose or wrinkled

8 After making a closed bed
   a Unlock the bed wheels (release the brakes)
   b Leave the bed in the high position
   c Leave used linens in the room on the chair
   d Attach the call light to the bed

9 When making an occupied bed
   a Explain that the person will roll over a "bump" of linens
   b Remove the top sheet and leave the person uncovered
   c Lower the far bed rail if working alone
   d Fan-fold bottom linens to the foot of the bed

10 You are making an occupied bed. You just tucked the used linens under the person. Next, you should
   a Have the person roll back onto the uncovered mattress
   b Apply a clean drawsheet before applying a clean bottom sheet
   c Remove gloves and practice hand hygiene before touching clean linens
   d Fold and remove the bath blanket

11 What is the purpose of a toe pleat?
   a It keeps the feet warm.
   b It keeps the feet cool.
   c It prevents pressure on the toes from top linens.
   d It keeps the toes from touching the foot-board.

12 For a surgical bed
   a Do not secure the bottom linens
   b Fan-fold top linens to the side of the bed
   c Fan-fold top linens to the foot of the bed
   d Do not apply top linens

Answers to Chapter 22 questions are on p. 902.

FOCUS ON PRACTICE

Problem Solving

You need to give a person a bath in bed (Chapter 24). The person must remain in bed. Which type of bed will you make? Will you change linens or give the bath first? While changing linens, when will you apply and remove gloves and practice hand hygiene?

Oral Hygiene

OBJECTIVES

- Define the key terms and key abbreviations in this chapter.
- Explain the purposes of oral hygiene.
- Explain why flossing is important.
- Describe the safety measures for giving mouth care to unconscious persons.

- Explain how to care for dentures.
- Identify the observations related to oral hygiene.
- Perform the procedures described in this chapter.
- Explain how to promote PRIDE in the person, the family, and yourself.

KEY TERMS

aspiration Breathing fluid, food, vomitus, or an object into the lungs
denture A removable replacement for missing teeth
hygiene The cleanliness practices that promote health and prevent disease
mouth care See "oral hygiene"

oral hygiene The practices that promote healthy tissues and structures of the mouth; mouth care
plaque A thin film that sticks to the teeth; it contains saliva, microbes, and other substances
tartar Hardened plaque

KEY ABBREVIATIONS

ADA	American Dental Association	ID	Identification

The teeth and mucous membranes of the mouth must be kept clean and intact. Otherwise teeth can decay. Microbes can enter the body.

Illness, disease, and some drugs often cause:
- A bad taste in the mouth.
- A whitish coating in the mouth and on the tongue.
- Redness and swelling in the mouth and on the tongue.
- Dry mouth. Dry mouth is common from oxygen, smoking, decreased fluid intake, and anxiety.

See *Body Structure and Function Review: The Teeth and Gums*. For greater detail, see Chapters 10 and 12.

BODY STRUCTURE AND FUNCTION REVIEW
The Teeth and Gums

Structure and Function

The *teeth* cut, chop, and grind food into small bits for swallowing and digestion. A tooth has 3 main parts (Fig. 23-1):

- The *crown* is the outer part.
- The *neck* is surrounded by *gums (gingivae)*.
- The *root* fits into the bone of the lower or upper jaw.

Teeth are covered with *enamel*. Enamel is a hard, outer coating. Below the enamel is a softer layer called *dentin*. The inner tooth contains nerves and blood vessels.

Changes With Aging

With age, *primary teeth* (baby teeth) are replaced with *permanent teeth* (adult teeth). Normally, adults have 32 permanent teeth.

Older persons may have decreased saliva production, loss of teeth, and difficulty chewing and swallowing. The number of taste buds decreases. Changes with aging can affect the person's appetite, eating, and speaking.

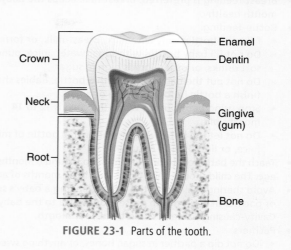

FIGURE 23-1 Parts of the tooth.

PURPOSE OF ORAL HYGIENE

Hygiene involves the cleanliness practices that promote health and prevent disease. *Oral hygiene (mouth care)* relates to the practices that promote healthy tissues and structures of the mouth.

Oral hygiene:
- Keeps the mouth and teeth clean.
- Prevents mouth odors and infections.
- Increases comfort.
- Makes food taste better.
- Reduces the risk for *tooth decay (cavities, dental caries)* and *periodontal disease (gum disease)*.
- Is an important part of infection prevention and overall health promotion.

Plaque and tartar build up from poor oral hygiene.
- *Plaque* is a thin film that sticks to the teeth. It contains saliva, microbes, and other substances.
- *Tartar* is hardened plaque. Tartar builds up at the gum line near the neck of the tooth.

Microbes in plaque produce acids that can damage enamel and cause tooth decay (cavities, dental caries). Brushing and flossing can prevent decay. However, once a cavity forms, a dentist needs to fill it to prevent more damage.

Tartar buildup causes periodontal disease (gum disease). *Gingivitis* is a mild form of gum disease. Tissues around the teeth are inflamed. The gums are red and swollen and bleed easily. *Periodontitis* is severe disease. Gums separate from the teeth. Bone is destroyed and teeth loosen. Tooth loss is common.

The nurse assesses the person's oral care needs. So may the speech-language pathologist and the dietitian.

See *Focus on Children and Older Persons: Purpose of Oral Hygiene.*
See *Delegation Guidelines: Purpose of Oral Hygiene*, p. 344.
See *Promoting Safety and Comfort: Purpose of Oral Hygiene*, p. 345.

FOCUS ON **CHILDREN AND OLDER PERSONS**
Purpose of Oral Hygiene

Children

Infants and young children need mouth care to remove food and bacteria. This helps prevent early childhood tooth decay *(baby bottle tooth decay, early childhood caries)*. Common in the upper and lower front teeth, it can occur in all teeth (Fig. 23-2). Prolonged teeth exposure to liquids containing sugar is the usual cause. Breast-milk, milk, formula, fruit juice, and other sweetened drinks contain sugar. Sugar coats the teeth. Bacteria in the mouth use sugars in such drinks for nourishment. The bacteria produce acids that cause tooth decay.

For early childhood oral hygiene, see Box 23-1 (p. 344).

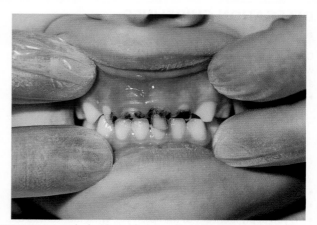

FIGURE 23-2 Baby bottle tooth decay. (From Eisen D, Lynch DP: *The mouth: diagnosis and treatment*, St Louis, 1998, Mosby.)

BOX 23-1	Oral Hygiene: Early Childhood

Preventing Tooth Decay
- Breast-feeding is preferred. Breast-milk keeps the baby's mouth healthy.
- Bottle-feeding:
  - Fill baby bottles only with milk, breast-milk, or formula.
  - Do not fill baby bottles with sugar water, juice, punch, soft drinks, or other liquids high in sugar.
  - Do not put the baby to bed with a bottle. Babies should finish a bottle before bedtime or a nap.
  - Stop using baby bottles when the child is 12 to 14 months old.
  - Do not let the baby walk around with a bottle of milk, juice, or liquids high in sugar.
- Teach the baby how to drink from a cup around 6 months of age. The child should drink from a cup by 12 months of age.
- Avoid sharing saliva with the baby. Cleaning a baby's spoon or pacifier in your mouth passes your saliva to the baby. Cavity-causing bacteria could be in your mouth.
- Pacifiers:
  - Do not dip a pacifier in sugar, honey, or anything sweet.
  - Do not let a baby suck on a pacifier all the time.

Care of Gums and Teeth
- Wipe the baby's gums after each feeding. Use a gauze pad or washcloth that is clean and damp.
- Start brushing when the first tooth erupts. (*Erupt* means to break through and become visible.)
- Use fluoride toothpaste (Fig. 23-3):
  - Until age 3—Use a smear (the size of a grain of rice) of fluoride toothpaste and a child-sized toothbrush.
  - Ages 3 to 6—Use a pea-sized amount of fluoride toothpaste.
- Brush gently.
- Supervise brushing until the child can spit out toothpaste. This is usually until age 6 or 7.
- Have a brushing routine for the child. For example, you and the child brush together at the same time.
- See "Flossing."
- Consult a dentist about when to schedule the baby's first dental visit. Do so after the first tooth erupts.

Modified from National Institutes of Health: Tooth decay—early childhood, Bethesda, Md., page updated January 24, 2022, and American Dental Association: Mouth healthy™: tooth decay with baby bottles, 2024.

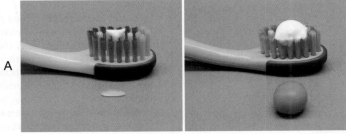

FIGURE 23-3 Toothpaste amounts in early childhood. **A,** A smear of toothpaste (the size of a grain of rice) is used until age 3. **B,** A pea-sized amount is used from ages 3 to 6. (ADA content –Toothpaste Amount image in early childhood; depicting pea sized. Copyright © 2020 American Dental Association. All rights reserved. Reprinted with permission.)

DELEGATION GUIDELINES

Purpose of Oral Hygiene

Oral hygiene procedures are routine nursing tasks. To assist with oral hygiene, you need this information from the nurse and the care plan.
- The type of oral hygiene to give. See procedures:
  - *Brushing and Flossing the Person's Teeth*, p. 346
  - *Assisting the Person to Brush and Floss the Teeth*, p. 348
  - *Providing Mouth Care for the Unconscious Person*, p. 350
  - *Providing Denture Care*, p. 352
- If flossing is needed.
- What cleaning agent and equipment to use.
- If you apply lubricant to the lips. If yes, what lubricant to use.
- How often to give oral hygiene.

- How much help the person needs.
- What observations to report and record:
  - Dry, cracked, swollen, or blistered lips
  - Mouth or breath odor
  - Redness, swelling, irritation, sores, or white patches in the mouth or on the tongue
  - Bleeding, swelling, or redness of the gums
  - Painful areas
  - Loose teeth
  - Rough, sharp, or chipped areas on dentures
  - Dentures that fit poorly
- When to report observations.
- What patient or resident concerns to report at once.

PROMOTING SAFETY AND COMFORT
Purpose of Oral Hygiene

Safety

You may have contact with the person's mucous membranes. Gums may bleed during mouth care. Also, the mouth has many microbes. Pathogens spread through sexual contact may be in the mouths of some persons. Follow Standard Precautions and the Bloodborne Pathogen Standard. Follow the rules of hand hygiene and the guidelines for glove use in Chapters 17 and 18.

In nursing centers, follow agency policies and procedures for using Enhanced Barrier Precautions for high-contact tasks. See Chapter 18.

Brush gently and carefully. Brushing hard can cause the gums to bleed. Inserting the toothbrush too far can stimulate the gag reflex.

Comfort

Follow the person's care plan and preferences for how often to perform oral hygiene. The American Dental Association (ADA) recommends brushing for 2 minutes 2 times daily. Some persons need or want oral care more often—after sleep, after meals, and at bedtime. Many people practice oral hygiene before meals. Some persons need mouth care every 2 hours or more often.

FLOSSING

Flossing cleans between the teeth. Flossing removes plaque from areas brushing cannot reach and removes food from between the teeth. It helps prevent periodontal disease and cavities.

Dental floss is commonly used. It is a soft thread used to clean between teeth. Other devices *(interdental cleaners)* may be used. *Inter* means between. Small brushes and plastic picks threaded with floss are examples. Some persons use powered air or water flossers to clean between teeth.

The ADA recommends flossing at least once a day. Flossing can be done before or after brushing. The person can choose the best time for thorough flossing—in the morning, after a meal, at bedtime, or when convenient. You need to floss for persons who cannot do so themselves.

See *Focus on Children and Older Persons: Flossing*.

FOCUS ON **CHILDREN AND OLDER PERSONS**
Flossing

Children

The ADA recommends that flossing start when 2 baby teeth touch. You need to floss for babies, toddlers, and pre-schoolers. You may need to remind and supervise older children when flossing.

EQUIPMENT

A toothbrush, toothpaste, floss or other interdental cleaner, and mouthwash are needed. A toothbrush with soft bristles is best. Using a toothpaste with fluoride helps protect the teeth from decay.

Sponge swabs (p. 349) are used for sore, tender mouths and for unconscious persons. Use sponge swabs with care. Make sure the foam pad is tight on the stick. The person could choke on the foam pad if it comes off.

You also need a kidney basin, water cup, straw, tissues, towels, and gloves. Many persons bring oral hygiene equipment from home. Electric toothbrushes are common.

▉ BRUSHING AND FLOSSING TEETH

Many people perform oral hygiene themselves. Others need help gathering and setting up oral hygiene equipment. You perform oral hygiene for persons who:

- Are very weak.
- Cannot move or use their arms.
- Are too confused to brush their teeth.

See procedure: *Brushing and Flossing the Person's Teeth*, p. 346.

See procedure: *Assisting the Person to Brush and Floss the Teeth*, p. 348.

Brushing and Flossing the Person's Teeth

QUALITY OF LIFE

- Knock before entering the person's room.
- Address the person by name.
- Introduce yourself by name and title.

- Explain the procedure before starting and during the procedure.
- Protect the person's rights during the procedure.
- Handle the person gently during the procedure.

PRE-PROCEDURE

1 Follow *Delegation Guidelines: Purpose of Oral Hygiene*, p. 344. See *Promoting Safety and Comfort: Purpose of Oral Hygiene*, p. 345.
2 Practice hand hygiene and get the following supplies.
   - Toothbrush with soft bristles
   - Toothpaste
   - Mouthwash (or solution noted on the care plan)
   - Floss or other interdental cleaner (if used)
   - Water cup with cool water
   - Straw
   - Kidney basin
   - Hand towel
   - Towel or paper towels (as a barrier for supplies)
   - Gloves
   - Laundry bag
3 Arrange items in the person's room. Place the barrier (towel, paper towels) on the over-bed table. Arrange items on top.
4 Practice hand hygiene.
5 Identify the person. Check the identification (ID) bracelet against the assignment sheet. Use 2 identifiers (Chapter 14). Also call the person by name.
6 Provide for privacy.
7 Raise the bed for body mechanics. Bed rails are up if used.

PROCEDURE

8 Lower the bed rail near you if up.
9 Assist the person to a sitting position or to a side-lying position near you. (NOTE: Some state competency tests require that the person is at a 60- to 90-degree angle. Other states require a 75- to 90-degree angle.)
10 Place the towel across the chest.
11 Adjust the over-bed table so you can reach it with ease.
12 Practice hand hygiene. Put on gloves.
13 Hold the toothbrush over the kidney basin. Pour some water over the brush.
14 Apply toothpaste to the toothbrush.
15 Brush the teeth gently with short strokes (Fig. 23-4). Brush the inner, outer, and chewing surfaces of upper and lower teeth.
16 Brush the tongue gently (see Fig. 23-4). Also gently brush the roof of the mouth, inside of the cheeks, and gums.
17 Let the person rinse the mouth with water. Hold the kidney basin under the chin (Fig. 23-5). Repeat this step as needed.
18 Floss the person's teeth (optional). See Figure 23-6.
   a Break off about an 18-inch piece of floss from the dispenser.
   b Wrap most of the floss around one of your middle fingers. Wrap a small amount around the middle finger on the other hand (see Fig. 23-6, *A*). (As floss is used, unwrap clean floss from the first middle finger. Wrap used floss around the middle finger on the other hand.)

   c Stretch the floss with your thumbs. Hold the floss firmly between your thumbs and index fingers (see Fig. 23-6, *B*).
   d Start at the back side of an upper back tooth. Work around to the other side of the mouth.
   e Gently insert the floss between the teeth with a rubbing motion. Do not jerk or snap the floss.
   f Gently slide the floss into the space between the gum and the tooth (see Fig. 23-6, *C*).
   g Rub the floss gently against the side of the tooth. Move away from the gum with slow back-and-forth and up-and-down motions (see Fig. 23-6, *D*).
   h Use a new section of floss for each tooth. Remember to floss the back side of the last tooth.
   i Floss the lower teeth. Start on one side. Work around to the other side. Remember to floss the back side of the last tooth.
   j Discard the floss.
19 Let the person use mouthwash or other solution. Hold the kidney basin under the chin.
20 Wipe the person's mouth. Remove the towel. Place the towel in the laundry bag.
21 Remove and discard the gloves. Practice hand hygiene.
22 Return the person to a safe and comfortable position.

POST-PROCEDURE

23 Provide for comfort. (See the inside of the back cover.)
24 Lower the bed to a safe and comfortable level. Raise or lower bed rails. Follow the care plan.
25 Clean up and store supplies and equipment. (Wear gloves. Change gloves as needed.)
   a Discard disposable items.
   b Rinse the toothbrush and return it to its proper place.
   c Follow agency procedures to clean and disinfect re-usable equipment. Return supplies and equipment to their proper place.
   d Follow agency policy for used linens.
   e Clean and dry the over-bed table. Dry with paper towels. Discard paper towels. Position the over-bed table as the person prefers.
   f Remove and discard gloves. Practice hand hygiene.
26 Place the call light and other needed items within reach.
27 Follow the care plan and the person's preferences for privacy measures to maintain. Leaving the privacy curtain, window coverings, and door open or closed are examples.
28 Complete a safety check of the room. (See the inside of the back cover.)
29 Practice hand hygiene.
30 Report and record your care and observations.

Upper teeth   Lower teeth

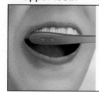
Hold the brush at a 45-degree angle to the gums.
Brush back and forth gently with short strokes.

Brush the inner, outer, and chewing surfaces of the upper and lower teeth.
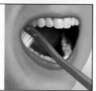

Tilt the brush to clean the inside of the front teeth.
Brush gently with up-and-down strokes.
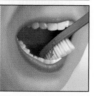

Brush the tongue.

FIGURE 23-4 Brushing the teeth and tongue.

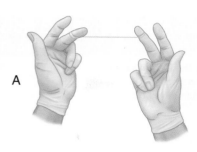
A   Wrap the floss around the middle fingers on both hands.

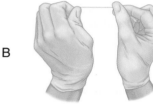
B   Hold the floss between your thumbs and index fingers.

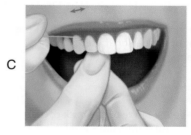
C   Insert the floss between the teeth with a gentle rubbing motion.
Slide the floss into the space between the gum and the tooth.

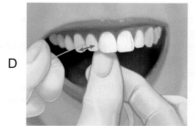
D   Rub the floss gently against the side of the tooth.
Move away from the gum.

FIGURE 23-6 Flossing with dental floss. **A** and **B,** Holding the floss. **C** and **D,** Flossing along the gum line and side of the tooth.

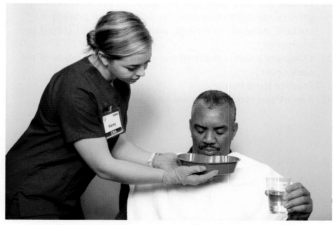

FIGURE 23-5 The kidney basin is held under the person's chin.

Assisting the Person to Brush and Floss the Teeth

QUALITY OF LIFE

- Knock before entering the person's room.
- Address the person by name.
- Introduce yourself by name and title.

- Explain the procedure before starting and during the procedure.
- Protect the person's rights during the procedure.
- Handle the person gently during the procedure.

PRE-PROCEDURE

1 Follow *Delegation Guidelines: Purpose of Oral Hygiene*, p. 344. See *Promoting Safety and Comfort: Purpose of Oral Hygiene*, p. 345.
2 Practice hand hygiene and get the following supplies.
   - Toothbrush with soft bristles
   - Toothpaste
   - Mouthwash (or solution noted on the care plan)
   - Floss or other interdental cleaner (if used)
   - Water cup with cool water
   - Straw
   - Kidney basin (if needed)
   - Hand towel
   - Towel or paper towels (as a barrier for supplies)
   - Gloves
   - Laundry bag

3 Arrange items in the person's room or bathroom. Place the barrier (towel, paper towels) on the over-bed table or bathroom counter. Arrange items on top.
4 Practice hand hygiene.
5 Identify the person. Check the ID bracelet against the assignment sheet. Use 2 identifiers (Chapter 14). Also call the person by name.
6 Provide for privacy.

PROCEDURE

7 Position the person for oral hygiene (sitting up in bed or at the bathroom sink).
8 Place the towel over the chest. This protects garments from spills.
9 Be sure the person can reach needed supplies. Adjust the over-bed table in front of the person if used.
10 Have the person perform hand hygiene (Chapter 17).

11 Have the person perform oral hygiene. This includes brushing the teeth and tongue, rinsing the mouth, flossing, and using mouthwash or other solution. In bed, the person spits into a kidney basin.
12 Remove the towel when the person is done. Place the towel in the laundry bag.
13 Return the person to a comfortable position. Assist the person out of the bathroom if needed.

POST-PROCEDURE

14 Provide for comfort. (See the inside of the back cover.)
15 Return the bed to a safe and comfortable level if it was adjusted. Follow the care plan.
16 Check that bed rails are raised or lowered following the care plan.
17 Clean up and store supplies and equipment. (Wear gloves. Change gloves as needed.)
   a Discard disposable items.
   b Rinse the toothbrush and return it to its proper place.
   c Follow agency procedures to clean and disinfect re-usable equipment. Return supplies and equipment to their proper place.
   d Follow agency policy for used linens.
   e Clean and dry the over-bed table. Dry with paper towels. Discard paper towels. Position the over-bed table as the person prefers.
   f Remove and discard gloves. Practice hand hygiene.

18 Place the call light and other needed items within reach.
19 Follow the care plan and the person's preferences for privacy measures to maintain. Leaving the privacy curtain, window coverings, and door open or closed are examples.
20 Complete a safety check of the room. (See the inside of the back cover.)
21 Practice hand hygiene.
22 Report and record your care and observations.

Mouth Care for the Unconscious Person

Unconscious (comatose) persons cannot eat or drink. Some breathe with their mouths open. Many receive oxygen. These factors cause mouth dryness. They also cause crusting on the tongue and mucous membranes. Oral hygiene keeps the mouth clean and moist. It also helps prevent infection.

The care plan states what cleaning agent to use. Apply the cleaning agent with sponge swabs (Fig. 23-7, *A*). To prevent the lips from cracking, apply a lubricant (check the care plan) after cleaning.

Unconscious persons usually cannot swallow. Protect them from choking and aspiration. *Aspiration* is breathing fluid, food, vomitus, or an object into the lungs. It can cause pneumonia and death. To prevent aspiration:

* Position the person on the side with the head turned well to the side (Fig. 23-8). In this position, excess fluid can run out of the mouth.
* Use a small amount of fluid to clean the mouth.
* Do not insert dentures. Unconscious persons do not wear dentures.

Do not use your fingers to keep the person's mouth open. The person can bite down on them. The bite breaks the skin, allowing microbes to enter the body. Infection is a risk. Using a bite block or plastic tongue depressor (bite stick) is a safe way to open the mouth (Fig. 23-7, *B*).

Mouth care is given at least every 2 hours. Follow the nurse's directions and the care plan.

See *Focus on Communication: Mouth Care for the Unconscious Person.*

See *Promoting Safety and Comfort: Mouth Care for the Unconscious Person.*

See procedure: *Providing Mouth Care for the Unconscious Person,* p. 350.

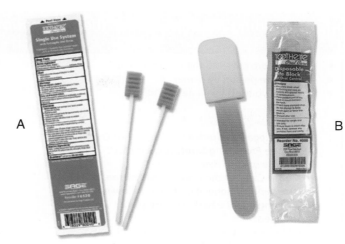

FIGURE 23-7 **A,** Oral sponge swabs. **B,** Bite block. (Courtesy Sage Products, LLC.)

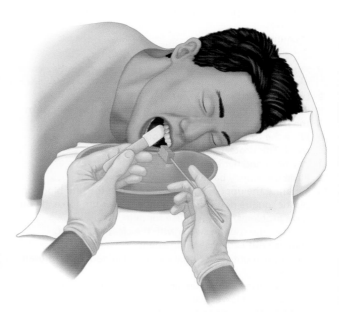

FIGURE 23-8 The unconscious person's head is turned well to the side to prevent aspiration. A bite block keeps the mouth open while cleaning the mouth with swabs.

FOCUS ON **COMMUNICATION**
Mouth Care for the Unconscious Person

Unconscious persons cannot speak or respond to you. However, some can hear. Always assume that unconscious persons can hear. Tell the person who you are. Call the person by name. Explain what you are doing step-by-step. Also, tell the person when you are done, when you are leaving, and when you will return.

PROMOTING SAFETY AND COMFORT
Mouth Care for the Unconscious Person

Safety
Use sponge swabs with care. Make sure the sponge pad is tight on the stick. The person could aspirate or choke on the sponge if it comes off the stick.

Press the sponge swab against the side of the cup to squeeze out excess cleaning agent. A small amount of fluid is used to prevent aspiration.

Comfort
Unconscious persons are re-positioned at least every 2 hours. Combine mouth care with skin care, re-positioning, and other comfort measures.

Providing Mouth Care for the Unconscious Person

QUALITY OF LIFE

- Knock before entering the person's room.
- Address the person by name.
- Introduce yourself by name and title.

- Explain the procedure before starting and during the procedure.
- Protect the person's rights during the procedure.
- Handle the person gently during the procedure.

PRE-PROCEDURE

1 Follow *Delegation Guidelines: Purpose of Oral Hygiene*, p. 344. See *Promoting Safety and Comfort:*
   a *Purpose of Oral Hygiene*, p. 345
   b *Mouth Care for the Unconscious Person*, p. 349
2 Practice hand hygiene and get the following supplies.
   - Cleaning agent (check the care plan)
   - Sponge swabs
   - Bite block or plastic tongue depressor
   - Water cup with cool water
   - Hand towel
   - Kidney basin
   - Lip lubricant (check the care plan)
   - Towel or paper towels (as a barrier for supplies)
   - Gloves
   - Laundry bag

3 Arrange items in the person's room. Place the barrier (towel, paper towels) on the over-bed table. Arrange items on top.
4 Practice hand hygiene.
5 Identify the person. Check the ID bracelet against the assignment sheet. Use 2 identifiers (Chapter 14). Also call the person by name.
6 Provide for privacy.
7 Raise the bed for body mechanics. Bed rails are up.

PROCEDURE

8 Lower the bed rail near you.
9 Position the person in a side-lying position near you. Turn the person's head well to the side.
10 Place the towel under the person's face and along the chest. This protects the person and bed.
11 Practice hand hygiene. Put on gloves.
12 Place the kidney basin under the chin.
13 Separate the upper and lower teeth. Use the bite block or plastic tongue depressor. Be gentle. Never use force. If you have problems, ask the nurse for help.
14 Moisten the sponge swabs with the cleaning agent. Squeeze out excess cleaning agent.
15 Clean the mouth. (Use new swabs as needed. Discard used swabs.)
   a Clean the inner, outer, and chewing surfaces of the upper and lower teeth.
   b Clean the gums and tongue.
   c Swab the roof of the mouth, inside of the cheeks, and the lips.

16 Moisten and squeeze out a clean swab. Swab the mouth to rinse. Discard the swab.
17 Remove the kidney basin.
18 Wipe the person's mouth. Remove the towel. Place the towel in the laundry bag.
19 Apply lubricant to the lips.
20 Remove and discard the gloves. Practice hand hygiene.
21 Return the person to a safe and comfortable position.

POST-PROCEDURE

22 Provide for comfort. (See the inside of the back cover.)
23 Lower the bed to a safe level. Follow the care plan.
24 Follow the care plan for bed rail use.
25 Clean up and store supplies and equipment. (Wear gloves. Change gloves as needed.)
   a Discard disposable items.
   b Follow agency procedures to clean and disinfect re-usable equipment. Return supplies and equipment to their proper place.
   c Follow agency policy for used linens.
   d Clean and dry the over-bed table. Dry with paper towels. Discard paper towels. Position the over-bed table near the bed for staff use.
   e Remove and discard the gloves. Practice hand hygiene.

26 Place the call light and other needed items within reach for staff and visitor use.
27 Follow the care plan for privacy measures to maintain. Leaving the privacy curtain, window coverings, and door open or closed are examples.
28 Complete a safety check of the room. (See the inside of the back cover.)
29 Tell the person that you are leaving the room. Say when you will return.
30 Practice hand hygiene.
31 Report and record your care and observations.

DENTURES

A *denture* is a removable replacement for missing teeth (Fig. 23-9). Tooth loss occurs from gum disease, tooth decay, or injury. Often called *false teeth*, complete and partial dentures are common.

- *Complete (full) dentures.* Dentures replace all of the upper or lower teeth.
- *Partial dentures.* The person has some teeth. The partial denture replaces the missing teeth. Natural teeth still need to be brushed and flossed. See procedure: *Brushing and Flossing the Person's Teeth*, p. 346. Or see procedure: *Assisting the Person to Brush and Floss the Teeth*, p. 348.

Some people do not wear their dentures. Others wear them only for eating. Remind patients and residents not to wrap dentures in tissues or napkins. Otherwise, they are easily discarded.

Denture Care Equipment

For cleaning, you need a denture cleaner, denture cup (see Fig. 23-9), and a denture brush with soft bristles. Use only denture cleaning products to avoid damaging dentures. Do not use toothpaste. Many types of toothpaste can damage dentures. Use a cleaner intended for use on dentures.

Dentures must be removed for cleaning. Do not use denture cleaning products on dentures while they are still in the mouth.

The manufacturer's instructions tell how to use the cleaning agent and what water temperature to use. Hot water causes warping—dentures lose their shape. When not worn, store them in a denture cup with cool or warm water or a denture soaking solution. Otherwise they can dry out and warp.

A denture adhesive may be used to hold dentures in place and keep food out of the inner part of the denture. The product (paste, cream, powder, pad, or strip) is applied to clean dentures. Follow the manufacturer's instructions for how to apply and the amount to use. Do not use too much adhesive. When cleaning dentures, gently brush to remove the adhesive. Adhesives are not used to fix dentures that fit poorly. Tell the nurse if dentures are loose.

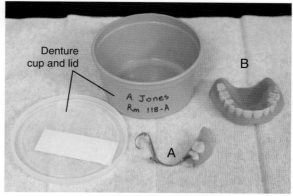

FIGURE 23-9 Dentures and a denture cup. **A**, Partial denture. **B**, Complete (full) denture.

Denture Care

Mouth care is given and dentures cleaned as often as natural teeth. Dentures are slippery when wet. They easily break or chip if dropped onto a hard surface (floor, sink, counter). Hold them firmly when removing or inserting them. During cleaning, firmly hold them over a sink filled half-way with water. Line the sink with a towel. This prevents the dentures from falling onto a hard surface.

Dentures are removed at bedtime. They are soaked over-night in a denture cleaning solution or water. Rinse the dentures before they are inserted.

If able, the person cleans the dentures. You clean dentures for persons who cannot do so.

See *Promoting Safety and Comfort: Denture Care.*
See procedure: *Providing Denture Care*, p. 352.

PROMOTING SAFETY AND COMFORT
Denture Care

Safety

Dentures are costly. Handle them very carefully. Label the denture cup and lid with the person's name and room and bed number (see Fig. 23-9). Report lost or damaged dentures at once.

Never carry dentures in your hands. Always use a denture cup or kidney basin. You could easily drop the dentures if holding them.

Faucets are contaminated. Use a clean, dry paper towel to turn the faucet on and off and to adjust the faucet. Or use your wrist. If you contaminate your gloves, remove them. Practice hand hygiene. Apply clean gloves.

Never place dentures on a contaminated surface. Place dentures in a clean kidney basin or denture cup.

Dentures are rinsed under running water. Do not rinse dentures in the water used to fill the sink. The sink is contaminated.

Providing Denture Care

QUALITY OF LIFE

- Knock before entering the person's room.
- Address the person by name.
- Introduce yourself by name and title.

- Explain the procedure before starting and during the procedure.
- Protect the person's rights during the procedure.
- Handle the person gently during the procedure.

PRE-PROCEDURE

1 Follow *Delegation Guidelines: Purpose of Oral Hygiene*, p. 344. See *Promoting Safety and Comfort:*
   a *Purpose of Oral Hygiene*, p. 345
   b *Denture Care*, p. 351
2 Practice hand hygiene and get the following supplies.
   • Denture brush
   • Denture cup and lid labeled with the person's name and room and bed number
   • Denture cleaning agent
   • Denture adhesive as noted in the care plan (if needed)
   • Mouthwash (or other noted solution)
   • Kidney basin
   • 2 hand towels
   • Gauze squares
   • Sponge swabs
   • Towel or paper towels (as a barrier for supplies)
   • Gloves
   • Laundry bag

3 Arrange items in the person's room and near the sink as needed.
   a Place a barrier (towel, paper towels) on the over-bed table if items will be used at the bedside. Arrange needed items on top—gloves, hand towel, gauze squares, kidney basin, sponge swabs, mouthwash (or other solution), denture adhesive (if needed).
   b Place a barrier (towel, paper towels) on the counter near the sink. Arrange needed items on top—denture cup and lid, hand towel, denture brush, denture cleaning agent.
4 Practice hand hygiene.
5 Identify the person. Check the ID bracelet against the assignment sheet. Use 2 identifiers (Chapter 14). Also call the person by name.
6 Provide for privacy.

PROCEDURE

7 Position the person for oral hygiene (sitting up in bed or at the sink). (For this procedure, the person is in bed.)
8 Place a towel over the person's chest.
9 Have the person practice hand hygiene if he or she will handle dentures. Practice hand hygiene. Put on gloves.
10 Have the person remove the dentures and place them in the kidney basin (if able).
11 Remove the dentures if the person cannot do so. Use gauze squares for a good grip on the slippery dentures.
   a Grasp the upper denture with your thumb and index finger (Fig. 23-10). Move it up and down slightly to break the seal. Gently remove the denture. Place it in the kidney basin.
   b Grasp and remove the lower denture with your thumb and index finger. Turn it slightly and lift it out of the person's mouth. Place it in the kidney basin.
12 Take the kidney basin with dentures to the sink.
13 Rinse the denture cup and lid.
14 Line the bottom of the sink with a towel. Do not use paper towels. Fill the sink half-way with water.
15 Rinse each denture under cool or warm running water. Follow agency policy for water temperature.
16 Return dentures to the kidney basin.
17 Apply the denture cleaning agent to the brush.
18 Brush each denture. Brush the inner, outer, and chewing surfaces and all surfaces that touch the gums (Fig. 23-11).
19 Rinse the dentures under running water. Use cool or warm water as directed by the cleaning agent manufacturer.
20 Place dentures in the denture cup. Cover the dentures with cool or warm water if they will be stored. Follow agency policy for water temperature. Close the lid tightly.

21 *If dentures will not be worn*, store them in a safe place. Follow agency policy and the person's preference for where to store dentures. Dentures must be in water or in a denture soaking solution.
22 Rinse the kidney basin. Take the kidney basin to the over-bed table. Take the denture cup if dentures will be worn.
23 Use sponge swabs to clean the gums, tongue, roof of the mouth, and inside of the cheeks. Discard used sponge swabs. Have the person use mouthwash (or noted solution). Hold the kidney basin under the chin. Wipe the person's mouth.
24 *If dentures will be worn:*
   a Apply denture adhesive if used. Some products are applied to wet dentures. Others are applied to dry dentures. Follow the manufacturer's instructions for how to apply and the amount to use.
   b Have the person insert the dentures. Insert them if the person cannot.
     1) Hold the upper denture firmly with your thumb and index finger. Raise the upper lip with the other hand. Insert the denture. Gently press on the denture with your index finger to make sure it is in place.
     2) Hold the lower denture with your thumb and index finger. Pull the lower lip down slightly. Insert the denture. Gently press down on it to make sure it is in place.
25 Wipe the person's mouth if needed. Remove the towel. Place it in the laundry bag.
26 Remove and discard the gloves. Practice hand hygiene.

Providing Denture Care—cont'd

POST-PROCEDURE

27 Provide for comfort. (See the inside of the back cover.)
28 Return the bed to a safe and comfortable level if it was adjusted. Follow the care plan.
29 Check that bed rails are raised or lowered following the care plan.
30 Drain the sink.
31 Clean up and store supplies and equipment. (Wear gloves. Change gloves as needed.)
 a Discard disposable items.
 b Rinse the brush. Empty and rinse the denture cup if dentures are worn. Return items to their proper place.
 c Follow agency procedures to clean and disinfect re-usable equipment. Return supplies and equipment to their proper place.
 d Clean and dry the over-bed table. Dry with paper towels. Discard paper towels. Position the over-bed table as the person prefers.
 e Remove the towel from the sink. Squeeze to remove excess water. Place the towel in the laundry bag.
 f Follow agency policy for used linens.
 g Remove and discard gloves. Practice hand hygiene.

32 Place the call light and other needed items within reach.
33 Follow the care plan and the person's preferences for privacy measures to maintain. Leaving the privacy curtain, window coverings, and door open or closed are examples.
34 Complete a safety check of the room. (See the inside of the back cover.)
35 Practice hand hygiene.
36 Report and record your care and observations.

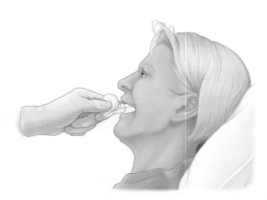

FIGURE 23-10 Removing dentures. Use a piece of gauze to grasp the denture.

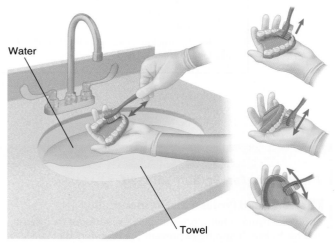

FIGURE 23-11 Cleaning dentures. Hold the dentures over a sink lined with a towel and filled half-way with water. Brush the inner, outer, and chewing surfaces. Brush the surfaces that touch the gums.

REPORTING AND RECORDING

You make many observations while assisting with oral hygiene.

- Dry, cracked, swollen, or blistered lips
- Mouth or breath odor
- Redness, swelling, irritation, sores, or white patches in the mouth or on the tongue
- Bleeding, swelling, or redness of the gums
- Reports of painful areas
- Loose teeth
- Rough, sharp, or chipped areas on dentures
- Loose dentures
- Reports of discomfort from dentures

Report and record your observations and the oral hygiene given (Fig. 23-12, p. 354). If not recorded, it is assumed that oral hygiene was not given. This can cause serious legal problems. Tell the nurse if the person refuses oral hygiene or if it was not given for another reason.

ORAL HYGIENE

Observations

Lips
- ☒ Dry, cracked
- ☐ Swelling
- ☐ Blisters
- ☐ Pain
- ☐ Other:

Teeth
- ☒ Pain
- ☐ Loose teeth
- ☐ Other:

Gums
- ☐ Bleeding
- ☐ Swelling
- ☐ Redness
- ☐ Pain or irritation
- ☐ Other:

Dentures
- ☐ Rough or sharp area(s)
- ☐ Chipped area(s)
- ☐ Loose denture(s)

Mouth and tongue
- ☐ Mouth or breath odor
- ☐ Swelling
- ☐ Redness
- ☐ Pain or irritation
- ☐ Sores
- ☐ White patches
- ☐ Other:

Nurse notified: M. Rhodes, RN

Care Measures

Oral hygiene
- ☒ Teeth brushed
- ☒ Mouth structures brushed (tongue, roof of mouth, inside of cheeks, gums)
- ☒ Teeth flossed
- ☐ Mouth structures cleaned with sponge swabs
- ☒ Lip lubricant applied

Denture care
- ☐ Upper denture
- ☐ Lower denture
- ☐ Denture(s) cleaned
- ☐ Adhesive applied
- ☐ Denture(s) placed in mouth
- ☐ Denture(s) soaked in cleaning solution

FIGURE 23-12 Charting sample.

FOCUS ON PRIDE
The Person, Family, and Yourself

Personal and Professional Responsibility

Good oral hygiene helps prevent cavities, periodontal disease, and tooth loss. It also helps prevent breath odors that can be offensive to patients and residents. Good oral hygiene is important for the person's overall health as well. You have a personal and professional responsibility to practice thorough brushing and flossing.

Rights and Respect

Many people do not like being seen without their dentures. The person has the right to privacy. Allow privacy when the person cleans dentures. If you clean dentures, return them to the person as soon as possible.

Independence and Social Interaction

Poor oral hygiene can affect appearance and cause breath odors. When self-esteem is affected, the person may avoid social contact with others. Follow the care plan to meet the person's social needs.

Delegation and Teamwork

Some persons use special equipment for oral care. For example, a person uses a powered water flossing device. Or swabs that connect to suction are used for an unconscious person. (Suction equipment withdraws fluid [Chapter 45].) Knowing how to use equipment is part of safe delegation (Chapter 4). Do not perform a task using equipment you are not trained to use or are not comfortable using. Ask the nurse for needed help.

Ethics and Laws

Thorough oral hygiene takes time. Follow the person's preferences for when to assist with or perform oral hygiene. Do not neglect oral hygiene.

FOCUS ON PRIDE: Application

What are your oral hygiene practices? How do you feel after performing oral hygiene? How can you improve your practices?

REVIEW QUESTIONS

Circle the BEST answer.

1 You perform oral hygiene to
   a Prevent aspiration
   b Keep the mouth dry
   c Prevent mouth odors and infection
   d Remove cavities

2 Which is a sign of periodontal disease?
   a Chapped lips
   b Difficulty swallowing
   c Yellow teeth
   d Red and swollen gums

3 A person's gums bleed. This may be caused by
   a Using a toothbrush with soft bristles
   b Brushing too firmly
   c Inserting dental floss gently
   d Using mouthwash

4 A person should floss
   a Every morning
   b Before meals
   c Before brushing
   d At least once a day

5 You are flossing correctly if you
   a Rub the floss gently against the side of each tooth
   b Only floss the front teeth
   c Rub the floss against the gums firmly
   d Re-use floss

6 When giving mouth care to an unconscious person, you should
   a Replace dentures in the mouth after cleaning
   b Use your fingers to keep the person's mouth open
   c Position the person supine to prevent aspiration
   d Remove excess cleaning agent from the sponge swab

7 How often is mouth care given to an unconscious person?
   a At least every 2 hours
   b At least every 4 hours
   c At least every 8 hours
   d At least twice daily

8 A person has a full upper denture and a partial lower denture. You need to
   a Leave the dentures in the mouth at bedtime
   b Leave the partial denture in the mouth for cleaning
   c Clean the dentures and brush and floss the remaining natural teeth
   d Place the upper denture in the sink while cleaning the lower denture

9 When cleaning dentures
   a Rinse the dentures in the water in the sink
   b Carry the dentures in your hands
   c Line the sink with a towel
   d Rinse the dentures in hot water

10 Which statement about denture care is *correct*?
    a Only use denture cleaning products on dentures.
    b Dentures can be stored in a dry denture cup over-night.
    c You do not need to rinse dentures after they soak in a cleaning solution.
    d Dentures do not break or chip easily.

11 A resident tells you that her dentures are loose. You should
    a Call the person's dentist
    b Tell the nurse
    c Line the denture with gauze
    d Apply a thick layer of adhesive

12 Which must you report to the nurse?
    a Clean dentures
    b Moist and intact lips
    c Bleeding gums
    d Food between the teeth

Answers to Chapter 23 questions are on p. 902.

FOCUS ON PRACTICE

Problem Solving

Two residents share a bathroom. You are gathering supplies for oral care. Two toothbrushes and tubes of toothpaste are in the bathroom. The items are not labeled. What will you do? How can you be sure that residents use their own equipment?

CHAPTER 24

Daily Hygiene and Bathing

OBJECTIVES

- Define the key terms and key abbreviations in this chapter.
- Explain why daily hygiene and bathing are important.
- Describe the care given before and after breakfast, in the afternoon, and in the evening.
- Describe the rules for bathing.
- Identify safety measures for tub baths and showers.
- Explain why perineal care is important.
- Identify the observations to report and record related to daily hygiene and bathing.
- Perform the procedures described in this chapter.
- Explain how to promote PRIDE in the person, the family, and yourself.

KEY TERMS

AM care See "early morning care"

bath blanket A covering used for privacy and warmth during bathing, hygiene, and other care measures

circumcised The fold of skin (foreskin) covering the glans of the penis was surgically removed

diaphoresis Profuse (excessive) sweating

early morning care Routine care given before breakfast; AM care

evening care Care given in the evening at bedtime; PM care

morning care Care given after breakfast; hygiene measures are more thorough at this time

pericare See "perineal care"

perineal care Cleaning the genital and anal areas; pericare

PM care See "evening care"

uncircumcised Foreskin covers the head of the penis

KEY ABBREVIATIONS

C	Centigrade	ID	Identification
F	Fahrenheit		

Daily hygiene and bathing practices promote comfort, safety, and health. The skin is the body's first line of defense against disease. Intact skin prevents microbes from entering the body and causing an infection. Besides cleansing, hygiene measures prevent body and breath odors, are relaxing, and increase circulation.

Many factors affect daily hygiene needs—perspiration (sweating), elimination, vomiting, drainage from wounds or body openings, bed rest, and activity. Illness and aging can affect self-care abilities. The amount of assistance needed varies. Culture and personal choice also affect hygiene needs. Bathing frequency (how often), time of day, and method (shower, tub bath, bed bath) vary. The person's needs and preferences are part of the care plan.

See *Body Structure and Function Review: The Skin*. For greater detail, see Chapters 10 and 12.

See *Caring About Culture: Daily Hygiene and Bathing*.

See *Focus on Communication: Daily Hygiene and Bathing*.

See *Promoting Safety and Comfort: Daily Hygiene and Bathing*.

BODY STRUCTURE AND FUNCTION REVIEW

The Skin

Structure and Function

The *skin* is the body's natural covering. There are 2 skin layers (Fig. 24-1).
- The *epidermis* is the outer layer.
- The *dermis* is the inner layer. Blood vessels, nerves, sweat glands, oil glands, and hair roots are found in the dermis.

Sweat glands (sudoriferous glands) secrete sweat through pores in the skin. Sweat helps regulate body temperature. *Oil glands (sebaceous glands)* secrete an oily substance near the hair shafts. The oil helps to keep the hair and skin soft and shiny.

The skin:
- Provides the body's protective covering. It protects organs from injury. It prevents microorganisms from entering the body.
- Contains nerve endings that sense pleasant and unpleasant stimulation. They sense cold, pain, touch, and pressure to protect the body from injury.
- Helps regulate body temperature. The dilation (widening) and constriction (narrowing) of blood vessels near the surface allows for cooling and heat retention. The secretion of sweat helps the body regulate temperature.

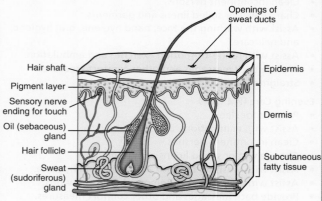

FIGURE 24-1 Structures of the skin.

Changes With Aging

In older persons, the skin becomes less elastic. It thins, sags, and loses strength. Skin is fragile and easily injured or burned. Brown spots *(age spots, liver spots)* are common on the wrists and hands. Folds, lines, and wrinkles appear. There is decreased secretion of oil. Dryness and itching occur.

There are fewer blood vessels and blood vessels become more fragile. Sweat production is decreased. Temperature regulation is affected. The fatty tissue layer thins. The person is more sensitive to cold. Fewer nerve endings affect temperature, pressure, and pain sensation.

There is whitening or graying of hair. Some women begin to have facial hair. Thinning and loss of hair is common. Hair is drier. Nails may become thick and tough.

✿ CARING ABOUT CULTURE

Daily Hygiene and Bathing

Personal hygiene is very important to *East Indian Hindus*. For religious duty, at least 1 bath a day is required. Some believe bathing after a meal is harmful. Another belief is that a cold bath prevents a blood disease. Some believe that eye injuries can occur if bath water is too hot. Hot water can be added to cold water. However, cold water is not added to hot water for a bath. After bathing, the body is carefully dried with a towel.

> NOTE: *Each person is unique. A person may not follow all of the beliefs and practices of his or her culture. Follow the care plan.*

Modified from Giger JN, Haddad L: Transcultural nursing: assessment and intervention, ed 8, St Louis, 2021, Elsevier.

FOCUS ON COMMUNICATION

Daily Hygiene and Bathing

During hygiene and bathing procedures, the person must be warm enough. You can ask:
- "Is the room warm enough?"
- "Is the water comfortable?" "Is it too hot?" "Is it too cold?"
- "Are you warm enough?"
- "Is the water starting to cool?"

PROMOTING SAFETY AND COMFORT

Daily Hygiene and Bathing

Safety
Hygiene and bathing measures often involve exposing and touching private areas—breasts, perineum, rectum. Sexual abuse has occurred in health care settings. The person may feel threatened or actually be abused. The person needs to be able to call for help. Keep the call light within the person's reach at all times. And always act in a professional manner.

You make observations while assisting with daily hygiene and bathing. The *Delegation Guidelines* in this chapter list the observations to report and record. Also report the following at once.
- Bleeding
- Signs of skin breakdown
- Discharge from the vagina, urinary tract, or rectum
- Unusual odors
- Changes from prior observations

DAILY CARE

Daily care includes the hygiene measures performed throughout the day (Box 24-1).

- *Early morning care (AM care)* includes routine care given before breakfast.
- *Morning care* includes care given after breakfast. Hygiene measures are more thorough at this time.
- *Evening care (PM care)* includes care given in the evening, at bedtime.

Most people have hygiene routines and habits. The care plan includes the person's specific needs and preferences, how much help the person needs, and what adaptive (assistive) devices to use (Fig. 24-2). You assist with hygiene as needed. Always protect the right to privacy and to personal choice.

See *Focus on Children and Older Persons: Daily Care.*

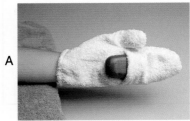
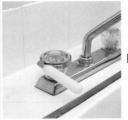

FIGURE 24-2 Adaptive (assistive) devices for hygiene. **A,** A wash mitt holds a bar of soap. **B,** A tap turner makes round knobs easy to turn. **C,** A long-handled sponge is used for hard-to-reach body parts. (Courtesy ElderStore, Alpharetta, Ga.)

FOCUS ON CHILDREN AND OLDER PERSONS

Daily Care

Older Persons

Some older persons resist daily care. Illness, disability, dementia, and personal choice are common reasons. Follow the care plan. Also see Chapter 54.

Bending and reaching may be hard for older and disabled persons. Some have weak hand grips. Adaptive (assistive) devices for hygiene promote independence (see Fig. 24-2). Let the person do as much as safely possible.

BOX 24-1 Daily Care

Before Breakfast (Early Morning Care or AM Care)
- Prepare for breakfast or morning tests.
- Assist with elimination.
- Clean incontinent persons.
- Change wet or soiled linens and garments.
- Assist with washing the face and with hand hygiene.
- Assist with oral hygiene. Insert dentures if worn.
- Assist with dressing and hair care.
- Assist with eyeglasses or contact lenses, hearing aids, and other needed devices. Clean eyeglasses.
- Position for breakfast—dining room, bedside chair, or in bed.
- Make beds and straighten units.

After Breakfast (Morning Care)
- Assist with elimination.
- Clean incontinent persons.
- Change wet or soiled linens and garments.
- Assist with washing the face, hand hygiene, oral hygiene, bathing, and perineal care.
- Assist with hair care, shaving, and changing garments.
- Assist with range-of-motion exercises and ambulation.
- Make beds and straighten rooms.

Afternoon Care
- Prepare for naps, visitors, or activity programs.
- Assist with elimination.
- Clean incontinent persons.
- Change wet or soiled linens and garments.
- Assist with washing the face, hand hygiene, oral hygiene, and hair care.
- Assist with range-of-motion exercises and ambulation.
- Provide back massages and other comfort measures.
- Straighten beds and units.

Evening Care (PM Care)
- Prepare for sleep.
- Assist with elimination.
- Clean incontinent persons.
- Change wet or soiled linens and garments.
- Assist with washing the face and with hand hygiene.
- Assist with oral hygiene. Remove dentures if worn.
- Provide back massages and other comfort measures.
- Help with changing into sleepwear.
- Store eyeglasses or contact lenses, hearing aids, and other devices.
- Straighten beds and units.

BATHING

Bathing cleans the skin and the genital and anal areas. Microbes, dead skin, perspiration (sweat), and excess oils are removed. A bath is refreshing and relaxing. Circulation is stimulated. Body parts are exercised. Observations are made. You have time to talk to the person.

The bathing method depends on the person's condition, self-care abilities, and personal choice. Complete or partial bed baths, tub baths, or showers are given.

Bathing frequency is a personal matter. Some people bathe daily. Others bathe weekly, every other day, or 2 to 3 times a week. Partial baths (p. 366) may be performed on days complete bathing is not done.

In hospitals, bathing is common after breakfast. In nursing centers, bathing is usually before or after breakfast or after the evening meal. The person's choice of bath time is respected when possible.

The rules for bed baths, tub baths, and showers are listed in Box 24-2. Safety, comfort, privacy, independence, and personal choice are important for bathing procedures.

See *Focus on Children and Older Persons: Bathing*, p. 360.
See *Delegation Guidelines: Bathing*, p. 360.
See *Promoting Safety and Comfort: Bathing*, p. 361.

BOX 24-2 Rules for Bathing

Bathing Method and Time
- Follow the care plan and personal preference for bathing method—bed bath, tub bath, shower.
- Follow the care plan and personal preference for bathing time.
- Clean the skin any time urine or feces (stools) are present. Bathe areas that had contact with urine or feces. This prevents skin breakdown and odors.

Safety
- Follow Standard Precautions and the Bloodborne Pathogen Standard.
- Collect needed items before the procedure.
- Use good body mechanics at all times.
- Follow the rules to safely move and transfer the person (Chapters 20 and 21).
- Protect the person from falling.
- Know what water temperature to use. (NOTE: Some states have regulations on the maximum temperature allowed in agencies.) Water temperature must be safe and comfortable. Use the following as a guide for adults. The °F symbol means degrees Fahrenheit and °C means degrees centigrade.
  - *Bed bath*—usually 110°F to 115°F (43.3°C to 46.1°C)
  - *Tub bath or shower*—usually 105°F (40.5°C)
  - *Perineal care*—usually 105°F to 109°F (40.5°C to 42.7°C)
- Remove hearing aids before bathing. Water will damage hearing aids.
- Do not place bar soap in the bath water (basin or tub). Keep bar soap in the soap dish between latherings. This prevents soapy water. It also prevents slipping and falls.

Comfort
- Provide for privacy. Screen the person (pull the privacy curtain). Close doors and window coverings—drapes, shades, blinds, shutters, and so on.
- Assist with elimination. Bathing stimulates the need to urinate. Comfort and relaxation increase if the person urinates first.
- Reduce drafts. Close doors and windows.
- Cover the person for privacy and warmth. Use a *bath blanket*—a covering used for privacy and warmth during bathing, hygiene, and other care measures.

Independence
- Allow personal choice when possible.
- Encourage the person to help as much as safely possible.

Skin Care Products
- Follow the care plan and personal preference for skin care products.
  - *Bar soaps.* Some bar soaps dry and irritate the skin. This can cause itching, discomfort, and skin injury. Rinse the skin thoroughly to remove all soap. Bar soap is not used regularly for older persons and persons with dry skin.
  - *Body washes and shower gels.* These are gentle on the skin. Many contain a moisturizer or skin softener. Rinse thoroughly after use.
  - *No-rinse cleansers.* Sprays and foams are common. Follow the manufacturer's instructions. Wash and pat dry. No rinsing is needed. Perineal cleansers are for perineal care (p. 372).
  - *Bath oils.* Bath oils keep the skin soft and can prevent dry skin. Bath oil may be added to a basin of water. Bath oils make showers and tubs slippery. Falls can occur.
  - *Lotions and creams.* These may be applied to the back, elbows, knees, and heels after bathing to protect the skin and prevent skin breakdown. Lotions (creams) are warmed before application. To warm, rub some lotion (cream) between your hands. Or place the bottle in warm water or run it under warm water.
  - *Powders.* Powders absorb moisture and prevent friction when surfaces rub together. Powder may be applied under the breasts, under the arms, between skin folds, or in the groin area (where a thigh and the abdomen meet). Apply in a thin, even layer after drying the skin well. Excessive amounts cause caking and crusts that irritate the skin.
  - *Deodorants and antiperspirants.* These are applied to the underarms to control body odors and perspiration (sweat). Do not apply to irritated skin.

Washing and Drying
- Wash from clean to dirty areas. Use a "head to toe" approach—eyes, face, neck, arms and hands, chest, abdomen, legs and feet. If you must turn the person to clean the back and buttocks, you may do so after cleaning the legs and feet. Otherwise, the back and buttocks can be cleaned after the chest and abdomen. Clean the genital and anal areas (perineal area) last (p. 372).
- Rinse the skin thoroughly. You must remove all soap.
- Pat the skin dry to avoid irritating or breaking the skin. Do not rub the skin.
- Dry well where skin has contact with skin—underarms, under the breasts, between skin folds, in the genital and anal areas, and between the toes.

FOCUS ON CHILDREN AND OLDER PERSONS

Bathing

Children

The care plan reflects the child's normal practices and needs during illness. Many older children enjoy showers. The nurse tells you how much help and supervision the child needs. Remember, independence and privacy are important to older children.

    See "Bathing an Infant" in Chapter 56.

Older Persons

Aging and soap dry the skin. Dry skin is easily damaged. Therefore older persons need a complete bed bath, tub bath, or shower only twice a week. They have partial baths on the other days. Some bathe daily without soap. Thorough rinsing is needed for soap. Lotion helps soften the skin.

    Bathing procedures can threaten persons with dementia. Confusion can increase. They may fear harm or danger. Some resist care and become agitated and combative. They may shout at you and cry out for help. Remain calm, patient, and soothing. The person may be calmer and less confused or agitated during a certain time of day. Bathing is scheduled for calm times.

    The nurse decides the best bathing procedure for the person. The rules in Box 24-2 apply. The care plan also has measures to help the person through the bath. For example:

- Say "cleaned up" or "washed," rather than "shower" or "bath."
- Complete pre-procedure activities. Ready supplies and linens and have everything you need.
- Provide for warmth. Prevent drafts. Have extra towels, an extra bath blanket, or a robe nearby.
- Provide good lighting.
- Draw bath water ahead of time. Test the water temperature and adjust as needed.
- Play soft music to help the person relax.
- Provide for safety.
  - Use a hand-held shower nozzle.
  - Have the person use a shower chair or shower bench.
  - Do not use bath oil. It can make the tub or shower slippery. And it may cause a urinary tract infection.
  - Do not leave the person alone in the tub or shower.
- Tell the person what you are doing step-by-step. Use clear, simple words and sentences.
- Let the person help as much as possible. For example, give the person a washcloth. Say what to wash step-by-step (face, arms, hands). Even if the person does not know what to do, let the person hold the washcloth if safe to do so.
- Put a towel over the shoulders (tub bath) or lap (shower). This helps the person feel less exposed.
- Do not rush the person.
- Use a calm, pleasant voice.
- Distract the person if needed.
- Calm the person.
- Handle the person gently.
- Try a partial bath if a shower or tub bath agitates the person.
- Try the bath later if the person continues to resist care.

DELEGATION GUIDELINES

Bathing

Bathing procedures are routine nursing tasks. To assist with bathing, you need this information from the nurse and the care plan.

- What bath to give—complete bed bath, partial bath, tub bath, or shower.
- If a towel bath or bag bath is needed for a bed bath (p. 366).
- How much help the person needs.
- Activity or position limits.
- What water temperature to use (see Box 24-2).
- What skin care products the person prefers (see Box 24-2).
- What observations to report and record:
  - The color of the skin, lips, nail beds, and sclera (whites of the eyes)
  - If the skin appears pale, gray-ish, yellow *(jaundice),* or bluish *(cyanotic)*
  - The location and description of rashes (Fig. 24-3).
  - Skin texture—smooth, rough, scaly, flaky, dry, moist
  - *Diaphoresis*—profuse (excessive) sweating
  - Bruises or open skin areas
  - Pale, reddened, or discolored areas, particularly over bony parts
  - Drainage or bleeding from wounds or body openings
  - Swelling of the feet and legs
  - Corns or calluses on the feet (Chapter 41)
  - Skin temperature (cold, cool, warm, hot)
  - Complaints of pain or discomfort
- When to report observations.
- What patient or resident concerns to report at once.

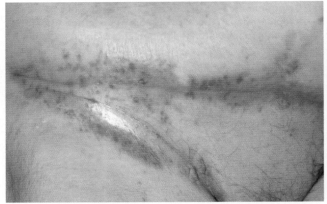

FIGURE 24-3 Rash in a skin fold. Moisture can collect between skin folds, causing irritation. Dry between skin folds thoroughly. (From Dinulos JGH: *Habif's clinical dermatology: a color guide to diagnosis and therapy,* ed 7, London, 2021, Elsevier.)

PROMOTING SAFETY AND COMFORT

Bathing

Safety

Water

Hot water can burn the skin. Measure water temperature according to agency policy. If unsure if the water is too hot, ask the nurse to check it.

Falls and Injuries

Protect the person from falls and other injuries. Follow the care plan for bed rail use. Ask a co-worker to help if needed. Make sure bed wheels are locked. When working alone, lower the bed to a safe level before leaving the bedside. Practice the safety measures in Chapters 14 and 15.

Safe Handling

Use good body mechanics to protect yourself from injury (Chapter 19). For the procedure that follows, you work on 1 side of the bed. To avoid straining and reaching, move the person to the side of the bed near you. Or wash 1 side of the body and then move to the other side to finish the bath. If room space allows, wash the side of the body near you (eyes and face, arm, hand, chest, abdomen, leg, foot). Then move the over-bed table with equipment and supplies to the other side of the bed. Finish the bath (arm, hand, leg, foot, back, and perineal care) on that side.

Preventing Infection

Follow Standard Precautions and the Bloodborne Pathogen Standard. Follow the rules of hand hygiene and the guidelines for glove use in Chapters 17 and 18. Wear gloves when contact with blood or body fluids, mucous membranes, or non-intact skin is likely. (For skills tested in your state, wear gloves as required by your state's competency exam. The procedures in this chapter include glove use.) Remove contaminated gloves and practice hand hygiene before moving to a clean body site or touching clean items or surfaces. Apply clean gloves if needed.

In nursing centers, follow agency policies and procedures for using Enhanced Barrier Precautions for high-contact tasks. See Chapter 18.

Bathing Equipment

Bathing equipment must be clean. A wash basin is used for 1 person. Tubs and showers may be used by many persons. See "Tub Bath and Shower Safety" on p. 369.

Foot Care

Ask the nurse if you should clean under the person's toenails. The device used (orangewood stick or nail file) has a sharp tip that could injure the person. Foot injuries can be very serious for some persons. See Chapter 25 for nail care.

Drying

Pat the skin dry. Dry well where skin has contact with skin— underarms, under the breasts, between skin folds, in the genital and anal areas, and between the toes. Moisture can collect between skin folds, providing a place for microbes to live and grow. Skin irritation and a rash can occur (see Fig. 24-3).

Powder

Apply powder with caution. Do not use powders near persons with respiratory disorders. Inhaling powder can irritate the airway and lungs. Before using powder, check with the nurse and the care plan. To safely apply powder:

*   Turn away from the person.
*   Sprinkle a small amount onto your hand or a cloth. Do not shake or sprinkle powder onto the person.
*   Apply the powder in a thin layer.
*   Make sure powder does not get on the floor. Powder is slippery and can cause falls.

Bedmaking

For an occupied bed, make the bed after the bath. See Chapter 22.

Comfort

Elimination

Before bathing, let the person meet elimination needs (Chapters 27 and 29). Bathing stimulates the need to urinate. Comfort is greater with an empty bladder. Also bathing is not interrupted.

Warmth

Provide for warmth. Cover the person with a bath blanket. Protect the person from drafts. Make sure the water is warm enough. Cool water causes chilling.

Oral Hygiene and Grooming

Oral hygiene is common before or after bathing (Chapter 23). Grooming measures often occur with bathing (Chapter 25). Allow personal choice and follow the care plan.

Clothing and Sleepwear

If the person prefers, remove clothing or sleepwear after washing the eyes, face, ears, and neck. Removing clothing or sleepwear at this time helps the person feel less exposed and provides more mental comfort with the bath. See Chapter 26 for changing garments (undressing and dressing).

Perineal Care

If able, have the person wash the genital and anal areas. This promotes privacy and helps prevent embarrassment. See "Perineal Care" on p. 372.

Persons With Bariatric Needs

Persons with bariatric needs may need help with hygiene. They may not be able to reach body parts. Skin folds are common. Good hygiene and skin care promote comfort and prevent pressure injuries and other skin problems.

The rules for bathing in Box 24-2 apply. Always follow the person's care plan for:

- How often to bathe the person.
- The bathing method.
- The number of staff needed.
- The equipment needed. A bariatric shower chair is an example.
- The cleaning agent to use. Soaps that dry and irritate the skin are avoided.
- How often to clean under skin folds. Such care may be needed several times a day. The person may perspire heavily. Moisture can collect between skin folds, providing a place for microbes to live and grow. Skin irritation and a rash can occur (see Fig. 24-3).
- How to dry under skin folds. Dry well to prevent skin irritation. The nurse may have you use a hand-held hair dryer on the "cool" setting.
- What product to place under skin folds. The nurse may have you place gauze or cotton-fabric under the folds. The material reduces friction and absorbs moisture.
- What skin care products to use and where to use them—powder, lotion, and so on.

See *Teamwork and Time Management: Persons With Bariatric Needs.*

The Complete Bed Bath

For a complete bed bath, you wash the person's entire body in bed. Bed baths are usually needed by persons who are:

- Unconscious
- Paralyzed
- In casts or traction
- Weak from illness or surgery
- Unable to bathe themselves

A bed bath is new to some people. Some are embarrassed to have their bodies seen. Some fear exposure. Explain how you give the bath and provide for privacy.

Bath water for bed baths cools rapidly. Heat is lost to the wash basin, over-bed table, washcloth, and your hands. Therefore water temperature for bed baths is usually between 110°F and 115°F (43.3°C and 46.1°C) for adults. Older persons have fragile skin. They need lower water temperatures.

See procedure: *Giving a Complete Bed Bath.*

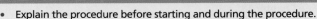

Giving a Complete Bed Bath

QUALITY OF LIFE

- Knock before entering the person's room.
- Address the person by name.
- Introduce yourself by name and title.
- Explain the procedure before starting and during the procedure.
- Protect the person's rights during the procedure.
- Handle the person gently during the procedure.

PRE-PROCEDURE

1. Follow *Delegation Guidelines: Bathing,* p. 360. See *Promoting Safety and Comfort:*
   a. *Daily Hygiene and Bathing,* p. 357
   b. *Bathing,* p. 361
2. Practice hand hygiene.
3. Identify the person. Check the identification (ID) bracelet against the assignment sheet. Use 2 identifiers (Chapter 14). Also call the person by name.
4. Collect clean linens. (See procedure: *Making a Closed Bed* in Chapter 22.) Place linens on a clean surface.
5. Get the following supplies:
   - Wash basin (if available, a second basin can be used—1 for washing and 1 for rinsing)
   - Soap or body wash
   - Water thermometer
   - Orangewood stick or nail file (if needed)
   - Washcloths—1 or more for washing and rinsing (some state competency tests specify a clean, "soap-free" washcloth for rinsing) and at least 4 washcloths for perineal care (p. 372)
   - Towels—at least 1 hand towel, 2 bath towels, and a separate towel for perineal care (p. 372)
   - Bath blanket
   - Clothing or sleepwear
   - Skin care products (as needed)—lotion, powder, deodorant (antiperspirant)
   - Brush and comb
   - Other grooming items as requested
   - Towel or paper towels (as a barrier for supplies)
   - Gloves
   - Laundry bag
6. Place a barrier (towel, paper towels) on the over-bed table. Arrange items on top. Adjust the height as needed.
7. Provide for privacy.
8. Raise the bed for body mechanics. Bed rails are up if used. Lower the bed rail near you if up.

Giving a Complete Bed Bath—cont'd

PROCEDURE

9 Cover the person with a bath blanket. Remove top linens (see procedure: *Making an Occupied Bed* in Chapter 22).

10 Remove clothing or sleepwear. Do not expose the person. Follow agency policy for used clothing or sleepwear. (Wear gloves if clothing is wet or soiled. Practice hand hygiene after removing and discarding gloves.)

11 Fill the wash basin ⅔ (two-thirds) full with water. (Follow the care plan for bed rail use. Raise the rail if used. Lower the bed to a safe level.) Follow the care plan for water temperature. Water temperature is usually 110°F to 115°F (43.3°C to 46.1°C) for adults. Measure water temperature. Use the water thermometer. Or dip your elbow or inner wrist into the basin to test the water.

12 Have the person check the water temperature. Adjust the water temperature as needed.

13 Place the basin on the over-bed table.

14 Raise the bed for body mechanics. Lower the bed rail near you if up.

15 Lower the head of the bed. It is as flat as possible. The person has at least 1 pillow.

16 Practice hand hygiene. Put on gloves.

17 Place a hand towel over the person's chest.

18 Make a mitt with the washcloth (Fig. 24-4, p. 364). Use a mitt for the entire bath. (NOTE: Some state competency tests require that the corners of the washcloth be contained during bathing. This is one method.)

19 Have the person close the eyes. Wash the eyelids and around the eyes with water. Do not use soap.

  a Clean the far eye. Gently wipe from the inner to the outer aspect of the eye with a corner of the mitt (Fig. 24-5, p. 364).

  b Clean the eye near you. Use a clean part of the washcloth for each stroke.

20 Wash, rinse, and dry the face, ears, and neck.

  a Ask if the person wants soap or body wash used on the face. If so, apply soap or body wash to the washcloth. If not, just use water. Wash the face and ears.

  b Wash the neck using soap or body wash.

  c Rinse all areas. Use a soap-free washcloth.

  d Pat dry with the towel on the chest.

21 Help the person move to the side of the bed near you.

22 Wash, rinse, and dry the far arm.

  a Expose the arm. Place a bath towel length-wise under the arm.

  b Apply soap or body wash to the washcloth.

  c Support the arm with your palm under the person's elbow. The person's forearm rests on your forearm.

  d Wash the arm, shoulder, and underarm. Use long, firm strokes (Fig. 24-6, p. 365).

  e Rinse all areas.

  f Pat dry. Dry well under the underarm.

23 Wash, rinse, and dry the far hand.

  a *Method 1*—Place the basin on the towel. Put the person's hand into the water (Fig. 24-7, p. 365). Have the person exercise the hand and fingers. Wash the hand well. Remove the basin.

  b *Method 2*—Apply soap or body wash to the washcloth. Wash the hand well.

  c Clean under the nails if nail care is done during the bath. Or perform nail care separately (Chapter 25). Use an orangewood stick or nail file.

  d Rinse the hand. Use a soap-free washcloth.

  e Pat dry.

  f Remove the towel under the arm. Cover the arm with the bath blanket.

24 Repeat steps 22 and 23 for the near arm and hand.

25 Wash, rinse, and dry the chest.

  a Place a bath towel over the chest cross-wise. Hold the towel in place. Pull the bath blanket from under the towel to the waist.

  b Apply soap or body wash to the washcloth.

  c Lift the towel slightly and wash the chest (Fig. 24-8, p. 365). Do not expose the person.

  d Rinse the chest. Use a soap-free washcloth.

  e Pat dry. Dry well under breasts.

26 Wash, rinse, and dry the abdomen.

  a Move the towel length-wise over the chest and abdomen. Do not expose the person. Pull the bath blanket down to the pubic area.

  b Apply soap or body wash to the washcloth.

  c Lift the towel slightly and wash the abdomen (Fig. 24-9, p. 365).

  d Rinse the abdomen. Use a soap-free washcloth.

  e Pat dry. Dry well under abdominal skin folds.

27 Pull the bath blanket up to the shoulders. Cover both arms. Remove the towel.

28 Change soapy or cool water as needed. Follow these safety measures.

  a Raise the bed rail if used. Lower the bed to a safe level.

  b Measure bath water temperature as in step 11. Have the person check the water temperature.

  c Raise the bed for body mechanics and lower the bed rail if used when you return.

29 Wash, rinse, and dry the far leg.

  a Uncover the far leg. Do not expose the genital area. Place a towel length-wise under the foot and leg.

  b Apply soap or body wash to a washcloth.

  c Bend the knee and support the leg with your arm. Wash it with long, firm strokes. Wash the skin fold area of the groin.

  d Rinse the leg. Use a soap-free washcloth.

  e Pat dry. Dry the groin area well.

30 Wash, rinse, and dry the far foot.

  a *Method 1*—Place the basin on the towel near the foot. Bend the knee and lift the leg slightly. Slide the basin under the foot. Place the foot in the basin (Fig. 24-10, p. 366). Wash the foot well. Carefully separate the toes. Remove the basin.

  b *Method 2*—Apply soap or body wash to the washcloth. Wash the foot well. Carefully separate the toes.

  c Clean under the nails if instructed to do so and if nail care is done during the bath. Or perform nail care separately (Chapter 25). Use an orangewood stick or nail file.

  d Rinse the foot. Use a soap-free washcloth.

  e Pat dry. Dry well between the toes.

  f Apply lotion to the foot if directed by the nurse and the care plan. Do not apply lotion between the toes.

  g Cover the leg with the bath blanket. Remove the towel.

31 Repeat steps 29 and 30 for the near leg and foot.

32 Change the water. Follow the safety measures in step 28.

Continued

Giving a Complete Bed Bath—cont'd

PROCEDURE—cont'd

33 Wash, rinse, and dry the back and buttocks.
  a Turn the person onto the side away from you. The person is covered with the bath blanket.
  b Uncover the back and buttocks. Do not expose the person. Place a towel length-wise on the bed along the back.
  c Apply soap or body wash to a washcloth.
  d Wash the back. Work from the back of the neck to the lower end of the buttocks. Use long, firm, continuous strokes (Fig. 24-11, p. 366).
  e Rinse the back and buttocks. Use a soap-free washcloth.
  f Pat dry.
34 Place used washcloths and towels in the laundry bag.
35 Turn the person onto the back.
36 Wash, rinse, and dry the genital and anal areas (p. 372).
  a Change the water. Follow the safety measures in step 28. Water temperature for perineal care is lower (usually 105°F to 109°F [40.5°C to 42.7°C]).
  b Allow the person to clean the genital and anal areas if able. If the person cannot do so, perform perineal care with clean gloves (p. 372). At least 4 washcloths and a clean towel are needed. Place each washcloth in the laundry bag after 1 use. Washcloths are not re-used for perineal care.

37 Remove and discard the gloves. Practice hand hygiene.
38 Give a back massage (Chapter 36).
39 Apply lotion, powder, and deodorant or antiperspirant as requested. See *Promoting Safety and Comfort: Bathing* (p. 361) for how to safely apply powder.
40 Put clean garments on the person (Chapter 26).
41 Comb and brush the person's hair (Chapter 25).
42 Make the bed (Chapter 22). Remove the bath blanket and place it in the laundry bag.

POST-PROCEDURE

43 Provide for comfort. (See the inside of the back cover.)
44 Lower the bed to a safe and comfortable level. Raise or lower bed rails. Follow the care plan.
45 Clean up and store supplies and equipment. (Wear gloves. Change gloves as needed.)
  a Discard disposable items.
  b Empty the wash basin.
  c Follow agency procedures to clean and disinfect re-usable equipment. Return supplies and equipment to their proper place.
  d Follow agency policy for used linens.
  e Clean and dry the over-bed table. Dry with paper towels. Discard paper towels. Position the over-bed table as the person prefers.
  f Remove and discard gloves. Practice hand hygiene.

46 Place the call light and other needed items within reach.
47 Follow the care plan and the person's preferences for privacy measures to maintain. Leaving the privacy curtain, window coverings, and door open or closed are examples.
48 Complete a safety check of the room. (See the inside of the back cover.)
49 Practice hand hygiene.
50 Report and record your care and observations.

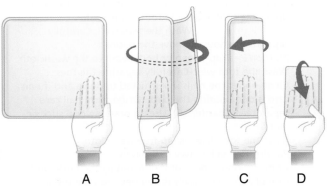

FIGURE 24-4 Making a mitted washcloth. **A,** Grasp the near side of the washcloth with your thumb. **B,** Bring the washcloth around and behind your hand. **C,** Fold the side of the washcloth over your palm as you grasp it with your thumb. **D,** Fold the top of the washcloth down and tuck it under next to your palm.

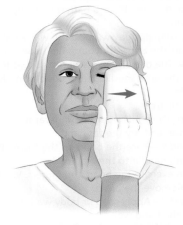

FIGURE 24-5 Washing the eyelids. Soap is not used. Eyes are gently wiped from the inner to the outer aspect. A clean part of the washcloth is used for each stroke. A clean part of the washcloth is used for the other eye.

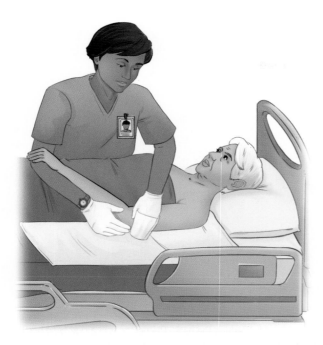

FIGURE 24-6 Washing the arm. The arm is washed with firm, long strokes using a mitted washcloth.

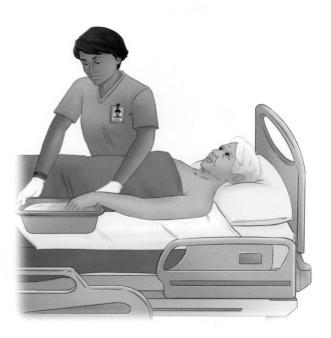

FIGURE 24-7 Washing the hand. The hand can be washed in the wash basin.

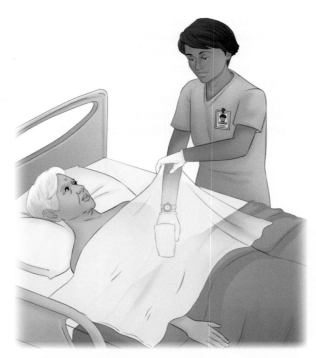

FIGURE 24-8 Washing the chest. A bath towel is placed horizontally over the chest area. The towel is lifted slightly to reach under and wash the chest. Breasts are not exposed.

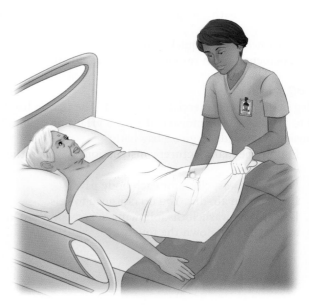

FIGURE 24-9 Washing the abdomen. The bath towel is turned so that it is vertical to cover the chest and abdomen. The towel is lifted slightly to bathe the abdomen. The bath blanket covers the pubic area.

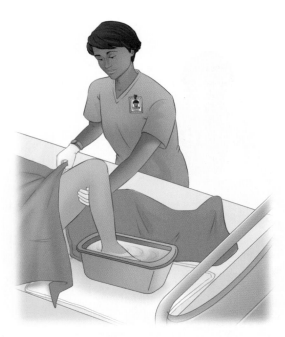

FIGURE 24-10 Washing the foot. The foot can be washed in the wash basin.

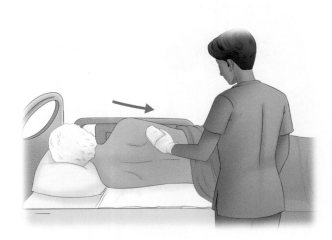

FIGURE 24-11 Washing the back. The person is in a side-lying position. A towel is length-wise on the bed to protect the linens from water. The back is washed with long, firm, continuous strokes.

Towel Baths

For a towel bath, an over-sized towel covers the person from the neck to the feet. The towel is wet with a solution of water and cleaning, skin-softening, and drying agents. The drying agent lets the skin dry fast. No rinsing is needed. The nurse and care plan tell you when to give a towel bath. To give a towel bath, follow agency policy.

The towel bath is quick, soothing, and relaxing. Persons with dementia often respond well to towel baths.

Bag Baths

Bag baths are commercially prepared. The plastic bag has 8 to 10 washcloths moistened with a cleansing agent. No rinsing is needed. To give a bag bath:

• Follow the manufacturer's instructions to warm the washcloths.
• Use a new washcloth for each body part.
• Let the skin air-dry. You do not need towels.
• Discard the washcloths following agency policy. Do not flush them down the toilet.

The Partial Bath

For a *partial bath*, the face, hands, underarms, back, buttocks, and perineal area are washed. Bathing prevents odors and discomfort in those areas. Some persons can wash in bed, at the bedside, or at the sink with warm running water (Fig. 24-12). You assist as needed. Most persons need help washing the back. You give partial baths to persons who cannot bathe themselves.

The rules for bathing apply (see Box 24-2). So do the complete bed bath considerations.

See procedure: *Assisting With the Partial Bath*.

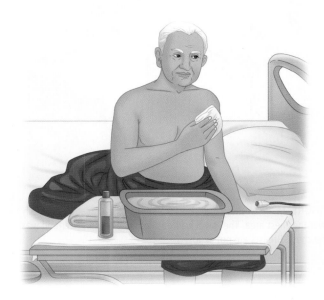

FIGURE 24-12 The person is bathing while sitting on the side of the bed. Needed equipment is within reach.

Assisting With the Partial Bath

QUALITY OF LIFE

- Knock before entering the person's room.
- Address the person by name.
- Introduce yourself by name and title.

- Explain the procedure before starting and during the procedure.
- Protect the person's rights during the procedure.
- Handle the person gently during the procedure.

PRE-PROCEDURE

1   Follow *Delegation Guidelines: Bathing*, p. 360. See *Promoting Safety and Comfort*:
    a   *Daily Hygiene and Bathing*, p. 357
    b   *Bathing*, p. 361

2   Follow steps 2 through 7 in procedure: *Giving a Complete Bed Bath*, p. 362. (This procedure explains how to assist with a partial bath in bed when the person can be left alone.)

PROCEDURE

3   Make sure the bed is in a low position.
4   Cover the person with a bath blanket. Remove top linens.
5   Fill the wash basin ⅔ (two-thirds) full with water. Water temperature is usually 110°F to 115°F (43.3°C to 46.1°C) or as directed by the nurse. Measure water temperature with the water thermometer. Or test bath water by dipping your elbow or inner wrist into the basin.
6   Have the person check the water temperature. Adjust the water temperature as needed.
7   Place the basin on the over-bed table.
8   Position the person in Fowler's position or sitting at the bedside.
9   Adjust the over-bed table so the person can reach the basin and supplies.
10 Help the person undress. (Wear gloves if clothing is wet or soiled. Practice hand hygiene after removing and discarding gloves.) Use the bath blanket for privacy and warmth.
11 Have the person wash easy-to-reach body parts. Explain that you will wash the back and areas the person cannot reach.
12 Be sure the call light is within reach. Have the person signal when help is needed or bathing is complete.
13 Practice hand hygiene. Then leave the room.

14 Return when the call light is on. Knock before entering. Practice hand hygiene.
15 Wash and dry areas the person could not reach.
    a   Change the bath water. Measure bath water temperature as in step 5. Have the person check the water temperature.
    b   Raise the bed for body mechanics. The far bed rail is up if used.
    c   Put on gloves.
    d   Ask what was washed. Wash and dry areas the person could not reach. The face, hands, underarms, back, buttocks, and perineal area are washed for the partial bath.
16 Place used washcloths and towels in the laundry bag.
17 Remove and discard gloves. Practice hand hygiene.
18 Give a back massage (Chapter 36).
19 Apply lotion, powder, and deodorant or antiperspirant as requested.
20 Help the person put on clean garments (Chapter 26).
21 Assist with hair care and other grooming needs (Chapter 25).
22 Make the bed. Remove the bath blanket and place it in the laundry bag.

POST-PROCEDURE

23 Provide for comfort. (See the inside of the back cover.)
24 Lower the bed to a safe and comfortable level. Raise or lower bed rails. Follow the care plan.
25 Clean up and store supplies and equipment. (Wear gloves. Change gloves as needed.)
    a   Discard disposable items.
    b   Empty the wash basin.
    c   Follow agency procedures to clean and disinfect re-usable equipment. Return supplies and equipment to their proper place.
    d   Follow agency policy for used linens.
    e   Clean and dry the over-bed table. Dry with paper towels. Discard paper towels. Position the over-bed table as the person prefers.
    f   Remove and discard gloves. Practice hand hygiene.

26 Place the call light and other needed items within reach.
27 Follow the care plan and the person's preferences for privacy measures to maintain. Leaving the privacy curtain, window coverings, and door open or closed are examples.
28 Complete a safety check of the room. (See the inside of the back cover.)
29 Practice hand hygiene.
30 Report and record your care and observations.

▌Tub Baths and Showers

Some people like tub baths. Others like showers. Follow the nurse's directions and the care plan for the method used and the amount of help the person needs.

Tub Baths. Tub baths are relaxing. However, a tub bath can make a person feel faint, weak, or tired. These are great risks for persons who were on bed rest. A tub bath lasts no longer than 20 minutes.

To get in and out of the tub, the person may use:
- A tub with a side entry door (Fig. 24-13).
- Bathing lift. The device transports and lifts the person into the tub (Fig. 24-14).
- Mechanical lift (Chapter 21).

Whirlpool (jetted) tubs have a cleansing action. You wash the upper body. Carefully wash under breasts and between skin folds. Also wash the perineal area. Pat the person dry with towels after the bath.

Showers. Some people can stand during a shower. Grab bars (safety bars) are used for support. Showers have slip-resistant surfaces. If not, a rubber bath mat is used. Weak or unsteady persons use:
- *Shower benches.* Some showers contain benches that fold down (Fig. 24-15). The person sits on the bench during the shower.
- *Shower chairs.* Water drains through an opening (Fig. 24-16). You may use the chair to transport the person to and from the shower. Or the person transfers to the shower chair in the bathroom or shower room. Lock (brake) the wheels during transfers and during the shower to prevent falls. Shower chairs come in different sizes. Use the correct size.
- *Shower trolleys (portable tubs).* The person has a shower lying down (Fig. 24-17). Lower the sides to transfer the person from the bed to the trolley. Then raise the side rails for transport to the tub or shower room. Use the hand-held nozzle for the shower.

Some shower rooms have 2 or more stations. Provide for privacy. Properly screen and cover the person. Also close doors and shower curtains.

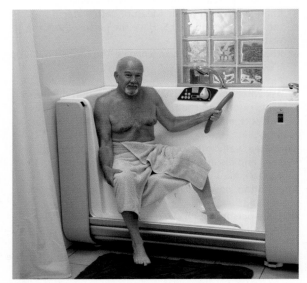

FIGURE 24-13 Tub with a side entry door. (Image used with permission of Arjo Inc.)

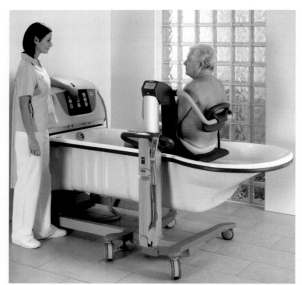

FIGURE 24-14 The lift lowers the person into the tub. (Image used with permission of Arjo Inc.)

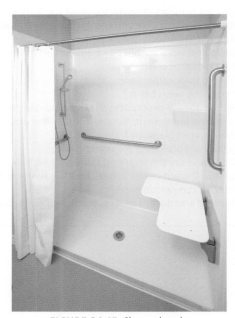

FIGURE 24-15 Shower bench.

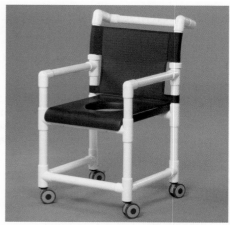

FIGURE 24-16 Shower chair. (Courtesy Innovative Products Unlimited, Niles, Mich.)

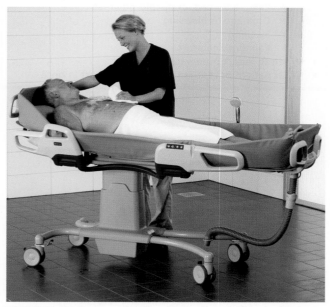

FIGURE 24-17 Shower trolley. The sides are lowered for transfers into and out of the trolley. (Image used with permission of Arjo Inc.)

Tub Bath and Shower Safety. Falls, burns, and chilling from water are risks during tub baths and showers. Safety is important (Box 24-3). The measures in Box 24-2 also apply.

See *Focus on Long-Term Care and Home Care: Tub Baths and Showers*, p. 370.

See *Teamwork and Time Management: Tub Baths and Showers*, p. 370.

See *Delegation Guidelines: Tub Baths and Showers*, p. 370.

See *Promoting Safety and Comfort: Tub Baths and Showers*, p. 370.

See procedure: *Assisting With a Tub Bath or Shower*, p. 371.

BOX 24-3 Tub Bath and Shower Safety

Tub Baths and Showers
- Follow agency procedures to clean and disinfect the tub, shower, and shared equipment before and after use.
- Make sure hand rails, grab bars (safety bars), lifts, and other safety aids are in working order.
- Place a rubber bath mat in the tub or on the shower floor if needed. This is not needed if there are slip-resistant strips or a slip-resistant surface.
- Provide for warmth and privacy. This includes during transport to and from the tub or shower room.
- Place the call light and other needed items within reach. Show how to use the call light.
- Have the person use grab bars (safety bars) to get in and out of the tub or shower.
- Follow the safety measures and transfer procedures for wheelchairs when using wheeled shower chairs. See Chapter 21.
- Know what water temperature to use (usually 105°F/40.5°C).
- Turn cold water on first, then hot water (for a 2-handled faucet). Turn hot water off first, then cold water. This helps prevent burns.
- Keep bar soap in the soap dish between latherings if used. This helps prevent slipping and falls in tubs and showers. It also prevents soapy tub water.
- Avoid bath oils. They make tub and shower surfaces slippery.
- Do not leave weak or unsteady persons unattended.
- Stay within hearing distance if the person can be left alone. Wait outside the door or shower curtain. You must be nearby if the person calls for you or has an accident.

Tub Baths
- Fill the tub before the person gets into it. For a tub with a side entry door, fill the tub with the person in it. Follow the manufacturer's instructions.
- Monitor water temperature as the tub fills.
- Use the digital display or a water thermometer to measure water temperature.
- Have the person check the water temperature. Adjust as needed.
- Drain the tub before the person gets out of the tub. Cover the person for warmth.

Showers
- Adjust water temperature to prevent chilling and burns.
- Use the digital display when checking water temperature.
- Have the person check the water temperature. Adjust as needed.
- Direct water away from the person when adjusting water temperature and pressure.
- Keep the water spray directed toward the person during the shower. This provides for warmth.
- Do not direct water spray toward the face. This can frighten the person.
- Turn off the shower before the person gets out of the shower. Cover the person for warmth.

FOCUS ON LONG-TERM CARE AND HOME CARE
Tub Baths and Showers

Home Care
Many homes have shower stalls or bathtub-shower units. To step into the tub or shower, have the person use the grab bars (safety bars). Help the person in and out of the tub or shower as needed.

The person may need a shower chair. The nurse helps the person and family find a safe chair for shower use.

The bathtub unit may not have a shower. A hand-held shower nozzle can be installed.

TEAMWORK AND TIME MANAGEMENT
Tub Baths and Showers

You need to reserve the tub or shower room and equipment for the person. Your co-workers do the same for their patients and residents. Consider the needs of others. For example:
- You reserve the shower room from 0945 to 1030. Do your best to follow the schedule. Have the shower room clean and ready for the next person.
- You and a co-worker schedule a shower for the same time. Plan new times with your co-worker.

All bed linens are changed on the person's bath or shower day. Co-workers can work together. For example, a co-worker makes the bed and straightens the person's room while you assist with the person's shower. The person returns to a clean bed and unit. Be willing to work with and help others.

Shower chairs are often shared. Clean and disinfect the chair after use. Return the shower chair to its proper place. Other staff know where to find it. Staff do not waste time looking for equipment.

DELEGATION GUIDELINES
Tub Baths and Showers

Before assisting with a tub bath or shower, you need this information from the nurse and the care plan.
- If the person takes a tub bath or shower
- What water temperature to use (usually 105°F/40.5°C)
- What equipment is needed—bathing lift, mechanical lift, shower chair, shower bench, shower trolley, and so on
- What size shower chair to use (if needed)—standard or bariatric
- How much help the person needs
- If the person can be left alone
- What observations to report and record:
  - Dizziness
  - Light-headedness
  - The observations listed in *Delegation Guidelines: Bathing*, p. 360:
    - Skin color, texture, moisture, and temperature
    - Bruises, rashes, or open skin areas
    - Pale, reddened, or discolored areas
    - Drainage or bleeding
    - Swelling
    - Pain or discomfort
- When to report observations
- What patient or resident concerns to report at once

PROMOTING SAFETY AND COMFORT
Tub Baths and Showers

Safety
Follow the safety measures for transfers (Chapter 21). Follow the care plan for the transfer method and number of staff needed. Remember:
- Slip-resistant footwear is worn for transfers.
- Be sure the floor is dry.
- Have the person use grab bars (safety bars) for support.
- Lock (brake) the wheels on a wheelchair and shower chair.
- Apply a transfer belt (gait belt) over clothing.

Follow the manufacturer's instructions for devices used—tub with a side entry door, bathing lift, mechanical lift, shower chair, and others.

Protect the person from chilling and burns. Remember to measure water temperature. Ask the person if the water is comfortable.

Clean and disinfect the tub or shower before and after use. This prevents the spread of microbes and infection.

Comfort
Warmth and privacy promote comfort during tub baths and showers.
- Make sure the tub or shower room is warm.
- Provide for privacy. The room door, window coverings, and shower curtain are closed for privacy.
- Make sure the water is comfortable for the person.
- Have the person remove clothing or robe and footwear just before getting into the tub or shower. Do not have the person exposed longer than necessary.
- Stay nearby (within hearing distance) if the person can be left alone. Provide as much privacy as possible.

Assisting With a Tub Bath or Shower

QUALITY OF LIFE

- Knock before entering the person's room.
- Address the person by name.
- Introduce yourself by name and title.

- Explain the procedure before starting and during the procedure.
- Protect the person's rights during the procedure.
- Handle the person gently during the procedure.

PRE-PROCEDURE

1 Follow *Delegation Guidelines:*
   a *Bathing*, p. 360
   b *Tub Baths and Showers*
   See *Promoting Safety and Comfort:*
   a *Daily Hygiene and Bathing*, p. 357
   b *Bathing*, p. 361
   c *Tub Baths and Showers*
2 Reserve the tub or shower room.
3 Practice hand hygiene.
4 Identify the person. Check the ID bracelet against the assignment sheet. Use 2 identifiers (Chapter 14). Also call the person by name.

5 Get the following supplies.
   - Washcloths—at least 1 for bathing or showering and washcloths for perineal care (p. 372)
   - Bath towels—at least 2
   - Bath blanket
   - Soap or body wash
   - Water thermometer (for a tub bath)
   - Clothing or sleepwear
   - Grooming items as requested
   - Robe and slip-resistant footwear
   - Rubber bath mat if needed
   - Disposable bath mat if needed
   - Gloves
   - Laundry bag
   - Wheelchair, shower chair, and so on as needed

PROCEDURE

6 Place items in the tub or shower room. Use the space provided or a chair.
7 Follow agency procedures to clean and disinfect the tub or shower and shared equipment (for example, a shower chair). (Wear gloves for this step. Practice hand hygiene after removing and discarding the gloves.)
8 Place a rubber bath mat in the tub or on the shower floor if needed. Do not block the drain.
9 Place the disposable bath mat on the floor in front of the tub or shower if needed.
10 Put the *OCCUPIED* sign on the door.
11 Return to the person's room. Provide for privacy. Practice hand hygiene.
12 Help the person sit on the side of the bed.
13 Help the person put on a robe and slip-resistant footwear. Or the person can leave on clothing.
14 Assist or transport the person to the tub or shower room.
15 Have the person sit on a chair if the person walked to the tub or shower room.
16 Provide for privacy.
17 *For a tub bath:*
   a Fill the tub half-way with warm water (usually 105°F/40.5°C). Follow the care plan for water temperature.
   b Measure water temperature. Use the water thermometer or check the digital display.
   c Have the person check the water temperature. Adjust the water temperature as needed.
18 *For a shower:*
   a Turn on the shower.
   b Adjust water temperature and pressure. Check the digital display. Water temperature is usually 105°F/40.5°C.
   c Have the person check the water temperature. Adjust the water temperature as needed.
19 Help the person undress and remove footwear.
20 Help the person into the tub or shower. Position the shower chair (if used) and lock (brake) the wheels.

21 Assist with washing as necessary. (Wear gloves.)
   a Wash the face, neck, arms, hands, chest, abdomen, back, buttocks, legs, and feet.
   b Provide perineal care if the person is not able. Wear clean gloves and use clean washcloths. Remove and discard gloves. Practice hand hygiene.
   c Follow the care plan and the person's preference for shampooing hair (Chapter 25). Assist with shampooing as needed.
22 Have the person use the call light when done or when help is needed. Remind the person that a tub bath lasts no longer than 20 minutes.
23 Place a towel across the chair.
24 Stay in the room or nearby if the person can be left alone. Check the person at least every 5 minutes.
25 Respond when the person signals for you.
26 Turn off the shower or drain the tub. Cover the person with the bath blanket.
27 Help the person out of the shower or tub and onto the chair.
28 Help the person dry off. Pat gently. Dry well under the underarms, under breasts, between skin folds, between the toes, and in the perineal area.
29 Place used washcloths and towels in the laundry bag.
30 Apply lotion, powder, and deodorant or antiperspirant as requested.
31 Help the person dress and put on footwear. Place the bath blanket in the laundry bag.
32 Practice hand hygiene.
33 Help the person return to his or her room. Provide for privacy.
34 Assist the person to a chair or into bed.
35 Provide a back massage if the person returns to bed (Chapter 36).
36 Assist with hair care and other grooming needs (Chapter 25).

Continued

Assisting With a Tub Bath or Shower—cont'd

POST-PROCEDURE

37 Provide for comfort. (See the inside of the back cover.)

38 Make sure the bed is at a safe and comfortable level. Follow the care plan.

39 Check that bed rails are raised or lowered following the care plan.

40 Place the call light and other needed items within reach.

41 Follow the care plan and the person's preferences for privacy measures to maintain. Leaving the privacy curtain, window coverings, and door open or closed are examples.

42 Complete a safety check of the room. (See the inside of the back cover.)

43 Practice hand hygiene. Return to the tub or shower room.

44 Clean up and store supplies and equipment. (Wear gloves. Change gloves as needed.)

  a Discard disposable items.

  b Follow agency procedures to clean and disinfect the tub or shower and shared equipment. Return supplies and equipment to their proper place.

  c Follow agency policy for used linens.

  d Remove and discard gloves. Practice hand hygiene.

45 Put the *UNOCCUPIED* sign on the door.

46 Report and record your care and observations.

PERINEAL CARE

Perineal care (pericare) involves cleaning the genital and anal areas. These areas provide a warm, moist, and dark place for microbes to grow. Cleaning prevents infection and odors and promotes comfort.

Perineal care is done daily during the bath. It also is done when the area is soiled with urine or feces (stools). Perineal care is very important for persons who:

- Have urinary catheters (Chapter 28).
- Have had rectal or genital surgery.
- Are menstruating (Chapter 10).
- Are incontinent of urine or feces (stools) (Chapters 27 and 29).
- Are uncircumcised (Fig. 24-18). Being *circumcised* means that the fold of skin (foreskin) covering the glans of the penis was surgically removed. Being *uncircumcised* means foreskin covers the head of the penis.

The person does perineal care if able. Otherwise, the nursing staff does so. This procedure can embarrass the person and staff, especially when it involves another gender.

Work from *front to back* or *top to bottom*. The urethral area (front or top) is the cleanest. The anal area (back or bottom) is the dirtiest. Therefore clean from the urethra to the anal area. This prevents spreading bacteria from the anal area to the vagina and urinary system.

The perineal area is delicate and easily injured. Use warm water, not hot. Use washcloths, towelettes, or swabs according to agency policy. Rinse off soap thoroughly. No-rinse perineal cleansers (sprays, foams) are common. These products do not require rinsing. Follow the manufacturer's instructions. Pat the area dry after rinsing. Dry well. This reduces moisture, prevents skin irritation, and promotes comfort.

See *Focus on Communication: Perineal Care.*

See *Delegation Guidelines: Perineal Care.*

See *Promoting Safety and Comfort: Perineal Care.*

See procedure: *Giving Female Perineal Care*, p. 374.

See procedure: *Giving Male Perineal Care*, p. 376.

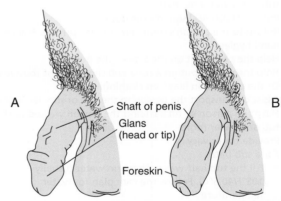

FIGURE 24-18 **A,** Circumcised penis. **B,** Uncircumcised penis.

FOCUS ON COMMUNICATION
Perineal Care

Perineal and *perineum* are not common terms. Most people understand *privates*, *private parts*, *crotch*, *genitals*, or *the area between your legs*. Use terms the person understands and that sound professional. Do not use slang or vulgar terms.

Talking to the person about perineal care may be difficult. You may be embarrassed. However, you must explain the procedure. You can say:

- "I'll give you some privacy to finish your bath. Can you reach everything you need? Please call for me if you need help. Here is your call light."
- "I'll give you time to finish your bath. Please wash your genital and rectal areas. Signal for me when you're done or need help."
- "Next I'll clean between your legs. I'll keep you covered with the bath blanket. I'll tell you before I touch you. Please tell me if you feel any pain or discomfort."
- "I'll clean your private parts now. Please let me know if you feel any pain or discomfort."

DELEGATION GUIDELINES
Perineal Care

Before giving perineal care, you need this information from the nurse and the care plan.
- When to give perineal care.
- What terms the person understands—perineum, privates, private parts, crotch, area between the legs, and so on.
- How much help the person needs.
- What water temperature to use—usually 105°F to 109°F (40.5°C to 42.7°C). Water in a basin cools rapidly.
- What cleaning agent to use.
- Any position restrictions or limits.
- What observations to report and record:
  - Odors
  - Redness, swelling, discharge, bleeding, or irritation
  - Complaints of pain, burning, or other discomfort
  - Signs of urinary or fecal incontinence
  - If you cannot retract the foreskin on an uncircumcised penis
- When to report observations.
- What patient or resident concerns to report at once.

PROMOTING SAFETY AND COMFORT
Perineal Care

Safety
Hot water can burn perineal tissues. To prevent burns, measure water temperature according to agency policy. Adjust the water temperature as needed. Notify the nurse if you have concerns about water temperature.

Contact with body fluids is likely during perineal care. Contact with blood may occur. Follow Standard Precautions and the Bloodborne Pathogen Standard. Follow the rules of hand hygiene and the guidelines for glove use in Chapters 17 and 18. Wear clean gloves for perineal care.

In nursing centers, follow agency policies and procedures for using Enhanced Barrier Precautions for high-contact tasks. See Chapter 18.

Persons who are incontinent need perineal care. Waterproof under-pads (Chapter 22) and incontinence products (Chapter 27) are commonly used. Remove wet or soiled items. Place a clean, dry waterproof under-pad under the person before cleaning. See "Applying Incontinence Products" in Chapter 27.

Comfort
Explain how you protect privacy. Close doors and window coverings. Drape (cover) the person with a bath blanket.

Perineal care involves touching the genital and anal areas. The person may prefer someone of the same gender for this care. Or the person may fear sexual assault. Always obtain the person's consent before providing perineal care. For mental comfort, the person may want a family member or another staff member present for the procedure. Ask if the person wants someone present and that person's name. Also keep the call light within the person's reach. If feeling threatened, the person can call for help.

If able, the person performs perineal care. This promotes privacy and helps prevent embarrassment. You need to:

1 Provide clean water. See step 12 in procedure: *Giving Female Perineal Care*, p. 374.
2 Adjust the over-bed table so the person can reach the supplies with ease.
3 Make sure the person understands what to do.
4 Place the call light and other needed items within reach. Have the person signal when finished.
5 Lower the bed to a safe and comfortable level. Follow the care plan.
6 Practice hand hygiene.
7 Leave the room.
8 Answer the call light promptly. Knock before entering the room.
9 Raise the bed for body mechanics.
10 Practice hand hygiene. Put on gloves.
11 Make sure the person has cleaned thoroughly. Assist the person with hand hygiene.
12 Finish the bathing procedure.

Giving Female Perineal Care

QUALITY OF LIFE

- Knock before entering the person's room.
- Address the person by name.
- Introduce yourself by name and title.

- Explain the procedure before starting and during the procedure.
- Protect the person's rights during the procedure.
- Handle the person gently during the procedure.

PRE-PROCEDURE

1 Follow *Delegation Guidelines: Perineal Care,* p. 373. See *Promoting Safety and Comfort:*
   a *Daily Hygiene and Bathing,* p. 357
   b *Perineal Care,* p. 373
2 Practice hand hygiene and get the following supplies.
   - Soap, body wash, or other cleansing agent as directed
   - At least 4 washcloths
   - Bath towel
   - Bath blanket
   - Water thermometer
   - Wash basin
   - Waterproof under-pad

   - Gloves
   - Laundry bag
   - Towel or paper towels (as a barrier for supplies)
3 Place the barrier (towel, paper towels) on the over-bed table. Arrange items on top.
4 Practice hand hygiene.
5 Identify the person. Check the ID bracelet against the assignment sheet. Use 2 identifiers (Chapter 14). Also call the person by name.
6 Provide for privacy.
7 Raise the bed for body mechanics. Bed rails are up if used. Lower the bed rail near you if up.

PROCEDURE

8 Position the person on the back.
9 Cover the person with a bath blanket. Move top linens to the foot of the bed.
10 Drape the person for comfort and privacy. See Figure 24-19 for 1 method.
11 Raise the bed rail if used. Lower the bed to a safe level.
12 Fill the wash basin. Water temperature is usually 105°F to 109°F (40.5°C to 42.7°C). Follow the care plan for water temperature. Measure water temperature according to agency policy. Have the person check the water temperature. Adjust the water temperature as needed.
13 Place the basin on the over-bed table.
14 Raise the bed for body mechanics. Lower the bed rail if up.
15 Practice hand hygiene. Put on gloves.
16 Place a waterproof under-pad under the buttocks. Have the person raise the hips or turn from side to side. Position the person on the back.
17 Help the person bend the knees and spread the legs. Or help the person spread the legs as much as possible with the knees straight.
18 Fold the corner of the bath blanket between the legs onto the abdomen.
19 Wet the washcloths.
20 Squeeze out water from a washcloth. Make a mitted washcloth. Apply soap, body wash, or other cleansing agent. (Squeeze out water every time you change washcloths. Put used washcloths in the laundry bag. *Do not place used washcloths back in the basin.*)
21 Clean the perineum. Change washcloths as needed.
   a Separate the labia.
   b Clean 1 side of the labia. Clean downward from front to back (top to bottom) with 1 stroke (Fig. 24-20, A). Use 1 part of a washcloth.
   c Clean the other side of the labia. Clean downward from front to back (top to bottom) with 1 stroke (Fig. 24-20, B). Use a clean part of a washcloth.
   d Clean the vaginal area. Clean downward from front to back (top to bottom) with 1 stroke (Fig. 24-20, C). Use a clean part of a washcloth.

22 Rinse the perineum with a clean washcloth. Change washcloths as needed.
   a Separate the labia.
   b Rinse 1 side of the labia. Rinse downward from front to back (top to bottom) with 1 stroke. Use 1 part of a washcloth.
   c Rinse the other side of the labia. Rinse downward from front to back (top to bottom) with 1 stroke. Use a clean part of a washcloth.
   d Rinse the vaginal area. Rinse downward from front to back (top to bottom) with 1 stroke. Use a clean part of a washcloth.
23 Pat dry the perineal area with the towel. Dry from front to back (top to bottom).
24 Fold the blanket back between the legs.
25 Help the person lower the legs and turn onto the side away from you.
26 Apply soap, body wash, or other cleansing agent to a clean mitted washcloth.
27 Clean and rinse the rectal area.
   a Clean from the vagina to the anus with 1 stroke (Fig. 24-21, p. 376). Use 1 part of the washcloth.
   b Repeat steps 26 and 27 (a) until the area is clean. Use a clean part of the washcloth for each stroke. Change washcloths as needed.
   c Rinse the rectal area with a clean washcloth. Rinse from the vagina to the anus. Repeat as necessary. Use a clean part of the washcloth for each stroke. Change washcloths as needed.
28 Pat dry the rectal area with the towel. Dry from the vagina to the anus. Place the towel in the laundry bag.
29 Fold and tuck the waterproof under-pad under the person. The wet side is inside. Have the person turn toward you or lay on the back and lift the buttocks. Remove the waterproof under-pad. Place it in the laundry bag. Position the person on the back. The person is covered with the bath blanket.
30 Remove and discard the gloves. Practice hand hygiene.
31 Apply clean and dry garments and linens as needed. Remove the bath blanket. Place it in the laundry bag.
32 Position the person for comfort.

Giving Female Perineal Care—cont'd

POST-PROCEDURE

33 Provide for comfort. (See the inside of the back cover.)

34 Lower the bed to a safe and comfortable level. Raise or lower bed rails. Follow the care plan.

35 Clean up and store supplies and equipment. (Wear gloves. Change gloves as needed.)
  a Discard disposable items.
  b Empty the wash basin.
  c Follow agency procedures to clean and disinfect re-usable equipment. Return supplies and equipment to their proper place.
  d Follow agency policy for used linens.
  e Clean and dry the over-bed table. Dry with paper towels. Discard paper towels. Position the over-bed table as the person prefers.
  f Remove and discard gloves. Practice hand hygiene.

36 Place the call light and other needed items within reach.

37 Follow the care plan and the person's preferences for privacy measures to maintain. Leaving the privacy curtain, window coverings, and door open or closed are examples.

38 Complete a safety check of the room. (See the inside of the back cover.)

39 Practice hand hygiene.

40 Report and record your care and observations.

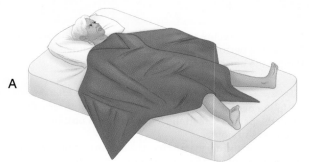 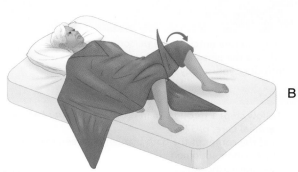

FIGURE 24-19 Draping for perineal care. **A,** Position the bath blanket like a diamond: 1 corner is at the neck, there is a corner at each side, and 1 corner is between the legs. **B,** Wrap the blanket around a leg by bringing the corner around the leg and over the top. Tuck the corner under the hip. Repeat for the other leg.

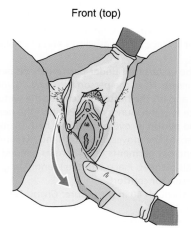

Front (top) Front (top) Front (top)

Back (bottom) Back (bottom) Back (bottom)

A B C

FIGURE 24-20 Cleaning the perineum. **A,** Separate the labia with 1 hand. Use a mitted washcloth to clean 1 side of the labia with a downward stroke. **B,** Clean the other side of the labia with a clean part of the washcloth. Use a downward stroke. **C,** Clean the vaginal area with a clean part of the washcloth. Use a downward stroke. (Note: Used areas of the washcloth are marked with Xs.)

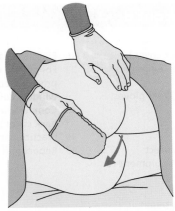

FIGURE 24-21 Clean the rectal area by wiping from front to back. The side-lying position allows thorough cleaning of the anal area.

Giving Male Perineal Care

QUALITY OF LIFE

- Knock before entering the person's room.
- Address the person by name.
- Introduce yourself by name and title.

- Explain the procedure before starting and during the procedure.
- Protect the person's rights during the procedure.
- Handle the person gently during the procedure.

PROCEDURE

1. Follow steps 1 through 16 in procedure: *Giving Female Perineal Care*, p. 374.
2. Fold the corner of the bath blanket between the legs onto the person's abdomen.
3. Wet the washcloths.
4. Squeeze out water from a washcloth. Make a mitted washcloth. Apply soap, body wash, or other cleansing agent. (Squeeze out water every time you change washcloths. Put used washcloths in the laundry bag. *Do not place used washcloths back in the basin.*)
5. Grasp the penis.
6. Retract the foreskin if the person is uncircumcised (Fig. 24-22).
7. Clean the tip. Start at the meatus. Use a circular motion (Fig. 24-23, *A*). Repeat as needed. Use a clean part of the washcloth each time.
8. Rinse the tip with another washcloth. Use the same circular motion.
9. Dry the tip (uncircumcised). Return the foreskin to its natural position.
10. Clean the shaft of the penis. Clean from the tip to the base of the shaft (Fig. 24-23, *B*). Use a clean part of a washcloth for each stroke.
11. Rinse the shaft. Use the same downward motion as in step 10. Use a clean part of a washcloth for each stroke.

12. Help the person bend the knees and spread the legs. Or help the person spread the legs as much as possible with the knees straight.
13. Clean, rinse, and dry the scrotum. Use a clean part of a washcloth.
14. Rinse the scrotum. Use a clean part of a washcloth. Observe for redness and irritation of the skin folds.
15. Pat dry the penis and the scrotum. Use the towel.
16. Fold the bath blanket back over the legs.
17. Help the person lower the legs and turn onto the side away from you.
18. Clean, rinse, and dry the rectal area. Clean from the scrotum (front) to the anus (back) (see Fig. 24-21). Use a clean part of the washcloth for each stroke. Change washcloths as needed. Rinse and dry well. Place used washcloths and the towel in the laundry bag.
19. Fold and tuck the waterproof under-pad under the person. The wet side is inside. Have the person turn toward you or lay on the back and lift the buttocks. Remove the waterproof under-pad. Place it in the laundry bag. Position the person on the back. The person is covered with the bath blanket.
20. Remove and discard the gloves. Practice hand hygiene.
21. Provide clean and dry garments and linens as needed. Remove the bath blanket. Place it in the laundry bag.
22. Position the person for comfort.
23. Follow steps 33 through 40 in procedure: *Giving Female Perineal Care*, p. 375.

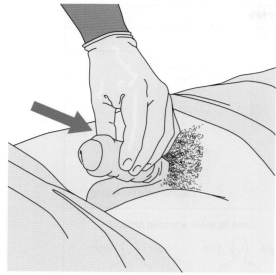

FIGURE 24-22 Retracting foreskin. Pull back the foreskin for perineal care. Return it to the normal position after cleaning, rinsing, and drying the tip of the penis.

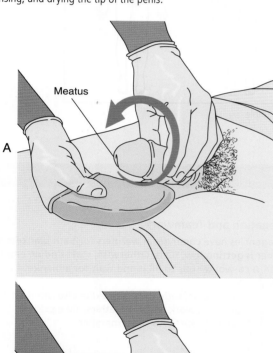

Meatus

A

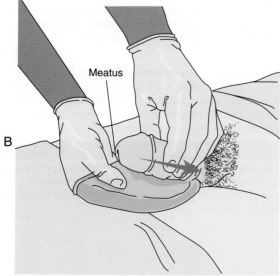

Meatus

B

FIGURE 24-23 Cleaning the penis. **A,** Clean the tip with a circular motion starting at the meatus. **B,** Clean the shaft. Clean from the tip to the base of the shaft.

REPORTING AND RECORDING

You make many observations while assisting with daily hygiene and bathing. See Box 24-4 for a summary of the observations to report and record.

Report and record the care given (Fig. 24-24, p. 378). If not recorded, it is assumed that care was not given. Tell the nurse if the person refuses care or if care is not given for another reason.

BOX 24-4	Daily Hygiene and Bathing Observations

Report the Following at Once
- Bleeding
- Signs of skin breakdown
- Discharge from the vagina or urinary tract
- Unusual odors
- Changes from prior observations

Bathing
- The color of the skin, lips, nail beds, and sclera (whites of the eyes)
- If the skin appears pale, gray-ish, yellow *(jaundice),* or bluish *(cyanotic)*
- The location and description of rashes
- Skin texture—smooth, rough, scaly, flaky, dry, moist
- *Diaphoresis*—profuse (excessive) sweating
- Bruises or open skin areas
- Pale, reddened, or discolored areas, particularly over bony parts
- Drainage or bleeding from wounds or body openings
- Swelling of the feet and legs
- Corns or calluses on the feet (Chapter 41)
- Skin temperature (cold, cool, warm, hot)
- Complaints of pain or discomfort

Perineal Care
- Odors
- Redness, swelling, discharge, bleeding, or irritation
- Complaints of pain, burning, or other discomfort
- Signs of urinary or fecal incontinence
- Foreskin that will not retract on an uncircumcised penis

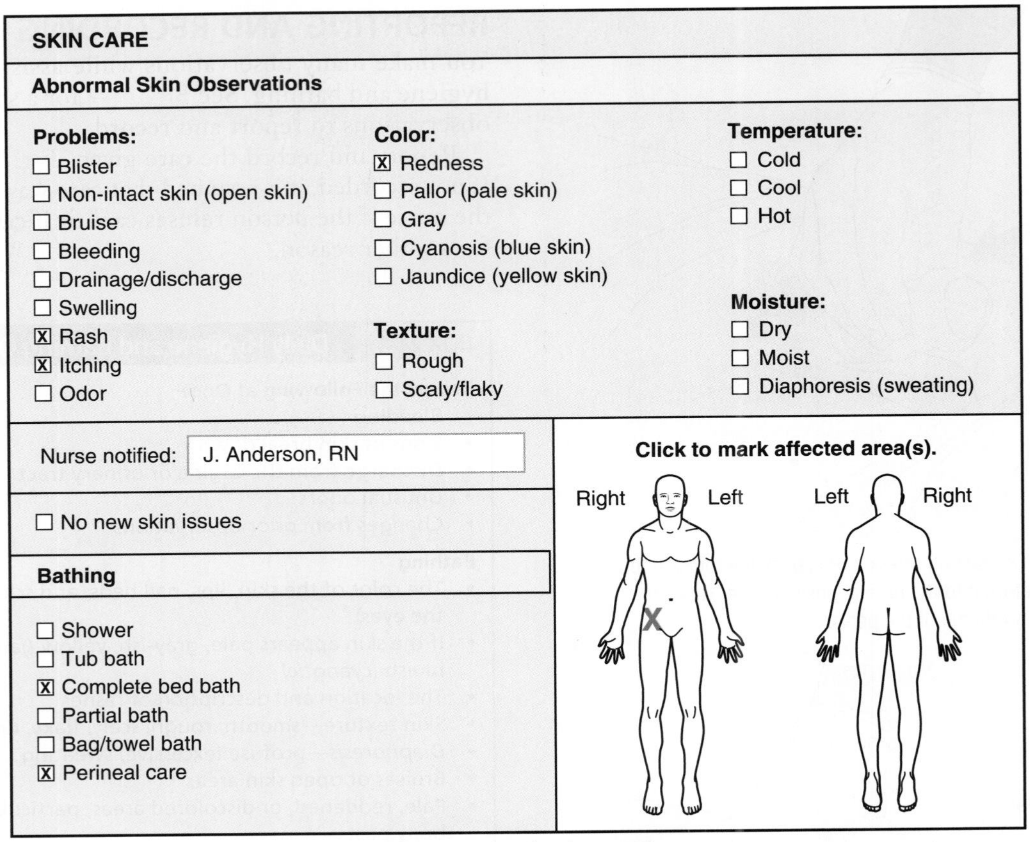

SKIN CARE		
Abnormal Skin Observations		

Problems:
☐ Blister
☐ Non-intact skin (open skin)
☐ Bruise
☐ Bleeding
☐ Drainage/discharge
☐ Swelling
☒ Rash
☒ Itching
☐ Odor

Color:
☒ Redness
☐ Pallor (pale skin)
☐ Gray
☐ Cyanosis (blue skin)
☐ Jaundice (yellow skin)

Texture:
☐ Rough
☐ Scaly/flaky

Temperature:
☐ Cold
☐ Cool
☐ Hot

Moisture:
☐ Dry
☐ Moist
☐ Diaphoresis (sweating)

Nurse notified: J. Anderson, RN

☐ No new skin issues

Bathing

☐ Shower
☐ Tub bath
☒ Complete bed bath
☐ Partial bath
☐ Bag/towel bath
☒ Perineal care

Click to mark affected area(s).
Right / Left   Left / Right

FIGURE 24-24 Charting sample.

FOCUS ON PRIDE
The Person, Family, and Yourself

Personal and Professional Responsibility

At first, you may be embarrassed to perform the procedures in this chapter. This improves with practice and experience. Practice perineal care in your classroom on a manikin. Do the full procedure as if it were a real person. Explain each step as you would with a patient or resident. Do not just practice once. Practice until you are comfortable.

Rights and Respect

Patients and residents have the right to choose schedules and routines. They also have the right to refuse care. Some persons refuse if it does not meet their preferences. For example:
• Preferring a bath, a person refuses a shower.
• A patient prefers to bathe at night, not in the morning.
• A male resident prefers perineal care by a male nursing assistant, not a female.
Refusing care for these reasons does not mean the person refuses to be clean. The person may accept if preferences are met. Tell the nurse of any refusal. Adjust as needed to respect the person's preferences.

Independence and Social Interaction

Bathing is a personal matter. Allow personal choice for bath time, products used, what to wear, and so on. Encourage self-care to the extent possible. Self-care promotes independence and improves self-esteem.

Delegation and Teamwork

Some agencies have commercial warmers for bath blankets. If a warmer is getting low, fill it. Otherwise, staff find an empty warmer. A co-worker has to fill it and wait for a blanket to heat up.

Avoid having the attitude that "someone else can do it." This shows poor teamwork and work ethics. Take pride in being a helpful and courteous team member.

Ethics and Laws

You will perform some tasks often. Bathing is an example. Over time, some staff become less careful with routine tasks. They may forget about dangers. Or they think that nothing bad will happen. This is very unsafe. Always be careful. Harm can result from routine care measures.

FOCUS ON PRIDE: Application

The care measures in this chapter are private and personal. What concerns do you have about performing these procedures? How will you stay calm and professional and ease the person's worries?

REVIEW QUESTIONS

Circle the BEST answer.

1 When assisting with daily care, you
   a Discourage the use of adaptive (assistive) devices
   b Provide for privacy if there is time
   c Follow the person's routines and habits
   d Change soiled linens in the afternoon

2 You are planning for early morning care and morning care. Which should you do *after* breakfast?
   a Apply eyeglasses and insert hearing aids
   b Give complete bed baths
   c Remove sleepwear and dress residents
   d Provide oral care and insert dentures

3 A person is incontinent. You should plan to
   a Give perineal care often throughout the day
   b Give a complete bed bath twice a day
   c Shower the person once a week
   d Give a tub bath when the person is soiled

4 To apply powder
   a Turn the person toward you
   b Sprinkle a small amount onto your hand
   c Apply a thick layer of powder
   d Shake the powder onto the person

5 You are giving a complete bed bath. Which is *correct?*
   a You use soap to wash the eye from the outer to the inner part.
   b You keep the person covered with a bath blanket as much as possible.
   c You continue washing with soapy, cool water.
   d You use another person's wash basin.

6 When bathing a person
   a Keep bar soap in the wash basin or tub
   b Wash from the dirtiest to the cleanest area
   c Assist with elimination after a bath
   d Rinse the skin well to remove all soap

7 You are preparing to give a complete bed bath. The water in the basin is 110°F (43.3°C). You should
   a Add cold water to the basin
   b Add hot water to the basin
   c Have the person check if the water is comfortable
   d Report the hot water concern to the nurse

8 When drying the person
   a Dry well between skin folds
   b Rub the skin dry
   c Avoid drying between the toes
   d Allow the person to air dry

9 A person can wash the face, arms, hands, chest, and abdomen. You should
   a Wash all areas for the person
   b Leave the other areas unwashed
   c Allow the person to wash the face and hands
   d Wash areas the person cannot reach

10 Which is helpful when showering a person with confusion?
   a Gather supplies after the person is in the shower.
   b Do not explain what you are doing.
   c Put a towel over the lap and have the person hold a washcloth.
   d Work quickly if the person resists.

11 When assisting with a shower in a shower room
   a Direct the water spray at the person's face
   b Allow a weak person to stand if you provide support
   c Go to the person's room to make the bed during the shower
   d Clean and disinfect the shower before and after use

12 You are transferring a person to a shower chair in the shower room. Which is *unsafe?*
   a The floor is wet.
   b The person has shoes on the feet.
   c The person holds the grab bar (safety bar).
   d The shower chair wheels are locked (braked).

13 You are filling a tub for a tub bath. You ask the person to check the water temperature. The person says it is cool. You should
   a Bathe the person quickly in the cool water
   b Give a shower instead
   c Drain the tub fully and refill it
   d Add warm water and ask if it feels better

14 A person asks you to rinse again at the end of a shower. Which reply is *best?*
   a "Which areas would you like rinsed?"
   b "We need to be done. I have other residents to bathe."
   c "I already rinsed you. Once is good enough."
   d "I can't. We have used enough water."

15 Water temperature for perineal care is between
   a 90°F and 95°F (32.2°C and 35.0°C)
   b 105°F and 109°F (40.5°C and 42.7°C)
   c 110°F and 115°F (43.3°C and 46.1°C)
   d 120°F and 125°F (48.8°C and 51.6°C)

16 Which action during perineal care is *correct?*
   a You rinse and re-use washcloths.
   b You do not retract foreskin on an uncircumcised penis.
   c You wear gloves.
   d You place washcloths in a sink full of water.

17 These statements are about perineal care. Which is *correct?*
   a Do not explain the procedure to avoid embarrassment.
   b The person does perineal care if able.
   c Clean from the back (bottom) to the front (top).
   d Draping the person is not needed.

18 You see a rash under a breast during a bath. You should
   a Ask the nurse to observe the area
   b Scrub the skin
   c Apply lotion to the area
   d Avoid drying the skin

Answers to Chapter 24 questions are on p. 902.

FOCUS ON PRACTICE

Problem Solving

A person has abdominal skin folds that are hard for 1 person to lift and clean under alone. The person has redness and itching under the skin folds. The nurse needs to apply a medicated powder to the area after bathing and drying well. Why is it important to dry the area well? How will you plan to provide care using teamwork and communication?

CHAPTER
25

Grooming

OBJECTIVES

- Define the key terms and key abbreviations in this chapter.
- Explain why grooming is important.
- Explain how to safely provide grooming measures—hair care, shaving, and nail and foot care.

- Perform the procedures described in this chapter.
- Explain how to promote PRIDE in the person, the family, and yourself.

KEY TERMS

alopecia Hair loss
anticoagulant A drug that prevents or slows down *(anti)* blood clotting *(coagulate)*
dandruff Excessive amounts of dry, white flakes from the scalp
hirsutism Excessive body hair
infestation Being in or on a host
lice See "pediculosis"
mite A very small spider-like organism

pediculosis Infestation with wingless insects that feed on blood; lice
pediculosis capitis Infestation of the scalp *(capitis)* with lice
pediculosis corporis Infestation of the body *(corporis)* with lice
pediculosis pubis Infestation of the pubic *(pubis)* hair with lice
scabies A skin disorder caused by a female mite

KEY ABBREVIATIONS

C	Centigrade	ID	Identification
F	Fahrenheit		

Hair care, shaving, and nail and foot care prevent infection and promote comfort. Such measures affect love, belonging, and self-esteem needs.

Grooming measures are matters of personal choice. Hair and nail care preferences vary. Culture also influences grooming practices.

The person performs grooming measures to the extent possible. This promotes independence and quality of life. The person may use adaptive (assistive) devices (Fig. 25-1).

See *Focus on Surveys: Grooming.*

See *Teamwork and Time Management: Grooming.*

See *Focus on Long-Term Care and Home Care: Grooming.*

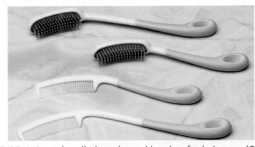

FIGURE 25-1 Long-handled combs and brushes for hair care. (Courtesy North Coast Medical Inc., Morgan Hill, Calif.)

HAIR CARE

The look and feel of hair affect mental well-being. The nursing process reflects the person's culture, personal choice, skin and scalp conditions, health history, and self-care ability. You assist with hair care as needed.

Skin and Scalp Conditions

Skin and scalp conditions include:

- *Alopecia*—hair loss. Hair loss may be complete or partial. Caused by heredity, male pattern baldness occurs with aging. Hair thins in some women with aging. Cancer treatments (radiation therapy to the head and chemotherapy) may cause alopecia in all age-groups. Skin disease, stress, poor nutrition, pregnancy, some drugs, and hormone changes are other causes. Except for hair loss from aging, hair usually grows back.
- *Hirsutism*—excessive body hair. It can occur in men, women, and children. Causes are heredity and abnormal amounts of male hormones.
- *Dandruff*—excessive amounts of dry, white flakes from the scalp. Itching is common. Sometimes eyebrows and ear canals are involved. Medicated shampoos may be ordered.

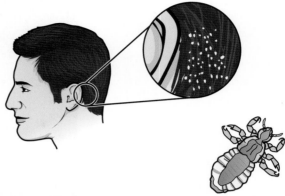

FIGURE 25-2 Head lice. (Redrawn from Medline Plus: *Head lice,* Bethesda, Md., National Institutes of Health.)

Infestations can also occur. *Infestation* means being in or on a host.

- *Pediculosis (lice)*—infestation with wingless insects that feed on blood (Fig. 25-2). Lice attach their eggs *(nits)* to hair shafts. Nits are oval and yellow to white in color. They hatch in about 1 week. After hatching, they bite the scalp or skin to feed on blood. About the size of a sesame seed, adult lice are tan to grayish white in color. Lice crawl. They do not hop or fly. They are transmitted by close person-to-person contact. Lice easily spread to others through clothing, head coverings, furniture, beds, towels, bed linens, combs, brushes, and sexual contact. Pets do not transmit human lice. Lice are treated with medicated shampoos, lotions, and creams specific for lice. Thorough bathing is needed. So is washing clothing and linens in hot water. Lice bites cause severe itching.
  - *Pediculosis capitis*—infestation of the scalp *(capitis)* with lice. It is commonly called "head lice."
  - *Pediculosis pubis*—infestation of the pubic *(pubis)* hair with lice. This form is also called "pubic lice" or "crabs."
  - *Pediculosis corporis*—infestation of the body *(corporis)* with lice. It is also called "body lice" or "clothes lice."
- *Scabies*—a skin disorder caused by a female mite (Fig. 25-3, p. 382). A *mite* is a very small spider-like organism. The female mite burrows into the skin and lays eggs. After hatching, the females produce more eggs. Infested with mites, the person has a rash and intense itching. Common sites are between the fingers, the wrists, underarms, thighs, and genital area. Other sites include the breasts, waist, and buttocks. Highly contagious, scabies is transmitted to others by close contact. Special creams are ordered to kill the mites. The person's room is cleaned. Clothing and linens are washed in hot water.

See *Focus on Communication: Skin and Scalp Conditions,* p. 382.

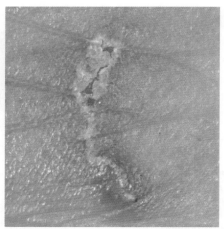

FIGURE 25-3 Scabies. (From Marks JG, Miller JJ: *Lookingbill & Marks' principles of dermatology,* ed 4, St Louis, 2006, Saunders.)

FOCUS ON COMMUNICATION

Skin and Scalp Conditions

Some skin or scalp conditions may alarm you. Remain professional. Do not say things that may embarrass the person.

Report an abnormal skin or scalp condition. Describe your observations. For example:
- "There are small red dots on Mr. Olson's right underarm. Would you please look at them?"
- "I saw some small white specks in Ms. Smith's hair. Would you please look at them before I wash her hair?"

Brushing and Combing Hair

The frequency and timing of brushing and combing hair are personal. Brushing and combing hair may be part of early morning care, morning care, or afternoon care (Chapter 24). Some people brush and comb hair before meals, before visitors arrive, and at bedtime.

Encourage patients and residents to do their own hair care. The person chooses how to brush, comb, and style hair. Assist as needed.

Brushing increases blood flow to the scalp. And it brings scalp oils along the hair shaft to help keep hair soft and shiny. Daily brushing and combing prevent matted and tangled hair. So does braiding. You need the person's consent to braid hair. *Never cut the person's hair.*

The procedure that follows gives instructions for brushing and combing hair that:
- *Is not matted or tangled.* Work from the scalp to the hair ends.
- *Is matted or tangled.* Work in small sections. Start at the hair ends. Hold the hair above the area being combed or brushed. Gently comb or brush through the matting or tangling to the hair ends. Have the person tell you if there is pain or discomfort. Gradually work up toward the scalp. Report matted or tangled hair to the nurse.

Special measures are needed for curly, coarse, or dry hair. Curly hair is often not brushed. Instead, it may be combed with a wide-tooth comb when wet. Apply hair care products as directed.

The person's hair care practices and products are part of the care plan. Let the person guide hair care.

See *Caring About Culture: Brushing and Combing Hair.*

See *Focus on Children and Older Persons: Brushing and Combing Hair.*

See *Delegation Guidelines: Brushing and Combing Hair.*

See *Promoting Safety and Comfort: Brushing and Combing Hair.*

See procedure: *Brushing and Combing Hair.*

🌸 CARING ABOUT CULTURE

Brushing and Combing Hair

Small braids (corn-rows) are common in some cultural groups. The braids are left intact for shampooing. To undo these braids, the nurse obtains the person's consent.

FOCUS ON CHILDREN AND OLDER PERSONS

Brushing and Combing Hair

Children
Hair-styles are important to older children and teenagers. Do not make judgments about hair-styles. Style hair in a way that pleases the child and parents. Do not style hair according to your standards or customs.

DELEGATION GUIDELINES
Brushing and Combing Hair

Brushing and combing hair are routine nursing tasks. To brush and comb hair, you need this information from the nurse and the care plan.

- How much help the person needs
- What to do for matted or tangled hair
- What to do for curly, coarse, or dry hair
- What hair care products to use
- The person's preferences and routine hair care measures
- What observations to report and record:
  - Scalp sores
  - Flaking
  - Itching
  - Rash
  - Hair falling out in patches; patches of hair loss
  - Very dry or very oily hair
  - Matted or tangled hair
  - The presence of nits or lice
    - Nits (lice eggs attached to hair shafts)—oval and yellow to white in color
    - Lice—about the size of a sesame seed and gray-ish white in color
    - Itching
    - Complaints of a tickling feeling or something moving in the hair
    - Irritability
    - Sores on the head or body caused by scratching
    - Rash
- When to report observations
- What patient or resident concerns to report at once

PROMOTING SAFETY AND COMFORT
Brushing and Combing Hair

Safety
Sharp brush bristles can injure the scalp. So can sharp or broken teeth on a comb. Report concerns about the person's brush or comb.

Wear gloves if the person has scalp sores, nits, lice, or other hair or scalp problems. Follow Standard Precautions and the Bloodborne Pathogen Standard.

Comfort
Protect garments from falling hair with a towel across the back and shoulders. For the person in bed, give hair care before changing linens and the pillowcase. If after a linen change, place a towel across the pillow to collect falling hair.

Combing or brushing matted or tangled hair can be painful. Do not rush. Do not comb or brush forcefully. Remind the person to tell you about any pain or discomfort during the procedure.

Brushing and Combing Hair

QUALITY OF LIFE

- Knock before entering the person's room.
- Address the person by name.
- Introduce yourself by name and title.
- Explain the procedure before starting and during the procedure.
- Protect the person's rights during the procedure.
- Handle the person gently during the procedure.

PRE-PROCEDURE

1 Follow *Delegation Guidelines: Brushing and Combing Hair.* See *Promoting Safety and Comfort: Brushing and Combing Hair.*
2 Practice hand hygiene.
3 Identify the person. Check the identification (ID) bracelet against the assignment sheet. Use 2 identifiers (Chapter 14). Also call the person by name.
4 Ask the person how to style hair.

5 Get the following supplies.
  - Comb and brush
  - Bath towel
  - Other hair care items as requested
  - Laundry bag
6 Arrange items nearby.
7 Provide for privacy.

Continued

Brushing and Combing Hair—cont'd

PROCEDURE

8 Position the person.
  a *In a chair*—Help the person to the chair. The person wears slip-resistant footwear for a transfer. Clothing properly covers the person. Or a robe is applied.
  b *In bed*—Raise the bed for body mechanics. Bed rails are up if used. Lower the bed rail near you. Assist the person to a semi-Fowler's position if allowed.
9 Place a towel across the back and shoulders or across the pillow.
10 Have the person remove eyeglasses if worn. Put them in the eyeglass case. Put the case inside the bedside stand.
11 *Hair that is not matted or tangled:*
  a Use the comb to part the hair.
    1) Part hair down the middle into 2 sides (Fig. 25-4, *A*).
    2) Divide 1 side into 2 smaller sections (Fig. 25-4, *B*).
  b Brush 1 of the small sections of hair. Start at the scalp and brush toward the hair ends (Fig. 25-5). Do the same for the other small section of hair. If the person prefers, brush long hair starting at the hair ends.
  c Repeat step 11 (a-2 and b) for the other side.

12 *Matted or tangled hair:*
  a Take a small section of hair near the ends. Hold above the area to be combed or brushed.
  b Comb or brush through to the hair ends.
  c Add small sections of hair as you work up to the scalp.
  d Comb or brush through each longer section to the hair ends.
13 Style the hair as the person prefers.
14 Remove the towel. Place it in the laundry bag.
15 Have the person put on the eyeglasses if worn.

POST-PROCEDURE

16 Provide for comfort. (See the inside of the back cover.)
17 Lower the bed to a safe and comfortable level. Raise or lower bed rails. Follow the care plan.
18 Clean up and store supplies and equipment. (Wear and change gloves as needed.)
  a Remove hair from the brush or comb. Discard hair.
  b Follow agency procedures to clean equipment. Return hair care items to their proper place.
  c Follow agency policy for used linens.
  d Clean and dry the over-bed table (if used). Dry with paper towels. Discard paper towels. Position the over-bed table as the person prefers.
  e Remove and discard gloves if worn. Practice hand hygiene.

19 Place the call light and other needed items within reach.
20 Follow the care plan and the person's preferences for privacy measures to maintain. Leaving the privacy curtain, window coverings, and door open or closed are examples.
21 Complete a safety check of the room. (See the inside of the back cover.)
22 Practice hand hygiene.
23 Report and record your care and observations.

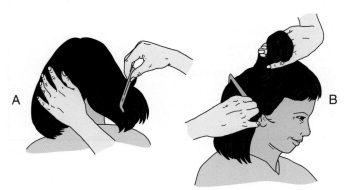

FIGURE 25-4 Parting hair. **A,** Part hair down the middle. Divide it into 2 sides. **B,** Then part 1 side into 2 smaller sections.

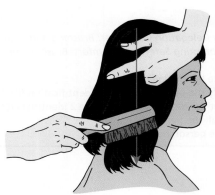

FIGURE 25-5 Brush hair that is not matted or tangled by starting at the scalp. Brush down to the hair ends.

Shampooing

People shampoo 1, 2, 3, or more times a week. Some people shampoo daily. Hair and scalp condition, hair-style, and personal choice affect frequency.

Shampoo method depends on the person's condition, safety factors, and personal choice. The nurse tells you what method to use.

- *Shampoo during the shower or tub bath.* Use a hand-held nozzle for persons in shower chairs or taking tub baths. Direct a spray of water at the hair.
- *Shampoo at the sink.* The person sits or lies facing away from the sink. A folded towel placed over the sink edge protects the neck. The person's head is tilted back over the sink edge. Or a shampoo tray is used (Fig. 25-6). Use a water pitcher or hand-held nozzle to wet and rinse the hair.
- *Shampoo in bed.* A shampoo basin under the head protects the linens and mattress from water. The device drains into a basin on a chair by the bed (Fig. 25-7). Use a water pitcher to wet and rinse the hair.

Dry and style hair as soon as possible after the shampoo. Women may want hair curled or rolled up before drying. Check with the nurse before doing so.

Shampoo Caps. Commercial shampoo caps have a cleaning agent that does not need rinsing. Some caps also have a conditioner. To use a shampoo cap:

1 Warm the package following the manufacturer's instructions.
2 Check the temperature. The cap should be warm. Do not use a cap that is too hot.
3 Apply the cap to the person's head.
4 Massage the hair and scalp gently through the cap. Follow the manufacturer's instructions for how long to massage—usually 1 to 3 minutes. Longer hair may require more time.
5 Remove the cap. Do not rinse the hair. Dry the hair with a towel if needed.
6 Comb the hair.

See *Focus on Long-Term Care and Home Care: Shampooing.*
See *Focus on Children and Older Persons: Shampooing,* p. 386.
See *Delegation Guidelines: Shampooing,* p. 386.
See *Promoting Safety and Comfort: Shampooing,* p. 386.
See procedure: *Shampooing the Person's Hair in Bed,* p. 386.

FOCUS ON LONG-TERM CARE AND HOME CARE

Shampooing

Long-Term Care
Beauty and barber shops are common in nursing centers (Fig. 25-8). Residents can have their hair shampooed, cut, and styled. Men can have their mustaches and beards groomed.

In nursing centers, shampoos are usually done on bath days. If done by a hairdresser or barber, do not shampoo hair. Provide a shower cap for the bath or shower.

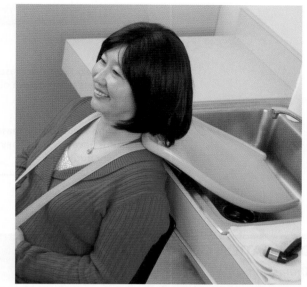
FIGURE 25-6 Shampooing at the sink with a shampoo tray. (Courtesy SP Ableware – Maddak, Wayne, NJ.)

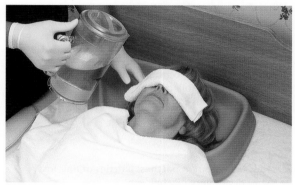
FIGURE 25-7 A shampoo basin is used for a shampoo in bed. Water drains into a collecting basin.

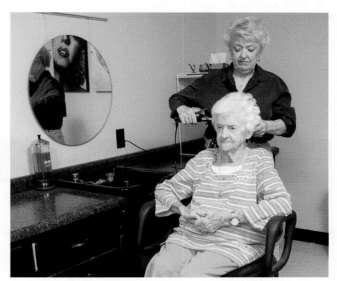
FIGURE 25-8 Beauty shop in a nursing center.

FOCUS ON CHILDREN AND OLDER PERSONS

Shampooing

Children
Oil gland secretion increases with puberty. Therefore adolescents tend to have oily hair. They may need to shampoo often.

Older Persons
Oil gland secretion decreases with aging. Therefore older persons have dry hair. They may shampoo less often than younger adults do.

DELEGATION GUIDELINES

Shampooing

Shampooing is a routine nursing task in many agencies. To shampoo a person, you need this information from the nurse and the care plan.
- When to shampoo the person's hair
- What method to use
- What shampoo and conditioner to use
- How to use and store medicated products if allowed by the state and agency
- The person's position restrictions or limits
- What water temperature to use—usually 105°F (Fahrenheit) (40.5°C [centigrade])
- If hair is curled or rolled up before drying
- What observations to report and record:
  - Scalp sores
  - Flaking
  - Itching
  - Rash
  - Hair falling out in patches; patches of hair loss
  - Very dry or very oily hair
  - Matted or tangled hair
  - The presence of nits or lice (p. 381)
  - How the person tolerated the procedure
- When to report observations
- What patient or resident concerns to report at once

PROMOTING SAFETY AND COMFORT

Shampooing

Safety
Remove hearing aids before shampooing. Water will damage hearing aids.

Wear gloves if the person has scalp sores, nits, lice, or other hair or scalp problems. Follow Standard Precautions and the Bloodborne Pathogen Standard. Follow the rules of hand hygiene and the guidelines for glove use in Chapters 17 and 18.

Keep shampoo away from and out of the eyes. Have the person hold a washcloth over the eyes. To rinse, cup your hand at the person's forehead. This keeps soapy water from running down the forehead and into the eyes.

For a shampoo on a stretcher at a sink, see Chapter 21 for stretcher safety. Lock (brake) the wheels. Use the safety straps (if present) and side rails. Keep the far side rail raised during the procedure.

Some people shampoo themselves during a tub bath or shower. Place an extra towel and requested shampoo products within the person's reach. Assist as needed.

Comfort
For a shampoo during the tub bath or shower, the person tips the head back to keep shampoo and water out of the eyes. Support the back of the head with 1 hand. Shampoo with your other hand. Some persons cannot tip their heads back. They lean forward and hold a folded washcloth over the eyes. Support the forehead with 1 hand as you shampoo with the other. Make sure that the person can breathe easily.

Many people have limited range of motion in their necks. They are not shampooed at the sink or on a stretcher.

Shampooing the Person's Hair in Bed

QUALITY OF LIFE

- Knock before entering the person's room.
- Address the person by name.
- Introduce yourself by name and title.
- Explain the procedure before starting and during the procedure.
- Protect the person's rights during the procedure.
- Handle the person gently during the procedure.

Shampooing the Person's Hair in Bed—cont'd

PRE-PROCEDURE

1 Follow *Delegation Guidelines: Shampooing.* See *Promoting Safety and Comfort: Shampooing.*
2 Practice hand hygiene and get the following supplies.
   - 2 bath towels
   - Washcloth
   - Shampoo
   - Hair conditioner (if requested)
   - Water thermometer
   - Water pitcher
   - Shampoo basin
   - Collecting basin
   - Waterproof under-pad
   - Gloves (if needed)
   - Comb and brush
   - Hair dryer
   - Laundry bag

3 Arrange items nearby. Place the collecting basin on a chair by the bed.
4 Practice hand hygiene.
5 Identify the person. Check the ID bracelet against the assignment sheet. Use 2 identifiers (Chapter 14). Also call the person by name.
6 Provide for privacy.
7 Raise the bed for body mechanics. Bed rails are up if used. Lower the bed rail near you if up.

PROCEDURE

8 Brush and comb hair to remove tangles. See procedure: *Brushing and Combing Hair* on p. 383.
9 Position the person for a shampoo in bed:
   a Lower the head of the bed. Remove the pillow.
   b Place the waterproof under-pad and shampoo basin under the head and shoulders.
   c Support the head and neck with a folded towel if necessary.
10 Cover the person's chest with a bath towel.
11 Fill the water pitcher. Follow these safety measures.
   a Raise the bed rail if used. Lower the bed to a safe level.
   b Measure water temperature following agency policy. Water temperature is usually 105°F (40.5°C). Have the person check the water temperature. Adjust water temperature as needed.
   c Raise the bed for body mechanics. Lower the bed rail if used when you return.
12 Put on gloves (if needed).
13 Have the person hold a washcloth over the eyes. It should not cover the nose and mouth. (NOTE: A damp washcloth is easier to hold and will not slip. However, your agency may require a dry washcloth.)
14 Use the water pitcher to wet the hair. Ask if the water temperature is comfortable. Adjust as needed.

15 Apply a small amount of shampoo.
16 Work up a lather with both hands. Start at the hairline. Work toward the back of the head.
17 Massage the scalp with your fingertips. Do not scratch the scalp with your fingernails.
18 Rinse the hair until the water runs clear.
19 Repeat steps 15 through 18 as needed.
20 Apply conditioner if used. Follow the directions on the container.
21 Squeeze water from the hair.
22 Cover the hair with a bath towel.
23 Remove the shampoo basin, collecting basin, and waterproof under-pad.
24 Dry the person's face with the towel on the chest.
25 Rub the hair and scalp with the towel. Rub gently. Use the second towel if the first one is wet.
26 Place towels in the laundry bag. Remove and discard gloves (if worn). Practice hand hygiene after removing and discarding gloves.
27 Raise the head of the bed.
28 Comb the hair to remove tangles. Dry and style hair as the person prefers. (Wear gloves if needed. Remove and discard gloves [if worn]. Practice hand hygiene after removing and discarding gloves.)

POST-PROCEDURE

29 Provide for comfort. (See the inside of the back cover.)
30 Lower the bed to a safe and comfortable level. Raise or lower bed rails. Follow the care plan.
31 Clean up and store supplies and equipment. (Wear gloves. Change gloves as needed.)
   a Discard disposable items.
   b Remove hair from the brush or comb. Discard hair.
   c Follow agency procedures to clean and disinfect re-usable equipment. Return supplies and equipment to their proper place.
   d Follow agency policy for used linens.
   e Clean and dry the over-bed table (if used). Dry with paper towels. Discard paper towels. Position the over-bed table as the person prefers.
   f Remove and discard gloves. Practice hand hygiene.

32 Place the call light and other needed items within reach.
33 Follow the care plan and the person's preferences for privacy measures to maintain. Leaving the privacy curtain, window coverings, and door open or closed are examples.
34 Complete a safety check of the room. (See the inside of the back cover.)
35 Practice hand hygiene.
36 Report and record your care and observations.

SHAVING

Shaving is a matter of personal preference. Facial shaving is common among men. Many women shave their legs and underarms. Some women shave facial hair. Other hair removal methods include waxing, hair removal products, plucking, and threading.

Electric shavers or safety razors are used (Fig. 25-9). Usually persons have their own electric shavers. Or the agency has a shaver. The shaver must be clean before and after use. Follow the manufacturer's instructions and agency procedures.

Safety razors (blade razors) have razor blades. They can cause nicks and cuts. Do not use safety razors on persons with healing problems or on those taking anticoagulant drugs. An *anticoagulant* is a drug that prevents or slows down *(anti)* blood clotting *(coagulate)*. Bleeding occurs easily and is hard to stop. A nick or cut can cause serious bleeding. Electric shavers are used instead.

Follow the rules in Box 25-1 for shaving. If you do not know how to use a person's shaving equipment, ask the nurse for help.

See *Focus on Children and Older Persons: Shaving.*
See *Delegation Guidelines: Shaving.*
See *Promoting Safety and Comfort: Shaving.*
See procedure: *Shaving the Person's Face With a Safety Razor,* p. 390.
See procedure: *Shaving the Person's Face With an Electric Shaver,* p. 391.

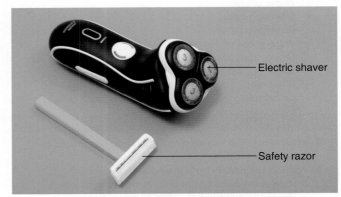

Electric shaver

Safety razor

FIGURE 25-9 Electric shaver and safety razor.

BOX 25-1	Rules for Shaving

- Follow Standard Precautions and the Bloodborne Pathogen Standard. Follow the rules of hand hygiene and the guidelines for glove use in Chapters 17 and 18.
- Protect bed linens and clothing. Place a towel under the part to be shaved. Or place a towel across the person's chest and shoulders to protect clothing.
- Encourage the person to do as much as safely possible.
- Hold the skin taut.
- Do not cut, nick, or irritate the skin. If nicks or cuts occur, apply direct pressure (Chapter 58). Report nicks, cuts, or irritation at once.

Safety Razors
- Do not use a safety razor on a person taking anticoagulant drugs. Use an electric shaver.
- Soften facial hair before shaving. Apply a warm, moist washcloth or towel to the face for a few minutes.
- Lather the area with shaving cream (shaving gel).
- Shave in the correct direction.
  - *Shaving the face*—Shave in the direction of hair growth (Fig. 25-10).
  - *Shaving the underarms*—Shave in the direction of hair growth.
  - *Shaving the legs*—Shave up from the ankles. This is against hair growth.
- Rinse the razor often to remove hair and lather.
- Rinse the skin thoroughly after shaving. Pat dry.

Electric Shavers
- Be sure the device is clean before use. Clean the device after use.
  - Open or remove the cutting head. Empty the razor into a wastebasket. If the razor has a cleaning brush, use it to remove hair. Brush gently. Do not tap the razor on the counter or on the side of the wastebasket. This can damage the razor.
  - Follow the manufacturer's instructions for cleaning and drying the cutting head after use.
- Use on a clean, dry face. Some persons use a pre-electric shave product (oil, lotion, powder) to prevent irritation. Follow the instructions on the product. (Follow the manufacturer's instructions for a razor that can be used with water.)
- Follow the manufacturer's instructions for the motion to use and the direction of the shave (Fig. 25-11).
- Shave sensitive areas first if the skin is tender and sensitive. See *Promoting Safety and Comfort: Shaving.* Press lightly. You may need to go over the same area more than once. However, avoid going over the same area many times. This can cause irritation.
- Follow safety measures for using electrical equipment (Chapter 14).
  - Charge a battery-powered device following the manufacturer's instructions.
  - Do not use near water.
  - Do not use when oxygen is in use.
  - Follow the care plan for what to use on a person with a pacemaker (Chapter 50). (A *pacemaker* is an implanted device that monitors and regulates heart rhythm.) Persons with pacemakers require extra precautions with electrical devices. Battery-powered electric shavers are safe for use when they are in good condition and used as intended. An electric shaver with a cord is to be kept at least 6 inches away from the pacemaker.

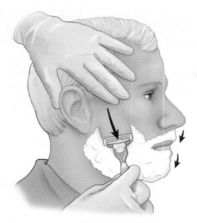

FIGURE 25-10 Shaving with a safety razor. Shave the face in the direction of hair growth. Use long strokes on the larger areas of the face. Use short strokes around the chin and lips.

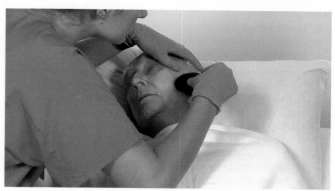

FIGURE 25-11 Shaving with an electric shaver. This rotary-type is moved in small circles over the face. (Mosby's Nursing Assistant Video Skills, 2015.)

FOCUS ON **CHILDREN AND OLDER PERSONS**
Shaving

Older Persons
Older persons with wrinkled skin are at risk for nicks and cuts. Safety razors are not used for them or persons with dementia. Persons with dementia may not understand what you are doing. They may resist care and move suddenly. Serious nicks and cuts can occur. Use electric shavers for these persons.

DELEGATION GUIDELINES
Shaving

Facial shaving is a routine nursing task. Shaving mustaches and beards is not a routine nursing task. See "Caring for Mustaches and Beards" on p. 392. Shaving legs and underarms may be delegated to you.

To shave a person's face, you need this information from the nurse and the care plan.
- What shaver to use—safety razor or electric shaver
- If the person takes anticoagulant drugs
- When to shave the person
- What facial hair to shave
- If there are tender or sensitive areas on the person's face
- What observations to report and record:
  - Nicks (report at once)
  - Cuts (report at once)
  - Bleeding (report at once)
  - Irritation
- When to report observations
- What patient or resident concerns to report at once

PROMOTING SAFETY AND COMFORT
Shaving

Safety
Safety razors are very sharp. Protect the person and yourself from nicks and cuts. Wear gloves. Follow Standard Precautions and the Bloodborne Pathogen Standard. Follow the rules of hand hygiene and the guidelines for glove use in Chapters 17 and 18. Discard used razor blades and disposable shavers in a sharps container. Do not re-cap the razor.

After rinsing a safety razor, wipe it to avoid dripping on the person. To protect yourself from cuts:
- Place a towel or several thicknesses of paper towels on the over-bed table. Do not hold them in your hand.
- Wipe the razor on the towel or paper towels.

For an electric shaver, follow the safety measures for electrical equipment (Chapter 14). Follow the manufacturer's instructions for use and cleaning. See Box 25-1.

Comfort
The neck area below the jaw may be tender and sensitive. Some electric shavers become warm or hot during use. The heat can irritate the skin. Shave tender areas first while the shaver is cool. Then move to other areas of the face.

Some people apply lotion or after-shave to the skin after shaving. Lotion softens the skin. After-shave closes skin pores. Do not apply if there are nicks, cuts, or irritation. Notify the nurse.

Shaving the Person's Face With a Safety Razor

QUALITY OF LIFE

- Knock before entering the person's room.
- Address the person by name.
- Introduce yourself by name and title.

- Explain the procedure before starting and during the procedure.
- Protect the person's rights during the procedure.
- Handle the person gently during the procedure.

PRE-PROCEDURE

1 Follow *Delegation Guidelines: Shaving*, p. 389. See *Promoting Safety and Comfort: Shaving*, p. 389.
2 Practice hand hygiene and get the following supplies.
   - Wash basin
   - Bath towel
   - Washcloth or hand towel
   - Towel or paper towels (to wipe the razor on)
   - Safety razor
   - Mirror
   - Shaving cream or shaving gel
   - Shaving brush if used

   - After-shave or lotion if used
   - Towel or paper towels (as a barrier for supplies)
   - Gloves
   - Laundry bag
3 Place the barrier (towel, paper towels) on the over-bed table. Arrange supplies on top.
4 Practice hand hygiene.
5 Identify the person. Check the ID bracelet against the assignment sheet. Use 2 identifiers (Chapter 14). Also call the person by name.
6 Provide for privacy.

PROCEDURE

7 Fill the wash basin with warm water. Place the basin on the over-bed table.
8 Raise the bed for body mechanics. Bed rails are up if used. Lower the bed rail near you if up.
9 Assist the person to semi-Fowler's position if allowed or to the supine position.
10 Adjust lighting to clearly see the person's face.
11 Place the towel over the person's chest and shoulders.
12 Adjust the over-bed table for easy reach.
13 Put on gloves.
14 Attach the razor blade to the shaver if necessary.
15 Wash the person's face. Do not dry.
16 Wet the washcloth or hand towel. Wring it out.
17 Apply the washcloth or towel to the face for a few minutes.
18 Apply shaving cream with your hands. If using gel, lather it before applying it. (If needed, change gloves or wipe excess shaving cream from your gloves using a towel or paper towel. Or use a shaving brush to apply lather.)

19 Hold the skin taut with 1 hand.
20 Shave in the direction of hair growth. Use shorter strokes around the chin and lips (see Fig. 25-10).
21 Rinse the razor often. Wipe it on a towel or paper towels.
22 Apply direct pressure to any bleeding areas (Chapter 58).
23 Wash off any remaining lather. Pat dry with the towel on the person's chest.
24 Apply after-shave or lotion if requested. (If there are nicks or cuts, do not apply after-shave or lotion.)
25 Remove the towel. Place the towel and washcloth (or hand towel) in the laundry bag. Remove and discard gloves. Practice hand hygiene.

POST-PROCEDURE

26 Provide for comfort. (See the inside of the back cover.)
27 Lower the bed to a safe and comfortable level. Raise or lower bed rails. Follow the care plan.
28 Clean up and store supplies and equipment. (Wear gloves. Change gloves as needed.)
   a Discard disposable items. Discard the razor blade or disposable razor into the sharps container.
   b Empty the wash basin.
   c Follow agency procedures to clean and disinfect re-usable equipment. Return supplies and equipment to their proper place.
   d Follow agency policy for used linens.
   e Clean and dry the over-bed table. Dry with paper towels. Discard paper towels. Position the over-bed table as the person prefers.
   f Remove and discard gloves. Practice hand hygiene.

29 Place the call light and other needed items within reach.
30 Follow the care plan and the person's preferences for privacy measures to maintain. Leaving the privacy curtain, window coverings, and door open or closed are examples.
31 Complete a safety check of the room. (See the inside of the back cover.)
32 Practice hand hygiene.
33 Report and record your care and observations. Report nicks, cuts, irritation, or bleeding to the nurse at once.

Shaving the Person's Face With an Electric Shaver

QUALITY OF LIFE

- Knock before entering the person's room.
- Address the person by name.
- Introduce yourself by name and title.

- Explain the procedure before starting and during the procedure.
- Protect the person's rights during the procedure.
- Handle the person gently during the procedure.

PRE-PROCEDURE

1 Follow *Delegation Guidelines: Shaving*, p. 389. See *Promoting Safety and Comfort: Shaving*, p. 389.
2 Practice hand hygiene and get the following supplies.
   - Wash basin
   - Bath towel
   - Washcloth or hand towel
   - Electric shaver
   - Mirror
   - Pre-electric shave product if used
   - After-shave or lotion if used

   - Towel or paper towels (as a barrier for supplies)
   - Gloves
   - Laundry bag
3 Place the barrier (towel, paper towels) on the over-bed table. Arrange supplies on top.
4 Practice hand hygiene.
5 Identify the person. Check the ID bracelet against the assignment sheet. Use 2 identifiers (Chapter 14). Also call the person by name.
6 Provide for privacy.

PROCEDURE

7 Be sure the shaver is clean. Follow the manufacturer's instructions. The shaver needs to be clean and dry before use.
8 Follow steps 7 through 13 in the procedure: *Shaving the Person's Face With a Safety Razor.*
9 Wash and dry the person's face.
10 Apply a pre-electric shave product (if used). Follow the instructions on the product.
11 Hold the skin taut with 1 hand.
12 Turn on the shaver. Shave facial hair (see Fig. 25-11). Follow the manufacturer's instructions for the motion to use and the direction of the shave. Shave any sensitive areas first. Press lightly. Avoid going over the same area many times.
   a *Rotary-type shaver*—Move the shaver in small circles over the face.
   b *Foil (oscillating blade) shaver*—Move the shaver in straight lines up and down or across the face. Follow the manufacturer's instructions and the person's preference. Use short strokes.

13 Apply direct pressure to any bleeding areas (Chapter 58). The risk of bleeding with electric shavers is low. However, irritation and breaks in the skin are possible.
14 Apply after-shave or lotion if requested. (If there are irritated areas, do not apply after-shave or lotion.)
15 Remove the towel. Place the towel and washcloth (or hand towel) in the laundry bag. Remove and discard gloves. Practice hand hygiene.

POST-PROCEDURE

16 Provide for comfort. (See the inside of the back cover.)
17 Lower the bed to a safe and comfortable level. Raise or lower bed rails. Follow the care plan.
18 Clean up and store supplies and equipment. (Wear gloves. Change gloves as needed.)
   a Discard disposable items.
   b Empty the wash basin.
   c Empty hair from the shaver. Follow the manufacturer's instructions and agency procedures to clean and dry the device. Return the shaver to its proper place.
   d Follow agency procedures to clean and disinfect re-usable equipment. Return supplies and equipment to their proper place.
   e Follow agency policy for used linens.
   f Clean and dry the over-bed table. Dry with paper towels. Discard paper towels. Position the over-bed table as the person prefers.
   g Remove and discard gloves. Practice hand hygiene.

19 Place the call light and other needed items within reach.
20 Follow the care plan and the person's preferences for privacy measures to maintain. Leaving the privacy curtain, window coverings, and door open or closed are examples.
21 Complete a safety check of the room. (See the inside of the back cover.)
22 Practice hand hygiene.
23 Report and record your care and observations. Report irritation or bleeding to the nurse at once.

Caring for Mustaches and Beards

Mustaches and beards need daily care. Food and mouth and nose drainage can collect in the whiskers. Daily washing and combing are needed. Ask the person how to groom a mustache or beard. *Never shave or trim a mustache or beard.*

Shaving Legs and Underarms

Shaving legs and underarms varies among cultures. Some persons shave only the lower legs. Others shave to mid-thigh or the entire leg.

To shave legs and underarms:

- Follow the rules in Box 25-1.
- Collect shaving items with bath items.
- Shave after bathing while the skin is soft.
- Use soap and water, shaving cream (gel), or lotion for the lather. Follow the care plan and the person's preferences.
- Use the kidney basin to rinse the razor. Do not use bath water.

▌ NAIL AND FOOT CARE

Nail and foot care prevents infection, injury, and odors. Hangnails, ingrown nails (nails that grow in at the side), and nails torn away from the skin cause skin breaks. Skin breaks are portals of entry for microbes. Long or broken nails can scratch the skin and snag clothing.

Dirty feet, socks, or stockings harbor microbes and cause odors. Shoes and socks provide a warm, moist place for microbes to grow. Injuries occur from stubbing toes, stepping on sharp objects, or being stepped on. Poorly fitting shoes cause blisters.

Poor circulation prolongs healing. Diabetes and vascular diseases cause poor circulation. Foot injuries or infections are very serious for older persons and those with circulatory disorders. Gangrene and amputation are serious complications (Chapter 49).

Nails are easier to clean and trim right after soaking or bathing. Use nail clippers to trim fingernails. *Never use scissors.* Use extreme caution to prevent damage to nearby tissues.

Clipping toenails can easily cause injuries. Some agencies do not let nursing assistants cut toenails. Follow agency policy.

See *Teamwork and Time Management: Nail and Foot Care.*

See *Focus on Long-Term Care and Home Care: Nail and Foot Care.*

See *Delegation Guidelines: Nail and Foot Care.*

See *Promoting Safety and Comfort: Nail and Foot Care.*

See procedure: *Giving Nail and Foot Care*, p. 394.

TEAMWORK AND TIME MANAGEMENT
Nail and Foot Care

Use your time well when giving nail and foot care. The fingernails soak for 5 to 10 minutes. The feet soak for 15 to 20 minutes. Make the person's bed or straighten the person's unit during soak time. Or assist with brushing and combing hair. Check your assignment sheet for other ways to meet the person's needs.

FOCUS ON LONG-TERM CARE AND HOME CARE
Nail and Foot Care

Home Care

Follow the care plan and the nurse's directions for how to position the person for nail and foot care. Fingernails may be soaked in a clean bowl or small basin. Feet may be soaked during a tub bath. Or the person may sit on a shower chair or bench as the feet soak in the tub. Otherwise, soak the feet in a basin or a whirlpool foot bath.

DELEGATION GUIDELINES
Nail and Foot Care

The procedure that follows is a routine nursing task. Clipping toenails is a nursing responsibility that may be delegated to you in some agencies.

To give nail and foot care, you need this information from the nurse and the care plan.

- What water temperature to use (usually 105°F/40.5°C)
- How long to soak fingernails (usually 5 to 10 minutes)
- How long to soak feet (usually 15 to 20 minutes or less)
- If fingernails should be filed but not trimmed
- How to position the person
- What observations to report and record:
  - Dry, irritated, or callused areas
  - Breaks in the skin
  - Redness, swelling
  - Corns (Chapter 41) on top of and between the toes
  - Blisters
  - Very thick nails
  - Loose nails
- When to report observations
- What patient or resident concerns to report at once

PROMOTING SAFETY AND COMFORT

Nail and Foot Care

Safety

To trim fingernails, use nail clippers. Clip straight across (Fig. 25-12). Then file the nails to smooth and round the corners. File in 1 direction. Filing back and forth can weaken the nail.

Some states and agencies do not let nursing assistants clip toenails. A nurse or podiatrist (foot [pod] doctor) cuts toenails and provides foot care for the following persons. *You do not clip the fingernails or toenails for persons who:*

- Have diabetes
- Have poor circulation
- Take drugs that affect blood clotting
- Have nail fungus, very thick nails, or ingrown nails (Chapter 41)

Check between the toes for cracks and sores. If not treated, a serious infection could occur.

The feet are easily burned. Persons with decreased sensation or circulatory problems may not feel hot temperatures.

Do not apply lotion between the toes. Also, lotion on the feet can be slippery. Slip-resistant footwear is applied before transferring or walking.

Breaks in the skin and bleeding can occur. Some persons do not practice proper hand hygiene after elimination. Some confused persons grab or scratch at under-garments or incontinence products. Feces (stools) may be under the fingernails. Provide frequent hand hygiene for such persons. Wear gloves for nail care. Follow Standard Precautions and the Bloodborne Pathogen Standard. Follow the rules of hand hygiene and the guidelines for glove use in Chapters 17 and 18.

Comfort

Sometimes you just trim the fingernails. Sometimes you just give foot care. To do both, the person sits at the over-bed table (Fig. 25-13). Provide for warmth and comfort.

Provide for your comfort during nail and foot care. Sit in front of the over-bed table to clean and trim fingernails. For foot care, rest the person's lower leg and foot on your lap. Or position the feet on the floor and kneel on the floor. Lay a towel across your lap or put a disposable waterproof pad (disposable bed protector—Chapter 22) on the floor to protect your uniform. Use good body mechanics. Always support the person's foot and ankle during foot care.

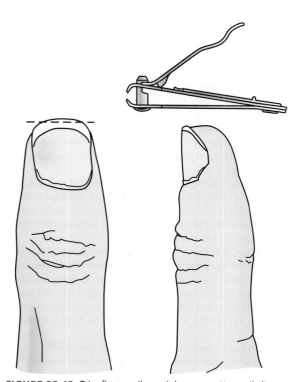

FIGURE 25-12 Trim fingernails straight across. Use nail clippers.

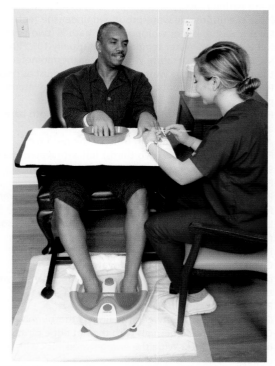

FIGURE 25-13 Nail and foot care. The feet soak in a whirlpool foot bath. The fingers are soaking in a kidney basin.

Giving Nail and Foot Care

QUALITY OF LIFE

- Knock before entering the person's room.
- Address the person by name.
- Introduce yourself by name and title.

- Explain the procedure before starting and during the procedure.
- Protect the person's rights during the procedure.
- Handle the person gently during the procedure.

PRE-PROCEDURE

1 Follow *Delegation Guidelines: Nail and Foot Care*, p. 392. See *Promoting Safety and Comfort: Nail and Foot Care*, p. 393.
2 Practice hand hygiene and get the following supplies.
   - Wash basin or whirlpool foot bath
   - Kidney basin
   - Soap
   - Water thermometer
   - Bath towel
   - Washcloth and hand towel (if needed)
   - Nail clippers
   - Orangewood stick
   - Emery board or nail file
   - Lotion for the hands
   - Lotion or petroleum jelly for the feet
   - Towel or paper towels (as a barrier for supplies)
   - Disposable waterproof pad
   - Gloves
   - Laundry bag

3 Place the barrier (towel, paper towels) on the over-bed table. Arrange supplies on top.
4 Practice hand hygiene.
5 Identify the person. Check the ID bracelet against the assignment sheet. Use 2 identifiers (Chapter 14). Also call the person by name.
6 Provide for privacy.

PROCEDURE

7 Assist the person to the bedside chair. Remove footwear and socks or stockings. Place the call light and other needed items within reach.
8 Place the disposable waterproof pad under the feet.
9 Fill the wash basin or whirlpool foot bath ⅔ (two-thirds) full with water. Water temperature is usually 105°F (40.5°C). Measure the temperature with a water thermometer. Have the person check the water temperature. Adjust as needed.
10 Place the basin or foot bath on the disposable waterproof pad.
11 Help the person put the feet into the water. Both bare feet are covered by water.
12 Adjust the over-bed table in front of the person.
13 Fill the kidney basin ⅔ (two-thirds) full with water. See step 9 for water temperature.
14 Place the kidney basin on the over-bed table.
15 Place the person's fingers into the basin. Position the arms for comfort (see Fig. 25-13).
16 Let the fingers soak for 5 to 10 minutes. Let the feet soak for 15 to 20 minutes. Re-warm water as needed.
17 Put on gloves.
18 Clean the hands with soap and water if needed or if required by your state's competency exam. Clean between the fingers. Rinse the hands.
19 Remove the kidney basin.
20 Dry the hands and between the fingers thoroughly.
21 Clean under the fingernails with the flat edge of the orangewood stick. Wipe the orangewood stick with a towel or paper towel after each nail.

22 Push cuticles back gently with the orangewood stick or a washcloth if requested by the person.
23 Trim fingernails straight across with the nail clippers (see Fig. 25-12). You may carefully round the corners slightly.
24 File and shape nails with an emery board or nail file. Nails are smooth with no rough edges. Check each nail for smoothness. File as needed. File in 1 direction.
25 Apply lotion to the hands. Warm the lotion first. To warm lotion, rub some between your hands or hold the bottle under warm water.
26 Move the over-bed table to the side. (NOTE: If your agency or state competency test requires clean gloves for foot care, remove and discard gloves. Practice hand hygiene. Put on clean gloves.)
27 Lift a foot out of the water. Support the foot and ankle with 1 hand. With your other hand, wash the foot and between the toes with soap and a washcloth. Return the foot to the water to rinse the foot and between the toes.
28 Repeat step 27 for the other foot.
29 Remove the feet from the water. Dry thoroughly, especially between the toes. Support the foot and ankle as needed.
30 Apply lotion or petroleum jelly to the tops, soles, and heels of the feet. Do not apply between the toes. Warm lotion or petroleum jelly first (see step 25). Remove excess lotion or petroleum jelly with a towel. Support the foot and ankle as needed.
31 Place the used towels and washcloth in the laundry bag. Remove and discard the gloves. Practice hand hygiene.
32 Help the person put on slip-resistant footwear.

Giving Nail and Foot Care—cont'd

POST-PROCEDURE

33 Provide for comfort. (See the inside of the back cover.)

34 Make sure the bed is at a safe and comfortable level. Follow the care plan.

35 Check that bed rails are raised or lowered following the care plan.

36 Clean up and store supplies and equipment. (Wear gloves. Change gloves as needed.)
   a Discard disposable items.
   b Empty the kidney basin and wash basin (whirlpool foot bath).
   c Follow agency procedures to clean and disinfect re-usable equipment. Return supplies and equipment to their proper place.
   d Follow agency policy for used linens.
   e Clean and dry the over-bed table. Dry with paper towels. Discard paper towels. Position the over-bed table as the person prefers.
   f Remove and discard gloves. Practice hand hygiene.

37 Place the call light and other needed items within reach.

38 Follow the care plan and the person's preferences for privacy measures to maintain. Leaving the privacy curtain, window coverings, and door open or closed are examples.

39 Complete a safety check of the room. (See the inside of the back cover.)

40 Practice hand hygiene.

41 Report and record your care and observations.

FOCUS ON PRIDE

The Person, Family, and Yourself

Personal and Professional Responsibility

Grooming promotes comfort, self-esteem, and body image. Clean hair and nails help mental well-being. So does a clean-shaven face or a well-groomed beard or mustache. Families and visitors notice how patients or residents are groomed. If not groomed well, they may question the quality of care you provide. Grooming is important.

Rights and Respect

Grooming preferences vary. Do not judge the person by your standards or impose your choices on the person. Respect the right to choose. Assist with grooming in a way that improves the person's self-esteem.

Independence and Social Interaction

Some family members want to help with grooming. For example, they want to style the person's hair. Or they want to apply lotion to the person's hands and feet.

With the person's permission, allow family to assist with grooming as much as safely possible. This promotes social interaction. It also involves the family in the person's care.

Delegation and Teamwork

Grooming takes time. You, the person, the nurse, and other team members work together to plan and organize care. For example, a resident had a stroke. Breakfast is at 0800, speech therapy is at 0930, and family visits during lunch. The resident prefers to comb hair, shave, and change clothes after breakfast but before visitors arrive. You plan to assist with grooming after breakfast and before speech therapy.

Do not neglect grooming because of a busy schedule. Plan to meet the person's needs at a time best for the person and the team.

Ethics and Laws

Patients and residents have the right to be free from mistreatment and restraint (Chapter 2). The following is a case where a nurse did not follow these ethical principles.

A nurse told a patient that she was going to cut his hair and trim his beard. The patient repeatedly stated that he did not want a haircut or his beard trimmed. The patient protested and resisted the nurse's actions. She continued her actions while 2 other staff members restrained the patient.

The patient reported the incident to his social worker. An investigation was conducted.

The nurse lost her job. The United States Court of Appeals agreed that the nurse's termination was warranted because of:

- *The nature and seriousness of the offense*
- *The restraint of the patient after he repeatedly objected (L. Taylor v. Department of Veterans Affairs, 2006.)*

Never force a care measure on a person. If a person resists or refuses care, stop. Do not proceed. Politely ask the person for the reason. Tell the nurse. You, the nurse, and the person can discuss a solution.

FOCUS ON PRIDE: Application

The family may notice when grooming differs from usual. The family may tell you what they expect. Why are their comments important? How can you show that you value their input?

REVIEW QUESTIONS

Circle the BEST answer.

1 A person with alopecia has
   a Excessive body hair
   b Dry, white flakes from the scalp
   c An infestation with lice
   d Hair loss

2 Which should you report before giving hair care?
   a Braided hair
   b White specks in the hair
   c Dry hair
   d Dirty hair

3 A person has tangled hair. You should
   a Cut out the tangled sections
   b Brush through small sections starting at the hair ends
   c Comb firmly from the scalp to the hair ends
   d Not brush the hair

4 A person's hair is *not* matted or tangled. When brushing hair, start at
   a The forehead and brush backward
   b The hair ends
   c The scalp
   d The back of the neck and brush forward

5 Brushing keeps the hair
   a Soft and shiny
   b Clean
   c Free of lice
   d Long

6 A person requests a shampoo. You should
   a Shampoo hair during the person's shower
   b Shampoo hair at the sink
   c Shampoo the person in bed
   d Follow the care plan for the shampoo method

7 To keep shampoo out of the eyes during a shower
   a Do not rinse the top of the head
   b Wipe off the shampoo with a washcloth
   c Have the person wear eyeglasses
   d Place a washcloth over the eyes and tip the head back

8 A person is able to shave himself. He needs help setting up and cleaning up. Which should you do?
   a Set up supplies and then clean up supplies after he shaves.
   b Set up supplies, shave him, and clean up supplies.
   c Refuse to set up and clean up supplies because he can shave himself.
   d Set up supplies but tell him to clean up when finished.

9 A resident needs to be shaved. The nurse tells you the resident takes an anticoagulant drug. You need to
   a Use a safety razor and shaving cream
   b Use a safety razor without shaving cream
   c Use the resident's electric shaver
   d Refuse to shave the resident

10 When shaving a person's face with a safety razor
   a Discard the razor in the wastebasket when done
   b Start at the jaw and shave upward
   c Hold the skin taut
   d Shave when the skin is dry

11 A person is nicked during shaving. Your *first* action is to
   a Wash your hands
   b Apply direct pressure
   c Tell the nurse
   d Apply a bandage

12 To trim fingernails, use
   a An emery board
   b Scissors
   c A nail file
   d Nail clippers

13 Which is *correct* when performing nail care?
   a Trim nails straight across and then file them.
   b Trim and file nails before cleaning them.
   c Do not clean under the fingernails.
   d File nails with a firm back-and-forth motion.

14 A person has poor circulation in the legs and feet. You should
   a Trim the person's toenails
   b Use hot water to soak the feet
   c Check the toes for cracks and sores
   d Not perform foot care

15 When giving foot care
   a Dry well between the toes
   b Apply lotion between the toes
   c Do not wash between the toes
   d Do not use soap

Answers to Chapter 25 questions are on p. 902.

FOCUS ON PRACTICE

Problem Solving

A resident with dementia has long fingernails. Some are broken and have rough edges. As you begin nail care, the resident resists by pulling away and yelling at you. How will you respond? Why is nail care important for this resident? What *cannot* be done?

Changing Garments

OBJECTIVES

- Define the key terms and key abbreviations in this chapter.
- Identify when garments need to be changed.
- Explain the rules for dressing and undressing.
- Explain how to safely change a patient gown on a person with an IV.

- Perform the procedures described in this chapter.
- Explain how to promote PRIDE in the person, the family, and yourself.

KEY TERMS

affected side The side of the body with weakness from illness or injury; weak side
garment An item of clothing

unaffected side The side of the body opposite the affected side; strong side
under-garment An item of clothing worn next to the skin under clothing

KEY ABBREVIATIONS

ID	Identification	IV	Intravenous

Clothing affects comfort and body image. The ability to dress and undress oneself promotes dignity and independence. You will assist patients and residents with dressing needs.

GARMENTS

A *garment* is an item of clothing. Age, gender, culture, comfort, season, and personal preference affect garment choices. An *under-garment* is an item of clothing worn next to the skin under clothing. Bras, undershirts, underwear (underpants, panties, briefs, boxer shorts), and slips are examples. Incontinence products may be worn (Chapter 27).

Hospital patients wear gowns (patient gowns) that open in the back (p. 405). For some examinations and procedures, the opening is in front (Chapter 38).

Nursing center residents wear street clothes during the day and sleepwear at bedtime. Resident clothing is labeled with the person's name in a way that respects dignity. For example, labels are inside clothing or shoes. Or a color-coded system is used. Know your agency's policy. Residents must be dressed in their own clothing. The person chooses what to wear.

See *Focus on Communication: Garments.*
See *Focus on Surveys: Garments.*

FOCUS ON **COMMUNICATION**

Garments

There are many types of and names for under-garments. For example, a person may refer to underwear as "drawers," "skivvies," or "britches." Persons in cold climates may wear "long johns." Use terms the person uses and understands. Be respectful and professional.

FOCUS ON **SURVEYS**

Garments

Surveyors will observe if residents:
- Are dressed in their own clothes.
- Are dressed in clothing of their choice.
- Are wearing the correct clothing for the time of day.

⚓ Changing Garments

In nursing centers, garments are often changed in the morning and at bedtime. They are changed for bathing and when wet or soiled.

In hospitals, the patient changes into a patient gown (p. 405) on admission. The gown is changed daily and as needed. When discharged, the patient changes into his or her own clothing.

The procedures that follow describe how to change garments that:

- *Open in the back.* Patient gowns and bras that fasten in the back are examples.
- *Are pulled over the head (pullover garments).* T-shirts, undershirts, and sweatshirts are examples.
- *Open in the front.* Shirts with buttons, vests, and coats and jackets are examples.

There is more than 1 method to remove and apply a garment. For example, one person prefers to remove a pullover garment from the head first. Another person needs 1 sleeve removed before bringing the garment over the head. Use the method that is best for the person. Areas of weakness, joint range of motion (Chapter 35), and personal preference are considered.

Health problems can cause weakness or affect function on 1 side of the body. Stroke and hip fracture are examples (Chapter 49). When changing garments, you need to know about areas of weakness.

- The *affected side* (*weak side*) is the side of the body with weakness from illness or injury.
- The *unaffected side* (*strong side*) is the side of the body opposite the affected side.

Some persons dress and undress themselves. Others need help. Allow the person to do as much as is safely possible. This promotes independence. Adaptive (assistive) devices may be used (Fig. 26-1). To assist with dressing and undressing, follow the rules in Box 26-1.

See *Focus on Communication: Changing Garments.*

See *Focus on Children and Older Persons: Changing Garments.*

See *Delegation Guidelines: Changing Garments.*

See *Promoting Safety and Comfort: Changing Garments.*

See procedure: *Undressing the Person*, p. 400.

See procedure: *Dressing the Person*, p. 402.

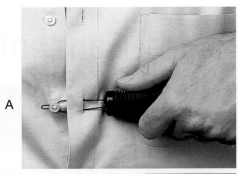
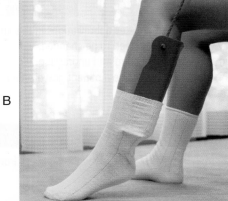
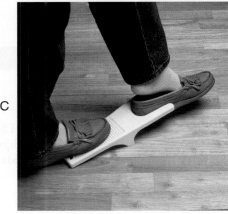

FIGURE 26-1 Dressing aids. **A,** A button hook to button and zip clothing. **B,** A sock assist to pull on socks and stockings. **C,** A shoe remover to take off shoes. (Courtesy North Coast Medical, Inc., Morgan Hill, Calif.)

BOX 26-1	Rules for Undressing and Dressing

- Provide for privacy. Do not expose the person.
- Encourage the person to do as much as possible.
- Let the person choose what to wear. Have the person choose the right under-garments.
- Make sure garments are the person's. (They do not belong to another patient or resident.)
- Make sure garments and footwear are the correct size.
- Consider areas of weakness.
  - Remove clothing from the *unaffected side (strong side)* first.
  - Put clothing on the *affected side (weak side)* first.

- Support the arm or leg to remove or put on a garment.
- Move and handle the body gently. Do not force a joint beyond its range of motion or to the point of pain. See Chapter 35.
- Follow the person's care plan and agency policy for removed garments. The agency or the person's family will launder (wash, dry, and return) the person's clothing. If the family does the laundry, removed clothing is usually kept in the person's room. It is not placed in the agency's hamper for used linens (Chapter 22).

FOCUS ON COMMUNICATION

Changing Garments

When changing garments, promote personal choice and independence. You can ask:
- "What would you like to wear today?"
- "There's a concert today. Do you want to wear something special?"
- "Do you need help with your buttons?"
- "Would you like help with your zipper?"

FOCUS ON CHILDREN AND OLDER PERSONS

Changing Garments

Older Persons

Persons with dementia may take longer to dress. Choosing clothing may be hard. Wearing the wrong clothing for the season and wearing clothes that do not match are common. Or they forget to put on a piece of clothing.

Allow the person to do as much as possible. The Alzheimer's and Related Dementias Education and Referral Center (ADEAR) suggests the following.
- Try to assist with dressing at the same time each day. Dressing becomes part of the daily routine.
- Allow extra time. Do not rush the person.
- Let the person choose from 2 or 3 outfits. The family may buy several of the same outfit. Dressing is easier if the person insists on wearing the same thing.
- Choose comfortable, easy to get on and off clothes. Garments with elastic waistbands and Velcro closures are examples. There are no zippers, buttons, hooks, snaps, or other closures.
- Stack clothes in the order they are put on. The person sees 1 item at a time. For example, an under-garment is put on first. The item is on top of the stack.
- Give clear, simple, and step-by-step directions. Give the person 1 item at a time.

DELEGATION GUIDELINES

Changing Garments

Changing garments is a routine nursing task. To assist with undressing and dressing, you need this information from the nurse and the care plan.
- How much help the person needs
- If the person can sit up and lean forward
- If the person can raise the hips to lift the buttocks off of the bed
- If the person has an affected side (weak side)
- If the person has limited range of motion in any joints
- If certain garments are needed
- If adaptive (assistive) devices are used
- What observations to report and record:
  - How much help was given
  - How the person tolerated the procedure
  - Complaints by the person
  - Changes in the person's behavior
- When to report observations
- What patient or resident concerns to report at once

PROMOTING SAFETY AND COMFORT

Changing Garments

Safety

To change garments in bed, you may need to turn the person from side to side. If the person uses bed rails, raise the far bed rail. If bed rails are not used, ask a co-worker to help turn and position the person. This protects the person from falling.

If contact with blood or body fluids is likely, wear gloves. Remove gloves and practice hand hygiene before touching clean garments. Follow Standard Precautions and the Bloodborne Pathogen Standard. Follow the rules of hand hygiene and the guidelines for glove use in Chapters 17 and 18.

In nursing centers, follow agency policies and procedures for using Enhanced Barrier Precautions for high-contact tasks. See Chapter 18.

Some persons have limited range of motion in 1 or more joints (Chapter 35). Pain can occur if the affected joint is moved too far. There is stiffness and difficulty moving the joint. Use caution when changing garments. Never force a joint beyond its present range of motion or to the point of pain.

Follow the safety measures for transfers (Chapter 21) and tub baths and showers (Chapter 24) when undressing and dressing in a tub or shower room. Follow the care plan for the transfer method and number of staff needed. Remember these safety measures if the person will stand.
- Slip-resistant footwear is worn for transfers.
- The floor is dry.
- The person uses grab bars (safety bars) for support.
- Wheelchair and shower chair wheels are locked (braked).
- A transfer belt (gait belt) is applied over clothing.

Comfort

Keep the person covered with the bath blanket as much as possible. This provides warmth and privacy.

Check that clothing is applied correctly. For example, the front of the shirt is in front. Adjust clothing for comfort and a neat appearance.

Undressing the Person

QUALITY OF LIFE

- Knock before entering the person's room.
- Address the person by name.
- Introduce yourself by name and title.

- Explain the procedure before starting and during the procedure.
- Protect the person's rights during the procedure.
- Handle the person gently during the procedure.

PRE-PROCEDURE

1 Follow *Delegation Guidelines: Changing Garments*, p. 399. See *Promoting Safety and Comfort: Changing Garments*, p. 399.
2 Ask a co-worker to help turn and position the person if needed.
3 Practice hand hygiene.
4 Identify the person. Check the identification (ID) bracelet against the assignment sheet. Use 2 identifiers (Chapter 14). Also call the person by name.

5 Get the following supplies.
  - Bath blanket
  - Laundry bag
  - Clothing requested by the person
6 Provide for privacy.
7 Raise the bed for body mechanics. Bed rails are up if used.

PROCEDURE

8 Stand on the person's affected (weak) side if the person has one. Lower the bed rail near you if up.
9 Position the person for the procedure. The head of the bed is raised if the person will sit up and lean forward. The head of the bed is flat if the person will turn from side to side.
10 Cover the person with a bath blanket. Fan-fold linens to the foot of the bed. Keep the person covered as much as possible throughout the procedure.
11 Remove garments that open in the back (Fig. 26-2).
  a *If the person can sit up and lean forward* (see Fig. 26-2, *A*):
    1) Have the person lean forward.
    2) Undo buttons, zippers, ties, snaps, or other closures.
    3) Bring the sides of the garment to the sides of the person.
    4) Have the person sit back.
  b *If the person cannot sit up and lean forward* (see Fig. 26-2, *B*):
    1) Turn the person away from you.
    2) Undo buttons, zippers, ties, snaps, or other closures.
    3) Tuck the far side of the garment under the person. Fold the near side onto the chest.
    4) Position the person supine.
  c Slide the garment off of the shoulder and arm on the unaffected (strong) side. Remove the garment from the affected (weak) side.
12 Remove pullover garments (Fig. 26-3).
  a Undo any buttons, zippers, ties, snaps, or other closures.
  b Remove the garment from the arm and shoulder on the unaffected (strong) side (see Fig. 26-3, *A*).
  c Have the person lean forward if able or turn the person toward you to bring the garment up to the neck. Have the person sit back. Or position the person supine.
  d Bring the garment over the head (see Fig. 26-3, *B*).
  e Remove the garment from the affected (weak) side (see Fig. 26-3, *C*).

13 Remove garments that open in the front.
  a Undo buttons, zippers, ties, snaps, or other closures.
  b Slide the garment off of the shoulder and arm on the unaffected (strong) side.
  c *If the person can sit up and lean forward:*
    1) Have the person lean forward.
    2) Bring the garment around the back to the affected (weak) side.
    3) Have the person sit back.
  d *If the person cannot sit up and lean forward:*
    1) Turn the person toward you.
    2) Tuck the removed part of the garment under the person.
    3) Turn the person away from you.
    4) Pull the side of the garment out from under the person. Make sure the person will not lie on it when supine.
    5) Position the person supine.
  e Remove the garment from the affected (weak) side.
14 Remove pants or slacks.
  a Remove footwear and socks.
  b Position the person supine.
  c Undo buttons, zippers, ties, snaps, or buckles. Remove a belt if worn.
  d *If the person can raise the hips to lift the buttocks off of the bed:*
    1) Have the person raise the hips.
    2) Bring the pants down over the hips and buttocks.
    3) Have the person lower the hips.
  e *If the person cannot raise the hips:*
    1) Turn the person toward you.
    2) Slide the pants off of the hip and buttock on the unaffected (strong) side.
    3) Turn the person away from you.
    4) Slide the pants off of the hip and buttock on the affected (weak) side.
    5) Position the person supine.
  f Slide the pants down the legs and over the feet.
15 Dress the person and complete the post-procedure steps. See procedure: *Dressing the Person*, p. 402.

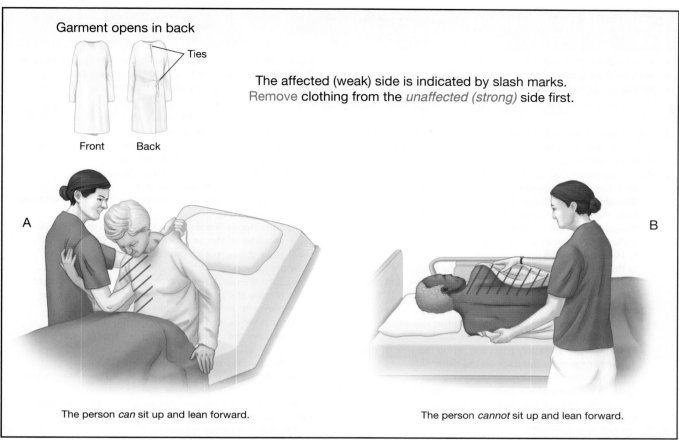

FIGURE 26-2 Removing a gown that opens in the back. **A,** The person can sit up and lean forward. The gown is untied and removed. **B,** The person cannot sit up and lean forward. The person is turned to untie and remove the gown.

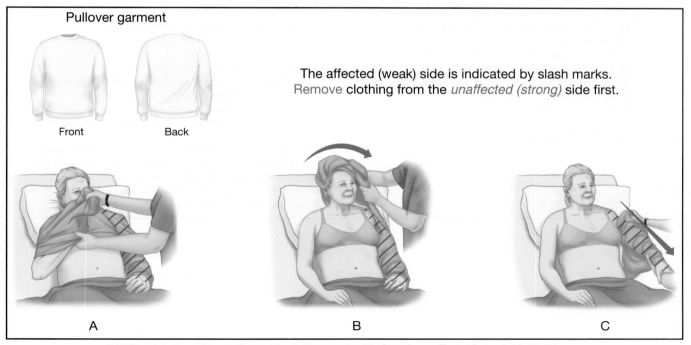

FIGURE 26-3 Removing a pullover shirt. **A,** Remove the shirt from the unaffected (strong) side. **B,** Bring the shirt over the head. **C,** Remove the shirt from the affected (weak) side. (NOTE: Reverse this order when dressing the person. Keep the person covered as much as possible.)

Dressing the Person

QUALITY OF LIFE

- Knock before entering the person's room.
- Address the person by name.
- Introduce yourself by name and title.

- Explain the procedure before starting and during the procedure.
- Protect the person's rights during the procedure.
- Handle the person gently during the procedure.

PROCEDURE

1 Follow steps 1 through 14 in the procedure: *Undressing the Person*, p. 400. Remain on the person's affected (weak) side if the person has one.
2 Put on garments that open in the back (Fig. 26-4).
   a Slide the correct sleeve of the garment onto the arm and shoulder of the affected (weak) side.
   b Slide the garment's other sleeve onto the arm and shoulder of the unaffected (strong) side.
   c *If the person can sit up and lean forward:*
      1) Have the person lean forward.
      2) Bring the sides of the garment to the back.
      3) Fasten buttons, zippers, ties, snaps, or other closures.
      4) Have the person sit back.
   d *If the person cannot sit up and lean forward:*
      1) Turn the person toward you. Bring the side of the garment around the back (Fig. 26-4, *A*).
      2) Turn the person away from you. Bring the side of the garment around the back on the other side (see Fig. 26-4, *B*).
      3) Bring the sides of the garment together. Fasten buttons, zippers, ties, snaps, or other closures.
      4) Position the person supine.
3 Put on pullover garments.
   a Slide the correct sleeve of the garment onto the arm and shoulder on the affected (weak) side.
   b Bring the garment over the head.
   c Slide the garment's other sleeve onto the arm and shoulder of the unaffected (strong) side.
   d Bring the garment down.
      1) *If the person can sit up and lean forward,* have the person lean forward. Pull the garment down. Have the person sit back.
      2) *If the person cannot sit up and lean forward:*
         a) Turn the person away from you.
         b) Pull the garment down on the affected (weak) side.
         c) Turn the person toward you.
         d) Pull the garment down on the unaffected (strong) side.
         e) Position the person supine.

4 Put on garments that open in the front (Fig. 26-5, p. 404).
   a Slide the correct sleeve of the garment onto the arm and shoulder on the affected (weak) side (see Fig. 26-5, *A*).
   b *If the person can sit up and lean forward:*
      1) Have the person lean forward.
      2) Bring the garment around the back to the unaffected (strong) side.
      3) Slide the garment's other sleeve onto the arm and shoulder of the unaffected (strong) side.
      4) Have the person sit back.
   c *If the person cannot sit up and lean forward:*
      1) Turn the person away from you. Bring the garment around the person's back. Tuck the far side of the garment under the person (see Fig. 26-5, *B*).
      2) Turn the person toward you. Bring the garment around the person's unaffected (strong) side (see Fig. 26-5, *C*).
      3) Position the person supine.
      4) Slide the garment onto the arm and shoulder on the unaffected (strong) side (see Fig. 26-5, *D*).
   d Fasten buttons, zippers, ties, snaps, or other closures.
5 Put on pants or slacks (Fig. 26-6, p. 405).
   a Position the person supine.
   b Slide the pants over the feet and up the legs.
   c *If the person can raise the hips to lift the buttocks off of the bed* (see Fig. 26-6, *A*):
      1) Have the person raise the hips.
      2) Bring the pants up over the hips and buttocks.
      3) Have the person lower the hips.
   d *If the person cannot raise the hips* (see Fig. 26-6, *B*):
      1) Turn the person away from you.
      2) Slide the pants over the hip and buttock on the affected (weak) side.
      3) Turn the person toward you.
      4) Slide the pants over the hip and buttock on the unaffected (strong) side.
      5) Position the person supine.
   e Fasten buttons, zippers, ties, snaps, a belt buckle, or other closures.
6 Put socks on the person. Socks are up all the way and smooth. See Chapter 40 for how to apply elastic stockings. Apply slip-resistant footwear if the person will get out of bed.
7 Remove the bath blanket. Place it in the laundry bag.
8 Cover the person or help the person out of bed.

Dressing the Person—cont'd

POST-PROCEDURE

9 Provide for comfort. (See the inside of the back cover.)
10 Lower the bed to a safe and comfortable level. Raise or lower bed rails. Follow the care plan.
11 Follow agency policy for removed clothing and used linens.
12 Place the call light and other needed items within reach.
13 Follow the care plan and the person's preferences for privacy measures to maintain. Leaving the privacy curtain, window coverings, and door open or closed are examples.

14 Complete a safety check of the room. (See the inside of the back cover.)
15 Practice hand hygiene.
16 Report and record your care and observations.

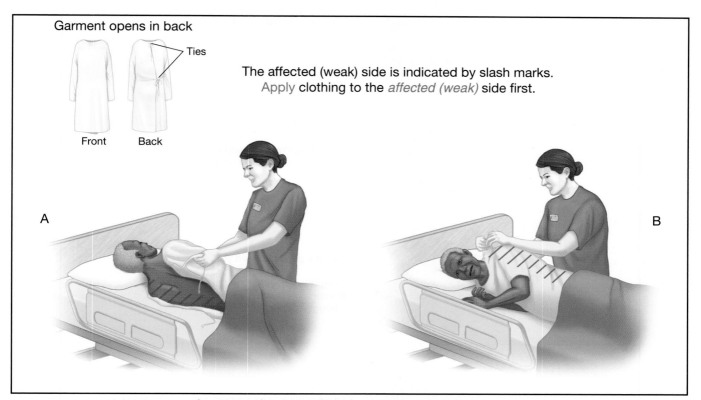

FIGURE 26-4 Applying a gown that opens in the back with the person lying down. **A,** Turn the person toward you after putting the gown on the arms. Bring the side of the gown to the person's back. **B,** Turn the person away from you. Bring the other side of the gown to the back and fasten.

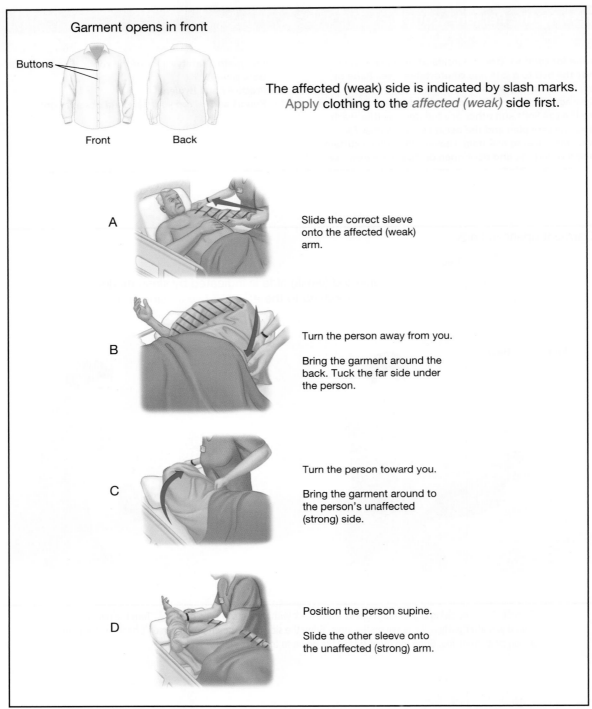

Garment opens in front

Buttons

Front   Back

The affected (weak) side is indicated by slash marks.
Apply clothing to the *affected (weak)* side first.

A — Slide the correct sleeve onto the affected (weak) arm.

B — Turn the person away from you.

Bring the garment around the back. Tuck the far side under the person.

C — Turn the person toward you.

Bring the garment around to the person's unaffected (strong) side.

D — Position the person supine.

Slide the other sleeve onto the unaffected (strong) arm.

FIGURE 26-5 Applying a shirt that opens in the front with the person lying down. **A,** Apply the garment to the affected (weak) arm. **B** and **C,** Turn the person to bring the garment around the back to the unaffected (strong) side. **D,** Position the person supine. Apply the garment to the unaffected (strong) arm. (NOTE: Reverse this order when undressing the person. Keep the person covered as much as possible.)

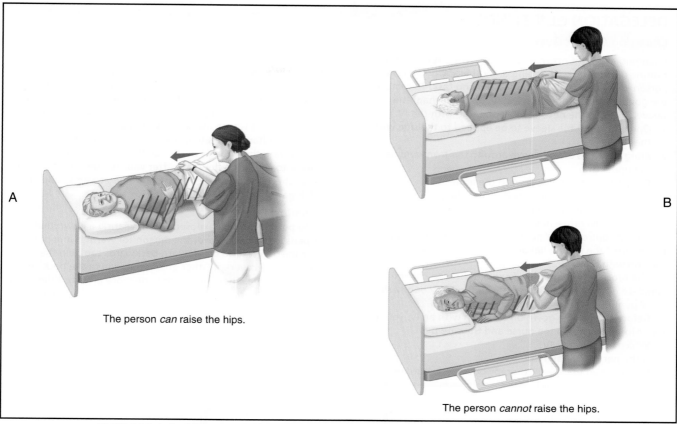

FIGURE 26-6 Applying pants. **A,** The person can raise the hips and buttocks off of the bed. The pants are slid over the hips and buttocks. **B,** The person cannot raise the hips. The person is turned to pull the pants up over the hip and buttock on the affected (weak) side and the unaffected (strong) side.

CHANGING PATIENT GOWNS

Patient gowns are designed for comfort and to allow treatment (Fig. 26-7).

- An *intravenous (IV) therapy gown* is used for IV therapy (Chapter 32). The gown opens along the sleeves and closes with ties, snaps, or Velcro.
- A *standard gown* does not open along the sleeves.

For injury or paralysis, remove the gown from the unaffected (strong) arm first. Support the affected (weak) arm while removing the gown. Put the clean gown on the affected (weak) arm first and then on the unaffected (strong) arm.

See *Delegation Guidelines: Changing Patient Gowns*, p. 406.

See *Promoting Safety and Comfort: Changing Patient Gowns*, p. 406.

See procedure: *Changing a Standard Patient Gown on a Person With an IV*, p. 407.

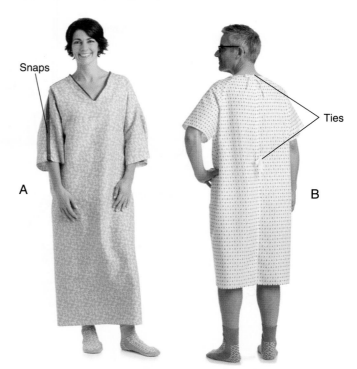

FIGURE 26-7 Patient gowns. **A,** IV therapy gown. Snaps on the sleeves allow for easy changing. **B,** Standard gown. This gown ties at the neck and back. (Courtesy Medline Industries, Inc. © Medline Industries, Inc. 2019.)

DELEGATION GUIDELINES
Changing Patient Gowns

Changing a patient gown on a person without an IV is a routine nursing task. Changing an IV therapy gown on a person with an IV is also a routine nursing task. To remove the gown from the side with the IV, open (unsnap) the sleeve. To apply the new gown to the side with the IV:

1 Open (unsnap) the sleeve to be applied to the side with the IV.
2 Bring the sides of the sleeve around the front and back of the upper arm.
3 Close (snap) the sleeve around the arm.

If a person has an IV attached to an IV bag (Fig. 26-8), you need to know if an IV pump is used (Chapter 33). IV pumps control the *flow rate*—how fast fluid enters the vein. You do not adjust controls on IV pumps. Do not use the following procedure if the person has an IV pump. The nurse handles the arm with the IV.

The procedure that follows explains how to change a standard gown when an IV is attached to an IV bag *without* an IV pump. This task may be delegated to you.

Before changing a gown on a person with an IV, you need this information from the nurse and the care plan.

- Which arm has the IV
- If the person has an IV pump
- Which gown to use—IV therapy gown, standard gown

PROMOTING SAFETY AND COMFORT
Changing Patient Gowns

Safety
In the procedure that follows, you need to lift the IV bag from the IV pole (see Fig. 26-8). Do not disconnect or remove any other parts of the IV set-up. Hold the bag up. Blood can enter the IV tubing if you lower the bag below the IV site. (The *IV site* is where the IV is inserted into the body—usually an arm or hand. The site is covered by a clear dressing.)

Moving the IV bag can change the flow rate. Ask the nurse to check the flow rate after you change the gown. You may check the flow rate if you are trained to do so and are delegated the task. See Chapter 33.

Comfort
The person can feel exposed when wearing a gown that opens in the back. Cover the person for warmth and privacy. A robe or a second gown worn backwards can help the person feel covered. Other gowns over-lap in the back and tie at the side. These gowns provide more privacy. When tied at the side, uncomfortable bows and knots at the back are avoided.

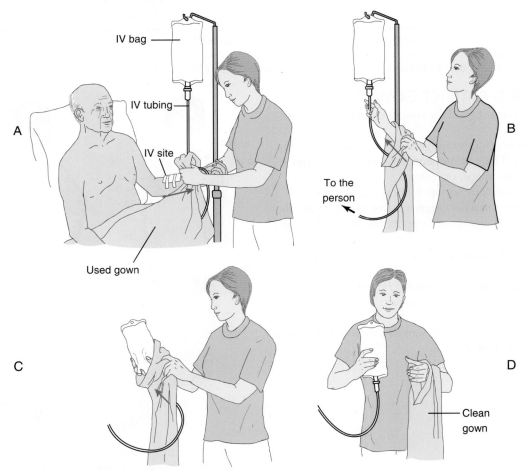

FIGURE 26-8 Changing a gown. **A,** Remove the gown from the arm with no IV. Gather up the sleeve on the arm with the IV. Slip it over the IV site and tubing. Remove it from the arm and hand. **B,** Slip the gathered sleeve along the IV tubing to the bag. **C,** Remove the IV bag from the pole. Pass it through the sleeve. **D,** Slip the gathered sleeve of the clean gown over the IV bag at the shoulder part of the gown.

Changing a Standard Patient Gown on a Person With an IV

QUALITY OF LIFE

- Knock before entering the person's room.
- Address the person by name.
- Introduce yourself by name and title.

- Explain the procedure before starting and during the procedure.
- Protect the person's rights during the procedure.
- Handle the person gently during the procedure.

PRE-PROCEDURE

1 Follow *Delegation Guidelines*:
  a *Changing Garments*, p. 399
  b *Changing Patient Gowns*
  See *Promoting Safety and Comfort*:
  c *Changing Garments*, p. 399
  d *Changing Patient Gowns*
2 Practice hand hygiene.
3 Identify the person. Check the ID bracelet against the assignment sheet. Use 2 identifiers (Chapter 14). Also call the person by name.

4 Get the following supplies.
  • Clean gown
  • Bath blanket
  • Laundry bag
5 Provide for privacy.
6 Raise the bed for body mechanics. Bed rails are up if used.

PROCEDURE

7 Lower the bed rail near you if up.
8 Cover the person with the bath blanket. Fan-fold linens to the foot of the bed.
9 Untie the gown. Free parts that the person is lying on.
10 Remove the gown from the arm with *no IV.*
11 Gather up the sleeve of the arm *with the IV.* Slide it over the IV site and tubing. Remove the arm and hand from the sleeve (see Fig. 26-8, *A*).
12 Keep the sleeve gathered. Slide the gathered sleeve along the tubing to the bag (see Fig. 26-8, *B*).
13 Remove the bag from the pole. Slide the bag and tubing through the sleeve (see Fig. 26-8, *C*). Do not pull on the tubing. Keep the bag above the IV site.

14 Hang the IV bag on the pole.
15 Place the used gown in the laundry bag.
16 Gather the sleeve of the clean gown that will go on the arm with the IV.
17 Remove the bag from the pole. Slip the sleeve over the bag at the shoulder part of the gown (see Fig. 26-8, *D*). Hang the bag.
18 Slide the gathered sleeve over the tubing, hand, arm, and IV site. Then slide it onto the shoulder.
19 Put the other side of the gown on the person. Fasten the gown.
20 Cover the person. Remove and store the bath blanket. Or place it in the laundry bag.

POST-PROCEDURE

21 Provide for comfort. (See the inside of the back cover.)
22 Lower the bed to a safe and comfortable level. Raise or lower bed rails. Follow the care plan.
23 Follow agency policy for used linens.
24 Place the call light and other needed items within reach.
25 Follow the care plan and the person's preferences for privacy measures to maintain. Leaving the privacy curtain, window coverings, and door open or closed are examples.

26 Complete a safety check of the room. (See the inside of the back cover.)
27 Practice hand hygiene.
28 Ask the nurse to check the flow rate.
29 Report and record your care and observations.

FOCUS ON PRIDE

The Person, Family, and Yourself

Personal and Professional Responsibility

Care measures are not just tasks to be completed. Show that you value the person.
- Be pleasant. Talk with the person.
- Avoid seeming rushed.
- Do a good job. Be thorough and careful.
- Compliment the person after dressing.

Rights and Respect

Appearance affects self-esteem. Garments should be clean, not wrinkled, and comfortable. Matching clothes and clothes for the correct season are worn. If a garment does not fit well, change it. Dress the person in a way that promotes dignity and respect.

Independence and Social Interaction

Ask what clothing the person prefers. Ask about comfort and appearance. Also ask if the person wants other items applied. Jewelry is an example. Personal choice promotes independence and quality of life.

Delegation and Teamwork

Some garments are worn as part of the person's treatment. Elastic stockings and binders or compression garments are examples (Chapters 40 and 41). You need more information from the nurse and the care plan before applying such garments.

Ethics and Laws

Special care measures are needed for persons with confusion or dementia who resist care (Chapter 54). Forcing care and neglecting care are wrong. Patience and problem solving are needed. A co-worker or family member may help with dressing. Or garments are changed at another time. Follow the person's routine. Be kind and gentle.

FOCUS ON PRIDE: Application

How does clothing affect your self-image? How will you promote dignity and independence when assisting with dressing and undressing?

REVIEW QUESTIONS

Circle the BEST answer.

1 In long-term care
   a Patient gowns are worn
   b Sleepwear is worn during the day
   c Garments are changed every other day
   d Street clothes are worn during the day

2 For spilled coffee on a shirt, you should
   a Give the person a sweater to cover the spill
   b Wipe the stain with a damp towel
   c Change the shirt at bedtime
   d Change the shirt right away

3 A person has weakness on the right side. Garments are removed
   a From the affected (weak) side first
   b From the unaffected (strong) side first
   c From either side first
   d In the same way they are applied

4 A person has limited range of motion in the left shoulder. Apply the person's shirt
   a To the affected side first
   b To the unaffected side first
   c To either side first
   d In the same way it was removed

5 When dressing
   a Do as much for the person as possible
   b Choose clothing for the person
   c Support the arm or leg
   d Move the person quickly

6 When dressing a person with dementia
   a Choose clothing with buttons
   b Give more than 1 direction at a time
   c Offer many clothing options
   d Follow the person's routine

7 An IV therapy gown
   a Opens at the sleeves
   b Does not have sleeves
   c Must be changed by the nurse
   d Provides less privacy than a standard gown

8 When changing a gown on a person with an IV, which should you do?
   a Hold the IV bag below the IV site.
   b Stop an IV pump to change a gown.
   c Have the nurse check the flow rate afterward.
   d Disconnect an IV to change a gown.

Answers to Chapter 26 questions are on p. 902.

FOCUS ON PRACTICE

Problem Solving

A person needs assistance with changing garments. The person is learning to use adaptive (assistive) devices to dress herself to the extent possible. Even though it takes more time, what do you promote when you allow the person to do as much as possible? Today, you feel busy and rushed. What will you do?

Urinary Needs

- Define the key terms and key abbreviations in this chapter.
- Describe the rules for normal urination.
- Describe normal urine.
- Identify the observations to report to the nurse.
- Describe urinary incontinence and the care required.

- Describe bladder training methods.
- Perform the procedures described in this chapter.
- Explain how to promote PRIDE in the person, the family, and yourself.

KEY TERMS

dysuria Painful or difficult *(dys)* urination *(uria)*; burning on urination

enuresis Lack of bladder control when past the usual age of toilet training

functional incontinence The person has bladder control but cannot use the toilet in time

groin Where a thigh and the abdomen meet

hematuria Blood *(hemat)* in the urine *(uria)*

mixed incontinence The combination of stress incontinence and urge incontinence

nocturia Frequent urination *(uria)* at night *(noc)*

oliguria Scant amount *(olig)* of urine *(uria)*; less than 500 mL in 24 hours

over-flow incontinence Small amounts of urine leak from a full bladder

polyuria Abnormally large amounts *(poly)* of urine *(uria)*

reflex incontinence Urine is lost at predictable intervals when a specific amount of urine is in the bladder

stress incontinence When urine leaks during exercise and certain movements that cause pressure on the bladder

transient incontinence Temporary or occasional incontinence that is reversed when the cause is treated

urge incontinence The loss of urine in response to a sudden, urgent need to void; the person cannot get to a toilet in time

urinary frequency Voiding at frequent intervals

urinary incontinence (UI) The involuntary loss or leakage of urine

urinary retention Not being able to completely empty the bladder

urinary urgency The need to void at once

urination The process of emptying urine from the bladder; voiding

voiding See "urination"

KEY ABBREVIATIONS

BM	Bowel movement	OAB	Over-active bladder
ID	Identification	UI	Urinary incontinence
mL	Milliliter	UTI	Urinary tract infection

Eliminating waste is a physical need. The urinary system removes waste products from the blood. It also maintains the body's water and electrolyte balance.

See *Body Structure and Function Review: The Urinary System*, p. 410.

See *Teamwork and Time Management: Urinary Needs*, p. 410.

See *Promoting Safety and Comfort: Urinary Needs*, p. 410.

BODY STRUCTURE AND FUNCTION REVIEW

The Urinary System

Structure and Function

The 2 *kidneys* (Fig. 27-1) lie in the upper abdomen against the back muscles on each side of the spine. Blood passes through the 2 kidneys. *Urine* is formed in the kidneys. Urine consists of wastes and excess fluids filtered out of the blood. Urine flows through the 2 *ureters* to the urinary *bladder*. Urine is stored in the bladder. The *urethra* connects the bladder to the outside of the body. The opening at the end of the urethra is called the *meatus.* Urine passes from the body through the meatus. Urine is a clear, yellowish fluid.

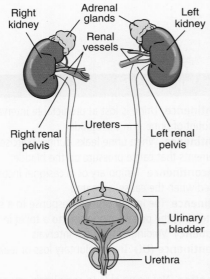

FIGURE 27-1 The urinary system.

Changes With Aging

In older persons, there is reduced blood supply to the kidneys, and the kidneys *atrophy* (shrink). Kidney function decreases. Bladder muscles weaken, and the tissues are less able to stretch. The bladder may hold less urine and not empty completely. Urinary problems may occur. In men, the prostate gland enlarges and can obstruct (block) urine flow (Chapter 52).

TEAMWORK AND TIME MANAGEMENT

Urinary Needs

Urinary needs may be urgent. Answer call lights promptly. Also, answer call lights for co-workers. Otherwise, incontinence may result (p. 420). The person is wet and embarrassed. Skin breakdown and infection are risks. Your co-worker has extra work—changing wet linens and garments. You like help when busy. So do your co-workers.

PROMOTING SAFETY AND COMFORT

Urinary Needs

Safety

Urinary elimination measures often involve exposing and touching private areas—the perineum and rectum. Sexual abuse has occurred in health care settings. The person may feel threatened or is actually being abused. The person needs to be able to call for help. Keep the call light within the person's reach at all times. Always act in a professional manner.

NORMAL URINATION

The healthy adult produces about 1500 mL (milliliters), or 3 pints, of urine a day. Many factors affect urine production—age, disease, the amount and kinds of fluid ingested, salt, body temperature, perspiration (sweating), and some drugs. Some substances increase urine production—coffee, tea, alcohol, and some drugs. A diet high in salt and some drugs cause the body to retain water. When water is retained, less urine is produced.

Urination (voiding) means the process of emptying urine from the bladder. The amount of fluid intake, habits, and available toilet facilities affect frequency. So do activity, work, bladder problems, and illness. People usually void at bedtime, after sleep, and before meals. Some void more often. Voiding at night disturbs sleep.

Some persons need help getting to the bathroom. Others use bedpans, urinals, or commodes. Follow the rules in Box 27-1 and the person's care plan.

See *Focus on Communication: Normal Urination.*
See *Focus on Children and Older Persons: Normal Urination.*

FOCUS ON COMMUNICATION

Normal Urination

Patients and residents may not use the terms "voiding" or "urinating." Do not ask: "Do you need to void?" or "Do you need to urinate?" if the person does not understand these words. Instead, you can ask these questions.
- "Do you need to use the bathroom (toilet)?"
- "Do you need the bedpan (urinal)?"
- "Do you need to pass urine (pass water)?"
- "Do you need to go potty?" (Some children use the term "potty.")
- "Do you need to pee?"

The word "pee" may offend some persons. Choose age-appropriate words that the person understands and uses. Follow the care plan.

FOCUS ON CHILDREN AND OLDER PERSONS

Normal Urination

Children

Infants produce 200 to 300 mL of urine a day. The amount increases as the baby grows older. An infant can have 6 to 20 wet diapers a day. Tell the nurse at once if an infant does not have a wet diaper for several hours. This signals dehydration (Chapter 32). It is very serious in infants.

BOX 27-1	Rules for Normal Urination

- Practice medical asepsis.
- Follow Standard Precautions. Follow the Bloodborne Pathogen Standard if blood is present.
- Provide fluids as the nurse and care plan direct.
- Follow voiding routines and habits. Check with the nurse and the person's care plan.
- Help the person to the bathroom upon request. Or provide the bedpan, urinal, or commode. The need to void may be urgent.
- Assist the person with urinary needs at regular times. Some people are embarrassed or are too weak to ask for help.
- Help the person assume a normal position for voiding if possible. Women sit or squat. Men stand.
- Warm the bedpan or urinal if time permits. The need may be urgent. (This is important if the item is metal.)
- Cover the person for warmth and privacy.
- Provide for privacy. Pull the privacy curtain around the bed, close room and bathroom doors, and close window coverings.
- Leave the room if the person can be alone. Stay nearby if the person is weak, unsteady, or at risk for falling (Chapter 15). Do not leave persons with dementia alone (Chapter 54).
- Tell the person that running water in the sink, flushing the toilet, or playing music can mask voiding sounds. Voiding with others nearby embarrasses some people.
- Place the call light and toilet paper within reach.
- Allow enough time. Do not rush the person.
- Promote relaxation. Some people like to read.
- Run water slowly in a sink if the person cannot start the urine stream. Hearing the sound of a water stream may help. Or place the person's fingers in warm water.
- Provide perineal care as needed (Chapter 24).
- Assist with hand hygiene after voiding. Provide a wash basin (or sink), soap, washcloth, and towel. Some agencies provide hand-wipes.

Observations

Normal urine color ranges from pale yellow (straw-colored) to light amber (Fig. 27-2). It is clear (not cloudy) with no particles. A faint odor is normal. Observe urine for color, clarity, odor, amount (output), particles, and blood.

Some foods change urine color. Red food dyes, beets, blackberries, and rhubarb cause red-colored urine. Carrots and sweet potatoes cause bright yellow urine. Asparagus causes a urine odor. Certain drugs change urine color. B vitamins cause bright yellow urine. Other drugs can cause reddish-orange, orange, blue, or green urine.

Dark urine is a sign of dehydration (Chapter 32). Dark brown or orange urine may signal a liver disorder. Cloudy urine, green urine, or urine with particles can occur with infection. Report such changes and the problems in Table 27-1. Ask the nurse to observe urine that looks or smells abnormal.

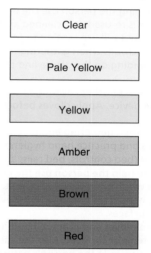

FIGURE 27-2 Color chart for urine.

TABLE 27-1	Urinary Elimination Problems	
Problem	Definition	Some Causes
Dysuria	Painful or difficult (*dys*) urination (*uria*); burning on urination	Urinary tract infection (UTI), trauma, urinary tract obstruction
Hematuria	Blood (*hemat*) in the urine (*uria*)	Kidney disease, UTI, trauma
Nocturia	Frequent urination (*uria*) at night (*noc*)	Excess fluid intake, kidney disease, prostate problems
Oliguria	Scant amount (*olig*) of urine (*uria*); less than 500 mL in 24 hours	Poor fluid intake, shock, burns, kidney disease, heart failure
Polyuria	Abnormally large amounts (*poly*) of urine (*uria*)	Drugs, excess fluid intake, diabetes, hormone imbalance
Urinary frequency	Voiding at frequent intervals	Excess fluid intake, UTI, pressure on the bladder, drugs
Urinary incontinence (UI)	The involuntary loss or leakage of urine	Trauma, disease, UTI, reproductive or urinary tract surgeries, aging, fecal impaction, constipation, not getting to the bathroom in time
Urinary retention	Not being able to completely empty the bladder	Prostate problems, nerve damage, UTI, drugs, surgery, kidney stones, constipation, trauma
Urinary urgency	The need to void at once	UTI, fear of incontinence, full bladder, stress

VOIDING EQUIPMENT

If the person is unable to use the toilet, other equipment is used for voiding. Bedpans, urinals, and commodes are common.

See *Promoting Safety and Comfort: Voiding Equipment.*

PROMOTING SAFETY AND COMFORT

Voiding Equipment

Safety

Urine is a body fluid. Follow Standard Precautions when handling urinary devices and their contents. This includes bedpans, urinals, commodes, urinary drainage bags (Chapter 28), and incontinence products. Follow the Bloodborne Pathogen Standard if blood is present. Follow the rules of hand hygiene and the guidelines for glove use in Chapters 17 and 18.

If the device (bedpan, urinal, commode) is new, gloves do not need to be worn when gathering equipment. Apply gloves before helping the person use the device.

When a device is re-used, it is cleaned and disinfected after use. You should still use caution to prevent the transmission of microbes when gathering re-used equipment. Depending on the device and the situation, you can:

- Use paper towels or other covering as a barrier when collecting the device. Apply gloves before helping the person use it.
- Apply gloves when gathering equipment. Remove and discard gloves and practice hand hygiene before touching other surfaces (bed controls, bed rails, and so on). Apply clean gloves to help the person use the device.
- Apply gloves when gathering equipment. Keep 1 hand "clean." This hand does not touch the device. Use it to touch other surfaces.

Remove soiled gloves and practice hand hygiene before touching clean items or surfaces. Also use caution to avoid contaminating surfaces in the person's bathroom. A paper towel can be used to turn a faucet on and off.

Do not place bedpans or urinals on over-bed tables and bedside stands. These are used for eating, as a work surface, and for personal items and supplies. These surfaces must not be contaminated with urine or feces (stools).

Patients and residents have their own voiding equipment. Some states and agencies require labeling the device with the person's name and room and bed number. Equipment is not shared among patients and residents.

In nursing centers, follow agency policies and procedures for using Enhanced Barrier Precautions for high-contact tasks. See Chapter 18.

Bedpans

Bedpans are used when the person cannot be out of bed. Women use bedpans for voiding and bowel movements (BMs). Men use them for BMs.

A *standard bedpan* is shown in Figure 27-3, *A.* The wide rim at the back goes under the buttocks.

A *fracture pan* has a thin rim. It is only about ½-inch deep at one end (Fig. 27-3, *B*). The smaller end (flat end) goes under the buttocks (Fig. 27-4). The person lies flat. Fracture pans are used:

- By persons with casts
- By persons in traction
- By persons with limited back motion
- By older persons with osteoporosis (fragile bones) or arthritis
- After spinal cord injury or surgery
- After a hip fracture or hip replacement surgery

Like a fracture pan, the small end (flat end) of a *bariatric bedpan* is placed under the buttocks (Fig. 27-3, *C*). Some have a weight capacity of 1200 pounds.

See *Delegation Guidelines: Bedpans.*
See *Promoting Safety and Comfort: Bedpans.*
See procedure: *Giving the Bedpan.*

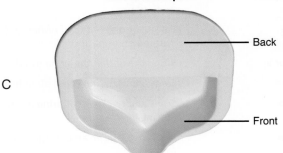

FIGURE 27-3 Bedpans. **A,** Standard bedpan. **B,** Fracture pan. **C,** Bariatric bedpan. (C, Courtesy AliMed, Inc., Dedham, Mass.)

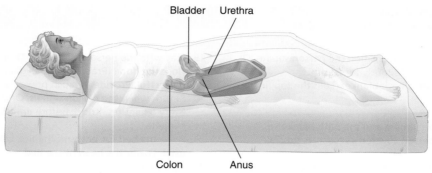

FIGURE 27-4 A person positioned on a fracture pan. The small end (flat end) is under the buttocks.

DELEGATION GUIDELINES

Bedpans

Assisting with a bedpan is a routine nursing task. To assist with a bedpan, you need this information from the nurse and the care plan.
- What bedpan to use—standard bedpan, fracture pan, bariatric bedpan
- Position or activity limits
- If the person can raise the hips to place the bedpan
- If you can leave the room or if you need to stay with the person
- If the nurse will observe the results before you flush the contents
- What observations to report and record:
  - Urine color, clarity, and odor
  - Amount
  - Presence of particles
  - Blood in the urine
  - Cloudy urine
  - Complaints of urgency, burning, dysuria, or other problems (see Table 27-1)
  - For bowel movements, see Chapter 29
- When to report observations
- What patient or resident concerns to report at once

PROMOTING SAFETY AND COMFORT

Bedpans

Safety
Remember to raise the bed as needed for good body mechanics. Lower the bed to a safe level before leaving the bedside. Raise or lower bed rails according to the care plan.

Comfort
Most bedpans are plastic. Metal bedpans are often cold. Warm a metal bedpan with warm water and dry it before use. Use clean, dry paper towels for drying.

The person's need to use the bedpan may be urgent. You will need to prioritize what measures to do. For example, raising the bed is a safety measure for you. Placing a bath blanket is a privacy measure. If time does not permit such measures before placing the bedpan, do not neglect them after it is placed.

The person must not sit on a bedpan for a long time. Bedpans are uncomfortable. They can lead to pressure injuries (Chapter 42).

Giving the Bedpan

QUALITY OF LIFE

- Knock before entering the person's room.
- Address the person by name.
- Introduce yourself by name and title.

- Explain the procedure before starting and during the procedure.
- Protect the person's rights during the procedure.
- Handle the person gently during the procedure.

PRE-PROCEDURE

1 Follow *Delegation Guidelines: Bedpans*. See *Promoting Safety and Comfort*:
  a *Urinary Needs*, p. 410
  b *Voiding Equipment*
  c *Bedpans*
2 Practice hand hygiene.
3 Provide for privacy.
4 Get the following supplies.
  - Bedpan
  - Bedpan cover (if used)
  - Toilet paper

  - Waterproof under-pad
  - Disposable waterproof pad (as a barrier for the bedpan)
  - Bath blanket
  - Gloves
  - Laundry bag
5 Arrange equipment nearby. Place the bedpan on the chair or bed. Use the disposable waterproof pad as a barrier between the bedpan and the surface.
6 Raise the bed for body mechanics. Bed rails are up if used. Lower the bed rail near you if up.

Continued

Giving the Bedpan—cont'd

PROCEDURE

7 Lower the head of the bed. Position the person supine. Or raise the head of the bed slightly for comfort.

8 Cover the person with a bath blanket. Fold the top linens out of the way.

9 Apply gloves.

10 Fold back the person's gown and the bath blanket as needed. Keep the person covered as much as possible.

11 Place the bedpan.
  a *If the person can raise the hips to lift the buttocks off of the bed:*
    1) Have the person flex (bend) the knees and raise the buttocks. The person pushes against the mattress with the feet.
    2) Slide your hand under the lower back. Help raise the buttocks.
    3) Place a waterproof under-pad under the buttocks if not already in place.
    4) Slide the bedpan under the person (Fig. 27-5).
    5) Have the person lower the buttocks onto the bedpan.
  b *If the person cannot raise the hips:*
    1) Turn the person to position a waterproof under-pad if not already in place.
    2) Turn the person onto the side away from you.
    3) Place the bedpan firmly against the buttocks. Push downward on the bedpan and toward the person (Fig. 27-6).
    4) Hold the bedpan securely. Turn the person onto the back.
  c Make sure the bedpan is centered under the person. When the person sits up, the urethra and anus should be over the opening (Fig. 27-7).

12 Cover the person with the bath blanket.

13 Remove and discard the gloves. Practice hand hygiene.

14 Raise the head of the bed so the person is in a sitting position (Fowler's position) for a standard bedpan. Or raise the head of the bed to a comfortable level for the person.

15 Check that the person is correctly positioned on the bedpan (see Fig. 27-7).

16 Raise the bed rail if used. Lower the bed.

17 Place the toilet paper and call light within reach.

18 Ask the person to signal when done or when help is needed. (NOTE: For some state competency tests, you ask the person to use hand-wipes for hand hygiene after wiping with toilet paper.)

19 Stay with the person as needed. Or leave the room and close the door. (Practice hand hygiene before leaving.) Be respectful. Provide as much privacy as possible.

20 Return when the person signals. Or check on the person every 5 minutes. Knock before entering. Practice hand hygiene.

21 Raise the bed for body mechanics. Lower the bed rail if used. Lower the head of the bed.

22 Apply gloves.

23 Have the person raise the buttocks. Remove the bedpan. Or hold the bedpan and turn the person onto the side away from you. Place the bedpan on the disposable waterproof pad or in the cover (if used).

24 Clean the genital area if the person cannot do so.
  a Clean from the meatus (front or top) to the anus (back or bottom) with toilet paper. Use fresh toilet paper for each wipe. Place used toilet paper in the bedpan.
  b Provide perineal care if needed (Chapter 24).
  c Remove the waterproof under-pad if needed. Place it in the laundry bag.
  d Cover the person with the bath blanket.
  e Remove and discard the gloves. Practice hand hygiene. Apply clean gloves.
  f Lower the person's gown. Cover the person with the top linens. Remove the bath blanket. Place it in the laundry bag.

25 Raise the bed rail if used. Lower the bed.

26 Take the bedpan to the bathroom. Note the color, amount (output), and character of urine or feces (stools). See "Measuring Intake and Output" in Chapter 32.

27 Empty the bedpan contents into the toilet. Rinse the bedpan. Pour the rinse into the toilet and flush.

28 Follow agency procedures to clean and disinfect the bedpan. Return the bedpan to its proper place.

29 Remove and discard the gloves. Practice hand hygiene. Apply clean gloves.

30 Help the person with hand hygiene.

31 Remove and discard the gloves. Practice hand hygiene.

POST-PROCEDURE

32 Provide for comfort. (See the inside of the back cover.)

33 Lower the bed to a safe and comfortable level. Raise or lower bed rails. Follow the care plan.

34 Clean up and store supplies and equipment. (Wear gloves. Change gloves as needed.)
  a Discard disposable items.
  b Follow agency procedures to clean and disinfect re-usable equipment. Return supplies and equipment to their proper place.
  c Follow agency policy for used linens.
  d Clean and dry the over-bed table if used. Dry with paper towels. Discard paper towels. Position the over-bed table as the person prefers.
  e Remove and discard gloves. Practice hand hygiene.

35 Place the call light and other needed items within reach.

36 Follow the care plan and the person's preferences for privacy measures to maintain. Leaving the privacy curtain, window coverings, and door open or closed are examples.

37 Complete a safety check of the room. (See the inside of the back cover.)

38 Practice hand hygiene.

39 Report and record your care and observations.

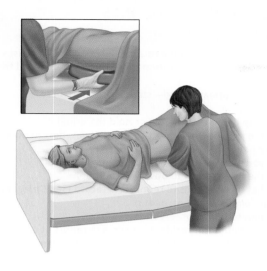

The person *can* raise the hips

FIGURE 27-5 Placing the bedpan when the person *can* raise the hips. Help the person raise the buttocks off of the bed if needed. Slide the bedpan under the person.

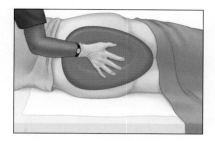
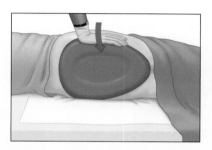

The person *cannot* raise the hips.

FIGURE 27-6 Placing the bedpan when the person *cannot* raise the hips. Turn the person to the side. Place the bedpan firmly against the buttocks. Push downward on the bedpan and toward the person. Turn the person onto the back.

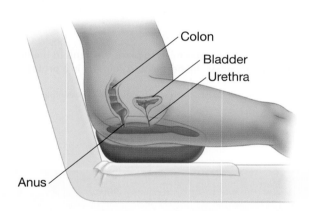

FIGURE 27-7 The person is positioned on the bedpan so the urethra and anus are directly over the opening.

Urinals

Urinals are used for voiding. Plastic urinals designed for men are common (Fig. 27-8). They have caps and hook-type handles. Men use urinals when standing (preferred), sitting, or lying in bed. Some men need support when standing. Urinals designed for females are less common. See "Female Urinals" on p. 418.

After use, the urinal cap is closed to prevent urine spills. Remind the person to use the call light after voiding. The urinal needs to be emptied as soon as possible to prevent spills, slipping and falls, and the growth of microbes. Remind the person not to place the urinal on the over-bed table or bedside stand. Follow agency policy for where to

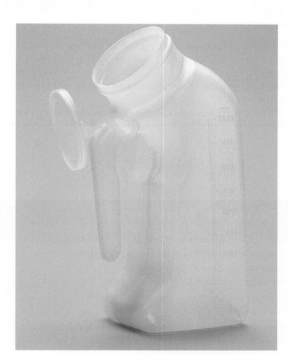

FIGURE 27-8 Urinal designed for males.

place the clean urinal. It may be hung on the bed rail or placed in a urinal holder attached to a bed rail, wheelchair, or walker (Fig. 27-9, p. 416).

See *Focus on Communication: Urinals*, p. 416.
See *Delegation Guidelines: Urinals*, p. 416.
See *Promoting Safety and Comfort: Urinals*, p. 416.
See procedure: *Giving the Male Urinal*, p. 416.

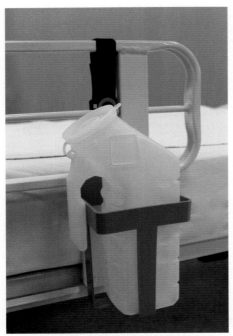

FIGURE 27-9 Urinal holder.

FOCUS ON COMMUNICATION

Urinals

You may need to assist some men with urinals. Or you may need to stay with the person. For comfort, explain why you must help. You can say:

- "I'll help you use the urinal. I need to stay with you so you don't fall."
- "I'll help you place and remove the urinal so it doesn't spill."

DELEGATION GUIDELINES

Urinals

Assisting with a urinal is a routine nursing task. To assist with a urinal, you need this information from the nurse and the care plan.

- How the urinal is used—standing, sitting, or lying in bed.
- If help is needed to place or hold the urinal.
- If the man needs support to stand. If yes, how many staff are needed.
- If you need to stay with the person.
- If the nurse needs to observe the urine.
- What observations to report and record (See *Delegation Guidelines: Bedpans*, p. 413).
- When to report observations.
- What patient or resident concerns to report at once.

PROMOTING SAFETY AND COMFORT

Urinals

Safety
Empty urinals promptly to prevent odors and the spread of microbes. A filled urinal spills easily, causing hazards. Also, it is an unpleasant sight and causes odor. Urinals are cleaned and disinfected after use.

Comfort
For some men, you may need to place the penis in the urinal. This may embarrass the person and you. Act in a professional manner.

Giving the Male Urinal

QUALITY OF LIFE

- Knock before entering the person's room.
- Address the person by name.
- Introduce yourself by name and title.

- Explain the procedure before starting and during the procedure.
- Protect the person's rights during the procedure.
- Handle the person gently during the procedure.

PRE-PROCEDURE

1 Follow *Delegation Guidelines: Urinals.* See *Promoting Safety and Comfort*:
   a *Urinary Needs*, p. 410
   b *Voiding Equipment*, p. 412
   c *Urinals*
2 Practice hand hygiene.
3 Provide for privacy.

4 Determine if the man will stand, sit, or lie in bed.
5 Get the following supplies.
   - Urinal
   - Slip-resistant footwear for standing (if needed)
   - Transfer belt (if needed)
   - Gloves

Giving the Male Urinal—cont'd

PROCEDURE

6 Apply gloves.
7 *Standing to use the urinal* (Fig. 27-10, *A*):
  a Prepare the person to stand. Help the person sit on the side of the bed. Apply slip-resistant footwear. Apply a transfer belt if needed (Chapter 15).
  b Help the person stand. Provide support if the person is unsteady.
  c Give the person the urinal.
8 *Using the urinal in bed* (Fig. 27-10, *B*):
  a Give the person the urinal.
  b Remind the person to tilt the bottom down to prevent spills.
9 Position the urinal and place the penis in the urinal if the person cannot do so.
10 *If the person can be left alone:*
  a Remove and discard the gloves. Practice hand hygiene.
  b Place the call light within reach. Ask the person to signal when done or when help is needed.
  c Maintain privacy measures. Cover the person for privacy if in bed.
  d Stay in the room or leave the room and close the door. Follow the care plan. Be respectful. Provide as much privacy as possible. (Practice hand hygiene before leaving the room.)
  e Return when the person signals. Or check on the person every 5 minutes. Knock before entering the room.
  f Practice hand hygiene. Apply gloves.

11 Close the urinal cap.
12 Assist with clothing and sitting as needed.
13 Take the urinal to the bathroom.
14 Note the color, amount (output), and clarity of urine.
15 Empty the urinal into the toilet. Rinse the urinal with cold water. Pour rinse into the toilet and flush.
16 Follow agency procedures to clean and disinfect the urinal. Return the urinal to its proper place.
17 Remove and discard the gloves. Practice hand hygiene. Apply clean gloves.
18 Assist with hand hygiene.
19 Remove and discard the gloves. Practice hand hygiene.

POST-PROCEDURE

20 Provide for comfort. (See the inside of the back cover.)
21 Make sure the bed is at a safe and comfortable level. Raise or lower bed rails. Follow the care plan.
22 Return supplies to their proper place.
23 Follow agency policy for any used linens.
24 Place the call light and other needed items within reach.

25 Follow the care plan and the person's preferences for privacy measures to maintain. Leaving the privacy curtain, window coverings, and door open or closed are examples.
26 Complete a safety check of the room. (See the inside of the back cover.)
27 Practice hand hygiene.
28 Report and record your care and observations.

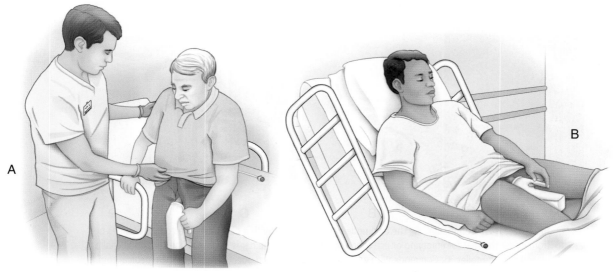

FIGURE 27-10 Using the male urinal. **A,** Standing. **B,** In bed.

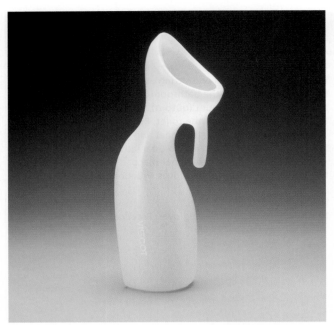

FIGURE 27-11 Urinal designed for females. (Courtesy Viscot Medical, LLC, East Hanover, NJ.)

Female Urinals. Female urinals are shaped to fit against a woman's body (Fig. 27-11). They can be used standing, sitting, or lying down (supine or lateral position). The device is positioned snugly under the urethra. The woman tilts her pelvis forward to the device when urinating. Proper positioning of the urinal is important to prevent leaking when voiding or removing the device.

Commodes

A commode (bedside commode) is a chair or wheelchair with an opening for a container (Fig. 27-12). Persons unable to walk to the bathroom often use commodes. The commode allows a normal position for elimination. The commode arms and back provide support and help prevent falls.

Some commodes, with the containers removed, are placed over toilets (see Fig. 27-12, *B*). The person uses the commode arms for support to sit and stand. And the commode serves as a higher toilet seat. If the commode has wheels (see Fig. 27-12, *C*), lock (brake) the wheels after properly positioning the commode.

See *Delegation Guidelines: Commodes*.
See *Promoting Safety and Comfort: Commodes*.
See procedure: *Helping the Person to the Commode*.

DELEGATION GUIDELINES
Commodes

Assisting with a commode is a routing nursing task. You need this information from the nurse and care plan when assisting with commode use.

- If the commode is used at the bedside or over the toilet
- How much help the person needs
- If you can leave the room or if you need to stay with the person
- If the nurse needs to observe urine or BMs before you flush the contents
- What observations to report and record (see *Delegation Guidelines: Bedpans*, p. 413)
- When to report observations
- What patient or resident concerns to report at once

PROMOTING SAFETY AND COMFORT
Commodes

Safety
You will transfer the person to and from the commode. Practice safe transfer procedures (Chapter 21). Use the transfer belt. Lock (brake) the wheels. Remove the transfer belt after the transfer. See "Transfer/Gait Belts" in Chapter 15.

Commodes are not shared among patients and residents. When no longer needed, the commode is returned to the supply department for disinfection.

Comfort
After transfer to the commode, cover the person's lap and legs with a bath blanket. This promotes warmth and privacy.

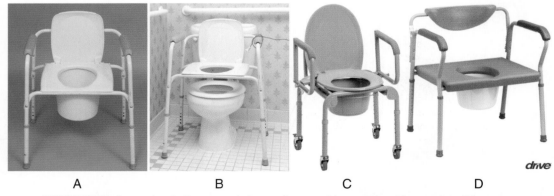

A   B   C   D

FIGURE 27-12 Commodes. **A,** The commode has a toilet seat with a container. The container slides out from under the seat for emptying or use over a toilet. **B,** The container is removed. The commode chair is placed over the toilet. **C,** Commode with wheels. **D,** Bariatric commode. (C, Courtesy drivemedical.com. D, Courtesy Medical Depot, Inc., Port Washington, NY.)

Helping the Person to the Commode

QUALITY OF LIFE

- Knock before entering the person's room.
- Address the person by name.
- Introduce yourself by name and title.

- Explain the procedure before starting and during the procedure.
- Protect the person's rights during the procedure.
- Handle the person gently during the procedure.

PRE-PROCEDURE

1 Follow *Delegation Guidelines: Commodes.* See *Promoting Safety and Comfort*:
  a *Urinary Needs,* p. 410
  b *Voiding Equipment,* p. 412
  c *Commodes*
2 Practice hand hygiene.
3 Provide for privacy.

4 Get the following supplies.
  - Commode
  - Toilet paper
  - Bath blanket
  - Transfer belt
  - Slip-resistant footwear
  - Gloves
  - Laundry bag
5 Arrange equipment. The commode is next to the bed. Check that the wheels are locked (braked) if present.

PROCEDURE

6 Help the person sit on the side of the bed. Follow the care plan for raising or lowering the bed rail.
7 Help the person put on slip-resistant footwear.
8 Apply the transfer belt.
9 Apply gloves if contact with urine or feces (stools) may occur.
10 Assist the person to the commode. Use the transfer belt. Help the person lower clothing as needed.
11 Remove and discard the gloves if worn and soiled. Practice hand hygiene after removing and discarding gloves.
12 Cover the person's lap and legs with a bath blanket for warmth and privacy. Remove the transfer belt.
13 Place the toilet paper within reach. (Provide hand-wipes if they are to be used for hand hygiene. Ask the person to use them after wiping with toilet paper.)
14 *If the person can be left alone:*
  a Place the call light within reach. Ask the person to signal when done or when help is needed.
  b Maintain privacy measures.
  c Stay in the room or leave the room and close the door. Follow the care plan. Be respectful. Provide as much privacy as possible. (Practice hand hygiene before leaving the room.)
  d Return when the person signals. Or check on the person every 5 minutes. Knock before entering.
  e Practice hand hygiene.

15 Apply gloves.
16 Remove the bath blanket. Place it in the laundry bag.
17 Help the person clean the genital area as needed. Remove and discard the gloves. Practice hand hygiene.
18 Apply the transfer belt. Help the person stand and fasten clothing as needed. Help the person back to bed using the transfer belt. Remove the transfer belt and footwear. Raise the bed rail if used.
19 Apply gloves. Remove and cover the commode container.
20 Take the container to the bathroom.
21 Observe urine and feces (stools) for color, amount (output), and character.
22 Empty the contents into the toilet. Rinse the container. Pour the rinse into the toilet and flush.
23 Follow agency procedures to clean and disinfect the container. Return the container to the commode. Close the lid.
24 Disinfect other parts of the commode if necessary.
25 Remove and discard the gloves. Practice hand hygiene. Apply clean gloves.
26 Assist with hand hygiene.
27 Remove and discard the gloves. Practice hand hygiene.

POST-PROCEDURE

28 Provide for comfort. (See the inside of the back cover.)
29 Make sure the bed is at a safe and comfortable level. Raise or lower bed rails. Follow the care plan.
30 Return supplies to their proper place.
31 Follow agency policy for used linens.
32 Place the call light and other needed items within reach.
33 Follow the care plan and the person's preferences for privacy measures to maintain. Leaving the privacy curtain, window coverings, and door open or closed are examples.

34 Complete a safety check of the room. (See the inside of the back cover.)
35 Practice hand hygiene.
36 Report and record your care and observations.

URINARY INCONTINENCE

Persons with urinary incontinence (UI) pass urine without intending to. Older persons are at risk for UI because of urinary tract changes, medical and surgical conditions, and drug therapy. Incontinence is not a normal part of aging.

Types of Urinary Incontinence

UI may be temporary or permanent. See Box 27-2 for risk factors and causes. Some factors can be reversed. Others cannot. Common types of incontinence are:

- *Stress incontinence*—Urine leaks during exercise and certain movements that cause pressure on the bladder. Urine loss is small. Often called *dribbling*, it occurs with laughing, sneezing, coughing, lifting, or other activities.
- *Urge incontinence*—Urine is lost in response to a sudden, urgent need to void. The person cannot get to a toilet in time. Urinary frequency, urinary urgency, and night-time voiding are common.
- *Mixed incontinence*—The person has a combination of stress incontinence and urge incontinence. Many older women have this type.
- *Over-flow incontinence*—Small amounts of urine leak from a full bladder. The person feels like the bladder is not empty. The person dribbles and may have a weak urine stream.
- *Functional incontinence*—The person has bladder control but cannot use the toilet in time. Immobility, restraints, unanswered call lights, no call light within reach, and difficulty removing clothing are causes. Not knowing where to find the bathroom, confusion, and disorientation are other causes.
- *Reflex incontinence*—Urine is lost at predictable intervals when a specific amount of urine is in the bladder. The person does not feel the need to void. Nervous system disorders and injuries are common causes.
- *Transient incontinence*—The person has temporary or occasional incontinence that is reversed when the cause is treated. (*Transient* means for a short time.)

BOX 27-2	Urinary Incontinence: Risk Factors and Causes

Risk Factors

- Women—pregnancy, childbirth, menopause
- Men—prostate problems
- Age—bladder muscles lose strength; the bladder holds less urine
- Over-weight—pressure on the bladder increases
- Smoking—coughing increases pressure on the bladder; irritates the bladder leading to over-active bladder
- *Over-active bladder (OAB)*—a condition in which there is a nearly constant urge to urinate; the person usually does not leak urine, but urge incontinence may develop
- Diabetes—nerve damage affects the bladder
- Kidney disease
- Immobility
- Restraint use
- Delays in voiding—see "Functional incontinence"
- Confusion and disorientation

Temporary Incontinence—Causes

- Alcohol and caffeine—increased urine production, stimulates the bladder leading to urge incontinence.
- Bladder irritation—some drinks and foods irritate the bladder. Sodas, tea, coffee, spicy foods, citrus fruits, and tomatoes are examples.
- Constipation or fecal impaction—irritates the nerves shared by the bladder and rectum. See Chapter 29.
- Delirium—see Chapter 54.
- Drug therapies.
- Increased fluid intake—urine production increases.
- Urinary tract infection (UTI)—irritates the bladder causing an urgent need to void.

Permanent Incontinence—Causes

- Aging changes
- Alzheimer's disease and other dementias (Chapter 54)
- Bladder cancer
- Hysterectomy—removal (*ectomy*) of the uterus (*hyster*) causing damage to the pelvic muscles
- Menopause
- Nervous system disorders (Chapter 49)
- Obstruction of the urinary tract
- Pregnancy and childbirth
- Prostate problems—prostatitis (inflammation [*itis*] of the prostate [*prostat*]), enlarged prostate, prostate cancer

Managing Urinary Incontinence

The goals of managing UI are to:
- Prevent urinary tract infections (UTIs).
- Restore as much bladder function as possible.

The person's care plan may include some of the measures listed in Box 27-3. *Good skin care and dry garments and linens are essential.* Promoting normal urinary elimination prevents incontinence in some people (see Box 27-1). Others need bladder training (p. 427). Sometimes catheters are needed (Chapter 28).

UI is embarrassing and uncomfortable. Garments are wet and odors develop. Skin irritation, infection, and pressure injuries are risks. Falls are a risk from trying to get to the bathroom quickly. Pride, dignity, and self-esteem are affected. Social isolation, loss of independence, and depression are common. Quality of life suffers.

UI is linked to abuse, mistreatment, and neglect. Frequent care is needed. The person may wet again right after skin care and changing wet garments and linens. Remember, the person does not choose to be incontinent. The person has the right to be free from abuse, mistreatment, and neglect. Kindness, empathy, understanding, and patience are needed.

See *Focus on Surveys: Managing Urinary Incontinence.*

See *Focus on Children and Older Persons: Managing Urinary Incontinence,* p. 422.

FOCUS ON SURVEYS

Managing Urinary Incontinence

Surveyors observe how incontinence is prevented, improved, or managed. They observe if staff:
- Follow the person's care plan.
- Keep call lights within reach.
- Answer call lights promptly.
- Provide a clear pathway to the bathroom.
- Provide good lighting for voiding.
- Assist with bedpans, urinals, and commodes as needed.
- Assist the person to the bathroom as needed.
- Respond appropriately when incontinence occurs.
- Protect the person's dignity when incontinence occurs.
- Check incontinent persons often.
- Change wet incontinence products and clothing promptly.
- Prevent prolonged exposure of the skin to urine.
- Provide hygiene measures to prevent skin breakdown.

BOX 27-3 Urinary Incontinence: Nursing Measures

- Record the person's voidings:
  - Incontinent
  - Successful use of the toilet, bedpan, urinal, or commode
- Record the amount voided (Chapter 32).
- Answer call lights promptly. The need to void may be urgent.
- Promote normal urinary elimination (see Box 27-1).
- Promote normal bowel elimination (Chapter 29).
- Assist with elimination at regular times—after sleep, before and after meals, at bedtime. Follow the person's routine. Assist promptly when help is requested.
- Encourage pelvic floor muscle exercises as instructed by the nurse (p. 427).
- Follow the person's bladder training program (p. 427).
- Provide a clear path to the bathroom.
- Have the person wear easy-to-remove clothing. UI can occur while dealing with buttons, zippers, other closures, and under-garments.
- Check the person often. Make sure the person is clean and dry.
- Help prevent UTIs.
  - Promote fluid intake as the nurse directs.
  - Have the person wear cotton underwear.
  - Keep the perineal area clean and dry.
  - Clean from front to back (top to bottom) during perineal care (Chapter 24).
- Decrease fluid intake at bedtime.
- Provide good skin care.
- Apply a barrier cream (ointment) to the skin or perineum as directed by the nurse. The application prevents irritation and skin damage.
- Provide dry garments and linens.
- Observe for signs of skin breakdown (Chapters 41 and 42).
- Use incontinence products as the nurse directs. Follow the manufacturer's instructions.
- Do not leave urinals in place to collect urine for persons who are incontinent.
- Keep the perineal area clean and dry (Chapter 24).
  - Protect the person and dry garments and linens from the wet incontinence product.
  - Remove wet incontinence products, garments, and linens.
  - Expose only the perineal area.
  - Use soap (or body wash) and water or a no-rinse product (perineal cleanser). Follow the care plan. For soap (or body wash) and water, use a safe and comfortable water temperature.
  - Dry the perineal area and buttocks.
  - Apply a clean, dry incontinence product and clean, dry garments and linens.
- Follow Standard Precautions. Follow the Bloodborne Pathogen Standard if blood is present. Follow the rules of hand hygiene and the guidelines for glove use in Chapters 17 and 18.

FOCUS ON CHILDREN AND OLDER PERSONS

Managing Urinary Incontinence

Children

Wetting in young children is normal. Diapers are worn until the child has bladder control (Chapters 11 and 56). Most children achieve day-time bladder control (dryness) between ages 2 and 4. Night-time bladder control comes later—usually by age 7.

Lack of bladder control when past the usual age of toilet training is called *enuresis*. Day-time enuresis is usually diagnosed around 5 or 6 years of age and night-time enuresis *(nocturnal enuresis; bed-wetting)* after age 7. Night-time enuresis is more common than day-time enuresis.

Bed-wetting can be caused by:

- Slower physical development. A small bladder holds less urine.
- Longer sleeping periods. More urine collects in the bladder over time.
- Producing more urine at night. The bladder over-fills.
- Not sensing a full bladder. The child does not wake up to void.
- Anxiety. Anxiety-causing events include moving, starting a new school, family events (a new baby, death, divorce), and abuse.
- Family history of bed-wetting.

Some health problems can cause enuresis. Constipation puts pressure on the bladder and can cause loss of bladder control. Other causes include UTI and other urinary tract problems, diabetes (Chapter 51), hormone problems, sleep apnea (Chapter 36), and nerve problems.

Other causes of day-time enuresis include:

- Over-active bladder. The child has urgency, urge incontinence, or urinary frequency—voids 8 or more times a day and at least 2 times at night.
- Infrequent voiding. The child holds urine for a long time. The urge to void is ignored, letting the bladder over-fill and leak. UTIs can develop.
- Incomplete voiding. The child does not relax enough to allow the bladder to empty. UTIs can develop.

Treatment depends on the cause. When caused by a health problem, the problem is treated. Treatment may also involve bladder training (p. 427), moisture alarms, and drug therapy. Rewarding the child for following the treatment plan, rather than staying dry, is important.

Older Persons

Complications from incontinence pose serious problems for older persons. These include falls, pressure injuries, and UTIs. Hospital or long-term care stays are often necessary.

Persons with dementia may void in the wrong places. Trash cans, planters, and closets are examples. Some persons throw incontinence products on the floor or in the toilet. Others resist staff efforts to stay clean and dry.

Provide safe care. The care plan may include measures recommended by the Alzheimer's Disease and Related Dementias Education and Referral Center (ADEAR).

- Remind the person to go to the bathroom every 2 to 3 hours during the day. Do not wait for the person to ask.
- Show the way or take the person to the bathroom.
- Keep pathways to the bathroom clear.
- Keep the bathroom clutter-free.
- Keep lights on in the pathway and bathroom.
- Have the person wear clothing and under-garments that are easy to remove.
- Post a big sign on the bathroom door that says "Toilet" or "Bathroom."
- Help the person in the bathroom.
- Observe for signs of needing to void. Restlessness and pulling at clothes are examples. Respond promptly.
- Stay calm when the person is incontinent. Give reassurance if the person is upset. (This means to help the person feel less upset and worried.)
- Report incontinence. Report the time, what the person was doing, and other observations. An incontinence pattern may emerge. If so, measures are planned to prevent the problem.
- Prevent incontinence during sleep. Limit the type and amount of fluids in the evening. Follow the care plan.
- Plan ahead for the person leaving the agency. Have the person wear easy-to-remove clothing. Pack extra clothing, incontinence products, and hygiene supplies. Know where to find restrooms.

You may need help to keep the person clean and dry. Ask your co-workers or the nurse for help. Remember, everyone has the right to privacy and safe care. They also have the right to be treated with dignity.

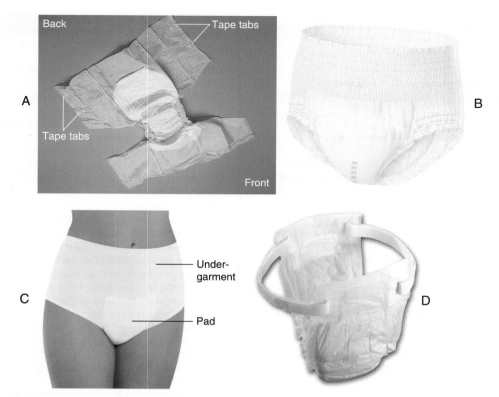

FIGURE 27-13 Disposable incontinence products. **A,** Complete incontinence brief. **B,** Pull-on underwear. **C,** Pad and under-garment. **D,** Belted under-garment. (B, Courtesy Hartmann, Inc., Heidenheim, Germany. C, Courtesy Hartmann USA, Inc., Rock Hill, SC. D, Courtesy Principle Business Enterprises, Dunbridge, Ohio.)

▥ Applying Incontinence Products

Incontinence products help keep the person dry. They usually have 2 layers and a waterproof back. Fluid passes through the top layer. It is absorbed by the bottom layer. Products come in various types and sizes.

Common incontinence products are shown in Figure 27-13. The nurse helps the person select products for his or her needs. To apply them, follow the manufacturer's instructions and agency procedures.

See *Focus on Communication: Applying Incontinence Products.*

See *Delegation Guidelines: Applying Incontinence Products.*

See *Promoting Safety and Comfort: Applying Incontinence Products*, p. 424.

See procedure: *Applying Incontinence Products*, p. 424.

FOCUS ON **COMMUNICATION**

Applying Incontinence Products

Incontinence products are often called "adult diapers." The word "diaper" may offend the person or lower self-esteem. Instead, say "brief," "pad," or "underwear." Some persons use the product's brand name. Use a term that promotes dignity and self-esteem.

DELEGATION GUIDELINES

Applying Incontinence Products

Changing incontinence products is a routine nursing task. To apply an incontinence product, you need this information from the nurse and the care plan.

- What product to use.
- What size to use.
- If a barrier cream (ointment) is needed. If yes, what product to use and how to apply it.
- What observations to report and record:
  - Complaints of pain, burning, irritation, or the need to void
  - Signs and symptoms of skin breakdown:
    - Redness, irritation, blisters
    - Complaints of pain, burning, tingling, or itching
  - The amount of urine—small, moderate, large
  - Urine color
  - Blood in the urine
  - Leakage
  - A poor product fit
- When to report observations.
- What patient or resident concerns to report at once.

PROMOTING SAFETY AND COMFORT
Applying Incontinence Products

Safety

To safely apply an incontinence product, follow the manufacturer's instructions. The guidelines in Box 27-4 will help prevent:

- Leakage
- Skin irritation, skin damage, and pressure injuries
- Tearing of the product

  Remove the soiled incontinence product from front to back (top to bottom). Apply the new product from front to back (top to bottom). In the procedure that follows, a new brief-style product is inserted between the legs from front to back while in the side-lying position. An alternative is to spread the back panel to cover the buttocks first, position the person supine, spread the legs, and bring the front of the product through the legs to spread the front panel. Use caution to prevent spreading bacteria from the anal area to the urinary system.

  Provide for safety if the person will stand for the procedure.

- Make sure the bed is in a low position that is safe and comfortable for the person.
- Lock (brake) the bed wheels.
- Have the person wear slip-resistant footwear.
- Provide something for the person to hold on to for balance and stability.

Comfort

For comfort, use the correct size. If the product is too large, urine can leak. If too small, the product will be too tight and uncomfortable.

BOX 27-4   Applying Incontinence Products

- Follow the manufacturer's instructions and the person's care plan.
- Use the correct size. The nurse or care plan tells you what size to use.
- Note the front and back of the product.
- Position the product correctly.
  - Center the product in the perineal area. For a male, the penis is downward.
  - Position the sides in the groin areas. The *groin* is where a thigh and the abdomen meet.
- Check for proper placement. The product should fit the shape of the body.
- Note the amount of urine (small, moderate, large). Also note how often you change the product. Large amounts of urine may require an extended-wear product.
- Do not let the plastic backing touch the person's skin.
- Provide perineal care after each incontinent episode.
- Do not use the product as a turning or lift sheet.
- Attach the tabs correctly. Some products will tear if you try to unfasten the tape or change the tape's position. Other products have adjustable tabs.
  - Attach the lower tab first. Attach it at a slightly upward angle. Do so for both sides.
  - Attach the upper tab after the lower tab is fastened. Attach it horizontally or at a slightly downward angle. Do so for both sides.

Applying Incontinence Products

QUALITY OF LIFE

- Knock before entering the person's room.
- Address the person by name.
- Introduce yourself by name and title.

- Explain the procedure before starting and during the procedure.
- Protect the person's rights during the procedure.
- Handle the person gently during the procedure.

PRE-PROCEDURE

1. Follow *Delegation Guidelines: Applying Incontinence Products*, p. 423. See *Promoting Safety and Comfort:*
   a *Urinary Needs*, p. 410
   b *Voiding Equipment*, p. 412
   c *Applying Incontinence Products*
2. Practice hand hygiene.
3. Provide for privacy.
4. Get the following supplies.
   - Incontinence product as directed by the nurse
   - Barrier cream (ointment) as directed by the nurse
   - Soap, body wash, or perineal cleanser
   - Items for perineal care (Chapter 24)
   - Waterproof under-pad—1 or 2 as needed
   - Bath blanket
   - Slip-resistant footwear if the person will stand
   - Towel or paper towels (as a barrier for supplies)
   - Plastic trash bag
   - Gloves
   - Laundry bag

5. Place the barrier (towel, paper towels) on the over-bed table. Arrange items on top.
6. Practice hand hygiene.
7. Identify the person. Check the identification (ID) bracelet against the assignment sheet. Use 2 identifiers (Chapter 14). Also call the person by name.
8. Mark the date, time, and your initials on the new product.
9. Fill the wash basin and place it on the over-bed table. Water temperature is usually 105°F to 109°F (Fahrenheit) (40.5°C to 42.7°C [centigrade]). Measure water temperature according to agency policy. Have the person check the water temperature. Adjust as needed.
10. Raise the bed for body mechanics (unless the person will stand). Bed rails are up if used. Lower the bed rail near you if up.

Applying Incontinence Products—cont'd

PROCEDURE

11 Position the person for the procedure. For this procedure, a brief is changed in bed. The person is on the back. The head of the bed is lowered as much as possible. (Note: Other products may be used. See step 17 [b and c] and step 24 [b and c] for others. The product may be changed in the bathroom. Have the person sit and stand as needed.)

12 Apply gloves.

13 Cover the person with a bath blanket. Lower top linens to the foot of the bed. If linens are wet, remove them and place them in the laundry bag.

14 Place a waterproof under-pad under the buttocks if not already in place. Replace a soiled under-pad. Have the person raise the buttocks off of the bed. Or turn the person from side to side. Position the person supine.

15 Move or remove clothing as needed. Lower or remove pants (slacks) if worn. Raise the person's gown if worn. Remove any wet garments. Follow agency policy for removed clothing.

16 Fold back the bath blanket. Keep the person covered as much as possible. Have the person spread the legs.

17 Remove the used product.
   a See Figure 27-14 (p. 426) for removal of a brief with the person in bed.
   b See Figure 27-15 (p. 426) for removal of a pad worn with an under-garment.
   c See Figure 27-16 (p. 427) for removal of pull-on underwear with the person standing.

18 Observe the urine during removal. Estimate the amount (small, medium, large). Observe for urine color and blood.

19 Place the used product in the trash bag. Tie or seal the bag and set it aside.

20 Perform perineal care (Chapter 24) wearing clean gloves. Clean all areas that had contact with urine. Wash, rinse, and dry the skin fold areas of the groin. Apply barrier cream (ointment) as directed.

21 Remove a wet waterproof under-pad. Place it in the laundry bag.

22 Remove and discard gloves. Practice hand hygiene. Apply clean gloves.

23 Place a clean waterproof under-pad under the buttocks if needed.

24 Apply the new product.
   a See Figure 27-14 (p. 426) for application of a brief with the person in bed.
   b See Figure 27-15 (p. 426) for application of a pad worn with an under-garment.
   c See Figure 27-16 (p. 427) for application of pull-on underwear with the person standing.

25 Smooth out all wrinkles and folds. Make sure the product is positioned correctly. It is centered in the perineal area with the sides in the groin areas. It fits the shape of the body.

26 Ask about comfort. Ask if the product feels too loose or too tight. Check for wrinkles or creases. Make sure the product does not rub or irritate the groin. Adjust the product as needed.

27 Raise or put on pants or slacks if worn. Or lower the person's gown.

28 Position the person for comfort. Cover the person. Remove the bath blanket. Place it in the laundry bag.

29 Assist the person with hand hygiene if needed. Remove and discard gloves. Practice hand hygiene.

POST-PROCEDURE

30 Provide for comfort. (See the inside of the back cover.)

31 Lower the bed to a safe and comfortable level. Raise or lower bed rails. Follow the care plan.

32 Clean up and store supplies and equipment. (Wear gloves. Change gloves as needed.)
   a Discard disposable items.
   b Empty the wash basin.
   c Follow agency procedures to clean and disinfect re-usable equipment. Return supplies and equipment to their proper place.
   d Follow agency policy for used linens.
   e Clean and dry the over-bed table. Dry with paper towels. Discard paper towels. Position the over-bed table as the person prefers.
   f Remove and discard gloves. Practice hand hygiene.

33 Place the call light and other needed items within reach.

34 Follow the care plan and the person's preferences for privacy measures to maintain. Leaving the privacy curtain, window coverings, and door open or closed are examples.

35 Complete a safety check of the room. (See the inside of the back cover.)

36 Practice hand hygiene.

37 Report and record your care and observations.

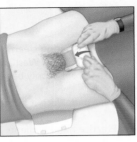 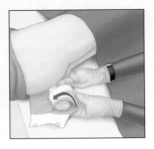

Remove the used brief.

1. Loosen all of the tabs on the brief. Tuck the far side of the back panel under the person.
    Roll the front of the product toward the back.
2. Have the person turn onto the side away from you. Continue rolling the product from front to back.
    Remove the used brief.

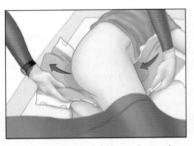 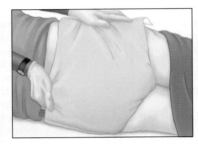 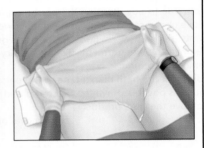

Apply a new brief. (Wear clean gloves.)

1. Position the person on the side facing away from you. Unfold the brief.
    Insert the brief between the legs from front to back.
2. Unfold and spread the back panel to cover the buttocks.
3. Position the person supine. Unfold and spread the front panel. Over-lap the back side panels over the front side panels.
4. Check the brief's alignment. The brief is centered in the perineal area and positioned high in the groin areas.
    The buttocks are covered. The brief fits the shape of the body. For a man, the penis is downward.

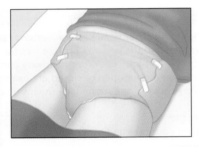

Secure the brief.

1. Attach the lower tabs at a slightly upward angle.
2. Attach the upper tabs horizontally or at a slightly downward angle.

FIGURE 27-14 Removing and applying an incontinence brief.

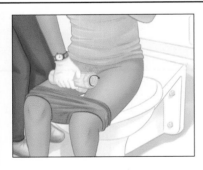 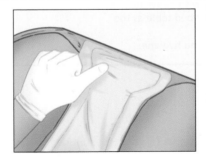 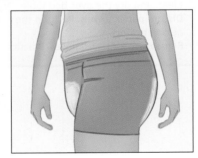

Remove the used pad.
1. Pull the under-garment down.
2. Roll the used pad from front to back.
    Remove the pad.

Apply a new pad. (Wear clean gloves.)
1. Unfold the new pad. Remove the covering from the pad's adhesive strip (if present).
    Insert the pad in the under-garment.
2. Have the person stand. Pull the under-garment up. Check that the pad is centered in the
    perineal area and is spread out smoothly.

FIGURE 27-15 Changing a pad worn with an under-garment.

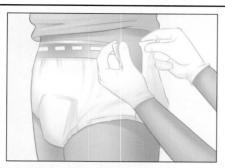
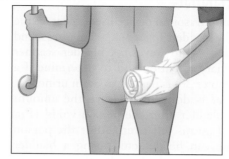

Remove the used underwear.
1. Tear the side seams of the used underwear.
2. Remove the used underwear from front to back. Roll the product with the soiled side inside.

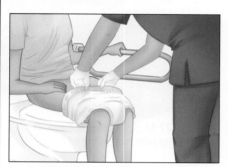
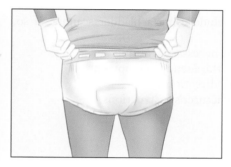

Apply new underwear. (Wear clean gloves.)
1. With the person sitting, slide the new underwear on. Pull them up over the feet to past the knees.
2. Have the person stand. Pull the underwear up.

FIGURE 27-16 Removing and applying pull-on underwear.

BLADDER TRAINING

Bladder training may help with incontinence. Control of urination is the goal. Bladder control promotes comfort and quality of life. It also increases self-esteem. Successful bladder training may take several weeks.

These methods may be used to help the person gain control of urination:

- *Pelvic floor muscle exercises (Kegel exercises).* The person is taught to contract pelvic muscles as if trying to stop a urine stream. The person contracts the muscles for about 3 to 5 seconds, relaxes, and contracts again. This is done 5 to 10 times. The exercises are done 3 to 4 times daily.
- *Bladder re-training (bladder rehabilitation).* The goal is to increase the time between the urge to void and voiding. The person is taught to:
  - Urinate following a schedule rather than the urge to void.
  - Resist the urge to urinate if it is not yet time to void.
  - Slowly increase the time between voids.

Some methods rely more on staff than the person. Such methods may be helpful for persons with confusion or dementia. Follow the person's care plan and the nurse's instructions to assist with the following methods.

- *Scheduled (timed) voiding.* Voiding is scheduled at regular times to match the person's voiding habits. Staff assist the person to void at scheduled times—every 2 hours during the day is common.
- *Prompted voiding.* The person learns to recognize the need to void and ask for help or void without help. Staff monitor, prompt, and provide positive feedback at regular times based on the person's voiding habits.
  - *Monitoring*—Staff ask about the need to void. Staff also may ask if the person feels wet or dry. The person is checked for incontinence and cleaned if needed.
  - *Prompting*—Staff ask the person to void. The person is never forced to try to void.
  - *Positive feedback*—Staff encourage correct awareness of being wet or dry and normal urination. Staff use positive words. Negative feedback is not given.

For persons preparing to stop the use of a urinary catheter (Chapter 28), the catheter may be clamped (pinched closed). This allows the bladder to fill. The catheter is unclamped (released) at scheduled times to empty the bladder. A bladder training method is used after catheter removal.

BLADDER SCANNING

A *bladder scanner* is an ultrasound device used to detect the amount of urine in the bladder (Fig. 27-17). (An ultrasound device functions using sound waves.) A bladder scanner may be used for urinary retention and to determine if a urinary catheter (Chapter 28) is needed to drain urine.

A *post-void residual* is done to measure the amount of urine left in the bladder after the person voids. (*Post* means after. *Residual* means left over.) After the person voids, residual urine can be detected using a bladder scanner. Ultrasound gel is applied on the abdomen over the bladder. A hand-held probe is placed over the site. The device scans and displays a measurement (volume in mL).

Your role may include using a bladder scanner. If so, make sure that you:

- Have received the necessary training.
- Know how to use the agency's equipment.
- Follow the nurse's directions.
- Follow the manufacturer's instructions.

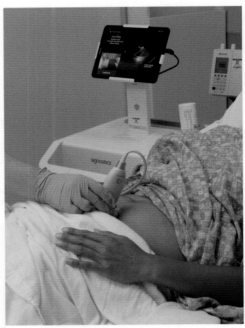

FIGURE 27-17 A bladder scanner. (From Williams P: *Fundamental concepts and skills for nursing,* ed 6, St Louis, 2023, Elsevier.)

FOCUS ON PRIDE

The Person, Family, and Yourself

Personal and Professional Responsibility

Some persons easily talk about urinary elimination. Others are shy or embarrassed. Note the person's verbal and nonverbal communication (Chapter 7). Watch for discomfort with words or topics. Be professional and speak with confidence. This puts the person at ease.

Rights and Respect

Illness and aging can affect voiding in private. Respect the right to privacy. Allow as much privacy as safely possible. If you must stay in the room, stand just outside the bathroom door in case the person needs you. Or stand on the other side of the privacy curtain if safe to do so. Follow the nurse's directions and the care plan.

Flush toilets and empty urinals, bedpans, and commodes promptly. The person has the right to a neat and clean setting. Do your best to promote comfort, dignity, and respect when assisting with elimination needs.

Independence and Social Interaction

Some persons can meet their own voiding needs. Others need some help but can be left alone to void. For persons needing some help, check on them often. Make sure the call light is within reach. Respond promptly.

Delegation and Teamwork

Accurate reporting and recording are important parts of delegation. See "Observations" on p. 411. Changes in urination may require changes in care. Report urinary problems and abnormal urine to the nurse. If unsure what to report or record, ask the nurse.

Ethics and Laws

Negligence occurs when a person does not act in a reasonable and careful manner and the person or the person's property is harmed (Chapter 5). The error is not intentional, but the negligent person is responsible. The following is a real example of negligent care.

A patient was admitted to the hospital with a diagnosis of mild pneumonia. He was to be in the hospital for 24 to 48 hours. While in the hospital, he was left on the bedpan for 4 hours. Pressure injuries resulted. He died of pneumonia after 41 days in the hospital.

His family sued the hospital. The jury awarded the family $800,000.

(Estate of D. Roberts v. William Beaumont Hospital, Mich., 2002.)

FOCUS ON PRIDE: *Application*

How does incontinence affect the person's dignity? How can it be prevented? Explain how your words and actions promote dignity when a person is incontinent.

REVIEW QUESTIONS

Circle the BEST answer.

1 Which is abnormal?
 a Clear, pale yellow urine
 b Urine with a faint odor
 c Cloudy urine with particles
 d Urine output of 1500 mL in 24 hours

2 Which prevents normal elimination?
 a Helping the person assume a normal position for voiding
 b Providing privacy
 c Helping the person to the bathroom as soon as requested
 d Staying with the person who uses a bedpan

3 Which definition is *correct?*
 a Dysuria means painful or difficult urination.
 b Oliguria means a large amount of urine.
 c Urinary retention means the need to void at once.
 d Urinary incontinence means the inability to void.

4 The person using a standard bedpan is in
 a Fowler's position
 b The supine position
 c The prone position
 d The side-lying position

5 When using a fracture pan
 a The person is in Fowler's position
 b The smaller end (flat end) is under the buttocks
 c The nurse must position the pan
 d The pan can be left in place for a long time

6 After using the urinal, the person should
 a Put it on the bedside stand
 b Use the call light
 c Put it on the over-bed table
 d Empty it

7 A person is at risk for falling. What should you explain before commode use?
 a "Do not use the armrests on the commode for support."
 b "The wheels on the commode are unlocked for your safety."
 c "I will leave the room while you use the commode."
 d "I need to apply a transfer belt."

8 After a person uses a commode, you should
 a Empty, rinse, clean, and disinfect the container
 b Return the commode to the supply area
 c Get a new container
 d Get a new commode

9 Urinary incontinence
 a Cannot be treated
 b Does not have mental or social effects
 c Is a normal part of aging
 d Requires good skin care

10 Which is a cause of functional incontinence?
 a A nervous system disorder
 b Sneezing
 c Unanswered call light
 d UTI

11 A resident with dementia is restless and pulling at the pants. What should you do *first?*
 a Distract the person with an activity
 b Help the person to use the bathroom
 c Play calming music
 d Take the person for a walk

12 When applying an incontinence product
 a Make sure the product is loose in the groin area
 b Remove the old product from back to front
 c Use the correct size
 d Use the product to turn and position the person

13 The goal of bladder training is to
 a Control the amount voided daily
 b Promote voiding at times best for staff
 c Allow the person to walk to the bathroom
 d Gain control of urination

14 Bladder re-training involves
 a Resisting the urge to void
 b Voiding every time the urge is felt
 c Negative feedback when incontinence occurs
 d Frequent voiding throughout the day and night

15 A person is incontinent. Which statement promotes dignity?
 a "You are doing this on purpose."
 b "Why didn't you ask for help like I told you to?"
 c "I will help you get clean and dry."
 d "This is the last time I am going to clean you today."

Answers to Chapter 27 questions are on p. 902.

FOCUS ON **PRACTICE**
Problem Solving

You assist a patient onto the commode. The person is unsteady and cannot be left alone. The person says: "I can't go if you stand here." What do you do? How will you provide privacy and safe care?

Urinary Catheters

OBJECTIVES

- Define the key terms and key abbreviations in this chapter.
- Explain why urinary catheters are used.
- Describe 4 types of urinary catheters.
- Explain the purpose and rules for catheter care.
- Describe 2 urine drainage systems.
- Explain how to re-connect a catheter and drainage tubing.

- Explain how to remove an indwelling catheter.
- Explain how to apply a condom catheter.
- Perform the procedures described in this chapter.
- Explain how to promote PRIDE in the person, the family, and yourself.

KEY TERMS

catheter A tube used to drain or inject fluid through a body opening
catheterization The process of inserting a catheter
condom catheter A soft sheath that slides over the penis and is used to drain urine
Foley catheter See "indwelling catheter"
gravity A natural force that pulls things downward

indwelling catheter A catheter left in the bladder so urine drains constantly into a drainage bag; retention or Foley catheter
retention catheter See "indwelling catheter"
straight catheter A catheter that drains the bladder and then is removed
supra-pubic catheter A catheter surgically inserted into the bladder through an incision above *(supra)* the pubis bone *(pubic)*

KEY ABBREVIATIONS

BM	Bowel movement		IV	Intravenous
CAUTI	Catheter-associated urinary tract infection		mL	Milliliter
ID	Identification		UTI	Urinary tract infection

A *catheter* is a tube used to drain or inject fluid through a body opening. A urinary catheter drains urine. *Catheterization* is the process of inserting a catheter. You need to understand your role and the measures needed to safely care for urinary catheters.

See *Focus on Surveys: Urinary Catheters.*
See *Promoting Safety and Comfort: Urinary Catheters.*

FOCUS ON SURVEYS

Urinary Catheters

Surveys are done to check the quality of treatments and services. The surveyor may ask you about:
- Your training in handling catheters, catheter tubing, drainage bags, catheter care, urinary tract infections (UTIs), catheter-related injuries, dislodgment (moving out of place), and skin breakdown
- What observations to report, when to report them, and to whom you should report

Answer questions the best you can. If you do not know an answer, tell the surveyor who you would ask or where you would find the answer.

PROMOTING SAFETY AND COMFORT

Urinary Catheters

Safety
Urinary catheter procedures often involve exposing and touching the perineum. Sexual abuse has occurred in health care settings. The person may feel threatened or is actually being abused. The person needs to be able to call for help. Keep the call light within the person's reach at all times. Always act in a professional manner.

Urine is a body fluid. Follow Standard Precautions for the procedures in this chapter. Follow the Bloodborne Pathogen Standard if blood is present. Follow the rules of hand hygiene and the guidelines for glove use in Chapters 17 and 18.

In nursing centers, follow agency policies and procedures for using Enhanced Barrier Precautions when the person has an indwelling medical device. A urinary catheter is an indwelling medical device. High-contact tasks and tasks involving the catheter require routine gown and glove use. See Chapter 18.

CATHETERS

There are different types of catheters:

- A *straight catheter* drains the bladder and then is removed.
- An *indwelling catheter* (*retention* or *Foley catheter*) is left in the bladder. Urine drains constantly into a drainage bag. A balloon by the tip is inflated with sterile water after the catheter is inserted. The balloon prevents the catheter from coming out of the bladder (Fig. 28-1). Tubing connects the catheter to a urine drainage bag. See Figure 28-2 for parts of an indwelling catheter and urine drainage system.
- A *supra-pubic catheter* is surgically inserted into the bladder through an incision above *(supra)* the pubis bone *(pubic)*. See Figure 28-3. Less common than the others, a supra-pubic catheter may be placed when the urethra is blocked or when a catheter is needed long-term.
- An *external catheter* is not inserted into the bladder. Used for men, a *condom catheter* is a soft sheath that slides over the penis. See "Condom Catheters" on p. 443. For women, see "Female External Catheters" on p. 446.

See *Focus on Long-Term Care and Home Care: Catheters*, p. 432.

See *Delegation Guidelines: Catheters*, p. 432.

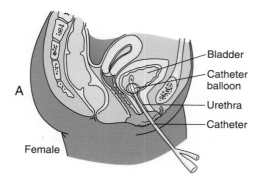
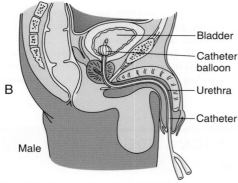

FIGURE 28-1 Indwelling catheter. **A**, Indwelling catheter in the female bladder. The inflated balloon at the tip prevents the catheter from slipping out through the urethra. **B**, Indwelling catheter with the balloon inflated in the male bladder.

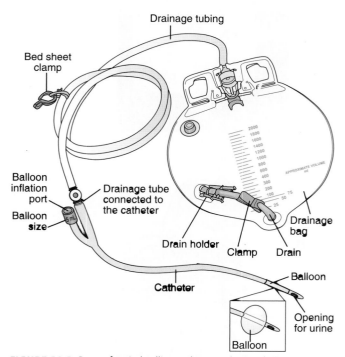

FIGURE 28-2 Parts of an indwelling catheter and urine drainage system.

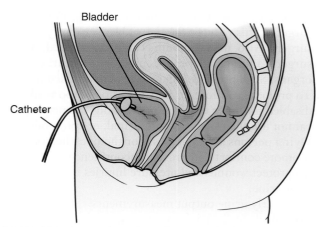

FIGURE 28-3 Supra-pubic catheter. (From Kostelnick C: *Mosby's textbook for long-term care nursing assistants*, ed 8, St Louis, 2020, Elsevier.)

Purposes of Catheters

Catheters are used:
- To keep the bladder empty before, during, and after surgery. This reduces the risk of bladder injury during surgery. Also, urine amounts can be monitored. After surgery, a full bladder causes pressure on nearby organs. Such pressure can lead to pain or discomfort.
- To promote comfort for persons who are too weak or disabled for other elimination methods. Some people cannot use the toilet, bedpan, urinal, or commode. Dying persons are examples. For them, catheters can promote comfort and prevent incontinence.
- To protect wounds and pressure injuries from contact with urine.
- For hourly urine output measurements.
- To collect sterile urine specimens.
- For urinary retention.
- To measure the amount of urine in the bladder after the person voids *(residual urine)*.

Catheters do not treat the cause of incontinence. They are a last resort for incontinence.

Catheter-Associated UTIs

The urinary system is sterile. Infection can occur if microbes enter. Catheters create a high risk for UTIs. A *catheter-associated urinary tract infection (CAUTI)* occurs when microbes enter the urinary tract through the catheter and cause an infection. Microbes travel up the catheter into the bladder and kidneys. CAUTIs can cause severe illness and death. Short-term use and proper catheter care can reduce the risk of a CAUTI.

◼ CATHETER CARE

You will care for persons with indwelling catheters. Follow the rules in Box 28-1 to promote safety and comfort.

See *Delegation Guidelines: Catheter Care*, p. 434.
See *Promoting Safety and Comfort: Catheter Care*, p. 434.
See procedure: *Giving Catheter Care*, p. 435.

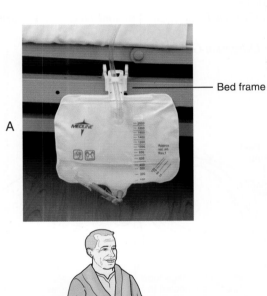

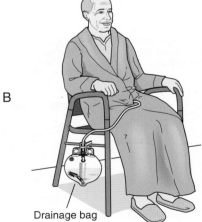

FIGURE 28-4 A, Urine drainage bag secured to the bed frame. The bag does not touch the floor. **B,** Urine drainage bag secured to a chair.

BOX 28-1	Indwelling Catheter Care

Preventing Infection
- Follow the rules of medical asepsis.
- Follow Standard Precautions. Follow the Bloodborne Pathogen Standard if blood is present.
- Encourage fluid intake as directed by the nurse and care plan.

The Drainage System
- Allow urine to flow freely through the catheter and drainage tube. Tubing should not have kinks. The person should not lie on the tubing.
- Keep the catheter connected to the drainage tube. Follow the measures on p. 436 if the catheter and drainage tube are disconnected.
- Keep the drainage tube and bag below the bladder. This prevents urine from flowing backward into the bladder. For a bed or chair transfer, keep the drainage bag lower than the bladder. Secure the drainage bag to the bed frame or chair after the transfer. See Figure 28-4.
- Move the drainage bag to the other side of the bed for turning and re-positioning on the other side.
- Hang the bag from the bed frame, lower part of the chair or wheelchair, or lower part of the IV (intravenous) pole.
- *Do not hang the drainage bag on a bed rail*. The bag is higher than the bladder when the bed rail is raised.
- Position tubing so it will not get tangled in wheelchair wheels.
- Hold the bag lower than the bladder when the person walks.
- *Do not let the drainage bag touch or rest on the floor*. This can contaminate the system.
- Position drainage tubing in a straight line or coil it on the bed. Secure it to the bottom linens (Fig. 28-5). Follow the nurse's directions and agency policy. Use a clip, bed sheet clamp, or other device as the nurse directs. Tubing must not loop below the drainage bag.

The Catheter
- Secure the catheter as the nurse directs.
  - Females: to the thigh (see Fig. 28-5, *A*).
  - Males:
    - To the thigh (see Fig. 28-5, *B*).
    - To the lower abdomen (see Fig. 28-5, *C*). This site may be used for long-term catheter use. The drainage bag remains below the bladder. Drainage is not affected.

The Catheter—cont'd
- Use a tube holder, tape, leg band, or other device to secure the catheter to the thigh or abdomen (Fig. 28-6, p. 434). The nurse tells you what to use. Securing the catheter prevents excess movement and friction at the insertion site (meatus). Catheter movement and friction can damage the meatus.
- Check for leaks. Check the connections to the drainage tube and the drainage bag. Report any leaks at once.
- Provide perineal care and catheter care according to the care plan—daily, twice a day, after bowel movements (BMs), or when vaginal discharge is present. (See procedure: *Giving Catheter Care*, p. 435.)

Measuring Urine (Output)
- Empty the drainage bag and measure urine:
  - At the end of the shift
  - To change to and from a leg bag and a standard drainage bag (p. 436)
  - When the bag is becoming full
  - Before measuring the person's weight (Chapter 37)
- Report an increase or decrease in urine amount.
- Provide a measuring container (graduate) for each person. This prevents the spread of microbes from 1 person to another.
- Do not let the drain on the drainage bag touch any surface.
- See procedure: *Emptying a Urine Drainage Bag*, p. 437.

Observations
- Report complaints at once—pain, burning, the need to void, or irritation. Also report the color, clarity, and odor of urine and the presence of particles or blood.
- Observe for signs and symptoms of a UTI. Report the following at once.
  - Fever.
  - Chills.
  - Flank pain or tenderness. The flank area is in the back between the ribs and the hip.
  - Change in the urine—blood, foul smell, particles, cloudiness, *oliguria* (scant [small] amount of urine).
  - Change in mental or functional status—confusion, decreased appetite, falls, decreased activity, tiredness, and so on.
  - Urine leakage around the catheter.

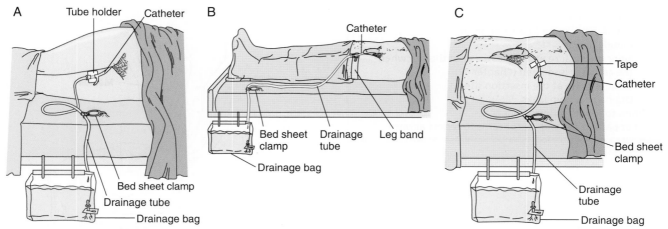

FIGURE 28-5 Securing catheters. **A,** This catheter is secured to the woman's thigh with a tube holder. The drainage tube is coiled on the bed and secured to bottom linens with a bed sheet clamp. **B,** This catheter is secured to the man's thigh with a leg band. Drainage tubing is in a straight line and secured to bottom linens with a bed sheet clamp. The drainage bag is at the foot of the bed. **C,** This catheter is secured to the man's lower abdomen with tape. Drainage tubing is secured to bottom linens with a bed sheet clamp.

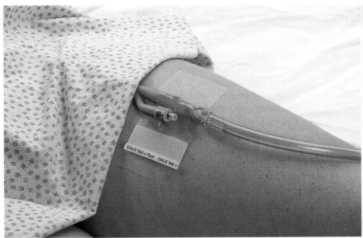 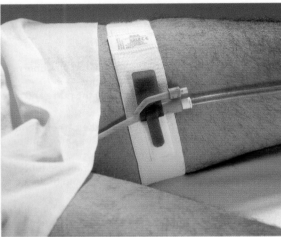

FIGURE 28-6 Catheter securing devices. **A,** Tube holder. **B,** Leg band. (© 2013–2016 Dale Medical Products, Inc. All rights reserved.)

DELEGATION GUIDELINES

Catheter Care

Catheter care is a routine nursing task. You need this information from the nurse and the care plan.

- When to give catheter care—daily, twice a day, after BMs, or because of vaginal discharge
- What water temperature to use for perineal care
- Where to secure the catheter—which thigh (sites are rotated to prevent skin breakdown) or the lower abdomen (for some males)
- How to secure the catheter—tube holder, leg band, tape, or other device
- How to position the drainage tubing—straight line or coiled on the bed
- Where to secure the drainage tubing and hang the drainage bag—bed, chair, or wheelchair
- How to secure drainage tubing—clip, bed sheet clamp, or other device
- What observations to report and record:
  - Complaints of pain, burning, irritation, or the need to void (report at once)
  - Crusting, abnormal drainage, or secretions
  - The color, clarity, and odor of urine
  - Particles in the urine
  - Blood in the urine (report at once)
  - Cloudy urine
  - Signs of pressure at the meatus or at the site where the catheter is secured (Chapter 42)
  - Urine leaking at the insertion site
  - Drainage system leaks
- When to report observations
- What patient or resident concerns to report at once

PROMOTING SAFETY AND COMFORT

Catheter Care

Safety

In some agencies, perineal care (Chapter 24) is sufficient hygiene for indwelling catheters. If so, step 17 in the procedure that follows is not performed. Follow agency policy and the care plan when a person has a catheter.

When giving catheter care, clean, rinse, and dry the catheter from the meatus down at least 4 inches. Move in 1 direction (away from the meatus). If needed, repeat with a clean area of the washcloth (towel) or a clean washcloth (towel).

Comfort

The catheter must not pull at the insertion site. This causes discomfort and irritation. Hold the catheter securely during catheter care. Then properly secure the catheter. Make sure the tubing is not under the person. Besides blocking urine flow, lying on the tubing is uncomfortable. It can also cause skin breakdown. To promote comfort, see Box 28-1.

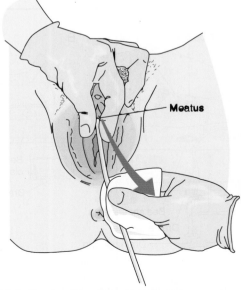

FIGURE 28-7 Cleaning the catheter. Hold the catheter at the meatus. Start at the meatus. Clean downward, away from the meatus. Clean at least 4 inches of the catheter.

Giving Catheter Care

QUALITY OF LIFE

- Knock before entering the person's room.
- Address the person by name.
- Introduce yourself by name and title.

- Explain the procedure before starting and during the procedure.
- Protect the person's rights during the procedure.
- Handle the person gently during the procedure.

PRE-PROCEDURE

1 Follow *Delegation Guidelines:*
  - *Perineal Care* (Chapter 24)
  - *Catheter Care*
  See *Promoting Safety and Comfort:*
  - *Perineal Care* (Chapter 24)
  - *Urinary Catheters,* p. 430
  - *Catheter Care*
2 Practice hand hygiene and get the following supplies.
  - Items for perineal care (Chapter 24)
  - At least 2 washcloths and 1 towel for catheter care
  - Bath blanket
  - Towel or paper towels (as a barrier for supplies)
  - Gloves
  - Laundry bag

3 Place the barrier (towel, paper towels) on the over-bed table. Arrange items on top.
4 Practice hand hygiene.
5 Identify the person. Check the identification (ID) bracelet against the assignment sheet. Use 2 identifiers (Chapter 14). Also call the person by name.
6 Fill the wash basin and place it on the over-bed table. Water temperature is about 105°F to 109°F (Fahrenheit) (40.5°C to 42.7°C [centigrade]). Measure water temperature according to agency policy. Have the person check the water temperature and adjust as needed.
7 Provide for privacy.
8 Raise the bed for body mechanics. Bed rails are up if used. Lower the bed rail near you if up.

PROCEDURE

9 Cover the person with a bath blanket. Fan-fold top linens to the foot of the bed.
10 Place the waterproof under-pad under the buttocks. To do so, have the person raise the buttocks off of the bed. Or turn the person from side to side.
11 Position and drape the person for perineal care (Chapter 24).
12 Practice hand hygiene. Apply gloves.
13 Fold back the bath blanket to expose the perineal area.
14 Check the drainage tubing. Make sure it is not kinked and that urine can flow freely.
15 Separate the labia (female). In an uncircumcised male, retract the foreskin (Chapter 24). Check for crusts, abnormal drainage, or secretions. Check for signs of pressure at the meatus (Chapter 42).
16 Give perineal care (Chapter 24). Keep the foreskin of the uncircumcised male retracted until step 19.
17 Clean, rinse, and dry the catheter.
  a Apply soap, body wash, or other cleansing agent to a clean, wet washcloth.
  b Hold the catheter at the meatus (Fig. 28-7). Do so for all of step 17.
  c Clean the catheter from the meatus down the catheter at least 4 inches. Clean downward, away from the meatus, with 1 stroke. See Figure 28-7. Do not tug or pull on the catheter. Repeat as needed with a clean area of the washcloth. Use another clean washcloth if needed.

  d Wet a clean, soap-free washcloth.
  e Rinse from the meatus down the catheter at least 4 inches. Rinse downward, away from the meatus, with 1 stroke. Do not tug or pull on the catheter. Repeat as needed with a clean area of the washcloth. Use another clean washcloth if needed.
  f Dry from the meatus down the catheter at least 4 inches. Do not tug or pull on the catheter.
18 Pat dry the perineal area. Dry from front to back (top to bottom).
19 Return the foreskin (uncircumcised male) to its natural position.
20 Secure the catheter. Position the tubing in a straight line or coiled on the bed. Follow the nurse's directions. Secure the tubing to the bottom linens (see Fig. 28-5).
21 Cover the person with the bath blanket. Remove the waterproof under-pad. Place it in the laundry bag.
22 Remove and discard the gloves. Practice hand hygiene.
23 Cover the person. Remove the bath blanket. Place it in the laundry bag.

POST-PROCEDURE

24 Provide for comfort. (See the inside of the back cover.)
25 Lower the bed to a safe and comfortable level. Raise or lower bed rails. Follow the care plan.
26 Clean up and store supplies and equipment. (Wear gloves. Change gloves as needed.)
  a Discard disposable items.
  b Empty the wash basin.
  c Follow agency procedures to clean and disinfect re-usable equipment. Return supplies and equipment to their proper place.
  d Follow agency policy for used linens.

  e Clean and dry the over-bed table. Dry with paper towels. Discard paper towels. Position the over-bed table as the person prefers.
  f Remove and discard gloves. Practice hand hygiene.
27 Place the call light and other needed items within reach.
28 Follow the care plan and the person's preferences for privacy measures to maintain. Leaving the privacy curtain, window coverings, and door open or closed are examples.
29 Complete a safety check of the room. (See the inside of the back cover.)
30 Practice hand hygiene.
31 Report and record your care and observations.

URINE DRAINAGE SYSTEMS

A closed drainage system is used for indwelling catheters. Only urine should enter the system. See Box 28-1 to prevent infection and for proper care of the drainage system.

There are 2 types of urine drainage bags.

- *Standard drainage bags* usually hold at least 2000 mL (milliliters) of urine (see Fig. 28-4).
- *Leg bags* attach to the thigh or calf with elastic bands or Velcro (Fig. 28-8). Leg bags hold less than 1,000 mL of urine.

Drainage systems can become disconnected. If that happens, tell the nurse at once. Do not touch the ends of the catheter or tubing. Box 28-2 describes how to re-connect the catheter and tubing.

A graduate (measuring container for fluid) is used when emptying drainage bags. You will learn how to measure liquids using a graduate in Chapter 32.

See *Delegation Guidelines: Urine Drainage Systems*.
See *Promoting Safety and Comfort: Urine Drainage Systems*.
See procedure: *Emptying a Urine Drainage Bag*.
See procedure: *Changing a Leg Bag to a Standard Drainage Bag*, p. 438.

BOX 28-2	Re-Connecting a Catheter and Drainage Tube

1 Practice hand hygiene. Put on gloves.
2 Wipe the end of the drainage tube with an antiseptic wipe.
3 Wipe the end of the catheter with another antiseptic wipe.
4 Do not put the ends down. Do not touch the ends after you clean them.
5 Connect the drainage tubing to the catheter.
6 Discard the wipes following agency policy.
7 Remove the gloves. Practice hand hygiene.

DELEGATION GUIDELINES
Urine Drainage Systems

Some persons use a standard drainage bag overnight and a leg bag during the day. Some agencies allow nursing assistants to change the drainage bag. If the task is delegated to you, make sure that:

- Your state allows you to perform the task.
- The task is in your job description (Chapter 3).
- You have the necessary education and training.
- The agency has determined that you are competent to perform the task safely.
- You know how to use the supplies and equipment.
- You review the procedure with the delegating nurse.
- The delegating nurse is available to answer questions and to guide and assist you as needed.

Emptying a urine drainage bag is a routine nursing task. You need this information from the nurse and the care plan to perform routine emptying or to change a drainage bag.

- What type of bag is used—standard drainage bag or leg bag
- When to empty or change the urine drainage bag
- What observations to report and record:
  - The amount of urine measured (Chapter 32)
  - The color, clarity, and odor of urine
  - Particles in the urine
  - Blood in the urine
  - Cloudy urine
  - Complaints of pain, burning, irritation, or the need to void
  - Drainage system leaks
- When to report observations
- What patient or resident concerns to report at once

To change a urine drainage bag, you also need this information.

- When to switch a standard drainage bag and leg bag
- What leg bag straps to use for application—elastic or Velcro
- Where to secure a leg bag—thigh or calf
- If you should clean and disinfect or discard the drainage bag
- What product to use and the procedure to follow for cleaning, disinfection, and storing

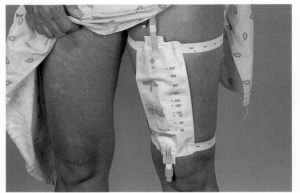

FIGURE 28-8 A leg bag. (From Elkin MK, Perry AG, Potter PA: *Nursing interventions and clinical skills*, ed 3, St Louis, 2004, Mosby.)

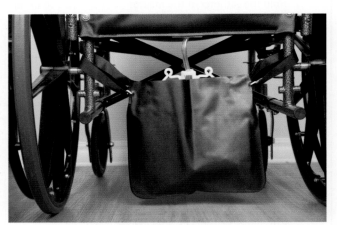

FIGURE 28-9 Drainage bag holder.

PROMOTING SAFETY AND COMFORT

Urine Drainage Systems

Safety
Urine drains from the bladder through the catheter and into a drainage bag. Gravity allows urine to drain. *Gravity* is a natural force that pulls things downward. Always keep the drainage bag below bladder level. This allows urine to flow downward from the force of gravity.

For the procedure: *Changing a Leg Bag to a Standard Drainage Bag* (p. 438), you will open sterile packages and the closed drainage system. You must keep sterile items free from contamination. You must prevent microbes from entering the system. Aseptic practices are required (Chapter 17). Follow the drainage bag manufacturer's instructions and agency procedures.

Leg bags hold less urine than standard drainage bags. Check leg bags often. Empty the leg bag if it is becoming half full. Measure, report, and record the amount of urine.

Comfort
Urine in a drainage bag embarrasses some people. Visitors can see the urine. To promote mental comfort, have visitors sit on the side away from the drainage bag. Try to empty the bag before visitors arrive. Measure, report, and record the amount of urine.

Some agencies have drainage bag holders (privacy bags) (Fig. 28-9). The drainage bag is placed inside the holder. The holder promotes privacy and keeps the drainage bag off of the floor.

Emptying a Urine Drainage Bag

QUALITY OF LIFE
- Knock before entering the person's room.
- Address the person by name.
- Introduce yourself by name and title.
- Explain the procedure before starting and during the procedure.
- Protect the person's rights during the procedure.
- Handle the person gently during the procedure.

PRE-PROCEDURE
1 Follow *Delegation Guidelines: Urine Drainage Systems.* See *Promoting Safety and Comfort:*
- *Urinary Catheters*, p. 430
- *Urine Drainage Systems*
2 Practice hand hygiene and get the following supplies.
- Graduate (measuring container)
- Gloves
- Paper towels or a disposable waterproof pad
- Antiseptic wipe
3 Arrange items in the person's room.
4 Practice hand hygiene.
5 Identify the person. Check the ID bracelet against the assignment sheet. Use 2 identifiers (Chapter 14). Also call the person by name.
6 Provide for privacy.

PROCEDURE
7 Apply gloves.
8 Place a paper towel or disposable waterproof pad on the floor. Place the graduate on top of it.
9 Place the graduate under the drainage bag.
10 Open the clamp on the drain.
11 Let all urine drain into the graduate. The drain does not touch the graduate (Fig. 28-10, p. 438).
12 Clean the end of the drain with an antiseptic wipe. Discard the wipe following agency policy.
13 Clamp and position the drain in the holder (Fig. 28-11, p. 438).
14 Measure urine. See procedure: *Measuring Intake and Output* in Chapter 32.
15 Remove and discard the paper towel or disposable waterproof pad.
16 Empty the graduate into the toilet. Rinse the graduate. Empty the rinse into the toilet and flush.
17 Follow agency procedures to clean and disinfect the graduate. Return the graduate to its proper place.
18 Remove and discard the gloves. Practice hand hygiene.
19 Record the time and amount of urine on the intake and output (I&O) record (Chapter 32).

POST-PROCEDURE
20 Provide for comfort. (See the inside of the back cover.)
21 Place the call light and other needed items within reach.
22 Follow the care plan and the person's preferences for privacy measures to maintain. Leaving the privacy curtain, window coverings, and door open or closed are examples.
23 Complete a safety check of the room. (See the inside of the back cover.)
24 Practice hand hygiene.
25 Report and record your care and observations.

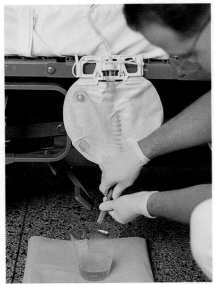

FIGURE 28-10 The clamp on the drainage bag is opened. The drain is directed into the graduate. The drain does not touch the inside of the graduate. (From Potter PA, Perry AG, Stockert PA, Hall AM: *Fundamentals of nursing*, ed 10, St Louis, 2021, Elsevier.)

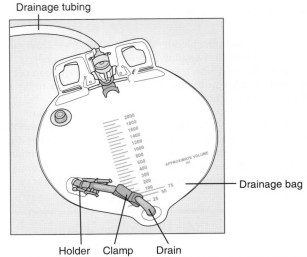

FIGURE 28-11 The clamp is closed and positioned in the holder on the drainage bag.

Changing a Leg Bag to a Standard Drainage Bag

QUALITY OF LIFE

- Knock before entering the person's room.
- Address the person by name.
- Introduce yourself by name and title.

- Explain the procedure before starting and during the procedure.
- Protect the person's rights during the procedure.
- Handle the person gently during the procedure.

PRE-PROCEDURE

1 Follow *Delegation Guidelines: Urine Drainage Systems*, p. 436. See *Promoting Safety and Comfort*:
  - *Urinary Catheters*, p. 430
  - *Urine Drainage Systems*, p. 437
2 Practice hand hygiene and get the following supplies.
  - Standard drainage bag and tubing
  - Antiseptic wipes
  - Sterile cap and plug (Fig. 28-12)
  - Catheter clamp
  - Items to empty the drainage bag (p. 437)
  - Waterproof under-pad
  - Bath blanket
  - Bedpan and cover (if used)
  - Disposable waterproof pad (as a barrier for the bedpan)

  - Paper towels
  - Towel or paper towels (as a barrier for supplies)
  - Gloves
  - Laundry bag
3 Place the barrier (towel, paper towels) on the over-bed table. Arrange items on top. Place the bedpan on the chair or bed. Use the disposable waterproof pad as a barrier between the bedpan and the surface.
4 Practice hand hygiene.
5 Identify the person. Check the ID bracelet against the assignment sheet. Use 2 identifiers (Chapter 14). Also call the person by name.
6 Provide for privacy.

PROCEDURE

7 Raise the bed to a safe height for dangling (Chapter 20) and for body mechanics. Have the person sit on the side of the bed. To assist, see procedure: *Sitting on the Side of the Bed (Dangling)* in Chapter 20. Follow the care plan for bed rail use.
8 Practice hand hygiene. Apply gloves.
9 Expose the catheter and leg bag.
10 Empty the drainage bag. See procedure: *Emptying a Urine Drainage Bag*, p. 437.
11 Clamp the catheter (Fig. 28-13). This prevents urine from draining from the catheter into the drainage tubing.
12 Let urine drain from below the clamp into the drainage tubing. This empties the lower end of the catheter.
13 Have the person lie down.
14 Cover the person with a bath blanket. Fold back the bath blanket to expose the catheter and leg bag.

15 Unfasten the straps on the leg bag. Place the waterproof under-pad under the catheter and leg bag.
16 Open the package with the standard drainage bag and tubing.
17 Attach the standard drainage bag to the bed frame.
18 Open the package with the sterile cap and plug (see Fig. 28-12, *A*). Do not let anything touch the sterile cap or plug.
19 Disconnect the catheter from the drainage tubing. Do not let anything touch the ends.
20 Insert the sterile plug into the catheter end (Fig. 28-14). Handle the end of the plug. Do not touch the part that goes inside the catheter. (If you contaminate the end of the catheter, wipe the end with an antiseptic wipe. Do so before inserting the sterile plug.)

Changing a Leg Bag to a Standard Drainage Bag—cont'd

PROCEDURE—cont'd

21 Place the sterile cap on the end of the leg bag drainage tube (see Fig. 28-12, *B*). (If you contaminate the tubing end, wipe the end with an antiseptic wipe. Do so before you put on the sterile cap.) Put the leg bag in the bedpan if the bag will be re-used.

22 Remove the cap from the new standard drainage bag tubing.

23 Remove the sterile plug from the catheter.

24 Insert the end of the drainage tubing into the catheter.

25 Remove the clamp from the catheter.

26 Position drainage tubing in a straight line or coiled on the bed. Follow the nurse's directions. Secure the tubing to the bottom linens.

27 Remove the waterproof under-pad. Place it in the laundry bag.

28 Remove and discard the gloves. Practice hand hygiene.

29 Cover the person. Remove the bath blanket. Place it in the laundry bag.

POST-PROCEDURE

30 Provide for comfort. (See the inside of the back cover.)

31 Lower the bed to a safe and comfortable level. Raise or lower bed rails. Follow the care plan.

32 Clean up and store supplies and equipment. (Wear gloves. Change gloves as needed.)

  a Discard disposable items.

  b Clean and disinfect re-usable equipment. Return supplies and equipment to their proper place.

  c Follow the manufacturer's instructions and agency policy to discard or re-use the leg bag. Follow agency procedures to clean, disinfect, and store a re-used leg bag. Or discard following agency policy.

  d Follow agency policy for used linens.

  e Clean and dry the over-bed table. Dry with paper towels. Discard paper towels. Position the over-bed table as the person prefers.

  f Remove and discard gloves. Practice hand hygiene.

33 Place the call light and other needed items within reach.

34 Follow the care plan and the person's preferences for privacy measures to maintain. Leaving the privacy curtain, window coverings, and door open or closed are examples.

35 Complete a safety check of the room. (See the inside of the back cover.)

36 Practice hand hygiene.

37 Report and record your care and observations.

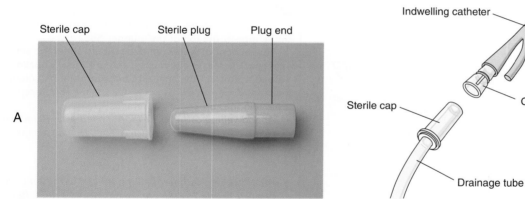

FIGURE 28-12 A, Sterile cap and catheter plug. Handle the outside of the cap and the end of the plug. The inside of the cap and the tip of the plug need to remain sterile. **B,** The plug goes into the end of the catheter. The cap goes on the leg bag (drainage tube).

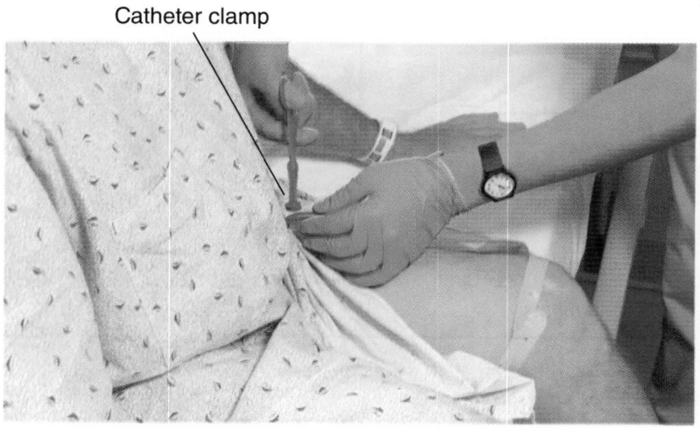

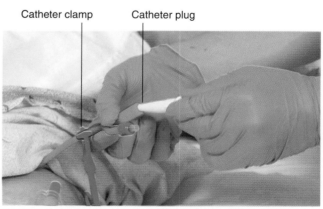

FIGURE 28-13 The catheter is clamped. This prevents urine from draining past the clamp. The clamp is applied directly to the catheter—not to the drainage tube. (From *Mosby's nursing assistant video skills 4.0*, St Louis, 2015, Elsevier.)

FIGURE 28-14 A catheter plug is inserted into the end of the catheter. (From *Mosby's nursing assistant video skills 4.0*, St. Louis, 2015, Elsevier.)

REMOVING INDWELLING CATHETERS

An indwelling catheter has 2 lumens (passage-ways). Sterile water is injected through 1 lumen (balloon inflation port) to inflate the balloon (Fig. 28-15). The water is injected with a syringe. Urine drains from the bladder through the other lumen.

To remove the catheter, the balloon is deflated—the water is removed. You need a syringe large enough to hold all the water in the balloon. The nurse tells you what size syringe to use.

The doctor orders catheter removal. The person may need bladder training first (Chapter 27). Dysuria and urinary frequency are common after removing catheters (Chapter 27).

See *Focus on Communication: Removing Indwelling Catheters.*
See *Focus on Math: Removing Indwelling Catheters.*
See *Delegation Guidelines: Removing Indwelling Catheters.*
See *Promoting Safety and Comfort: Removing Indwelling Catheters.*
See procedure: *Removing an Indwelling Catheter*, p. 442.

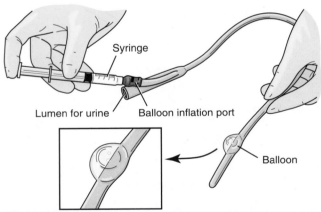

FIGURE 28-15 The balloon of an indwelling catheter is inflated with water. A syringe is used to inject the water. A syringe also is used to remove the water.

Labels: Syringe; Lumen for urine; Balloon inflation port; Balloon

---

FOCUS ON COMMUNICATION

Removing Indwelling Catheters

Explain the procedure to the person before starting and during the procedure. Also, tell the person about possible discomfort and when it might be felt. Have the person tell you at once if pain is felt or if you should stop. For example:

> I'm going to remove your catheter. I will explain the procedure step-by-step. You may feel a little pressure or discomfort when I remove the tube. I will tell you before I remove it. I will ask you to slowly breathe out as I remove it. This helps you to relax. Please tell me right away if you feel pain or if you need me to stop.

Ask the person to take a deep breath in through the nose and then to breathe out (exhale) through pursed lips. (See Chapter 44 for deep breathing.) Remove the catheter as the person exhales. This distracts the person and promotes relaxation. Explain each step in a calm and professional way to reduce anxiety and provide comfort. Avoid seeming bossy or hurried. Politely say what you will do and what the person needs to do.

FOCUS ON MATH

Removing Indwelling Catheters

To remove indwelling catheters, you must know how to measure liquid using a syringe. Syringes are marked in milliliters (mL). An mL is a unit used to measure liquid. Read the syringe at the top of the plunger. See Figure 28-16.

The amount of water removed should equal the amount injected. The nurse tells you the amount used for balloon inflation. Subtract the amount removed from the amount injected. If there is a difference, tell the nurse before removing the catheter. For example:

- *An indwelling catheter balloon is filled with 10 mL. You remove 7 mL. The difference is 3 mL. Do not remove the catheter. Call for the nurse.*

$$10 \text{ mL} - 7 \text{ mL} = 3 \text{ mL}$$

- *An indwelling catheter balloon is filled with 10 mL. You remove 10 mL. The difference is 0 mL. You can safely remove the catheter.*

$$10 \text{ mL} - 10 \text{ mL} = 0 \text{ mL}$$

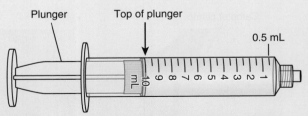

FIGURE 28-16 A syringe is read at the top of the plunger. This syringe measures 10 mL. Short lines mark 0.5 (one-half) mL measurements.

Labels: Plunger; Top of plunger; 0.5 mL

DELEGATION GUIDELINES
Removing Indwelling Catheters

In some agencies, removal of indwelling catheters is a delegated nursing task. If the task is delegated to you, make sure that:

- Your state allows you to perform the task.
- The task is in your job description (Chapter 3).
- You have the necessary education and training.
- The agency has determined that you are competent to perform the task safely.
- You know how to use the supplies and equipment.
- You review the procedure with the delegating nurse.
- The delegating nurse is available to answer questions and to guide and assist you as needed.

If the above conditions are met, you need this information from the nurse.

- When to remove the catheter
- The amount of water used for balloon inflation
- Syringe size needed
- What observations to report and record:
  - Amount of water removed from the balloon
  - The amount of urine in the drainage bag
  - Color, clarity, and odor of urine
  - Particles in the urine
  - Blood in the urine
  - Signs of pressure at the meatus (Chapter 42)
  - How the person tolerated the procedure
  - Complaints of pain, burning, irritation, or the need to void
  - The time and amount voided after catheter removal
  - Any other observations
- When to report observations
- What patient or resident concerns to report at once

PROMOTING SAFETY AND COMFORT
Removing Indwelling Catheters

Safety
The catheter package prescribes the amount of water needed to inflate the balloon. For proper inflation, the amount of water used may be greater than the balloon size. See Figure 28-17. Before removing the catheter, you must know the amount of water in the balloon. The nurse tells you the amount.

You must remove all water from the balloon. If the balloon is filled with 10 mL, 10 mL must be removed. Otherwise, injury to the urethra is likely as the catheter is removed. Do not remove the catheter if water remains in the balloon. Call for the nurse at once.

Comfort
To deflate the balloon, allow the water to flow out into the syringe. Pulling on the plunger to remove the water can cause ridges in the balloon and discomfort during catheter removal. Also, forceful pulling can collapse the tube. If pulling is needed, pull gently and slowly.

Properly Inflated **Under Inflated**

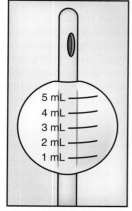
5 mL urinary catheter balloon inflated with 10 mL of water

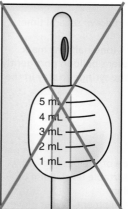
5 mL urinary catheter balloon inflated with 5 mL of water

FIGURE 28-17 The balloon must be inflated properly to avoid drainage and deflation problems. The balloon size marked on the catheter may not equal the amount of water in the balloon. The nurse tells you the amount of water in the balloon.

Removing an Indwelling Catheter

QUALITY OF LIFE

- Knock before entering the person's room.
- Address the person by name.
- Introduce yourself by name and title.

- Explain the procedure before starting and during the procedure.
- Protect the person's rights during the procedure.
- Handle the person gently during the procedure.

PRE-PROCEDURE

1 Follow *Delegation Guidelines: Removing Indwelling Catheters*, p. 441. See *Promoting Safety and Comfort:*
- *Urinary Catheters*, p. 430
- *Removing Indwelling Catheters*, p. 441
2 Practice hand hygiene and get the following supplies.
- Disposable waterproof pad
- Syringe in the size as directed by the nurse
- Towel
- Bath blanket
- Disposable bag
- Items to empty the drainage bag (p. 437)
- Gloves
- Laundry bag

3 Arrange items in the person's room.
4 Practice hand hygiene.
5 Identify the person. Check the ID bracelet against the assignment sheet. Use 2 identifiers (Chapter 14). Also call the person by name.
6 Provide for privacy.
7 Raise the bed for body mechanics. Bed rails are up if used. Lower the bed rail near you if up.

PROCEDURE

8 Position and drape the person as for perineal care (Chapter 24).
9 Check the size of the syringe. Know the amount of water in the balloon. Make sure the syringe is large enough to withdraw all the water from the balloon.
10 Practice hand hygiene. Apply gloves.
11 Fold back the bath blanket to expose the catheter.
12 Remove the tube holder, leg band, or tape securing the catheter to the person.
13 Position the disposable waterproof pad.
    a Female—between the legs
    b Male—over the thighs
14 Remove all of the water from the balloon. (NOTE: You must know how much water is in the balloon. For example, if the balloon is filled with 10 mL of water, you must remove 10 mL of water.)
    a Slide the syringe plunger up and down several times. This loosens the plunger.
    b Pull the plunger back to the 0.5 (one-half) mL mark.
    c Attach the syringe to the catheter's balloon port gently. Use only enough force to get the syringe to stay in the port.

d Allow the water to drain into the syringe. Wait at least 30 seconds to allow the full amount to drain. Do not pull back on the plunger. Pressure in the balloon will force the plunger back and fill the syringe. If the water is draining slowly or not at all, call for the nurse. Do not remove the catheter if there is water in the balloon. The nurse may have you:
    1) Gently re-position the syringe in the port.
    2) Re-position the person.
    3) Pull back on the syringe gently and slowly. Forceful pulling can collapse the tube.
15 Pull the catheter straight out once all of the water is removed. Have the person breathe out slowly during removal. Remove the catheter gently.
16 Wrap the catheter in the disposable waterproof pad.
17 Dry the perineal area with the towel. Place the towel in the laundry bag.
18 Cover the person with the bath blanket.
19 Lift the drainage tubing to ensure that all urine has drained from the tubing into the drainage bag. Empty the drainage bag. Note the amount of urine. Unhook the bag from the bed. Place the used catheter, tubing, and drainage bag in the disposable bag.
20 Remove and discard the gloves. Practice hand hygiene.
21 Cover the person. Remove the bath blanket. Place it in the laundry bag.

POST-PROCEDURE

22 Provide for comfort. (See the inside of the back cover.)
23 Lower the bed to a safe and comfortable level. Raise or lower bed rails. Follow the care plan.
24 Clean up and store supplies and equipment. (Wear gloves. Change gloves as needed.)
    a Discard disposable items. Discard the used catheter, tubing, and drainage bag following agency policy.
    b Empty the graduate into the toilet. Rinse the graduate. Empty the rinse into the toilet and flush. Follow agency procedures to clean and disinfect the graduate. Return supplies and equipment to their proper place.
    c Follow agency policy for used linens.

d Clean and dry the over-bed table if used. Dry with paper towels. Discard paper towels. Position the over-bed table as the person prefers.
    e Remove and discard gloves. Practice hand hygiene.
25 Place the call light and other needed items within reach.
26 Follow the care plan and the person's preferences for privacy measures to maintain. Leaving the privacy curtain, window coverings, and door open or closed are examples.
27 Complete a safety check of the room. (See the inside of the back cover.)
28 Practice hand hygiene.
29 Report and record your care and observations.

CONDOM CATHETERS

Condom catheters may be used for incontinent men (Fig. 28-18). They also are called *external catheters, Texas catheters,* and *urinary sheaths*. A *condom catheter* is a soft sheath that slides over the penis and is used to drain urine. Tubing connects the condom catheter to the drainage bag. Many men prefer leg bags (see Fig. 28-8).

Condom catheters are changed daily after perineal care. Thoroughly wash and dry the penis before applying the catheter.

Condom catheters come in different sizes and styles. The nurse measures the person for the correct size. The catheter is either self-adhesive or non-adhesive.

- *Self-adhesive catheters* have adhesive inside the catheter. The adhesive secures the catheter to the penis.
- *Non-adhesive catheters* require an adhesive strip or other securing method provided by the manufacturer. *If an adhesive strip is used, do not apply it completely around the penis in a circle. Apply the adhesive strip in a spiral* (Fig. 28-19). *This allows blood flow to the penis. Do not use other types of tape.* They do not expand. Blood flow to the penis will be cut off, injuring the penis.

Follow the manufacturer's instructions for how to secure the catheter. The procedure that follows is used as a guide.

See *Delegation Guidelines: Condom Catheters*, p. 444.

See *Promoting Safety and Comfort: Condom Catheters*, p. 444.

See procedure: *Applying a Condom Catheter*, p. 444.

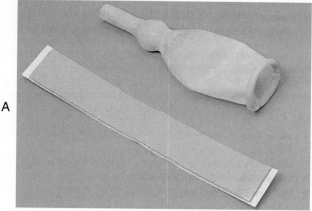

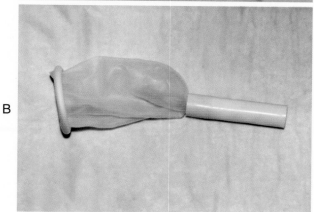

FIGURE 28-18 A, Condom catheter with an adhesive strip. **B,** Self-adhesive condom catheter. (A, From Elkin MK, Perry AG, Potter PA: *Nursing interventions and clinical skills*, ed 4, St. Louis, 2008, Mosby. B, From Gosnell K, Cooper K: *Foundations of nursing*, ed 9, St Louis, 2023, Elsevier.)

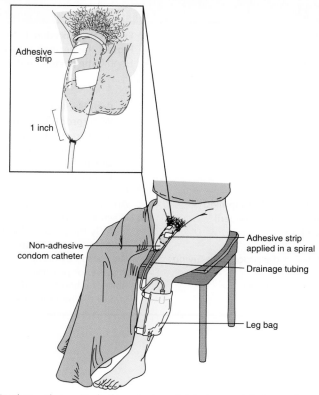

FIGURE 28-19 Condom catheter attached to a leg bag. A 1-inch space is between the penis and the end of the catheter. Elastic tape is applied in a *spiral* to secure a non-adhesive condom catheter to the penis.

DELEGATION GUIDELINES
Condom Catheters

Depending on the agency, removing and applying a condom catheter may be a routine task or a delegated nursing task. Before removing and applying a condom catheter, you need to be trained and comfortable using your agency's supplies. You also need this information from the nurse and the care plan.
- What type of condom catheter to use
- What size condom catheter to use
- When to remove the catheter and apply a new one
- If a leg bag or standard drainage bag is used
- What leg bag straps to use—elastic or Velcro
- What water temperature to use for perineal care
- What observations to report and record:
  - Reddened or open areas on the penis
  - Swelling of the penis
  - Color, clarity, and odor of urine
  - Particles in the urine
  - Blood in the urine
  - Cloudy urine
- When to report observations
- What patient or resident concerns to report at once

PROMOTING SAFETY AND COMFORT
Condom Catheters

Safety
Do not apply a condom catheter if the penis is red, irritated, or shows signs of skin breakdown. Report your observations at once.

If you do not know how to use a certain condom catheter, ask for help. Have the nurse show you the correct application. Then ask the nurse to observe you applying the catheter.

Blood must flow to the penis. If an adhesive strip is needed, use what is packaged with the catheter. Apply it in a spiral.

Comfort
To apply a condom catheter, you need to touch and handle the penis. This can embarrass the person. Explain the procedure. Provide privacy. Keep the person covered as much as possible. Act in a professional manner.

The penis may begin to become erect when touched. Cover the person. Allow time for the penis to return to its relaxed state. Give reassurance that this is a normal response. If needed, allow privacy and say when you will return. Or ask the person to signal for you to finish the procedure. Provide for safety. Place the urinal and call light in reach. Knock before entering the room.

Applying a Condom Catheter

QUALITY OF LIFE
- Knock before entering the person's room.
- Address the person by name.
- Introduce yourself by name and title.
- Explain the procedure before starting and during the procedure.
- Protect the person's rights during the procedure.
- Handle the person gently during the procedure.

PRE-PROCEDURE
1 Follow *Delegation Guidelines:*
  - *Perineal Care* (Chapter 24)
  - *Condom Catheters*
  See *Promoting Safety and Comfort:*
  - *Perineal Care* (Chapter 24)
  - *Urinary Catheters,* p. 430
  - *Condom Catheters*
2 Practice hand hygiene and get the following supplies.
  - Condom catheter (with adhesive strip if needed)
  - Standard drainage bag or leg bag
  - Cap for the drainage bag
  - Basin of warm water (see step 6 in the procedure: *Giving Catheter Care,* p. 435)
  - Soap, body wash, or other cleansing agent
  - Towel and washcloths
  - Bath blanket
  - Waterproof under-pad
  - Items to empty the drainage bag (p. 437)
  - Towel or paper towel (as a barrier for supplies)
  - Gloves
  - Laundry bag
3 Place a barrier (towel, paper towels) on the over-bed table. Arrange items on top.
4 Practice hand hygiene.
5 Identify the person. Check the ID bracelet against the assignment sheet. Use 2 identifiers (Chapter 14). Also call the person by name.
6 Provide for privacy.
7 Raise the bed for body mechanics. Bed rails are up if used. Lower the bed rail near you if up.

Applying a Condom Catheter—cont'd

PROCEDURE

8 Cover the person with a bath blanket. Lower top linens.
9 Position the waterproof under-pad under the person. Have the person raise the buttocks off of the bed. Or turn the person from side to side.
10 Position and drape the person for perineal care (Chapter 24).
11 Practice hand hygiene. Apply gloves.
12 Secure the standard drainage bag to the bed frame. Or have a leg bag ready. Close the drain.
13 Fold back the bath blanket to expose the genital area. Keep the person covered as much as possible.
14 Remove the used condom catheter.
   a *For a catheter with a single-sided adhesive strip (outside)*—Remove the adhesive strip.
   b *For a self-adhesive catheter*—If needed, wet a washcloth with warm water. Apply it to the penis for a few minutes. This helps release the adhesive.
   c Roll the sheath off of the penis.
   d *For a catheter with a double-sided adhesive strip (inside)*—Remove the adhesive strip after rolling the sheath off of the penis.
15 Disconnect the used tubing from the condom catheter. Cap the drainage tube.
16 Discard the condom catheter and adhesive strip (if used).
17 Provide perineal care (Chapter 24). Be sure the penis is dried well. For an uncircumcised male, the foreskin is returned to its natural position before the new condom catheter is applied.
18 Observe the penis for reddened areas, skin breakdown, and irritation. If present, do not apply a new catheter. Call for the nurse.
19 Remove and discard the gloves. Practice hand hygiene. Put on clean gloves.

20 Apply the new condom catheter. Follow the manufacturer's instructions.
   a Grasp the penis.
   b *For a catheter with a double-sided adhesive strip (inside):*
      1) Remove the paper liner from 1 side of the adhesive strip.
      2) Apply the adhesive strip in a spiral on the penis. Begin just behind the penis head. Do not apply the adhesive strip completely around the penis.
      3) Remove the paper liner from the other side of the adhesive strip.
      4) Roll the condom onto the penis. Follow the manufacturer's instructions for the amount of space to leave between the catheter and the penis tip. A 1-inch space is common.
      5) Gently press the condom to the adhesive strip on the penis.
   c *For a catheter with a single-sided adhesive strip (outside):*
      1) Roll the condom onto the penis. Follow the manufacturer's instructions for the amount of space to leave between the catheter and the penis tip. A 1-inch space is common.
      2) Remove the paper liner from the adhesive strip.
      3) Apply the adhesive strip in a spiral over the condom catheter (see Fig. 28-19). Begin at the penis head. Do not apply the adhesive strip completely around the penis.
   d *For a self-adhesive catheter:* Roll the condom onto the penis. Follow the manufacturer's instructions for the amount of time to hold. About 1 minute is common.
21 Make sure the penis tip does not touch the condom. Make sure the condom is not twisted.
22 Connect the condom catheter to the new drainage tubing. Secure excess tubing on the bed. Or attach a leg bag.
23 Cover the person with the bath blanket. Remove the waterproof under-pad. Place it in the laundry bag.
24 Empty the used drainage bag. See procedure: *Emptying a Urine Drainage Bag*, p. 437. Measure and record the urine amount (Chapter 32).
25 Remove and discard the gloves. Practice hand hygiene.
26 Cover the person. Remove the bath blanket. Place it in the laundry bag.

POST-PROCEDURE

27 Provide for comfort. (See the inside of the back cover.)
28 Lower the bed to a safe and comfortable level. Raise or lower bed rails. Follow the care plan.
29 Clean up and store supplies and equipment. (Wear gloves. Change gloves as needed.)
   a Discard disposable items.
   b Follow the manufacturer's instructions and agency policy to discard or re-use the drainage bag. Follow agency procedures to clean, disinfect, and store a re-used bag. Or discard following agency policy.
   c Empty the wash basin.
   d Follow agency procedures to clean and disinfect re-usable equipment. Return supplies and equipment to their proper place.

   e Follow agency policy for used linens.
   f Clean and dry the over-bed table. Dry with paper towels. Discard paper towels. Position the over-bed table as the person prefers.
   g Remove and discard gloves. Practice hand hygiene.
30 Place the call light and other needed items within reach.
31 Follow the care plan and the person's preferences for privacy measures to maintain. Leaving the privacy curtain, window coverings, and door open or closed are examples.
32 Complete a safety check of the room. (See the inside of the back cover.)
33 Practice hand hygiene.
34 Report and record your care and observations.

FEMALE EXTERNAL CATHETERS

For women, external catheter systems have been developed that use a flexible device with soft gauze (fabric). The device is placed between the labia and connected to suction to draw urine away from the body. (*Suction* involves withdrawing or sucking up fluid.) Such systems may be used when bed rest (Chapter 35) is required.

If your agency uses female external catheters, you will be trained to use the system properly. Follow the manufacturer's instructions and the nurse's directions. Good skin care and pressure injury precautions (Chapter 42) are required.

FOCUS ON **PRIDE**

The Person, Family, and Yourself

Personal and Professional Responsibility

With urinary catheters, the risk of UTIs is high. How you give care can lower the risk of UTI. Do you:
- Prevent urine from flowing back into the bladder when moving the drainage bag?
- Use a clean area of the washcloth for each stroke during catheter care?
- Keep the drain from touching the graduate or other surface?
- Use a clean, separate graduate to empty each person's drainage bag?

Rights and Respect

Respect the right to privacy. Simple actions make a difference. For example, knock before entering a room. Before any procedure, explain how you will provide privacy. This is very important for procedures that involve exposing and touching private areas.

Independence and Social Interaction

Urinary catheters are short-term or long-term. Some persons manage their own catheters. The nurse teaches the person to provide catheter care. You:
- Give encouragement. Be kind, patient, and professional.
- Reinforce the nurse's instructions.
- Tell the nurse if the person has questions or if you think more teaching is needed.

Delegation and Teamwork

Tasks become more complex as more care equipment is needed. For example, you need to transfer a person from the chair to bed. The person has a urinary catheter. You must:
- Keep the catheter and drainage tube free of kinks.
- Keep the drainage bag below bladder level.
- Avoid resting the bag on the floor.
- Make sure the person is not lying on the drainage tube.

Ethics and Laws

With more training, some states and agencies allow nursing assistants to insert indwelling catheters. Others do not. Follow state and agency rules. Never perform a task outside your role limits.

FOCUS ON **PRIDE**: *Application*

How might needing a urinary catheter affect the person mentally? How can you promote mental comfort?

REVIEW QUESTIONS

Circle the BEST answer.

1 Urinary catheters are used
  a To prevent urinary tract infections
  b To treat the cause of incontinence
  c To keep the bladder empty for surgery
  d For staff convenience with incontinent persons

2 A person has a catheter. Which is *safe?*
  a Keeping the drainage bag above the bladder level
  b Taping a leak at the connection site
  c Attaching the drainage bag to the bed rail
  d Removing a kink from the drainage tubing

3 A person has a catheter. Which is *correct?*
  a Report pain, burning, or irritation at once.
  b Allow the tubing to hang below the drainage bag.
  c Empty the drainage bag once daily.
  d Use the same graduate for all persons.

4 A person has a catheter. You are going to turn the person from the left to the right side. What should you do with the drainage bag?
  a Move it to the right side.
  b Keep it on the left side.
  c Hang it from an IV pole.
  d Remove it.

5 For a female, a catheter is secured to
  a The abdomen
  b The gown with a safety pin
  c The thigh with a tube holder
  d The bottom linens with tape

6 For catheter care
  a Clean from the drainage tube connection up the catheter at least 4 inches
  b Clean from the meatus down the catheter at least 4 inches
  c Pull on the catheter to make sure it is secure
  d Clamp the catheter to prevent leaking

7 Which statement about drainage systems is *true?*
  a A leg bag holds about 2000 mL.
  b A standard drainage bag holds less than a leg bag.
  c A closed drainage system means the drain cannot be opened.
  d Microbes in the drainage system can cause a UTI.

8 A drainage system becomes disconnected. You need
  a A new drainage bag and paper towels
  b A sterile cap and catheter plug
  c Gloves and antiseptic wipes
  d A waterproof under-pad and a catheter clamp

9 When emptying a standard drainage bag
  a Do not let the drain touch the graduate
  b Gloves are not needed
  c Clamp the catheter
  d Disconnect the catheter and drainage bag

10 You are going to remove a urinary catheter. You plan to
  a Attach a needle to the syringe
  b Ask the nurse how much water is in the balloon
  c Pull the catheter with more force if there is resistance
  d Use an antiseptic swab to clean the meatus

11 You are removing an indwelling catheter. The balloon is filled with 10 mL. You withdraw 6 mL. What should you do?
  a Call for the nurse.
  b Inject the water.
  c Pull the catheter out.
  d Cut the catheter.

12 A condom catheter requires an adhesive strip to secure it to the penis. Apply the adhesive strip
  a Completely around the penis
  b To the thigh
  c To the abdomen
  d In a spiral

Answers to Chapter 28 questions are on p. 902.

FOCUS ON PRACTICE

Problem Solving

A patient with a urinary catheter tells you: "I feel like I have to pee, and I feel pressure down there." The patient points to the lower abdomen. There is no urine in the drainage bag. Is this normal? What do you do?

Bowel Needs

See *Body Structure and Function Review: The Gastro-Intestinal Tract.*

See *Delegation Guidelines: Bowel Needs.*

See *Promoting Safety and Comfort: Bowel Needs.*

OBJECTIVES

- Define the key terms and key abbreviations in this chapter.
- Describe normal defecation and the observations to report.
- Identify the factors affecting bowel elimination.
- Explain how to promote comfort and safety during bowel movements.
- Describe the common bowel problems.
- Describe bowel training.

- Explain why enemas are given.
- Describe the common enema solutions.
- Describe the rules for giving enemas.
- Describe how to care for a person with an ostomy.
- Perform the procedures described in this chapter.
- Explain how to promote PRIDE in the person, the family, and yourself.

KEY TERMS

colostomy A surgically created opening *(stomy)* between the colon *(colo)* and the body's surface

constipation The passage of a hard, dry stool

defecation The process of excreting feces from the rectum through the anus; bowel movement

dehydration A decrease in the amount of water in the body

diarrhea The frequent passage of liquid stools

enema The introduction of fluid into the rectum and lower colon

fecal impaction The prolonged retention and buildup of feces in the rectum

fecal incontinence The inability to control the passage of feces and flatus through the anus

feces The semi-solid mass of waste products in the colon that is expelled through the anus; stool or stools

flatulence The excessive formation of gas or air in the stomach and intestines

flatus Gas or air passed through the anus

ileostomy A surgically created opening *(stomy)* between the ileum (small intestine *[ileo]*) and the body's surface

melena A black, tarry stool

ostomy A surgically created opening that connects an internal organ to the body's surface; see "colostomy" and "ileostomy"

peristalsis The alternating contraction and relaxation of muscles that moves food through the digestive system

stoma A surgically created opening seen on the body's surface; see "colostomy" and "ileostomy"

stool Excreted feces; stools

suppository A cone-shaped, solid drug that is inserted into a body opening; it melts at body temperature

KEY ABBREVIATIONS

BM	Bowel movement	IV	Intravenous
C. diff	*Clostridioides difficile; Clostridium difficile*	mL	Milliliter
GI	Gastro-intestinal	SSE	Soapsuds enema
ID	Identification		

Bowel elimination is a basic physical need. Wastes are excreted from the gastro-intestinal (GI) system (Chapter 10). Normal bowel elimination is important. Problems easily occur. You assist patients and residents to meet bowel needs.

BODY STRUCTURE AND FUNCTION REVIEW
The Gastro-Intestinal Tract

Structure and Function

Bowel elimination is the excretion of wastes through the gastro-intestinal (GI) tract (Chapter 10). The digestive system (GI system) is shown in Figure 29-1. Food and fluids are normally taken in through the *mouth.* They are partially digested in the *stomach.* The partially digested food and fluids are called *chyme.*

Chyme passes from the stomach into the *small intestine (small bowel)—duodenum, jejunum,* and *ileum.* Movement occurs because of peristalsis. (*Peristalsis* is the alternating contraction and relaxation of muscles that moves food through the digestive system.) Further digestion and absorption of nutrients occur in the small bowel. Next, the chyme enters the *large intestine (large bowel* or *colon)* where fluid is absorbed. Chyme becomes less fluid and more solid in consistency as it passes through the large intestine. *Feces (stool; stools)* refers to the semi-solid mass of waste products in the colon that is expelled through the anus.

Feces are stored in the *rectum* and excreted from the body. *Defecation (bowel movement)* is the process of excreting feces from the rectum through the anus. *Stool (stools)* refers to excreted feces.

Changes With Aging

With age, secretion of saliva and digestive juices decreases. Some foods are difficult to chew, swallow, and digest. Peristalsis decreases, causing flatulence (gas) (p. 454) and constipation (p. 452).

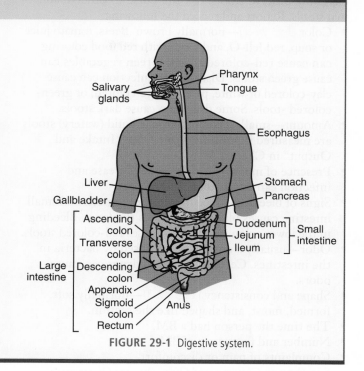

FIGURE 29-1 Digestive system.

DELEGATION GUIDELINES
Bowel Needs

Most procedures in this chapter are not routine nursing tasks. They may be delegated nursing tasks in some states and agencies. Before performing a procedure, make sure that:

- Your state allows you to perform the task.
- The task is in your job description (Chapter 3).
- You have the necessary education and training.
- The agency has determined that you are competent to perform the task safely.
- You know how to use the supplies and equipment.
- You review the procedure with the delegating nurse.
- The delegating nurse is available to answer questions and to guide and assist you as needed.

PROMOTING SAFETY AND COMFORT
Bowel Needs

Safety

Assisting with bowel needs may involve exposing and touching the rectum, a private area. And you may have to give perineal care. Always keep the call light within the person's reach. And always act in a professional manner.

Contact with feces (stools) is likely when assisting with bowel needs. Follow Standard Precautions. Follow the Bloodborne Pathogen Standard if blood is present. Follow the rules of hand hygiene and the guidelines for glove use in Chapters 17 and 18.

In nursing centers, follow agency policies and procedures for using Enhanced Barrier Precautions. See Chapter 18.

NORMAL BOWEL ELIMINATION

Bowel movements (BMs) vary from person to person. Frequency varies—daily, 2 to 3 times a day, every 2 to 3 days for adults. Time of day also varies.

See *Focus on Communication: Normal Bowel Elimination.*

See *Focus on Children and Older Persons: Normal Bowel Elimination.*

FOCUS ON COMMUNICATION
Normal Bowel Elimination

The term *bowel movement* and the abbreviation *BM* are commonly used. For some people, *poop* is a common word. For others, it is embarrassing. In this chapter, *stool* or *stools* refers to excreted feces. The word *feces* may be less familiar to patients and residents. Use a term the person understands and uses. Be professional.

FOCUS ON **CHILDREN AND OLDER PERSONS**
Normal Bowel Elimination

Children

Newborns who are breast-fed usually have a BM with every feeding. Formula-fed babies have fewer BMs. Frequency changes as children grow older. Infants usually have 2 or 3 BMs a day. Toddlers usually have 1 or 2 a day. One BM a day is normal for older children.

Observations

Carefully observe stools. Ask the nurse to observe abnormal stools. Report and record the following:

- Color (Fig. 29-2)—normally brown. Beets, tomato juice or soup, red Jell-O, and foods with red food coloring can cause red-colored stools. Green vegetables can cause green stools. Diseases and infection can cause clay-colored or white, pale, orange-colored, or green-colored stools. Some drugs can cause dark stools.
- Amount—small, medium, large. Liquid (watery) stools are measured in milliliters (mL). See "Intake and Output" in Chapter 32.
- Presence of mucus—usually none. Disease and infection can cause stools with mucus.
- Signs of bleeding—bleeding in the stomach and small intestine causes black, tarry stools *(melena)*. Bleeding in the lower colon and rectum causes red-colored stools.
- Odor—usually a normal odor caused by bacteria in the intestines. Certain foods and drugs can cause odors.
- Shape and consistency (Fig. 29-3)—normally soft, formed, moist, and shaped like the rectum.
- The time the person had a BM.
- Number and frequency of BMs.
- Complaints of pain or discomfort.
  See *Focus on Children and Older Persons: Observations.*
  See *Focus on Communication: Observations.*

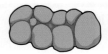 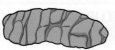

Formed with lumps   Formed with cracks   Smooth and soft

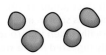 

Small hard lumps   Small soft lumps

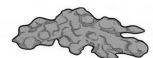 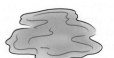

Loose and unformed   Watery

FIGURE 29-3 Stool shapes and consistencies.

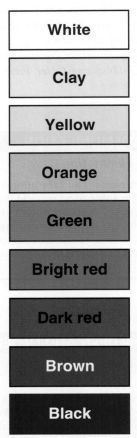

FIGURE 29-2 Color chart for stools.

White

Clay

Yellow

Orange

Green

Bright red

Dark red

Brown

Black

FOCUS ON CHILDREN AND OLDER PERSONS

Observations

Children
Breast-fed babies have yellow and seedy-looking stools that are soft or runny. Formula-fed babies have yellow to brown stools that are firmer (like the consistency of peanut butter). Stool color and consistency change with solid foods.

FOCUS ON COMMUNICATION

Observations

Many patients and residents tend to their own bowel needs. Information is needed for the person's record and the nursing process. To ask about BMs, you can say:
- "Did you have a BM today?"
- "Please tell me about your BM."
- "When did you have a BM?"
- "What was the amount?"
- "Were the stools soft or hard?"
- "Were the stools formed or loose?"
- "What was the color?"
- "Did you have bleeding, pain, or problems having a BM?"
- "Have you been passing gas?"
- "Do you need to pass more gas?"
- "Do you need help cleaning yourself?"

Follow agency policy to report and record what the person said or what you observed. Use the agency's form to record BMs (Fig. 29-4). Or record in the person's chart. For example:

Resident reported a medium-sized, soft, formed, brown BM after breakfast today. Denied bleeding, pain, straining, or other problems. Resident performed perineal care.

DATE: 01/21	TIME: 1015

BOWEL ELIMINATION: OBSERVATIONS

Shape & consistency	Color	Amount
☐ Watery	☐ White	☐ None
☐ Loose and unformed	☐ Clay	☐ Small
	☐ Yellow	☒ Medium
☐ Lumps	☐ Orange	☐ Large
☐ Small soft	☐ Green	**Volume:**
☐ Small hard	☐ Bright red	☐☐☐ mL
☐ Smooth and soft	☐ Dark red	**Pain**
☒ Formed	☒ Brown	☒ No
☒ With cracks	☐ Black	☐ Yes
☐ With lumps		Rating ☐ /10

Notes	Odor
Denied straining or other problems. Observed stools and reported observations to the nurse. ▲ ▼	☒ Normal
	☐ Abnormal
	Flatus
Nurse notified: C. Yung, RN	☒ Passing flatus
	☐ No flatus

FIGURE 29-4 Bowel elimination record.

FACTORS AFFECTING BMs

These factors affect BM frequency, consistency, color, and odor. Normal, regular elimination is a goal of the nursing process.

- *Privacy.* Lack of privacy can prevent a BM despite the urge. Odors and sounds are embarrassing. Some people ignore the urge when people are present.
- *Habits.* After breakfast is a common time for a BM. Being relaxed, not tense, is helpful. To relax, some people drink a hot beverage, read, or take a walk.
- *Diet—high-fiber foods.* High-fiber foods leave a residue, creating bulk to prevent constipation (p. 452). Fruits, vegetables, and whole-grain cereals and breads are high in fiber. Intake of such foods may be poor. Digestion problems and chewing difficulties (loss of teeth, poorly fitting dentures) are causes. Bran may be added to cereal, prunes, or prune juice to promote BMs.
- *Diet—other foods.* Milk and milk products may cause constipation or diarrhea. Chocolate and other foods cause similar reactions. Spicy foods can irritate the intestines, causing frequent BMs or diarrhea. Gas-forming foods stimulate peristalsis, aiding BMs. Such foods include onions, beans, cabbage, cauliflower, radishes, and cucumbers.
- *Fluids.* Feces contain water. Stool consistency depends on how much water is absorbed by the colon. Feces harden and dry when large amounts of water are absorbed or from poor fluid intake or vomiting. Hard, dry feces move slowly through the colon, leading to constipation. Drinking 6 to 8 glasses of water daily promotes normal BMs. Warm fluids—coffee, tea, hot cider, warm water—increase peristalsis.
- *Activity.* Exercise and activity maintain muscle tone and stimulate peristalsis. Constipation may result from inactivity or bed rest.

- *Drugs.* Some drugs are used to prevent constipation or diarrhea. Other drugs have constipation or diarrhea as side effects. Pain-relief drugs can slow peristalsis, causing constipation. Antibiotics (used to fight or prevent infections) often cause diarrhea. Diarrhea occurs when the antibiotics kill normal flora in the colon. Normal flora is needed to form feces. (See "Normal Flora" in Chapter 17.)
- *Disability.* Some people have a BM whenever feces enter the rectum. They have no control. A bowel training program is needed (p. 454).
- *Aging.* Age affects bowel elimination.

See *Focus on Children and Older Persons: Factors Affecting BMs.*

FOCUS ON CHILDREN AND OLDER PERSONS

Factors Affecting BMs

Children
Infants and toddlers cannot control BMs. They have a BM whenever feces enter the rectum. Bowel training usually begins between 2 and 3 years of age.

Older Persons
Aging causes GI changes. Peristalsis slows. Constipation is a risk. Some older persons lose bowel control. Older persons are at risk for GI tumors and disorders.

Older persons may not completely empty the rectum. They may have a BM about 30 to 60 minutes after the first BM.

Many older persons are very concerned if they do not have a BM every day. The nurse assesses the person's regular patterns and instructs about normal elimination. Tell the nurse if the person is concerned about regularity.

Safety and Comfort

The care plan has measures to meet bowel needs. It may involve diet, fluids, and exercise. The measures in Box 29-1 (p. 452) promote safety and comfort.

See *Focus on Communication: Safety and Comfort.*
See *Teamwork and Time Management: Safety and Comfort.*

FOCUS ON COMMUNICATION

Safety and Comfort

Odors and sounds are common with BMs. Control your verbal and nonverbal responses. Be professional. Do not laugh at or make fun of a person. Your words and actions must promote comfort, dignity, and self-esteem.

TEAMWORK AND TIME MANAGEMENT

Safety and Comfort

BM needs may be urgent. Answer call lights promptly. Also help co-workers answer call lights. Listen closely for bathroom call lights. The sound and light color are different from call lights in rooms. Respond at once. Do not leave patients and residents sitting on toilets, commodes, or bedpans. Do not leave them sitting or lying in stools.

BOX 29-1	Safety and Comfort: Bowel Needs

- Assist the person promptly. BM needs may be urgent.
- Practice medical asepsis.
- Follow Standard Precautions. Follow the Bloodborne Pathogen Standard if blood is present.
- Provide for privacy.
  - Ask visitors to leave the room.
  - Close doors, privacy curtains, and window coverings.
- Help the person to the toilet or commode. Or provide the bedpan. For greater privacy, a commode with wheels may be used in the bathroom. Follow these privacy and safety measures to wheel a person into a bathroom on a commode.
  - Follow the safety measures to prevent equipment accidents (Chapter 14). Do not exceed the weight capacity of the commode.
  - Follow the commode manufacturer's instructions for use and a safe moving distance.
  - Cover the person during the transport.
  - Remove the container before use over a toilet.
  - Use caution when moving a person on a commode over a toilet. For males, be sure that the genitals will not be hit or pinched as the commode is moved in place.
  - Lock (brake) the wheels when not moving the commode.

- Warm a bedpan (if used). This is important if the bedpan is metal.
- Position the person in a sitting or squatting position.
- Cover the person for warmth and privacy.
- Allow enough time for a BM.
- Place the call light and toilet paper within reach.
- Leave the room if the person can be alone. Check on the person at least every 5 minutes.
- Stay nearby if the person is weak or unsteady.
- Be sure the person is wiped and cleaned well. Provide perineal care as needed.
- Flush stools promptly. This reduces odors and prevents the spread of microbes.
- Assist the person with hand hygiene after elimination.
- Follow the care plan for fecal incontinence.

COMMON PROBLEMS

Common problems include constipation, fecal impaction, diarrhea, fecal incontinence, and flatulence.

Constipation

When feces move slowly through the bowel, more water is absorbed. Constipation can occur. *Constipation* is the passage of a hard, dry stool. The person strains to have a BM. Stools are large or marble-sized. Large stools cause pain as they pass through the anus.

Common causes of constipation include:
- A low-fiber diet
- Ignoring the urge to have a BM
- Decreased fluid intake
- Inactivity
- Drugs
- Aging
- Certain diseases

Diet changes, fluids, and activity prevent or relieve constipation. The doctor may order 1 or more of the following:
- Stool softeners—drugs that soften feces. A BM is easier when feces are soft.
- Laxatives—drugs that promote bowel elimination. They increase the bulk of feces, soften feces, and lubricate the intestinal wall.
- Suppositories (p. 455).
- Enemas (p. 455).

Fecal Impaction

A *fecal impaction* is the prolonged retention and buildup of feces in the rectum. Feces are hard or putty-like. Fecal impaction results from un-relieved constipation. The person cannot have a BM. More water is absorbed from the already hard feces. Liquid feces pass around the hardened fecal mass in the rectum and seep from the anus.

Signs and symptoms of fecal impaction include:
- Trying many times to have a BM
- Abdominal discomfort
- Abdominal distention (swelling)
- Nausea
- Cramping
- Rectal pain
- Poor appetite (especially older persons)
- Confusion (especially older persons)
- Fever (especially older persons)

Fecal impaction is a serious problem. It must be prevented. Follow agency policy for recording BMs. Report large stools or difficulty passing stools. Also tell the nurse if the person is concerned about constipation.

The nurse does a digital (finger) exam to check for an impaction. A lubricated, gloved finger is inserted into the rectum to feel for a hard mass in the lower rectum (Fig. 29-5). The feces may be out of reach higher in the colon. The digital exam often causes the urge to have a BM. Drugs, suppositories, or enemas may be ordered to remove the impaction.

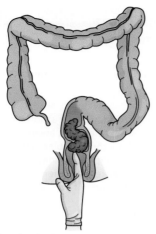

FIGURE 29-5 A gloved index finger is used to check for and remove a fecal impaction.

Sometimes *digital removal of an impaction* is done (see Fig. 29-5). A lubricated, gloved finger is inserted into the rectum and hooked around a piece of feces. Then the finger and feces are removed. The stool is dropped into the bedpan. The process is repeated as needed.

See *Delegation Guidelines: Fecal Impaction.*

DELEGATION GUIDELINES

Fecal Impaction

Checking for and removing impactions present dangers. The vagus nerve can be stimulated, which slows the heart rate. The heart rate can slow to unsafe levels in some persons. Rectal bleeding can also occur. Removing an impaction is painful. The nurse gives a pain-relief drug before the procedure.

You do not check for or remove fecal impactions. You may be asked to assist the nurse. If so, you need to know:

- What supplies are needed. Lubricant, gloves, a bedpan, toilet paper, a bath blanket, and items for perineal care are gathered.
- How to position the person. A left side-lying or left semi-prone position is used.
- When to check the person's pulse. Check the pulse before, during, and after the procedure. Know how often to check the pulse during the procedure (the interval). Check the rate and rhythm (Chapter 34). Know what change is significant.
- If you need to cue the person to relax during the procedure. Having the person take slow, deep breaths can help. (See Chapter 44 for deep breathing.)
- What to use for elimination after the procedure. The toilet, bedpan, or commode may be used.
- If the nurse needs to observe stools after the procedure.
- What observations to report and record:
  - The pulse rates measured
  - Color, amount, consistency, shape, and odor of stools
  - Complaints of cramping, pain, or discomfort
- When to report observations
- What patient or resident concerns to report at once

Diarrhea

Diarrhea is the frequent passage of liquid stools. Feces move through the intestines rapidly. This reduces the time for fluid absorption. The need for a BM is urgent. Some people cannot get to a bathroom in time. Abdominal cramping, nausea, and vomiting may occur.

Causes of diarrhea include infections, some drugs, irritating foods, and microbes in food and water. Diet and drugs are ordered to reduce peristalsis. You need to:

- Assist with elimination needs promptly.
- Dispose of stools promptly. This prevents odors and the spread of microbes.
- Give good skin care. Liquid stools irritate the skin. So does frequent wiping with toilet paper. Skin breakdown and pressure injuries are risks.

Dehydration is a risk from fluid loss. *Dehydration* is a decrease in the amount of water in the body. The person has pale or flushed skin, dry skin, and a coated tongue. Urine is dark and scant in amount (*oliguria*). Thirst, weakness, dizziness, and confusion also occur. Falling blood pressure and increased pulse and respirations are serious signs. Death can occur. The nursing process is used to meet fluid needs. The doctor may order intravenous (IV) fluids (Chapter 33).

Microbes can cause diarrhea. Preventing their spread is important. Always follow Standard Precautions when in contact with stools.

See *Focus on Children and Older Persons: Diarrhea.*
See *Promoting Safety and Comfort: Diarrhea.*

FOCUS ON **CHILDREN AND OLDER PERSONS**

Diarrhea

Children
Infants and children have large amounts of body water. Dehydration can quickly become severe. Report a liquid or watery stool at once. Ask the nurse to observe the stool. Note the number of wet diapers. Infants void less when dehydrated.

Older Persons
Older persons are at risk for dehydration. The amount of body water decreases with aging. Many diseases affect body fluids. So do many drugs. Report signs of diarrhea at once. Ask the nurse to observe the stool. Death is a risk when dehydration is not recognized and treated.

PROMOTING SAFETY AND COMFORT

Diarrhea

Safety
A gown protects your clothes and body from contact with body fluids. If stools are not contained or may have contact with your clothes or body, wear a gown and gloves for the task (Chapter 18).

Comfort
The need for a BM is urgent when the person has diarrhea. Answer call lights promptly. Some people cannot get to a bathroom in time. Soiling results. Assist the person with hygiene needs and garment changes as needed. Be patient and kind. The person cannot control BMs.

C. diff and Norovirus. *Clostridioides difficile* (*C. difficile*; formerly *Clostridium difficile*) is a bacterium that causes diarrhea and inflammation of the colon (*colitis*). Commonly called *C. diff*, it can cause death. Persons at risk are those who are older, have weakened immune systems, have been taking antibiotics, or have had exposure to *C. diff*. Older persons in hospitals and nursing centers are at high risk. Signs and symptoms include watery diarrhea, fever, loss of appetite, nausea, and abdominal pain or tenderness.

Norovirus is a virus that causes inflammation of the stomach and intestines (*gastroenteritis*). The person usually has diarrhea, nausea, vomiting, and abdominal pain. Fever, headache, and body aches can occur. Signs and symptoms begin within 1 to 2 days of exposure and can last for 1 to 3 days. Young children, older persons, and persons with chronic illnesses are at high risk for dehydration.

C. diff and norovirus are highly contagious. A person can become infected by touching items or surfaces contaminated with the microbe and then touching the mouth or mucous membranes. You can spread the microbe if your contaminated hands or gloves:

- Touch a person
- Contaminate surfaces

Standard Precautions and Contact Precautions (Chapter 18) are required when caring for a person with *C. diff* or norovirus. Wear a gown and gloves when entering the person's room and giving care. Alcohol-based hand sanitizers are not as effective against *C. diff* and norovirus as soap and water. *Hand-washing with soap and water is required.* Care items and surfaces are disinfected with a bleach solution.

Fecal Incontinence

Fecal incontinence is the inability to control the passage of feces and flatus through the anus. Causes include:

- Intestinal diseases.
- Nervous system diseases and injuries.
- Fecal impaction or diarrhea.
- Some drugs.
- Chronic illness.
- Aging.
- Mental health disorders or dementia (Chapters 53 and 54). The person may not recognize needing to or having a BM.
- Unanswered call lights.
- Not getting to the bathroom in time. The person may have mobility problems or may walk slowly. The bathroom may be too far away or in use.
- Problems removing clothes.
- Not finding the bathroom in a new setting.

Fecal incontinence has emotional effects. Frustration, embarrassment, anger, and humiliation are common. The person needs good skin care and may need:

- Bowel training
- Help with elimination after meals and every 2 to 3 hours
- Incontinence products (Chapter 27) to keep garments and linens clean

See *Focus on Children and Older Persons: Fecal Incontinence.*

FOCUS ON CHILDREN AND OLDER PERSONS

Fecal Incontinence

Children
Infants and toddlers have fecal incontinence until toilet trained.

Older Persons
Persons with dementia may smear stools on themselves, furniture, and walls. Some are not aware of having BMs. Some resist care. Follow the care plan. The measures for urinary incontinence (Chapter 27) may be part of the care plan for fecal incontinence. Be patient. Ask for help from co-workers. Talk to the nurse if you have problems keeping the person clean.

Flatulence

Gas and air are normally in the stomach and intestines. They are expelled through the mouth (burping, belching, eructating) and anus. Gas or air passed through the anus is called *flatus*. *Flatulence* is the excessive formation of gas or air in the stomach and intestines. Causes include:

- Swallowing air while eating and drinking. This includes chewing gum, eating fast, drinking through a straw, and drinking carbonated beverages.
- Bacterial action in the intestines.
- Gas-forming foods—onions, beans, cabbage, cauliflower, radishes, and cucumbers.
- Constipation.
- Certain digestive disorders.
- Bowel and abdominal surgeries.
- Drugs that decrease peristalsis.

If flatus is not expelled, the intestines swell or enlarge (*distend*) from the pressure of gases. Abdominal cramping or pain, shortness of breath, and a swollen abdomen (*bloating*) occur. Exercise, walking, moving in bed, and the left side-lying position help to expel flatus. Enemas and drugs may be ordered to relieve flatulence.

BOWEL TRAINING

Bowel training has 2 goals.

- To gain control of BMs.
- To develop a regular pattern of elimination. Fecal impaction, constipation, and fecal incontinence are prevented.

Meals, especially breakfast, stimulate peristalsis and the urge for a BM. The person's usual time for a BM is noted on the care plan. So is toilet, commode, or bedpan use. The care plan includes a high-fiber diet, increased fluids, warm fluids, activity, and privacy. Follow the person's care plan for bowel training.

Suppositories

A *suppository* is a cone-shaped, solid drug that is inserted into a body opening; it melts at body temperature. A nurse inserts a rectal suppository into the rectum (Fig. 29-6).

A suppository may be ordered for constipation, fecal impaction, or bowel training. A BM occurs about 30 minutes later.

See *Delegation Guidelines: Suppositories*.

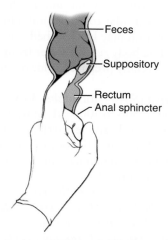

FIGURE 29-6 A rectal suppository is inserted along the rectal wall. It is not inserted into feces. (Modified from Williams P: *deWit's fundamental concepts and skills for nursing*, ed 6, St Louis, 2022, Elsevier.)

DELEGATION GUIDELINES

Suppositories

Rectal suppositories are drugs. You do not administer (give) suppositories without additional training. You may be asked to assist the nurse. If so, you need to know:

- What supplies are needed. Lubricant, gloves, toilet paper, and a bath blanket are gathered. The nurse is responsible for the suppository.
- How to position the person for the procedure. A left side-lying or left semi-prone position is used.
- How to position the person after the procedure and for how long. A comfortable left side-lying or left semi-prone position for 15 to 20 minutes is common.
- How soon to expect the urge for a BM.
- What to use for elimination after the procedure. The toilet, bedpan, or commode may be used.
- If the nurse needs to observe stools after the procedure.
- What observations to report and record:
  - How long the person retained the suppository
  - Color, amount, consistency, shape, and odor of stools
  - Complaints of cramping, pain, or discomfort
  - Complaints of nausea or weakness
- When to report observations
- What patient or resident concerns to report at once

ENEMAS

An *enema* is the introduction of fluid into the rectum and lower colon. Enemas are ordered to:

- Remove feces.
- Relieve constipation, fecal impaction, or flatulence.
- Clean the bowel of feces before certain surgeries and diagnostic procedures.

Safety and comfort measures for bowel needs are practiced when giving enemas (see Box 29-1). So are the rules in Box 29-2.

The enema ordered depends on the purpose—cleansing, constipation, fecal impaction, or flatulence. Consult with the nurse and use the agency's procedure manual to safely prepare and give enemas. You do not give enemas that contain drugs. Nurses give them.

See *Delegation Guidelines: Enemas*, p. 456.
See *Promoting Safety and Comfort: Enemas*, p. 456.

BOX 29-2   Giving Enemas

- Have the person void first. This increases comfort during the procedure.
- Assist with or give the enema ordered.
  - Cleansing enema (p. 456)—tap water enema, saline enema, or soapsuds enema (SSE)
  - Small-volume enema (p. 459)
  - Oil-retention enema (p. 460)
- Follow agency procedures to warm the solution and measure the temperature (if applicable). See *Delegation Guidelines: Cleansing Enemas* (p. 457). A cold solution can cause cramping. A hot solution can burn tissues. Saline may be warmed in a basin of warm water before being added to the enema bag.
- Position the person as the nurse directs. The left semi-prone or left side-lying position is preferred. Lying on the left side aids retention of the solution because of gravity and the natural curve of the colon.
- Know how far to insert the enema tip or tubing. Check your agency's procedure manual or ask the nurse. Depending on the enema type, it is usually inserted 2 to 4 inches in adults.
- Lubricate the enema tip or tubing before insertion.
- Stop insertion if there is resistance, the person complains of pain, or bleeding occurs.
- Ask the nurse how high to raise the enema bag for a cleansing enema. For adults, it is usually positioned 12 inches above the anus.
- Give the amount of solution ordered. Give the solution slowly. Usually it takes 10 to 15 minutes to give 750 to 1000 mL.
  - Raising the bag speeds up the flow.
  - Lowering the bag slows the flow.
  - Clamping the tube stops the flow.
- Hold the enema tube in place while giving the solution.
- Ask the nurse how long the person should try to retain the solution. The length of time depends on the amount and type of solution.
- Make sure the bathroom will be vacant when the person needs to have a BM. Make sure that another person will not use the bathroom. If the person uses the bedpan or commode, have the device ready.
- Ask the nurse to observe the enema results.

DELEGATION GUIDELINES

Enemas

You may be asked to assist the nurse with giving enemas. In some states and agencies, giving enemas can be delegated to nursing assistants. If the task is delegated to you, make sure the conditions in *Delegation Guidelines: Bowel Needs* (p. 449) are met. If those conditions are met, you need the following information from the nurse.

- What enema to give—cleansing, small-volume, or oil-retention
- What lubricant to use
- When to give the enema
- What position to use—left semi-prone or left side-lying position
- How far to insert the enema tube or tip
- How long the person should try to retain the solution
- What observations to report and record:
  - The amount of solution given
  - Bleeding or resistance when inserting the enema tube or tip
  - How long the person retained the enema solution
  - Color, amount, consistency, shape, and odor of stools
  - Complaints of cramping, pain, or discomfort
  - Complaints of nausea or weakness
  - How the person tolerated the procedure
- When to report observations
- What patient or resident concerns to report at once

PROMOTING SAFETY AND COMFORT

Enemas

Safety
Enemas are usually safe procedures. Many people give themselves enemas at home. However, enemas are dangerous for older persons and those with certain heart and kidney diseases. Also, enemas should not be used repeatedly.

Comfort
Before an enema, make sure that the bathroom is ready for use. Or have the bedpan or commode ready. Always keep a bedpan nearby in case the enema solution and stools are expelled. You promote mental comfort when the person knows the bathroom, commode, or bedpan is ready.

The person should retain the solution for as long as possible. Provide for a comfortable left semi-prone or left side-lying position. When comfortable, it is easier to tolerate the procedure.

To prevent cramping:
- Use the correct water temperature (if applicable). Cool water causes cramping.
- Give the solution slowly.

Cleansing Enemas

Cleansing enemas clean the bowel of feces and flatus. They relieve constipation and fecal impaction. They are given before certain surgeries and diagnostic procedures. Cleansing enemas take effect in a short time—usually within 10 minutes.

A tap water, saline, or soapsuds enema is ordered. An *enemas until clear* order means that enemas are given until the return solution is clear and free of stools. Agency policy may allow repeating certain enemas 2 or 3 times. You may be asked to assist the nurse with cleansing enemas. If allowed by the state and agency, the procedure may be delegated. Follow your agency's policies and procedures.

The following are different types of cleansing enemas.
- *Tap water enema*—is obtained from a faucet. The colon may absorb some of the water into the bloodstream. This creates a fluid imbalance. *Only 1 tap water enema is given. Do not repeat the enema.* Repeated tap water enemas increase the risk of excessive fluid absorption.
- *Saline enema*—saline is a solution of salt and water. The solution is similar to body fluid. However, some of the salt solution may be absorbed, causing a fluid imbalance. The body retains water from the excess salt. A commercially prepared solution (normal saline) is used.
- *Soapsuds enema (SSE)*—for adults, 3 to 5 mL of castile soap is added to 500 to 1000 mL of water or saline. Castile soap is gentle and less irritating than stronger soaps. The SSE irritates the bowel's mucous lining. Repeated enemas can damage the bowel. So can using more than 3 to 5 mL of castile soap or stronger soaps.

See *Focus on Math: Cleansing Enemas.*
See *Focus on Children and Older Persons: Cleansing Enemas.*
See *Delegation Guidelines: Cleansing Enemas.*
See procedure: *Giving a Cleansing Enema to an Adult.*

FOCUS ON MATH

Cleansing Enemas

Cleansing enemas are given over 10 to 15 minutes. The nurse tells you the amount of solution to give and the amount of time to give it in. While giving the solution, monitor how fast the fluid flows. To calculate the amount to give per minute, divide the total amount (in milliliters [mL]) by the time (in minutes). Each minute as you give the enema, subtract this amount to check if the rate is too fast or too slow.

For example, you are to give a 750-mL saline enema over 15 minutes. Divide 750 mL by 15 minutes. The fluid in the bag should decrease by about 50 mL each minute.

750 mL ÷ 15 minutes = 50 mL/minute

Note the start time. Check the amount at least each minute. After 1 minute, the solution should be at the 700 mL mark.

750 mL – 50 mL = 700 mL (after 1 minute)

After 2 minutes, the solution should be about half-way between the 700 mL and 600 mL marks (650 mL).

700 mL – 50 mL = 650 mL (after 2 minutes)

After 3 minutes, the solution should be at the 600 mL mark, and so on.

650 mL – 50 mL = 600 mL (after 3 minutes)

If the solution is flowing too fast or too slow, follow the nurse's directions. If too fast, the bag is lowered to slow the flow. If too slow, the bag is raised to increase the flow. Clamp the tube and call for the nurse if you need help with the flow rate.

FOCUS ON CHILDREN AND OLDER PERSONS
Cleansing Enemas

Children
Saline enemas are used for cleansing enemas in children. The nurse tells you the amount of solution to give. These are guidelines:

- Infants—120 to 240 mL
- Children 2 to 4 years—240 to 360 mL
- Children 4 to 10 years—360 to 480 mL
- Children 11 years and older—480 to 720 mL

How far to insert the tube depends on the child's age and needs. For example, no more than 1 inch for infants and no more than 4 inches for older children. The nurse tells you how far to insert the tube.

Infants cannot tell you they hurt. If cramping occurs, the child draws up the knees. The child's cry is higher-pitched than normal.

In children, cleansing enemas take effect in about 2 to 5 minutes.

DELEGATION GUIDELINES
Cleansing Enemas

See Box 29-2 and *Delegation Guidelines: Enemas* for the guidelines for giving enemas. Giving a cleansing enema requires additional information from the nurse. You need to know:

- What solution to use—tap water or saline
- What the solution temperature should be—usually 98.6°F to 100°F (Fahrenheit) (37.0°C to 37.8°C [centigrade]); sometimes warmer temperatures (105°F/40.5°C) are used for adults
- The amount of solution ordered—usually 500 to 1000 mL for adults
- If an additive is needed and how much—3 to 5 mL of castile soap for an SSE
- What size enema tube to use
- How far to insert the enema tubing—usually 2 to 4 inches for adults
- How high to hold the solution container—usually 12 inches above the anus
- How fast to give the solution—750 to 1000 mL are usually given over 10 to 15 minutes (See *Focus on Math: Cleansing Enemas*)
- How many times to repeat the enema

Giving a Cleansing Enema to an Adult
QUALITY OF LIFE

- Knock before entering the person's room.
- Address the person by name.
- Introduce yourself by name and title.

- Explain the procedure before starting and during the procedure.
- Protect the person's rights during the procedure.
- Handle the person gently during the procedure.

PRE-PROCEDURE

1 Follow *Delegation Guidelines*:
  a *Bowel Needs*, p. 449
  b *Enemas*
  c *Cleansing Enemas*
  See *Promoting Safety and Comfort*:
  a *Bowel Needs*, p. 449
  b *Enemas*
2 Practice hand hygiene and get the following supplies.
  - Disposable enema kit as directed by the nurse (enema bag and tube with clamp)
  - Enema solution as directed by the nurse
  - Additive (if needed)—3 to 5 mL (1 teaspoon) castile soap for an SSE
  - Graduate (measuring container)
  - Water thermometer or other means of measuring solution temperature as directed by agency procedure
  - Lubricant
  - IV (intravenous) pole

  - Commode or bedpan as needed (this procedure uses a commode)
  - Toilet paper
  - Bath blanket
  - Waterproof under-pad
  - Slip-resistant footwear
  - Robe (if needed)
  - Transfer/gait belt (if needed)
  - Disposable bag
  - Gloves
  - Laundry bag
3 Arrange items in the person's room and bathroom.
4 Practice hand hygiene.
5 Identify the person. Check the identification (ID) bracelet against the assignment sheet. Use 2 identifiers (Chapter 14). Also call the person by name.
6 Provide for privacy.

Continued

Giving a Cleansing Enema to an Adult—cont'd

PROCEDURE

7 Position the IV pole so the enema bag will be 12 inches above the anus. Or it is at the height directed by the nurse.

8 Prepare the enema.
   a Close the clamp on the tube.
   b Fill the enema bag with the correct amount of solution. Follow agency procedures for warming and checking the temperature. (Add castile soap for an SSE as directed by the nurse. Add it to the bag after the water to reduce suds.)
   c Seal the bag.
   d Hang the bag on the IV pole.
   e Remove air from the tubing. Hold the opening of the tube over a receptacle (graduate, sink, bedpan). Release the clamp. Let the solution flow to the end of the tubing. Clamp the tube.

9 Position the person. Cover the person for warmth and privacy.
   a Raise the bed for body mechanics. Bed rails are up if used. Lower the bed rail near you if up.
   b Cover the person with a bath blanket. Fan-fold top linens to the foot of the bed.
   c Place a waterproof under-pad under the buttocks.
   d Position the person in the left semi-prone or left side-lying position.

10 Apply gloves.

11 Give the enema.
   a Lubricate the tip of the tube. Lubricate 2 to 4 inches of the tube.
   b Fold back the bath blanket to expose the anal area. Separate the buttocks to see the anus.
   c Ask the person to take a deep breath in through the nose and breathe out slowly through the mouth.
   d Insert the tube gently 2 to 4 inches into the adult's rectum (Fig. 29-7). Do this when the person is exhaling. Stop if the person complains of pain, you feel resistance, or bleeding occurs.
   e Check the amount of solution in the bag.
   f Unclamp the tube. Give the solution slowly (Fig. 29-8).
   g Ask the person to take slow, deep breaths. This helps the person relax.
   h Clamp the tube if the person needs to have a BM, has cramping, or starts to expel the solution. Also, clamp the tube if the person is sweating or complains of nausea or weakness. Unclamp when symptoms subside.
   i Give the amount of solution ordered. Stop if the person cannot tolerate the procedure.
   j Clamp the tube before it is empty. This prevents air from entering the bowel.
   k Hold toilet paper around the tube and against the anus. Remove the tube. Place the enema bag and tube in a bag for disposal.

12 Cover the person with the bath blanket.

13 Remove and discard gloves. Practice hand hygiene.

14 Encourage retention of the enema for the time ordered. Maintain the left semi-prone or left side-lying position.

15 Lower the bed to a safe and comfortable level. Raise or lower bed rails. Follow the care plan. Provide for comfort.

16 Discard disposable items. Discard the enema bag and tube following agency policy.

17 Assist the person to the commode when the person requests. Follow these privacy and safety measures.
   a Be sure the person's clothing properly covers the person or apply a robe when up.
   b Apply slip-resistant footwear.
   c Use a transfer/gait belt as needed.
   d Be sure the bed is at a level that is safe for a transfer.
   e Raise or lower bed rails according to the care plan.
   f Wear gloves as needed. Practice hand hygiene after removing and discarding gloves.
   g Replace the waterproof under-pad on the bed if it is soiled.
   h Stay with the person as needed. Or leave the room and close the door. (Place the call light and toilet paper in reach. Practice hand hygiene before leaving.) Be respectful. Provide as much privacy as possible. Return when the person signals. Or check on the person every 5 minutes. Knock before entering the room. Practice hand hygiene after returning.

18 Apply gloves.

19 Assist with wiping and perineal care (Chapter 24) as needed. Remove and discard the gloves. Practice hand hygiene.

20 Assist the person back to bed. Cover the person. Place the bath blanket in the laundry bag.

21 Observe enema results for amount, color, consistency, shape, and odor. Call the nurse to observe the results.

22 Assist with hand hygiene. (Wear gloves. Practice hand hygiene after removing and discarding the gloves.)

POST-PROCEDURE

23 Provide for comfort. (See the inside of the back cover.)

24 Lower the bed to a safe and comfortable level. Raise or lower bed rails. Follow the care plan.

25 Clean up and store supplies and equipment. (Wear gloves. Change gloves as needed.)
   a Discard disposable items.
   b Empty the commode after the nurse observes the results (Chapter 27).
   c Follow agency procedures to clean and disinfect the commode and other re-usable equipment. Return supplies and equipment to their proper place.
   d Follow agency policy for used linens.
   e Clean and dry the over-bed table if used. Dry with paper towels. Discard paper towels. Position the over-bed table as the person prefers.
   f Remove and discard gloves. Practice hand hygiene.

26 Place the call light and other needed items within reach.

27 Follow the care plan and the person's preferences for privacy measures to maintain. Leaving the privacy curtain, window coverings, and door open or closed are examples.

28 Complete a safety check of the room. (See the inside of the back cover.)

29 Practice hand hygiene.

30 Report and record your care and observations.

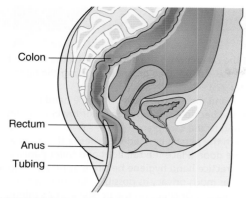

FIGURE 29-7 Enema tubing inserted into the adult rectum.

Small-Volume Enemas

Small-volume enemas irritate and distend the rectum to cause a BM. They are ordered for constipation or when the bowel does not need complete cleansing.

The enema is commercially prepared and ready to use. The solution is usually given at room temperature. To give the enema, insert the lubricated tip 2 inches into the rectum for an adult (Fig. 29-9). Gently squeeze and roll up the plastic container from the bottom. Do not release pressure on the bottle. Otherwise, solution is drawn from the rectum back into the bottle.

Urge the person to retain the solution until the need to have a BM is felt. This usually takes 1 to 5 minutes or as long as 10 minutes. Staying in the left semi-prone or left side-lying position helps retain the enema.

See procedure: *Giving a Small-Volume Enema.*

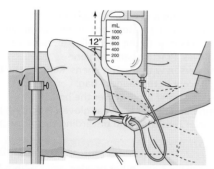

FIGURE 29-8 Giving a cleansing enema to an adult. The person is in a left semi-prone position. The enema bag hangs from an IV pole. The height of the bag determines the speed of the flow. Begin with the bag 12 inches above the anus. Raise the bag to increase the flow. Lower the bag to slow the flow. Clamp the tube to stop the flow.

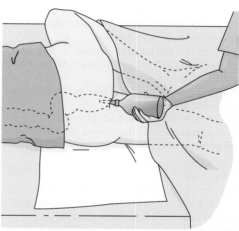

FIGURE 29-9 The small-volume enema tip is inserted 2 inches into the rectum.

Giving a Small-Volume Enema

QUALITY OF LIFE

- Knock before entering the person's room.
- Address the person by name.
- Introduce yourself by name and title.

- Explain the procedure before starting and during the procedure.
- Protect the person's rights during the procedure.
- Handle the person gently during the procedure.

PRE-PROCEDURE

1 Follow *Delegation Guidelines*:
  a *Bowel Needs*, p. 449
  b *Enemas*, p. 456
  See *Promoting Safety and Comfort*:
  a *Bowel Needs*, p. 449
  b *Enemas*, p. 456
2 Practice hand hygiene and get the following supplies.
  • Small-volume enema
  • Commode or bedpan (this procedure uses a bedpan)
  • Bedpan cover (if used)
  • Disposable waterproof pad
  • Toilet paper

  • Bath blanket
  • Waterproof under-pad
  • Gloves
  • Laundry bag
3 Arrange items in the person's room.
4 Practice hand hygiene.
5 Identify the person. Check the ID bracelet against the assignment sheet. Use 2 identifiers (Chapter 14). Also call the person by name.
6 Provide for privacy.
7 Raise the bed for body mechanics. Bed rails are up if used. Lower the bed rail near you if up.

Continued

Giving a Small-Volume Enema—cont'd

PROCEDURE

8 Position the person. Cover the person for warmth and privacy.
  a Cover the person with a bath blanket. Fan-fold top linens to the foot of the bed.
  b Place a waterproof under-pad under the buttocks.
  c Position the person in the left semi-prone or left side-lying position.
9 Apply gloves.
10 Position the bedpan nearby. Use the disposable waterproof pad as a barrier.
11 Give the enema.
  a Fold back the bath blanket to expose the anal area.
  b Remove the cap from the enema tip.
  c Separate the buttocks to see the anus.
  d Ask the person to take a deep breath in through the nose and breathe out slowly through the mouth.
  e Insert the enema tip 2 inches into the adult's rectum (see Fig. 29-9). Do this as the person exhales. Insert the tip gently. Stop if the person complains of pain, you feel resistance, or bleeding occurs.
  f Squeeze and roll up the container gently. Do not release pressure on the bottle until after you remove the tip from the rectum.
  g Put the container into the box, tip first. Discard the container and box.
12 Cover the person with the bath blanket.
13 Encourage retention of the enema. Maintain the left semi-prone or left side-lying position. Provide for comfort.
14 Assist the person onto the bedpan when the person has the urge to have a BM. (See procedure: *Giving the Bedpan* in Chapter 27.)
15 Remove and discard the gloves. Practice hand hygiene.
16 Lower the bed to a safe level. Raise or lower bed rails according to the care plan.
17 Stay with the person as needed. Or leave the room and close the door. (Place the call light and toilet paper in reach. Practice hand hygiene before leaving.) Be respectful. Provide as much privacy as possible. Return when the person signals. Or check on the person every 5 minutes. Knock before entering the room. Practice hand hygiene after returning.
18 Raise the bed for body mechanics. Lower the bed rail if up.
19 Apply gloves.
20 Remove the bedpan. Observe enema results for amount, color, consistency, shape, and odor. Call the nurse to observe the results.
21 Assist with wiping and perineal care (Chapter 24) as needed. Remove the waterproof under-pad as needed. Cover the person with the bath blanket. Remove and discard gloves. Practice hand hygiene.
22 Cover the person with the top linens. Remove the bath blanket. Place it in the laundry bag.
23 Raise the bed rail if used. Lower the bed.
24 Assist with hand hygiene. (Wear gloves. Practice hand hygiene after removing and discarding the gloves.)

POST-PROCEDURE

25 Provide for comfort. (See the inside of the back cover.)
26 Be sure the bed is at a safe and comfortable level. Raise or lower bed rails. Follow the care plan.
27 Clean up and store supplies and equipment. (Wear gloves. Change gloves as needed.)
  a Discard disposable items.
  b Empty the bedpan after the nurse observes the results (Chapter 27).
  c Follow agency procedures to clean and disinfect the bedpan and other re-usable equipment. Return supplies and equipment to their proper place.
  d Follow agency policy for used linens.
  e Clean and dry the over-bed table if used. Dry with paper towels. Discard paper towels. Position the over-bed table as the person prefers.
  f Remove and discard gloves. Practice hand hygiene.
28 Place the call light and other needed items within reach.
29 Follow the care plan and the person's preferences for privacy measures to maintain. Leaving the privacy curtain, window coverings, and door open or closed are examples.
30 Complete a safety check of the room. (See the inside of the back cover.)
31 Practice hand hygiene.
32 Report and record your care and observations.

Oil-Retention Enemas

Oil-retention enemas relieve constipation and fecal impaction. The oil softens feces and lubricates the rectum so feces pass with ease. Depending on the type, the oil-retention enema may act quickly. For others, the oil is retained for 30 minutes to 1 to 3 hours. Most oil-retention enemas are ready to use. Follow the manufacturer's instructions.

See *Promoting Safety and Comfort: Oil-Retention Enemas.*
See procedure: *Giving an Oil-Retention Enema.*

PROMOTING SAFETY AND COMFORT
Oil-Retention Enemas

Safety
An oil-retention enema may be retained for at least 30 minutes. Leave the room after giving the enema. Check on the person often. Say when you will return. Remind the person to signal if help is needed. Report any problems at once.

Giving an Oil-Retention Enema

QUALITY OF LIFE

- Knock before entering the person's room.
- Address the person by name.
- Introduce yourself by name and title.

- Explain the procedure before starting and during the procedure.
- Protect the person's rights during the procedure.
- Handle the person gently during the procedure.

PRE-PROCEDURE

1 Follow *Delegation Guidelines*:
   a *Bowel Needs*, p. 449
   b *Enemas*, p. 456
   See *Promoting Safety and Comfort*:
   a *Bowel Needs*, p. 449
   b *Enemas*, p. 456
   c *Oil-Retention Enemas*
2 Practice hand hygiene and get the following supplies.
   - Oil-retention enema
   - Commode or bedpan as needed (this procedure uses a toilet)
   - Slip-resistant footwear and transfer/gait belt (if needed)

- Waterproof under-pads
- Bath blanket
- Gloves
- Laundry bag
3 Arrange items in the person's room.
4 Practice hand hygiene.
5 Identify the person. Check the ID bracelet against the assignment sheet. Use 2 identifiers (Chapter 14). Also call the person by name.
6 Provide for privacy.
7 Raise the bed for body mechanics. Bed rails are up if used. Lower the bed rail near you if up.

PROCEDURE

8 Follow steps 8 through 13 in procedure: *Giving a Small-Volume Enema*. (Eliminate use of a bedpan if not needed. Or keep a bedpan nearby for prompt use.)
9 Remove and discard gloves. Practice hand hygiene.
10 Complete the usual post-procedure steps if the enema is to be retained for a long period (see steps 15 through 22).
11 Check the person often. Replace the waterproof under-pad on the bed as needed if there is leakage. (Wear gloves. Practice hand hygiene after removing and discarding gloves.) Remind the person to call before flushing if the person uses the bathroom without help.

12 Return when the person signals. Practice hand hygiene.
13 Assist the person to and from the bathroom if help is needed. Practice safety measures for transfers (Chapter 21) and walking (Chapter 35). Provide as much privacy as possible. Assist with wiping, perineal care, and hand hygiene as needed. (Wear gloves. Change gloves as needed. Remove and discard gloves and practice hand hygiene.)
14 Observe enema results for amount, color, consistency, shape, and odor. Call the nurse to observe the results. (Flush after the nurse observes the results.)

POST-PROCEDURE

15 Provide for comfort. (See the inside of the back cover.)
16 Be sure the bed is at a safe and comfortable level. Raise or lower bed rails. Follow the care plan.
17 Clean up and store supplies and equipment. Follow agency policy for used linens.
18 Place the call light and other needed items within reach.
19 Follow the care plan and the person's preferences for privacy measures to maintain. Leaving the privacy curtain, window coverings, and door open or closed are examples.

20 Complete a safety check of the room. (See the inside of the back cover.)
21 Practice hand hygiene.
22 Report and record your care and observations.

THE PERSON WITH AN OSTOMY

Sometimes part of the intestines is removed surgically. Cancer, bowel disease, and trauma (stab or bullet wounds) are common reasons. An ostomy is sometimes necessary. An *ostomy* is a surgically created opening that connects an internal organ to the body's surface. The surgically created opening seen on the body's surface is called a *stoma* (Fig. 29-10). An ostomy pouch is worn over the stoma to collect stools and flatus.

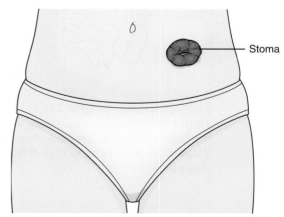

FIGURE 29-10 A stoma on the surface of the body.

Colostomy

A *colostomy* is a surgically created opening *(stomy)* between the colon *(colo)* and the body's surface. Part of the colon is brought out onto the body's surface and a stoma is made. Feces and flatus pass through the stoma instead of the anus.

With a permanent colostomy, the diseased part of the colon is removed. A temporary colostomy gives the diseased or injured bowel time to heal. After healing, the bowel is surgically re-connected.

The colostomy site depends on the site of disease or injury (Fig. 29-11). Stool consistency—liquid to formed—depends on the colostomy site. The more colon remaining to absorb water, the more solid and formed the stool. If the colostomy is near the end of the colon, stools are formed.

Stools irritate the skin. Skin care prevents skin breakdown around the stoma. The skin is washed and dried. A skin barrier applied around the stoma protects the skin from contact with stools. The skin barrier is part of the pouch or a separate device.

Ileostomy

An *ileostomy* is a surgically created opening *(stomy)* between the ileum (small intestine *[ileo]*) and the body's surface. Part of the ileum is brought out onto the body's surface and a stoma is made. The entire colon is removed (Fig. 29-12).

Liquid stools drain constantly from an ileostomy. Water is not absorbed because the colon was removed. Feces in the small intestine contain digestive juices that are very irritating to the skin. The ostomy pouch must fit well. Stools must not touch the skin. Good skin care is required.

Ostomy Pouches

A plastic ostomy pouch with an adhesive back is applied to the skin. Some pouches are secured to ostomy belts (Fig. 29-13). The pouch bulges when stools or flatus pass into it. An outlet (drain) is opened to empty the pouch of stools or to release flatus.

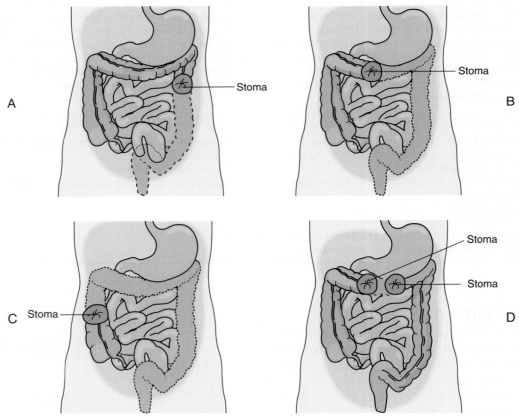

FIGURE 29-11 Colostomy sites. *Shading* shows the part of the bowel surgically removed. **A,** Sigmoid or descending colostomy. **B,** Transverse colostomy. **C,** Ascending colostomy. **D,** Double-barrel colostomy has 2 stomas. One allows for the excretion of feces. The other is for drugs to help the bowel heal. This type is usually temporary.

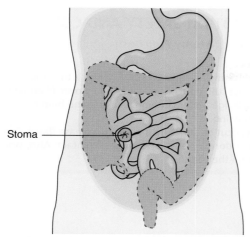

FIGURE 29-12 An ileostomy. The entire large intestine is removed. *Shading* shows the part of the bowel surgically removed.

Stoma

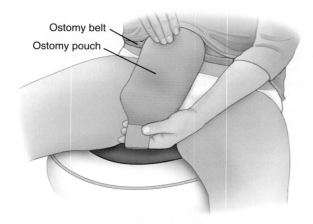

Ostomy belt
Ostomy pouch

FIGURE 29-13 An ostomy pouch secured to an ostomy belt. The pouch is emptied by directing it into the toilet and opening the outlet.

The pouch is changed every 2 to 7 days and when it leaks. Frequent pouch changes can damage the skin.

Odors are prevented by:

- Using odor-free pouches.
- Performing good hygiene.
- Emptying the pouch.
- Avoiding gas-forming foods.
- Putting deodorants into the pouch.

The person wears normal clothes. Tight garments can prevent feces from entering the pouch. Also, bulging from stools and flatus can be seen with tight clothes.

Peristalsis decreases during sleep and increases after eating and drinking. After sleep, the stoma is less likely to expel feces. If the person showers or bathes with the pouch off, it is best done before breakfast. Showers and baths are delayed for 1 to 2 hours after a new pouch is applied. This gives adhesive time to seal to the skin.

See *Delegation Guidelines: Ostomy Pouches.*

DELEGATION GUIDELINES

Ostomy Pouches

Nurses are responsible for changing pouches. You do not change ostomy pouches without additional training. If delegated to you, the conditions in *Delegation Guidelines: Bowel Needs* (p. 449) must be met to accept the task.

The nurse may ask you to remove an ostomy pouch before the person's shower or bath. The stoma may bleed slightly. You will not cause the person discomfort if you touch the stoma. The stoma does not have sensation.

Follow agency policy for pouch disposal. Pouches are not flushed down the toilet.

Emptying Ostomy Pouches. An ostomy pouch is emptied when it is about one-third (⅓) to one-half (½) full with stools. It is also opened to release flatus. Depending on the person, ostomy type, and ostomy location, pouches are usually emptied 2 to 6 times a day. Because ileostomies constantly drain liquid feces, ileostomy pouches are emptied more often than colostomy pouches.

Pouches are emptied into the toilet (see Fig. 29-13) or a bedpan. Before emptying, toilet paper is placed in the toilet to prevent splashing. The outlet is wiped with toilet paper or a pre-moistened wipe after emptying. The pouch is closed with a clip, clamp, or other closure (Fig. 29-14).

See *Delegation Guidelines: Emptying Ostomy Pouches*, p. 464.

See *Promoting Safety and Comfort: Emptying Ostomy Pouches*, p. 464.

See procedure: *Assisting the Person to Empty an Ostomy Pouch*, p. 464.

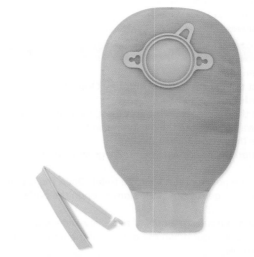

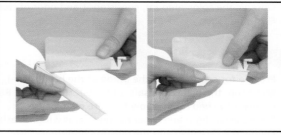

FIGURE 29-14 An ostomy pouch with a clamp. The clamp is used to close the pouch. (Courtesy Hollister Incorporated, Libertyville, Ill.)

DELEGATION GUIDELINES

Emptying Ostomy Pouches

Assisting the person to empty an ostomy pouch may be a routine nursing task. To empty a pouch, you need this information from the nurse and the care plan.

- If the person has a colostomy or ileostomy
- When to empty the pouch
- What special equipment and supplies to use
- What observations to report and record:
  - Color, amount, consistency, and odor of stools
  - Complaints of pain or discomfort
- When to report observations
- What patient or resident concerns to report at once

PROMOTING SAFETY AND COMFORT

Emptying Ostomy Pouches

Comfort

Empty ostomy pouches promptly when ⅓ to ½ full. Otherwise, the pouch can leak. And an over-filled pouch can cause a bulge under clothing. Leaking and bulging can be embarrassing.

Never cut or puncture a pouch to release flatus. The pouch's odor barrier will no longer be intact. Also, stools can leak from the pouch.

Assisting the Person to Empty an Ostomy Pouch

QUALITY OF LIFE

- Knock before entering the person's room.
- Address the person by name.
- Introduce yourself by name and title.
- Explain the procedure before starting and during the procedure.
- Protect the person's rights during the procedure.
- Handle the person gently during the procedure.

PRE-PROCEDURE

1 Follow *Delegation Guidelines*:
  a *Bowel Needs*, p. 449
  b *Emptying Ostomy Pouches*
  See *Promoting Safety and Comfort*:
  a *Bowel Needs*, p. 449
  b *Emptying Ostomy Pouches*
2 Practice hand hygiene and get the following supplies.
  - Toilet paper
  - Pre-moistened wipes
  - Plastic bag (for wipes)
  - Gloves

3 Arrange items in the person's bathroom. Make a cuff on the plastic bag (if used). (Fold down the top portion of the bag.) Place the bag within reach. Place a few sheets of toilet paper in the toilet bowl. This helps prevent splashing when the pouch is emptied.
4 Practice hand hygiene.
5 Identify the person. Check the ID bracelet against the assignment sheet. Use 2 identifiers (Chapter 14). Also call the person by name.
6 Provide for privacy.

PROCEDURE

7 Put on gloves.
8 Assist the person to the bathroom. Close the bathroom door for privacy.
9 Help the person sit on the toilet and move garments out of the way. Make sure the person is comfortable.
10 Have the person spread the legs.
11 Position the pouch between the legs and over the toilet.
12 Hold the pouch outlet over the toilet. Open the clip or clamp and gently pinch the sides to open the outlet (see Fig. 29-13).
13 Allow the pouch to empty. If necessary, slide your thumb and index finger down the outside of the pouch to push out stools.
14 Observe the color, amount, consistency, and odor of stools. Flush the toilet.

15 Clean the inside of the pouch outlet with toilet paper or a pre-moistened wipe (Fig. 29-15). Make sure the inside is thoroughly clean. Discard toilet paper into the toilet. Discard the wipe into the plastic bag.
16 Clean the outside of the pouch outlet. Clean the clip (clamp) if soiled. Make sure the outside and the clip (clamp) are thoroughly clean. Use toilet paper or a pre-moistened wipe. Discard the toilet paper or wipe as in step 15.
17 Close the pouch outlet with the clip (clamp). See Figure 29-14. Follow the manufacturer's instructions.
18 Remove and discard gloves. Practice hand hygiene. Apply clean gloves.
19 Assist with hand hygiene.
20 Tie or seal the plastic bag (if used). Follow agency policy for disposal.
21 Remove and discard gloves. Practice hand hygiene.
22 Help the person back to bed.

POST-PROCEDURE

23 Provide for comfort. (See the inside of the back cover.)
24 Make sure the bed is at a safe and comfortable level. Raise or lower the bed rails. Follow the care plan.
25 Place the call light and other needed items within reach.
26 Follow the care plan and the person's preferences for privacy measures to maintain. Leaving the privacy curtain, window coverings, and door open or closed are examples.

27 Complete a safety check of the room. (See the inside of the back cover.)
28 Practice hand hygiene.
29 Report and record your care and observations.

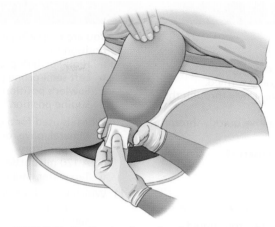

FIGURE 29-15 Cleaning the outlet of an ostomy pouch.

FOCUS ON **PRIDE**
The Person, Family, and Yourself

Personal and Professional Responsibility
Skin care needs after bowel elimination vary. Some persons are independent. Others require help with wiping and hand hygiene. If the person is soiled, provide perineal care. For persons with diarrhea or fecal incontinence, more frequent care is needed.

Follow the person's care plan. Give care as often as needed with a helpful attitude. Allow as much independence as possible.

Rights and Respect
Bowel needs require privacy. Some persons are embarrassed to have a BM in a strange setting. To promote comfort and privacy:
- Ask others to leave the room.
- Close doors, privacy curtains, and window coverings.
- Turn on water or music to mask sounds.
- Cover the person.
- Allow enough time. Place the call light nearby and ask the person to call if help is needed.
- Knock before entering the room. Tell the person who you are. Ask if you can enter before opening the door completely.
- Use an agency-approved spray for odors.

Independence and Social Interaction
Some persons have had ostomies for a long time. They may have special routines or care measures. When you assist, ask what they prefer. To promote independence, allow personal choice and control as much as safely possible.

Delegation and Teamwork
You will have situations that require problem solving and help. You may be asked to do something you have not done alone before. Communicate your questions or concerns to the nurse. For example, you can say: "I have practiced this procedure, but I have not done it on my own. Are you available to supervise me?"

Guidance and assistance are part of the nurse's role in delegation. The nurse needs to know your comfort level with tasks. Never be ashamed to ask for guidance and assistance.

Ethics and Laws
All persons must be protected from abuse, mistreatment, and neglect. Examples include:
- Leaving a person sitting or lying in urine or stools
- Leaving a person on a toilet, commode, or bedpan for a long time
- Telling a person to void or have a BM in bed (soil the bed)

Federal and state laws require the reporting and investigating of abuse, mistreatment, and neglect. Protect the person and yourself. Check patients or residents often. Be careful and focused. Always treat the person with dignity.

FOCUS ON **PRIDE**: *Application*
You are asked to do an unfamiliar task. Do you seek help? Do you try to do it alone? Does asking for help bother you? Explain why being able to ask for help is a strength.

REVIEW QUESTIONS

Circle the BEST answer.

1 Which is *true?*
   a A person must have a BM every day.
   b Stools are normally brown, soft, and formed.
   c Diarrhea occurs when feces move slowly through the bowel.
   d Constipation occurs when feces move quickly through the bowel.

2 Which should you ask the nurse to observe?
   a A black and tarry stool
   b The person's first BM of the day
   c Stool with an odor
   d Smooth and soft stool from a colostomy

3 A person is worried about constipation. You should
   a Decrease the person's fluid intake
   b Help the person to the bathroom every hour
   c Tell the person not to worry
   d Report the concern to the nurse

4 The prolonged retention and buildup of feces in the rectum is called
   a Constipation
   b Fecal impaction
   c Diarrhea
   d Fecal incontinence

5 These measures promote normal BMs. Which is outside your role limits?
   a Provide oral fluids according to the care plan.
   b Assist with activity according to the care plan.
   c Give drugs to control diarrhea.
   d Provide privacy for bowel elimination.

6 Dehydration is a risk from
   a Fecal impaction
   b Flatulence
   c Constipation
   d Diarrhea

7 A person has *C. difficile.* You should
   a Disinfect care items with soap and water
   b Use an alcohol-based hand sanitizer for hand hygiene
   c Wear a gown and gloves when giving care
   d Refuse to care for the person

8 Bowel training is aimed at
   a Bowel control and regular elimination
   b Ostomy control
   c Promoting toilet use
   d Preventing bleeding

9 You are preparing a person for an enema. You need to position the person in the
   a High-Fowler's position
   b Left semi-prone position
   c Fowler's position
   d Supine position

10 Which is used for a cleansing enema?
   a Mineral, olive, or cottonseed oil
   b A suppository
   c A 120-mL bottle of solution
   d Tap water, saline, or a soapsuds enema

11 Which is used for cleansing enemas in children?
   a Soapsuds
   b Saline
   c Oil
   d Tap water

12 When giving an enema
   a Use a cool solution
   b Give the solution slowly
   c Have the person void after giving the enema
   d Insert the tube until you feel resistance

13 A small-volume enema is retained
   a For 2 minutes
   b At least 10 to 20 minutes
   c At least 30 minutes
   d Until the urge to have a BM is felt

14 A person has an ileostomy. Which is *normal?*
   a Stools are liquid and drain constantly into the pouch.
   b Stools are small hard lumps that pass every 2 to 4 hours.
   c Stools are large and formed and pass every 1 to 2 days.
   d The person has pain when stools pass.

15 When emptying an ostomy pouch, you should
   a Wait until the pouch is full to empty it
   b Wipe the outlet clean after emptying the pouch
   c Remove the pouch to empty it
   d Empty the contents into the wastebasket

Answers to Chapter 29 questions are on p. 902.

FOCUS ON PRACTICE

Problem Solving

You respond to a resident's call light. The resident needs to have a BM urgently. The bathroom is occupied by the roommate. What do you do?

Nutrition

- Define the key terms and key abbreviations in this chapter.
- Explain the purpose and use of the MyPlate symbol.
- Describe the functions and sources of nutrients.
- Explain how to read and use food labels.

- Describe the special diets and between-meal snacks.
- Explain how to assist with measuring food intake.
- Explain how to promote PRIDE in the person, the family, and yourself.

calorie The fuel or energy value of food
cholesterol A soft, waxy substance found in the bloodstream and all body cells
dysphagia Difficulty *(dys)* swallowing *(phagia)*

nutrient A substance that is ingested, digested, absorbed, and used by the body
nutrition The processes involved in the ingestion, digestion, absorption, and use of food and fluids by the body

FDA	Food and Drug Administration		mg	Milligram
GI	Gastro-intestinal		oz	Ounce
HHS	U.S. Department of Health and Human Services		USDA	U.S. Department of Agriculture

Food is a basic need. The person's diet affects physical and mental well-being and function. A poor diet and poor eating habits:

- Increase the risk for disease and infection.
- Cause chronic illnesses to become worse.
- Cause healing problems.
- Increase the risk for accidents and injuries.

Many factors affect dietary needs and practices. Culture, finances, age, illness, food allergies, weight and height, physical activity, and personal choice are examples. The health team includes these and other factors in planning the person's nutrition needs.

NOTE: Federal agencies often issue and revise nutrition-related guidelines. *Dietary Guidelines for Americans, Physical Activity Guidelines for Americans* (p. 468), MyPlate (p. 468), and food labels (p. 472) are examples. The Internet provides access to the most current information.

BASIC NUTRITION

Nutrition is the processes involved in the ingestion, digestion, absorption, and use of food and fluids by the body. Foods and fluids contain nutrients.

A *nutrient* is a substance that is ingested, digested, absorbed, and used by the body. Nutrients are grouped into fats, proteins, carbohydrates, vitamins, minerals, and water. See "Nutrients" on p. 470.

Fats, proteins, and carbohydrates provide fuel for energy. A *calorie* is the fuel or energy value of food.

- 1 gram of fat—9 calories
- 1 gram of protein—4 calories
- 1 gram of carbohydrate—4 calories

A well-balanced diet and correct calorie intake are needed for growth, healing, and body function. A high-fat, high-calorie diet causes weight gain and obesity. A low-calorie diet promotes weight loss.

Dietary and Activity Guidelines

Dietary Guidelines for Americans are issued every 5 years by the U.S. Department of Agriculture (USDA) and the U.S. Department of Health and Human Services (HHS). The guidelines help promote health, reduce the risk of chronic diseases, and meet nutrient needs. For the most current dietary guidelines, search the Internet for *Dietary Guidelines for Americans*.

The HHS also issues *Physical Activity Guidelines for Americans.* These guidelines are used along with the dietary guidelines to promote health. For the most current activity guidelines, search the Internet for *Physical Activity Guidelines for Americans.*

MyPlate. The MyPlate symbol (Fig. 30-1) encourages healthy eating from 5 food groups. Issued by the USDA, MyPlate is based on the *Dietary Guidelines for Americans.* MyPlate helps people:
* Learn how much to eat from each food group.
* Look at their eating routine and make choices that are rich in nutrients.
* Develop a healthy eating routine that can improve current and future health.
* Eat a variety of grains, vegetables, fruits, dairy foods, and protein foods. Added sugars, saturated fat (p. 470), and sodium are limited.

See *Focus on Children and Older Persons: MyPlate.*

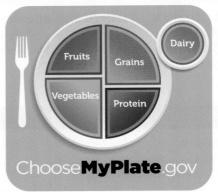

FIGURE 30-1 The MyPlate symbol. (Courtesy U.S. Department of Agriculture, Center for Nutrition and Policy Promotion.)

FOCUS ON CHILDREN AND OLDER PERSONS
MyPlate

Children
Toddlers are exploring new foods and learning to communicate needs and preferences. Pre-schoolers are learning independence. "Picky eating" is a common behavior. The USDA offers these suggestions.
* Try serving a new food with a familiar food at the same meal. It may take 8 to 10 or more tries to accept a new food.
* Balance recommended amounts over a few days or a week if the child will not eat the suggested amounts every day.
* Offer different foods from all food groups each day. Offer different foods from day to day. Encourage choices from a variety of foods.
* Serve foods in small portions.
* Watch that the child is not filling up on drinks between meals. Offer water between meals if the child is thirsty.
* Include the child in meal preparation. Young children can rinse fruits and vegetables, tear lettuce, and stir ingredients. They enjoy tasting foods that they helped prepare.

Physical Activity. The HHS recommends that adults do at least 1 of the following weekly.
* 2 hours and 30 minutes of moderate-intensity physical activity
* 1 hour and 15 minutes of vigorous-intensity physical activity

Activities should be *aerobic.* Aerobic activities make the heart beat faster. To determine if an activity is moderate or vigorous, a person can try talking while being active.
* An activity is *moderate-intensity* if breathing is harder than normal but the person can still have a conversation.
* An activity is *vigorous-intensity* if the person can say only a few words before needing to take a breath.

Adults also should do muscle-strengthening activities at least 2 days a week. Push-ups, sit-ups, and weight-lifting are examples.

See *Focus on Children and Older Persons: Physical Activity.*

FOCUS ON CHILDREN AND OLDER PERSONS
Physical Activity

Children
Physical activity promotes healthy growth and development. The HHS recommends that caregivers of pre-schoolers encourage active play throughout the day. Play should involve a variety of activities of all intensities (light, moderate, and vigorous). Hopping, skipping, jumping, and tumbling are examples. Being active 3 hours a day is a healthy goal for pre-school-age children.

For children 6 to 17 years of age, the HHS recommends:
* 1 hour or more of moderate or vigorous physical activity each day.
* Vigorous activity at least 3 days a week.
* Muscle and bone strengthening activities at least 3 days a week. Climbing and jumping are examples.

Older Persons
Physical activity can help older persons maintain strength and independence. Activity also can help manage many health problems, including diabetes and high blood pressure. Exercises that maintain or improve balance are helpful for persons at risk for falls.

Food Groups

The 5 food groups are:
* Grains group
* Vegetable group
* Fruit group
* Dairy group
* Protein foods group

The amount needed from each food group depends on age, biological sex, height and weight, and physical activity. See Table 30-1 for sources, general recommendations for daily servings and serving sizes for adults, and health benefits.

TABLE 30-1 Food Groups

Food Sources	Daily Servings and Serving Sizes	Health Benefits
Grains <ul><li>Grains are foods made from wheat, rice, oats, cornmeal, barley, or other cereal grains. Bread, pasta, oatmeal, breakfast cereals, tortillas, and grits are examples.</li><li>*Whole grains* have the entire grain kernel. Whole-wheat flour, bulgur (cracked wheat), oatmeal, and brown rice are examples.</li><li>*Refined grains* are processed to remove parts of the grain kernel. White flour, white bread, corn grits, and white rice are examples. They have less dietary fiber than whole grains.</li></ul>	**Daily Servings**<ul><li>Adult women: 5 to 8 ounces (oz) with at least 3 to 4 oz from whole grains</li><li>Adult men: 6 to 10 oz with at least 3 to 5 oz from whole grains</li></ul>**Serving Sizes**<ul><li>1 oz = 1 slice of bread</li><li>1 oz = 1 cup breakfast cereal</li><li>1 oz = ½ cup cooked rice, oatmeal, or pasta</li></ul>	<ul><li>May lower cholesterol (p. 470) and reduce the risk of heart disease, including heart attack and stroke.</li><li>May help digestion and prevent constipation. (Fiber is important for proper bowel function.)</li><li>May help with weight management.</li><li>May prevent certain birth defects.</li><li>Contain dietary fiber, several B vitamins (thiamin, riboflavin, niacin, folate [folic acid]), and minerals (iron, magnesium, and selenium).</li></ul>
Vegetables <ul><li>Vegetables can be raw, cooked, fresh, frozen, canned, dried, or juiced.</li><li>*Dark green vegetables*—broccoli, collard greens, dark green leafy lettuce, kale, mustard greens, romaine lettuce, spinach, turnip greens, watercress.</li><li>*Red and orange vegetables*—acorn, butternut, and Hubbard squashes; carrots; pumpkin; red and orange peppers; sweet potatoes; tomatoes; tomato juice.</li><li>*Beans, peas, and lentils*—black beans, black-eyed peas, garbanzo beans (chickpeas), kidney beans, pinto beans, split peas, lentils.</li><li>*Starchy vegetables*—corn, green peas, hominy, potatoes.</li><li>*Other vegetables*—avocado, bean sprouts, cabbage, cauliflower, celery, cucumbers, green beans, green peppers, iceberg (head) lettuce, mushrooms, onions, summer squash, zucchini.</li></ul>	**Daily Servings**<ul><li>Adult women: 2 to 3 cups</li><li>Adult men: 2½ to 4 cups</li></ul>**Serving Sizes**<ul><li>1 cup = 1 cup raw or cooked vegetables or vegetable juice</li><li>1 cup = 2 cups raw leafy greens</li></ul>	<ul><li>May lower cholesterol and reduce the risk of heart disease, including heart attack and stroke.</li><li>May protect against certain cancers.</li><li>May help lower calorie intake. Most vegetables are low in fat and calories.</li><li>May prevent certain birth defects.</li><li>Contain potassium, dietary fiber, folate (folic acid), and vitamins A and C.</li></ul>
Fruits <ul><li>Any fruit or 100% fruit juice counts as part of the fruit group.</li><li>Fruits may be fresh, frozen, canned, or dried. They may be whole, cut up, pureed, or cooked.</li><li>Avoid fruits canned in syrup. Syrup contains added sugar. Choose fruits canned in 100% fruit juice or water.</li></ul>	**Daily Servings**<ul><li>Adult women: 1½ to 2 cups</li><li>Adult men: 2 to 2½ cups</li></ul>**Serving Sizes**<ul><li>1 cup = 1 cup fruit</li><li>1 cup = 1 cup fruit juice</li><li>1 cup = ½ cup dried fruit</li></ul>	<ul><li>May lower cholesterol and reduce the risk of heart disease, including heart attack and stroke.</li><li>May protect against certain cancers.</li><li>May help bowel function.</li><li>May help lower fat and calorie intake. Most fruits are low in fat and calories.</li><li>Contain no cholesterol.</li><li>Are low in sodium (salt).</li><li>Contain potassium, dietary fiber, vitamin C, and folate (folic acid).</li></ul>
Dairy <ul><li>All fluid milk products are part of the dairy group. So are many foods made from milk. Yogurt and cheese are examples.</li><li>Low-fat or fat-free choices are best.</li><li>Cream, cream cheese, and butter are not in this group.</li></ul>	**Daily Servings**<ul><li>Adult women: 3 cups</li><li>Adult men: 3 cups</li></ul>**Serving Sizes**<ul><li>1 cup = 1 cup milk, yogurt, or soy milk</li><li>1 cup = 1½ oz natural cheese</li><li>1 cup = 1 oz processed cheese</li></ul>	<ul><li>Help build bones and teeth and maintain bone mass. This may reduce the risk of osteoporosis.</li><li>May reduce the risk of high blood pressure.</li><li>Contain calcium, potassium, vitamin D, and protein.</li></ul>

Continued

TABLE 30-1	Food Groups—cont'd	
Food Sources	Daily Servings and Serving Sizes	Health Benefits

Protein Foods
• All foods made from meat, poultry, seafood, eggs, processed soy products, nuts, and seeds are protein foods.
• Beans, peas, and lentils are in this group and the vegetable group.
• Some protein foods are high in saturated fat. For healthy choices, remember:
  • Choose lean or low-fat meat and poultry.
  • Limit foods high in saturated fat. Fatty cuts of beef, pork, and lamb; regular (75% to 85% lean) ground beef; regular sausages, hot dogs, and bacon are examples.
  • Seafood like salmon, trout, and anchovies contain healthy fats.
  • Processed meats (ham, sausage, hot dogs, luncheon and deli meats) have added sodium (salt).
  • Vary the kinds of protein foods eaten. Include seafood, nuts, seeds, and soy products throughout the week.
	Daily Servings
	• Adult women: 5 to 6½ oz
	• Adult men: 5½ to 7 oz
	
	Serving Sizes
	• 1 oz = 1 oz lean meat, poultry, or fish
	• 1 oz = 1 egg
	• 1 oz = 1 tablespoon peanut butter
	• 1 oz = ¼ cup cooked beans
	• 1 oz = ½ oz nuts or seeds
		• Contain nutrients needed for health and body maintenance—protein, B vitamins (niacin, thiamin, riboflavin, and B_6), vitamin E, iron, zinc, and magnesium.
		• Proteins are building blocks needed for body structure and function.

Modified from U.S. Department of Agriculture: Eat Healthy.

Nutrients

No food or food group has every essential nutrient. A well-balanced diet ensures an adequate intake of essential nutrients.

- *Protein*—is a component of all body cells. It is essential for tissue growth and repair. It provides energy and is important for many body processes. Sources include meat, fish, poultry, eggs, milk and milk products, beans, peas, lentils, nuts, seeds, soy products, whole grains, and vegetables.
- *Carbohydrates*—provide energy and fiber for bowel elimination.
  - *Dietary fiber (fiber)*. Fiber is not digested. It provides the bulky part of chyme for elimination. Good sources include whole grains, fruits, vegetables, beans and peas, and nuts and seeds.
  - *Sugars*. Sugars are broken down by the body into glucose. Glucose is used for energy. Sugars are naturally present in many nutritious foods and drinks (dairy products, fruits, vegetables). Consuming *added sugars* increases calories without important nutrients. See "Food Labels" on p. 472.
- *Fats*—provide energy. They add flavor and help the body use certain vitamins. Fat is a basic part of cell membranes and supports important body processes. Unneeded dietary fat is stored as body fat (*adipose tissue*) to be a source of energy later when calories from carbohydrates are used up. Some fats are healthy. Others are not. See "Fats and Oils."

- *Vitamins*—are needed for certain body functions. The body stores vitamins A, D, E, and K. Vitamin C and the B complex vitamins are not stored. They must be ingested daily. The lack of a certain vitamin results in illness. See Table 30-2.
- *Minerals*—are needed for bone and tooth formation, nerve and muscle function, fluid balance, and other body processes. Foods containing calcium help prevent musculo-skeletal changes. See Table 30-3.
- *Water*—is essential for all body processes (Chapter 32).

Fats and Oils

Solid fats are solid at room temperature. Butter, beef fat (tallow, suet), chicken fat, pork fat (lard), stick margarine, and shortening are examples. Desserts and baked goods, many cheeses, and whole milk also contain solid fats. Solid fats contain more unhealthy fats called saturated fats and *trans* fats. (No longer recognized as safe, the major source of artificial *trans* fat in the U.S. food supply was removed as of June 2018.)

Saturated fats affect cholesterol levels. *Cholesterol* is a soft, waxy substance found in the bloodstream and all body cells. When certain cholesterol levels are high, the risk for heart disease increases. Eating less saturated fat can improve cholesterol and lower the risk for heart disease.

Oils are liquid fats. Oils come from plants and fish. Oils are not a food group, but they do provide nutrients (unsaturated fats and vitamin E). Oils (including vegetable oils [canola, corn, olive] and oils in foods such as seafood and nuts) are part of a healthy diet.

TABLE 30-2	Common Vitamins	
Vitamin	Major Functions	Sources
Vitamin A	Growth and development, immune function, reproduction, red blood cell formation, skin and bone formation, vision	Cantaloupe, carrots, dairy products, eggs, fortified cereals, green leafy vegetables, pumpkin, red peppers, sweet potatoes
Vitamin B$_1$ (thiamin)	Changing food into energy, nervous system function	Beans and peas, enriched grain products (bread, cereal, pasta, rice), nuts, pork, sunflower seeds, whole grains
Vitamin B$_2$ (riboflavin)	Changing food into energy, growth and development, red blood cell formation	Eggs, enriched grain products, meats, milk, mushrooms, poultry, seafood, spinach
Vitamin B$_3$ (niacin)	Cholesterol production, changing food into energy, digestion, nervous system function	Beans, beef, enriched grain products, nuts, pork, poultry, seafood, whole grains
Vitamin B$_{12}$	Changing food into energy, nervous system function, red blood cell formation	Dairy products, eggs, fortified cereals, meats, poultry, seafood
Folate (folic acid)	Prevention of birth defects, protein metabolism, red blood cell formation	Asparagus, avocado, beans and peas, enriched grain products, green leafy vegetables, orange juice
Vitamin C (ascorbic acid)	*Antioxidant* (substance that prevents cell damage), formation of substances that hold tissues together, immune function, wound healing	Broccoli, Brussels sprouts, cantaloupe, citrus fruits and juices, kiwi, peppers, strawberries, tomatoes and tomato juice
Vitamin D	Blood pressure control, bone growth, calcium balance, hormone production, immune and nervous system function	Egg yolks; fish; fish oil; fortified cereals, dairy products, orange juice, and soy drinks; mushrooms
Vitamin E	Antioxidant, formation of blood vessels, immune function	Fortified cereals and juices, green vegetables, nuts and seeds, peanuts and peanut butter, vegetable oils
Vitamin K	Blood clotting, strong bones	Green vegetables

Modified from U.S. Food and Drug Administration, *Vitamins and Minerals Chart.*

TABLE 30-3	Common Minerals	
Mineral	Major Functions	Sources
Calcium	Blood clotting, bone and teeth formation, blood vessel function, hormone secretion, muscle contraction, nervous system function	Canned seafood with bones; dairy products; fortified cereals, orange juice, and soy drinks; green vegetables; tofu
Phosphorus	Acid-base balance, bone formation, energy production and storage, hormone function	Beans and peas; dairy products; meats; nuts and seeds; poultry; seafood; whole-grain, enriched, and fortified cereals and breads
Iron	Energy production, growth and development, immune function, red blood cell formation, reproduction, wound healing	Beans, peas, and lentils; cantaloupe; eggs; green vegetables (asparagus, beet greens, broccoli, spinach, Swiss chard); meats; nuts; poultry; raisins; seafood; seeds; soy products; whole-grain, enriched, and fortified breads, cereals, pasta, and rice
Iodine	Growth and development, metabolism, reproduction, thyroid hormone function	Breads and cereals, dairy products, iodized salt, potatoes, seafood, seaweed, turkey
Sodium	Acid-base balance, blood pressure control, fluid balance, muscle and nerve function	Almost all foods, table salt (see p. 475)
Potassium	Blood pressure control, carbohydrate metabolism, fluid balance, growth and development, heart function, muscle and nervous system function, protein formation	Beans, nuts, dairy products (milk, yogurt), fruits (oranges, apricots, bananas, kiwi, cantaloupe, grapefruit), juices (orange, pomegranate, prune, carrot and other vegetable juices), seafood, tomato products, vegetables (potatoes, sweet potatoes, beet greens, spinach)

Modified from U.S. Food and Drug Administration, *Vitamins and Minerals Chart.*

Food Labels

Food labels are used to make informed food choices for a healthy diet (Fig. 30-2). Food labels contain information about:

- *Serving size and the number of servings in each package.* Nutrition information on the label is based on 1 serving. The serving size is not a recommendation on how much to eat or drink.
- *Calories.* The number of calories in 1 serving. The number of servings eaten determines the number of calories eaten.
- *Nutrients.* The U.S. Food and Drug Administration (FDA) recommends eating:
  - Less saturated fat, sodium, and added sugars
  - More dietary fiber, vitamin D, calcium, iron, and potassium
- *Percent Daily Value (%DV).* The %DV shows how much of a nutrient is in 1 serving of the food. The %DV helps you decide if a food is high or low in a nutrient. The value is based on a 2000-calorie daily diet. According to the FDA, a 5% DV is low. A DV of 20% or more is high. See *Focus on Math: Food Labels.*

SPECIAL DIETS

Doctors may order special diets (therapeutic diets) (Table 30-4):

- For a nutritional deficiency or a disease
- For weight gain or loss
- To remove or decrease certain substances in the diet

Persons with diseases of the heart, kidneys, gallbladder, pancreas, liver, stomach, or intestines often need special diets. High-protein diets are needed to heal wounds and pressure injuries. Adding bran to the diet provides fiber for bowel elimination. Allergies, excess weight, and other disorders also require special diets.

The sodium-controlled diet is often ordered (p. 475). So is a diabetes meal plan (p. 475). Persons with swallowing problems may need a dysphagia diet (p. 476 and Chapter 31). *Regular diet (general diet)* means there are no dietary limits or restrictions.

Surgery and some tests, procedures, and treatments require that nothing is eaten. The person has an NPO order. *NPO* stands for nothing by mouth *(nil per os)* (Chapter 33).

The health team considers the need for dietary changes, personal choices, religion, culture, and eating problems. They also consider food allergies and intolerances (sensitivities) (Chapter 31). The nurse and dietitian teach the person and family about the diet.

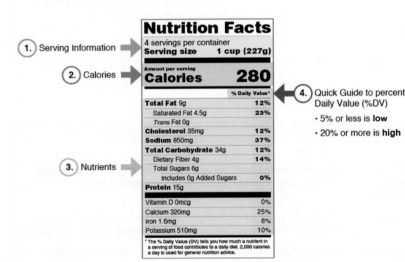

FIGURE 30-2 Parts of the Nutrition Facts Label. (From U.S. Food and Drug Administration, 2023.)

FOCUS ON MATH

Food Labels

The nutrition information on a food label is based on 1 serving. When reading a label, note the serving size amount. The number of calories and nutrients listed is based on that amount. If less is eaten, less calories and nutrients are consumed. If more is eaten, more calories and nutrients are consumed.

See the following table for how to calculate the number of calories, total fat, and sodium for different serving amounts of the food label shown in Figure 30-2.

	Calories	Total Fat	Sodium
1 Serving = 1 cup	280 calories	9 grams	850 milligrams
½ Serving = ½ cup (divide by 2)	140 calories	4½ grams	425 milligrams
2 Servings = 2 cups (multiply by 2)	560 calories	18 grams	1700 milligrams

TABLE 30-4	Special Diets	
Diet	**Use**	**Foods Allowed/Restricted**
Clear liquid—foods liquid at room temperature and clear or able to see through; non-irritating; non-gas forming; leave a small amount of residue	After surgery; for acute illness, infection, nausea, and vomiting; and to prepare for gastro-intestinal (GI) exams	Water, tea, and coffee *(without milk or cream)*; carbonated drinks; gelatin; fruit juices *without pulp* (apple, grape, cranberry); fat-free broth; hard candy, sugar, and Popsicles; *may need to avoid liquids with red coloring*
Full liquid—foods liquid at room temperature	Advance from clear-liquid diet after surgery; for stomach irritation, fever, nausea, and vomiting; for persons unable to chew, swallow, or digest solid foods	Foods on the clear-liquid diet; custard; strained soups; strained fruit and vegetable juices; milk and milk-shakes; cooked cereals; plain ice cream and sherbet; plain pudding; yogurt
Mechanical soft—semi-solid foods that are easily digested	Advance from full-liquid diet; chewing and swallowing problems, GI disorders, and infections	All liquids; eggs *(not fried)*; broiled, baked, or roasted meat, fish, or poultry that is chopped or shredded; mild cheeses (American, Swiss, cheddar, cream, cottage); strained fruit juices; refined bread *(no crust)* and crackers; cooked cereal; cooked or pureed vegetables; cooked or canned fruit *without skin or seeds*; plain pudding; plain cakes and soft cookies *without fruit or nuts*
Pureed—foods with a smooth, uniform texture that hold their shape on a spoon	Chewing and swallowing problems	All liquids (thickened—Chapter 31); pureed meat, fish, poultry, eggs; cooked and pureed vegetables; soft or cooked and pureed fruits *without skin or seeds*; plain yogurt and pudding; cooked cereal; pureed pasta and other grains that can be pureed smooth; strained or pureed soups; *foods that must be chewed are not allowed*
Fiber- and residue-restricted—foods that leave a small amount of residue in the colon	Diseases of the colon and diarrhea	Coffee, tea, milk, carbonated drinks, strained fruit and vegetable juices; refined bread and crackers; creamed and refined cereal; rice; cottage and cream cheese; eggs *(not fried)*; plain puddings and cakes; gelatin; custard; sherbet and ice cream; canned or cooked fruit *without skin or seeds*; potatoes *(not fried)*; strained cooked vegetables; plain pasta; *no raw fruits or vegetables*
High-fiber—foods that increase residue and fiber in the colon to stimulate peristalsis	Constipation and GI disorders	All fruits and vegetables, whole-wheat bread, whole-grain cereals, whole-grain rice, beans, and nuts are promoted; other foods (dairy, meat) are allowed but are not high-fiber
Bland—foods that are non-irritating and low in roughage; foods served at moderate temperatures; no strong spices or condiments	Ulcers, gallbladder disorders, and some intestinal disorders; after abdominal surgery	Lean meats; white bread; creamed and refined cereals; cream or cottage cheese; gelatin; plain puddings, cakes, and cookies; eggs *(not fried)*; butter and cream; canned fruits and vegetables *without skin and seeds*; strained fruit juices; potatoes *(not fried)*; pastas and rice; strained or soft cooked carrots, peas, beets, spinach, squash, and asparagus tips; creamed soups from allowed vegetables; *no fried or spicy foods*
High-calorie—3000 to 4000 calories daily; includes 3 full meals and between-meal snacks	Weight gain and some thyroid problems	Dietary increases in all foods; large portions of regular diet with 3 between-meal snacks

Continued

TABLE 30-4	Special Diets—cont'd	
Diet	Use	Foods Allowed/Restricted
Calorie-controlled—adequate nutrients while controlling calories to promote weight loss and reduce body fat	Weight loss	Foods low in fats and carbohydrates and lean meats; *avoid butter, cream, rice, gravies, salad oils, noodles, cakes, pastries, carbonated and alcoholic drinks, candy, potato chips, and similar foods*
High-iron—foods high in iron	Anemia; after blood loss; for women during the reproductive years	Liver and other organ meats; lean meats; egg yolks; shellfish; dried fruits; dried beans; green leafy vegetables; lima beans; peanut butter; enriched breads and cereals
Fat-controlled (low cholesterol)—foods low in fat and prepared without adding fat	Heart, gallbladder, and liver diseases; disorders of fat digestion; diseases of the pancreas	Skim milk (fat-free) or buttermilk; cottage cheese *(no other cheeses allowed);* gelatin; sherbet; fruit; lean meat, poultry, and fish (baked, broiled, or roasted); fat-free broth; soups made with skim milk (fat-free); soft (tub) margarine; rice, pasta, breads, and cereals; vegetables; potatoes
High-protein—aids and promotes tissue healing	Burns, high fever, infection, and some liver diseases	Meat, milk, eggs, cheese, fish, poultry; breads and cereals; green leafy vegetables
Sodium-controlled—a certain amount of sodium is allowed	Heart disease, fluid retention, liver diseases, and some kidney diseases	Fruits and vegetables and unsalted butter are allowed; *adding salt at the table is not allowed; highly salted foods and foods high in sodium are not allowed; the use of salt during cooking may be restricted*
Gluten-free—foods without the gluten protein	Celiac disease	Beans; seeds; nuts; eggs; meats, fish, and poultry *(without breading, batter, or marinade);* fruits and vegetables; most dairy foods; gluten-free grains and starches (arrowroot, corn, cornmeal, hominy, flax, millet, rice, soy, and tapioca); gluten-free flours (rice, soy, corn, potato, bean); *no foods containing wheat, barley, triticale, or rye*
Lactose restricted—foods with little to no lactose (a sugar in milk and milk products)	Lactose intolerance	Lactose-free or lactose-reduced milk and milk products; vegetables, fruits, and breads and cereals not prepared with milk or milk products; plain meat, fish, poultry, and eggs; *reduce or avoid milk and milk products (yogurt, cheese) as directed; avoid boxed, canned, frozen, packaged, or prepared foods containing milk or milk products;* include other sources of calcium and vitamin D (see Tables 30-2 and 30-3)
Diabetes meal plan—food and fluids are balanced with physical activity and drugs to manage blood glucose levels	Diabetes (Chapter 51)	Determined by nutritional and energy requirements and drugs to treat diabetes; *limit fried foods, foods high in fat and sodium, foods and drinks with added sugars;* sugar substitutes are allowed
Renal diet—low in sodium and phosphorus; certain amounts of protein and potassium; restricted fluids (Chapter 32)	Chronic kidney disease (Chapter 52)	*Avoid foods high in sodium and phosphorus; include or limit protein foods and foods high in potassium as directed* (see Table 30-3)

The Sodium-Controlled Diet

According to the American Heart Association (AHA), the average amount of sodium in the daily diet is greater than 3400 mg (milligrams). Lowering sodium (commonly called *salt*) in the diet reduces the risk of high blood pressure, heart disease, and stroke. For most adults, the AHA recommends limiting sodium intake to no more than 2300 mg a day. The AHA says that no more than 1500 mg daily is a better goal.

With too much sodium, the body retains (holds) water. Tissues swell. There is excess fluid in the blood vessels. The heart works harder. With heart disease, the extra workload can cause serious problems or death.

Sodium control lowers the amount of sodium in the body. Less water is retained. Less water in the tissues and blood vessels reduces the heart's workload.

The doctor orders the amount of sodium allowed. Sodium-controlled diets involve:

- Omitting high-sodium foods (Box 30-1)
- Not adding salt to food at the table
- Limiting the amount of salt used in cooking
- Diet planning

Diabetes Meal Plan

Diabetes is a chronic illness in which the body cannot produce or use insulin properly (Chapter 51). The pancreas produces and secretes insulin. Insulin lets the body use sugar. Without enough insulin, sugar builds up in the bloodstream. It is not used by cells for energy. Treatment usually involves insulin or other drugs, diet, and exercise.

A meal plan for healthy eating is developed. It often involves:

- Food preferences (likes, eating habits, meal times, culture, and life-style). Food amounts and preparation methods may be restricted.
- Portion control. Healthy foods from each food group are eaten. The person's meal plan states the amounts allowed from each group.
- Carbohydrate counting (carb counting). The person keeps track of the amount of carbohydrates eaten each day.
- Eating meals and snacks at regular times. The person may need to eat at regular times to maintain a certain blood glucose (blood sugar) level.

BOX 30-1 High-Sodium Foods

Grains
- Baked goods—biscuits, muffins, cakes, cookies, pies, pastries, sweet rolls, donuts, and so on
- Breads and rolls
- Cereals—cold, instant hot
- Noodle mixes
- Pancakes
- Salted snack foods—pretzels, corn chips, popcorn, crackers, chips, and so on
- Stuffing mixes
- Waffles

Vegetables
- Canned vegetables
- Olives
- Pickles and other pickled vegetables
- Relish
- Sauerkraut
- Tomato sauce or paste
- Vegetable juices—tomato, V8, Bloody Mary mixes
- Vegetables with sauces, creams, or seasonings

Fruits
- None—fruits are not high in sodium

Dairy Group
- Buttermilk
- Cheese
- Commercial dips made with sour cream

Protein Foods
- Bacon and Canadian bacon
- Canned meats and fish—chicken, tuna, salmon, anchovies, sardines
- Caviar
- Chipped, dried, and corned beef and other meats
- Deli meats—turkey, ham, bologna, salami, pastrami, and so on
- Dried fish

Protein Foods—cont'd
- Ham
- Herring
- Hot dogs (frankfurters)
- Liverwurst
- Lox and smoked salmon
- Mackerel
- Pepperoni
- Salt pork
- Sausages
- Scrapple
- Shellfish—shrimp, crab, clams, oysters, scallops, lobster

Other
- Asian foods—Chinese, Japanese, East Indian, Thai, Vietnamese
- Baking soda and baking powder
- Catsup (ketchup)
- Cocoa mixes
- Commercially prepared dinners—frozen, canned, boxed, and so on
- Mayonnaise
- Mexican foods
- Mustard
- Pasta dishes—lasagna, manicotti, ravioli
- Peanut butter
- Pizzas
- Pot pies
- Salad dressings
- Salted nuts or seeds
- Sauces—soy, teriyaki, Worcestershire, steak, barbecue, pasta, chili, cocktail
- Seasoning salts—garlic, onion, celery, meat tenderizers, monosodium glutamate (MSG), and so on
- Soups—canned, packaged, instant, dried, bouillon

Serve meals and snacks on time. Always check what was eaten. Report what the person did and did not eat. A between-meal snack makes up for what was not eaten. The nurse tells you what to provide. The amount of insulin given depends on food intake and physical activity. Report changes in the person's eating habits.

The Renal Diet

When the kidneys do not function normally, waste products build up in the body. Fluid is retained. See "Chronic Kidney Disease" in Chapter 52.

Dietary changes are often needed to manage kidney (renal) disease. A healthy meal plan is developed. The plan varies depending on the person's treatment and individual needs. A renal diet involves:

- Eating less sodium (p. 475) and restricting fluids (Chapter 32).
- Planning what types of protein and how much protein to eat. Protein is an important nutrient. However, excess protein can strain the kidneys and cause wastes to build up.
- Limiting phosphorus. Excess phosphorus can damage the bones and blood vessels.
- Knowing whether to include or avoid foods high in potassium. Nerve and muscle function are affected when potassium levels are outside the normal range.

See "The Sodium-Controlled Diet" on p. 475. See Table 30-1 for protein sources. See Table 30-3 for foods high in phosphorus and potassium.

The Dysphagia Diet

Dysphagia means difficulty *(dys)* swallowing *(phagia)*. Breathing food and fluids into the lungs *(aspiration)* is a risk. Food thickness and texture are changed to ease swallowing.

Liquids are often thickened to meet the person's needs. See "Dysphagia" in Chapter 31.

Between-Meal Snacks

Many special diets involve between-meal snacks. Snacks provide extra nutrients. Common snacks are crackers, milk, juice, a milk-shake, wafers, a sandwich, gelatin, and custard.

FOOD INTAKE

Food intake is measured in different ways. Follow agency policy for the method used.

- *Percentage of food eaten.* Food intake ranges from 0 to 100 percent (%). Some agencies record the percentage of the whole meal tray. Others record the percentage of each food item eaten. See Figure 30-3.
- *Words to describe estimated intake.* Words such as *all, good, fair, poor,* and *refused* may be listed as options in the medical record. You need to know how the agency defines words like *good, fair,* and *poor.* The following is a guide.
  - All—all (100%) or almost all of the food was eaten
  - Good—about 75% was eaten
  - Fair—about half (50%) was eaten
  - Poor—about 25% was eaten
  - Refused—none (0%) was eaten or the meal was refused after 1 or 2 bites
- *Calorie counts.* Note what the person ate and how much. For example, a chicken breast, rice, beans, fruit salad, and pudding were served. The person ate all the chicken, half the rice, and the fruit salad. The beans and pudding were not eaten. Note these on the flow sheet. A nurse or dietitian converts these portions into calories. See *Focus on Math: Food Intake.*

See *Focus on Communication: Food Intake.*

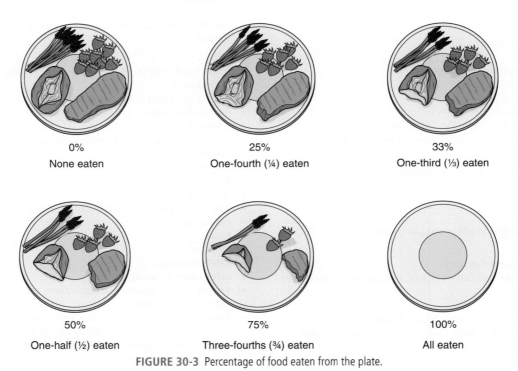

FIGURE 30-3 Percentage of food eaten from the plate.

FOCUS ON MATH

Food Intake

 To measure food intake, you need to understand percents. Percents measure parts of a whole (Fig. 30-4). The "whole" is written as 100%.

To measure food intake, compare the food left to that served. Depending on agency policy and the food type, *estimate* or *calculate* food intake. *To estimate,* record the approximate amount of food eaten. See Figure 30-3. *To calculate:*

1 Subtract the amount left from the amount served. (This is the amount the person ate.)
2 Divide the number from step 1 by the amount served (the number of pieces making up the whole).
3 Multiply the number from step 2 by 100 for a percent. (*Percent* means out of 100.)
   For example, 8 apple slices were served; 2 remain on the plate.

   8 slices − 2 slices = 6 slices

   The person ate 6 apple slices; 8 were served.

   6 slices (number eaten) ÷ 8 slices (number served) = 0.75

   0.75 × 100 = 75%

   75% of the apple slices were eaten.

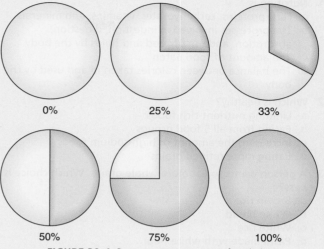

FIGURE 30-4 Percents measure parts of a whole.

FOCUS ON COMMUNICATION

Food Intake

The person may not eat everything served. Asking why gives information about the person—likes, dislikes, how the person feels. Report what you learn to the nurse.

When you ask, ask with interest. Do not use words or a tone that sound like the person did something wrong.

You can ask:
- "Did your food taste okay?"
- "Do you like mashed potatoes (or other food not eaten)?"
- "Was the food too hot or too cold?"
- "Was the food seasoned well?"
- "Would you like something else?"
- "Do you not feel like eating today?"
- "How are you feeling today?"

FOCUS ON **PRIDE**

The Person, Family, and Yourself

Personal and Professional Responsibility

Your nutrition choices matter. The food and drinks you choose regularly over time make up your eating pattern. Healthy patterns and regular physical activity promote health. You need to be healthy in order to care for others.

Rights and Respect

People often comment about food likes and dislikes. People have the right to express what they prefer. Do not say the person is complaining or being picky. Learning the person's likes and dislikes can improve nutrition. It also shows interest and concern for the person.

Independence and Social Interaction

Physical activity can be a social experience. Walking with a friend, riding bicycles as a family, or golfing with others are examples. Regular physical activity has long-term health benefits. Choose activities you enjoy.

Delegation and Teamwork

Measuring food intake takes practice. You may have questions. Do not guess. Ask for help. During your training, ask your instructor. At work, ask the nurse or dietary staff.

Ethics and Laws

Each person is different. A person may have a special diet or food allergy (Chapter 31). You must know what each person can and cannot have. Know each person's needs. Protect the person from harm. If unsure, ask the nurse.

FOCUS ON **PRIDE**: Application

Consider your life-style choices. Do you try to eat a healthy diet? What do you do for regular physical activity? What goals do you have? Even small changes can improve health.

REVIEW QUESTIONS

Circle the BEST answer.

1 Nutrition is
   a Fats, proteins, carbohydrates, vitamins, and minerals
   b The processes involved in ingestion, digestion, absorption, and use of food and fluids by the body
   c The amount of food eaten
   d The balance between calories taken in and used by the body

2 Which is healthy?
   a Limiting nutrient-rich foods
   b Eating from all 5 food groups
   c Increasing the amount of high-sodium foods
   d Eating more refined grains

3 A person wants to eat more whole grains. Which choice is *best*?
   a Brown rice
   b White bread
   c White rice
   d Pasta made with white flour

4 Which would meet an adult male's daily dairy needs?
   a 1 slice of bread, 1 cup of cheese, and ½ oz of nuts
   b 2 cups of milk and 1 cup of cooked rice
   c 1 cup of milk, 1 cup of yogurt, and 1½ oz of cheese
   d 2 tablespoons of peanut butter and 1 egg

5 In which food group does saturated fat need to be considered?
   a Grains
   b Vegetables
   c Fruit
   d Protein foods

6 Protein is needed for
   a Tissue growth and repair
   b Fiber for bowel elimination
   c Fluid balance
   d Improved food taste

7 Which foods provide the *most* protein?
   a Butter and cream
   b Tomatoes and potatoes
   c Meats and fish
   d Corn and lettuce

8 A person needs more fiber to promote bowel elimination. Which choice is *best*?
   a Refined grains
   b Fruits and vegetables
   c Meats
   d Dairy foods

9 These statements are about fats and oils. Which is *true*?
   a Vegetable oils and oils in fish and nuts are healthy choices.
   b Butter, beef fat, and chicken fat are healthy choices.
   c Saturated fats do not affect heart disease risk.
   d Oils are a food group.

10 The serving information on a food label tells you
   a The serving size and number of servings in the package
   b How much you should eat of the product
   c How the product needs to be stored before serving
   d How to cook and serve the product

11 These statements are about special diets. Which is *true*?
   a A person on a full liquid diet can have rice and bread.
   b Meats on a mechanical soft diet are chopped or shredded.
   c A person on a gluten-free diet can have whole-wheat bread.
   d A lactose-restricted diet includes more milk products.

12 The sodium-controlled diet involves
   a Omitting high-sodium foods
   b Adding salt to food at the table
   c Using 3000 mg of salt in cooking
   d A sodium-intake flow sheet

13 Diabetes meal planning involves
   a Changing the thickness of foods
   b Eating larger food portions
   c Controlling sodium
   d Eating at regular times

14 A person with kidney failure requires a renal diet. The person needs to limit potassium. Which choice for breakfast is *best*?
   a A cup of orange juice
   b A banana
   c A cup of yogurt
   d White toast

15 A dysphagia diet is used for persons with
   a High blood pressure
   b Nausea
   c Difficulty swallowing
   d A decreased appetite

16 A resident eats half of the food on the meal tray. Food intake for this meal is
   a 25%
   b 33%
   c 50%
   d 75%

Answers to Chapter 30 questions are on p. 902.

FOCUS ON **PRACTICE**

Problem Solving

A resident with diabetes has an order for a diabetes meal plan. You serve the person coffee. The person says: "I like it sweetened." The agency has sugar packets and sugar substitute packets available. What will you do? What will you do if you do not know what a person can have?

Meeting Nutrition Needs

CHAPTER
31

OBJECTIVES

- Define the key terms and key abbreviations in this chapter.
- Describe the factors that affect eating and nutrition.
- Identify the signs and symptoms of dysphagia and aspiration.
- Identify the safety measures to prevent aspiration.
- Describe CMS requirements for the food served.

- Explain how to assist with nutrition needs.
- Explain how to prevent foodborne illnesses.
- Perform the procedures described in this chapter.
- Explain how to promote PRIDE in the person, the family, and yourself.

KEY TERMS

anorexia The loss of appetite
aspiration Breathing fluid, food, vomitus, or an object into the lungs

dysphagia Difficulty *(dys)* swallowing *(phagia)*

KEY ABBREVIATIONS

CMS	Centers for Medicare & Medicaid Services	**ID**	Identification
GI	Gastro-intestinal	**USDA**	U.S. Department of Agriculture

A team approach is needed to meet a person's nutrition needs. The person, nursing team, doctor, and dietitian are involved. A speech therapist and occupational therapist may also be a part. So is the family if necessary. The person's likes, dislikes, abilities, individual needs, and life-long habits are part of the care plan.

You help meet nutritional needs by preparing patients and residents for meals and serving meal trays. When necessary, you may need to feed a person.

See *Focus on Surveys: Meeting Nutrition Needs.*

FOCUS ON SURVEYS

Meeting Nutrition Needs

The health team develops a care plan to meet the person's nutrition needs. Surveyors may ask you:
- How food and fluid intake are observed and reported (Chapters 30 and 32).
- How eating ability is observed and reported.
- About the measures to prevent or meet changes in nutrition needs. Snacks and frequent meals are examples.
- About the goals for nutrition in the care plan.

FACTORS AFFECTING EATING AND NUTRITION

Many factors affect eating and nutrition. They begin in childhood and continue throughout life.

Culture and Religion

Culture influences dietary practices, food choices, and food preparation. Frying, baking, smoking, or roasting food and eating raw food are some cultural practices. So is using sauces, herbs, and spices.

Many cultural groups have their main meal at mid-day. They eat light meals in the evening. Others have lighter meals in the morning and mid-day and have the larger meal in the evening.

Selecting, preparing, and eating food often involve religion. For example, certain foods are not allowed. Or only certain foods or no foods are eaten during a *fast*. A person may follow all, some, or none of the dietary practices of his or her faith. Respect the person's practices.

See *Caring About Culture: Food Practices*, p. 480.

479

Personal Choice and Finances

Food likes and dislikes are influenced by foods served in the home. Food choices depend on how food looks, how it is prepared, its smell, and ingredients. Usually food likes change with age and social experiences.

Personal choice may involve a vegetarian diet. The focus is on plants for food—fruits, vegetables, dried beans and peas, grains, seeds, and nuts. Vegetarian eating patterns vary. For example:

- Vegan diet—excludes all meat and animal products.
- Lacto-vegetarian diet—includes dairy *(lacto)* products.
- Lacto-ovo vegetarian diet—includes dairy *(lacto)* products and eggs *(ovo)*.

People with limited incomes may buy cheaper carbohydrate foods. Their diets often lack protein and certain vitamins and minerals.

Appetite and Body Reactions

Appetite relates to the desire for food. The loss of appetite is called *anorexia*. Changes in appetite can occur because of illness, drugs, level of activity, stress, anxiety, depression, and pain. The person's setting is another factor. Unpleasant sights, thoughts, and smells can cause appetite loss.

Food allergies cause an immune response. The person may react with a rash, swelling, or itching. Some reactions are life-threatening (Chapter 58). Foods that cause allergic reactions are avoided.

A *food intolerance (food sensitivity)* occurs when there are problems digesting certain foods. There are negative body reactions. But the immune system is not activated. Nausea, vomiting, diarrhea, indigestion, gas, or headaches may occur. Some reactions can be treated or prevented.

Aging

Gastro-intestinal (GI) changes occur with aging. Taste and smell dull. Appetite decreases. Secretion of digestive juices decreases. Fried and fatty foods may cause indigestion.

Some people avoid the high-fiber foods needed for bowel elimination—apricots, celery, and fruits and vegetables with skins and seeds. High-fiber foods are hard to chew and can irritate the intestines.

Foods providing soft bulk are often ordered for chewing problems or constipation. Whole-grain cereals and cooked fruits and vegetables are examples.

Calorie needs are lower. Energy and activity levels are lower. Foods that contain calcium help prevent musculoskeletal changes. Protein is needed for tissue growth and repair. Because of cost, diets may lack high-protein foods.

Illness and Disability

Appetite often decreases during illness and recovery from injuries. However, nutrition needs increase. The body must fight infection, heal tissue, and replace lost blood cells. Nutrients lost through vomiting and diarrhea need to be replaced.

Drugs can cause appetite loss, dry mouth, impaired taste, confusion, nausea, constipation, or changes in GI function. They can cause inflammation of the mouth, throat, esophagus, and stomach.

Disease or injury can affect the hands, wrists, and arms. Some persons can eat independently with the use of adaptive equipment (assistive devices) (Fig. 31-1). The speech

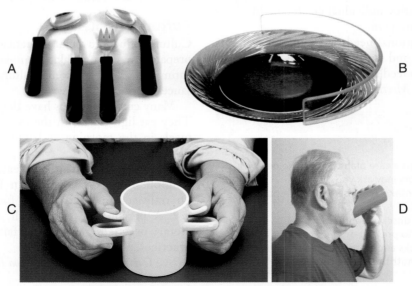

FIGURE 31-1 Adaptive equipment (assistive devices) for meals. **A,** Eating utensils have tapered and angled handles. The knife cuts with slicing and rocking motions. **B,** The plate guard helps keep food on the plate. **C,** The thumb grips on the cup help prevent spilling. **D,** A "Nosey Cup" allows for drinking without tilting the head back. (A, B, and C, Courtesy Elderstore, Alpharetta, Ga. D, From Barney K, Perkinson M: *Occupational therapy with aging adults,* St Louis, 2016, Mosby.)

therapist and occupational therapist teach the person how to use them. Make sure each person has needed devices.

Special diets (Chapter 30) are required to manage some health problems. There may be dietary restrictions—the limiting or elimination of certain foods. Or the person needs to increase the intake of certain foods to provide needed nutrients. Or foods may need to be prepared in a certain way so the person can eat them. A dietitian teaches about special diets and helps with meal planning.

Chewing and Swallowing Problems

Mouth, teeth, and gum problems can affect chewing. Examples include oral pain, dry or sore mouth, gum disease (Chapter 23), dental problems, and dentures that fit poorly. Broken, decayed, or missing teeth also affect chewing (especially meats).

Stroke; pain; confusion; dry mouth; and diseases of the mouth, throat, and esophagus can affect swallowing. See "Dysphagia."

DYSPHAGIA

Dysphagia means difficulty *(dys)* swallowing *(phagia)*. A *slow swallow* means the person has difficulty getting enough food and fluids for good nutrition and fluid balance. An *unsafe swallow* means that food enters the airway (aspiration). *Aspiration* is breathing fluid, food, vomitus, or an object into the lungs.

When feeding a person with dysphagia, you must:
- Know the signs and symptoms of dysphagia (Box 31-1).
- Feed the person according to the care plan.
- Follow the person's ordered diet. A dysphagia diet is common. Food and fluid thicknesses are changed to meet the person's needs (see Box 31-1).
- Follow aspiration precautions (see Box 31-1) and the care plan.
- Report changes in how the person eats.
- Report signs and symptoms of aspiration at once (see Box 31-1).

BOX 31-1   Dysphagia

Dysphagia Signs and Symptoms
- Avoids foods that need chewing.
- Avoids foods with certain textures and temperatures.
- Tires during a meal.
- Has food spill out of the mouth while eating.
- "Pockets" or "squirrels" food in the cheeks. This means that food remains or is hidden in the mouth.
- Eats slowly, especially solid foods.
- Reports difficulty swallowing or pain with swallowing.
- Coughs or chokes before, during, or after swallowing.
- Makes gurgling sounds while talking or breathing after swallowing.
- Clears the throat often during a meal.
- Has hoarseness—especially after eating.
- Spits out food suddenly and almost violently.
- Regurgitates food after eating. (Food comes back up into the mouth.)
- Has food come up through the nose.
- Has a runny nose, sneezes, or has excessive drooling.
- Complains of frequent heartburn.
- Has a decreased appetite.

Dysphagia Diet
- The doctor, speech therapist, occupational therapist, dietitian, and nurse choose food and liquid thicknesses.
- Food thickness and texture are changed to ease swallowing.
  - *Mechanical soft*—foods have a moist, soft texture. Meats are chopped, blended, or ground. Vegetables are cooked well.
  - *Pureed*—foods have a smooth, uniform texture and hold their shape on a spoon. Foods are "pudding-like" and have no lumps.

Dysphagia Diet—cont'd
- Liquids are thickened as needed (Fig. 31-2, p. 482).
  - *Nectar-thick liquid*—mildly thick. The liquid coats and drips off of a spoon. It can flow through a straw.
  - *Honey-thick liquid*—moderately thick. The liquid flows off of a spoon like honey. The person can drink it from a cup.
  - *Pudding-thick (spoon-thick) liquid*—extremely thick. The liquid stays on a spoon in a soft mound. It can be sipped or served with a spoon.

Aspiration Precautions
- Help the person with meals and snacks. Follow the care plan.
- Position the person upright as the nurse and care plan direct. The person remains upright for at least 1 hour after eating.
- Support the upper back, shoulders, and neck with a pillow.
- Do not rush.
- Avoid distractions.
- Offer or encourage small bites and frequent drinks.
- Follow the care plan for straw use. A straw may not be allowed.
- Place food in the mouth on the unaffected side if there is weakness on 1 side.
- Make sure food or fluids are swallowed before giving more.
- Check the person's mouth after eating for pocketing. Check inside the cheeks, under the tongue, and on the roof of the mouth. Remove any food (p. 485).
- Provide mouth care after eating.
- Observe for signs and symptoms of aspiration. Report the following at once.
  - Choking
  - Coughing
  - Difficulty breathing during or after meals or snacks
  - Abnormal breathing or respiratory sounds
- Report and record your observations.

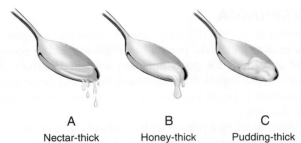

A	B	C
Nectar-thick	Honey-thick	Pudding-thick

FIGURE 31-2 **A,** Nectar-thick liquid. **B,** Honey-thick liquid. **C,** Pudding-thick (spoon-thick) liquid.

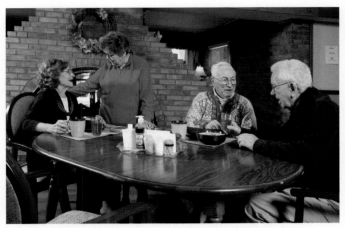

FIGURE 31-3 Residents eating in the dining room. Volunteers help as needed.

NUTRITION AND FOOD REQUIREMENTS

Health care agencies have requirements for assessing and meeting the dietary needs of patients and residents.

See *Focus on Long-Term Care and Home Care: Nutrition and Food Requirements.*

FOCUS ON LONG-TERM CARE AND HOME CARE

Nutrition and Food Requirements

Long-Term Care
The Centers for Medicare & Medicaid Services (CMS) requires that the health team assess the resident's nutritional status and factors affecting eating and nutrition (p. 479). The person's appearance, height and weight (Chapter 37), food intake (Chapter 30), and fluid balance (Chapter 32) are assessed. A care plan is developed to set goals and meet needs. Goals may relate to:
- Weight management—gain, loss, maintenance
- Fluid balance (Chapter 32)
- Management of a health problem
The CMS also has requirements for the food served in nursing centers.
- Each person's nutrition needs are met.
- The person's religious and cultural needs and preferences are met.
- The person's diet is well balanced. It is nourishing and tastes good. Food is well seasoned. It is not too salty or too sweet.
- Food is appetizing. It has an appealing aroma (smell) and is attractive.
- Hot food is served hot. Cold food is served cold.
- Food is served promptly. If not, hot food cools and cold food warms.
- Food is prepared to meet each person's needs. Special diets are followed (Chapter 30). Food is cut, ground, chopped, or pureed to meet the person's individual needs.
- Food that is served accommodates the person's food allergies or intolerances.
- Other foods are offered if the food served is refused. The substituted food must have a similar nutritional value to the first foods served.
- Each person receives at least 3 meals a day. A bedtime snack is offered.
- The center provides needed adaptive equipment (assistive devices) and utensils (see Fig. 31-1). They promote independence. Make sure the person has needed equipment.

Dining Programs

Agency dining programs vary. The method used depends on the setting and the person's needs. The following are examples.
- *Social dining.* Common in nursing centers, a dining area has many tables. A table seats 4 to 6 residents (Fig. 31-3). Food items are selected from a daily menu. Persons who are able feed themselves. Staff help with feeding as needed.
- *Restaurant-style menus.* Common in hospitals, food is selected from a menu to allow more food choices. Meals may be served at scheduled times. Or the person can order food any time.
- *Open dining.* A buffet is open for several hours.
- *Family dining.* Common in home settings, food is served in bowls and on platters. Persons serve themselves.

Nursing centers usually serve meals at scheduled times. If a person prefers to eat outside of the scheduled times, the agency provides alternative meals and snacks that are suitable and nourishing. This is included in the person's care plan.

Some nursing center residents eat in their rooms by choice. If *low-stimulation dining* is needed, staff plan seating to prevent distractions. The person's setting needs to be suitable for dining. A pleasant dining experience is important.

Hospitals usually have "room service" meal programs. A full menu including breakfast, lunch, and dinner options is kept in the person's room. When ready to eat, the person calls the dietary department to place an order. Food is served a short while later. This program allows the person to eat when hungry. For a fee, visitors can order food to dine with the person.

▐ PREPARING FOR MEALS

Preparing patients and residents for meals promotes comfort. To promote comfort:

- Provide oral hygiene. Make sure dentures are in place.
- Make sure eyeglasses and hearing aids are in place.
- Assist with elimination needs.
- Make sure incontinent persons are clean and dry.
- Position the person in a comfortable, upright position.
- Reduce or remove unpleasant odors, sights, and sounds. See Chapter 13.
- Follow the care plan for pain-relief measures. See Chapter 36.
- Assist the person with hand hygiene.

See *Focus on Long-Term Care and Home Care: Preparing for Meals.*

See *Delegation Guidelines: Preparing for Meals.*
See *Promoting Safety and Comfort: Preparing for Meals.*
See procedure: *Preparing the Person for a Meal.*

FOCUS ON LONG-TERM CARE AND HOME CARE

Preparing for Meals

Home Care

Nursing assistants in home care settings may need to shop for groceries, plan meals, or cook. These roles require an understanding of:

- A balanced diet and food labels (Chapter 30).
- Special diet orders (Chapter 30).
- The person's food likes, dislikes, and eating habits.
- Meal planning. Recipe ingredients are included on a shopping list.
- Responsible shopping. Receipts and any money are handled following agency policy.
- How to follow a recipe.
- Safe food preparation and storage. See "Foodborne Illness" on p. 488.

DELEGATION GUIDELINES

Preparing for Meals

Preparing for meals is a routine nursing task. You need this information from the nurse and the care plan.

- How much help the person needs
- Where the person will eat—room or dining room
- What the person uses for elimination—toilet, commode, bedpan, or urinal
- What type of oral hygiene to give
- If the person wears dentures
- If the person wears eyeglasses or hearing aids
- How to position the person—in bed, a chair, or wheelchair
- If the person needs help to the dining room
- If the person uses a wheelchair, walker, or cane
- When to report observations
- What patient or resident concerns to report at once

PROMOTING SAFETY AND COMFORT

Preparing for Meals

Safety

Before meals, the person needs to eliminate and have oral hygiene. Follow the practices of medical asepsis and Standard Precautions. Follow the rules of hand hygiene and the guidelines for glove use in Chapters 17 and 18.

In nursing centers, follow agency policies and procedures for using Enhanced Barrier Precautions for high-contact tasks. See Chapter 18.

▐ Preparing the Person for a Meal

QUALITY OF LIFE

- Knock before entering the person's room.
- Address the person by name.
- Introduce yourself by name and title.

- Explain the procedure before starting and during the procedure.
- Protect the person's rights during the procedure.
- Handle the person gently during the procedure.

PRE-PROCEDURE

1 Follow *Delegation Guidelines: Preparing for Meals.* See *Promoting Safety and Comfort: Preparing for Meals.*
2 Practice hand hygiene and get the following supplies.
  - Supplies for oral hygiene (Chapter 23)
  - Supplies for elimination (Chapter 27)
  - Supplies for hand hygiene—hand-wipes or soap, water, washcloth, and towel
  - Supplies for a transfer if needed (Chapter 21)
  - Gloves

3 Arrange items in the person's room.
4 Practice hand hygiene.
5 Identify the person. Check the identification (ID) bracelet against the assignment sheet. Use 2 identifiers (Chapter 14). Also call the person by name.
6 Provide for privacy.

Continued

Preparing the Person for a Meal—cont'd

PROCEDURE

7 Make sure eyeglasses and hearing aids are in place.

8 Assist with oral hygiene as needed. Make sure dentures are in place. Wear gloves and practice hand hygiene after removing and discarding them.

9 Assist with elimination as needed. Make sure the person is clean and dry if incontinent. Wear gloves and practice hand hygiene after removing and discarding them.

10 Assist with hand hygiene. Wear gloves and practice hand hygiene after removing and discarding them.

11 Clean up and store supplies and equipment. (Wear gloves. Change gloves as needed.)
  a Discard disposable items.
  b Follow agency procedures to clean and disinfect re-usable equipment. Return supplies and equipment to their proper place.
  c Follow agency policy for used linens.
  d Clean and dry the over-bed table. Dry with paper towels. Discard paper towels. Leave items off of the over-bed table if it will be used for the meal. Or position the over-bed table with needed items as the person prefers for a meal in the dining room.
  e Remove and discard gloves. Practice hand hygiene.

12 *For the person who will eat in bed:*
  a Raise the head of the bed to a comfortable position—Fowler's (45 to 60 degrees) or high-Fowler's (60 to 90 degrees). (Note: Some state competency tests require at least 45 degrees. Others require 75 to 90 degrees.)
  b Adjust the over-bed table in front of the person.

13 *For the person who will sit in a chair:*
  a Position the person in a chair or wheelchair.
  b Adjust the over-bed table in front of the person.

14 *For the person who eats in the dining room,* assist the person to the dining room.

POST-PROCEDURE

15 *For the person who will eat in the room:*
  a Provide for comfort. (See the inside of the back cover.)
  b Straighten the room. Eliminate unpleasant noise, odors, or equipment.
  c Place the call light and other needed items within reach.
  d Follow the care plan and the person's preferences for privacy measures to maintain. Leaving the privacy curtain, window coverings, and door open or closed are examples.
  e Complete a safety check of the room. (See the inside of the back cover.)

16 Practice hand hygiene.

17 Report and record your care and observations.

SERVING MEALS

Food is served in covered containers to keep foods at the correct temperature. Hot food is kept hot. Cold food is kept cold. Uncover food just before the person eats. Uncovered food changes temperature quickly.

Prepare persons for meals before food is served. If they are ready to eat, you can serve meals promptly. Food is kept at the correct temperature.

Serve meals in the assigned order. In nursing centers, residents seated at tables are served at the same time.

If food is not served within 15 minutes, re-check food temperatures. Follow agency policy. If not at the correct temperature, get fresh food. Temperature guides and food thermometers are in dining rooms and in nursing unit kitchens. Some agencies allow re-heating in microwave ovens.

Snacks are served upon arrival on the nursing unit. Provide needed utensils, a straw, and a napkin. Follow the same considerations and procedures for serving meals and feeding the person (p. 486).

See *Focus on Communication: Serving Meals.*
See *Teamwork and Time Management: Serving Meals.*
See *Delegation Guidelines: Serving Meals.*
See *Promoting Safety and Comfort: Serving Meals.*
See procedure: *Serving Meal Trays.*

FOCUS ON COMMUNICATION

Serving Meals

A dietary card is a common method used to communicate each person's needs and the items served. Dietary staff place the person's card on the person's tray. Dietary cards often include:
- Identification information
- The person's ordered diet—regular or special (therapeutic) (Chapter 30)
- Any food allergies or intolerances
- If adaptive equipment (assistive devices) are needed
- The food items served on the meal tray

The procedures in this chapter for serving meal trays and feeding the person include use of a dietary card. If your agency uses dietary cards, check the card carefully. If you have a question, ask the nurse. Follow agency practices to be sure the person is given the correct meal.

TEAMWORK AND TIME MANAGEMENT
Serving Meals

Meal trays are served in the order set by the health team. You will serve trays to your patients and residents and to those assigned to other nursing assistants. Your co-workers do the same. The goal is to serve trays promptly. This keeps food at the desired temperature.

DELEGATION GUIDELINES
Serving Meals

Serving meal trays is a routine nursing task. You need this information from the nurse and the care plan.
- The person's food allergies or intolerances (if any)
- What adaptive equipment (assistive devices) are needed
- If the person needs help opening cartons, cutting food, buttering bread, and so on
- If the person's food intake (Chapter 30) and fluid intake (Chapter 32) are measured
- When to report observations
- What patient or resident concerns to report at once

PROMOTING SAFETY AND COMFORT
Serving Meals

Safety
Always check food temperature if re-heating is required. Food that is too hot can cause burns.

After eating, check the person's mouth for food (pocketing). Remove any food. Follow these safety measures.
- Use sponge swabs (Chapter 23) as needed. Wear gloves. Practice hand hygiene after removing and discarding them.
- Have the person tip the chin downward (toward the chest) to prevent aspiration.
- Call for the nurse if you cannot remove food easily.

Comfort
Check the person's position when serving a meal. The position may have changed after the person was prepared to eat. Provide other comfort measures as needed. See the inside of the back cover.

Some agencies offer clothing protectors that can be worn at meal times. A clothing protector resembles a "bib" and can lower dignity. Do not assume the person wants to wear one. Respect the person's choice. Use of a napkin is an age-appropriate alternative.

Serving Meal Trays

QUALITY OF LIFE

- Knock before entering the person's room.
- Address the person by name.
- Introduce yourself by name and title.

- Explain the procedure before starting and during the procedure.
- Protect the person's rights during the procedure.
- Handle the person gently during the procedure.

PRE-PROCEDURE

1 Follow *Delegation Guidelines: Serving Meals.* See *Promoting Safety and Comfort: Serving Meals.*
2 Practice hand hygiene.

3 Prepare the person for the meal if not already done. See procedure: *Preparing the Person for a Meal*, p. 483.

PROCEDURE

4 Check items on the tray with the dietary card. Make sure the tray is complete and has needed adaptive equipment (assistive devices).
5 Identify the person. Check the ID bracelet against the dietary card. Use 2 identifiers (Chapter 14). Also call the person by name.
6 Place the tray within the person's reach. Adjust the over-bed table as needed (if used).
7 Remove food covers. Open cartons, cut food into bite-sized pieces, butter bread, and so on as needed (Fig. 31-4, p. 486). Season food as the person prefers and the care plan allows.
8 Place the napkin, adaptive equipment (assistive devices), and eating utensils within reach. Help the person apply a clothes protector (towel, napkin) if needed.
9 Place the call light within reach for persons eating in their rooms.

10 Do the following when the person is done eating.
  a Measure and record fluid intake if ordered (Chapter 32).
  b Note the amount and type of foods eaten (Chapter 30).
  c Check for and remove any food in the mouth (pocketing). See *Promoting Safety and Comfort: Serving Meals.*
  d Remove the item used to protect clothing if worn. Follow agency policy for used linens. Discard a disposable napkin.
  e Remove the tray.
  f Clean spills. Clean and dry the over-bed table if used. Dry with paper towels. Discard the paper towels.
  g Change any soiled clothing. Follow agency policy for removed clothing.
  h Assist with oral hygiene and hand hygiene. Provide for privacy. Wear gloves. Practice hand hygiene after removing and discarding the gloves.
  i Help the person return to bed if needed.

POST-PROCEDURE

11 Provide for comfort. (See the inside of the back cover.)
12 Raise or lower bed rails. Follow the care plan.
13 Place the call light and other needed items within reach.
14 Follow the care plan and the person's preferences for privacy measures to maintain. Leaving the privacy curtain, window coverings, and door open or closed are examples.

15 Complete a safety check of the room. (See the inside of the back cover.)
16 Practice hand hygiene.
17 Report and record your care and observations.

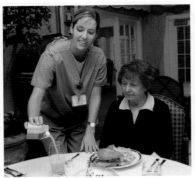

FIGURE 31-4 Cartons and containers are opened for the person.

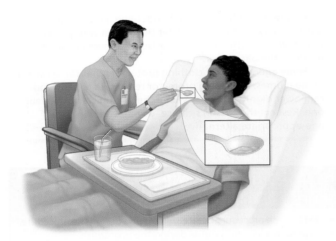

FIGURE 31-5 A spoon is used to feed the person. The spoon is one-third (⅓) full.

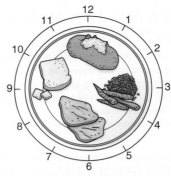

FIGURE 31-6 The numbers on a clock are used to help a visually impaired person locate food.

FEEDING THE PERSON

Weakness, paralysis, casts, confusion, and other limits can make self-feeding impossible. These persons are fed.

Serve food and fluids in the order the person prefers. Offer fluids during the meal. Fluids help the person chew and swallow.

Use teaspoons to feed the person. They are safer than forks. The teaspoon should be only one-third (⅓) full (Fig. 31-5). This portion is chewed and swallowed easily. Some people need smaller portions. Follow the care plan.

Persons who need to be fed may feel angry or embarrassed. Some are depressed, resentful, or refuse to eat. Let them do what they can. Some can handle "finger foods" (bread, cookies, crackers). If strong enough, let them hold milk or juice cups (never hot drinks). Follow ordered activity limits. Provide support. Encourage them to try, even if food is spilled.

Visually impaired persons often recognize foods from their aromas. Describe what is on the plate and what you are offering. For persons who feed themselves, describe foods and fluids and their place on the plate. Use the numbers on a clock for the location of foods (Fig. 31-6).

Many people pray before eating. Allow time and privacy for prayer. This shows respect and caring.

Meals provide social contact with others. Talk with the person. Allow time to chew and swallow. Sit facing the person. Sitting is more relaxing. It shows that you have time. You can also see how well the person is eating and watch for swallowing problems.

See *Focus on Children and Older Persons: Feeding the Person*.
See *Focus on Surveys: Feeding the Person*.
See *Delegation Guidelines: Feeding the Person*.
See *Promoting Safety and Comfort: Feeding the Person*.
See procedure: *Feeding the Person*.

FOCUS ON CHILDREN AND OLDER PERSONS
Feeding the Person

Older Persons
Persons with dementia may become distracted during meals. Some do not sit long enough to eat. Others forget how to use eating utensils. Some persons resist efforts to help them eat. A confused person may throw or spit food.

These measures may be helpful for persons with dementia. Follow the person's care plan.
- Keep meal times and the setting consistent.
- Provide a calm, quiet setting. Limit noise and distractions. This helps the person focus.
- Limit the number of food choices.
- Offer several small meals during the day instead of larger ones.
- Use straws or cups with lids. These make drinking easier.
- Provide finger foods if the person has problems with utensils. A bowl may be easier to use than a plate.
- Provide healthy snacks. Keep snacks where the person can see them.

Be patient. Tell the nurse if you feel upset or impatient. The person has the right to be treated with dignity and respect.

FOCUS ON SURVEYS
Feeding the Person

Surveyors observe if staff:
- Provide help with eating.
- Encourage the person to eat.
- Help the person use adaptive equipment (assistive devices).
- Feed the person if necessary.

DELEGATION GUIDELINES
Feeding the Person

Feeding patients and residents is a routine nursing task. Before feeding a person, you need this information from the nurse and the care plan.

- The person's food allergies or intolerances (if any)
- Why the person needs help
- How much help the person needs
- How to position the person
- If the person can manage finger foods
- The person's activity limits
- If the person has a special diet order or dietary restrictions
- Feeding portion size—⅓ teaspoonful or less
- Needed safety measures if the person has dysphagia
- If the person can use a straw
- What observations to report and record:
  - The amount and kind of food eaten
  - Complaints of nausea or dysphagia
  - Signs and symptoms of dysphagia
  - Signs and symptoms of aspiration
- When to report observations
- What patient or resident concerns to report at once

PROMOTING SAFETY AND COMFORT
Feeding the Person

Safety
Check food temperature. Very hot foods and fluids can burn the person. If food needs cooled, do not blow on it. Foods can be cooled by stirring them, spreading them out, or cutting them into small pieces.

Prevent aspiration. Check the person's mouth before offering more food or fluids. The mouth must be empty between bites and swallows.

The person must be alert enough to eat. Health problems, drug side effects, and fatigue can affect level of consciousness. *Do not try to feed a person who is drowsy.* Tell the nurse right away.

Some training programs do not allow students to assist with feeding in patient or resident rooms without staff or the instructor present. Some training programs only allow students to assist with feeding in the dining area. Follow the rules for your training program.

Comfort
The person will eat better if not rushed. Sit to show that you have time. Standing communicates being in a hurry.

Wipe the person's hands, face, and mouth as needed during the meal. Use the napkin or a wet washcloth. Then dry the person with a towel.

Feeding the Person

QUALITY OF LIFE

- Knock before entering the person's room.
- Address the person by name.
- Introduce yourself by name and title.

- Explain the procedure before starting and during the procedure.
- Protect the person's rights during the procedure.
- Handle the person gently during the procedure.

PRE-PROCEDURE

1 Follow *Delegation Guidelines: Feeding the Person.* See *Promoting Safety and Comfort:*
   a *Serving Meals*, p. 485
   b *Feeding the Person*
2 Practice hand hygiene.

3 Position the person in a comfortable position for eating—sitting in a chair or in Fowler's (45 to 60 degrees) or high-Fowler's (60 to 90 degrees). (NOTE: Some state competency tests require at least 45 degrees. Others require 75 to 90 degrees.)
4 Get the tray. Place the tray on the over-bed table or dining table where the person can reach it.

PROCEDURE

5 Check items on the tray with the dietary card. Make sure the tray is complete.
6 Identify the person. Check the ID bracelet against the dietary card. Use 2 identifiers (Chapter 14). Also call the person by name.
7 Drape a napkin across the person's chest and underneath the chin. Or apply a clothes protector or towel if needed.
8 Clean the person's hands. (NOTE: Some state competency tests require soap and water. Others allow hand sanitizer or a hand-wipe.)
9 Place the chair where you can sit comfortably. Sit facing the person at eye level.
10 Tell the person what foods and fluids are on the tray.
11 Prepare food for eating. Cut food into bite-sized pieces. Season food as the person prefers and as the care plan allows.

12 Serve foods in the order the person prefers. Identify foods as you serve them. Alternate between solid and liquid foods. Use a spoon for safety (see Fig. 31-5). Allow enough time to chew and swallow. Do not rush the person.
13 Offer fluids (water, coffee, milk, juice, tea, or other fluid) frequently. (NOTE: Some state competency tests require that a drink is offered for at least every 2 to 3 bites of food.) Use straws (if allowed) for liquids if the person cannot drink out of a glass or cup. Have 1 straw for each liquid. Provide short straws for weak persons. Follow the care plan for using straws.
14 Follow the care plan if the person has dysphagia. Give thickened liquid with a spoon if needed.
15 Check the person's mouth before offering more food or fluids. Make sure the mouth is empty between bites and swallows. Ask if the person is ready for the next bite or drink.

Continued

Feeding the Person—cont'd

PROCEDURE—cont'd

16 Wipe the person's hands, face, and mouth as needed during the meal. Use the napkin or a hand-wipe.
17 Talk with the person in a pleasant manner.
18 Encourage the person to eat as much as possible.
19 Wipe the person's mouth with a napkin or a hand-wipe when finished. Discard the napkin or hand-wipe.
20 Note how much and which foods were eaten (Chapter 30).
21 Measure and record fluid intake if ordered (Chapter 32).

22 Remove the item used to protect clothing if worn. Follow agency policy for used linens. Discard a disposable napkin.
23 Remove the tray.
24 Take the person to his or her room (if in a dining area). Clean and dry the over-bed table (if used in the person's room). Dry with paper towels. Discard the paper towels.
25 Assist with oral hygiene and hand hygiene. Provide for privacy. Wear gloves. Practice hand hygiene after removing and discarding gloves.

POST-PROCEDURE

26 Provide for comfort. (See the inside of the back cover.)
27 Raise or lower bed rails. Follow the care plan.
28 Place the call light and other needed items within reach.
29 Follow the care plan and the person's preferences for privacy measures to maintain. Leaving the privacy curtain, window coverings, and door open or closed are examples.

30 Complete a safety check of the room. (See the inside of the back cover.)
31 Return a food tray from a room to the food cart.
32 Practice hand hygiene.
33 Report and record your care and observations.

FOODBORNE ILLNESS

Fresh produce and raw (uncooked) meat, poultry, seafood, and eggs are not sterile. Pathogens may be present on food when purchased. Cooked and ready-to-eat foods can become contaminated from the environment or from other food. For example, meat juices spill or splash onto other food. Food handlers with poor hygiene can contaminate food.

If contaminated food is ingested, a foodborne illness (food poisoning) can occur. Signs and symptoms vary depending on the pathogen. Nausea, vomiting, diarrhea, abdominal pain, and fever are common. Report signs and symptoms of foodborne illness to the nurse at once.

There are measures you can take to prevent foodborne illness. To keep food safe, the U.S. Department of Agriculture (USDA) recommends these 4 safety tips.

- *Clean.* Wash hands, utensils, and counter tops often.
- *Separate.* Avoid cross-contamination. Do not let raw meat, poultry, seafood, eggs, or their juices touch other foods that will not be cooked.
- *Cook.* Cook food to a safe internal temperature (Fig. 31-7). Use a food thermometer to check the internal temperature. When re-heating cooked food, re-heat to 165°F (Fahrenheit).
- *Chill.* Refrigerate or freeze food that can spoil within 2 hours. If the air is 90°F or above, chill food within 1 hour.

Pathogens grow rapidly between 40°F and 140°F. This range is called the "danger zone" by the USDA. You must keep food out of the "danger zone." To do so, keep cold food cold and hot food hot.

See *Focus on Long-Term Care and Home Care: Foodborne Illness.*

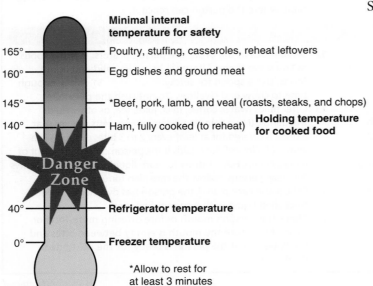

FIGURE 31-7 Food temperature guide. (Modified from U.S. Department of Agriculture: "Danger Zone" [40 °F–140 °F].)

FOCUS ON LONG-TERM CARE AND HOME CARE
Foodborne Illness

Home Care
You need to protect the patient and family from foodborne illnesses. Follow the clean, separate, cook, and chill safety tips.

Clean
- Practice hand-washing with soap and water (Chapter 17):
  - Before, during, and after preparing food
  - After handling raw meat, poultry, seafood, or their juices; or uncooked eggs
  - Before eating
  - After elimination
  - After changing a diaper or helping a child who has used the toilet
  - After touching an animal, animal feed, or animal waste
  - After touching garbage
  - Before and after caring for an ill person
  - Before and after treating a cut or wound
  - After blowing your nose, coughing, or sneezing
- Wash surfaces and utensils after each use.
  - Use hot, soapy water to wash cutting boards, dishes, utensils, and countertops. Do so especially if they held raw meat, poultry, seafood, or eggs.
  - Wash dish cloths often in the hot cycle of a washing machine.
- Wash fruits and vegetables.
  - Rinse under running water. Do not use soap, bleach, or commercial produce washes.
  - Rinse before peeling, removing skin, or cutting away damaged or bruised areas.
  - Scrub firm produce (melons, cucumbers) with a clean produce brush.
  - Dry produce with a paper towel or clean cloth towel.
  - Do not wash bagged produce marked "pre-washed."
- Do not wash meat, poultry, seafood, or eggs.

Separate: Do Not Cross Contaminate
- Use separate cutting boards, plates, and utensils for foods that will not be cooked and for raw foods (meat, poultry, seafood, eggs). For example, use 1 cutting board for fresh produce. Use another for raw meat.
  - Replace cutting boards when worn.
  - Wash thoroughly all plates, utensils, and cutting boards that have touched raw meat, poultry, seafood, eggs, or flour. Do so before re-use with hot, soapy water.
- Keep certain types of food separate.
  - While shopping:
    - Separate raw meat, poultry, seafood, and eggs from other foods.
    - Place raw meat, poultry, and seafood in plastic bags while shopping if available.
    - Place raw meat, poultry, and seafood in separate bags from other foods when checking out.
  - At home:
    - Place raw meat, poultry, and seafood in containers or plastic bags. Bags should be leak-proof and sealed.
    - Freeze raw meat, poultry, and seafood if not to be used within a few days.
  - Refrigerator:
    - Keep eggs in their original carton.
    - Store eggs in the main section of the refrigerator. Do not store them in the door.

Cook to the Right Temperature
- Use a food thermometer to make sure food is safe. Food is safely cooked when the internal temperature is high enough to kill pathogens. Place the food thermometer in the thickest part of the food. The thermometer should not touch bone, fat, or gristle.
- Use a cooking chart or food temperature guide to make sure food has reached a safe temperature (see Fig. 31-7).
- Keep food hot (140°F or above) after cooking.
  - Serve food right after cooking.
  - Keep food out of the danger zone (see Fig. 31-7) if not serving it right after cooking. Use a heat source—chafing dish, warming tray, slow cooker.
- Microwave food thoroughly (165°F or above).
  - Follow package directions for cooking to make sure food is thoroughly cooked.
  - Stir food in the middle of the cooking time. Follow package directions for commercially prepared foods that are not designed for stirring during heating.
  - Follow package directions after cooking. For example, "Let stand for 2 minutes after cooking." Letting food sit for a few minutes allows colder areas to absorb heat from hotter areas.

Chill: Refrigerate and Freeze Food Properly
- Remember that microbes causing food poisoning multiply the fastest between 40°F and 140°F.
- Check that the refrigerator is set to 40°F or below and the freezer to 0°F. Use an appliance thermometer.
- Do not leave foods that will spoil out of the refrigerator for more than 2 hours.
- Refrigerate food within 1 hour if it was exposed to temperatures above 90°F.
- Place left-overs in shallow containers. Refrigerate promptly for quick cooling.
- Never thaw or marinate foods on the counter. Thaw or marinate meat, poultry, and seafood in the refrigerator.
- Check a cold food storage chart for when to throw out food.

Modified from U.S. Department of Health and Human Services: 4 steps to food safety, last reviewed September 18, 2023.

FOCUS ON **PRIDE**

FOCUS ON **PRIDE**

The Person, Family, and Yourself

Personal and Professional Responsibility

You can help make meal time pleasant. Smile and greet each person as you serve food. Ask if help is needed. Talk with the person as you prepare food. When feeding, focus on the person. Meal time should be as pleasant as possible.

Rights and Respect

The person has the right to refuse a food or drink because of personal preference. If refused, a substitute (alternative) should be offered.

Independence and Social Interaction

Meals provide a time for social contact. A friendly, social setting is important. Some nursing centers have areas for residents to dine with guests. Families and friends may bring food from home. This helps meet love and belonging needs. Tell the nurse when the person receives food. The food must not interfere with the person's diet.

Delegation and Teamwork

Meals are a busy time. Teamwork is important. Staff work together to help residents to the dining area and serve food promptly. Staff must make sure everyone is served and nutrition needs are met. Have a helpful attitude.

Ethics and Laws

A person's nutrition needs can change. Poor appetite, decreased food intake, and weight loss signal a change. The health team must address changes in nutrition needs. Neglect can result from unmet needs. Tell the nurse about any changes or concerns.

FOCUS ON **PRIDE**: *Application*

How do sights, sounds, smells, and personal preferences affect meal time? How can you help make it pleasant?

REVIEW QUESTIONS

Circle the BEST answer.

1 These statements are about factors affecting eating and nutrition. Which is *true?*
   a Culture and religion do not affect dietary practices.
   b Negative body reactions affect food choices.
   c Less nutrients are needed during illness and recovery.
   d Food appearance and smell are not important factors.

2 Persons with dysphagia
   a Are fed in the semi-Fowler's position
   b Have a regular diet
   c Are fed according to the care plan
   d Eat alone in their rooms

3 A person coughs and drools while eating. You should
   a Give the person a drink
   b Puree the person's food
   c Give mouth care and continue feeding
   d Tell the nurse

4 A person requires pudding-thick liquid. This liquid should be
   a Mildly thick and able to flow through a straw
   b Moderately thick and flow off of a spoon
   c Moderately thick with lumps
   d Extremely thick and mound on a spoon

5 Nursing centers must
   a Serve food promptly
   b Serve 2 meals a day
   c Serve food at room temperature to avoid burns
   d Serve food under-seasoned to lower sodium intake

6 A resident refuses to eat pork. The person
   a Should be offered a different item of similar nutritional value
   b Cannot refuse menu items without a special diet order
   c Should have the family bring a meal when pork is served
   d Needs to try foods before refusing them

7 Which promotes comfort and preparation for a meal?
   a The urinal is nearby and contains urine.
   b The incontinent person is clean and dry.
   c Dentures are in the denture cup in the bathroom.
   d The person used the bathroom without hand hygiene afterward.

8 A person needs help opening cartons and cutting food. You should
   a Ask dietary staff to help the person
   b Tell the person you do not have time
   c Assist the person as needed
   d Refuse to help to promote independence

9 A person is served a meal tray. Which is a problem?
   a The food was served in a covered container.
   b The tray contains adaptive equipment (assistive devices).
   c The dietary card lists "strawberries" as an allergy. Pears were served.
   d The dietary card lists "pureed diet." A whole pork chop was served.

10 You are assisting with feeding in the dining room. A person is drowsy and will not drink from a straw. You should
   a Yell to awaken the person
   b Tell the nurse right away
   c Try to give the person bites of food
   d Go feed someone else

11 When feeding a person
   a Ask in what order the person likes foods served
   b Use a fork
   c Stand facing the person
   d Talk with your co-workers

12 After feeding a person
   a Leave the person's clothing protector in place
   b Use your fingers to remove food left in the mouth
   c Clean the person's face and hands
   d Position the person supine if aspiration is a risk

13 You are re-heating cooked food. The food temperature should be
   a 40°F
   b 90°F
   c 140°F
   d 165°F

14 Which can cause foodborne illness?
   a Washing fruits before serving them
   b Keeping cooked foods at or above 140°F until served
   c Storing eggs in the main section of the refrigerator
   d Using 1 cutting board for raw meat and then for vegetables that will not be cooked

15 You should
   a Wash poultry before cooking it
   b Thaw ground beef on a counter top
   c Wash kitchen surfaces with hot, soapy water
   d Refrigerate left-over food within 4 hours

Answers to Chapter 31 questions are on p. 902.

FOCUS ON **PRACTICE**

Problem Solving

After receiving a breakfast tray, a resident says: "I didn't ask for eggs this morning." You check the dietary card and notice the tray is for another person. What will you do? Why is this a problem?

OBJECTIVES

- Define the key terms and key abbreviations in this chapter.
- Describe fluid requirements.
- Identify the causes, signs and symptoms, and care measures for dehydration and fluid overload.
- Explain how to assist with special fluid orders.
- Explain the purpose of intake and output records.
- Identify what to count as fluid intake and output.

- Explain how to measure intake and output.
- Explain how to provide drinking water and assist with meeting fluid needs.
- Perform the procedures described in this chapter.
- Explain how to promote PRIDE in the person, the family, and yourself.

KEY TERMS

dehydration A decrease in the amount of water in the body
edema The swelling of body tissues with water
electrolytes Minerals dissolved in water

graduate A measuring container for fluid
intake The amount of fluid taken in; input
output The amount of fluid lost

KEY ABBREVIATIONS

ID	Identification	mL	Milliliter
I&O	Intake and output	NPO	*Nil per os;* nothing by mouth
IV	Intravenous	oz	Ounce

Water is needed to live. Death can result from too much or too little water. You will help meet fluid needs. Measuring intake and output and providing drinking water are examples.

FLUID BALANCE

Water is ingested through fluids and foods. Water is normally lost through urine and feces (stools). It is also lost through the skin (perspiration) and the lungs (expiration).

The words *hydrated* and *hydration* relate to normal fluid balance. When a person is hydrated, the body has enough water to function normally. For normal hydration, fluid intake must roughly equal output.

- *Intake (input)* is the amount of fluid taken in.
- *Output* is the amount of fluid lost.

Dehydration occurs when output exceeds intake. *Dehydration* is a decrease in the amount of water in the body.

Fluid overload occurs when fluid intake exceeds fluid output. Edema is often a sign. *Edema* is the swelling of body tissues with water. It is common in people with heart, kidney, and liver diseases. Edema often occurs in the legs, ankles, and feet (Fig. 32-1). *Pulmonary edema* is a severe form of edema affecting the lungs (Chapter 50).

Common causes and signs and symptoms of dehydration and fluid overload are listed in Table 32-1. Care measures that relate to the nursing assistant's role are also listed.

See *Focus on Children and Older Persons: Fluid Balance*, p. 494.

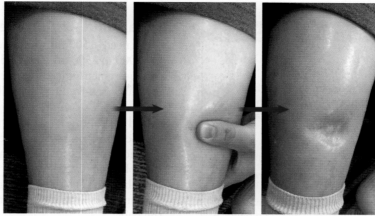

FIGURE 32-1 Edema in the lower leg. The nurse applies pressure to the body part to check for edema. (Courtesy Kellie White.)

TABLE 32-1	Dehydration and Fluid Overload	
Causes	**Signs and Symptoms**	**Care Measures**
Dehydration		
• Bleeding • Vomiting • Diarrhea • Sweating (perspiration): excess (*diaphoresis*) • Fever • Urine production: increased • Drug therapy • Fluid intake: poor, none • Fluid restriction • Function problems: difficulty drinking, reaching fluids, communicating fluid needs • Dementia • Level of consciousness: altered	• Blood pressure: low • Postural hypotension (Chapter 35) • Pulse: fast, weak • Respirations: fast • Weight loss • Confusion, delirium (Chapter 54) • Dizziness, feeling light-headed • Consciousness: altered • Irritability • Fatigue • Headache • Muscle cramps • Thirst • Dry, cool skin • Dry mouth and lips, coated tongue • Poor *skin turgor*—when pinched and released, skin slowly returns to its normal position • Urine changes: dark yellow or amber, strong smell, scant amount (*oliguria*) • Shock (Chapter 58)	• Observe for and report signs and symptoms of dehydration. • Measure weight accurately as often as directed (Chapter 37). Report weight change (loss). • Encourage fluids as ordered. See "Special Fluid Orders" on p. 494. • Keep the person's water mug (cup, pitcher) filled and within reach. • Ask about the person's fluid preferences. Provide preferred fluids. • Offer fluids each time you give care. • Measure intake and output accurately (p. 495). • Report low intake and excess fluid losses. (See "Normal Fluid Requirements" on p. 494.)
Fluid Overload		
• Heart disease • Liver disease • Kidney disease • Hormone disorders • Fluid intake: excess • Sodium intake: excess • Intravenous (IV) therapy • Tap water enemas (Chapter 29)	• Blood pressure: high • Pulse: fast or slow, strong • Respirations: fast • Weight gain: rapid • Confusion • Irritability • Fatigue • Skin changes: tight, smooth, shiny • Edema: feet, ankles, legs, abdomen, fingers, hands, face (see Fig. 32-1) • Dyspnea: worse with activity (exertion); worse lying down (*orthopnea*) • Lung sounds: crackling • Urine output: decreased	• Observe for and report signs and symptoms of fluid overload. • Measure weight accurately as often as directed (Chapter 37). Report weight change (gain)—2 pounds in 1 day. • Restrict fluids as ordered. See "Special Fluid Orders" on p. 494. • Provide frequent oral hygiene (Chapter 23). • Measure intake and output accurately (p. 495). • Follow the person's ordered diet (Chapter 30). A sodium-restricted diet is common. • Follow the care plan for positioning. Elevate swollen legs and arms as directed. Elevate the head of the bed for comfort. Turn and re-position at least every 2 hours. • Observe for signs of pressure injury (Chapter 42). • Handle body areas with edema carefully. • Balance activity and rest periods. • Apply elastic stockings or bandages as directed (Chapter 40). • Assist with elimination needs promptly. Drugs may be given to increase urine output.

Fluid Balance

Children

Infants and young children have more body water than adults do. Excess fluid losses cannot be tolerated. They quickly become severe in an infant or child. Death can occur.

Older Persons

The amount of body water decreases as people age. In older persons, the thirst sensation decreases. They need water but may not feel thirsty. Offer water often.

Older persons are at risk for diseases affecting fluid balance. They commonly take drugs that affect fluid balance. Dehydration and edema are risks. Some persons have special fluid orders.

Persons with dementia are at higher risk for dehydration (Chapter 54). In early dementia, the person may not remember to drink fluids regularly. As dementia progresses, the person may have trouble turning on a faucet or filling a cup. In the late stage, communicating needs is severely impaired. Follow the care plan to meet the person's needs. Observe closely for signs and symptoms of dehydration.

Normal Fluid Requirements

An adult needs 1500 mL (milliliters) of fluid daily to survive. About 2000 to 2500 mL are needed for normal fluid balance. Fluid requirements increase with hot weather, exercise, pregnancy and breast-feeding, fever, illness, and excess fluid losses.

Electrolytes. *Electrolytes* are minerals dissolved in water. Sodium, potassium, calcium, and magnesium are some electrolytes. Electrolytes are needed for:

- Fluid balance
- Acid-base (pH) balance (Chapter 10)
- Movement of nutrients into the cells and wastes out of the cells
- Nerve, muscle, heart, and brain function

An *electrolyte imbalance* occurs when an electrolyte level is too low or too high. Dehydration and fluid overload are causes. Heart, kidney, and liver disorders can affect electrolyte levels. So can certain drugs and intravenous (IV) therapy (Chapter 33). Normal fluid and electrolyte levels are needed for body function.

SPECIAL FLUID ORDERS

The person may need a special fluid order to meet fluid needs. The order is part of the person's care plan. The nurse teaches the person and family what the person is allowed to have. Common fluid orders are listed in Table 32-2.

TABLE 32-2	**Common Fluid Orders**		
Fluid Order	Description	Some Uses	Care Measures
Encourage fluids	The person drinks an increased amount of fluid.	Dehydration, urinary tract infections, kidney stones	• Follow the care plan for the amount. • Keep a variety of fluids within the person's reach. • Offer fluids often and help the person drink if not able to do so alone.
Restrict fluids	Fluids are limited to a certain amount.	Edema, kidney failure, heart failure	• Follow the care plan for the amount allowed. • Offer fluids in small amounts and in small containers. • Remove the water mug (cup, pitcher) or keep it out of sight. • Provide frequent oral hygiene to keep the mouth moist.
Nothing by mouth (NPO)	The person cannot eat or drink anything. NPO stands for *nil per os—* nothing *(nil)* by *(per)* mouth *(os)*.	Before and after surgery, before some laboratory tests and diagnostic procedures, to treat certain illnesses	• Post an NPO sign above the bed or at the room door. Follow agency policy. • Remove the water mug (cup, pitcher) from the room. • Provide frequent oral hygiene. The person must not swallow any fluid. • Follow the nurse's directions for how long the person will be NPO. The person is NPO for 6 to 12 hours before surgery and for some tests and procedures.
Thickened liquids	Water and all fluids are thickened by the dietary department.	Difficulty swallowing *(dysphagia)*	• Serve thickened liquids as directed by the nurse and the care plan. Thickened commercial fluids are used. Or the dietary department thickens fluids. • Follow agency policy for how to record intake for thickened liquids. • See "Dysphagia" in Chapter 31.

INTAKE AND OUTPUT

An intake and output (I&O) record monitors the amounts of fluid taken into (intake) and fluid leaving (output) the body. You will measure and record I&O.

- *Intake.* All oral fluids are measured and recorded—water, milk, coffee, tea, juices, soups, and soft drinks. So are foods that melt at room temperature—ice cream, sherbet, custard, gelatin, and Popsicles. The nurse measures and records IV fluids and tube feedings (Chapter 33).
- *Output.* Urine, vomitus, diarrhea, and wound drainage amounts are measured and recorded. Output from an ostomy (Chapter 29) and drainage from suction (Chapter 45) are also included as output. (*Suction* means to withdraw fluid. Fluid suctioned from the stomach through a naso-gastric [NG] tube is an example.)

I&O records are used to plan and evaluate treatment. They also are kept for special fluid orders.

Measuring Intake and Output

Intake and output are measured in milliliters (mL). See Box 32-1 for amounts to know.

You must know the serving sizes of bowls, dishes, cups, pitchers, mugs, glasses, and other containers. This information may be on the I&O record (Fig. 32-2). Or the serving size is on the container.

BOX 32-1	I&O Measures
1 cubic centimeter (cc) = 1 mL	
1 teaspoon = 5 mL	
1 tablespoon = 15 mL	
1 oz = 30 mL	
1 cup = 240 mL	
1 pint = about 500 mL	
1 quart = about 1000 mL	
1 liter (L) = 1000 mL	

FLUID INTAKE AND OUTPUT FLOW SHEET
DATE *Oct 12*

RECORD TOTALS IN PATIENT'S MEDICAL RECORD		DIET/FLUID ORDERS *Regular*	
Water glass	240 mL	Gelatin	120 mL
Juice glass	120 mL	Ice cream	90 mL
Milk carton	240 mL	Broth/strained soup	180 mL
Coffee cup	240 mL	Styrofoam cup	180 mL
Soft drink can	360 mL	Water mug	1000 mL
Tea glass	180 mL	Ice chips	½ amount of mL in cup

	TIME	ORAL	TYPE & AMOUNT	TIME	IV	ENTERAL	TIME	SOURCE	AMOUNT
			INTAKE				**OUTPUT**		
2300-0700		FLUIDS					2330	Void	225 mL
							0545	Void	325 mL
	0645	MUG/OTHER	Water 200 mL						
			8-HOUR SUB-TOTAL			200 mL	**8-HOUR SUB-TOTAL**		550 mL
0700-1500	0830	BREAKFAST	Coffee 240 mL Milk 160 mL				0750	Void	200 mL
							0930	Void	225 mL
							1145	Void	250 mL
							1330	Void	200 mL
	1015	SNACK	Juice 120 mL						
	1230	LUNCH	Soft drink 240 mL Ice cream 90 mL Soup 90 mL						
		SNACK							
	1450	MUG/OTHER	Water 300 mL						
			8-HOUR SUB-TOTAL			1240 mL	**8-HOUR SUB-TOTAL**		875 mL
1500-2300	1740	DINNER	Tea 180 mL Soft drink 100 mL				1505	Void	275 mL
							1655	Void	150 mL
							2010	Void	150 mL
							2115	Vomitus	100 mL
	1930	SNACK	Gelatin 120 mL						
	2230	MUG/OTHER	Water 325 mL						
			8-HOUR SUB-TOTAL			725 mL	**8-HOUR SUB-TOTAL**		675 mL
			24-HOUR TOTAL			2165 mL	**24-HOUR TOTAL**		2100 mL

FIGURE 32-2 A sample intake and output (I&O) record.

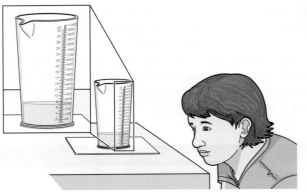

FIGURE 32-3 A graduate is on a flat surface. The amount is read at eye level.

A measuring container for fluid is called a *graduate*. Like a measuring cup, the graduate is marked in ounces (oz) and milliliters (mL). For an accurate measurement, place the device on a flat surface and read it at eye level (Fig. 32-3). Separate graduates are used for intake and for output.

The amount measured is recorded in the correct column on the I&O record (see Fig. 32-2). Amounts are totaled at the end of the shift and 24-hour day. The totals are entered into the person's medical record. They also are shared during the end-of-shift report.

The purpose of measuring I&O and how to help are explained to the person. Some persons measure and record their intake. Family members may help. The urinal, commode, bedpan, or specimen pan (Chapter 39) is used to void. Remind the person not to void in the toilet. Urine voided in the toilet cannot be measured. Also remind the person not to put toilet paper in the voiding container.

See *Focus on Math: Measuring Intake and Output.*
See *Delegation Guidelines: Measuring Intake and Output*, p. 498.
See *Promoting Safety and Comfort: Measuring Intake and Output*, p. 498.
See procedure: *Measuring Intake and Output*, p. 498.

FOCUS ON MATH

Measuring Intake and Output

 To measure I&O, you must accurately read and calculate measurements.

Reading Measuring Containers
Measuring containers (graduates, urinals, and specimen pans) are marked in mL (milliliters) and oz (ounces). The container may not have all lines labeled. To calculate unlabeled measurements (Fig. 32-4):

1 Choose the labeled line above the fluid level and the labeled line below it.

    400 mL and 300 mL

2 Subtract these 2 numbers. The result is called the *difference*.

    400 mL – 300 mL = 100 mL

3 Count the number of spaces between the 2 labeled lines in step 1.

    4 spaces

4 Divide the difference in step 2 by the number of spaces.

    100 mL ÷ 4 spaces = 25 mL
    Each line increases by 25 mL.

NOTE: Some state competency tests instruct to round up to the nearest 25 mL if the fluid level is between measurement lines. To *round up* means to choose the higher value.

Converting Ounces to Milliliters
In health care settings, intake is measured in mL (milliliters). Some containers show the serving amount in oz (ounces). You need to convert (change) the serving amount from oz to mL. One oz equals 30 mL (1 oz = 30 mL). To convert, multiply the number of oz by 30. For example:

A coffee cup holds 8 oz. Multiply 8 oz by 30 (the number of mL in each oz). The 8 oz coffee cup equals 240 mL.

    8 oz × 30 mL/oz = 240 mL
    (mL/oz is read as "milliliters per ounce")
    8 oz equals 240 mL.

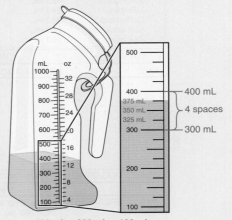

    400 mL – 300 mL = 100 mL
    100 mL ÷ 4 = 25 mL
    Each line increases by 25 mL.

FIGURE 32-4 Calculating unlabeled measurements. Divide the difference between 2 labeled lines by the number of spaces between the 2 lines. Each line on this urinal increases by 25 mL. The measurements between 300 mL and 400 mL are 325 mL, 350 mL, and 375 mL.

Measuring Intake
To measure intake, subtract the amount of liquid left (remaining amount) from the full amount of liquid served (full serving amount).

1 Check the full serving amount. This is found on the container or on the I&O record.

2 Measure the amount of liquid left in the container. Use a graduate.

3 Subtract the amount in step 2 from the amount in step 1.

FOCUS ON MATH—cont'd

Measuring Intake and Output

Measuring Intake—cont'd

The following is an example of how to measure intake.

A person was served a 120 mL glass of juice. You pour the liquid left in the glass into a graduate. You measure 90 mL in the graduate and calculate the intake amount.

120 mL (amount served) – 90 mL (amount left) = 30 mL (intake amount)

The person drank 30 mL of juice.

For total intake for a meal, measure the intake for each liquid served. Add the intake amounts from each liquid together. For example:

A person drank all of a cup of coffee (240 mL) and 30 mL of juice.

Liquid	Amount Served	Amount Left	Intake Amount
Coffee	240 mL	0 mL	240 mL
Juice	120 mL	90 mL	30 mL
		Total Intake	240 mL + 30 mL = 270 mL

The total intake for this meal was 270 mL.

Measuring Output

For output, measure the amount of liquid in the measuring device (graduate, urinal, specimen pan). See "Reading Measuring Containers" if you need to calculate an unlabeled measurement on the device.

Totaling I&O for a Shift

A shift total (sub-total) is calculated at the end of the shift. See Figure 32-2. The intake amounts during the shift are added together. The output amounts during the shift are added together. For example:

- *Intake for a shift—during your shift a person drank 270 mL at breakfast, 390 mL at lunch, 90 mL as a snack, and 400 mL of water. The total intake for your shift is 1150 mL.*

  270 mL + 390 mL + 90 mL + 400 mL = 1150 mL

- *Output for a shift—a person voided 3 times during your shift. The amounts were 200 mL, 250 mL, and 100 mL. The total output for your shift is 550 mL.*

  200 mL + 250 mL + 100 mL = 550 mL

Totaling 24-Hour I&O

Intake and output amounts are totaled at the end of the 24-hour day. See Figure 32-2. The intake amounts for the full day are added together. The output amounts for the full day are added together. For example:

- *24-hour intake—a person drank 125 mL during the first shift, 1150 mL during the second shift, and 600 mL during the third shift. The total 24-hour intake amount is 1875 mL.*

  125 mL + 1150 mL + 600 mL = 1875 mL

- *24-hour output—a person voided 450 mL during the first shift, 550 mL during the second shift, and 800 mL during the third shift. The total 24-hour output amount is 1800 mL.*

  450 mL + 550 mL + 800 mL = 1800 mL

Estimating Using Fractions

Measuring is the most accurate method to determine intake. However, as part of your training or work you may need to know how to estimate using fractions.

A *fraction* is used to communicate a certain part of a whole (Fig. 32-5). The bottom number (*denominator*) is the number of equal parts the whole is divided into. The top number (*numerator*) is the number of parts being measured. For example:

- In the fraction ½ (one-half), the whole is divided into 2 equal parts. One part is being measured.
- In the fraction ⅔ (two-thirds), the whole is divided into 3 equal parts. Two parts are being measured.
- In the fraction ¾ (three-fourths), the whole is divided into 4 equal parts. Three parts are being measured.

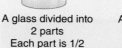

A glass divided into
2 parts
Each part is 1/2

A glass divided into
3 parts
Each part is 1/3

A glass divided into
4 parts
Each part is 1/4

FIGURE 32-5 Fractions measure parts of a whole. The fraction's bottom number (denominator) is the number of equal parts the whole is divided into.

To calculate intake using fractions:

1 Divide the full serving amount by the fraction's denominator. (This divides the whole into equal parts.) *For example, a person drank ¾ of a 4 oz (120 mL) cup of juice. Divide the whole (120 mL) by the fraction's denominator (4).*

   120 mL ÷ 4 = 30 mL

   Each part is 30 mL.

2 Multiply the amount in step 1 by the fraction's numerator. (This is the amount being measured.)

   30 mL × 3 = 90 mL

   ¾ of 120 mL = 90 mL.

   The person drank 90 mL of juice.

See Figure 32-6 (p. 498) for an example.

FOCUS ON MATH—cont'd

Measuring Intake and Output

Estimating Using Fractions—cont'd

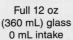

Full 12 oz (360 mL) glass 0 mL intake | 1/4 drank 90 mL intake | 1/3 drank 120 mL intake | 1/2 drank 180 mL intake | 2/3 drank 240 mL intake | 3/4 drank 270 mL intake | Empty 12 oz glass 360 mL intake

FIGURE 32-6 Estimating intake using fractions.

Figure 32-6 shows different intake amounts from a 12 oz (360 mL) glass. See the table below for different intake amounts for 4 oz, 6 oz, and 8 oz containers using fractions.

	1/4	1/2	3/4	1/3	2/3
4 oz = 120 mL	30 mL	60 mL	90 mL	40 mL	80 mL
6 oz = 180 mL	45 mL	90 mL	135 mL	60 mL	120 mL
8 oz = 240 mL	60 mL	120 mL	180 mL	80 mL	160 mL

DELEGATION GUIDELINES

Measuring Intake and Output

Measuring I&O is a routine nursing task. You need this information from the nurse and the care plan.
- If the person has a special fluid order (p. 494)
- When to report measurements—hourly or end-of-shift
- What the person uses for voiding—urinal, bedpan, commode, or specimen pan (Chapters 27 and 39)
- If the person has a catheter (Chapter 28)
- What patient or resident concerns to report at once

PROMOTING SAFETY AND COMFORT

Measuring Intake and Output

Safety
Urine, vomitus, diarrhea, and wound drainage are body fluids. Follow Standard Precautions when measuring output. Follow the Bloodborne Pathogen Standard if blood is present. Follow the rules of hand hygiene and the guidelines for glove use in Chapters 17 and 18.

Follow agency procedures to disinfect the graduate and device used for output collection after use. Remember to use separate graduates for intake and output.

Comfort
Promptly measure and empty the contents of urinals, bedpans, commodes, specimen pans, and kidney basins. This helps prevent or reduce odors. Odors can disturb the person.

Measuring Intake and Output

QUALITY OF LIFE

- Knock before entering the person's room.
- Address the person by name.
- Introduce yourself by name and title.

- Explain the procedure before starting and during the procedure.
- Protect the person's rights during the procedure.
- Handle the person gently during the procedure.

PRE-PROCEDURE

1 Follow *Delegation Guidelines: Measuring Intake and Output*. See *Promoting Safety and Comfort: Measuring Intake and Output*.
2 Practice hand hygiene and get the following supplies.
   - I&O record
   - 2 graduates:
     - A graduate for intake
     - A graduate for output
   - Needed supplies for urinary or bowel elimination (Chapters 27, 28, and 39)
   - Gloves
   - Paper towels or a disposable waterproof pad
3 Arrange items in the person's room.
4 Practice hand hygiene.
5 Identify the person. Check the identification (ID) bracelet against the I&O record. Use 2 identifiers (Chapter 14). Also call the person by name.
6 Provide for privacy.

Measuring Intake and Output—cont'd

PROCEDURE

7 Put on gloves.
8 Measure intake.
   a Pour liquid remaining in the container into the graduate used to measure intake. Avoid spills and splashes on the outside of the graduate.
   b Place the graduate on a flat surface. Measure the amount at eye level (see Fig. 32-3).
   c Check the serving amount on the I&O record. Or check the serving size of each container.
   d Subtract the remaining amount from the full serving amount. Note the amount. (For example, a cup holds 240 mL. The amount in the graduate is 50 mL. 240 mL – 50 mL = 190 mL.)
   e Pour fluid in the graduate back into the container.
   f Repeat step 8 (a-e) for each liquid.
   g Add the amounts from each liquid together.
   h Record the time and amount on the I&O record.
   i Discard the excess liquids. Follow agency procedures to clean the graduate. Return the graduate to its proper place.

9 Assist with elimination if needed. Measure output.
   a Pour the fluid into the graduate used to measure output. Avoid spills and splashes on the outside of the graduate.
   b Place the device on a paper towel (or disposable waterproof pad) on a flat surface. Measure the amount at eye level.
   c Dispose of fluid in the toilet. Avoid splashes.
   d Rinse the graduate. Pour the rinse into the toilet and flush. Follow agency procedures for cleaning and disinfection. Return the graduate to its proper place.
   e Rinse the voiding receptacle or other container. Pour the rinse into the toilet and flush. Follow agency procedures for cleaning and disinfection. Return the item to its proper place.
   f Remove and discard the gloves. Practice hand hygiene.
   g Record the output amount on the person's I&O record.

POST-PROCEDURE

10 Provide for comfort. (See the inside of the back cover.)
11 Place the call light and other needed items within reach.
12 Follow the care plan and the person's preferences for privacy measures to maintain. Leaving the privacy curtain, window coverings, and door open or closed are examples.
13 Complete a safety check of the room. (See the inside of the back cover.)
14 Practice hand hygiene.
15 Report and record your care and observations.

PROVIDING DRINKING WATER

You normally provide fresh drinking water each shift and when the person's water mug (cup, pitcher) is empty (Fig. 32-7). Follow the care plan and the nurse's instructions for persons with special fluid orders (p. 494).

• Fluid restriction—The person is not given more than the limited amount.
• NPO—The person is not given fluids.
• Thickened liquids—The person must be given liquids of a certain thickness (Chapter 31).

Some agencies do not use the following procedure. Instead, each mug is filled as needed. You take the mug to an ice and water dispenser. Fill the mug with ice first. Then add water. Follow the agency's procedure for providing fresh drinking water.

See *Focus on Communication: Providing Drinking Water*, p. 500.
See *Delegation Guidelines: Providing Drinking Water*, p. 500.
See *Promoting Safety and Comfort: Providing Drinking Water*, p. 500.
See procedure: *Providing Drinking Water*, p. 500.

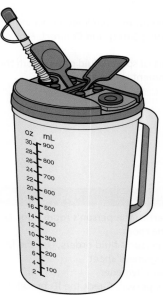

FIGURE 32-7 Water mug with straw. The mug is marked in milliliters (mL) and ounces (oz).

FOCUS ON COMMUNICATION

Providing Drinking Water

People vary about ice in their water. Ask what the person prefers. You can say:
- "Would you like ice in your water?"
- "How much ice do you prefer in your water?"
- "Do you like more ice or more water?"

Also ask where to place the mug. Be sure the person can reach it.

DELEGATION GUIDELINES

Providing Drinking Water

Providing drinking water is a routine nursing task. You need this information from the nurse and the care plan.
- The person's fluid orders
- How much ice to add
- If the person uses a straw

PROMOTING SAFETY AND COMFORT

Providing Drinking Water

Safety

Water mugs can spread microbes. To prevent the spread of microbes:
- Label the mug with the person's name and room and bed number.
- Do not touch the rim or inside of the mug or lid.
- Do not let the ice scoop touch the mug, lid, or straw.
- Place the ice scoop in the scoop holder or on a towel for the scoop. Do not place it in the ice container or dispenser.
- Keep the ice chest closed when not in use.
- Make sure the mug is clean. Also check for cracks and chips. Provide a new mug as needed.
- Practice hand hygiene between each mug. This prevents the spread of microbes from 1 person's mug to another person's mug.

Providing Drinking Water

QUALITY OF LIFE

- Knock before entering the person's room.
- Address the person by name.
- Introduce yourself by name and title.
- Explain the procedure before starting and during the procedure.
- Protect the person's rights during the procedure.
- Handle the person gently during the procedure.

PRE-PROCEDURE

1. Follow *Delegation Guidelines: Providing Drinking Water.* See *Promoting Safety and Comfort: Providing Drinking Water.*
2. Obtain a list of special fluid orders from the nurse. Or use your assignment sheet.
3. Practice hand hygiene and get the following supplies.
   - Cart
   - Ice chest filled with ice
   - Cover for the ice chest
   - Scoop
   - Paper towels
   - Water mugs
   - Water pitcher filled with cold water (optional depending on agency procedure)
   - Towel for the scoop (if there is no scoop holder)
4. Cover the cart with paper towels. Arrange equipment on top of the paper towels.

PROCEDURE

5. Take the cart to the person's room door. Do not take the cart into the room.
6. Check the person's fluid orders. Use the list from the nurse or your assignment sheet.
7. Practice hand hygiene.
8. Identify the person. Check the ID bracelet against the fluid orders sheet or your assignment sheet. Use 2 identifiers (Chapter 14). Also call the person by name.
9. Take the mug from the over-bed table. Empty it into the sink.
10. Determine if a new mug is needed.
11. Use the scoop to fill the mug with ice (Fig. 32-8). Do not let the scoop touch the mug, lid, or straw.
12. Place the ice scoop in the scoop holder or on a clean towel.
13. Fill the mug with water. Get water from the sink or the water pitcher on the cart.
14. Place the mug on the over-bed table. Make sure the mug is within the person's reach.

POST-PROCEDURE

15. Provide for comfort. (See the inside of the back cover.)
16. Place the call light and other needed items within reach.
17. Complete a safety check of the room. (See the inside of the back cover.)
18. Practice hand hygiene.
19. Repeats steps 5 through 18 for each person.

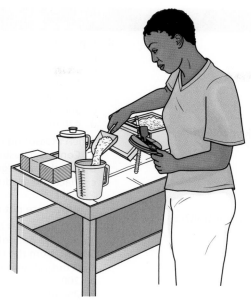

FIGURE 32-8 Providing drinking water.

FOCUS ON **PRIDE**

The Person, Family, and Yourself

Personal and Professional Responsibility

An *attentive* person is careful, alert, and thorough. These qualities are important when assisting with fluid needs. Follow each person's fluid order. Measure and record I&O correctly. Watch for signs and symptoms of dehydration and fluid overload. Report problems at once.

Rights and Respect

Patients and residents may complain about orders and treatments. For example, a resident does not like thickened liquids. Or a patient has an order to encourage fluids. The person is tired of being reminded to drink. Do not ignore complaints. They communicate needs. Listen and show respect.

Independence and Social Interaction

Personal choice promotes independence. Ask about the person's preferences. Drink choice, straw use, the amount of ice in drinks, and cream or sugar in coffee are examples.

Delegation and Teamwork

Some skills require math. Measuring I&O is an example. Math is hard for some persons. You may need extra practice. Tell your instructor. On the job, ask the nurse if you have a question. Do not be embarrassed to ask for help.

Ethics and Laws

The following is a real example of a court case involving fluid needs.

Mr. Phillip Caruso was admitted to a nursing center on January 22 after about 5 weeks of hospital care. On January 23, the doctor found him to be in stable condition. He showed signs of adequate hydration and responded to the doctor's commands.

The nursing center "did not keep a chart of Phillip's intake or output of fluids." According to the nurses, Mr. Caruso received:

- *3 meals a day.*
- *3 snacks [a day] with juice or milk.*
- *Drugs 4 times a day. He was given 4 oz of water with the drugs.*
- *Offers of something to drink every 2 hours during the night.*

Seven days later (January 29), Mr. Caruso was taken to the hospital. The emergency room doctor diagnosed severe dehydration. He was weak, was confused, had tremors, and had dry skin with poor turgor. In the hospital, Mr. Caruso was treated with IV fluids and a catheter and for a urinary tract infection caused by the catheter.

Mr. Caruso returned to the nursing center on February 19. He died on May 14.

His family sued and charged the nursing center with negligence, abuse, and neglect for failing to give Mr. Caruso enough water. They claimed that the dehydration led to declines in his physical and mental condition.

The jury found in favor of the family. The jury awarded the family $195,000 and attorney fees. The nursing center appealed the case. Because of a legal technicality, a judge ordered a new trial.

(I. Caruso v. Pine Manor Nursing Center, Ill., 1989.)

You can do your part to promote good fluid intake. Follow the person's care plan. Carefully record intake and output as ordered. Report and record concerns about the person's intake.

FOCUS ON **PRIDE**: *Application*

A person with an order to restrict fluids complains of thirst. How can you meet the person's needs?

REVIEW QUESTIONS

Circle the BEST answer.

1 Which is a source of fluid loss?
   a Edema
   b Hydration
   c Perspiration
   d IV therapy

2 A person with diarrhea has scant, dark yellow urine. This is a sign of
   a Normal hydration
   b Edema
   c Infection
   d Dehydration

3 A person has edema. Which should you question?
   a Encourage fluids.
   b Restrict fluids.
   c Provide frequent oral hygiene.
   d Monitor I&O.

4 A person is NPO. You should
   a Provide a variety of fluids
   b Remove the water mug from the room
   c Offer fluids in small amounts and in small containers
   d Remove oral hygiene equipment from the room

5 Which are counted as fluid intake?
   a Broths and ice cream
   b Sauces and melted cheese
   c Thick stews and mashed potatoes
   d Butter and syrup

6 A person drank all of an 8-oz carton of milk. How many mL of fluid would you chart on the I&O record?
   a 8 mL
   b 60 mL
   c 120 mL
   d 240 mL

7 A person drank ½ (one-half) of a 4-oz cup of juice. How many mL of fluid would you chart on the I&O record?
   a 2 mL
   b 4 mL
   c 60 mL
   d 120 mL

8 A person was served 240 mL of coffee and 120 mL of juice. You measure 50 mL of coffee and 60 mL of juice left. What do you chart for intake on the I&O record?
   a 110 mL
   b 250 mL
   c 360 mL
   d 470 mL

9 When measuring output
   a Convert measurements to ounces
   b Use the same graduate you used for intake
   c Place the graduate on a flat surface and read it at eye level
   d Gloves are not needed

10 During your shift a patient vomited twice—125 mL and 75 mL. The patient had diarrhea once—50 mL. You empty 500 mL from the urine drainage bag. What is the total shift output amount?
   a 200 mL
   b 250 mL
   c 500 mL
   d 750 mL

11 Before providing fresh drinking water, you need to know the person's
   a Food intake
   b Fluid orders
   c Diet
   d Preferred beverages

12 Which prevents contamination when passing drinking water?
   a Labeling the mug with the person's name
   b Keeping the ice chest open when not in use
   c Laying the ice scoop in the ice container
   d Touching the mug with the ice scoop

Answers to Chapter 32 questions are on p. 902.

FOCUS ON PRACTICE

Problem Solving

One patient is being treated for dehydration. Another has edema. How is your care of both similar? How is it different?

Nutritional Support and IV Therapy

OBJECTIVES

- Define the key terms and key abbreviations in this chapter.
- Identify the reasons for nutritional support and IV therapy.
- Explain how tube feedings are given.
- Describe scheduled and continuous feedings.
- Explain how to prevent aspiration.
- Describe the comfort measures for the person with a feeding tube.
- Describe parenteral nutrition.
- Describe the IV therapy sites.

- Identify the equipment used in IV therapy.
- Describe how to assist with the IV flow rate.
- Identify the safety measures for IV therapy.
- Identify the observations to report during nutritional support or IV therapy.
- Explain how to assist with nutritional support and IV therapy.
- Explain how to promote PRIDE in the person, the family, and yourself.

KEY TERMS

aspiration Breathing fluid, food, vomitus, or an object into the lungs

enteral nutrition Giving nutrients into the gastro-intestinal (GI) tract *(enteral)* through a feeding tube

flow rate The number of drops per minute (gtt/min) or milliliters per hour (mL/hr)

gastrostomy tube A feeding tube inserted through a surgically created opening *(stomy)* in the stomach *(gastro)*

gavage The process of giving a tube feeding

intravenous (IV) therapy Giving fluids through a needle or catheter inserted into a vein; IV and IV infusion

jejunostomy tube A feeding tube inserted into a surgically created opening *(stomy)* in the *jejunum* of the small intestine

naso-enteral tube A feeding tube inserted through the nose *(naso)* into the small bowel *(enteral)*

naso-gastric (NG) tube A feeding tube inserted through the nose *(naso)* into the stomach *(gastro)*

parenteral nutrition Giving nutrients through a catheter inserted into a vein; *para* means beyond; *enteral* relates to the bowel

percutaneous endoscopic gastrostomy (PEG) tube A feeding tube inserted into the stomach *(gastro)* through a small incision *(stomy)* made through *(per)* the skin *(cutaneous);* a lighted instrument *(scope)* is used to see inside a body cavity or organ *(endo)*

regurgitation The backward flow of stomach contents into the mouth

KEY ABBREVIATIONS

GI	Gastro-intestinal	NG	Naso-gastric
gtt	Drops	NPO	Nothing by mouth
gtt/min	Drops per minute	oz	Ounce
IV	Intravenous	PEG	Percutaneous endoscopic gastrostomy
mL	Milliliter	TPN	Total parenteral nutrition
mL/hr	Milliliters per hour		

Many persons cannot eat or drink because of illness, surgery, or injury. They may have chewing, swallowing, or digestion problems. Some persons have poor appetite or refuse to eat or drink. Others cannot eat enough to meet their nutritional needs. Nutritional support or intravenous (IV) therapy may be ordered to meet food and fluid needs.

See *Delegation Guidelines: Nutritional Support and IV Therapy*.

DELEGATION GUIDELINES
Nutritional Support and IV Therapy

The nurse is responsible for tasks involving nutritional support and IV therapy. Your state and agency may allow you to assist with some of the care measures in this chapter. Before doing so, make sure that:
- Your state allows you to perform the task.
- The task is in your job description (Chapter 3).
- You have the necessary education and training.
- The agency has determined that you are competent to perform the task safely.
- You know how to use the supplies and equipment.
- You review the procedure with the delegating nurse.
- The delegating nurse is available to answer questions and to guide and assist you as needed.
- An RN (registered nurse) has identified and labeled all tubes, catheters, and needles.

ENTERAL NUTRITION

Some persons cannot or will not ingest food. Or food cannot pass through the digestive system normally. Some persons have high nutritional needs. Poor nutrition can result. Common causes are:
- Cancer, especially cancers of the head, neck, and esophagus
- Trauma to the face, mouth, head, or neck
- Coma (Chapter 14)
- Chewing problems
- *Dysphagia* (difficulty swallowing)
- Dementia (Chapter 54)
- Eating disorders (Chapter 53)
- Nervous system disorders (Chapter 49)
- Prolonged vomiting or diarrhea
- Major burns, major trauma, or surgery
- Acquired immunodeficiency syndrome (AIDS) (Chapter 48)
- Delayed stomach emptying (*gastroparesis*) or bowel obstruction (blockage)
- Illnesses and disorders affecting eating and nutrition

Enteral nutrition is giving nutrients into the gastro-intestinal (GI) tract (*enteral*) through a feeding tube. Receiving nutrients through a tube (tube feeding) replaces or supplements (adds to) normal feeding.

Types of Feeding Tubes
These feeding tubes are common.
- *Naso-gastric (NG) tube.* A feeding tube is inserted through the nose (*naso*) into the stomach (*gastro*) (Fig. 33-1). A doctor or an RN inserts the tube.
- *Naso-enteral tube.* A feeding tube is inserted through the nose (*naso*) into the small bowel (*enteral*) (Fig. 33-2). A doctor or RN inserts the tube.
- *Gastrostomy tube.* A feeding tube is inserted through a surgically created opening (*stomy*) in the stomach (*gastro*). It is also called a G-tube. See Figure 33-3. A doctor inserts the tube.
- *Jejunostomy tube.* A feeding tube is inserted into a surgically created opening (*stomy*) in the *jejunum* of the small intestine. It is also called a J-tube. See Figure 33-4.
- *Percutaneous endoscopic gastrostomy (PEG) tube.* A feeding tube is inserted into the stomach (*gastro*) through a small incision (*stomy*) made through (*per*) the skin (*cutaneous*). A lighted instrument (*scope*) is used to see inside a body cavity or organ (*endo*). See Figure 33-5. A doctor inserts the tube.

NG and naso-enteral tubes are used for short-term nutritional support—usually less than 6 weeks. Gastrostomy, jejunostomy, and PEG tubes are used for long-term nutritional support—usually more than 6 weeks.

Formulas
The doctor orders the type of formula, the amount to give, and when to give tube feedings. Most formulas contain proteins, carbohydrates, fats, vitamins, and minerals. Commercial formulas are common.

See *Promoting Safety and Comfort: Formulas*.

PROMOTING SAFETY AND COMFORT
Formulas

Safety
Like food, microbes can grow in formula and cause illness if not stored properly. Un-opened formula is stored at room temperature. Open, un-used formula is stored in the refrigerator. The formula must be covered and labeled with the date and time. The formula is discarded after 24 hours.

Comfort
Cold fluids can cause cramping. Formula is given at room temperature. Refrigerated formula is warmed to room temperature. The manufacturer's instructions are followed for warming cold formula. The nurse may have you set the formula out at room temperature for 30 minutes before the feeding. Do not use a microwave or stove to warm formula.

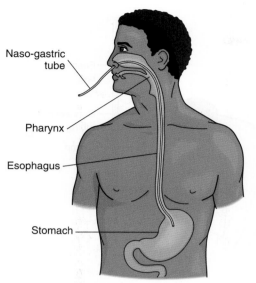

FIGURE 33-1 A naso-gastric (NG) tube is inserted through the nose and esophagus and into the stomach.

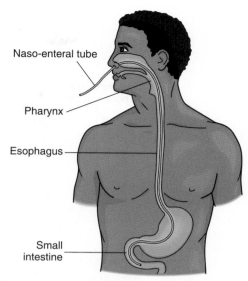

FIGURE 33-2 A naso-enteral tube is inserted through the nose and into the small intestine.

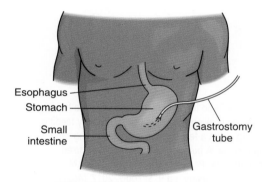

FIGURE 33-3 A gastrostomy tube.

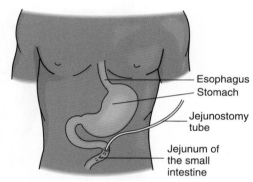

FIGURE 33-4 A jejunostomy tube.

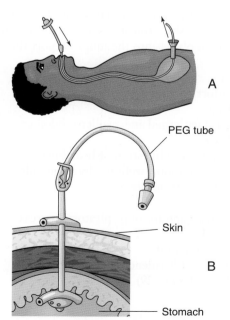

FIGURE 33-5 A, A percutaneous endoscopic gastrostomy (PEG) tube is inserted. **B,** PEG tube in place.

Feeding Methods

Gavage is the process of giving a tube feeding. Tube feedings can be given in 3 ways (Fig. 33-6, p. 506).

- *Syringe feeding* (Fig. 33-6, *A*)—Formula is poured into a syringe. The syringe attaches to the feeding tube. The height of the syringe controls how fast the formula flows.
- *Gravity feeding* (Fig. 33-6, *B*)—Formula is in a feeding bag. Tubing connects the bag to the feeding tube. The bag hangs on a pole. A clamp on the tubing and the height of the bag control how fast the formula flows.
- *Pump feeding* (Fig. 33-6, *C*)—A feeding pump is used. Formula is pumped from the bag, through connecting tubing, and into the feeding tube. Formula drips into the feeding tube at a certain rate.

After a feeding, the nurse removes the syringe or connecting tubing. The nurse caps or plugs the end of the feeding tube. This prevents air from entering the tube and fluid from leaking out.

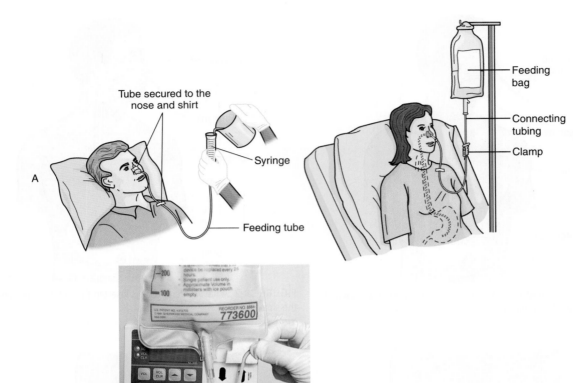

FIGURE 33-6 Tube feeding methods. **A,** Syringe feeding. A tube feeding is given with a syringe. **B,** Gravity feeding. Formula drips from a feeding bag into the feeding tube. **C,** Pump feeding. A pump for enteral feeding is used. (C, From Potter PA, Perry AG, Stockert PA, Hall AM: *Fundamentals of nursing,* ed 9, St Louis, 2017, Mosby.)

Feeding Times

Tube feedings are given at certain times. Or they are given over a 24-hour period.

Scheduled feedings (intermittent feedings) are given at certain times. (*Intermittent* means to start, stop, and then start again.) Between 3 and 8 feedings are given each day. Usually 8 to 12 ounces (oz) (240 to 360 milliliters [mL]) are given over about 30 minutes or less for an adult. The frequency, amount, and time are like a normal eating pattern.

Continuous feedings are usually given over 24 hours. A feeding pump is used (see Fig. 33-6, *C*). The person receives a certain amount each hour. A pump alarm sounds if something is wrong. When you hear an alarm, tell the nurse.

See *Teamwork and Time Management: Feeding Times.*

TEAMWORK AND TIME MANAGEMENT

Feeding Times

The nurse and manufacturer's instructions direct how long formula can hang. Note the time that a feeding started. Notify the nurse when the time limit is near. For example, a feeding started at 0800. It can hang for 8 hours (until 1600). At 1530 or 1545, tell the nurse how much time is left. Also report the amount of formula left.

Observations

Diarrhea, constipation, delayed stomach emptying, and aspiration are risks. *Aspiration* is breathing fluid, food, vomitus, or an object into the lungs. **Report the following at once.**

- Nausea
- Discomfort during the feeding
- Vomiting
- Distended (enlarged and swollen) abdomen
- Coughing
- Complaints of indigestion or heartburn
- Redness, irritation, swelling, drainage, odor, or pain at the tube's insertion site
- Fever
- Signs and symptoms of respiratory distress (Chapter 44)
- Increased pulse rate
- Complaints of flatulence (Chapter 29)
- Diarrhea (Chapter 29)

Regurgitation and Aspiration

Aspiration is a major risk from tube feedings. It can cause pneumonia and death. Aspiration can occur:

- *During insertion.* NG tubes and naso-enteral tubes are passed through the nose into the esophagus and then into the stomach or small intestine. The tube can slip into the airway. An x-ray is taken after insertion to check tube placement.
- *From the tube moving out of place.* Coughing, sneezing, vomiting, suctioning (the process of withdrawing or sucking up fluids), and poor positioning are common causes. A tube can move from the stomach or intestines into the esophagus and then into the airway. The RN checks tube placement before every scheduled tube feeding. With continuous feedings, the RN checks tube placement every 4 hours. The RN attaches a syringe to the tube. GI secretions are withdrawn through the syringe. Then the pH of the secretions is measured. *You never check feeding tube placement.*
- *From regurgitation.* *Regurgitation* is the backward flow of stomach contents into the mouth. Delayed stomach emptying and over-feeding are common causes.

Preventing Regurgitation and Aspiration. To help prevent regurgitation and aspiration:

- Position the person in Fowler's or semi-Fowler's position during feedings. Follow the care plan and the nurse's directions.
- Maintain Fowler's or semi-Fowler's position after feedings. Do so for 1 to 2 hours after the feeding or at all times. This allows formula to move through the GI tract. Follow the care plan and the nurse's directions.
- Avoid the left side-lying position. It prevents the stomach from emptying into the small intestine.

During digestion, food slowly passes from the stomach into the small intestine. The stomach handles larger amounts of food than the small intestine. With intestinal tubes, feedings are given at a slow rate. The risk of regurgitation is less with intestinal tubes than with NG or gastrostomy tubes.

Persons with NG or gastrostomy tubes are at high risk for regurgitation. Before a feeding, the nurse checks that the stomach is emptying normally. The nurse aspirates (pulls into a syringe) stomach contents and measures the amount. This is called *residual*. *Residual* means remaining (what remains). Depending on the amount, the nurse decides to give or delay the feeding. The intent is to prevent aspiration from regurgitation caused by over-feeding.

See *Focus on Children and Older Persons: Preventing Regurgitation and Aspiration.*

FOCUS ON CHILDREN AND OLDER PERSONS

Preventing Regurgitation and Aspiration

Older Persons
Digestion slows with aging. Stomach emptying also slows. Older persons are at risk for regurgitation and aspiration. Less formula and longer feeding times prevent over-feeding.

Comfort Measures

Some persons with feeding tubes are not allowed to eat or drink. The abbreviation *NPO* means nothing by mouth. Dry mouth, dry lips, and sore throat cause discomfort. Sometimes hard candy or gum is allowed. These measures are common every 2 hours while the person is awake.

- Oral hygiene
- Lubricant for the lips
- Mouth rinses

Feeding tubes in the nose can irritate and cause pressure on the nose. They can change the shape of the nostrils or cause pressure injuries. These measures are common.

- Clean the nose and nostrils every 4 to 8 hours.
- Secure the tube to the nose (Fig. 33-7). Use tape or a tube holder. Tube holders have foam cushions that prevent pressure on the nose. Re-taping is not needed. Re-taping irritates the nose.
- Secure the tube to the person's garment at the shoulder area (see Fig. 33-6, *A*). This prevents the tube from pulling or dangling. Both can cause pressure on the nose. Do 1 of the following according to agency policy.
  - Loop a rubber band around the tube. Then pin the rubber band to the garment with a safety pin.
  - Tape the tube to the garment.

Assisting With Tube Feedings

The nurse may ask you to assist with tube feedings. With more training, some states and agencies allow nursing assistants to give tube feedings and remove NG tubes. *Remember, you never insert feeding tubes, check their placement, or check residual stomach contents. They are the RN's responsibility.*

See *Delegation Guidelines: Assisting With Tube Feedings,* p. 508.

See *Promoting Safety and Comfort: Assisting With Tube Feedings,* p. 508.

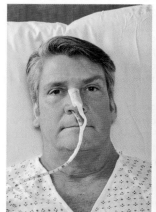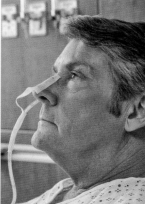

FIGURE 33-7 The feeding tube is secured to the nose. (From Perry AG, Potter PA, Ostendorf WR: *Clinical nursing skills & techniques,* ed 10, St Louis, 2022, Elsevier.)

DELEGATION GUIDELINES

Assisting With Tube Feedings

You may be asked to assist with tube feedings. In some states and agencies, giving tube feedings and removing NG tubes can be delegated to nursing assistants. If a task is delegated to you, make sure that the conditions in *Delegation Guidelines: Nutritional Support and IV Therapy* (p. 504) are met. If those conditions are met, you need this information from the nurse and the care plan.

- That the RN has checked tube placement and residual stomach contents
- The type of tube—NG, naso-enteral, gastrostomy, jejunostomy, or PEG
- What feeding method to use—syringe, gravity, or pump feeding
- What size syringe to use—usually 30 or 60 mL for an adult
- How to position the person for the feeding—Fowler's or semi-Fowler's
- How to position the person after the feeding—Fowler's or semi-Fowler's
- What formula to use
- How much formula to give
- How high to raise the syringe or hang the feeding bag (usually 18 to 24 inches above the stomach or intestines)
- The amount of flushing solution to use—usually 30 to 60 mL (1 to 2 oz) of water for an adult
- When to flush the feeding tube
- How fast to give the feeding if using a syringe—usually over 30 minutes or less
- The flow rate (in drops per minute) for a gravity feeding with a feeding bag (p. 512)
- The flow rate (in milliliters per hour) if a feeding pump is used (p. 512)
- If ice is kept around the bag for a continuous feeding
- If you are to remove an NG tube, when to remove the tube
- What observations to report and record
- When to report observations
- What patient or resident concerns to report at once

PROMOTING SAFETY AND COMFORT

Assisting With Tube Feedings

Safety

Besides a feeding tube, the person may have other tubes. An IV, a breathing tube (Chapter 45), and drainage tubes (Chapter 40) are examples. *Formula must enter only the feeding tube.* Otherwise, the person can die. The nurse labels each tube and its purpose. These safety measures are performed before a tube feeding is given.

- The room light is turned on. This is done even if the person is sleeping.
- The nurse checks and inspects the feeding tube and label.
- The nurse checks tube placement and residual.
- The feeding tube is traced back to the insertion site. For example, if the person has an NG tube, the tube ends at the nose. If the person has a gastrostomy tube, the tube ends at the abdomen. If you do not end at the correct place, do not give the tube feeding. Ask the nurse for help.

  Nasal secretions are body fluids. So is drainage at an ostomy site. Follow Standard Precautions. Follow the Bloodborne Pathogen Standard if blood is present. Follow the rules of hand hygiene and the guidelines for glove use in Chapters 17 and 18.

  In nursing centers, follow agency policies and procedures for using Enhanced Barrier Precautions when the person has an indwelling medical device. Feeding tubes are indwelling medical devices. High-contact tasks and tasks involving the feeding tube require routine gown and glove use. See Chapter 18.

  Remind visitors to call for a nurse if any tube becomes disconnected. They could connect the wrong tubes together.

PARENTERAL NUTRITION

Parenteral nutrition is giving nutrients through a catheter inserted into a vein (Fig. 33-8). (*Para* means beyond. *Enteral* relates to the bowel.) A *catheter* is a tube used to drain or inject *(infuse)* fluid. In parenteral nutrition, a nutrient solution is *infused*—put into the body. The solution is given directly into the bloodstream. Nutrients do not enter the GI tract. Parenteral nutrition is often called *total parenteral nutrition (TPN)* or *hyperalimentation*. (*Hyper* means high or excessive. *Alimentation* means nourishment.)

The solution contains water, proteins, carbohydrates, vitamins, and minerals. It drips through a catheter inserted into a large vein. TPN is used when the person cannot receive oral or enteral feedings. Or it is used when oral or enteral feedings are not enough to meet nutrition needs.

Common reasons for TPN include:
- Disease, injury, or surgery to the GI tract
- Severe trauma, infection, or burns
- NPO for more than 5 to 7 days
- GI side effects from cancer treatments (Chapter 48)
- Prolonged coma
- Prolonged *anorexia* (loss of appetite)

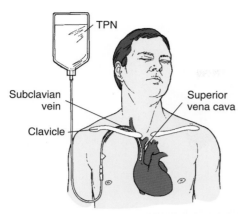

FIGURE 33-8 Parenteral nutrition. (From *Mosby's dictionary of medicine, nursing, and health professions*, ed 11, St Louis, 2022, Elsevier.)

Observations

TPN risks include infection, fluid imbalances, and blood sugar imbalances. Report the following to the nurse at once.
* Fever, chills, and other signs and symptoms of infection (Chapter 17)
* Signs and symptoms of sugar imbalances (see "Diabetes" in Chapter 51)
* Chest pain
* Difficulty breathing or shortness of breath
* Cough
* Nausea and vomiting
* Diarrhea
* Thirst
* Rapid heart rate or an irregular heartbeat
* Weakness or fatigue
* Sweating
* *Pallor* (pale skin)
* Trembling
* Confusion or behavior changes

Assisting With TPN

The nurse is responsible for all aspects of TPN. To assist, carefully observe the person. Also assist with basic needs and activities of daily living. The person may be NPO. Provide frequent oral hygiene, lubricant to the lips, and mouth rinses as the nurse and care plan direct. Also follow other aspects of the person's care plan. Many aspects of IV therapy apply to TPN.

IV THERAPY

Intravenous (IV) therapy (IV, IV infusion) is giving fluids through a needle or catheter inserted into a vein (Fig. 33-9). Fluid flows directly into the bloodstream.

IV therapy is ordered to:
* Provide fluids.
* Replace minerals and vitamins lost from illness or injury.
* Provide sugar for energy.
* Give drugs and blood.

RNs are responsible for IV therapy. They start and maintain the infusion as ordered. RNs also give IV drugs and administer blood. State laws vary about your role and that of LPNs/LVNs in IV therapy. See "Assisting With IV Therapy" on p. 513.

IV Equipment

The basic equipment used in IV therapy is shown in Figure 33-9.
* The fluid to be infused is in a plastic bag—*IV bag*.
* A needle is inserted into a vein. Usually, the needle retracts (is removed) and a small, flexible tube called a *catheter (cannula)* is left in the vein (*venous catheter, intravenous cannula*). See Figure 33-10 (p. 510).
* *Infusion tubing (IV tube)* connects the catheter (cannula) to the IV bag.
  * Fluid drips from the bag into a *drip chamber.*
  * A *clamp* is used to start, stop, or regulate (change) how fast the fluid flows (flow rate).
* The IV bag hangs from an *IV pole (IV standard)* or ceiling hook.

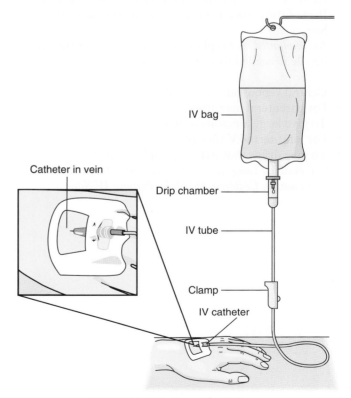

FIGURE 33-9 Equipment for IV therapy.

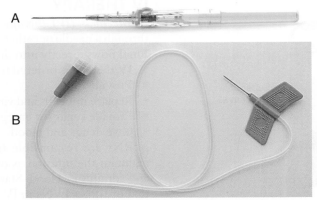

FIGURE 33-10 A, Intravenous catheter. **B,** Butterfly needle. (Courtesy and © Becton, Dickinson and Company.)

IV Sites

Peripheral and central venous sites are used. *Peripheral IV sites* are away from the center of the body. For adults, the back of the hand and inner forearm are useful sites (Fig. 33-11). *Central venous sites* are close to the heart. A catheter is threaded into a vein near the heart. The catheter is called a *central venous catheter* or a *central line.*

- A *peripherally inserted central catheter (PICC)* begins in a large peripheral vein in the upper arm. The catheter tip ends at the heart. See Figure 33-12, *A.*
- A *tunneled catheter* begins in a vein in the neck or chest. It is passed under the skin and ends at the heart. Part of the catheter remains outside the skin for use. See Figure 33-12, *B.*
- An *implanted port* is placed under the skin. A special needle is needed to access (use) the device. See Figure 33-12, *C.*

Central venous sites are used:
- For parenteral nutrition
- To give large amounts of fluid
- For long-term IV therapy
- To give drugs that irritate peripheral veins.
  See *Focus on Long-Term Care and Home Care: IV Sites.*
  See *Focus on Children and Older Persons: IV Sites.*

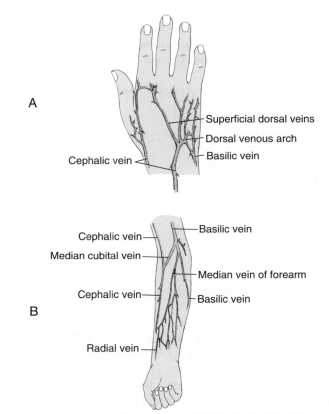

FIGURE 33-11 Peripheral IV sites. **A,** Back of the hand. **B,** Inner forearm. (From Potter PA, Perry AG, Stockert PA, Hall AM: *Fundamentals of nursing,* ed 10, St Louis, 2021, Elsevier.)

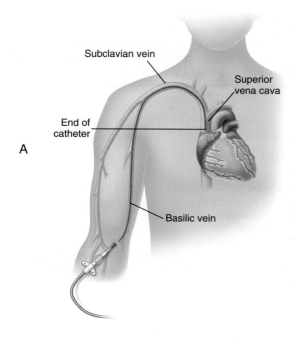

A

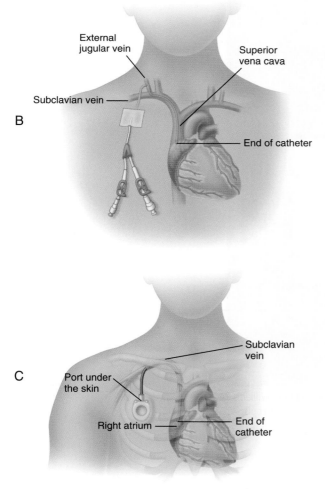

B

C

> ## FOCUS ON **LONG-TERM CARE AND HOME CARE**
> ### *IV Sites*
> #### Home Care
> Patients can receive IV therapy at home. They often have central venous catheters. The RN teaches the patient and family about giving drugs and managing the catheter.

> ## FOCUS ON **CHILDREN AND OLDER PERSONS**
> ### *IV Sites*
> #### Children
> See Figure 33-13 for the IV sites in children. The hand, wrist, and inner arm sites are commonly used. The site selected depends on:
> - The child's age. Scalp veins are sometimes used in infants. For a toddler, foot veins are avoided. IVs in foot veins prevent walking.
> - The amount and kind of fluid ordered.
> - How long the IV will be needed.

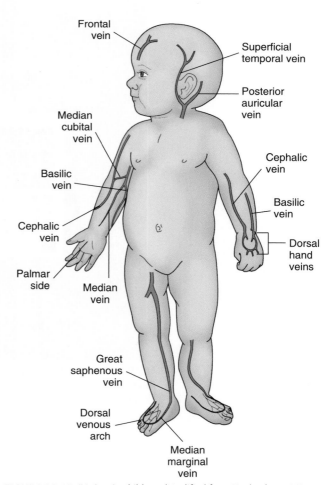

FIGURE 33-12 Central venous catheters. **A,** Peripherally inserted central catheter (PICC). **B,** Tunneled catheter. **C,** Implanted port. The device is under the skin. (Modified from Ignatavicious DD, Workman ML, Rebar C: *Medical-surgical nursing: patient-centered collaborative care,* ed 9, St Louis, 2018, Elsevier.)

FIGURE 33-13 IV sites in children. (Modified from Hockenberry MJ, Wilson D, Rodgers CC: *Wong's nursing care of infants and children,* ed 11, St Louis, 2019, Elsevier.)

Flow Rate

The doctor orders the amount of fluid to give *(infuse)* and the amount of time to give it in. With this information, the RN figures the flow rate. The *flow rate* is the number of drops per minute (gtt/min) or milliliters per hour (mL/hr). The abbreviation *gtt* (from the Latin word *guttae*) means drops.

An electronic pump is often used (Fig. 33-14). The flow rate is displayed in mL/hr. An alarm sounds if something is wrong. Tell the nurse at once if you hear an alarm. If a pump is not used, the RN sets the clamp for the flow rate. *Never adjust any controls on IV pumps or change the position of the clamp.*

See *Teamwork and Time Management: Flow Rate.*
See *Promoting Safety and Comfort: Flow Rate.*
See *Focus on Math: Flow Rate.*

TEAMWORK AND TIME MANAGEMENT

Flow Rate

Patients and residents cared for by you and other staff may have IVs. When near the person or walking past the person's room, make sure the IV is dripping. Also check the amount of fluid in the bag. Report any problems to a nurse at once.

PROMOTING SAFETY AND COMFORT

Flow Rate

Safety
The person can suffer serious harm if the flow rate is too fast or too slow. Flow rate changes can occur from:
- Position changes
- Kinked tubes
- Lying on the tube

Never change the position of the clamp or adjust any controls on infusion pumps. Tell the nurse at once about a problem with the flow rate.

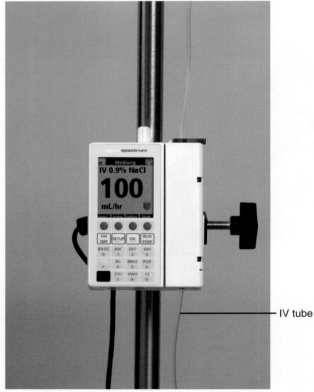

FIGURE 33-14 Electronic IV pump. (Modified from Williams PA: *Fundamental concepts and skills for nursing,* ed 6, St Louis, 2022, Elsevier.)

FOCUS ON MATH

Flow Rate

Counting Drops per Minute

You can check the flow rate when a pump is not used. The nurse tells you the number of drops per minute (gtt/min). Use a watch. Count the number of drops that fall in the drip chamber in 1 minute (60 seconds). See Figure 33-15. Tell the nurse at once if:

- No fluid is dripping.
- The rate is too fast or too slow.
- The bag is empty or close to being empty.

For example: The nurse tells you the number of drops per minute is to be 25 gtt/min. You count 31 gtt/min.

> *31 gtt/min (rate counted) is greater than 25 gtt/min (correct rate).*
> *The rate is too fast. You tell the nurse.*

Time Tape

A *time tape* tracks fluid given over a period of time (Fig. 33-16). The nurse marks the tape with times. If the rate is correct, the fluid level is at the nurse's mark on the tape at the correct time. To check the rate, compare the fluid level with the time on the tape.

- If the fluid is above the time line, the flow is too slow. Not enough fluid has been given.
- If the fluid is below the time line, the flow is too fast. Too much fluid has been given.

Tell the nurse at once if too little or too much fluid has been given.

For example, the doctor orders 1000 mL of fluid over 10 hours. The nurse calculates the flow rate and marks the time tape (see Fig. 33-16). The nurse starts the infusion at 0700 (7:00 AM). The nurse checks the fluid level for the first hour. You are asked to check the fluid level at 0900 (9:00 AM). At 0900, the fluid level is as shown in Figure 33-16. The fluid level is below the 0900 line. The flow is too fast. You tell the nurse.

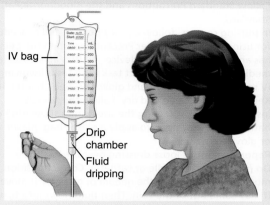

FIGURE 33-15 Counting drops per minute.

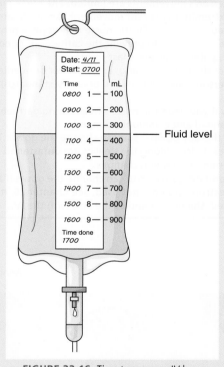

FIGURE 33-16 Time tape on an IV bag.

Assisting With IV Therapy

You help meet the safety, hygiene, and activity needs of persons with IVs. Follow the safety measures in Box 33-1 (p. 514). Report any sign or symptom listed in Box 33-1 at once.

You never start or maintain IV therapy. Nor do you regulate the flow rate or change IV bags. You never give blood or IV drugs.

With more training, your state and agency may allow you to discontinue (remove) a peripheral IV.

See *Focus on Communication: Assisting With IV Therapy,* p. 515.

See *Delegation Guidelines: Assisting With IV Therapy,* p. 515.

BOX 33-1	IV Therapy

Safety Measures

- Follow Standard Precautions and the Bloodborne Pathogen Standard.
- In nursing centers, follow agency policies and procedures for using Enhanced Barrier Precautions when the person has an indwelling medical device. An IV is an indwelling medical device. High-contact tasks and tasks involving the IV require routine gown and glove use. See Chapter 18.
- Keep the IV site clean and dry. Follow the nurse's instructions for protecting the site during showering or bathing. You may need to apply a plastic bag, plastic wrap, or glove to the site.
- Report a moist or loose dressing over the IV site.
- Do not move the needle or catheter. Correct position must be maintained. If the needle or catheter is moved, it may come out of the vein. Then fluid flows into tissues (*infiltration*). Or the flow stops.
- Follow the safety measures for restraints (Chapter 16) when the person's movements are limited. The nurse may splint the extremity to prevent movement. An armboard may be used (Fig. 33-17). Or the nurse may apply a protective device (Fig. 33-18) to prevent the catheter or needle from moving. Restraints are a last resort.
- Protect the IV bag, tubing, and catheter or needle when the person walks. Portable IV poles (IV standards) are used (Fig. 33-19).
- Know if you need the nurse's help during garment changes. Plan ahead and communicate needs.
  - IV therapy gown—You can change the gown. The snaps (ties, Velcro) along the sleeves are unfastened and fastened for gown changes.
  - Standard gown—You can change the gown if an electronic pump is not used. See Chapter 26. If a pump is used, the nurse handles the arm with the IV.

Safety Measures—cont'd

- Plan moving and transfer procedures to avoid pulling on the IV site. Allow enough slack in the tubing. Move the IV pole (IV standard) as needed. The catheter or needle can move from pressure on the tube.
- Tell the nurse if an IV pump alarm sounds. This may mean:
  - There is air in the tubing.
  - The infusion is done.
  - The pump's battery is low.
  - Fluid flow is blocked. Kinks in the tubing and closed clamps are common reasons.

Signs and Symptoms of Complications

- Report the following at once.
  - Local—at the IV site
    - Bleeding
    - Blood backing up into the IV tube
    - Puffiness or swelling
    - Pale or reddened skin
    - Complaints of pain at or above the IV site
    - Hot or cold skin near the site
  - Systemic—involving the whole body
    - *Fever* (elevated body temperature)
    - Itching
    - Changes in blood pressure: increase or decrease
    - Pulse rate greater than 100 beats per minute
    - Irregular pulse
    - *Cyanosis* (bluish color)
    - Confusion or changes in mental function
    - Loss of consciousness
    - Difficulty breathing or shortness of breath
    - Decreasing or no urine output
    - Chest pain
    - Nausea

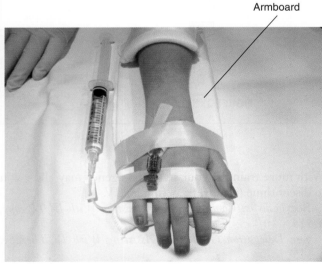

Armboard

FIGURE 33-17   An armboard prevents movement at an IV site. (Modified from Roberts JR, Custalow CB, Thomsen TW: *Roberts and Hedges' clinical procedures in emergency medicine and acute care*, ed 7, Philadelphia, 2019, Elsevier.)

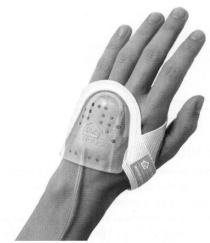

FIGURE 33-18   I.V. House Protective Device. (Courtesy I.V. House, St Louis, Mo.)

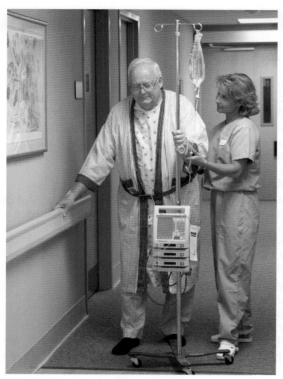

FIGURE 33-19 A person walking with an IV using a portable IV pole.

FOCUS ON COMMUNICATION

Assisting With IV Therapy

For an IV in the arm, arm position can affect fluid flow. You may need to remind the person:
- To position the arm a certain way
- About position limits
  For example, a bent arm causes the fluid flow to stop. You can say: "Please keep your arm straight. The fluid will not flow through your IV when your arm is bent."

DELEGATION GUIDELINES

Assisting With IV Therapy

The nurse is responsible for IV therapy. If discontinuing (removing) a peripheral IV is delegated to you, make sure that the conditions in *Delegation Guidelines: Nutritional Support and IV Therapy* (p. 504) are met. If those conditions are met, you need this information from the nurse and the care plan.
- When to discontinue the IV
- If the person has 2 or more IVs, which IV to discontinue
- What supplies to use
- What observations to report and record (see Box 33-1)
- When to report observations
- What patient or resident concerns to report at once

FOCUS ON **PRIDE**

The Person, Family, and Yourself

Personal and Professional Responsibility

An IV in the arm can limit hand and arm movement. You may need to assist with hygiene, grooming, food and fluid, or activity needs. Assist only to the extent needed. The person should do as much as safely possible.

Rights and Respect

Persons needing nutritional support or IV therapy may be very ill. Sometimes decisions are made to stop therapy and allow the person to die. The person or family makes the decision after talking to the doctor. See Chapter 59. Show respect for the person and family and their decision.

Independence and Social Interaction

Some persons with feeding tubes are still able to eat. Others are not. Some tubes are temporary. Others are permanent.

Emotional and social changes can occur especially when enteral nutrition replaces all feeding and is permanent. The person may miss the taste of food and social contact during meals. Feelings of sadness, loss, dependence, and loneliness can occur. You can:
- Listen.
- Provide emotional support.
- Encourage social contact.
- Tell the nurse about any concerns.

Delegation and Teamwork

Before any task, you must know how to protect IVs. For example:
- A person with an IV needs a shower. You must keep the IV site dry.
- A person receiving IV therapy needs to move from the bed to the chair. You must plan the move to avoid pulling on the IV site.

Planning is an important part of safe care. Think through tasks carefully before performing them. Ask for help if you are not sure what to do.

Ethics and Laws

When you hear an IV pump alarm (sound), tell the nurse. Do so even if not assigned to the person. You do not adjust controls on IV pumps. Working within your role limits protects the person from harm and yourself from losing your ability to work as a nursing assistant.

FOCUS ON **PRIDE**: Application

Consider the emotional impact of 1 treatment in this chapter. Describe how the person might feel. How can you provide mental comfort?

REVIEW QUESTIONS

Circle the BEST answer.

1 Enteral nutrition
   a Requires an NG tube
   b Is given into a central venous site
   c Is given into the GI tract
   d Requires an IV

2 The process of giving a tube feeding is called
   a Gavage
   b Parenteral nutrition
   c Aspiration
   d Infusion

3 For a tube feeding, the person is positioned in
   a Fowler's or semi-Fowler's position
   b The left side-lying position
   c The right side-lying position
   d The supine position

4 Formula for a tube feeding is given
   a At body temperature
   b At room temperature
   c Hot
   d Cold

5 Continuous enteral feedings are given
   a With a syringe
   b By gravity
   c With an IV infusion pump
   d With an enteral feeding pump

6 The nurse checks feeding tube placement to prevent
   a Aspiration
   b Bleeding
   c Over-feeding
   d Cramping

7 Which position prevents regurgitation after a tube feeding?
   a Fowler's or semi-Fowler's position
   b The supine position
   c The left or right side-lying position
   d The prone position

8 The risk of regurgitation is greatest with
   a Naso-enteral tubes
   b Total parenteral nutrition
   c NG and gastrostomy tubes
   d A jejunostomy tube

9 A person with a feeding tube is NPO. Which should you question?
   a Provide oral hygiene.
   b Provide mouth rinses.
   c Give clear liquids.
   d Apply lubricant to the lips.

10 A person has an NG tube. To prevent nasal irritation
   a Clean the tube every 8 hours
   b Replace the tape on the nose every 4 hours
   c Remove the tube every 4 hours
   d Secure the tube to the person's gown

11 A nurse asks you to give a tube feeding. You do not know how. Which response is *best?*
   a "I think I can do it!"
   b "I have not been trained to give tube feedings."
   c "Can you ask someone else to do it?"
   d "I am busy, but I can do it in a little while."

12 A person is receiving TPN. You know that TPN
   a Involves a nutrient solution
   b Is given through a feeding tube
   c Can cause pressure injuries on the nose
   d Requires that the person be NPO

13 A person is receiving TPN. The person complains of chest pain and difficulty breathing. What should you do?
   a Put the person in Fowler's position.
   b Call for the nurse.
   c Stop the TPN.
   d Provide oral hygiene.

14 Which is a peripheral IV site?
   a A PICC
   b An implanted port
   c A central line
   d An IV on the back of the hand

15 The IV flow rate is
   a The number of gtt/hr
   b The amount of fluid given in 1 minute
   c The number of gtt/min or mL/hr
   d The amount of fluid in the IV bag

16 What is the *correct* way to check an IV flow rate?
   a Count the drops in 30 seconds. Multiply the number by 2.
   b Count the drops for 1 minute.
   c Check if the fluid is dripping.
   d Measure the amount of fluid.

17 You note that the IV bag is almost empty. You should
   a Clamp the IV tubing
   b Tell the nurse
   c Remove the IV
   d Adjust the flow rate

18 You see swelling around an IV site. You should
   a Tell the nurse
   b Move the IV catheter
   c Remove the IV
   d Clamp the IV tubing

Answers to Chapter 33 questions are on p. 902.

FOCUS ON **PRACTICE**

Problem Solving

You enter the room to check on a patient receiving a continuous tube feeding. The head of the bed is flat and the person says: "My mouth is dry." The feeding pump alarm begins to sound. What do you do first? What do you do next? What can you do within your role limits? What does the nurse need to do?

Vital Signs

OBJECTIVES

- Define the key terms and key abbreviations in this chapter.
- Explain why vital signs are measured.
- List the factors affecting vital signs.
- Identify the sites used to measure body temperature.
- Explain when to use and avoid each temperature site.
- Identify normal ranges at different temperature sites.
- Define fever and how it can differ in older persons.
- Explain how to use thermometers.
- Identify the pulse sites.

- Describe a normal pulse and normal respirations.
- Describe the practices for measuring blood pressure.
- Identify the normal ranges for blood pressure.
- Explain your role in measuring, reporting, and recording vital signs.
- Perform the procedures described in this chapter.
- Explain how to promote PRIDE in the person, the family, and yourself.

KEY TERMS

afebrile Without *(a)* a fever *(febrile)*

apical-radial pulse Taking the apical and radial pulses at the same time

blood pressure (BP) The amount of force exerted against the walls of an artery by the blood

body temperature The amount of heat in the body that is a balance between the amount of heat produced and the amount lost by the body

bradycardia A slow *(brady)* heart rate *(cardia);* less than 60 beats per minute

diastole The period of heart muscle relaxation; the heart is at rest

diastolic pressure The pressure in the arteries when the heart is at rest

febrile With a fever

fever Elevated body temperature

hypertension High blood pressure

hypotension Low blood pressure

pulse The beat of the heart felt at an artery as a wave of blood passes through the artery

pulse deficit The difference between the apical and radial pulse rates

pulse rate The number of heartbeats or pulses in 1 minute

respiration Breathing air into (inhalation) and out of (exhalation) the lungs

sphygmomanometer A cuff and measuring device used to measure blood pressure

stethoscope An instrument used to listen to the sounds produced by the heart, lungs, and other body organs

systole The period of heart muscle contraction; the heart is pumping blood

systolic pressure The pressure in the arteries when the heart contracts

tachycardia A rapid *(tachy)* heart rate *(cardia);* more than 100 beats per minute

thermometer A device used to measure *(meter)* temperature *(thermo)*

vital signs Measurements of body function—temperature, pulse, respirations, and blood pressure; pulse oximetry and pain are included in some agencies

KEY ABBREVIATIONS

BP	Blood pressure	IV	Intravenous
C	Centigrade	mm	Millimeter
F	Fahrenheit	mm Hg	Millimeters of mercury
Hg	Mercury	TPR	Temperature, pulse, and respirations
ID	Identification		

Regulation of body temperature, heart function, and breathing are 3 vital body processes. *Vital signs* are measurements of body function. They include:

- Temperature
- Pulse
- Respirations
- Blood pressure
- Pulse oximetry (in some agencies)
- Pain (in some agencies)

Vital signs are often called TPR (temperature, pulse, and respirations) and BP (blood pressure). See "Pulse Oximetry" (p. 543 and Chapter 44) and "Pain" (p. 543 and Chapter 36).

MEASURING AND REPORTING VITAL SIGNS

A person's vital signs vary within certain limits. Box 34-1 lists factors that affect vital signs.

Vital signs detect even minor changes in normal body function. They tell about treatment response. They often signal life-threatening events. Part of the assessment step in the nursing process, vital signs are measured:

- During physical exams
- When the person is admitted to a health care agency
- When the person's condition requires
- Before and after surgery, complex procedures, and diagnostic tests
- After some care measures, such as ambulation (walking)
- After a fall or other injury
- When drugs affect the respiratory or circulatory system
- When the person complains of pain, dizziness, light-headedness, feeling faint, shortness of breath, a rapid heart rate, or not feeling well
- As stated on the care plan (usually daily, twice a day, or weekly in nursing centers)

You must accurately measure, record, and report vital signs. If unsure of your measurements, ask the nurse for help. Unless otherwise ordered, take vital signs with the person at rest—lying or sitting. Report the following at once.

- A vital sign that is changed from a prior measurement. The nurse tells you what change is important.
- An abnormal vital sign (a vital sign above or below the normal range).
  See "Reporting and Recording" on p. 544.
  See *Focus on Communication: Measuring and Reporting Vital Signs.*
  See *Focus on Children and Older Persons: Measuring and Reporting Vital Signs.*

BOX 34-1	Factors Affecting Vital Signs	
• Activity, exercise	• Biological sex (male, female)	• Sleep
• Age	• Drugs	• Smoking
• Anger	• Eating	• Stress
• Anxiety, fear	• Illness	• Weather
	• Pain	• Weight

FOCUS ON COMMUNICATION
Measuring and Reporting Vital Signs

Some persons like to know their vital signs. If agency policy allows, tell the person the measurements. With the person's consent, you can tell family members if they ask. This information is private and confidential. Roommates and visitors must not hear what you say. For greater privacy, write the measurements for the person.

A measurement may be abnormal. Or you are not able to feel a pulse or hear a blood pressure. Do not alarm the person. You can say:

- "It was difficult to hear your blood pressure. I need to try to take it again."
- "Your pulse is a little slow (fast). I'll have the nurse check it."
- "Your temperature is higher than normal. I'll check it again and tell the nurse."

FOCUS ON CHILDREN AND OLDER PERSONS
Measuring and Reporting Vital Signs

Children
How you measure vital signs varies with the child's age. Equipment also varies. Agency policy and the nurse direct what you do.

In young children, pulse and respirations are measured before procedures that may be frightening or uncomfortable. Such procedures may increase the pulse and respiratory rates. Measuring temperature and blood pressure are examples. The nurse tells you the order for vital signs. The nurse may have you measure temperature and blood pressure after pulse and respirations. If the child is crying, include that when reporting and recording measurements.

Older Persons
When measuring vital signs, the person with dementia may move, hit at you, or grab equipment. This is not safe for the person or you. Two staff members may be needed. One tries to calm and distract the person. The other measures the vital signs.

Try the procedure when the person is calmer. Or take the respirations and pulse at one time. Then take the temperature and blood pressure later.

Approach the person calmly. Use a soothing voice. Explain what you will do. Do not rush. Follow the care plan for the best way to calm and distract the person. If you cannot measure vital signs, tell the nurse.

BODY TEMPERATURE

Body temperature is the amount of heat in the body. It is a balance between the amount of heat produced and the amount lost by the body. Heat is produced as cells use nutrients for energy. It is lost through the skin, breathing, urine, and feces (stools).

You use thermometers to measure temperature. A *thermometer* is a device used to measure (*meter*) temperature (*thermo*). Thermometers have Fahrenheit (F) or centigrade (C) scales. The degrees symbol (°) is used to record temperatures.

A *baseline* is a person's usual measurement in a healthy state. A person's temperature is fairly stable. However, it does vary throughout the day. It is lower in the morning and higher in the afternoon and evening. Body temperature is affected by the factors listed in Box 34-1, pregnancy, and the menstrual cycle.

Temperature Sites and Measurements

Temperature sites are listed in Box 34-2. Temperature measurements vary depending on the site used. Thus, it is best to use the same site for a person's ongoing measurements. Record the measurement site along with the temperature measurement.

Normal body temperature varies from person to person. On average, in a healthy adult:

- The normal oral temperature is around 98.6°F (37.0°C).
- Rectal temperature is usually *higher* than the oral temperature—around 99.6°F (37.5°C).
- Axillary temperature is usually *lower* than the oral temperature—around 97.6°F (36.5°C).

See Table 34-1 for an average adult's baseline temperature with a range of normal daily variations.

Axillary, tympanic membrane, and temporal artery sites are often used to screen for an abnormal temperature. If abnormal, the measurement is confirmed with another site—oral or rectal.

Fever means an elevated body temperature. Fever is the body's response to infection. The body raises the temperature in an attempt to kill invading microbes. Usually, a body temperature of 100.4°F (38.0°C) or higher is considered a fever in an adult or child. Follow agency guidelines on fever by age and measurement site. These terms may be used to describe the person.

- *Febrile*—with a fever. (The Latin word *febris* means fever.)
- *Afebrile*—without (*a*) a fever (*febrile*).

Low and high body temperatures can occur from cold and heat exposure. Body temperatures lower than 95°F (35.0°C) and higher than 103°F (39.4°C) are dangerous. See "Cold and Heat-Related Illnesses" in Chapter 58.

The nurse and care plan direct which temperature site to use and the person's normal temperature range. Report and record temperatures accurately following agency policies and procedures.

BOX 34-2 Temperature Sites

Oral Site (Mouth)
Oral temperatures are *not* taken if the person:
- Is unable to hold the thermometer under the tongue. Young age (usually under 4 or 5) and paralysis are reasons.
- Is unconscious.
- Has had surgery or an injury to the face, neck, nose, or mouth.
- Is receiving oxygen.
- Breathes through the mouth.
- Is restless, confused, or disoriented.
- Has a sore mouth.
- Has a convulsive (seizure) disorder.

Rectal Site (Rectum)
The rectal site is used for infants (over 1 month) and young children (3 years and under). Rectal temperatures are taken when the oral site cannot be used. Rectal temperatures are *not* taken if the person:
- Has diarrhea.
- Has a rectal disorder or injury.
- Has heart disease.
- Had rectal surgery.
- Is confused or agitated.

Axillary Site (Underarm)
The axillary site is less reliable than the other sites. It is used when other sites cannot be used. Do *not* use this site right after bathing.

Tympanic Membrane Site (Ear)
The site has fewer microbes than the mouth or rectum. The risk of spreading infection is reduced. The route is comfortable and non-invasive. This site is not accurate in children younger than 6 months old.
Too much earwax can cause an incorrect measurement. This site is *not* used if the person has:
- An ear disorder
- Ear drainage
- Earwax buildup

Temporal Artery Site (Forehead)
Body temperature is measured at the temporal artery in the forehead. The site is non-invasive.

TABLE 34-1 Average Adult Body Temperatures

Site	Baseline	Normal Range
Oral	98.6°F 37.0°C	97.6°F to 99.6°F 36.5°C to 37.5°C
Rectal	99.6°F 37.5°C	98.6°F to 100.4°F 37.0°C to 38.0°C
Axillary	97.6°F 36.5°C	96.6°F to 98.6°F 36.0°C to 37.0°C

See *Focus on Children and Older Persons: Temperature Sites and Measurements*, p. 520.

See *Focus on Communication: Temperature Sites and Measurements*, p. 520.

See *Promoting Safety and Comfort: Temperature Sites and Measurements*, p. 520.

FOCUS ON CHILDREN AND OLDER PERSONS
Temperature Sites and Measurements

Children
The oral site is not used for infants and children younger than 4 to 5 years. Use other routes as directed by the nurse and the care plan. See Box 34-2.

Older Persons
Older persons have lower body temperatures than younger persons. Their average temperatures are usually lower. The temperature that is considered a fever is lower. For example, an older person's baseline oral temperature is around 97.6°F (36.5°C). The nurse directs you to report an oral temperature of 99.0°F (37.2°C) or higher right away.

Older persons may not respond to infection with a fever. Monitor closely for other signs and symptoms (Chapter 17). The following changes need to be reported right away.

- Confusion
- Agitation or failure to cooperate with staff
- A decline in the person's ability to perform activities of daily living (ADL)
- Incontinence
- Falling
- A poor appetite or decline in intake

Tympanic membrane and temporal artery sites are used for persons who are confused and resist care. Oral and rectal sites are unsafe. The person may move, resist care, or bite down on the thermometer. This can injure the mouth, teeth, or rectum.

FOCUS ON COMMUNICATION
Temperature Sites and Measurements

Some persons have difficulty keeping an oral thermometer in place correctly. The rectal site can be uncomfortable. The axillary site has a longer measurement time than the other sites. To promote comfort, talk the person through the procedure. You can say:
- "I'm almost done. Are you doing okay?"
- "The thermometer is working. Please hold it still under your tongue a little longer."

PROMOTING SAFETY AND COMFORT
Temperature Sites and Measurements

Safety
Rectal temperatures are dangerous for persons with heart disease. The thermometer can stimulate the vagus nerve and slow the heart rate to dangerous levels.

Thermometer Types
There are different types of thermometers. See Table 34-2 and Figure 34-1 (p. 522). Electronic thermometers display the temperature on the front of the device. Follow the manufacturer's instructions and agency procedures to use, disinfect, and store thermometers.

See *Teamwork and Time Management: Thermometer Types*, p. 522.

See *Promoting Safety and Comfort: Thermometer Types*, p. 522.

See *Focus on Long-Term Care and Home Care: Thermometer Types*, p. 522.

TABLE 34-2	Thermometer Types		
Thermometer Type	Description		Guidelines for Use
Standard electronic thermometer (see Fig. 34-1, A)	• Battery operated. • The *probe* is inserted at the measurement site. • Measures temperature in 4 to 15 seconds. **Measurement sites:** • Oral • Rectal • Axillary		• Oral and axillary probes are *blue*. • Rectal probes are *red*. • *Probe covers* are disposable sheaths used to prevent the spread of infection. • Apply a new cover for each use. Discard after use.
Tympanic membrane thermometer (see Fig. 34-1, B)	• Battery operated. • Measures temperature in 1 to 3 seconds. **Measurement site:** • Tympanic membrane (ear)		• Do not use if there is ear drainage. • Probe covers are used. Discard after use. • Remove hearing aid (if worn). Wait 5 to 10 minutes before the measurement or as directed by the thermometer manufacturer. • Gently insert the covered probe into the ear.

TABLE 34-2	Thermometer Types—cont'd	
Thermometer Type	Description	Guidelines for Use
Temporal artery thermometer (see Fig. 34-1, *C*)	• Battery operated. • Measures temperature in 3 to 4 seconds. **Measurement site:** • Temporal artery (forehead)	• Probe covers prevent the spread of infection. Discard after use. • Use the exposed side of the head. Do not use the side covered by hair, a dressing, a hat, or other covering. Do not use the side that was on a pillow.
Non-contact infrared thermometer (see Fig. 34-1, *D*)	• Battery operated • There is no contact between the person and the device. • Measures surface (skin) temperature and calculates body temperature. Best used for screening. Abnormal temperatures should be measured with another thermometer type. • Most measure temperature within 1 second.	• No contact prevents the spread of infection. • Use in a draft-free area that is out of direct sunlight and not near a heat source. • Room temperature and humidity may affect temperature readings. • Be sure the forehead is clean, dry, and exposed. Coverings (headbands, hats), hair, and sweat can affect measurements. • Hold the thermometer straight in front of the forehead. Follow the manufacturer's instructions for the angle and distance from the forehead. • Do not touch the sensor area.
Digital thermometer (see Fig. 34-1, *E*)	• Small and battery operated. • Measures temperature in 6 to 60 seconds. **Measurement sites:** • Oral • Rectal • Axillary	• Probe covers prevent the spread of infection. Discard after use.
Disposable oral thermometer (see Fig. 34-1, *F*)	• Measures temperature using small chemical dots that change color when heated. **Measurement site:** • Oral	• Each dot changes color at a certain temperature. • Temperature is measured in 45 to 60 seconds. • Disposable. Discard after use.
Glass thermometer (see Fig. 34-1, *G*)	• A hollow glass tube filled with a substance that expands and rises in the tube when heated. When cooled, the substance moves back down the tube. • Measurement time varies by site. **Measurement sites:** • Oral • Rectal • Axillary	• The *stem* part is held. The *tip* is inserted at the measurement site. • Oral and axillary thermometers have a *blue* or *green* stem. They may have long and slender, stubby, or pear-shaped tips. • Rectal thermometers have a *red* stem and a stubby tip. • Problems with use include: • Long measurement times—oral 2 to 3 minutes, rectal 2 minutes, axillary 5 to 10 minutes. • They break easily and can injure the measurement site. • Mercury thermometers are hazardous. See *Promoting Safety and Comfort: Thermometer Types*, p. 522. • See "Using a Glass Thermometer" (p. 525) and "Reading a Glass Thermometer" (p. 526).

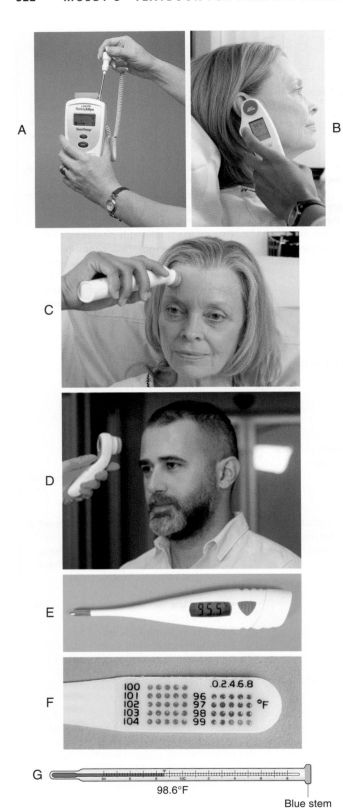

FIGURE 34-1 Thermometer types. **A,** Standard electronic thermometer. **B,** Tympanic membrane thermometer. **C,** Temporal artery thermometer. **D,** Non-contact infrared thermometer. **E,** Digital thermometer. **F,** Disposable oral thermometer. **G,** Glass thermometer with a blue stem (for oral or axillary temperatures). (D, Modified from U.S. Food and Drug Administration, 2020.)

Taking Temperatures

The nurse and care plan tell you:
- When to take the person's temperature
- What site to use
- What thermometer to use
- Normal values and significant changes to report

There are many types of electronic thermometers. Follow the manufacturer's instructions. The procedure that follows is used as a guide.

See *Delegation Guidelines: Taking Temperatures.*

See *Promoting Safety and Comfort: Taking Temperatures.*

See procedure: *Taking a Temperature With an Electronic Thermometer.*

DELEGATION GUIDELINES
Taking Temperatures

Taking a temperature is a routine nursing task. Before doing so, you need this information from the nurse and the care plan.

- What site to use for each person—oral, rectal, axillary, tympanic membrane, or temporal artery
- What thermometer to use for each person
- How long to leave a glass thermometer in place
- When to take temperatures
- Which persons are at risk for a fever
- Normal temperature range
- What observations to report and record
- When to report observations
- What patient or resident concerns to report at once:
  - A temperature changed from a past measurement
  - A temperature outside of the normal range

PROMOTING SAFETY AND COMFORT
Taking Temperatures

Safety
Probe covers (sheaths) are used on thermometers to prevent the spread of microbes from person to person. Or dedicated equipment is used (Chapter 18)—patients or residents have their own thermometers. Follow Standard Precautions when taking temperatures. Follow the Bloodborne Pathogen Standard if blood is present. Follow the rules of hand hygiene and the guidelines for glove use in Chapters 17 and 18. Wear gloves if contact with blood or body fluids is likely.

With rectal temperatures, gloved hands may have contact with feces (stools). Plan ahead to avoid contaminating other items (such as your note pad, assignment sheet, or pen). You can:

- Note the measurement with an unsoiled, gloved hand and then finish the procedure.
- Use the thermometer's "recall" or "memory" function if it has one. (This shows the last temperature measured.) Finish the procedure. Remove gloves and practice hand hygiene. Then view the measurement again to note accurately.
- Remove soiled gloves and practice hand hygiene. Note the measurement. Apply clean gloves to wipe the person and complete the procedure.

Comfort
Do not leave a thermometer in place longer than needed. This affects comfort.

Taking a Temperature With an Electronic Thermometer

QUALITY OF LIFE

- Knock before entering the person's room.
- Address the person by name.
- Introduce yourself by name and title.

- Explain the procedure before starting and during the procedure.
- Protect the person's rights during the procedure.
- Handle the person gently during the procedure.

PRE-PROCEDURE

1 Follow *Delegation Guidelines: Taking Temperatures*. See *Promoting Safety and Comfort: Taking Temperatures*.
2 For an oral temperature, ask the person not to eat, drink, smoke, or chew gum for at least 15 to 20 minutes before the measurement or as required by agency policy.
3 Practice hand hygiene and get the following supplies.
   - Thermometer—standard electronic, tympanic membrane, or temporal artery
   - Probe for a standard electronic thermometer:
     - Blue—oral or axillary
     - Red—rectal
   - Probe covers
   - Toilet paper and lubricant as directed by the nurse (rectal temperature)
   - Towel and laundry bag (axillary temperature)
   - Gloves as needed

4 Plug the probe into the thermometer if using a standard electronic thermometer.
5 Arrange items in the person's room if needed.
6 Practice hand hygiene.
7 Identify the person. Check the identification (ID) bracelet against the assignment sheet. Use 2 identifiers (Chapter 14). Also call the person by name.
8 Provide for privacy.

PROCEDURE

9 Position the person.
   a *For an oral, axillary, tympanic membrane, or temporal artery temperature*—Have the person sit or lie down.
   b *For a rectal temperature*—Assist the person into a semi-prone or side-lying position.
10 Put on gloves if contact with blood or body fluids is likely.
11 Insert the probe into a probe cover.

12 *For an oral temperature:*
   a Have the person open the mouth and raise the tongue.
   b Place the covered probe at the base of the tongue and to 1 side (Fig. 34-2, p. 524).
   c Have the person lower the tongue and close the mouth.
   d Start the thermometer if needed. Hold the probe in place until the thermometer indicates the temperature is measured. A tone or a flashing or steady light is common.

Continued

Taking a Temperature With an Electronic Thermometer—cont'd

PROCEDURE—cont'd

13 *For a rectal temperature:*
  a Lubricate the end of the covered probe.
  b Expose the anal area.
  c Raise the upper buttock (Fig. 34-3).
  d Insert the probe ½ inch into the rectum.
  e Start the thermometer if needed. Hold the probe in place until the thermometer indicates the temperature is measured. A tone or a flashing or steady light is common.

14 *For an axillary temperature:*
  a Help the person remove an arm from the gown. Do not expose the person.
  b Dry the axilla with the towel. Follow agency policy for used linens.
  c Place the covered probe in the center of the axilla (Fig. 34-4).
  d Place the person's arm over the chest.
  e Start the thermometer if needed. Hold the probe in place until the thermometer indicates the temperature is measured. A tone or a flashing or steady light is common.

15 *For a tympanic membrane temperature:*
  a Have the person turn the head so the ear is in front of you.
  b Pull up and back on the adult's ear to straighten the ear canal (Fig. 34-5). For children younger than 4 years of age, the nurse may have you pull the ear down and back.
  c Insert the covered probe gently.
  d Start the thermometer if needed. Hold the probe in place until the thermometer indicates the temperature is measured. A tone or a flashing or steady light is common.

16 *For a temporal artery temperature:*
  a Place the device in the center of the forehead.
  b Press the scan button.
  c Slide the device right or left across the temporal artery (p. 528) (see Fig. 34-1, *C*). Use the side of the head that is exposed. Keep the thermometer flat on the forehead and in contact with the skin.
  d Release the scan button when the thermometer reaches the hairline.

17 Remove the probe from the site. Read the temperature on the display.
18 Press the eject button to discard the cover.
19 Note the person's name, temperature, and temperature site on your note pad or assignment sheet.
20 Return the probe to the holder.
21 Help the person put the gown back on (axillary temperature). For a rectal temperature:
  a Wipe the anal area with toilet paper to remove lubricant.
  b Cover the person.
  c Dispose of used toilet paper.
  d Remove and discard gloves. Practice hand hygiene.

POST-PROCEDURE

22 Provide for comfort. (See the inside of the back cover.)
23 Follow the care plan and the person's preferences for privacy measures to maintain. Leaving the privacy curtain, window coverings, and door open or closed are examples.
24 Place the call light and other needed items within reach.
25 Complete a safety check of the room. (See the inside of the back cover.)

26 Practice hand hygiene.
27 Return the thermometer to the charging unit. Follow agency policy for disinfection.
28 Report and record the temperature. Note the temperature site. Report an abnormal temperature at once.

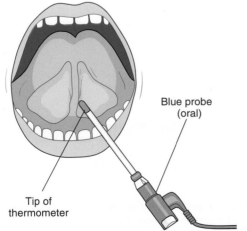

FIGURE 34-2 The thermometer is placed at the base of the tongue (under the tongue) and to 1 side.

Blue probe (oral)

Tip of thermometer

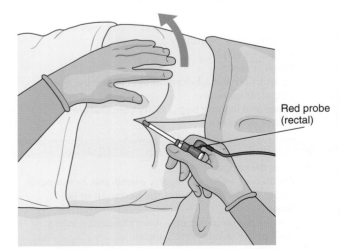

Red probe (rectal)

FIGURE 34-3 The rectal temperature is taken with the person in a side-lying position. The buttock is raised to expose the anus.

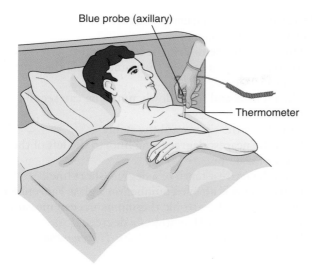

FIGURE 34-4 The thermometer is in the center of the axilla and the person's arm is over the chest.

Using a Glass Thermometer

Glass thermometers are not commonly used in health care settings. You may be taught how to use them in your training program. To use a glass thermometer:

1 Rinse the thermometer under cold, running water if it was soaking in a disinfectant. Do not use hot water. The substance inside can expand and break the thermometer. Dry the thermometer from the stem to the tip with tissues.
2 Check for breaks, cracks, or chips. Discard it following agency policy if it is broken, cracked, or chipped.
3 Shake down the thermometer below the lowest number. Hold the device by the stem. Stand away from walls, tables, and other hard surfaces. Flex and snap your wrist until the substance is below 94°F or 34°C (Fig. 34-6).
4 Insert it into a plastic cover if used (Fig. 34-7, p. 526).
5 Insert the thermometer at the measurement site. See Table 34-2 for the measurement times for each site.
6 After use, remove the plastic cover and read the thermometer. See "Reading a Glass Thermometer" on p. 526. Record the temperature.
7 Shake down the thermometer again. Clean, disinfect, and store the thermometer following agency policy.

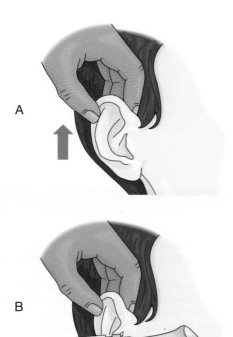

FIGURE 34-5 Tympanic membrane thermometer. **A,** The adult's ear is pulled up and back. **B,** The probe is inserted into the ear canal.

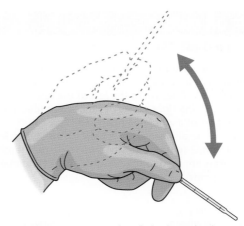

FIGURE 34-6 The wrist is snapped to shake down the thermometer. This moves the substance down the tube.

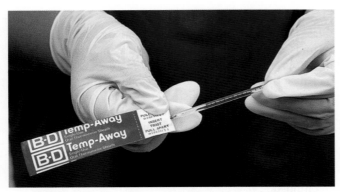

FIGURE 34-7 The thermometer is inserted into a plastic cover.

Reading a Glass Thermometer. Do the following to read a glass thermometer:
- Hold it at the stem. Bring it to eye level (Fig. 34-8).
- Turn it until you can see the numbers and the long and short lines.
- Turn it back and forth slowly until you can see the silver or red line.
- Read from the tip toward the stem.
- Read the nearest degree (long line) to the left of the silver or red line.
- Read the nearest tenth of a degree (short line). (NOTE: This is an even number on a glass Fahrenheit thermometer. Electronic thermometers can measure Fahrenheit to 0.1 [1-tenth] of a degree.)
See *Focus on Math: Reading a Glass Thermometer.*

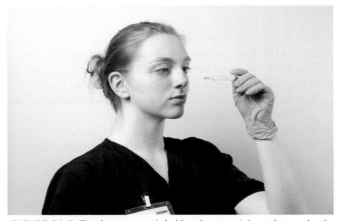

FIGURE 34-8 The thermometer is held at the stem. It is read at eye level.

FOCUS ON MATH

Reading a Glass Thermometer

To read a glass thermometer, you must understand whole numbers and decimals. Whole numbers are 0, 1, 2, 3, and so on. They are to the *left* of the decimal point. The numbers to the *right* of the decimal point (decimal place values) are part of a whole number. See Figure 34-9.

The first decimal place value is the "tenths" place. It is read as 1-tenth, 2-tenths, 3-tenths, and so on to 9-tenths. Thermometers are read to the "tenths" place (1 number past the decimal point).

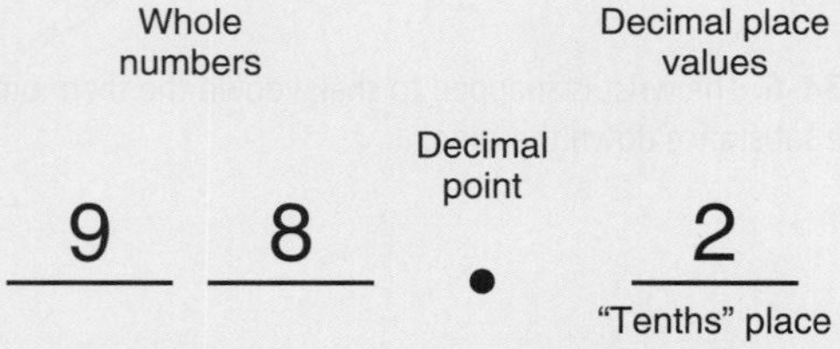

To read a glass thermometer (Fig. 34-10):
1 Read the nearest long line to the left of the silver or red line.
- Fahrenheit—each long line is 1 degree from 94°F to 108°F.
- Centigrade—each long line is 1 degree from 34°C to 42°C.
2 Read the nearest tenth of a degree (short line).
- Fahrenheit—each short line is 0.2 (2-tenths) of a degree (2-tenths, 4-tenths, 6-tenths, and 8-tenths).
- Centigrade—each short line is 0.1 (1-tenth) of a degree (1-tenth, 2-tenths, 3-tenths, and so on to 9-tenths).

Whole numbers   Decimal place values

Decimal point

9   8   •   2

"Tenths" place

FIGURE 34-9 Values used to read thermometers.

FOCUS ON MATH—cont'd
Reading a Glass Thermometer

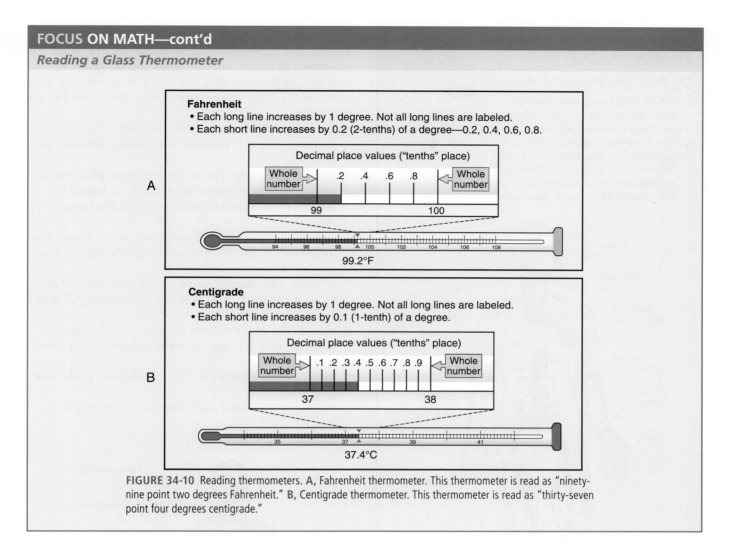

Fahrenheit
- Each long line increases by 1 degree. Not all long lines are labeled.
- Each short line increases by 0.2 (2-tenths) of a degree—0.2, 0.4, 0.6, 0.8.

Decimal place values ("tenths" place)

99.2°F

Centigrade
- Each long line increases by 1 degree. Not all long lines are labeled.
- Each short line increases by 0.1 (1-tenth) of a degree.

Decimal place values ("tenths" place)

37.4°C

FIGURE 34-10 Reading thermometers. **A,** Fahrenheit thermometer. This thermometer is read as "ninety-nine point two degrees Fahrenheit." **B,** Centigrade thermometer. This thermometer is read as "thirty-seven point four degrees centigrade."

PULSE

Arteries carry blood from the heart to all parts of the body. The *pulse* is the beat of the heart felt at an artery as a wave of blood passes through the artery. A pulse occurs when the heart beats.

See *Body Structure and Function Review: The Heart and Blood Vessels.*

BODY STRUCTURE AND FUNCTION REVIEW
The Heart and Blood Vessels

Structure and Function
The heart pumps blood through the blood vessels to the tissues and cells. The heart lies in the middle to lower part of the chest cavity toward the left side (Fig. 34-11).

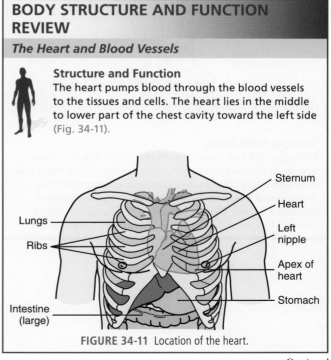

FIGURE 34-11 Location of the heart.

Continued

BODY STRUCTURE AND FUNCTION REVIEW—cont'd

The Heart and Blood Vessels

Structure and Function—cont'd

There are 2 phases of heart action. *Diastole* is the resting phase. Heart chambers (*atria* and *ventricles*) fill with blood. *Systole* is the working phase. The heart contracts. Blood is pumped through the blood vessels (Fig. 34-12).

- *Arteries* carry blood away from the heart.
- *Veins* return blood to the heart.
  See Chapter 10 for more information.

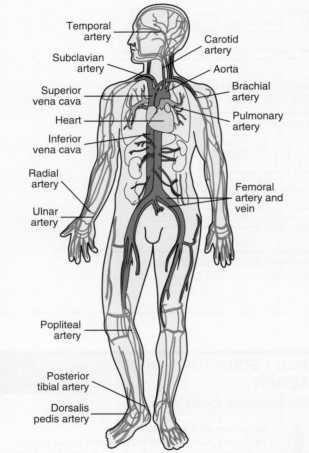

FIGURE 34-12 Blood vessels. Arteries are shown in *red*. Veins are *blue*.

Changes With Aging

With age, the heart pumps with less force. The heart rate may slow. Abnormal heart rhythms can occur. The heart may enlarge slightly. The arteries narrow and become stiffer. A weakened heart works harder to pump blood through narrowed vessels. Blood pressure (p. 537) and circulation changes can occur. See Chapter 12 for more information.

Pulse Sites

The temporal, carotid, brachial, radial, femoral, popliteal, posterior tibial, and dorsalis pedis (pedal) pulses are on each side of the body (Fig. 34-13). The arteries are close to the body surface and lie over a bone. Therefore they are easy to feel.

You use pulse sites in the following ways.

- *Temporal.* You may measure temperature over this site (p. 519).
- *Carotid.* The carotid pulse is taken on an adult during cardiopulmonary resuscitation (CPR) (Chapter 58). Never press on both carotid arteries at the same time.
- *Apical.* This site is over the tip (apex) of the heart. You use a stethoscope to listen and count the pulse at this site (p. 530).
- *Brachial.* This site is routinely used when measuring blood pressure (p. 537). It is also used during CPR on an infant (Chapter 58).
- *Radial.* The radial pulse is routinely used to measure pulse (p. 530). It is easy to reach and find. The person is not exposed.
- *Pedal.* This site is used to check blood flow in the foot (p. 534).
  See *Focus on Children and Older Persons: Pulse Sites.*

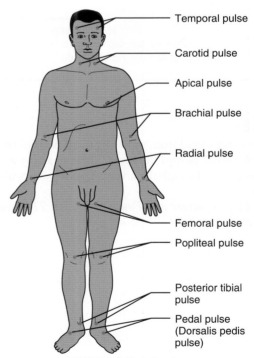

FIGURE 34-13 Pulse sites.

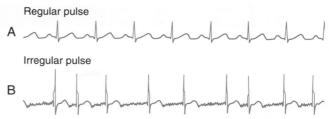

FIGURE 34-14 A, The electrocardiogram shows a regular pulse. The beats occur at regular intervals. (NOTE: Each tall spike is a beat.) **B,** These beats are at irregular intervals.

Pulse Rate

The *pulse rate* is the number of heartbeats or pulses in 1 minute. The rate varies for each age-group (Table 34-3). Pulse rate is affected by the factors in Box 34-1. Some drugs increase the pulse rate. Other drugs slow the pulse.

The adult pulse rate is normally between 60 and 100 beats per minute. A rate of less than 60 or more than 100 is abnormal. Report abnormal pulses at once.

- *Tachycardia* is a rapid *(tachy)* heart rate *(cardia)*. The heart rate is more than 100 beats per minute.
- *Bradycardia* is a slow *(brady)* heart rate *(cardia)*. The heart rate is less than 60 beats per minute.

Using a Stethoscope

A *stethoscope* is an instrument used to listen to the sounds produced by the heart, lungs, and other body organs (Fig. 34-15). You use it to hear apical pulses and for blood pressures. See Box 34-3 (p. 530) for how to use a stethoscope.

See *Focus on Communication: Using a Stethoscope*, p. 530.
See *Promoting Safety and Comfort: Using a Stethoscope*, p. 530.

TABLE 34-3	Normal Pulse Ranges by Age-Group
Age-Group	**Pulse Rate per Minute**
Infant	80 to 160
Toddler	80 to 130
Preschool	80 to 120
School Age to Late Childhood	70 to 110
Adolescent to Adult	60 to 100

Modified from Kliegman RM, et al: Nelson textbook of pediatrics, ed 21, St Louis, 2020, Elsevier. (NOTE: Rates reflect the pulse at rest. Age-groups are used to show the general narrowing of the normal pulse range with age.)

Pulse Rhythm and Force

The pulse *rhythm* should be in a regular pattern. The pause between beats is the same. An irregular pulse is when the beats are not evenly spaced or beats are skipped (Fig. 34-14).

Force relates to pulse strength. A forceful pulse is easy to feel. It is described as *strong, full,* or *bounding.* Hard-to-feel pulses are described as *weak, thready,* or *feeble.*

Electronic blood pressure equipment (p. 538) can also count pulses. The pulse rate and blood pressures are shown. Some show if the pulse is regular or irregular. However, you need to feel the pulse to determine its force.

Pulse oximetry equipment can also count pulses. See Chapter 44.

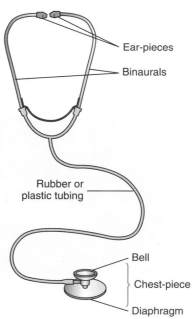

FIGURE 34-15 Parts of a stethoscope.

BOX 34-3	Using a Stethoscope

- Wipe the ear-pieces and chest-piece with antiseptic wipes before and after use. See Figure 34-15 for the parts of a stethoscope.
- Place the ear-piece tips in your ears. The bend of the tips points forward. Ear-pieces should fit snugly to block out noises. They should not cause ear pain or discomfort.
- Tap the diaphragm gently. You should hear the tapping. If not, turn the chest-piece at the tubing. Gently tap the diaphragm again. Proceed if you hear the tapping sound. Check with the nurse if you do not hear the tapping.
- Place the diaphragm over the pulse site. Hold it in place as in Figure 34-16.
- Prevent noise. Do not let anything touch the tubing. Ask the person to be silent. Make sure the room is quiet.

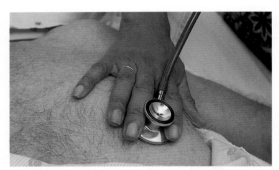

FIGURE 34-16 The stethoscope is held in place with the fingertips of the index and middle fingers.

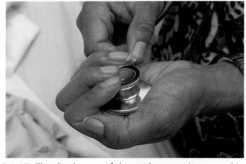

FIGURE 34-17 The diaphragm of the stethoscope is warmed in the palm of the hand.

Taking Pulses

You will take radial, apical, and apical-radial pulses. You must count, report, and record accurately.

The radial pulse is used for routine vital signs. Place the first 2 or 3 fingertips against the radial artery. The radial artery is on the thumb side of the wrist (Fig. 34-18). Follow agency policy for how long to count. The following is common.

- Regular pulse—count the pulse for 30 seconds. Multiply by 2 for the number of pulses in 1 minute.
- Irregular pulse—count the pulse for 1 minute.

The apical pulse is located 2 to 3 inches left of the lower part of the sternum (Fig. 34-19). Use a stethoscope and count the pulse for 1 minute. The heartbeat normally sounds like a *lub-dub*. Count each *lub-dub* as 1 beat. Do not count the *lub* as 1 beat and the *dub* as another.

Apical pulses are taken on infants, young children, and persons who:

- Have heart disease.
- Have irregular heart rhythms.
- Take drugs that affect the heart.

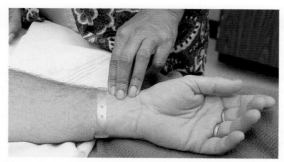

FIGURE 34-18 A radial pulse is felt using the first 2 or 3 middle fingertips.

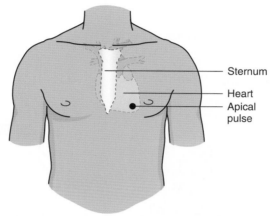

FIGURE 34-19 The apical pulse is located 2 to 3 inches to the left of the sternum (breastbone). A stethoscope is placed over the site to listen. A *lub-dub* sound is normally heard.

The apical and radial pulses should be the same. Sometimes heart contractions are not strong enough to create pulses in the radial artery. Then the radial rate is less than the apical rate. Heart disease is a common cause. To see if the apical and radial pulses are equal, 2 staff members are needed. One takes the radial pulse; the other takes the apical pulse (Fig. 34-20). Taking the apical and radial pulses at the same time is called the ***apical-radial pulse***. The ***pulse deficit*** is the difference between the apical and radial pulse rates.

(NOTE: State competency tests require the use of a watch with a second [sweep] hand when taking pulses.)

See *Focus on Math: Taking Pulses*, p. 532.

See *Delegation Guidelines: Taking Pulses*, p. 533.

See *Promoting Safety and Comfort: Taking Pulses*, p. 533.

See procedure: *Taking a Radial Pulse*, p. 533.

See procedure: *Taking an Apical Pulse and an Apical-Radial Pulse*, p. 534.

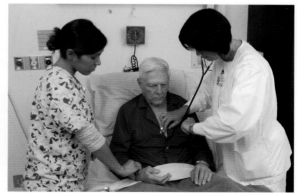

FIGURE 34-20 Taking an apical-radial pulse. One worker takes the apical pulse. The other takes the radial pulse.

FOCUS ON MATH

Taking Pulses

To count a pulse, use a watch with a second (sweep) hand. Start counting when the second (sweep) hand is at the 12, 3, 6, or 9 position. When counting a pulse for 30 seconds, do 1 of the following. See Figure 34-21.

- When starting at 12, count until position 6.
- When starting at 3, count until position 9.
- When starting at 6, count until position 12.
- When starting at 9, count until position 3.

For a 60-second pulse, count until the second (sweep) hand is back at the start position—12, 3, 6, or 9.

Radial Pulses

Pulse rate is measured in beats per minute. When you measure a regular pulse for 30 seconds, multiply the number by 2. This gives the number of beats per minute (60 seconds). For example: *You count 36 beats in 30 seconds. For the number of beats per minute, multiply 36 by 2.*

$$36 \text{ beats} \times 2 = 72 \text{ beats}$$
The pulse is 72 beats per minute.

Apical-Radial Pulses

For the *pulse deficit,* subtract the radial rate from the apical rate. (The radial rate is never greater than the apical rate.) For example:

- *The apical rate is 84 beats per minute. The radial rate is 84 beats per minute.*

$$84 \text{ apical beats} - 84 \text{ radial beats} = 0$$
The pulse deficit is 0.

- *The apical rate is 90 beats per minute. The radial rate is 86 beats per minute.*

$$90 \text{ apical beats} - 86 \text{ radial beats} = 4$$
The pulse deficit is 4.

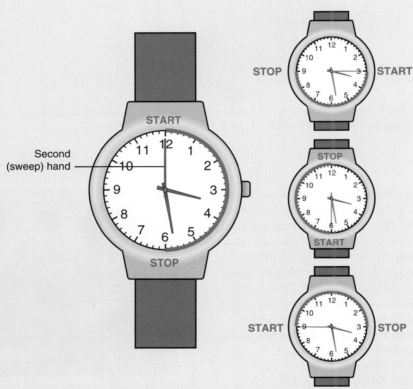

FIGURE 34-21 Using a watch with a second (sweep) hand to count for 30 seconds.

DELEGATION GUIDELINES
Taking Pulses

Taking a pulse is a routine nursing task. Before doing so, you need this information from the nurse and the care plan.

- What pulse to take for each person—radial, apical, or apical-radial
- When to take the pulse
- What other vital signs to measure
- How long to count the pulse—30 seconds or 1 minute
- If the nurse has concerns about certain patients or residents
- What observations to report and record:
  - The pulse site
  - The pulse rate—report a pulse rate less than 60 *(bradycardia)* or more than 100 *(tachycardia)* beats per minute at once
  - Pulse deficit for an apical-radial pulse
  - If the pulse is regular or irregular
  - Pulse force—strong (full, bounding) or weak (thready, feeble)
- When to report the pulse rate
- What patient or resident concerns to report at once

PROMOTING SAFETY AND COMFORT
Taking Pulses

Safety

Use your first 2 or 3 fingertips to take a pulse. Do not use your thumb. You could mistake the pulse in your thumb for the person's pulse. Reporting and recording the wrong pulse rate can harm the person.

Comfort

Position the person's arm so it is supported. Do not let the arm dangle.

Taking a Radial Pulse

QUALITY OF LIFE

- Knock before entering the person's room.
- Address the person by name.
- Introduce yourself by name and title.

- Explain the procedure before starting and during the procedure.
- Protect the person's rights during the procedure.
- Handle the person gently during the procedure.

PRE-PROCEDURE

1 Follow *Delegation Guidelines: Taking Pulses.* See *Promoting Safety and Comfort: Taking Pulses.*
2 Practice hand hygiene.

3 Identify the person. Check the ID bracelet against the assignment sheet. Use 2 identifiers (Chapter 14). Also call the person by name.
4 Provide for privacy.

PROCEDURE

5 Have the person sit or lie down.
6 Locate the radial pulse on the thumb side of the person's wrist. Use your first 2 or 3 middle fingertips (see Fig. 34-18).
7 Note if the pulse is strong or weak and regular or irregular.
8 Count the pulse for 30 seconds. Multiply the number of beats by 2 for the number of pulses in 60 seconds (1 minute). This is the pulse rate. For example:
  - You count 45 beats in 30 seconds.
  - Multiply 45 beats by 2.
  - 45 beats × 2 = 90 beats per minute.

9 Count the pulse for 1 minute if:
  - Directed by the nurse and the care plan.
  - Required by agency policy.
  - The pulse was irregular.
  - Required for your state competency test.
10 Note the following on your note pad or assignment sheet.
  a The person's name
  b Pulse site
  c Pulse rate
  d Pulse strength
  e If the pulse was regular or irregular

POST-PROCEDURE

11 Provide for comfort. (See the inside of the back cover.)
12 Place the call light and other needed items within reach.
13 Follow the care plan and the person's preferences for privacy measures to maintain. Leaving the privacy curtain, window coverings, and door open or closed are examples.

14 Complete a safety check of the room. (See the inside of the back cover.)
15 Practice hand hygiene.
16 Report and record the pulse rate and your observations. Report an abnormal pulse at once.

Taking an Apical Pulse and an Apical-Radial Pulse

QUALITY OF LIFE

- Knock before entering the person's room.
- Address the person by name.
- Introduce yourself by name and title.

- Explain the procedure before starting and during the procedure.
- Protect the person's rights during the procedure.
- Handle the person gently during the procedure.

PRE-PROCEDURE

1 Follow *Delegation Guidelines: Taking Pulses*, p. 533.
   See *Promoting Safety and Comfort:*
   a *Using a Stethoscope*, p. 530
   b *Taking Pulses*, p. 533
2 Ask a co-worker to help you (for an apical-radial pulse).
3 Practice hand hygiene and get the following supplies.
   - Stethoscope
   - Antiseptic wipes

4 Practice hand hygiene.
5 Identify the person. Check the ID bracelet against the assignment sheet. Use 2 identifiers (Chapter 14). Also call the person by name.
6 Provide for privacy.

PROCEDURE

7 Clean the stethoscope ear-pieces and chest-piece with an antiseptic wipe. Discard the wipe.
8 Have the person sit or lie down.
9 *For an apical pulse:*
   a Expose the upper part of the left chest. Expose a woman's breasts only to the extent necessary.
   b Warm the diaphragm in your palm.
   c Place the stethoscope ear-pieces in your ears. The bend of the tips points forward.
   d Find the apical pulse. Place the diaphragm 2 to 3 inches to the left of the breastbone (see Fig. 34-19).
   e Count the pulse for 1 minute. (Count each lub-dub as 1 beat.) Note if it was regular or irregular.
10 *For an apical-radial pulse:*
   a Perform step 9 (a-c).
   b Find the apical pulse. See step 9 (d). Your co-worker finds the radial pulse (see Fig. 34-20).
   c Give the signal to begin counting.
   d Count the apical pulse for 1 minute. Your co-worker counts the radial pulse for 1 minute.
   e Give the signal to stop counting. Ask your co-worker for the radial pulse rate.

11 Cover the person. Remove the stethoscope ear-pieces from your ears.
12 *For an apical-radial pulse,* subtract the radial pulse from the apical pulse for the pulse deficit. For example:
   - You counted 72 apical beats per minute.
   - Your co-worker counted 66 radial beats per minute.
   - Subtract 66 (radial pulse) from 72 (apical pulse).
   - 72 apical beats – 66 radial beats = 6. The pulse deficit is 6.
13 Note the person's name, pulse site(s), pulse rate(s), and pulse deficit on your note pad or assignment sheet. Note if the pulse was regular or irregular.

POST-PROCEDURE

14 Provide for comfort. (See the inside of the back cover.)
15 Place the call light and other needed items within reach.
16 Follow the care plan and the person's preferences for privacy measures to maintain. Leaving the privacy curtain, window coverings, and door open or closed are examples.
17 Complete a safety check of the room. (See the inside of the back cover.)
18 Clean the stethoscope ear-pieces and chest-piece with an antiseptic wipe. Discard the wipe.

19 Practice hand hygiene.
20 Return the stethoscope to its proper place. Follow agency policy for disinfection.
21 Report and record your observations. Note if the pulse was regular or irregular. Record the pulse rate with *Ap* for apical. For an apical-radial pulse, record the apical and radial pulse rates and the pulse deficit. Report an abnormal pulse at once.

Checking Pedal Pulses. The pedal (dorsalis pedis) pulse is used to check blood flow in the foot. The dorsalis pedis artery is over a foot bone (Fig. 34-22). Often a nurse will mark the skin with an X where the pulse is found. This is so that all staff use the same site.

When a pedal pulse cannot be felt, a *Doppler* is used (Fig. 34-23). A Doppler uses ultrasound (sound waves) to find a pulse. The device is named after Christian J. Doppler. He developed the ultrasound method. When held over the pulse site, the Doppler makes a "whooshing" sound for each pulse.

Your role may include using a Doppler. If so, make sure that you:
- Have received the necessary training.
- Know how to use the equipment.
- Follow the nurse's directions and the manufacturer's instructions.

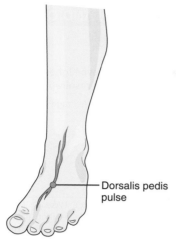

Dorsalis pedis pulse

FIGURE 34-22 The pedal pulse.

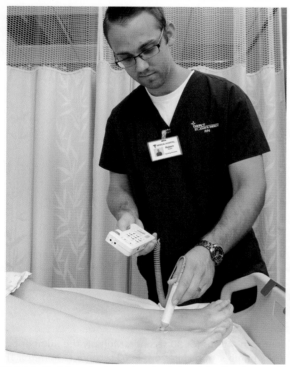

FIGURE 34-23 A Doppler is used to check a pedal pulse. (From Williams P: *Fundamental concepts and skills for nursing*, ed 6, St Louis, 2023, Saunders.)

RESPIRATIONS

Respiration involves breathing air into (inhalation) and out of (exhalation) the lungs. With each respiration there is:

- 1 inhalation—the chest rises. Air enters the lungs.
- 1 exhalation—the chest falls. Air leaves the lungs.

The healthy adult has 12 to 20 respirations per minute. See Box 34-1 for the factors affecting vital signs. Heart and respiratory diseases often increase the respiratory rate.

Respirations are normally quiet, effortless, and regular. Both sides of the chest rise and fall equally. See Chapter 44 for abnormal respiratory patterns.

See *Body Structure and Function Review: The Respiratory System*.

BODY STRUCTURE AND FUNCTION REVIEW

The Respiratory System

Structure and Function

Every cell needs oxygen. The respiratory system (Fig. 34-24) brings oxygen into the lungs and removes carbon dioxide. *Respiration* is the process of supplying the cells with oxygen and removing carbon dioxide from them. Respiration involves *inhalation* (breathing in) and *exhalation* (breathing out). The terms *inspiration* (breathing in) and *expiration* (breathing out) are also used.

Air enters the body through the mouth and nose. Air passes through the *pharynx* (throat), *larynx* (voice box), and *trachea*. The trachea divides at its lower end into the *right bronchus* and *left bronchus*. Each bronchus enters a *lung*. The bronchi divide many times into smaller branches called *bronchioles*. The bronchioles further divide and end in tiny 1-celled air sacs called *alveoli*. They are supplied by capillaries.

Oxygen and carbon dioxide are exchanged between the alveoli and capillaries. Blood in the capillaries picks up oxygen from the alveoli. Then the blood returns to the heart and is pumped to the rest of the body. Alveoli pick up carbon dioxide from the capillaries for exhalation.

The lungs are separated from the abdominal cavity by a muscle called the *diaphragm*. A bony framework made up of the ribs, sternum, and vertebrae protects the lungs.

See Chapter 10 for more information.

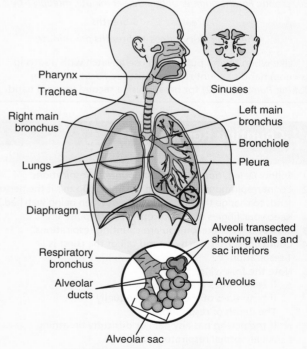

FIGURE 34-24 The respiratory system.

Changes With Aging

With age, respiratory muscles weaken. Some lung tissue is lost. Lung tissue becomes less elastic (more rigid). The chest is less able to expand and contract. Difficulty breathing and decreased strength for coughing and clearing the airway can occur. See Chapter 12 for more information.

Counting Respirations

Count respirations when the person is at rest. Position the person so you can see the chest rise and fall. To some extent, a person can control the rate and depth of breathing. People tend to change their breathing patterns when they know their respirations are being counted. Therefore do not tell the person that you are counting them.

Count respirations right after taking a pulse. Keep your fingers or stethoscope over the pulse site. The person assumes you are taking the pulse. To count respirations, watch the chest rise and fall. Count chest rises for 30 seconds. Multiply the number by 2 for the number of respirations in 1 minute. If you note an abnormal pattern, count respirations for 1 minute.

(NOTE: State competency tests require the use of a watch with a second [sweep] hand when counting respirations.)

See *Focus on Math: Counting Respirations*.

See *Focus on Children and Older Persons: Counting Respirations*.

See *Delegation Guidelines: Counting Respirations*.

See procedure: *Counting Respirations*.

FOCUS ON CHILDREN AND OLDER PERSONS
Counting Respirations

Children
Infants and young children have higher respiratory rates than adults. Count an infant's respirations for 1 minute.

Age-Group	Average Rate (Breaths per Minute)
Infant	30
Toddler	25
Preschool	23
School Age	20
Late Childhood	19
Adolescent	16 to 18

Modified from Hockenberry MJ, Rodgers CC, Wilson D: Wong's essentials of pediatric nursing, ed 11, St Louis, 2022, Elsevier. (NOTE: Rates reflect respirations at rest. Age-groups are used to show the general lowering of the rate with age.)

FOCUS ON MATH
Counting Respirations

Respirations are measured in breaths per minute. When you count regular respirations for 30 seconds, multiply the number by 2. This gives the number of respirations per minute (60 seconds). For example: *You count 8 breaths in 30 seconds. For the number of breaths per minute, multiply 8 by 2.*

$$8\ breaths \times 2 = 16\ breaths$$

The respiratory rate is 16 breaths per minute.

Like when taking pulses, you use a watch with a second (sweep) hand to count respirations. See *Focus on Math: Taking Pulses* (p. 532) for how to use a second (sweep) hand.

DELEGATION GUIDELINES
Counting Respirations

Counting respirations is a routine nursing task. Before doing so, you need this information from the nurse and the care plan.
- How long to count respirations for each person— 30 seconds or 1 minute
- When to count respirations
- If the nurse has concerns about certain patients or residents
- What other vital signs to measure
- What observations to report and record:
  - The respiratory rate
  - Equality and depth of respirations
  - If the respirations were regular or irregular
  - If the person has pain or difficulty breathing
  - Any respiratory noises
  - An abnormal respiratory pattern (Chapter 44)
- When to report observations
- What patient or resident concerns to report at once

Counting Respirations

PROCEDURE

1. Follow *Delegation Guidelines: Counting Respirations*.
2. Count respirations after taking the pulse. (Do this if the person tends to change the breathing pattern when being watched.) Keep your fingers or stethoscope over the pulse site.
3. Do not tell the person you are counting respirations.
4. Count chest rises. Each rise and fall of the chest is 1 respiration.
5. Note the following.
   - If respirations are regular
   - If both sides of the chest rise equally
   - The depth of respirations
   - If the person has any pain or difficulty breathing
   - An abnormal respiratory pattern
6. Count respirations for 30 seconds. Multiply the number by 2 for the number of respirations in 60 seconds (1 minute). This is the respiratory rate. For example:
   - You count 9 breaths in 30 seconds.
   - Multiply 9 breaths by 2.
   - 9 breaths × 2 = 18 breaths per minute.
7. Count respirations for 1 minute if:
   - Directed by the nurse and the care plan.
   - Required by agency policy.
   - They are abnormal or irregular.
   - Required for your state competency test.
8. Note the person's name, respiratory rate, and other observations on your note pad or assignment sheet.

POST-PROCEDURE

9. Provide for comfort. (See the inside of the back cover.)
10. Place the call light and other needed items within reach.
11. Follow the care plan and the person's preferences for privacy measures to maintain. Leaving the privacy curtain, window coverings, and door open or closed are examples.
12. Complete a safety check of the room. (See the inside of the back cover.)
13. Practice hand hygiene.
14. Report and record the respiratory rate and your observations. Report abnormal respirations at once.

BLOOD PRESSURE

Blood pressure (BP) is the amount of force exerted against the walls of an artery by the blood. BP is controlled by:

- The force of heart contractions
- The amount of blood pumped with each heartbeat
- How easily the blood flows through the blood vessels

Systole is the period of heart muscle contraction. The heart is pumping blood. *Diastole* is the period of heart muscle relaxation. The heart is at rest.

You measure systolic and diastolic pressures. The *systolic pressure* is the pressure in the arteries when the heart contracts. It is the higher pressure. The *diastolic pressure* is the pressure in the arteries when the heart is at rest. It is the lower pressure.

BP is measured in millimeters (mm) of mercury (Hg). The systolic pressure is recorded over the diastolic pressure. For example, a systolic pressure of 120 mm Hg (millimeters of mercury) and a diastolic pressure of 80 mm Hg are written as 120/80 mm Hg. This is read as "120 over 80 millimeters of mercury."

Normal and Abnormal Blood Pressures

BP can change from minute to minute. Factors affecting BP are listed in *Box 34-4*.

BP has normal ranges.

- *Systolic pressure*—90 mm Hg or higher but lower than 120 mm Hg
- *Diastolic pressure*—60 mm Hg or higher but lower than 80 mm Hg

Treatment is indicated for *hypertension* (high blood pressure) and *hypotension* (low blood pressure). Blood pressure is high when:

- The systolic pressure is 140 mm Hg or higher.
- The diastolic pressure is 90 mm Hg or higher.

When heart disease risk factors are present, a systolic pressure of 130 mm Hg or higher or a diastolic pressure of 80 mm Hg or higher may be considered hypertension. See Chapter 50.

Some people normally have low blood pressures. However, hypotension can signal a life-threatening problem. Blood pressure is low when:

- The systolic pressure is below 90 mm Hg.
- The diastolic pressure is below 60 mm Hg.

Report a systolic measurement at or above 120 mm Hg or below 90 mm Hg. Report a diastolic measurement at or above 80 mm Hg or below 60 mm Hg.

See *Focus on Communication: Normal and Abnormal Blood Pressures.*

See *Focus on Children and Older Persons: Normal and Abnormal Blood Pressures*, p. 538.

FOCUS ON COMMUNICATION

Normal and Abnormal Blood Pressures

If agency policy allows, you can tell the person the BP. If the BP is abnormal, the person may worry and say: "That is higher (lower) than normal for me." Be calm and professional. You can say: "Yes, it was a little high (low). I will tell your nurse."

Report abnormal blood pressures to the nurse. You must report some concerns at once. For example, a BP is 82/58 and the person is dizzy. You help the person lie down and press the call light to report your concern. You identify yourself and say: "Please have the nurse come to room 216 right away." When the nurse arrives, you say: "I measured the BP at 82/58 with the complaint of dizziness. How can I help?"

BOX 34-4   Factors Affecting Blood Pressure

- *Age.* BP increases with age. It is lowest in infants and children. It is highest in adults.
- *Biological sex (male or female).* Women usually have lower blood pressures than men do. Blood pressures rise in women after menopause.
- *Family history and heredity.* High blood pressure tends to run in families. Black persons generally have higher blood pressures than others. They tend to get high blood pressure earlier in life.
- *Blood volume.* This is the amount of blood in the circulatory system. Severe bleeding lowers the blood volume. Therefore BP lowers. Giving IV (intravenous) fluids rapidly increases the blood volume. The BP rises.
- *Stress.* Stress includes anxiety, fear, and emotions. BP increases as the body responds to stress.
- *Pain.* Pain can increase BP. However, severe pain can cause shock. BP is seriously low in the state of shock (Chapter 58).
- *Exercise.* BP increases. BP is usually measured at rest.
- *Weight.* BP is higher in over-weight persons. It lowers with weight loss.
- *Diet.* A high-sodium diet increases the amount of water in the body. The extra fluid volume increases BP.
- *Drugs.* Drugs can be given to raise or lower BP. Other drugs have the side effects of high or low BP. (A *side effect* is an undesirable reaction to a drug or therapy.)
- *Position.* BP is higher when lying down. It is lower in the standing position. Sudden changes in position can cause a drop in BP (postural hypotension). When the person stands BP may drop suddenly. Dizziness and fainting can occur.
- *Smoking.* BP increases. Nicotine in cigarettes causes blood vessels to narrow. The heart works harder to pump blood through narrowed vessels.
- *Alcohol.* Excessive alcohol intake can raise BP.
- *Certain health problems.* Some kidney diseases cause high blood pressure. High cholesterol, sleep apnea (Chapter 50), and diabetes (Chapter 51) are linked to high blood pressure.

Blood Pressure Equipment

A *sphygmomanometer* has a cuff and a measuring device for measuring blood pressure. (*Sphygmo* means pulse. A device for measuring pressure is called a *manometer*.) These types are common.

- The *aneroid type* is a manual device with a round dial and a needle that points to the numbers (Fig. 34-25, *A*). (*Manual* relates to being operated by hand.)
- The *electronic type* shows the systolic and diastolic pressures and the pulse rate (Fig. 34-25, *B*).
- A *wrist manometer* (Fig. 34-25, *C*) measures blood pressure at the wrist. Some also show the pulse rate. Also called *wrist monitors*, this type is less reliable and is sensitive to body position. However, the device may be used for persons with bariatric needs. When measuring BP, the arm and wrist must be at heart level. Follow the manufacturer's instructions for use.

For the aneroid and electronic types, you wrap the blood pressure cuff around the upper arm. Tubing connects the cuff to the manometer. When inflated (filled with air), the cuff causes pressure over the brachial artery. BP is measured as the cuff deflates (air is released).

- *Aneroid type.* A tube connects the cuff to a small, hand-held bulb. See Figure 34-26. To use the aneroid type:
  1 Hold the bulb with the air-release valve up.
  2 Turn the air-release valve clockwise (to the right) to close the valve.
  3 Squeeze the bulb. Squeezing the bulb inflates the cuff. (If you hear air leaking out and the cuff is not filling with air, the valve is not closed.)
  4 Turn the valve counter-clockwise (to the left) to deflate the cuff. Only turn the valve slightly. Turning the valve too much will cause the cuff to deflate too quickly.
  5 Use a stethoscope to listen over the brachial artery as the cuff slowly deflates. Blood flowing through the arteries produces sounds.
     - The first sound heard is the systolic pressure.
     - The last sound heard is the diastolic pressure.
- *Electronic type.* No stethoscope is needed. A button is pressed to inflate the cuff. The cuff deflates automatically. The BP is displayed. Follow the manufacturer's instructions.
  See *Promoting Safety and Comfort: Blood Pressure Equipment.*
  See *Focus on Children and Older Persons: Blood Pressure Equipment.*

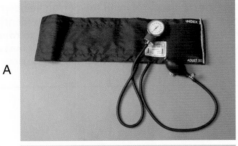
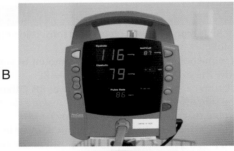
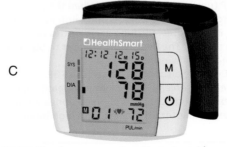

FIGURE 34-25 Blood pressure equipment. **A,** Aneroid manometer and cuff. **B,** Electronic manometer. **C,** Wrist manometer (monitor). (C, Courtesy Briggs Medical Service Company, Des Moines, Iowa.)

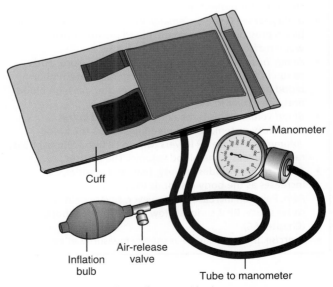

FIGURE 34-26 Parts of an aneroid sphygmomanometer.

PROMOTING SAFETY AND COMFORT

Blood Pressure Equipment

Safety

Manometers containing mercury are being phased out of health care (Fig. 34-27). Some agencies may still use them. Handle mercury manometers carefully. If one breaks, call for the nurse at once. Do not touch the mercury. Do not let the person touch it. The agency follows special procedures for handling hazardous substances. See Chapter 14.

Comfort

Inflate the cuff only to the extent necessary. (See procedure: *Measuring Blood Pressure With an Aneroid Manometer*, p. 541.) The inflated cuff causes discomfort. The higher the inflation, the greater the discomfort.

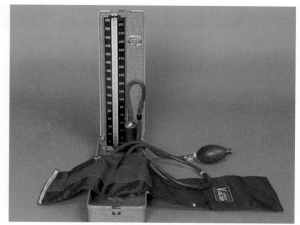

FIGURE 34-27 A mercury manometer.

FOCUS ON CHILDREN AND OLDER PERSONS

Blood Pressure Equipment

Children

Blood pressure cuffs are manufactured in different sizes (Fig. 34-28). Pediatric blood pressure cuffs are used for children. Infant and child sizes are available. The nurse tells you what size to use.

Measuring Blood Pressure

You measure blood pressure in the brachial artery. Correct cuff size, cuff placement, and arm position are needed for an accurate measurement. Box 34-5 lists the guidelines for measuring blood pressure.

See *Focus on Math: Measuring Blood Pressure*, p. 540.

See *Delegation Guidelines: Measuring Blood Pressure*, p. 541.

See procedure: *Measuring Blood Pressure With an Aneroid Manometer*, p. 541.

See procedure: *Measuring Blood Pressure With an Electronic Manometer*, p. 543.

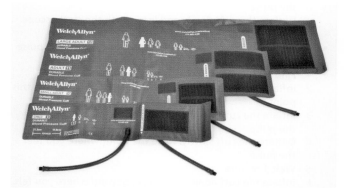

FIGURE 34-28 Blood pressure cuffs in different sizes. (From Niedzwiecki B, Pepper J, Weaver PA: *Kinn's the medical assistant: an applied learning approach*, ed 15, St Louis, 2023, Elsevier.)

BOX 34-5	Guidelines for Measuring Blood Pressure

- Do not take BP on an arm:
  - With an IV infusion
  - With an arm cast
  - With a dialysis access site
  - On the side of breast surgery
  - That is injured
- Ask the nurse if unsure of which arm to use.
- Let the person rest for 10 to 20 minutes before measuring BP.
- Measure BP with the person sitting or lying. Sometimes BP is measured in the standing position.
- Position the arm at the level of the heart. Support the arm with the palm up.

- Use the correct size cuff as directed by the nurse and the care plan (see Fig. 34-28). A cuff that is too small or too large causes a wrong reading.
- Apply the cuff to the bare upper arm. Clothing can affect the measurement.
- Make sure the cuff is snug. A loose cuff causes a wrong reading.
- Ask the person to be still during the measurement. Electronic BP manometers measure BP using sensors. Movement can affect accuracy.
- Ask the nurse for help if you have trouble measuring a BP. Frequent measurements at the same site can block blood flow and cause injury.

Continued

BOX 34-5	Guidelines for Measuring Blood Pressure—cont'd

Aneroid Type

- Make sure the room is quiet. Talking, TV, music, and sounds from the hallway can affect hearing through a stethoscope.
- Have the manometer where you can clearly see it.
- Place the diaphragm of the stethoscope firmly over the brachial artery. The entire diaphragm has contact with the skin.
- Use 1 of the following methods as directed by your instructor or the nurse. Methods 1 and 2 use the pulse as a guide for how much to inflate the cuff and at what point to listen for the systolic pressure. The systolic reading should be near the point where the pulse stops (Method 1) or returns (Method 2).
- *Method 1—Feel for the pulse to stop.*
    1 Find the radial pulse.
    2 Inflate the cuff until you cannot feel the pulse. Note this point.
    3 Inflate the cuff 30 mm Hg beyond where you last felt the pulse.
    4 Deflate the cuff slowly and listen with the stethoscope over the brachial artery.
- *Method 2—Feel for the pulse to stop. Check that the pulse returns at this point.*
    1 Find the radial pulse.
    2 Inflate the cuff until you cannot feel the pulse. Note this point.
    3 Inflate the cuff 30 mm Hg beyond where you last felt the pulse.
    4 Deflate the cuff slowly. Note the point where you feel the pulse.
    5 Wait 1 minute.
    6 Inflate the cuff again, 30 mm Hg beyond where you felt the pulse return.
    7 Deflate the cuff slowly and listen with the stethoscope over the brachial artery.

Aneroid Type—cont'd

- *Method 3—Inflate the cuff beyond the usual systolic pressure.*
    1 Inflate the cuff 160 mm Hg to 180 mm Hg.
    2 Deflate the cuff completely if you hear a blood pressure sound right away when listening with the stethoscope over the brachial artery.
    3 Re-inflate the cuff to 200 mm Hg if needed.
    4 Deflate the cuff slowly and listen with the stethoscope over the brachial artery.
- Measure the systolic and diastolic pressures.
    - The first sound is the systolic pressure.
    - The point where the sound disappears (the last sound heard) is the diastolic pressure.
- Take the BP again if you are not sure of accuracy. Wait at least 1 minute before repeating the measurement. Do not repeat the measurement multiple times using the same arm. Ask the nurse to take the BP if you are unsure of the measurement.
- Tell the nurse at once if you cannot hear the blood pressure.

FOCUS ON MATH

Measuring Blood Pressure

 Aneroid manometers have long and short lines (Fig. 34-29).

- Long lines mark 10 mm Hg values.
- Short lines mark 2 mm Hg values (2, 4, 6, and 8).

Read the manometer as the cuff deflates. The needle is dropping.

- If the needle is at a long line, note this value. Long line values end in 0. For example: 70, 80, 90, 100, 110, 120, and so on.
- If the needle is between 2 long lines:
    - Note the value of the long line below the needle.
    - Note the short line. Count up from the long line below by even numbers. Short line values end with 2, 4, 6, or 8. See Figure 34-29.

For example, *the needle is at the 3rd short line between 90 and 100. Count up by even numbers from 90. Line 1 is 92. Line 2 is 94. Line 3 is 96. The value is 96.*

If needed, round up to the nearest 2 mm Hg. When you *round up* you choose the higher value. For example, *the needle is between 82 and 80. Report and record the value as 82 mm Hg.*

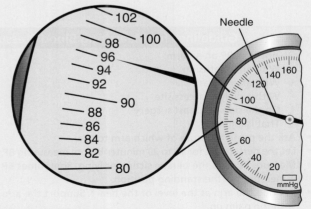

FIGURE 34-29 Reading the aneroid manometer. Long lines mark 10 mm Hg values. Short lines mark 2 mm Hg values.

DELEGATION GUIDELINES
Measuring Blood Pressure

Measuring BP is a routine nursing task. You need this information from the nurse and the care plan.

- When to measure BP
- What equipment to use (p. 538)
- What arm to use
- The person's normal blood pressure range
- If the nurse has concerns about certain patients or residents
- If the person needs to be lying down, sitting, or standing
- What size cuff to use—infant, child-sized, adult-small, adult-regular, adult-large
- What observations to report and record
- When to report the BP measurement
- What patient or resident concerns to report at once

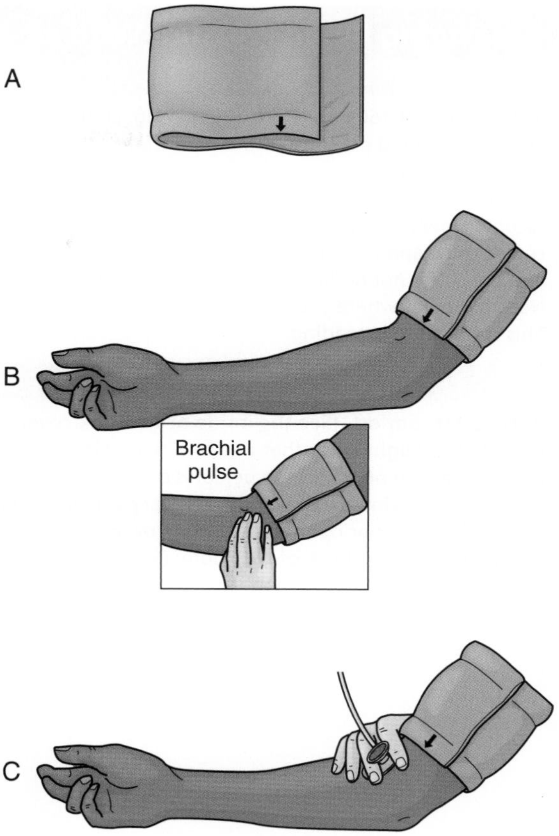

A

B

Brachial pulse

C

FIGURE 34-30 Measuring blood pressure. **A,** The arrow is used for correct cuff alignment. **B,** The cuff is placed so the arrow is aligned with the brachial artery. **C,** The diaphragm of the stethoscope is over the brachial artery.

Measuring Blood Pressure With an Aneroid Manometer

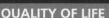

QUALITY OF LIFE

- Knock before entering the person's room.
- Address the person by name.
- Introduce yourself by name and title.

- Explain the procedure before starting and during the procedure.
- Protect the person's rights during the procedure.
- Handle the person gently during the procedure.

PRE-PROCEDURE

1 Follow *Delegation Guidelines: Measuring Blood Pressure.*
  See *Promoting Safety and Comfort:*
  a *Using a Stethoscope,* p. 530
  b *Blood Pressure Equipment,* p. 539
2 Practice hand hygiene and get the following supplies.
  - Aneroid sphygmomanometer
  - Stethoscope
  - Antiseptic wipes

3 Practice hand hygiene.
4 Identify the person. Check the ID bracelet against the assignment sheet. Use 2 identifiers (Chapter 14). Also call the person by name.
5 Provide for privacy.

PROCEDURE

6 Have the person sit or lie down.
7 Position the person's arm level with the heart. The palm is up.
8 Clean the stethoscope ear-pieces and chest-piece with an antiseptic wipe. Warm the diaphragm in your palm. Discard the wipe.
9 Stand no more than 3 feet away from the manometer.
10 Expose the upper arm.
11 Squeeze the cuff to expel (remove) any air. Close the valve on the bulb.
12 Find the brachial artery at the inner aspect of the elbow. (The brachial artery is on the little finger side of the arm.) Use your fingertips.

13 Locate the arrow on the cuff (Fig. 34-30, *A*). Align the arrow with the brachial artery (Fig. 34-30, *B*). Wrap the cuff around the upper arm at least 1 inch above the elbow. It is even and snug.
14 Use Method 1 or 2 if directed by your instructor or the nurse. See Box 34-5. These methods guide how much to inflate the cuff and at what point to listen for the systolic pressure. This procedure uses Method 3.
15 Place the stethoscope ear-pieces in your ears. Place the stethoscope's diaphragm over the brachial artery (Fig. 34-30, *C*). Do not place it under the cuff.

Continued

Measuring Blood Pressure With an Aneroid Manometer—cont'd

PROCEDURE—cont'd

16 Inflate the cuff 160 mm Hg to 180 mm Hg. Deflate the cuff if you hear a blood pressure sound. Re-inflate the cuff to 200 mm Hg if needed.

17 Deflate the cuff at an even rate of 2 to 4 millimeters per second. Slowly turn the valve counter-clockwise to deflate the cuff. If the manometer needle (see Fig. 34-29) stops dropping and the cuff is not deflating, you need to turn the valve more.

18 Note the point where you hear the first sound (Fig. 34-31, A). This is the systolic reading.

19 Continue to deflate the cuff. Note the point where the sound disappears (the last sound heard). This is the diastolic reading (Fig. 34-31, B).

20 Deflate the cuff completely. Remove the cuff. Remove the stethoscope ear-pieces from your ears.

21 Note the person's name and BP on your note pad or assignment sheet. The BP in Figure 34-31 is written as 130/84 mm Hg.

22 Return the cuff to the case or wall holder.

POST-PROCEDURE

23 Provide for comfort. (See the inside of the back cover.)

24 Place the call light and other needed items within reach.

25 Follow the care plan and the person's preferences for privacy measures to maintain. Leaving the privacy curtain, window coverings, and door open or closed are examples.

26 Complete a safety check of the room. (See the inside of the back cover.)

27 Clean the stethoscope ear-pieces and chest-piece with an antiseptic wipe. Discard the wipe.

28 Practice hand hygiene.

29 Return equipment to its proper place. Follow agency policy for disinfection.

30 Report and record the BP. Note which arm was used. Report an abnormal BP at once.

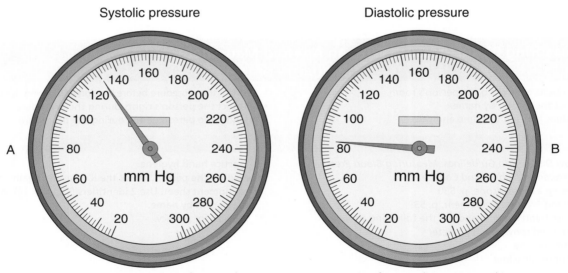

FIGURE 34-31 Manometer readings. **A,** This manometer is at 130 mm Hg for a systolic pressure. **B,** This manometer is at 84 mm Hg for a diastolic pressure. (NOTE: Both pressures are above the normal range.)

Measuring Blood Pressure With an Electronic Manometer

QUALITY OF LIFE

- Knock before entering the person's room.
- Address the person by name.
- Introduce yourself by name and title.

- Explain the procedure before starting and during the procedure.
- Protect the person's rights during the procedure.
- Handle the person gently during the procedure.

PRE-PROCEDURE

1 Follow *Delegation Guidelines: Measuring Blood Pressure*, p. 541.
2 Practice hand hygiene and get the following supplies.
   - Electronic BP manometer
   - BP cuff for use with the device (in the correct size for the person)

3 Practice hand hygiene.
4 Identify the person. Check the ID bracelet against the assignment sheet. Use 2 identifiers (Chapter 14). Also call the person by name.
5 Provide for privacy.

PROCEDURE

6 Have the person sit or lie down.
7 Position the arm level with the heart.
8 Expose the upper arm. The palm is up.
9 Squeeze the cuff to expel (remove) any air.
10 Turn on the electronic BP manometer.
11 Connect the cuff to the manometer's connection tubing.
12 Find the brachial artery at the inner aspect of the elbow. (The brachial artery is on the little finger side of the arm.) Use your fingertips.

13 Locate the arrow on the cuff. Align the arrow with the brachial artery. Wrap the cuff around the upper arm at least 1 inch above the elbow. It is even and snug.
14 Press the start button on the device. Leave the cuff in place while the device measures the BP. Ask the person to be still.
15 Remove the cuff after the BP is measured. The BP is displayed on the device.
16 Note the person's name and BP on your note pad or assignment sheet.
17 Follow agency policy for where to store the cuff (in the person's room or with the BP manometer).

POST-PROCEDURE

18 Provide for comfort. (See the inside of the back cover.)
19 Place the call light and other needed items within reach.
20 Follow the care plan and the person's preferences for privacy measures to maintain. Leaving the privacy curtain, window coverings, and door open or closed are examples.
21 Complete a safety check of the room. (See the inside of the back cover.)

22 Practice hand hygiene.
23 Return equipment to its proper place. Follow agency policy for disinfection.
24 Report and record the BP. Note which arm was used. Report an abnormal BP at once.

PULSE OXIMETRY

Pulse oximetry measures the oxygen level in the blood. This is often measured with temperature, pulse, respirations, and blood pressure. It may be a vital sign in some agencies. See "Pulse Oximetry" in Chapter 44.

PAIN

Pain is a warning sign from the body. It signals tissue damage. Therefore many agencies consider it to be a vital sign. See "Pain" in Chapter 36.

REPORTING AND RECORDING

You must report and record accurately. You also must know what to report at once. Report:

- A change in any vital sign from a prior measurement. Follow the nurse's guidelines for what change the nurse considers important.
- An abnormal vital sign. Normal values for an adult are:
  - Temperature—normal measurements vary by person and by site.
    - Average oral temperature is 98.6°F (37.0°C).
    - Average rectal temperature is 99.6 °F (37.5°C).
    - Average axillary temperature is 97.6°F (36.5°C).
  - Pulse—60 to 100 beats per minute.
  - Respirations—12 to 20 breaths per minute.
  - Blood pressure—90/60 mm Hg or higher but lower than 120/80 mm Hg.

Vital signs are recorded in the person's medical record. If measured often, a flow sheet or graphic sheet may be used (Fig. 34-32). Past and current measurements can be compared easily.

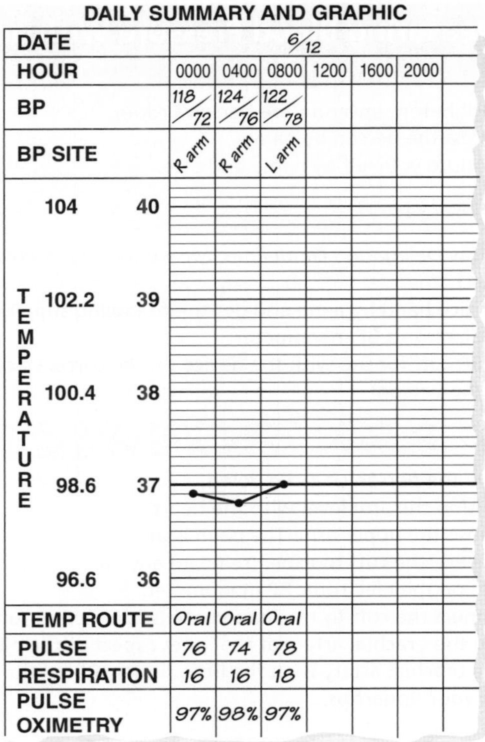

DAILY SUMMARY AND GRAPHIC

DATE	6/12					
HOUR	0000	0400	0800	1200	1600	2000
BP	118/72	124/76	122/78			
BP SITE	R arm	R arm	L arm			
TEMPERATURE (104 40; 102.2 39; 100.4 38; 98.6 37; 96.6 36)						
TEMP ROUTE	Oral	Oral	Oral			
PULSE	76	74	78			
RESPIRATION	16	16	18			
PULSE OXIMETRY	97%	98%	97%			

FIGURE 34-32 Charting sample on a graphic sheet.

FOCUS ON PRIDE

The Person, Family, and Yourself

Personal and Professional Responsibility

Learning to measure vital signs takes practice. Do not be upset if you struggle at first. Plan when and what you will practice. Use class time wisely. Tell your instructor if you need more practice. Never be ashamed to ask for more practice time. Practice builds confidence.

Rights and Respect

The nurse may ask you to re-take a measurement. Or the nurse may re-check the measurement. Do not be offended. Show respect. Avoid negative thoughts or statements about the nurse or yourself. It does not mean the nurse does not trust you or that you have done something wrong. The nurse checks the measurements for safe care.

Independence and Social Interaction

Personal choice promotes independence. The person may prefer a certain arm for pulses and blood pressures. If safe to do so, use the arm the person prefers. Unless directed otherwise, let the person choose to sit or lie when vital signs are measured.

Delegation and Teamwork

You may care for persons needing Transmission-Based Precautions (Chapter 18). You must prevent the spread of infection from equipment. Some agencies have isolation carts or kits with equipment for vital signs. The equipment is left in the person's room. Do not use your own stethoscope or bring other equipment into the room or home. If equipment must be brought in, disinfect it after use. Special disinfectants may be needed. Follow agency policy to protect others from infection.

Ethics and Laws

Measurements must be accurate. Tell the nurse if you are unsure of any measurement. For example, you cannot feel a pulse or hear a blood pressure. Never make up a measurement. Reporting or recording false measurements is wrong. The person can be harmed. Take pride in doing the right thing by honest reporting and recording.

FOCUS ON PRIDE: *Application*

Plan to practice vital signs at school and at home. Practice on classmates, family, and friends. Who will you practice with? What will you practice most at school? What can you practice at home?

REVIEW QUESTIONS

Circle the BEST answer.

1 A rectal temperature is taken when the person
   a Is unconscious
   b Has heart disease
   c Is confused
   d Has diarrhea

2 You use an electronic thermometer to measure an oral temperature in an adult. The measurement is 101.3°F (38.5°C). Which action is *correct?*
   a Use an oral glass thermometer to confirm the measurement.
   b Check the person's axillary temperature and report both measurements.
   c Record the measurement as normal in the person's medical record.
   d Report the fever to the nurse.

3 Which site is used to confirm a fever in a 1-year-old?
   a Oral site
   b Rectal site
   c Axillary site
   d Tympanic membrane site

4 Which statement about body temperature in older persons is *true?*
   a Older persons have lower body temperatures than younger persons.
   b Older persons have higher body temperatures than younger persons.
   c Body temperature does not change with age.
   d Older persons respond to infection with higher fevers.

5 To use an electronic thermometer
   a Shake down the thermometer before each use
   b Leave the thermometer in place for 2 minutes
   c Cover the probe with a probe cover
   d Use the blue probe for a rectal temperature

6 Which is usually used to take an adult's pulse?
   a The radial pulse
   b The apical pulse
   c The carotid pulse
   d The brachial pulse

7 For an adult, which pulse do you report at once?
   a A regular pulse at 64 beats per minute
   b A strong pulse at 78 beats per minute
   c A regular pulse at 90 beats per minute
   d An irregular pulse at 124 beats per minute

8 You count a regular pulse for 30 seconds. Which is *correct?*
   a Divide the number of beats by 2 for the pulse rate.
   b If you count 44 beats, record a pulse rate of 44.
   c If you count 44 beats, record a pulse rate of 88.
   d Ask the nurse to check a regular pulse.

9 Which statement about the apical-radial pulse is *true?*
   a The radial pulse can be greater than the apical pulse.
   b The apical pulse can be greater than the radial pulse.
   c The apical and radial pulses are always equal.
   d The pulse deficit is always 0.

10 Which statement about measuring respirations is *true?*
   a Count the rise and fall of the chest as 2 respirations.
   b Count an abnormal pattern for 30 seconds.
   c A rate of 14 is abnormal for an adult.
   d Respirations are normally quiet.

11 Respirations are usually counted
   a After taking the temperature
   b Before taking the pulse
   c After taking the pulse
   d After taking the blood pressure

12 Which adult blood pressure is normal?
   a 80/54 mm Hg
   b 140/90 mm Hg
   c 112/78 mm Hg
   d 130/82 mm Hg

13 When measuring BP
   a Apply the cuff to the bare upper arm
   b Use the arm with an IV infusion
   c Make sure the cuff is loose
   d Place the stethoscope under the cuff

14 You apply the BP cuff to the person's arm. You place the stethoscope over the brachial artery. What do you do next?
   a Listen for the pulse with the cuff deflated.
   b Inflate the cuff as much as possible.
   c Listen for sounds as you inflate the cuff.
   d Inflate the cuff and listen for sounds as you deflate the cuff.

15 When measuring BP, you hear the first sound at 116. You should
   a Re-check the measurement because it is abnormal
   b Record the pulse as 116 beats per minute
   c Record 116 as the top number (the systolic pressure)
   d Record 116 as the bottom number (the diastolic pressure)

16 When taking a BP, you hear the last sound at the 1st short line above 70. You record the
   a Systolic pressure as 70
   b Diastolic pressure as 71
   c Systolic pressure as 72
   d Diastolic pressure as 72

17 You are not sure you heard a BP correctly. You should
   a Record what you think you heard
   b Measure the BP again after 1 minute
   c Repeat the BP using the bell part of the stethoscope
   d Ask another nursing assistant to take the BP

18 When using electronic BP equipment, you need
   a A stethoscope and antiseptic wipes
   b A BP cuff in the correct size that connects to the device
   c An inflation bulb with an air-release valve
   d The nurse to operate the equipment

Answers to Chapter 34 questions are on p. 903.

FOCUS ON PRACTICE

Problem Solving

A person's pulse is 110. The respiratory rate is 24. The oral temperature is 100.8°F. You think you heard the BP at 86/52. You are unsure of the measurement. What will you do? Are any of the vital signs abnormal? What must you do?

Exercise and Activity

OBJECTIVES

- Define the key terms and key abbreviations in this chapter.
- Explain the difference between mobility and immobility.
- Identify the complications of immobility.
- Identify ways to prevent complications from immobility.
- Describe range-of-motion exercises.

- Identify devices used for positioning and support.
- Describe how to use different walking aids.
- Perform the procedures described in this chapter.
- Explain how to promote PRIDE in the person, the family, and yourself.

KEY TERMS

abduction Moving a body part away from the mid-line of the body

adduction Moving a body part toward the mid-line of the body

ambulation The act of walking

atrophy The decrease in size or wasting away of tissue

bed rest Restricting a person to bed and limiting activity for health reasons

contracture Decreased motion and stiffness of a joint caused by shortening (contracting) of a muscle

deconditioning The loss of muscle strength from inactivity

dorsiflexion Bending the toes and foot up at the ankle

extension Straightening a body part

external rotation Turning the joint outward

flexion Bending a body part

footdrop The foot falls down at the ankle; permanent plantar flexion

hyperextension Excessive straightening of a body part

immobility The inability to move

internal rotation Turning the joint inward

mobility A person's ability to move

opposition Touching an opposite finger with the thumb

orthostatic hypotension See "postural hypotension"

orthotic A device used to support a muscle, promote a certain motion, or correct a deformity; *ortho* means to straighten

plantar flexion Bending the foot down at the ankle

postural hypotension Abnormally low *(hypo)* blood pressure when the person suddenly stands up *(postural)*; orthostatic hypotension

pronation Turning the joint downward

range of motion (ROM) The movement of a joint to the extent possible without causing pain

rotation Turning the joint

supination Turning the joint upward

syncope A brief loss of consciousness; fainting

KEY ABBREVIATIONS

ADL	Activities of daily living		PROM	Passive range of motion
AFO	Ankle-foot orthosis		ROM	Range of motion
ID	Identification			

Exercise and activity are important for every body system. Illness, surgery, injury, pain, and aging can cause weakness and some activity limits.

You help promote exercise and activity in all persons to the extent possible. The care plan and your assignment sheet include the person's activity level and needed exercises.

The goal may be to:
- Improve independence for the home setting.
- Attain the highest level of function possible.
- Prevent loss of function.

See *Focus on Children and Older Persons: Exercise and Activity.*

MOBILITY AND IMMOBILITY

Mobility involves a person's ability to move. *Immobility* refers to the inability to move. Immobility (inactivity), whether mild or severe, affects every body system and mental well-being. *Deconditioning* is the loss of muscle strength from inactivity. When not active, deconditioning can occur quickly. See "Complications of Immobility."

Bed Rest

Bed rest means restricting a person to bed and limiting activity for health reasons. Bed rest is ordered for a health problem or because of a change in the person's condition. Common reasons are to:

- Reduce oxygen needs.
- Reduce pain.
- Reduce swelling.
- Promote healing.

These types of bed rest are common.

- *Strict (complete) bed rest.* Everything is done for the person. All activities of daily living (ADL) are done in bed.
- *Bed rest.* The person performs some ADL. Self-feeding, oral hygiene, bathing, shaving, and hair care are often allowed.
- *Bed rest with commode privileges.* The commode is used at the bedside for elimination.
- *Bed rest with bathroom privileges (bed rest with BRP).* The bathroom is used for elimination.

Bed rest definitions vary among agencies. Follow the person's care plan and your assignment sheet for the activities allowed. Ask the nurse if you have questions about a person's activity limits.

Complications of Immobility

Immobility can cause serious complications. Pressure injuries, constipation, and fecal impaction can result. Urinary tract infections and renal calculi (kidney stones) can occur. So can blood clots (thrombi) and pneumonia (inflammation and infection of the lung).

The musculo-skeletal system is affected too. For normal movement, you must help prevent the following.

- A *contracture* is decreased motion and stiffness of a joint caused by shortening (contracting) of a muscle. The contracted muscle is fixed into position, is deformed, and cannot stretch (Fig. 35-1). Common sites are the fingers, wrists, elbows, toes, ankles, knees, and hips. They can also occur in the neck and spine. The site is deformed and stiff.
- *Atrophy* is the decrease in size or the wasting away of tissue. Tissues shrink in size. *Muscle atrophy* is a decrease in size or a wasting away of muscle (Fig. 35-2).

Postural hypotension (orthostatic hypotension) is abnormally low *(hypo)* blood pressure when the person suddenly stands up *(postural)*. (*Orthostatic* relates to an upright posture.) When moving from lying to sitting to standing, the blood pressure drops. The person becomes dizzy, weak, and has spots before the eyes. Syncope can occur. *Syncope (fainting)* is a brief loss of consciousness (Chapter 58).

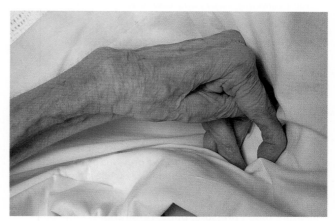

FIGURE 35-1 A contracture.

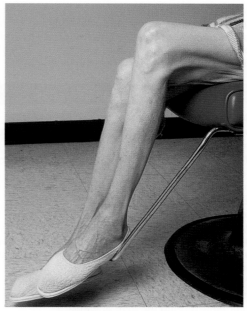

FIGURE 35-2 Muscle atrophy.

Preventing Complications

Good nursing care can prevent complications from immobility. Exercise helps prevent contractures, muscle atrophy, and other complications from immobility. Some exercise occurs with ADL. Range-of-motion exercises promote joint mobility. Weight-bearing exercises are needed to gain muscle strength. See "Ambulation" on p. 560.

Good alignment and frequent position changes are important measures. Devices may be used to support body parts and maintain proper position. See "Positioning Devices" on p. 553.

Increasing mobility to the extent possible is a goal. The person progresses in stages from:

1 Supine to Fowler's position
2 Fowler's position to sitting on the side of the bed
3 Sitting on the side of the bed to standing
4 Standing to walking or sitting in a chair

The person's care plan includes needed care measures to prevent complications and promote mobility.

See *Promoting Safety and Comfort: Preventing Complications*.

⫿ RANGE-OF-MOTION EXERCISES

The movement of a joint to the extent possible without causing pain is the ***range of motion (ROM)*** of the joint. Daily activities involve ROM movements. Bathing, hair care, eating, reaching, changing garments, and walking are examples.

Range-of-motion exercises involve moving the joints through their complete range of motion (Box 35-1). Depending on the person's abilities, ROM exercises are active, passive, or active-assistive.

- *Active* ROM exercises—are done by the person.
- *Passive* ROM (PROM) exercises—you move the joints through their range of motion.
- *Active-assistive* ROM exercises—the person does the exercises with some help.

See *Focus on Surveys: Range-of-Motion Exercises.*

See *Focus on Children and Older Persons: Range-of-Motion Exercises.*

See *Delegation Guidelines: Range-of-Motion Exercises.*

See *Promoting Safety and Comfort: Range-of-Motion Exercises.*

See procedure: *Performing Range-of-Motion Exercises.*

PROMOTING SAFETY AND COMFORT

Preventing Complications

Safety

Slowly changing positions is key to preventing postural hypotension. Give the person time to adjust to 1 position (supine, Fowler's position, sitting, standing) before moving to the next. Ask about weakness, dizziness, or spots before the eyes. Return the person to the previous position if any occur. For example, the person is dizzy while standing. Help the person sit.

Measure vital signs. While the person is lying down, measure blood pressure, pulse, respirations, and pulse oximetry (Chapters 34 and 44). Measure vital signs in other positions (sitting, standing) as directed by the nurse.

Report and record the person's vital signs and symptoms. Call for the nurse at once if you have concerns about the person's condition.

FOCUS ON SURVEYS

Range-of-Motion Exercises

The person's care plan includes the measures planned to maintain or improve mobility.

ROM exercises may be included 2 or more times a day. Persons on bed rest need more frequent ROM exercises. So do those who cannot walk, turn, or transfer themselves because of illness or injury. The goal may be 1 of the following.

- Increase range of motion.
- Prevent loss of or further decreases in range of motion. Surveyors may observe you performing ROM activities.

BOX 35-1   Range-of-Motion Exercises

Joint Movements

- *Abduction*—moving a body part away from the mid-line of the body
- *Adduction*—moving a body part toward the mid-line of the body
- *Opposition*—touching an opposite finger with the thumb
- *Flexion*—bending a body part
- *Extension*—straightening a body part
- *Hyperextension*—excessive straightening of a body part
- *Dorsiflexion*—bending the toes and foot up at the ankle
- *Plantar flexion*—bending the foot down at the ankle
- *Rotation*—turning the joint
- *Internal rotation*—turning the joint inward
- *External rotation*—turning the joint outward
- *Pronation*—turning the joint downward
- *Supination*—turning the joint upward

Safety Measures

- Cover the person with a bath blanket for warmth and privacy.
- Exercise only the joints the nurse tells you to exercise.
- Use good body mechanics.
- Expose only the body part being exercised.
- Support the part being exercised at all times.
- Move the joint slowly, smoothly, and gently.
- Do not force a joint beyond its present range of motion or to the point of pain. As each joint is exercised ask if the person:
  - Feels that the joint cannot move any farther.
  - Feels pain or discomfort in the joint.
  - Needs to stop or rest.
- Observe for signs of pain (Chapter 36). Restlessness and grimacing are examples.
- Stop if you meet resistance or suspect pain. Tell the nurse.

FOCUS ON CHILDREN AND OLDER PERSONS
Range-of-Motion Exercises

Children
Most play activities promote active ROM exercise. For example:
- Kicking a balloon or foam ball.
- Touching a balloon that is held or hung in different places.
- Playing basketball with bean-bags, wadded paper, or foam balls. Use a hoop or wastebasket as the target.
- Playing "pat-a-cake" or "Simon Says" (clap, kick, jump, and other motions).
- Having the child act like a bird, butterfly, spider, monkey, horse, or other animal.
- Playing video or computer games for finger and hand movements.
- Playing with finger paints, clay, or play dough.
- Having tricycle or wheelchair races.
- Playing "hide and seek." Hide a toy in the bed or room. Check with the nurse and care plan for the child's activity limits. Make sure the nurse approves of the play activity.

Modified from Hockenberry MJ et al: Wong's nursing care of infants and children, ed 11, St Louis, 2019, Elsevier.

DELEGATION GUIDELINES
Range-of-Motion Exercises

Performing range-of-motion exercises may be a routine nursing task in your agency. (See *Promoting Safety and Comfort: Range-of-Motion Exercises.*) When performing ROM exercises, you need this information from the nurse and the care plan.
- If ROM exercises are active, passive, or active-assistive
- Which joints to exercise
- What ROM exercises to do— see Box 35-1
- When to do the exercises
- How many times to repeat each exercise
- What observations to report and record:
  - The time the exercises were performed
  - The joints exercised and the exercises performed
  - The number of times the exercises were performed on each joint
  - Complaints of pain or signs of stiffness or spasm; specify the joint or body part involved
  - The degree to which the person took part in the exercises
- When to report observations
- What patient or resident concerns to report at once

PROMOTING SAFETY AND COMFORT
Range-of-Motion Exercises

Safety
ROM exercises can cause pain and injury if not done correctly. Practice the safety measures in Box 35-1. Remind the person to tell you about any pain during the procedure.

ROM exercises to the neck can cause serious injury if not done correctly. Some agencies give nursing assistants special training before doing such exercises. Other agencies do not let nursing assistants do them. Know your agency's policy.

Perform ROM exercises to the neck only if allowed by your agency, if you received needed training, and if they are delegated to you. In some agencies, only physical therapists do neck exercises.

Comfort
To promote physical comfort during ROM exercises, see Box 35-1. Provide privacy to promote mental comfort.

Performing Range-of-Motion Exercises

QUALITY OF LIFE
- Knock before entering the person's room.
- Address the person by name.
- Introduce yourself by name and title.
- Explain the procedure before starting and during the procedure.
- Protect the person's rights during the procedure.
- Handle the person gently during the procedure.

PRE-PROCEDURE
1 Follow *Delegation Guidelines: Range-of-Motion Exercises.* See *Promoting Safety and Comfort: Range-of-Motion Exercises.*
2 Practice hand hygiene.
3 Identify the person. Check the identification (ID) bracelet against the assignment sheet. Use 2 identifiers (Chapter 14). Also call the person by name.
4 Get a bath blanket.
5 Provide for privacy.
6 Raise the bed for body mechanics. Bed rails are up if used. Lower the bed rail near you if up.

Continued

Performing Range-of-Motion Exercises—cont'd

PROCEDURE

7 Position the person supine or in a position of comfort that allows for joint movement.

8 Cover the person with the bath blanket. Fan-fold top linens to the foot of the bed.

9 Exercise the neck *if allowed by your agency and if the nurse instructs you to do so* (Fig. 35-3).
   a Place your hands over the ears to support the head. Support the jaw with your fingers.
   b Flexion—Bring the head forward. The chin touches the chest.
   c Extension—Straighten the head.
   d Hyperextension—Bring the head backward until the chin points up. (Straighten the head to continue other exercises.)
   e Rotation—Turn the head from side to side.
   f Lateral flexion—Move the head to the right and to the left.
   g Repeat flexion, extension, hyperextension, rotation, and lateral flexion 5 times—or the number of times stated on the care plan.

10 Exercise the shoulder (Fig. 35-4).
   a Support the wrist with 1 hand. Support the elbow with the other hand.
   b Flexion—Raise the arm straight up in front and over the head.
   c Extension—Bring the arm down.
   d Hyperextension—Move the arm behind the body. (Do this if the person is in a straight-backed chair or is standing. Bring the arm back to the side of the body to continue other exercises.)
   e Abduction—Move the straight arm away from the side of the body.
   f Adduction—Move the straight arm to the side of the body.
   g Internal rotation—Bend the elbow. Place it at the same level as the shoulder. Move the forearm and hand so the fingers point down.
   h External rotation—Move the forearm and hand so the fingers point up.
   i Repeat flexion, extension, hyperextension, abduction, adduction, and internal and external rotation 5 times—or the number of times stated on the care plan.

11 Exercise the elbow (Fig. 35-5).
   a Support the wrist with 1 hand. Support the elbow with your other hand.
   b Flexion—Bend the arm so the same-side shoulder is touched.
   c Extension—Straighten the arm.
   d Repeat flexion and extension 5 times—or the number of times stated on the care plan.

12 Exercise the forearm (Fig. 35-6).
   a Continue to support the wrist and elbow.
   b Pronation—Turn the hand so the palm is down.
   c Supination—Turn the hand so the palm is up.
   d Repeat pronation and supination 5 times—or the number of times stated on the care plan.

13 Exercise the wrist (Fig. 35-7, p. 552).
   a Support the wrist with both of your hands.
   b Flexion—Bend the hand down.
   c Extension—Straighten the hand.
   d Hyperextension—Bend the hand back. (Straighten the hand to continue other exercises.)
   e Radial flexion (deviation)—Turn the hand toward the thumb.
   f Ulnar flexion (deviation)—Turn the hand toward the little finger.
   g Repeat flexion, extension, hyperextension, radial flexion (deviation), and ulnar flexion (deviation) 5 times—or the number of times stated on the care plan.

14 Exercise the thumb (Fig. 35-8, p. 552).
   a Support the person's hand with 1 hand. Support the thumb with your other hand.
   b Abduction—Move the thumb out from the inner part of the index finger.
   c Adduction—Move the thumb back next to the index finger.
   d Opposition—Touch each fingertip with the thumb.
   e Flexion—Bend the thumb into the hand.
   f Extension—Move the thumb out to the side of the fingers.
   g Repeat abduction, adduction, opposition, flexion, and extension 5 times—or the number of times stated on the care plan.

15 Exercise the fingers (Fig. 35-9, p. 552).
   a Abduction—Spread the fingers apart.
   b Adduction—Bring the fingers together.
   c Flexion—Make a fist.
   d Extension—Straighten the fingers so the fingers, hand, and arm are straight.
   e Repeat abduction, adduction, flexion, and extension 5 times—or the number of times stated on the care plan.

16 Exercise the hip (Fig. 35-10, p. 552).
   a Support the leg. Place 1 hand under the knee. Place your other hand under the ankle.
   b Flexion—Raise the leg.
   c Extension—Straighten the leg.
   d Hyperextension—Move the leg behind the body. (Do this if the person is standing. Bring the leg back to the side of the body to continue other exercises.)
   e Abduction—Move the leg away from the body.
   f Adduction—Move the leg toward the other leg.
   g Internal rotation—Turn the leg inward.
   h External rotation—Turn the leg outward.
   i Repeat flexion, extension, hyperextension, abduction, adduction, and internal and external rotation 5 times—or the number of times stated on the care plan.

17 Exercise the knee (Fig. 35-11, p. 552).
   a Support the knee. Place 1 hand under the knee. Place your other hand under the ankle.
   b Flexion—Bend the knee.
   c Extension—Straighten the knee.
   d Repeat flexion and extension 5 times—or the number of times stated on the care plan.

Performing Range-of-Motion Exercises—cont'd

PROCEDURE—cont'd

18 Exercise the ankle (Fig. 35-12, p. 552).
  a Support the foot and ankle. Place 1 hand under the foot. Place your other hand under the ankle.
  b Dorsiflexion—Pull the foot upward. Push down on the heel at the same time.
  c Plantar flexion—Turn the foot down. Or point the toes.
  d Repeat dorsiflexion and plantar flexion 5 times—or the number of times stated on the care plan.
19 Exercise the foot (Fig. 35-13, p. 552).
  a Continue to support the foot and ankle.
  b Pronation—Turn the outside of the foot up and the inside down.
  c Supination—Turn the inside of the foot up and the outside down.
  d Repeat pronation and supination 5 times—or the number of times stated on the care plan.

20 Exercise the toes (Fig. 35-14, p. 552).
  a Flexion—Curl the toes.
  b Extension—Straighten the toes.
  c Abduction—Spread the toes.
  d Adduction—Put the toes together.
  e Repeat flexion, extension, abduction, and adduction 5 times—or the number of times stated on the care plan.
21 Cover the leg. Raise the bed rail if used.
22 Go to the other side. Lower the bed rail near you if up.
23 Repeat steps 10 through 20.
24 Cover the person with the top linens. Remove the bath blanket. Fold and return the bath blanket to its proper place. Or follow agency policy for used linens.

POST-PROCEDURE

25 Provide for comfort. (See the inside of the back cover.)
26 Lower the bed to a safe and comfortable level. Raise or lower bed rails. Follow the care plan.
27 Place the call light and other needed items within reach.
28 Follow the care plan and the person's preferences for privacy measures to maintain. Leaving the privacy curtain, window coverings, and door open or closed are examples.

29 Complete a safety check of the room. (See the inside of the back cover.)
30 Practice hand hygiene.
31 Report and record your care and observations.

Flexion　Extension　Hyperextension　Rotation　Lateral flexion

FIGURE 35-3 Range-of-motion exercises for the neck.

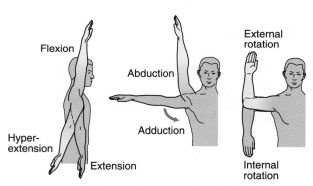

FIGURE 35-4 Range-of-motion exercises for the shoulder.

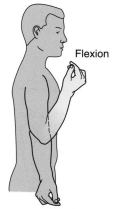

FIGURE 35-5 Range-of-motion exercises for the elbow.

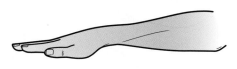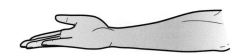

FIGURE 35-6 Range-of-motion exercises for the forearm.

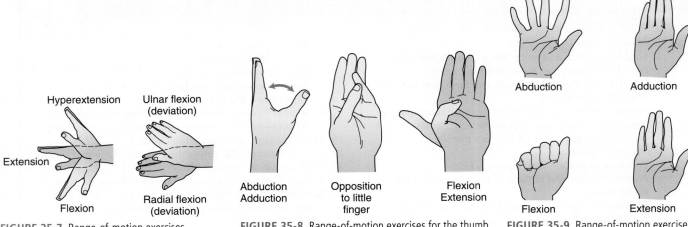

FIGURE 35-7 Range-of-motion exercises for the wrist.

FIGURE 35-8 Range-of-motion exercises for the thumb.

FIGURE 35-9 Range-of-motion exercises for the fingers.

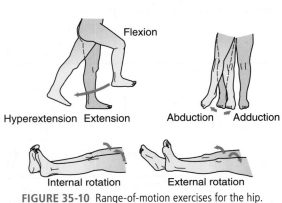

FIGURE 35-10 Range-of-motion exercises for the hip.

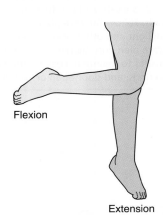

FIGURE 35-11 Range-of-motion exercises for the knee.

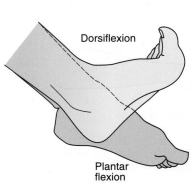

FIGURE 35-12 Range-of-motion exercises for the ankle.

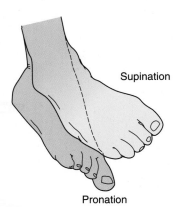

FIGURE 35-13 Range-of-motion exercises for the foot.

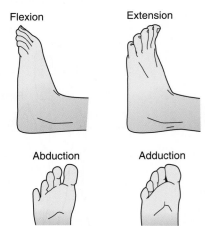

FIGURE 35-14 Range-of-motion exercises for the toes.

POSITIONING DEVICES

Body alignment and positioning were discussed in Chapter 19. Positioning (supportive) devices are often used to maintain a certain position. See Table 35-1.

An *orthotic* is a device used to support a muscle, promote a certain motion, or correct a deformity. (*Ortho* means to straighten.) Paralysis and muscle weakness are common reasons for orthotic devices. Braces and ankle-foot orthoses (AFOs) are examples (see Table 35-1).

Keep the skin and bony points in contact with positioning devices clean and dry. This prevents skin breakdown. Observe for skin changes during bathing and when a device is applied or removed. Report redness or signs of skin breakdown at once. Also report complaints of pain or discomfort. The care plan tells you when to use positioning devices.

A *trapeze* (Chapter 20) may be used for exercises to strengthen arm muscles. It is also used to move and re-position in bed.

TABLE 35-1	Positioning Devices	
Device	Description	Example
Foot-board	• Prevents plantar flexion that can lead to footdrop. *Footdrop is when the foot falls down at the ankle (permanent plantar flexion).* • The soles of the feet are flush against the foot-board. • Foot-boards also serve as bed cradles by keeping top linens off of the feet and toes.	
Bed cradle	• Keeps the weight of top linens off of the feet and toes. Heavy top linens can cause footdrop and pressure injuries (Chapter 42).	
Trochanter roll	• Prevents the hip and leg from turning outward (external rotation). • A bath blanket or bath towel is folded to the desired length and rolled up tightly. The flat end is placed under the person from the hip to the knee. The roll is tucked alongside the body.	

Continued

TABLE 35-1	Positioning Devices—cont'd	
Device	**Description**	**Example**
Hip abduction wedge	• Keeps the hips abducted (apart). • The wedge is placed between the person's legs. The device is common after hip replacement surgery.	
Hand roll (hand grip)	• Prevents contractures of the thumb, fingers, and wrist.	
Finger cushion	• Prevents contractures of the thumb, fingers, and wrist. The fingers are separated.	
Splint	• Keeps elbows, wrists, thumbs, fingers, ankles, or knees in the normal position. • Usually secured in place with Velcro.	

TABLE 35-1	Positioning Devices—cont'd	
Device	Description	Example
Brace	• Supports a weak body part. Prevents or corrects deformities or prevents joint movement. • Applied over the ankle, knee, or back.	
Ankle-foot orthosis (AFO)	• Provides support and alignment to the ankle and foot. Used for footdrop, an AFO is common after a stroke. • Worn with a sock and shoe and secured with a Velcro strap.	
Bed board	• Placed under the mattress to prevent mattress sagging. May be used in home settings by persons with back problems. • Covered with canvas or other material. • Split boards may be hinged in the middle for use with an adjustable bed (allowing the head of the bed to be raised).	

Splint image courtesy Ongoing Care Solutions, Inc., Pinellas Park, Fla. Knee brace image courtesy AliMed, Inc., Dedham, Mass.

WALKING AIDS

Some people are weak and unsteady and need help walking. Canes and walkers are common for safety. Sometimes crutches are needed. Orthotic devices (p. 553) may also be used.

The walking aid ordered depends on the person's condition, size, support needed, and type of disability. A physical therapist (PT) teaches the person how to use needed devices.

Canes

Canes are used for weakness on 1 side of the body. They help provide balance and support. Single-tip and 4-point (quad) canes are common (Fig. 35-15). A 4-point cane gives more support than a single-tip cane but can be harder to move.

A cane is held on the strong side (unaffected side) of the body. For example, if the left leg is weak, the cane is held in the right hand. The grip is level with the hip. The tip is positioned about 6 to 10 inches to the side of the strong foot.

When walking:

* The cane is moved forward along with the weak leg. It is even with the weak leg (Fig. 35-16, *A*).
* The cane is left in place as the strong leg is moved forward past the cane and the weak leg (Fig. 35-16, *B*). See *Promoting Safety and Comfort: Canes*.

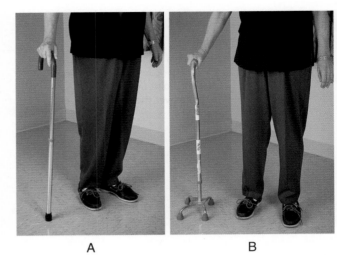

A   B

FIGURE 35-15 A, Single-tip cane. **B,** Four-point (quad) cane.

PROMOTING SAFETY AND COMFORT

Canes

Check that the person's cane is within reach and will not fall to the floor when not in use. A 4-point (quad) cane will stand freely. A single-tip cane needs to be securely propped in place. Otherwise, it will fall to the floor. The person can fall trying to reach the cane.

Cane handles are touched often. Microbes can live and grow on handles. Follow agency procedures for routine cleaning and disinfection of surfaces touched often. Also, help the person with hand hygiene before using a cane if the person's hands may be contaminated. This includes after elimination and after contact with blood or body fluids.

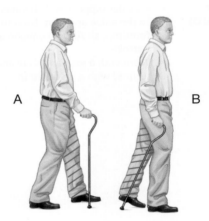

A   B

FIGURE 35-16 Walking with a cane. **A,** The cane is moved forward along with the weak leg. The cane is even with the weak leg. **B,** The cane is left in place. The strong leg is moved forward past the cane and the weak leg. (NOTE: The weak leg is indicated by slash marks.)

Walkers

A walker gives more support than a cane. Wheeled walkers have wheels on the front legs and rubber tips on the back legs (Fig. 35-17). Rubber tips on the back legs prevent the walker from moving while the person is standing. To walk, the person pushes the walker about 6 to 8 inches in front of the feet.

Walker accessories are common. Baskets, pouches, and trays can attach to the walker for needed items. This allows more independence. The hands are free to grip the walker. Gliders or walker tennis balls are also common. Placed on the rear legs, they allow the walker to glide more easily on carpets and other surfaces. See Figure 35-18.

See *Promoting Safety and Comfort: Walkers.*

PROMOTING SAFETY AND COMFORT
Walkers

Safety

Wheels are usually on the outside of the walker (see Fig. 35-17). With wheels on the outside, the walker is too wide for some doorways. Moving the wheels to the inside of the walker reduces the width. The person can go through narrower doorways.

Walkers vary in design. Some walkers have brakes and seats. The person sits to rest. Never push the walker when the person is seated.

Like canes, walker handles are touched often. They need to be cleaned and disinfected regularly. See *Promoting Safety and Comfort: Canes.*

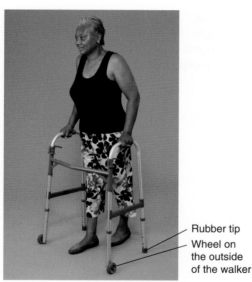

FIGURE 35-17 Wheeled walker.

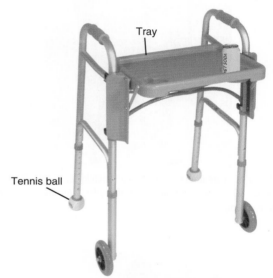

FIGURE 35-18 This walker has a tray and walker tennis balls on the rear legs. (Courtesy Drivemedical.com.)

Crutches

Crutches are used when the person cannot use 1 leg or when 1 or both legs need to gain strength. Injury, surgery, and deformity are some reasons for needing crutches. The need may be temporary or permanent.

Forearm crutches are shown in Figure 35-19. Underarm crutches extend from the underarm to the ground (Fig. 35-20).

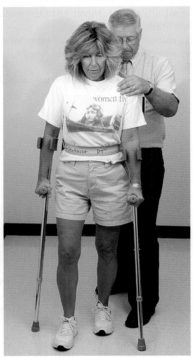

FIGURE 35-19 Forearm crutches. (From Fairchild SL, Kuchler R, Washington RD: *Pierson and Fairchild's principles & techniques of patient care*, ed 6, St Louis, 2018, Elsevier.)

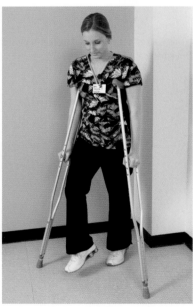

FIGURE 35-20 Underarm crutches.

The person learns to crutch walk, use stairs, and sit and stand. Falls are a risk. Follow these safety measures.

- Check the crutch tips. They must not be worn down, torn, or wet. Replace worn or torn crutch tips. Dry wet tips with a towel or paper towels.
- Check crutches for flaws. Check wooden crutches for cracks and metal crutches for bends.
- Tighten all bolts.
- Have the person wear street shoes. They must be flat and have slip-resistant soles.
- Make sure clothes fit well. Loose clothes may get caught between the crutches and underarms. Loose clothes and long skirts can hang forward and block the person's view of the feet and crutch tips.
- Practice safety measures to prevent falls (Chapter 15).
- Keep crutches within the person's reach. Put them by the person's chair or against a wall.
- Know which crutch gait the person uses.
  - 4-point gait (Fig. 35-21)
  - 3-point gait (Fig. 35-22)
  - 2-point gait (Fig. 35-23)
  - Swing-to gait (Fig. 35-24)
  - Swing-through gait (Fig. 35-25)

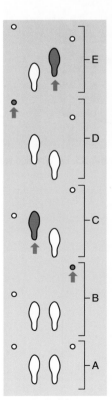

FIGURE 35-21 The 4-point gait. Both legs are used. The right crutch is moved forward and then the left foot. Then the left crutch is moved forward followed by the right foot.

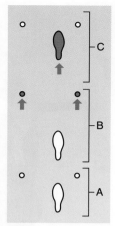

FIGURE 35-22 The 3-point gait. One leg is used. Both crutches are moved forward. Then the good foot is moved forward.

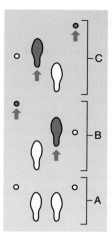

FIGURE 35-23 The 2-point gait. The person bears some weight on each foot. The left crutch and right foot are moved forward at the same time. Then the right crutch and left foot are moved forward.

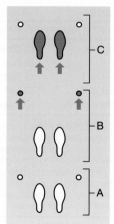

FIGURE 35-24 Swing-to gait. The person bears some weight on each leg. Both crutches are moved forward. Then the person lifts both legs and *swings to* the crutches.

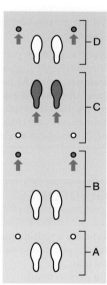

FIGURE 35-25 Swing-through gait. The person bears some weight on each leg. Both crutches are moved forward. Then the person lifts both legs and *swings through* the crutches.

AMBULATION

Ambulation is the act of walking. To walk, contractures and muscle atrophy must be prevented. After bed rest, activity increases in stages. First the person sits upright. Next the person stands. Then the person walks a few steps. Distance increases as the person gains strength.

Follow the care plan when helping a person walk (Fig. 35-26). Use a gait (transfer) belt (Chapter 15). Hand rails or a cane or walker provide support. Check the person for postural hypotension (p. 548).

See *Focus on Communication: Ambulation.*
See *Delegation Guidelines: Ambulation.*
See *Promoting Safety and Comfort: Ambulation.*
See procedure: *Assisting With Ambulation.*

FOCUS ON COMMUNICATION

Ambulation

Before ambulating, explain the activity. This promotes comfort and reduces fear. Explain:

- How far to walk
- What adaptive (assistive) devices are used
- That you will use a gait belt
- How you will assist
- What the person is to report to you
- How you will help if the person begins to fall
  For example, you can say:

I am going to help you walk from your bed to the doorway and back. This belt helps support you while you walk. I will be at your side holding the belt at all times. Tell me right away if you feel unsteady, dizzy, weak, or faint. Also tell me if you feel any pain or discomfort. If you begin to fall, I will use the belt to pull you close to me and gently lower you to the floor. Do you have any questions?

DELEGATION GUIDELINES

Ambulation

Assisting with ambulation is a routine nursing task. Before assisting with ambulation, you need this information from the nurse and the care plan.

- How much help the person needs
- If the person wears an orthotic device
- If the person uses a cane, walker, or crutches
- Areas of weakness—right arm or leg, left arm or leg
- How far to walk the person
- What observations to report and record (Fig. 35-27):
  - How well the person tolerated the activity
  - Shuffling, sliding, limping, or walking on tip-toes
  - Balance problems
  - Complaints of pain or discomfort
  - Complaints of postural hypotension—weakness, dizziness, spots before the eyes, feeling faint
  - The distance walked
- When to report observations
- What patient or resident concerns to report at once

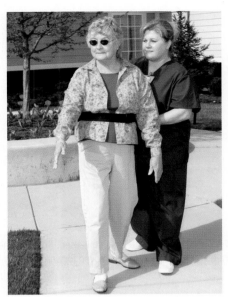

FIGURE 35-26 Assisting with ambulation. The nursing assistant walks at the person's side and slightly behind her. A gait belt is used for safety.

DATE: 06/16	TIME: 1415
ACTIVITY AND POSITIONING	
☒ Ambulate	☐ Chair
☐ Self	☒ Bed
☒ Assist of 1	☒ Right side
☐ Assist of 2	☐ Left side
☐ Mechanical lift	☐ Back

Ambulated 25 feet in the hallway with assist of 1 and use of a gait belt. Reminded not to shuffle the feet. Showed no signs of distress or discomfort. Denied feeling dizzy, light-headed, or weak. No c/o pain. Assisted to bed after ambulating. Positioned on right side with a pillow behind the back, under the head, and between the legs. Denied any other needs.

SAFETY	
☒ Gait belt	☒ Belongings in reach
☒ Slip-resistant shoes	☒ Bed rails raised
☒ Call light in reach	☐ Bed rails lowered
☒ Bed in low position	

FIGURE 35-27 Charting sample.

PROMOTING SAFETY AND COMFORT
Ambulation

Safety

Practice the safety measures to prevent falls (Chapter 15). Use a gait belt to help the person stand and during ambulation. When walking, stand at the side and slightly behind the person on the weak side. Support the weak side.

If a walker is used, remind the person not to pull on the walker to stand. The walker can tip. The person pushes on the mattress or the chair's armrests to stand (Chapter 21).

Remind the person to walk normally. Encourage the person to stand erect (upright) with the head up and the back straight. Discourage shuffling, sliding, and walking on tip-toes.

Comfort

The fear of falling affects mental comfort. Explain the purpose of the gait belt. Also explain how you will help the person if the person starts to fall (Chapter 15).

Assisting With Ambulation

QUALITY OF LIFE

- Knock before entering the person's room.
- Address the person by name.
- Introduce yourself by name and title.

- Explain the procedure before starting and during the procedure.
- Protect the person's rights during the procedure.
- Handle the person gently during the procedure.

PRE-PROCEDURE

1 Follow *Delegation Guidelines: Ambulation.* See *Promoting Safety and Comfort: Ambulation.*
2 Practice hand hygiene.
3 Identify the person. Check the ID bracelet against the assignment sheet. Use 2 identifiers (Chapter 14). Also call the person by name.

4 Get the following supplies.
  - Slip-resistant footwear
  - Paper towel or towel to protect bottom linens (if needed)
  - Gait (transfer) belt
  - Walker or cane (if needed)
5 Provide for privacy.

PROCEDURE

6 Adjust the bed to a safe and comfortable level for a transfer. Follow the care plan. Lock (brake) the bed wheels.
7 Fan-fold top linens to the foot of the bed.
8 Place the paper towel or towel under the person's feet to protect bottom linens. Put footwear on the person. Or apply footwear when the person is seated on the side of the bed (step 9).
9 Help the person sit on the side of the bed. (See procedure: *Sitting on the Side of the Bed [Dangling]* in Chapter 20.)
10 Make sure the person's feet are flat on the floor.
11 Make sure that the person is properly dressed.
12 Apply the gait belt at the waist over clothing. (See procedure: *Using a Transfer/Gait Belt* in Chapter 15.)
13 Position the walker (if used) in front of the person. Or have the person hold the cane (if used) on the strong side.
14 Help the person stand. (See procedure: *Transferring the Person to a Chair or Wheelchair* in Chapter 21.) Grasp the gait belt at each side.
15 Stand at the weak side while the person gains balance. Hold the belt at the side and back. Grasp the handles or grasp the belt from underneath. Hands are in an upward position (upward grasp).
16 Encourage the person to stand erect (upright) with the head up and the back straight.
17 *Positioning a walker or cane:*
  a Walker—The walker is 6 to 8 inches in front of the person.
  b Cane—The cane is held on the strong side. The tip is 6 to 10 inches to the side of the strong foot.

18 Help the person walk. Walk to the side and slightly behind the person on the person's weak side. Provide support with the gait belt (see Fig. 35-26). Have the person use the hand rail on the strong side (unless using a walker or cane).
19 *For a walker or cane:*
  a Walker—With both hands, the person pushes the walker 6 to 8 inches in front of the feet.
  b Cane:
    1) The cane (on the strong side) is moved forward along with the weak leg. It is even with the weak leg (see Fig. 35-16, *A*).
    2) The strong leg is moved forward past the cane and the weak leg (see Fig. 35-16, *B*).
20 Encourage the person to walk normally. The heel strikes the floor first. Discourage shuffling, sliding, or walking on tip-toes.
21 Walk the ordered distance if the person tolerates the activity. Do not rush the person.
22 Help the person return to bed. Remove the gait belt. (See procedure: *Transferring the Person From a Chair or Wheelchair to Bed* in Chapter 21.)
23 Remove the shoes. Remove the paper towel or towel over the bottom sheet (if used). Discard the paper towel or follow agency policy for used linens.
24 Lower the head of the bed. Help the person to the center of the bed. Cover the person with the top linens.

Continued

Assisting With Ambulation—cont'd

POST-PROCEDURE

25 Provide for comfort. (See the inside of the back cover.)
26 Lower the bed to a safe and comfortable level. Raise or lower bed rails. Follow the care plan.
27 Place the call light and other needed items within reach.
28 Return the shoes, gait belt, and walker or cane to their proper place.

29 Follow the care plan and the person's preferences for privacy measures to maintain. Leaving the privacy curtain, window coverings, and door open or closed are examples.
30 Complete a safety check of the room. (See the inside of the back cover.)
31 Practice hand hygiene.
32 Report and record your care and observations (see Fig. 35-27).

FOCUS ON PRIDE

The Person, Family, and Yourself

Personal and Professional Responsibility

Exercise and activity promote normal function of all body systems. Good conditioning has long-term effects. To promote activity, exercise, and well-being, you can:

- Encourage the person to be as active as possible.
- Resist the urge to do things that the person can safely do alone or with some help.
- Focus on the person's abilities.
- Give praise when the person is doing well, making progress, or giving a good effort.

Rights and Respect

Garments must provide privacy during exercise and activity. When ambulating, the person's gown must not be open in the back. During ROM exercises, cover the person with a bath blanket. Expose only the body part being exercised. Protect the right to privacy. Privacy promotes dignity and mental comfort.

Independence and Social Interaction

Nursing center activity programs promote physical, mental, and social well-being. Joints and muscles are exercised. Circulation is stimulated. Social interaction is mentally stimulating.

Bingo, movies, dances, exercise groups, shopping and museum trips, concerts, and guest speakers are common. Residents may tell you about favorite pastimes. Listen with interest. Suggest options that they may like. Allow personal choice to promote independence.

Delegation and Teamwork

To meet goals, all staff must follow the person's care plan. Progress slows or stops when only some staff follow the plan. For example, a person is to walk to and from the dining room at meal times. To save time, some staff push the person to the dining room in a wheelchair. Deconditioning results. All staff must do their part for the person's well-being.

Ethics and Laws

Persons with contractures must be moved slowly and carefully. Otherwise pain and injury can occur. This case shows the result of a disregard for safe care.

A licensed nursing assistant (LNA) cared for a person with Alzheimer's disease. The resident was severely contracted. Her ability to communicate was poor. And she could not make decisions. The LNA admitted to:

- *Being observed pulling the resident's arms away from her body and allowing them to snap back*
- *Being observed pulling the resident's legs upward from the bed and allowing them to fall back down*
- *Failing to remove a bowel movement while cleaning the resident*

The Board found that the LNA abused and improperly cared for the resident. The unprofessional conduct violated the Administrative Rules of the Board of Nursing because of:

- *Abusing or improperly caring for a patient*
- *Performing unsafe or unacceptable patient care*
- *Failing to conform to acceptable standards of practice*
- *Engaging in conduct likely to harm the public*

The LNA's license was suspended indefinitely. (State of Vermont Board of Nursing, 2000.)

Suspend indefinitely means that the LNA:

- Had to give her license to the Board.
- Could ask the Board to re-instate her license but had to prove that she:
  - Posed no danger to the public or practice of nursing.
  - Would safely and competently perform an LNA's duties.
  - Meets requirements for license renewal and re-instatement.

You can lose your ability to work as a nursing assistant for handling persons in ways that cause harm. Work carefully. Move patients and residents in a way that shows you care for their comfort, safety, and well-being.

FOCUS ON PRIDE: Application

How can you encourage independence and self-worth in persons needing help with exercise and activity?

REVIEW QUESTIONS

Circle the BEST answer.

1 You promote activity to the extent possible to
   a Maintain or improve function
   b Reduce swelling
   c Prevent pain
   d Reduce oxygen needs

2 The purpose of bed rest is to
   a Prevent postural hypotension
   b Reduce pain and promote healing
   c Prevent pressure injuries, constipation, and blood clots
   d Cause contractures and muscle atrophy

3 A contracture is
   a The loss of muscle strength from inactivity
   b A decrease in the size of a muscle
   c A blood clot in the muscle
   d Decreased motion and stiffness of a joint

4 Which statement about complications of immobility is *true?*
   a ROM exercises and frequent position changes can prevent complications.
   b Complications of immobility are minor.
   c It takes a long time for deconditioning to occur.
   d Complications cannot be prevented.

5 You sit a person up at the side of the bed to transfer to the commode. The person says: "I feel faint." What should you do?
   a Transfer the person to the commode.
   b Lay the person down in bed.
   c Have the person sit on the side of the bed longer.
   d Leave to get the nurse.

6 Before beginning passive range-of-motion (PROM) exercises, you need to explain that
   a The person will move the joints alone
   b You will uncover the person to prevent sweating
   c The person should tell you if there is pain
   d The goal is to push past points of resistance

7 When performing PROM exercises, which may cause injury?
   a Supporting the part being exercised
   b Moving the joint slowly, smoothly, and gently
   c Forcing the joint through its full range of motion
   d Exercising only the joints indicated by the nurse

8 Flexion involves
   a Bending the body part
   b Straightening the body part
   c Moving the body part toward the body
   d Moving the body part away from the body

9 Turning the joint downward is called
   a Dorsiflexion
   b Rotation
   c Supination
   d Pronation

10 Which prevents the hip from turning outward?
   a A cane
   b A foot-board
   c A trochanter roll
   d A knee brace

11 A person uses a finger cushion to prevent finger contractures. Which is *correct?*
   a Clean and dry the skin under the device before use.
   b Follow agency policies for restraint use while using the device.
   c Force the fingers to extend when placing the device.
   d Only use the device when the person has hand pain.

12 Which helps prevent permanent plantar flexion (footdrop)?
   a An abduction wedge
   b A foot-board
   c A trochanter roll
   d Crutches

13 A hip abduction wedge
   a Keeps the legs apart
   b Keeps the legs together
   c Keeps the legs crossed
   d Raises both legs

14 A person wears an ankle-foot orthosis (AFO). Which is *correct?*
   a Remind the person that a shoe is not worn with the device.
   b Remove the person's sock before application.
   c Check for redness on areas in contact with the AFO.
   d Do not remove the orthosis for bathing.

15 A person is using a cane. Which needs to be corrected?
   a The person moves the cane along with the weak leg.
   b The grip is level with the hip.
   c The cane's tip is about 10 inches to the side of the foot.
   d The person is holding the cane on the weak side.

16 Which provides the most support for walking?
   a Single-tip cane
   b Four-point (quad) cane
   c A knee brace
   d Walker

17 Which describes proper use of a wheeled walker?
   a The person pulls on the walker handles to stand.
   b The walker is pushed 6 to 8 inches in front of the feet.
   c The person's back is hunched (bent over) during use.
   d The walker is not used to walk short distances.

18 A person uses crutches. Which is a safety problem?
   a Crutch tips are wet.
   b The person wears slip-resistant shoes.
   c Crutches are within the person's reach.
   d Crutch bolts are tight.

19 When assisting with ambulation
   a Grasp the top of the gait belt with 1 hand
   b Have the person walk without footwear
   c Remind the person not to shuffle the feet
   d Walk on the person's strong side

20 What should you say to promote normal walking?
   a "Keep your back straight and your head up."
   b "Look down at your feet so you don't trip."
   c "Slide your feet if it is hard to lift them."
   d "You need to walk faster."

Answers to Chapter 35 questions are on p. 903.

FOCUS ON **PRACTICE**

Problem Solving

You are assisting a resident to ambulate in the hallway with a walker and gait belt. The resident says: "I feel dizzy." No chair is nearby. A wheelchair is at the nurses' station at the end of the hallway. What will you do? How might planning and teamwork help in this situation?

Comfort, Rest, and Sleep

- Define the key terms and key abbreviations in this chapter.
- Explain why comfort, rest, and sleep are important.
- List the Centers for Medicare & Medicaid Services (CMS) room requirements that promote comfort and well-being.
- Explain why pain is personal.
- Identify the factors affecting pain and the different types of pain.
- List the signs and symptoms of pain.
- List the nursing measures for comfort and pain relief.
- Explain the purposes of a back massage.

- Explain why meeting basic needs promotes rest.
- Identify when rest is needed.
- Describe the factors affecting sleep.
- Describe the sleep requirements of different age-groups.
- Explain how circadian rhythm affects sleep.
- Describe the common sleep disorders.
- List the nursing measures that promote rest and sleep.
- Perform the procedure described in this chapter.
- Explain how to promote PRIDE in the person, the family, and yourself.

KEY TERMS

acute pain Pain that is sharp or severe; felt suddenly from injury, disease, trauma, or surgery

chronic pain Pain that continues for a long time (longer than 12 weeks, occurs off and on, or is persistent [constant])

circadian rhythm Daily rhythm based on a 24-hour cycle that involves behavior, sleep, eating, and waking patterns; the day-night cycle or body rhythm

comfort A state of well-being; the person has no physical or emotional pain and is calm and at ease

discomfort See "pain"

distraction To focus the person's attention on something unrelated to pain

guided imagery Creating and focusing on a relaxing image

insomnia A chronic condition in which the person cannot sleep or stay asleep all night

pain To ache, hurt, or be sore; discomfort

phantom pain Pain that seems to come from a body part that is no longer there

radiating pain Pain felt at the site of tissue damage and that spreads to other areas

referred pain Pain from a body part that is felt in another body part

relaxation To be free from mental and physical stress

rest To be calm, at ease, and relaxed with no anxiety or stress

sleep A state of reduced consciousness, reduced voluntary muscle activity, and lowered metabolism

sleep apnea Pauses *(a)* in breathing *(pnea)* that occur during sleep

sleep deprivation The amount and quality of sleep are not adequate, causing reduced function and alertness

sleepwalking When the person leaves the bed and walks about while sleeping

KEY ABBREVIATIONS

CMS	Centers for Medicare & Medicaid Services	ID	Identification

Comfort, rest, and sleep are needed for well-being. The total person (physical, emotional, social, and spiritual) is affected by comfort, rest, and sleep. When problems occur, quality of life is affected.

Rest and sleep restore energy. Pain, illness, and injury increase the need for rest and sleep. The body needs more energy for healing, repair, and daily functions.

See *Focus on Long-Term Care and Home Care: Comfort, Rest, and Sleep.*

FOCUS ON LONG-TERM CARE AND HOME CARE

Comfort, Rest, and Sleep

Long-Term Care

The Centers for Medicare & Medicaid Services (CMS) requires care that promotes well-being. Chapter 13 describes the requirements for a safe and comfortable setting in nursing centers. Report problems that you cannot address to the nurse.

- Rooms are designed for 1 or 2 persons. (Some older facilities are allowed up to 4.)
- Rooms are designed and equipped for privacy.
- The person's setting accommodates individual needs and preferences.
- The bed is the proper height and size for the person.
- The person has a clean, comfortable mattress.
- Bed linens are correct for the weather and climate.
- Linens are clean, dry, and in good condition.
- The room is clean and orderly.
- The room temperature is between 71°F and 81°F (Fahrenheit).
- Water temperature is safe and comfortable.
- Ventilation, humidity, and odor levels are acceptable.
- Sound levels are comfortable.
- Lighting is adequate and comfortable.
- The person's room is home-like.
- Needed items are within reach.

FOCUS ON COMMUNICATION

Comfort

Do not assume the person is comfortable. For example, you can ask the following.

- "Are you comfortable?"
- "Are you warm enough?"
- "Do you need another blanket?"
- "Do you need another pillow?"
- "Should I adjust your pillow?"

Communication can promote mental comfort. It provides reassurance that needs will be met. You can say: "I want you to be comfortable. Please tell me how I can help you be more comfortable." Follow through with meeting the person's comfort needs. See "Comfort Measures" on p. 568.

COMFORT

Comfort is a state of well-being. The person has no physical or emotional pain and is calm and at ease. Age, illness, and activity affect comfort. So do temperature, ventilation, noise, odors, and lighting. Such factors are controlled to meet the person's needs (Chapter 13). Pain is a major factor affecting comfort.

See *Focus on Communication: Comfort.*

Pain

Pain (discomfort) means to ache, hurt, or be sore. Pain is a warning sign from the body. Often considered to be a vital sign (Chapter 34), it signals tissue damage. Pain often causes the person to seek health care.

Pain is subjective (Chapter 8). That means you cannot see, hear, touch or feel, or smell another person's pain or discomfort. You must rely on what the person says. If a person reports pain (discomfort), the person has pain (discomfort).

Pain is personal. That is, pain differs for each person. What *hurts* to one person may *ache* or be *sore* to another person. Many factors can affect pain and the person's response to pain (Box 36-1).

You must believe what patients and residents tell you about their pain. Report complaints of pain to the nurse for the nursing process.

See *Focus on Children and Older Persons: Pain,* p. 566.

See *Caring About Culture: Pain,* p. 566.

BOX 36-1	**Factors Affecting Pain**

Past and current experiences. One's experiences and those of others help in learning about pain and what to expect. Pain severity, its cause, how long it lasted, and pain relief affect the person's current response to pain.

Anxiety. Anxiety relates to feelings of fear, dread, worry, and concern. The person is uneasy and tense. Pain can cause anxiety, which makes pain worse. Helping the person understand the cause of pain and what to expect helps to reduce anxiety and lessen pain.

Rest and sleep needs. Such needs increase with illness and injury. Pain seems worse when rest and sleep are affected.

Attention. Pain seems worse when it is the person's main focus. Pain seems worse when there are no distractions—TV, visitors, activity, and so on. Especially at night when unable to sleep, the person has time to think about pain.

Support from others. Dealing with pain is often easier when family and friends offer comfort and support. Touch, encouragement, or being available or nearby helps the person deal with pain. Facing pain alone is hard, especially for children and older persons.

Personal and family duties. Some people try to ignore or deny pain because of a job; school; or caring for children, a partner, or parents.

The meaning of pain. Pain can have different meanings. For example, pain can:

- Be a sign of weakness.
- Signal the need for tests and treatment.
- Bring pleasure, such as the pain of childbirth.
- Be useful. For example, the person does not have to work or can avoid certain people.
- Lead to doting and pampering. The person likes the attention.

Culture. Culture affects pain responses. In some cultures, the person in pain is stoic. To be *stoic* means to show no reaction to joy, sorrow, pleasure, or pain. Strong verbal and nonverbal pain reactions are seen in other cultures. See *Caring About Culture: Pain,* p. 566.

Illness. Some diseases affect pain sensations. The person may not feel pain. If pain is not felt, the person does not know to seek health care. Disease or injury may go undetected.

Age. See *Focus on Children and Older Persons: Pain,* p. 566.

FOCUS ON CHILDREN AND OLDER PERSONS

Pain

Children

Children usually have had fewer pain experiences than adults. They rely on adults for pain relief. Children cannot manage pain like adults do. Adults can buy some pain-relief drugs and go to a doctor. They can distract attention away from pain with music, work, reading, and hobbies.

Older Persons

Some older persons have many painful health problems. Chronic (long-term) pain may mask new pain. Or new pain is ignored. They may think it involves a known problem. Or pain is denied or ignored because of what it may mean.

Some persons cannot tell you about pain. Behavior changes can signal pain. See "Signs and Symptoms." For example:
- An older person has increased confusion, restlessness, and loss of appetite.
- A person who normally moans and groans becomes quiet and withdrawn.
- A friendly and outgoing person becomes agitated and aggressive.
- A person who is normally quiet becomes restless and cries easily.

All persons have the right to correct pain management. Always report behavior changes. The nurse does a pain assessment when behavior changes.

✿ CARING ABOUT CULTURE

Pain

Some people of *Mexico* and the *Philippines* may appear stoic in reaction to pain. In the *Philippines,* some people view pain as the will of God and believe that God will give strength to bear the pain.

In *Vietnam,* pain may be severe before some people request pain-relief measures. In *China,* showing emotion may be viewed as a weakness of character. If so, pain is often suppressed.

Non-English-speaking persons may have problems describing pain in English. The agency uses interpreters to communicate with the person.

NOTE: *Each person is unique. A person may not follow all of the beliefs and practices of his or her culture. Follow the care plan.*

Modified from D'Avanzo CE: Pocket guide to cultural health assessment, ed 4, St Louis, 2008, Mosby.

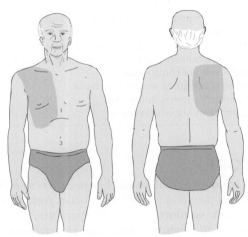

FIGURE 36-1 Gallbladder pain may radiate (spread) to the right upper abdomen, the right shoulder, and the back.

Types of Pain. Doctors use the type of pain for diagnosing. Nurses use the type for the nursing process. Pain can signal a new problem. Or it may be an ongoing symptom.

Acute pain is sharp or severe. It is felt suddenly from injury, disease, trauma, or surgery. Acute pain signals a new injury or a life-threatening event. There is tissue damage. Acute pain lasts a short time and lessens with healing.

Chronic pain continues for a long time (longer than 12 weeks, occurs off and on, or is persistent [constant]). Chronic pain is often a symptom of an ongoing health problem. Arthritis is an example. Sometimes healing has occurred. There is no longer tissue damage, but pain remains.

Sometimes pain is felt in areas other than the affected area. *Radiating pain* is felt at the site of tissue damage and spreads to other areas. For example, low back pain can radiate to the buttocks and legs. Gallbladder disease can cause pain in the right upper abdomen, the back, and the right shoulder (Fig. 36-1). *Referred pain* is pain from a body part that is felt in another body part. For example, pain from a heart attack may be felt in the left shoulder, left arm, neck, or jaw without chest pain.

Pain can also be sensed in areas no longer present. *Phantom pain* seems to come from a body part that is no longer there. For example, a person with an amputated leg may still sense leg pain.

Signs and Symptoms. Promptly report any information you collect about pain. Write down what the person says. Use the person's exact words to report and record. The nurse needs the following information.

- *Location.* Where is the pain? Ask the person to point to the area. Ask the person if the pain is anywhere else and to point to those areas.
- *Onset and duration.* When did the pain start? How long has it lasted?
- *Intensity.* Is the pain mild, moderate, or severe? Have the person rate the pain on a scale of 0 to 10, with 10 as the most severe (Fig. 36-2). Or use the *Wong-Baker FACES® Pain Rating Scale* (Fig. 36-3). Designed for children, the scale is useful for all age-groups. Explain that each face shows how a person feels. Ask which face best matches how the person feels.
- *Description.* Have the person describe the pain or discomfort. If necessary, offer some of the words listed in Box 36-2.
- *Factors causing pain.* These are called precipitating factors. To *precipitate* means to cause. Such factors include moving or turning in bed, coughing or deep breathing, and exercise. Ask what the person was doing before the pain started and when it started.
- *Factors affecting pain.* Ask what makes the pain better and what makes it worse.
- *Vital signs.* Measure pulse, respirations, and blood pressure (Chapter 34). Vital signs often increase with acute pain. They may be normal with chronic pain.
- *Other signs and symptoms.* Does the person have other symptoms—dizziness, nausea, vomiting, weakness, numbness or tingling, or others? Box 36-3 lists the signs and symptoms that often occur with pain.

See *Focus on Communication: Signs and Symptoms*, p. 568.

See *Focus on Children and Older Persons: Signs and Symptoms*, p. 568.

See *Focus on Surveys: Signs and Symptoms*, p. 568.

BOX 36-2	Words Used to Describe Pain
• Aching	• Radiating
• Burning	• Ripping
• Cramping	• Sharp
• Crushing	• Shooting
• Discomfort	• Soreness
• Dull	• Spasms
• Gnawing	• Squeezing
• Heaviness	• Stabbing
• Hurting	• Tearing
• Knife-like	• Tenderness
• Numbness	• Throbbing
• Piercing	• Tightness
• Pins and needles	• Tingling
• Pressure	• Vise-like

BOX 36-3   Pain: Signs and Symptoms

Body Responses
- Appetite: changes in
- Dizziness
- Nausea, vomiting
- Numbness, tingling
- Skin: pale (*pallor*)
- Sleep: difficulty with
- Sweating (*diaphoresis*)
- Vital signs (pulse, respirations, and blood pressure): increased
- Weakness
- Weight loss

Behaviors
- Clenching the jaw
- Crying
- Frowning
- Gait: changes in, limping
- Gasping
- Grimacing
- Groaning, grunting, moaning
- Holding the affected body part (splinting, guarding)
- Irritability
- Mood: changes in, depressed
- Pacing
- Positioning: maintaining 1 position, refusing to move, frequent position changes
- Pulling away when touched
- Quietness
- Resisting care
- Restlessness
- Rubbing a body part or area
- Screaming
- Speech: slow or rapid, loud or quiet
- Whimpering

Ask the person to rate the pain on a scale of 0 to 10.										
No pain									Worst pain imaginable	
0	1	2	3	4	5	6	7	8	9	10

FIGURE 36-2 Pain rating scale. (Modified from Williams P: *deWit's fundamental concepts and skills for nursing*, ed 6, St Louis, 2022, Elsevier.)

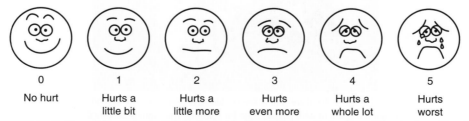

0	1	2	3	4	5
No hurt	Hurts a little bit	Hurts a little more	Hurts even more	Hurts a whole lot	Hurts worst

FIGURE 36-3 Wong-Baker FACES® Pain Rating Scale. (Modified from Hockenberry MJ and others: *Wong's nursing care of infants and children*, ed 11, St Louis, 2019, Elsevier.)

FOCUS ON COMMUNICATION

Signs and Symptoms

A person may use words like "hurt" or "discomfort" instead of "pain." Children may use "owie" or "boo boo." Use words that the person uses.

Some persons have trouble rating pain intensity on a 0 to 10 scale. Instead, you can ask if the pain is mild, moderate, or severe.

FOCUS ON CHILDREN AND OLDER PERSONS

Signs and Symptoms

Children
Be alert to behaviors that signal a child's pain. Infants cry, fuss, and are restless. Such behaviors also mean hunger and needing a diaper changed. Toddlers and pre-schoolers may not have the words to express pain. Older children may restrict play, school, and sports to lessen pain.

Older Persons
Some persons are no longer able to communicate about pain. This can occur with dementia (Chapter 54). Pain must still be assessed and managed. Observe closely for behavior and body changes. Report changes at once. Pay attention to:
- *Facial expressions and sounds.* Frowning, grimacing, looking tense, moaning, groaning, calling out, crying, and whimpering are examples.
- *Body movements.* Restlessness, pacing, fidgeting, pulling away when touched, and rubbing or holding a body part are examples.
- *Behavior and mood.* Sadness, agitation, aggression, resisting care, and being unusually quiet are examples.
- *Breathing.* Labored breathing, rapid breathing, and breathing at different rates are examples. See Chapter 44 for abnormal respirations.
- *Ability to be comforted (consoled).* The extent to which comfort measures help gives information about pain intensity and pain relief.

All persons have the right to correct pain management. The nurse does a pain assessment when behavior changes.

FOCUS ON SURVEYS

Signs and Symptoms

Pain interferes with well-being—function, mobility, mood, sleep, and quality of life. The agency must:
- Recognize when a person has pain.
- Identify when pain might occur.
- Evaluate pain and its causes.
- Manage or prevent pain.

You may be the first to observe signs and symptoms of pain. You must recognize and report a change in the person's behavior and function. You follow the care plan for pain-relief measures. Therefore a surveyor may ask you about pain. Examples are:
- What are the signs and symptoms of pain?
- How do you ask a person to rate the intensity of pain?
- What factors can cause pain or make it worse?
- When and how do you report observations about pain?
- How do you assist the nurse with pain-relief measures? (See "Comfort Measures.")

Comfort Measures

The nurse uses the nursing process to promote comfort and relieve pain (Fig. 36-4). The care plan may include the measures in Box 36-4.

Sometimes distraction, relaxation, and guided imagery are needed. If asked to assist, the nurse tells you what to do.
- *Distraction* means to focus the person's attention on something unrelated to pain. Music, games, singing, praying, TV, and needlework can distract attention.
- *Relaxation* means to be free from mental and physical stress. This state reduces pain and anxiety. The person is taught to breathe deeply and slowly and to contract and relax muscle groups. A comfortable position and a quiet room are important.
- *Guided imagery* is creating and focusing on a relaxing image. The person is coached to relax and focus on a pleasant scene. A calm, soft voice is used to help the person focus. Details are noted in the care plan so staff use the same image and methods. Soft music, a blanket for warmth, and a darkened room may help.

See *Focus on Children and Older Persons: Comfort Measures.*

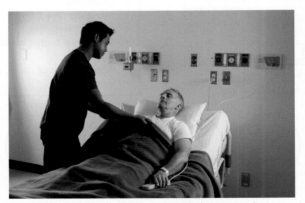

FIGURE 36-4 Measures are implemented to relieve pain. The person is in good alignment with pillows used for comfort. The room is darkened. Blankets provide warmth.

BOX 36-4 Comfort and Pain-Relief Measures

- Position the person in good alignment. Use pillows for support.
- Provide a calm, quiet, darkened setting (see Fig. 36-4).
- Keep bed linens clean, dry, tight, and wrinkle-free.
- Make sure the person is not lying on tubes.
- Assist with elimination needs.
- Adjust the room temperature to meet the person's needs.
- Provide blankets for warmth and to prevent chilling.
- Use correct moving and turning procedures.
- Wait 30 minutes after pain-relief drugs are given to give care or start activities.
- Give a back massage.
- Provide soft music to distract the person.
- Talk softly and gently.
- Use touch to provide comfort.
- Allow family and friends at the bedside as requested by the person.
- Avoid sudden or jarring movements of the bed or chair.
- Handle the person gently.
- Apply warm or cold applications as directed by the nurse (Chapter 43).
- Practice safety measures if the person takes strong pain-relief drugs or sedatives. See "Pain-Relief Drugs."

FOCUS ON CHILDREN AND OLDER PERSONS

Comfort Measures

Children
Pacifiers and favorite toys and blankets can comfort infants and young children. So can holding, rocking, touching, and talking or singing to them. Check with the nurse before you pick up and hold a child. Sometimes children are not held for treatment reasons.

Pain-Relief Drugs. Nurses give ordered pain-relief drugs. The intent is to reduce or relieve pain. Drugs often have side effects. *Side effects (adverse reactions)* are unintended effects that are usually not desired. Side effects depend on the drug used.

Some pain-relief drugs can cause postural hypotension (Chapter 35), drowsiness, dizziness, and coordination problems. Some can cause constipation or nausea and vomiting. Allergic reactions can occur. Severe allergic reactions are emergencies (Chapter 58).

Protect the person from injury and falls when strong pain-relief drugs are used.
- Keep the bed in a low position that is safe and comfortable for the person. Follow the care plan.
- Raise bed rails as directed. Follow the care plan.
- Check on the person every 10 to 15 minutes.
- Provide help when the person needs to stand and walk. Use a transfer/gait belt (Chapter 15).

Follow the care plan for other needed safety measures. Ask the nurse what side effects to report right away.

See *Promoting Safety and Comfort: Pain-Relief Drugs*.

PROMOTING SAFETY AND COMFORT

Pain-Relief Drugs

Safety
Certain pain-relief drugs have the potential to be mis-used. Addiction (Chapter 53) and overdose from use of opioid drugs (Chapter 58) is a growing concern. *Opioids* are a group of drugs that may be prescribed for pain relief. The prescription drugs fentanyl, oxycodone, hydrocodone, codeine, and morphine are examples. Taking too much of such drugs can slow or stop a person's breathing and cause death.

The Centers for Disease Control and Prevention (CDC) reports that nearly 92,000 people died from drug overdoses in 2020. Among those deaths, about 75% involved an opioid. See "Opioid Overdose" for emergency care in Chapter 58.

The Back Massage. The back massage (back rub) can promote comfort and help relieve pain. It relaxes muscles and stimulates circulation. Good times for back massages are after re-positioning, after baths or showers, and with evening care. Back massages last 3 to 5 minutes. Observe the skin before the massage. Look for breaks in the skin, bruises, reddened areas, and other signs of skin breakdown.

Lotion reduces friction during the massage and softens the skin. Warm the lotion before applying it. To warm, rub some lotion between your hands. Or place the bottle in warm water or run it under warm water.

Use firm strokes. Keep your hands in contact with the person's skin. After the massage, apply lotion to the elbows, knees, and heels. Those bony areas are at risk for skin breakdown.

See *Delegation Guidelines: The Back Massage.*
See *Promoting Safety and Comfort: The Back Massage*, p. 570.
See procedure: *Giving a Back Massage*, p. 570.

DELEGATION GUIDELINES

The Back Massage

Giving a back massage is a routine nursing task. Before giving a back massage, you need this information from the nurse and the care plan.
- If the person can have a back massage. See *Promoting Safety and Comfort: The Back Massage*, p. 570.
- How to position the person.
- If the person has position limits. If yes, what are they?
- When to give a back massage.
- If the person needs back massages often for comfort and to relax.
- What observations to report and record:
  - Breaks in the skin
  - Bruising
  - Reddened areas
  - Signs of skin breakdown
- When to report observations.
- What patient or resident concerns to report at once.

PROMOTING SAFETY AND COMFORT

The Back Massage

Safety

Back massages can harm persons with certain heart diseases, back injuries and surgeries, skin diseases, and lung disorders. Check with the nurse and the care plan before giving back massages.

Do not massage reddened bony areas. Reddened areas signal skin breakdown and pressure injuries (Chapter 42).

Do not massage non-intact skin (open skin, skin with breaks). Massage can cause more tissue damage.

Comfort

The prone position is best for a massage. The side-lying position is often used. Older and disabled persons usually find the side-lying position more comfortable.

Giving a Back Massage

QUALITY OF LIFE

- Knock before entering the person's room.
- Address the person by name.
- Introduce yourself by name and title.

- Explain the procedure before starting and during the procedure.
- Protect the person's rights during the procedure.
- Handle the person gently during the procedure.

PRE-PROCEDURE

1 Follow *Delegation Guidelines: The Back Massage*, p. 569. See *Promoting Safety and Comfort: The Back Massage*.
2 Practice hand hygiene.
3 Identify the person. Check the identification (ID) bracelet against the assignment sheet. Use 2 identifiers (Chapter 14). Also call the person by name.

4 Get the following supplies.
   - Bath blanket
   - Bath towel
   - Lotion
   - Laundry bag
5 Provide for privacy.
6 Raise the bed for body mechanics. Bed rails are up if used. Lower the bed rail near you if up.

PROCEDURE

7 Position the person in the prone or side-lying position. The back is toward you.
8 Cover the person with a bath blanket. Expose the back, shoulders, and upper arms.
9 Lay the towel on the bed along the back. Do this if the person is in a side-lying position.
10 Warm the lotion.
11 Explain that the lotion may feel cool and wet.
12 Apply lotion to the lower back area.
13 Stroke up from the lower back to the shoulders. Then stroke down over the upper arms. Stroke up the upper arms, across the shoulders, and down the back (Fig. 36-5). Use firm strokes. Keep your hands in contact with the person's skin.
14 Repeat step 13 for at least 3 minutes.

15 Knead the back (Fig. 36-6).
   a Grasp the skin between your thumb and fingers.
   b Knead half of the back. Start at the lower back and move up to the shoulder. Then knead down from the shoulder to the lower back.
   c Repeat on the other half of the back.
16 Apply lotion to bony areas. Use circular motions with the tips of your index and middle fingers. *(Do not massage reddened bony areas.)*
17 Use fast movements to stimulate. Use slow movements to relax the person.
18 Stroke with long, firm movements to end the massage. Tell the person when you are finishing.
19 Straighten and secure clothing or sleepwear.
20 Cover the person. Remove the towel and bath blanket. Place them in the laundry bag.

POST-PROCEDURE

21 Provide for comfort. (See the inside of the back cover.)
22 Lower the bed to a safe and comfortable level. Raise or lower bed rails. Follow the care plan.
23 Place the call light and other needed items within reach.
24 Return lotion to its proper place. Follow agency policy for used linens.

25 Follow the care plan and the person's preferences for privacy measures to maintain. Leaving the privacy curtain, window coverings, and door open or closed are examples.
26 Complete a safety check of the room. (See the inside of the back cover.)
27 Practice hand hygiene.
28 Report and record your care and observations.

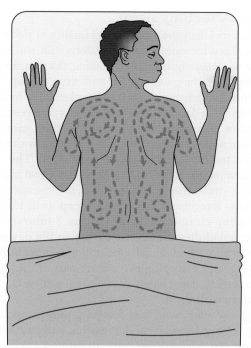

FIGURE 36-5 The person is in the prone position for a back massage. Stroke upward from the lower back to the shoulders, down over the upper arms, back up the upper arms, across the shoulders, and down to the lower back.

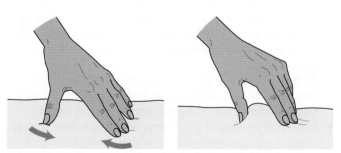

FIGURE 36-6 Knead by picking up tissue between the thumb and fingers.

BOX 36-5	Promoting Rest: Meeting Basic Needs

Physical needs. Thirst and hunger can affect rest. So can pain or discomfort. A comfortable position and good alignment are important. So is a quiet setting with clean, dry, and wrinkle-free linens. People usually rest easier in a clean, neat, and uncluttered room. Elimination needs are met before rest. Incontinent persons must be clean and dry.

Safety and security needs.
- The person must feel safe from injury and falling. Follow the care plan for safety measures (Chapters 14 and 15). Keep the call light and needed items within reach.
- Understanding care helps the person feel safe. Having questions answered can reduce worry. Explain when and how care will be given.
- Many people have rituals or routines before resting. Going to the bathroom, brushing teeth, and washing the face and hands are examples. Some people pray. Some have a snack, lock doors, or make sure loved ones are safe at home. The person may want a certain blanket or other covering. Follow routines and rituals whenever possible.
- Privacy promotes uninterrupted rest. Follow the care plan and the person's preferences for privacy measures.

Love and belonging needs. Visits or calls from family and friends may relax the person. The person knows that others care. Reading cards and letters may be relaxing and restful (Fig. 36-7).

Self-esteem needs.
- Maintaining control and promoting personal choice are important. The person chooses times of rest and how to rest.
- Clothing, hygiene, and grooming can affect dignity and comfort. Patient gowns embarrass some people. Others fear exposure. Many persons rest better in their own sleepwear. Good hygiene and grooming are important. This includes hair care and being clean and odor-free.
- A courteous comment and calling the person by name shows kindness and respect. For example: "Have a nice rest, Mary."

REST

Rest means to be calm, at ease, and relaxed with no anxiety or stress. Rest may involve no activity. Or the person does calming and relaxing things. Some people do crafts, work puzzles, play card games, listen to music, or watch TV. Hobbies can be restful and relaxing. Distraction, relaxation, and guided imagery also promote rest. So does a back massage.

A person is more relaxed when basic needs are met (Box 36-5). Meet food, fluid, and elimination needs before times of rest. The person needs to feel safe, secure, and comfortable. Proper positioning and good alignment promote rest. Provide a quiet and clean setting. Keep the call light within reach. It is comforting to know how to get help if needed.

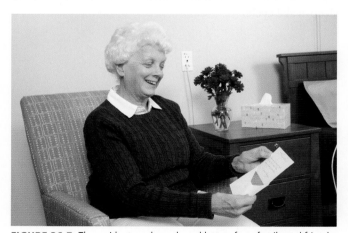

FIGURE 36-7 The resident reads cards and letters from family and friends.

Plan and organize care for uninterrupted rest. A 15- or 20-minute time of rest refreshes some people. Others need more time. Ill or injured persons need to rest often. Some persons need rest before or after a procedure. Some like to rest after meals. Health care routines usually allow for afternoon rest. Be aware of the person's limits. Allow rest when needed.

For some persons, bed rest is required for healing. See Chapter 35.

SLEEP

Sleep is a state of reduced consciousness, reduced voluntary muscle activity, and lowered metabolism. With reduced consciousness, the person can respond to loud noises or gentle shaking. There are no voluntary arm or leg movements during sleep. *Metabolism* is the burning of nutrients to produce energy for the body. Less energy is needed during sleep. Thus metabolism is reduced during sleep. People wake up from sleep.

Sleep is a basic need. The mind and body rest. The body saves energy. Body functions slow. Vital signs are lower than when awake. Tissue healing and repair occur. Sleep lowers stress, tension, and anxiety. It refreshes and renews the person. The person regains energy and mental alertness. The person thinks and functions better after sleep.

Circadian Rhythm

Sleep is part of circadian rhythm. (*Circa* means about. *Dies* means day.) *Circadian rhythm (day-night cycle, body rhythm)* is a daily rhythm based on a 24-hour cycle that involves behavior, sleep, eating, and waking patterns. Primarily a response to light and darkness, circadian rhythm affects functioning.

An important part of circadian rhythm is the sleep-wake cycle. The cycle signals when to sleep and when to wake up. It is why most people feel awake and active during the day and ready for sleep at night. Health care often interferes with a person's circadian rhythm and the sleep-wake cycle. Sleep problems easily occur. Many people work evening and night shifts. Their bodies must adjust to changes in the sleep-wake cycle.

Factors Affecting Sleep

Many factors affect the amount and quality of sleep.

- *Illness.* Illness increases the need for sleep. Pain, nausea, vomiting, coughing, difficulty breathing, diarrhea, frequent voiding, and itching can interfere with sleep. So can treatments and therapies and being awakened for treatments or drugs. Care devices can cause uncomfortable positions.
- *Nutrition.* Sleep needs increase with weight gain and decrease with weight loss. Drinks and foods with caffeine (coffee, tea, colas, chocolate) prevent sleep. The protein *tryptophan* tends to help sleep. It is found in protein sources—milk, cheese, red meat, fish, poultry, and peanuts.
- *Exercise.* Exercise helps people sleep well. However, exercising close to bedtime (within 3 hours) can cause wakefulness. Exercise earlier in the day is best.
- *Sleep setting.* The bed, pillows, noises, temperature, lighting, and a sleeping partner are part of the person's sleep setting. Any change in the usual setting can interfere with sleep.
- *Drugs and other substances.* Sleeping pills promote sleep. Drugs for anxiety, depression, and pain may cause sleep. Some drugs cause nightmares and frequent voiding. Alcohol can interfere with sleep. A stimulant, caffeine prevents sleep. Caffeine is found in some drugs and some drinks and foods. See "Nutrition" above.
- *Life-style changes.* Life-style relates to a person's daily routines and way of living. The person has usual sleep and wake times. Work, school, play, social events, and travel are some factors affecting the person's sleep-wake times.
- *Electronic devices.* Light from electronic devices (TV, computer, phone, tablet) can make falling asleep difficult. Content that is upsetting can keep a person awake.
- *Emotional problems.* Fear, worry, depression, and anxiety affect sleep. Causes include problems with health, money, work, family, and relationships.
- *Age.* Sleep needs vary for each age-group. The amount needed decreases with age. The average adult needs 7 or more hours of sleep per night. See *Focus on Children and Older Persons: Factors Affecting Sleep.*

FOCUS ON CHILDREN AND OLDER PERSONS

Factors Affecting Sleep

Children

Children need more sleep than adults. The table below is a guideline on the amount of sleep needed for each age-group.

Age-Group	Hours of Sleep per Day
Infant	12 to 16 hours
Toddler	11 to 14 hours
Preschool	10 to 13 hours
School Age and Late Childhood	9 to 12 hours
Teenage	8 to 10 hours

Modified from Centers for Disease Control and Prevention: How much sleep do I need?, *Atlanta, Ga., last reviewed September 14, 2022.*

Older Persons

Older adults need about 7 to 9 hours of sleep each night. Some older persons also nap during the day. Plan care for uninterrupted naps.

Sleep problems are common with Alzheimer's disease and other dementias. Night-time wandering is common. Restlessness and confusion often increase at night. This increases the risk of falls. Night-time wandering in a safe and supervised setting is useful for some persons. Others need to be quietly and calmly directed back to their rooms. Measures to promote sleep are tried. See "Promoting Sleep" and Chapter 54. Follow the care plan.

Sleep Disorders

Sleep disorders involve repeated sleep problems. The amount and quality of sleep are affected. Physical and behavioral problems can result. See Box 36-6 for some signs and symptoms of sleep disorders.

- *Insomnia* is a chronic condition in which the person cannot sleep or stay asleep all night.
- *Sleep deprivation* is when the amount and quality of sleep are not adequate, causing reduced function and alertness. Sleep is interrupted. See "Factors Affecting Sleep" for some causes of disrupted sleep.
- *Sleepwalking* is when the person leaves the bed and walks about while sleeping. The person is not aware of sleepwalking and has no memory of the event. The event lasts 3 to 4 minutes or longer. You need to:
  - Protect the person from injury. Falls are a risk. Care tubings (intravenous, catheters, feeding) can cause injury if pulled out of the body when the person gets out of bed.
  - Awaken a sleepwalker gently. The person is easily startled.
  - Guide the person back to bed.
- *Sleep apnea* is when pauses in breathing occur during sleep. *Apnea* is the lack or absence (*a*) of breathing (*pnea*). The usual cause is blockage of the airway from relaxed muscles and tissues. Sleep problems and day-time sleepiness can result. See Chapter 50.

See *Teamwork and Time Management: Sleep Disorders.*

TEAMWORK AND TIME MANAGEMENT

Sleep Disorders

You may find a person sleepwalking. Help the person back to bed even if not assigned to the person's care. Provide for comfort. Then tell the nurse what happened and what you did.

BOX 36-6	Sleep Disorders: Signs and Symptoms

- Agitation
- Attention: decreased
- Coordination: problems with
- Disorientation
- Eyes: red, puffy, dark circles under the eyes
- Fatigue
- Hallucinations (Chapters 53 and 54)
- Irritability
- Memory: reduced word memory; problems finding the right word
- Mood: moodiness; mood swings
- Pulse: irregular
- Reasoning and judgment: decreased
- Responses to questions, conversations, or situations: slowed
- Restlessness
- Sleepiness
- Speech: slurred
- Tremors: in the hands

Promoting Sleep

The nurse assesses the person's sleep patterns. Report any of the signs and symptoms listed in Box 36-6 and your observations about how the person slept. Measures are planned to promote sleep (Box 36-7, p. 574). Follow the care plan.

Bedtime rituals and routines are important. They are allowed if safe. The person may have a bedtime snack or perform hygiene in a certain order. Children and some adults enjoy being read to or reading themselves. Some watch TV if it does not disrupt sleep. Some pray or meditate before sleep.

The person is involved in care planning. The person chooses when to nap or go to bed. The person chooses the measures that promote comfort, rest, and sleep. Follow the care plan and the person's wishes.

See *Focus on Long-Term Care and Home Care: Promoting Sleep,* p. 574.

BOX 36-7	Promoting Sleep

- Plan care for uninterrupted rest.
- Encourage the person to avoid business or family matters before bedtime.
- Allow a flexible bedtime. Bedtime is when the person is tired, not a certain time.
- Provide a comfortable room temperature.
- Let the person take a warm bath or shower.
- Provide a bedtime snack.
- Avoid caffeine (coffee, tea, colas, chocolate).
- Avoid alcoholic beverages.
- Have the person void (urinate) before going to bed.
- Make sure incontinent persons are clean and dry. Change a baby's diaper.
- Have the person wear loose-fitting, comfortable sleepwear.
- Provide for extra warmth (blankets, socks) as needed.
- Make sure linens are clean, dry, and wrinkle-free.
- Position the person in good alignment and in a comfortable position.
- Support body parts as ordered.
- Give a back massage.
- Provide measures to relieve pain.
- Assist with relaxation exercises as ordered.
- Follow bedtime rituals and routines.
- Make sure needed items are within reach.
- Sit and talk with the person.
- Reduce noise.
- Darken the room—close window coverings and the privacy curtain. Shut off or dim lights.
- Dim lights in hallways and the nursing unit.

FOCUS ON LONG-TERM CARE AND HOME CARE

Promoting Sleep

Long-Term Care
Some persons like to check on other residents before going to bed. Some have the duty of turning off lights at bedtime. These actions promote the person's dignity and mental comfort.

FOCUS ON PRIDE

The Person, Family, and Yourself

Personal and Professional Responsibility
Unmanaged pain decreases quality of life. You have an important role in assisting with pain relief. You talk with patients and residents and listen to their needs. Report signs and symptoms of pain. Report what the person said and what you observed. The nurse uses this information to assess, plan, and evaluate pain relief.

Rights and Respect
Your care can either promote comfort and relaxation or cause stress, discomfort, and worry. For example:
- Are you prompt to meet needs?
- Do you ask about the person's preferences?
- Do you communicate in a respectful way?
- Do you allow time for rest?
- Do you leave the person's room clean, neat, and safe?

Take pride in providing care in a way that protects the right to quality of life.

Independence and Social Interaction
A person's emotional, spiritual, and social needs affect comfort. Visits or calls from family and friends can be comforting. Looking at photos of family and friends is enjoyable. For some, religious ceremonies or rituals promote peace and healing. Allow time and privacy for such needs.

Delegation and Teamwork
The health team coordinates care and therapies with pain-relief measures and rest periods. It is common to wait 30 minutes after a pain-relief drug is given to perform procedures and provide care. The nurse tells you how long to wait. The person is allowed to rest after tiring activities, procedures, and therapies. Planning and communication are needed for effective teamwork and quality care.

Ethics and Laws
Questioning what the person says about pain can be harmful. For example, a person rates headache pain as 7 on the 0 to 10 pain rating scale. The person is working on a crossword puzzle and listening to music. When you have a headache, you need to rest in a dark, quiet room. You doubt the person and decide not to tell the nurse. The person really had a bad headache. The person was using the crossword puzzle and music as distractions. Because you did not report the pain, the person did not receive pain-relief measures.

Ignoring a person's pain is wrong. Reporting a different pain rating is wrong. Avoid making judgments about the person's pain. Accurate reporting is needed for proper pain management.

FOCUS ON PRIDE: Application
Family and visitors often provide comfort. How will you welcome the person's visitors? How will you show you value them and their time with the person?

REVIEW QUESTIONS

Circle the BEST answer.

1 A resident says the bed's mattress is very uncomfortable. It disrupts sleep. Which action is *best*?
   a Assure the person that it will get better in time.
   b Suggest that the person sleep in the recliner instead.
   c Report the problem to the nurse.
   d Cover the mattress with pillows.

2 Which statement about pain is *true*?
   a Pain is a warning sign from the body.
   b Age and culture do not affect pain responses.
   c Pain experiences are the same for each person.
   d Pain can be measured with equipment.

3 A person is restless and complains of pain. You should
   a Rate the intensity based on the person's behavior
   b Give a pain-relief drug and tell the nurse
   c Tell the nurse only if you think the person has pain
   d Report the person's exact words

4 A person has had knee pain on and off for several years. This type of pain is
   a Acute pain
   b Chronic pain
   c Radiating pain
   d Not important

5 Moving causes a person pain. The nurse gave a pain-relief drug. When should you give care that involves moving the person?
   a Right before the drug is given
   b Right after the drug is given
   c 30 minutes after the drug is given
   d When you have time

6 A drug was given for pain relief. The nurse said the drug can cause drowsiness and dizziness. To promote safety
   a Keep the bed in the raised position
   b Quickly change positions to avoid dizziness
   c Check on the person every 2 hours
   d Provide help if the person needs to get up

7 Which measure promotes comfort and pain relief?
   a Providing a blanket
   b Speaking loudly
   c Keeping bright lights on in the room
   d Asking about comfort every 5 minutes

8 When giving a back massage
   a Massage for 15 to 20 minutes
   b Warm the lotion before applying it
   c Massage reddened areas
   d Position the person in Fowler's position

9 Which shows that you understand how basic needs affect rest?
   a You leave the call light out of the person's reach.
   b You let an alarm sound for 5 minutes before responding.
   c You help the person to the bathroom before rest.
   d You lay the person down on wet, wrinkled linens.

10 A person tires easily. You are giving morning care. When should the person rest?
   a After you complete morning care
   b After the bath and before hair care
   c After you make the bed
   d When the person needs to

11 A healthy 70-year-old person needs
   a To go to bed by 9:00 PM (2100)
   b To sleep more during the day than at night
   c 7 to 9 hours of sleep each night
   d 10 to 12 hours of sleep each night

12 Which statement about sleep is *true*?
   a Sleep increases stress, tension, and anxiety.
   b Persons with dementia usually sleep well at night.
   c The body does not heal during sleep.
   d Sleep deprivation can affect functioning.

13 Which can prevent sleep?
   a Cheese
   b Chocolate
   c Milk
   d Beef

14 Which measure before bedtime promotes sleep?
   a Following the person's routines
   b Asking the person about family matters
   c Providing hot tea
   d Leaving the hallway light on

Answers to Chapter 36 questions are on p. 903.

FOCUS ON PRACTICE

Problem Solving

Prioritize the following comfort needs. Which would you do first, second, third, and last? Explain the reasons for the order.
- Provide a blanket.
- Report chest pain that began suddenly.
- Help a person who received a pain-relief drug 1 hour ago to the bathroom.
- Provide a back massage before bedtime.

OBJECTIVES

- Define the key terms and key abbreviations in this chapter.
- Describe your role in admissions, transfers, discharges, and moving the person to a new room.
- Explain how to help the person and family feel safe in the health care setting.
- Identify the rules for measuring weight and height.

- Explain why a person is moved to a new room within the agency.
- Perform the procedures described in this chapter.
- Explain how to promote PRIDE in the person, the family, and yourself.

KEY TERMS

admission Official entry of a person into a health care setting
discharge Official departure of a person from a health care setting

transfer Moving the person to another health care setting; moving the person to a new room within the agency

KEY ABBREVIATIONS

CMS	Centers for Medicare & Medicaid Services	in	Inch; inches
ft	Foot; feet	lb	Pound; pounds
ID	Identification		

*A*dmission is the official entry of a person into a health care setting. It can cause anxiety and fear in patients, residents, and families. Worries and fears about serious health problems, treatments, surgeries, and pain are common.

The setting is new and strange. Patients, residents, and families may have concerns and fears about:
- Where to go, what to do, and what to expect
- Never returning home
- Who gives care, how care is given, and if the correct care is given
- Finding the bathroom
- Getting meals
- How to get help
- Being abused
- Strange sights and sounds
- Being apart from family and friends
- Making new friends
- Leaving homes and possessions behind

Moving to another room may cause similar concerns. So may a transfer to another hospital or nursing center. Discharge to a home setting is usually a happy time. However, the person may need home care.

Transfer and discharge are defined as follows.
- *Transfer* is moving the person to another health care setting. In some agencies it also means moving the person to a new room within the agency.
- *Discharge* is the official departure of a person from a health care setting.

Admission, transfer, and discharge are critical events. So is moving to a new room. The new room may be on another nursing unit. These events involve:
- Privacy and confidentiality
- Understanding and communicating with the person
- Communicating with the health team
- Respect for the person and the person's property
- Being kind, courteous, and respectful
- Reporting and recording

See *Focus on Long-Term Care and Home Care: Admissions, Transfers, and Discharges.*

See *Teamwork and Time Management: Admissions, Transfers, and Discharges.*

See *Delegation Guidelines: Admissions, Transfers, and Discharges.*

See *Promoting Safety and Comfort: Admissions, Transfers, and Discharges.*

FOCUS ON LONG-TERM CARE AND HOME CARE

Admissions, Transfers, and Discharges

Long-Term Care

The Centers for Medicare & Medicaid Services (CMS) has standards for nursing center transfers and discharges. The person's rights are protected. An ombudsman protects the person's interests.

Reasons for a transfer or discharge include:

- The person's needs cannot be met in the center. The move is necessary for the person's welfare (well-being).
- The person's health has improved. The center's services are no longer needed.
- The health or safety of others is in danger.
- The person has not paid to stay in the center.
- The center closes.

The person and family are told of the date and time of the transfer or discharge. They are given the name and location where the person will be going.

TEAMWORK AND TIME MANAGEMENT

Admissions, Transfers, and Discharges

Transfers, discharges, and changing rooms are easier when staff work together. When asking for help, politely share:

- What you need help with
- When you will need help
- How much time it will take

Remember to thank your co-worker for helping you.

DELEGATION GUIDELINES

Admissions, Transfers, and Discharges

Assisting with admissions, transfers, and discharges are routine nursing tasks. You need this information from the nurse.

- If the person is being admitted, transferred, discharged, or moved to a new room
- If moving to a new room, the person's new room and bed number
- The transportation method to or from the agency—car, ambulance, or wheelchair van
- How the person will move about within the agency—walking, wheelchair, stretcher, or bed
- The person's room and bed number
- What equipment and supplies are needed
- If the person will wear clothes, a patient gown, or sleepwear
- If the person stays in bed or can be in a chair
- When to report observations
- What patient or resident concerns to report at once

PROMOTING SAFETY AND COMFORT

Admissions, Transfers, and Discharges

Safety

The person may develop pain or distress during admission, transfer, discharge, or when moving to a new room. If so, call for the nurse at once. Stay with the person. Assist the nurse as needed.

Follow agency policies for transporting persons requiring Transmission-Based Precautions. See Chapter 18.

Comfort

Admission, transfer, or discharge may be stressful for the person. So may moving to a new room. Some persons are happy. Others are sad and fearful. Some anxiety is normal. To provide mental comfort:

- Explain what you are doing and why.
- Do not rush the person.
- Be sensitive to the person's needs and feelings.

ADMISSIONS

The admission process usually starts in the admitting office. It may start in a hospital emergency room (ER). Admitting staff or a nurse obtains identifying information for the admission record—full name, age, birth date, and so on.

The person is given an identification (ID) number and often an ID bracelet (Chapter 14). The person or legal representative signs admitting papers and a general consent for treatment.

The nursing unit is told when to expect a new patient or resident. The person's room and bed number are given. In some agencies, the person can walk to the room if able. Most persons require transport by wheelchair or stretcher.

Preparing the Room

You prepare the room for the person's arrival. Figure 37-1 shows a room ready for a new resident.

See procedure: *Preparing the Person's Room*, p. 578.

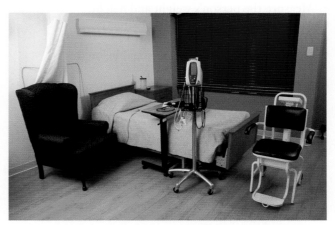

FIGURE 37-1 The room is ready for a new resident.

Preparing the Person's Room

PROCEDURE

1 Follow *Delegation Guidelines: Admissions, Transfers, and Discharges,* p. 577.
2 Practice hand hygiene and get the following supplies.
   - Admission kit—wash basin, soap, toothpaste, toothbrush, water mug, and so on
   - Nursing assistant admission checklist (if used) (Fig. 37-2)
   - Thermometer
   - Stethoscope and blood pressure equipment
   - Pulse oximeter (Chapter 44)
   - Patient gown or sleepwear (if needed)
   - Towels and washcloths
   - IV (intravenous) pole (if needed)
   - Bedpan and urinal (if needed)
   - Other items requested by the nurse
3 Place the following on the over-bed table.
   - Thermometer
   - Stethoscope and blood pressure equipment
   - Pulse oximeter (Chapter 44)
   - Nursing assistant admission checklist

4 Place the water mug on the bedside stand or over-bed table.
5 Place the following in the bedside stand.
   - Admission kit
   - Bedpan and urinal
   - Patient gown or sleepwear
   - Towels and washcloths
6 *If the person arrives by stretcher:*
   a Make a surgical bed (Chapter 22).
   b Raise the bed for a transfer from a stretcher.
   c Keep the call light off of the bed.
7 *If the person is ambulatory or arrives by wheelchair:*
   a Leave the bed closed.
   b Lower the bed to a safe and comfortable level as directed by the nurse.
   c Attach the call light to the bed linens.
8 Place the IV pole (if needed) next to the head of the bed.
9 Practice hand hygiene.

Admitting the Person

A nurse usually greets and escorts the person and family to the room. You might do so if the person has no discomfort or distress.

Admission is your first chance to make a good impression. You must:
- Greet the person by name and title. Use the admission record to find out the person's name.
- Introduce yourself by name and title to the person, family, and friends.
- Act in a professional manner.
- Treat the person with dignity and respect.

See *Focus on Long-Term Care and Home Care: Admitting the Person.*

The Admission Procedure.
During the admission procedure the nurse may ask you to:
- Measure the person's weight and height.
- Measure vital signs and pulse oximetry.
- Obtain a urine specimen.
- Complete a clothing and personal belongings list.
- Orient the person to the room, the nursing unit, and the agency.

See procedure: *Admitting the Person,* p. 580.

FOCUS ON LONG-TERM CARE AND HOME CARE

Admitting the Person

Long-Term Care

In nursing centers, admission procedures are often started 2 or 3 days before the person enters the center. Needed information is obtained from the person or family member.

Some residents arrive by ambulance or wheelchair van. The attendants take them to their assigned rooms. Some arrive by car. The nurses or nursing assistants take them to their rooms. Often a family member is present.

A nurse or social worker explains the resident's rights to the person and family. They also receive written matter explaining them.

The person's photo is taken. The person may receive an ID bracelet. Photos or ID bracelets are used to identify the person (Chapter 14).

Do not rush admission procedures. Rather, treat the person and family as guests in your home. Offer a beverage. Visit with them. Tell them nice things about the center.

Introduce roommates and other residents. Knowing other residents provides comfort and support. Residents understand, better than anyone else, what a nursing center is like.

The center is the person's home. Make the room as home-like as possible. You may help with unpacking and putting clothes away. The person may have pictures or photos to hang or display. Show care and compassion. Help the person feel safe, comfortable, and secure.

Persons with dementia and their families may need extra help during the admission process. Often confusion increases in a new setting. Fear, agitation, and wanting to leave are common. The family also is fearful. Many feel guilty about the need for nursing center care. You assist in helping the person and family feel safe and welcome.

Admission is often an emotional time for the person and family. They do not part until ready to do so. Remember, the center is now the person's home.

ADMISSION CHECKLIST

Preferred name *Sam*   ID *278-64593*

Measurements

Weight *195* **lb**

☐ Standing scale
☑ Chair scale
☐ Wheelchair scale
☐ Wheelchair weight _____ lb

Height *5* **ft** *10* **in**

Pain

Location ___*Low back*___
Intensity *3*
Description ___*Aching*___

Vital signs

Temperature *98.2* °F

☑ Oral   ☐ Axillary
☐ Rectal   ☐ Tympanic membrane

Pulse *78*
Respirations *20*
Blood pressure *122/84* mm Hg

☑ Right arm   ☑ Lying
☐ Left arm   ☐ Sitting

Pulse oximetry *98* %

Care Measures

Assist with garments

☑ Dressed
☐ Patient gown
☐ Sleepwear

Items within reach

☑ Filled water mug
☑ Call light
☑ TV and light controls
☑ Needed/requested items

Assist to

☑ Bed
☐ Chair
☐ Other _____

Belongings

☑ Label personal property and care items.
☑ Provide and label denture cup.
☑ Complete the clothing and personal belongings lists.
☑ Place clothes and personal items in closet, drawers, and bedside stand.

Orient Person and Family to Setting

Room

☑ Call light
☑ Bed, TV, and light controls
☑ Items in the bedside stand
☑ Over-bed table
☑ Electrical outlets for charging electronic devices
☑ Phone and phone calls
☑ Bathroom and bathroom call light

Agency

☑ Names of nurses, nursing assistants, and other staff
☑ Visiting hours and policies
☑ Internet access
☑ Nurses' station
☑ Lounge
☑ Chapel or quiet area
☑ Dining room
☑ Meal and snack times

Safety and Comfort

☑ Bed at a safe and comfortable level
☑ Bed rails raised
☐ Bed rails lowered
☑ Safety check of room

☑ Ask about comfort needs
☑ Comfort measures: *Provided a blanket, raised head of bed to level of comfort, reported pain to nurse*

Nursing assistant *C. Collins, CNA*   Checklist given to *J. Miller, RN*   Date *11/24* Time *1415*

FIGURE 37-2 A sample nursing assistant admission checklist.

Admitting the Person

QUALITY OF LIFE

- Knock before entering the person's room.
- Address the person by name.
- Introduce yourself by name and title.

- Explain the procedure before starting and during the procedure.
- Protect the person's rights during the procedure.
- Handle the person gently during the procedure.

PRE-PROCEDURE

1 Follow *Delegation Guidelines: Admissions, Transfers, and Discharges*, p. 577. See *Promoting Safety and Comfort: Admissions, Transfers, and Discharges*, p. 577.

2 Practice hand hygiene.
3 Prepare the room. See procedure: *Preparing the Person's Room*, p. 578.

PROCEDURE

4 Practice hand hygiene.
5 Identify the person. Use 2 identifiers (Chapter 14). Check the information in the admission record and on the ID bracelet.
6 Greet the person by name. Ask what name the person prefers.
7 Introduce yourself to the person and others present. Give your name and title. Explain that you assist the nurses in giving care.
8 Introduce the roommate.
9 Provide for privacy. Ask family or friends to leave the room unless the person prefers that someone stay. Tell them how much time you need and direct them to the waiting area.
10 Let the person stay dressed if the person's condition permits. Or help with changing into a patient gown or sleepwear.
11 Provide for comfort. The person is in bed or in a chair as directed by the nurse.
12 Assist the nurse with assessment.
  a Measure vital signs and pulse oximetry.
  b Measure weight and height.
  c Collect information on the nursing assistant admission checklist.
13 Orient the person and family to the area.
  a Give names of the nurses and nursing assistants (Fig. 37-3).
  b Explain the purpose of items in the bedside stand.
  c Explain how to use the over-bed table.

  d Show how to use the call light.
  e Show the person the bathroom. Explain how to use the call light in the bathroom.
  f Show how to use bed, TV, and light controls.
  g Explain how to use the agency's phone. Place the phone within reach.
  h Explain how to connect to the Internet.
  i Show the electrical outlets for charging electronic devices.
  j Explain where to find the nurses' station, lounge, chapel, dining room, and other areas.
  k Identify staff—housekeeping, dietary, physical therapy, and others. Also identify students who are in the agency.
  l Explain when meals and snacks are served.
  m Explain visiting hours and policies.
14 Fill the water mug if oral fluids are allowed.
15 Place the call light within reach.
16 Place other controls and needed items within reach.
17 Provide a denture cup if needed. Label it with the person's name and room and bed number.
18 Label the person's property and personal care items with the person's name (if not done by the family). Follow agency policy for labeling items.
19 Complete a clothing and personal belongings list (Chapter 14). Follow agency policy for labeling clothing.
20 Help the person put away clothes and personal items. Use the closet, drawers, and bedside stand. (The family may help with this step.)

POST-PROCEDURE

21 Provide for comfort. (See the inside of the back cover.)
22 Make sure the bed is at a safe and comfortable level. Check that bed rails are raised or lowered as needed. Follow the nurse's directions.
23 Remind the person that the call light is nearby to call for staff. Ask if the person has any other needs right away.

24 Follow the person's preferences for privacy measures to maintain.
25 Complete a safety check of the room. (See the inside of the back cover.)
26 Practice hand hygiene.
27 Report and record your care and observations.

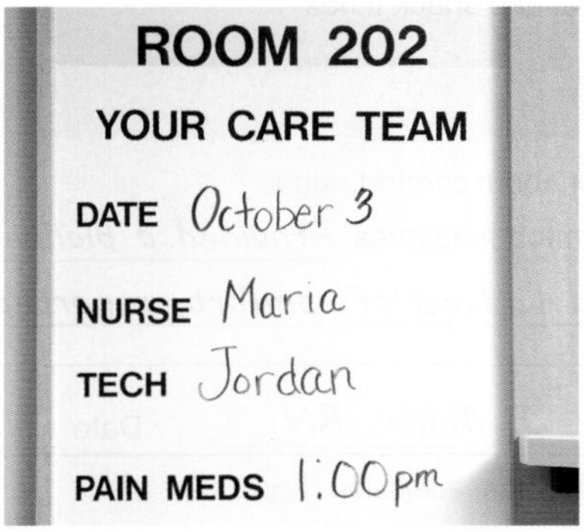

ROOM 202

YOUR CARE TEAM

DATE October 3

NURSE Maria

TECH Jordan

PAIN MEDS 1:00 pm

FIGURE 37-3 The names of nursing team members are posted on a marker board.

Weight and Height

Weight and height are measured on admission. Then the person is weighed daily, weekly, or monthly. This is done to measure weight gain or loss.

A standing scale (Fig. 37-4) is used for persons able to stand and walk. Wheelchair scales (Fig. 37-5) are also common. A person can sit in a chair scale (Fig. 37-6). Some beds and mechanical lifts (Chapter 21) contain scales.

Accurate measurements are important. Consistency matters. To measure weight and height, follow the guidelines in Box 37-1 (p. 582).

See *Teamwork and Time Management: Weight and Height*, p. 582.

See *Delegation Guidelines: Weight and Height*, p. 582.

See *Focus on Math: Weight and Height*, p. 582.

See procedure: *Measuring Weight and Height With a Standing Scale*, p. 584.

See procedure: *Measuring Height—The Person Is in Bed*, p. 585.

To use a wheelchair scale:

1. Weigh the person's wheelchair while the person is in bed or in a chair. Note the wheelchair's weight.

2. Weigh the person while seated in the wheelchair.

3. Subtract the weight of the wheelchair (weight from step 1) from the weight of the person in the wheelchair (weight from step 2). This is the person's weight.

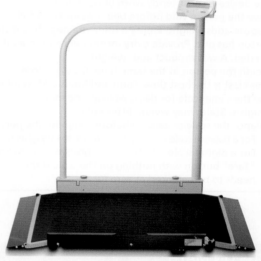

FIGURE 37-5 Wheelchair scale. (NOTE: This is a digital scale.) (Scale image courtesy Seca Corp., Chino, Calif.)

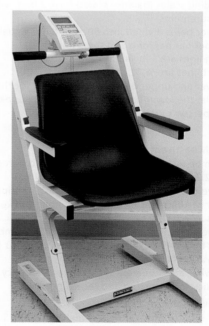

FIGURE 37-6 Chair scale.

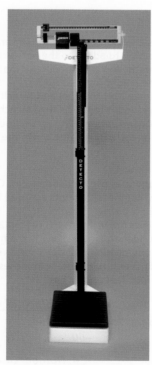

FIGURE 37-4 Standing scale. (NOTE: This is a balance scale.)

BOX 37-1   Measuring Weight and Height

- Follow the manufacturer's instructions for the scale used.
- Practice safety measures to prevent falls. See Chapter 15.
- Protect the person from chilling and drafts. See Chapter 13.
- Have the person wear similar clothing for repeated measurements. Wearing a patient gown or sleepwear is best. Clothes add weight. Footwear adds to the weight and height measurements.
- Know if the person wears or removes a prosthesis (Chapter 49) or other device for a weight measurement. The device is consistently worn or not worn.
- Have the person void before being weighed. A full bladder adds weight. Empty a urine drainage bag if the person has one. Provide a dry incontinence product if needed. A wet product adds weight.
- Weigh the person at the same time of day. Before breakfast is the best time. Food and fluids add weight.
- Use the same scale for daily, weekly, and monthly weights. Scales may weigh differently.
- Balance the scale at zero (0) before weighing the person.
  - For a balance scale (see Fig. 37-4), move the weights to zero.
  - For a digital scale (see Fig. 37-5), press the "Zero" or "Tare" button with nothing on the scale if the scale needs to be balanced at zero (0).

TEAMWORK AND TIME MANAGEMENT
Weight and Height

Nursing units usually have just 1 standing scale. In some agencies, chair, wheelchair, and lift scales are shared with other nursing units. Return the device to the storage area as soon as possible. Do not have your co-workers wait or look for the scale.

DELEGATION GUIDELINES
Weight and Height

Measuring weight and height are routine nursing tasks. You need this information from the nurse and the care plan.
- When to measure weight and height
- What scale to use
- If height is measured with the person in bed
- What measurements to use (see *Focus on Math: Weight and Height*)
- When to report the measurements
- What patient or resident concerns to report at once

FOCUS ON MATH
Weight and Height

Weight—Reading the Scale
Standing scales (balance scales) have 2 bars with measurements (Fig. 37-7).
- The lower bar is divided into 50 pound (lb) values.
- The upper bar has long and short lines.
  - Long lines are 1 lb values.
  - Short lines are ¼, ½, and ¾ lb values.

The lower and upper bar values are added for the weight. For example, *the lower bar is at 100 lb and the upper bar is at 34 lb. The person's weight is 134 lb.*

100 lb + 34 lb = 134 lb

Weight—Measurements
Weight can be measured in pounds (lb) or kilograms (kg). There are 2.2 pounds in 1 kilogram (2.2 lb = 1 kg).
- To convert (change) kilograms to pounds, multiply the number of kilograms by 2.2. For example: *100 kg is the same as 220 lb (100 kg × 2.2 = 220 lb).*
- To convert pounds to kilograms, divide the number of pounds by 2.2. For example: *32 lb is the same as 14.5 kg (32 lb ÷ 2.2 = 14.5 kg).*

Know what measurement is used in your agency. Follow agency policy for reporting and recording.

Weight—Wheelchair Scales
See Figure 37-5 for how to use a wheelchair scale. Subtract the weight of the wheelchair from the weight of the person in the wheelchair. For example, *the person's wheelchair weighs 35 lb. The weight of the person and the wheelchair is 200 lb.*

200 lb (weight of the person and wheelchair) – 35 lb (wheelchair's weight) = 165 lb

The person weighs 165 lb.

Height—Reading the Height Rod
The height rod has 2 sections—upper and lower. Raise or lower the upper section to adjust to the person's height. If the person is taller than the lower section, read the height at the movable part of the height rod.

The rod is marked with 1 inch (in) and ¼ inch values (¼, ½, and ¾). Read height to the nearest ¼ inch. The numbers on the lower section increase moving *up* the rod. The numbers on the upper section increase moving *down* the rod. See Figure 37-8.

Height—Measurements
For height, some agencies use feet and inches. Others only use inches. Know what measurements are used in your agency.

There are 12 inches (in) in 1 foot (ft) (1 ft = 12 in). To convert inches into feet and inches, divide the number of inches by 12. Use long division. If it does not divide evenly by 12, the number left over is the number of inches. *For example: Convert 64 inches into feet and inches.*

5 Number of feet
12 Inches per foot | 64 Inches
–60
4 Number of inches

64 inches = 5 ft 4 in

FOCUS ON MATH—cont'd

Weight and Height

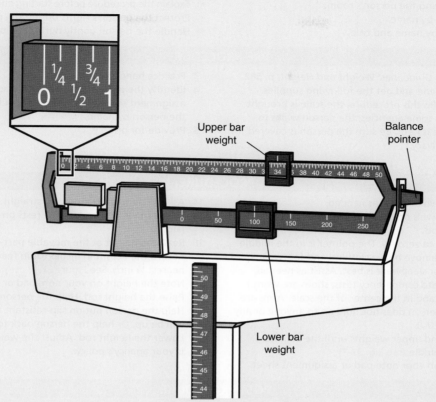

Upper bar weight

Balance pointer

Lower bar weight

FIGURE 37-7 A balance scale. The lower bar weight is at 100 lb. The upper bar weight is at 34 lb. The weight is 134 lb (100 lb + 34 lb = 134 lb).

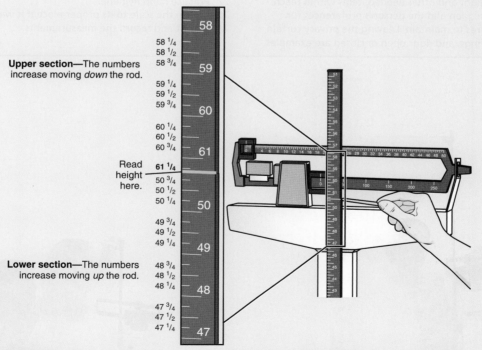

Upper section—The numbers increase moving *down* the rod.

Read height here.

Lower section—The numbers increase moving *up* the rod.

FIGURE 37-8 Height is read at the movable part of the height rod. (Note: The movable part of the height rod is marked with a yellow line.) This height rod measures 61¼ inches (5 feet 1¼ inches).

Measuring Weight and Height With a Standing Scale

QUALITY OF LIFE

- Knock before entering the person's room.
- Address the person by name.
- Introduce yourself by name and title.

- Explain the procedure before starting and during the procedure.
- Protect the person's rights during the procedure.
- Handle the person gently during the procedure.

PRE-PROCEDURE

1 Follow *Delegation Guidelines: Weight and Height*, p. 582.
2 Practice hand hygiene and get the following supplies.
   - Standing scale (In this procedure, the scale is brought to the room. In some agencies, the person walks to where the scale is kept. Be sure the person is covered for warmth and privacy.)
   - Paper towels

3 Practice hand hygiene.
4 Identify the person. Check the ID bracelet against the assignment sheet. Use 2 identifiers (Chapter 14). Also call the person by name.
5 Provide for privacy.

PROCEDURE

6 Ask the person to void. Assist as needed.
7 Place the paper towels on the scale platform.
8 Raise the height rod.
9 Move the weights to zero (0). The pointer is in the middle.
10 Have the person remove heavy clothing and footwear. Wearing a gown or sleepwear is best. Assist as needed. (NOTE: For some state competency tests, shoes are worn.)
11 Help the person stand in the center of the scale. Arms are at the sides. The person does not hold on to anyone or anything. See Figure 37-9.
12 Move the lower and upper weights until the balance pointer is in the middle (see Fig. 37-7).
13 Note the weight on your note pad or assignment sheet.

14 Ask the person to stand very straight.
15 Lower the height rod until it rests on the person's head (Fig. 37-10).
16 Read the height at the movable part of the height rod. Record the height in inches (or in feet and inches) to the nearest ¼ inch. See Figure 37-8.
17 Note the height on your note pad or assignment sheet.
18 Raise the height rod. Help the person step off of the scale.
19 Help the person put on slip-resistant footwear if the person will be up. Or help the person back to bed.
20 Lower the height rod. Adjust the weights to zero (0) if this is your agency's policy.

POST-PROCEDURE

21 Provide for comfort. (See the inside of the back cover.)
22 Make sure the bed is at a safe and comfortable level. Raise or lower bed rails. Follow the care plan.
23 Place the call light and other needed items within reach.
24 Follow the care plan and the person's preferences for privacy measures to maintain. Leaving the privacy curtain, window coverings, and door open or closed are examples.

25 Complete a safety check of the room. (See the inside of the back cover.)
26 Discard the paper towels.
27 Practice hand hygiene.
28 Return the scale to its proper place if it was moved.
29 Report and record the measurements.

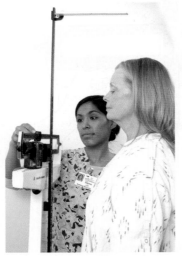

FIGURE 37-9 The person is weighed.

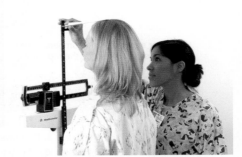

FIGURE 37-10 The height rod rests on the person's head.

Measuring Height—The Person Is in Bed

QUALITY OF LIFE

- Knock before entering the person's room.
- Address the person by name.
- Introduce yourself by name and title.

- Explain the procedure before starting and during the procedure.
- Protect the person's rights during the procedure.
- Handle the person gently during the procedure.

PRE-PROCEDURE

1 Follow *Delegation Guidelines: Weight and Height*, p. 582.
2 Practice hand hygiene and get a measuring tape and ruler.
3 Ask a co-worker to help you.
4 Practice hand hygiene.

5 Identify the person. Check the ID bracelet against the assignment sheet. Use 2 identifiers (Chapter 14). Also call the person by name.
6 Provide for privacy.
7 Raise the bed for body mechanics. Bed rails are up if used. Lower the bed rails (if up).

PROCEDURE

8 Position the person supine if the position is allowed. (Some persons cannot straighten due to contractures or abnormal curvature of the spine. Follow the nurse's directions for positioning and measurement.)
9 Position the tape measure and ruler (Fig. 37-11).
   a Have your co-worker place and hold the beginning of the tape measure at the person's heel.
   b Pull the other end of the tape measure along the person's body. Pull it until it extends a few inches past the head.
   c Place the ruler flat across the top of the person's head and across the tape measure. Make sure the ruler is level.

10 Read the height measurement. This is the point where the lower edge of the ruler touches the tape measure.
11 Note the height measurement on your note pad or assignment sheet.

POST-PROCEDURE

12 Provide for comfort. (See the inside of the back cover.)
13 Lower the bed to a safe and comfortable level. Raise or lower bed rails. Follow the care plan.
14 Place the call light and other needed items within reach.
15 Complete a safety check of the room. (See the inside of the back cover.)

16 Follow the care plan and the person's preferences for privacy measures to maintain. Leaving the privacy curtain, window coverings, and door open or closed are examples.
17 Practice hand hygiene.
18 Return equipment to its proper place.
19 Report and record the height.

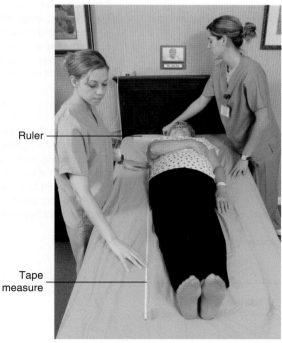

FIGURE 37-11 Height is measured in bed. The tape measure extends from the heel to the top of the head. The ruler is flat across the top of the person's head.

MOVING THE PERSON TO A NEW ROOM

Sometimes a person is moved to a new room. Reasons include:

- A change in condition.
- The person requests a room change.
- Roommates do not get along.
- Care needs change.

The doctor, nurse, or social worker explains the reasons for the move to the person and family. You assist with the move or perform the entire procedure. The person is transported by wheelchair, stretcher, or the bed.

Support and reassure the person. If the new room is on another nursing unit, the person does not know the staff. Use good communication skills.

- Avoid pat answers. "It will be okay" is an example.
- Use touch to provide comfort.
- Introduce the person to the staff and roommate.
- Wish the person well as you leave.
  See procedure: *Moving the Person to a New Room.*

Moving the Person to a New Room

QUALITY OF LIFE

- Knock before entering the person's room.
- Address the person by name.
- Introduce yourself by name and title.

- Explain the procedure before starting and during the procedure.
- Protect the person's rights during the procedure.
- Handle the person gently during the procedure.

PRE-PROCEDURE

1 Follow *Delegation Guidelines: Admissions, Transfers, and Discharges*, p. 577. See *Promoting Safety and Comfort: Admissions, Transfers, and Discharges*, p. 577.
2 Practice hand hygiene and get the following supplies.
   - Wheelchair or stretcher
   - Utility cart
   - Bags for belongings
   - Bath blanket

3 Ask a co-worker to help you.
4 Practice hand hygiene.
5 Identify the person. Check the ID bracelet against the assignment sheet. Use 2 identifiers (Chapter 14). Call the person by name.
6 Provide for privacy.

PROCEDURE

7 Place the person's belongings in bags if needed. Place the belongings and any care equipment to be transferred on the cart.
8 Transfer the person to a wheelchair or stretcher (Chapter 21). Cover the person with the bath blanket.
9 Transport the person to the new room. Your co-worker brings the cart.
10 Help transfer the person to the bed or chair. Help position the person (Chapters 19 and 21).

11 Help arrange the person's belongings and equipment.
12 Introduce yourself to the receiving nurse by name and title. Report the following.
   - How the person tolerated the transfer
   - Observations made during the transfer
   - That a nurse from the previous unit will communicate and answer questions about care
13 Practice hand hygiene.

POST-PROCEDURE

14 Return the wheelchair or stretcher and the cart to the storage area.
15 Report and record the following.
   - The time of the transfer
   - Who helped you with the transfer
   - Where the person was taken
   - How the person was transferred (bed, wheelchair, or stretcher)
   - How the person tolerated the transfer
   - Who received the person
   - Other observations

16 Remove bed linens and clean the unit if it is your job. Practice hand hygiene and wear gloves for this step. (The housekeeping staff may do this step.)
17 Remove and discard the gloves. Practice hand hygiene.
18 Make a closed bed (Chapter 22).
19 Follow agency policy for used linens.
20 Practice hand hygiene.

TRANSFERS AND DISCHARGES

Transfers and discharges are usually planned in advance. The person goes home or to another agency. If being discharged to home, the health team teaches the person and family about diet, exercise, drugs, procedures, and treatments. Home care, equipment, and therapies are arranged as needed. A doctor's appointment is given.

The nurse tells you when to start the transfer or discharge procedure and when the person is ready to leave. Usually a wheelchair is used. If leaving by ambulance, a stretcher is used.

Use good communication skills during a transfer or discharge. Wish the person and family well as they leave the agency.

A person may want to leave the agency without the doctor's permission. Tell the nurse at once. The nurse or social worker handles the matter.

See procedure: *Transferring or Discharging the Person.*

Transferring or Discharging the Person

QUALITY OF LIFE

- Knock before entering the person's room.
- Address the person by name.
- Introduce yourself by name and title.
- Explain the procedure before starting and during the procedure.
- Protect the person's rights during the procedure.
- Handle the person gently during the procedure.

PRE-PROCEDURE

1 Follow *Delegation Guidelines: Admissions, Transfers, and Discharges*, p. 577. See *Promoting Safety and Comfort: Admissions, Transfers, and Discharges*, p. 577.
2 Practice hand hygiene and get the following supplies as needed.
   - Wheelchair
   - Utility cart
   - Bags for belongings
3 Ask a co-worker to help you.
4 Practice hand hygiene.
5 Identify the person. Check the ID bracelet against the assignment sheet. Use 2 identifiers (Chapter 14). Also call the person by name.
6 Provide for privacy.

PROCEDURE

7 Help the person dress as needed.
8 Help the person pack. Place belongings in bags if needed. Check the bathroom and all drawers and closets. Make sure all items are collected.
9 Check off the clothing list and personal belongings list. Give the lists to the nurse.
10 Tell the nurse that the person is ready for the final visit. The nurse:
   a Gives needed prescriptions.
   b Provides discharge instructions.
   c Returns valuables from the safe.
   d Has the person sign the clothing and personal belongings lists.
11 *For the person leaving by wheelchair:*
   a Get a wheelchair and a utility cart for the person's items. Ask a co-worker to help you.
   b Help the person into the wheelchair.
   c Take the person to the exit area.
   d Lock (brake) the wheelchair wheels.
   e Help the person into the vehicle (Fig. 37-12, p. 588).
   f Help put the person's items into the vehicle.
12 *For the person leaving by ambulance:*
   a If you will leave the room, perform the usual post-procedure comfort and safety steps. Return to assist when the ambulance attendants arrive.
   b Raise the bed for a transfer to the stretcher. Assist with the transfer as directed (Chapter 21).
13 Practice hand hygiene.

POST-PROCEDURE

14 Return the wheelchair and cart to the storage area if used.
15 Report and record the following.
   - The time of the discharge
   - Who helped you with the procedure
   - How the person was transported
   - Who was with the person
   - The person's destination
   - Other observations
16 Remove bed linens and clean the unit if it is your job. Practice hand hygiene and wear gloves for this step. (The housekeeping staff may do this step.)
17 Remove and discard the gloves. Practice hand hygiene.
18 Make a closed bed (Chapter 22).
19 Follow agency policy for used linens.
20 Practice hand hygiene.

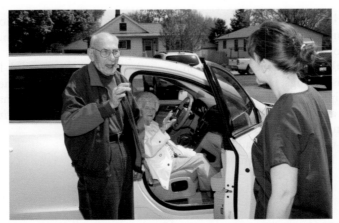

FIGURE 37-12 The resident in the car is being discharged.

FOCUS ON PRIDE

The Person, Family, and Yourself

Personal and Professional Responsibility

Admission to a hospital or nursing center is often hard for the person and family. Transfers and discharges also can cause fear and worry. To help the person adjust:

- Be courteous, caring, efficient, and competent.
- Be sensitive to fears and concerns.
- Handle the person's belongings carefully and with respect. Protect them from loss or damage.
- Focus on the person and family. Do not rush. Do not discuss other work you need to do.
- Treat the person and family like you want your loved ones treated.

Rights and Respect

Know your agency's rules for visitors. Do not assume that all units or agencies have the same rules. For example, psychiatric, intensive care, and pediatric units often have special rules. Give the person and visitors correct information. If you do not know, ask the nurse.

The person has the right to decide who can visit. Tell the nurse about the person's requests.

Independence and Social Interaction

A new setting brings social challenges. In a nursing center, the first hours and days can be lonely. The person can feel isolated and depressed.

You can help with these social challenges. Visit new residents and introduce them to other residents. Encourage them to take part in activities. Observe for and report social isolation or roommate troubles. Make sure your interactions are pleasant.

Delegation and Teamwork

The family often wants to be present during admissions, transfers, and discharges. They may have questions or need to answer questions. If the person consents, the family may be present.

Sometimes privacy is needed. For example, the nurse may need to ask about personal or embarrassing topics. Or the person needs to get dressed. The nurse may have you manage and assist the family when privacy is needed. The family is important. To show care and concern:

- Take them to the waiting area.
- Offer coffee or water while they wait.
- Show where they can get food and drinks.
- Tell them where they can make phone calls.
- Ask if there is anything they need.

Ethics and Laws

Before discharge, the person receives discharge instructions. Common information includes drugs to continue or stop, new prescriptions, activity, diet, appointments, and special care instructions. The nurse explains the information, provides teaching, and answers questions. The information is given orally and in writing.

You may be tempted to give the person the information. Discharge teaching is beyond the scope of your role. You may provide wrong information. The person can be harmed.

If a person asks you about discharge instructions, say: "The nurse will give you information and answer your questions before you leave." Take pride in following the limits of your role.

FOCUS ON PRIDE: Application

Admissions, transfers, and discharges take time. You may be busy and have other tasks to do. How will you show that the person is the most important at the time?

REVIEW QUESTIONS

Circle the BEST answer.

1 A person will be arriving by ambulance on a stretcher. You should
   a Make a closed bed and leave it in a low position
   b Make an open bed and raise the head of the bed
   c Make a surgical bed and assist with the transfer
   d Make an occupied bed after the person arrives

2 You are greeting a person during admission. Which greeting is *best*?
   a "Hi. You can put your things in the closet."
   b "Welcome, Mrs. Stone. I am Jesse, a nursing assistant. I'll help with your admission."
   c "Your family needs to wait in the waiting room."
   d "This is your room. It is nicer than some of the other rooms."

3 When the person arrives in the room, you
   a Record the person's identifying information
   b Measure vital signs
   c Explain the person's rights
   d Review the doctor's orders

4 A patient is being transferred to your unit. You arrive before the nurse to help the staff move the person to the bed. The person is restless and reports pain. Which should you do *first*?
   a Call for the nurse to report the pain.
   b Complete the admission checklist.
   c Orient the person to the room.
   d Measure the person's vital signs, height, and weight.

5 A new resident with dementia talks about wanting to go home. Which will you do?
   a Begin gathering the person's belongings.
   b Contact an ombudsman.
   c Explain that this is the person's new home.
   d Listen and meet needs to help the person feel safe and comfortable.

6 You are going to measure weight with a standing scale. Which should you correct before weighing the person?
   a The person's urine drainage bag is half full.
   b The scale is balanced at zero (0).
   c There is a paper towel on the scale platform.
   d The person is in the center of the scale with arms at the sides.

7 When measuring height with a standing scale
   a Balance the height rod at zero (0)
   b Read the height at the very top of the height rod
   c Have the person stand very straight
   d Record height to the nearest inch

8 What is 68 inches in feet and inches?
   a 4 ft 0 in
   b 5 ft 6 in
   c 5 ft 8 in
   d 6 ft 8 in

9 Before transferring a person to another nursing unit, you
   a Gather the person's belongings
   b Explain the reason for the move
   c Tell the staff on the new unit to come get the person
   d Reassure the person by saying: "You'll be fine."

10 When discharging a person, you
   a Teach the person about diet and drugs
   b Arrange for home care
   c Decide when the person can leave
   d Help the person into the vehicle

Answers to Chapter 37 questions are on p. 903.

FOCUS ON PRACTICE

Problem Solving

A person is waiting for a new room on another nursing unit. The room is not yet ready. Ready to move, the person is becoming anxious. How can you provide comfort and ease anxiety? How can you make the move efficient when the room is ready?

- Define the key terms in this chapter.
- Explain what to do before, during, and after an examination (exam).
- Identify the equipment used for an exam.
- Describe how to prepare and drape a person for an exam.

- Explain the rules for assisting with an exam.
- Perform the procedure described in this chapter.
- Explain how to promote PRIDE in the person, the family, and yourself.

dorsal recumbent position The supine position with the legs together (*dorsal* means the back of something; *recumbent* means to lie down); horizontal recumbent position
genupectoral position See "knee-chest position" (*genu* means knee; *pectoral* refers to the chest)
horizontal recumbent position See "dorsal recumbent position"
knee-chest position The person kneels and rests the body on the knees and chest; the head is turned to 1 side, the arms are above the head or flexed at the elbows, the back is straight, and the body is flexed about 90 degrees at the hips; genupectoral position
laryngeal mirror An instrument used to examine the mouth, teeth, and throat

lithotomy position The person lies on the back with the hips at the edge of the exam table, the knees are flexed, the hips are externally rotated, and the feet are in stirrups
nasal speculum An instrument (*speculum*) used to examine the inside of the nose (*nasal*)
ophthalmoscope A lighted instrument (*scope*) used to examine the internal eye (*ophthalmo*) structures
otoscope A lighted instrument (*scope*) used to examine the external ear (*oto*) and the eardrum (tympanic membrane)
percussion hammer An instrument used to tap body parts to test reflexes (*percussion* means to strike hard); reflex hammer
tuning fork An instrument vibrated to test hearing
vaginal speculum An instrument (*speculum*) used to open the vagina (*vaginal*) to examine it and the cervix

Doctors and advanced practice registered nurses (APRNs) perform physical examinations (exams). Exams are done to:
- Promote health.
- Determine fitness for work or sports.
- Diagnose disease.

YOUR ROLE
Your role depends on agency policies and on what the examiner prefers. You may be asked to:
- Collect linens, equipment, and supplies.
- Prepare the exam room or the person's room.
- Cover the exam table with a clean drawsheet or paper.
- Provide for lighting.
- Transport the person to and from the exam room.
- Prepare the person for the exam.
- Hand equipment and supplies to the examiner.
- Label specimen containers.
- Discard used supplies and clean equipment.
- Help the person dress or to a comfortable position after the exam.
- Follow agency policy for used linens.

EQUIPMENT
The instruments in Figure 38-1 are commonly used in exams.
- *Laryngeal mirror*—used to examine the mouth, teeth, and throat.
- *Nasal speculum*—an instrument (*speculum*) used to examine the inside of the nose (*nasal*).
- *Ophthalmoscope*—a lighted instrument (*scope*) used to examine the internal eye (*ophthalmo*) structures.
- *Otoscope*—a lighted instrument (*scope*) used to examine the external ear (*oto*) and the eardrum (tympanic membrane). Some otoscopes can be changed into an ophthalmoscope.
- *Percussion hammer (reflex hammer)*—used to tap body parts to test reflexes. *Percussion* means to strike hard.
- *Tuning fork*—vibrated to test hearing.
- *Vaginal speculum*—an instrument (*speculum*) used to open the vagina (*vaginal*) to examine it and the cervix.

Some agencies prepare exam trays. If not, collect the items listed in the procedure: *Preparing the Person for an Examination*, p. 592. Arrange them on a tray or table.

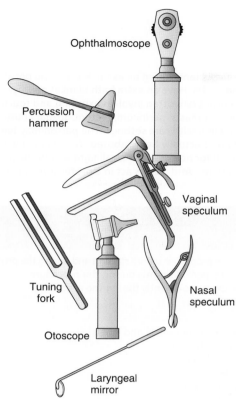

Ophthalmoscope

Percussion hammer

Vaginal speculum

Tuning fork

Nasal speculum

Otoscope

Laryngeal mirror

FIGURE 38-1 Physical exam instruments.

PREPARING THE PERSON

The physical exam can cause concerns. People may worry about findings. Some are confused or have fears about the procedure. Discomfort, embarrassment, exposure, and not knowing the procedure cause anxiety. Respect the person's feelings and concerns.

The nurse explains the exam's purpose and what to expect. Then the nurse obtains the person's consent. To assist the nurse:

- Provide for privacy.
  - Close the door.
  - Pull any privacy curtains.
  - Have the person put on a patient gown. Assist as needed. Usually all clothes are removed. The gown reduces the naked feeling and fear of exposure.
- Have the person void to empty the bladder. This lets the examiner feel the abdominal organs. A full bladder can change the normal position and shape of organs. It also causes discomfort, especially when feeling the abdominal organs.
- Obtain a urine specimen if needed. Explain how to collect the specimen (Chapter 39). Label the container.
- Measure and record vital signs, weight, height, and pulse oximetry.
- Drape the person. Use a paper drape, bath blanket, sheet, or drawsheet.
- Position the person for the exam.

See *Focus on Communication: Preparing the Person.*
See *Focus on Children and Older Persons: Preparing the Person.*
See *Delegation Guidelines: Preparing the Person.*
See *Promoting Safety and Comfort: Preparing the Person,* p. 592.
See procedure: *Preparing the Person for an Examination,* p. 592.

FOCUS ON COMMUNICATION

Preparing the Person

When preparing a person for an exam, do not assume the person knows what to do. Tell the person what clothing to remove, how to put on the gown (opening to the front or to the back), and where to sit. For example:

Please remove your clothes and put on this gown. The gown opens in the back. Under-garments can stay on. You can put your clothes on this chair. Here is a blanket to cover yourself. Please have a seat on the exam table after you change. Do you need help changing or have any questions?

FOCUS ON CHILDREN AND OLDER PERSONS

Preparing the Person

Children
Babies wear diapers for an exam. Toddlers, pre-school children, and school-age children can wear underpants. Diapers or underpants are removed or lowered as needed during the exam.

Older Persons
Nursing center residents have an exam at least once a year. The person has the right to personal choice. The doctor or nurse explains the reason for the exam. The person is told who will do the exam and when and how it will be done.

The exam requires the person's consent. The person may want a different examiner. Or the person may want a family member present for the exam and when the results are explained.

DELEGATION GUIDELINES

Preparing the Person

In some agencies, preparing persons for exams is a routine nursing task. In others it is a delegated nursing task. To prepare a person for an exam, you need this information from the nurse and the care plan.

- When to prepare the person.
- What room to prepare—an exam room or the person's room.
- How to position the person.
- The equipment and supplies needed.
- If a urine specimen is needed. If yes, should you collect a random urine specimen or a midstream specimen (Chapter 39)?
- What patient or resident concerns to report at once.

PROMOTING SAFETY AND COMFORT

Preparing the Person

Safety

Protect the person from falls and injuries. Use caution when an exam table is used. The person can fall getting on or off of the table or while seated on the table. Have help to get the person on or off of the table if needed. Do not leave persons who are at risk for falling unattended. Do not leave persons with dementia alone.

Comfort

Warmth is important during an exam. Protect the person from chilling and drafts. Have an extra bath blanket nearby.

The physical exam often involves exposing and touching private areas—breasts, perineum, rectum. Sexual abuse has occurred in health care settings. The person may feel threatened or is actually being abused. The person needs to be able to call for help. Keep the call light within the person's reach at all times. And always act in a professional manner.

Preparing the Person for an Examination

QUALITY OF LIFE

- Knock before entering the person's room.
- Address the person by name.
- Introduce yourself by name and title.

- Explain the procedure before starting and during the procedure.
- Protect the person's rights during the procedure.
- Handle the person gently during the procedure.

PRE-PROCEDURE

1 Follow *Delegation Guidelines: Preparing the Person*, p. 591. See *Promoting Safety and Comfort: Preparing the Person*.
2 Practice hand hygiene and get the following supplies as needed.
   - Exam form
   - Flashlight
   - Blood pressure equipment
   - Stethoscope
   - Thermometer
   - Pulse oximeter (Chapter 44)
   - Scale
   - Tongue depressors (blades)
   - Laryngeal mirror
   - Ophthalmoscope
   - Otoscope
   - Nasal speculum
   - Percussion (reflex) hammer
   - Tuning fork
   - Vaginal speculum (for a female)
   - Tape measure
   - Gloves
   - Water-soluble lubricant
   - Cotton-tipped applicators

   - Specimen containers and labels
   - Disposable bag
   - Kidney basin
   - Towel
   - Bath blanket
   - Tissues
   - Drape (sheet, bath blanket, drawsheet, or paper drape)
   - Paper towels
   - Cotton balls
   - Waterproof under-pad
   - Eye chart (Snellen chart)
   - Slides
   - Patient gown
   - Alcohol wipes
   - Wastebasket
   - Container for soiled instruments
   - Marking pencils or pens
   - Laundry bag
3 Practice hand hygiene.
4 Identify the person. Check the identification (ID) bracelet against the assignment sheet. Use 2 identifiers (Chapter 14). Also call the person by name.
5 Provide for privacy.

PROCEDURE

6 Have the person put on the gown. Tell the person what clothes to remove and where to place them. Assist as needed.
7 Ask the person to void. Collect a urine specimen if needed. Provide for privacy.
8 Transport the person to the exam room. (Omit this step for an exam in the person's room.)
9 Measure weight and height (Chapter 37). Record the measurements on the exam form.
10 Help the person onto the exam table. Provide a step stool if necessary. (Omit this step for an exam in the person's room.)
11 Raise the far bed rail (if used). Raise the bed to a safe and comfortable working height. (Omit this step if an exam table is used.)

12 Measure vital signs and pulse oximetry. Record them on the exam form.
13 Place a waterproof under-pad under the buttocks if not already present.
14 Position the person as directed.
15 Drape (cover) the person.
16 Raise the bed rail near you (if used).
17 Provide for adequate lighting.
18 Notify the examiner that the person is ready.
   a *If you will stay in the room*—Use the call light and stay with the person.
   b *If you will leave the room*—Lower the bed (if used) to a safe and comfortable level. Provide for comfort and safety. Maintain privacy measures. Practice hand hygiene. Leave the room to notify the examiner.

POSITIONING AND DRAPING

Before helping the person assume and maintain the position, explain:

- Why the position is needed
- How to assume the position
- How you will drape the person for warmth and privacy
- How long to expect to stay in the position

Some exam positions are uncomfortable and embarrassing. For such positions, wait until the examiner is present and ready to perform the part of the exam requiring the position. Then assist the person into the position.

Exam Positions

The examiner may request 1 of the following exam positions.

- *Dorsal recumbent position (horizontal recumbent position)*—the person is supine with the legs together. (*Dorsal* means the back of something; *recumbent* means to lie down.) The position is used to examine the abdomen, chest, and breasts. To examine the perineal area, the knees are flexed and hips externally rotated. Drape the person as in Figure 38-2, *A.*
- *Lithotomy position*—the person lies on the back. Hips are at the edge of the exam table. Knees are flexed and hips externally rotated. Feet are in stirrups. See Figure 38-2, *B.* The position is used to examine the vagina and cervix. See draping for perineal care in Chapter 24. Some agencies provide socks for the feet and calves.
- *Knee-chest position*—the person kneels and rests the body on the knees and chest. The head is turned to 1 side. The arms are above the head or flexed at the elbows. The back is straight. The body is flexed about 90 degrees at the hips. See Figure 38-2, *C.* The position is also called the *genupectoral position.* (*Genu* means knee. *Pectoral* refers to the chest.) The position is used to examine the rectum. Apply the drape in a diamond shape to cover the back, buttocks, and thighs.
- The *semi-prone position*—is sometimes used to examine the rectum or vagina. See Figure 38-2, *D* and Chapter 19. Apply the drape in a diamond shape. The examiner folds back the near corner to expose the rectum or vagina.

See *Focus on Children and Older Persons: Positioning and Draping.*

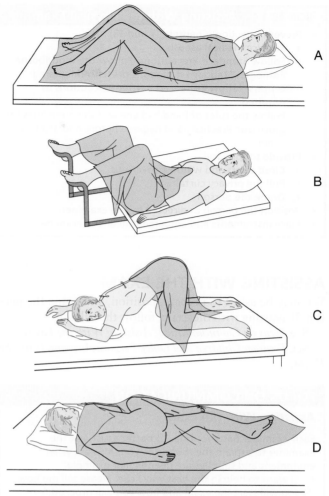

FIGURE 38-2 Positioning and draping for the physical exam. **A,** Dorsal recumbent position. **B,** Lithotomy position. **C,** Knee-chest position. **D,** Semi-prone position.

BOX 38-1	Assisting With the Physical Exam

- Prevent infection (Chapters 17 and 18).
  - Practice medical asepsis.
  - Follow Standard Precautions. Follow the Bloodborne Pathogen Standard if blood is present. In nursing centers, follow Enhanced Barrier Precautions as required.
  - Follow the rules of hand hygiene and the guidelines for glove use. Practice hand hygiene before and after the exam.
- Provide for privacy.
  - Close doors and window coverings.
  - Pull the privacy curtain.
  - Drape the person.
- Position the person as directed by the examiner.
- Place instruments and equipment near the examiner.
- Stay in the room for the legal protection of the person and the examiner if:
  - The examiner needs a staff member of the person's biological sex present. A male is present for a male's exam. A female is present for a female's exam.
  - The person requests.
  - The examiner requests. The person's consent is needed.
- Protect the person from falling.
- Reassure the person throughout the exam.
- Anticipate the examiner's need for equipment and supplies.
- Expose only the body part being examined.
- Place paper towels or a disposable waterproof pad on the floor if the person will stand without footwear.
- Keep the call light within the person's reach. Show the person where it is and how to use it.

ASSISTING WITH THE EXAM

You may be asked to prepare, position, and drape the person. If assisting with the exam, follow the rules in Box 38-1.

See *Focus on Communication: Assisting With the Exam.*

See *Focus on Children and Older Persons: Assisting With the Exam.*

FOCUS ON COMMUNICATION

Assisting With the Exam

Each examiner has a routine. To better assist, ask the examiner to explain the routine to you. Also ask what equipment and supplies are needed. For example:
- "I want to help in the best way I can. Please tell me how you will start the exam and how you will proceed."
- "Please ask for equipment and supplies as you need them. That way I can hand you the correct item."

FOCUS ON CHILDREN AND OLDER PERSONS

Assisting With the Exam

Children

A parent is present when children are examined. The parent may need to hold and keep a child still during some parts of the exam. Being kept still may frighten a child. A child may fear harm or separation from the parent. A calm, comforting manner helps the child and parent. The parent may have fears too.

The equipment is the same as for adult exams. Vaginal speculums are not used. Games and toys are used to assess development. Toys are also used to promote comfort and to show what will happen during the exam. For example, an examiner places a stethoscope on a doll before it is placed on a child.

Older Persons

Persons with dementia may resist the examiner's efforts. The person may be agitated and aggressive from confusion and fear. Do not restrain or force the person to have the exam. The exam is tried another time. Sometimes a family member can calm the person. The person's rights are always respected.

After the Exam

After the exam, the person dresses or returns to bed. If lubricant was used to examine the vagina or rectum, provide supplies to wipe or clean those areas. Assist and provide hand hygiene as needed.

You may need to label specimens and take them to the correct area with a requisition slip (Chapter 39). You also need to clean up and store supplies and equipment.
- Discard disposable items.
- Follow agency procedures to clean, disinfect, or sterilize re-usable items. This includes the otoscope and ophthalmoscope tips and stethoscope. Return items to the tray or storage area. Send a re-usable speculum to the supply department. It needs to be sterilized.
- Follow agency procedures to clean and disinfect the exam area if this is your job. Straighten the person's unit if the exam is performed in the person's room.
- Cover the exam table with a clean drawsheet or paper.
- Replace supplies on the exam tray.
- Follow agency policy for used linens.

Wear gloves and change them as needed during clean up. Follow Standard Precautions. Follow the Bloodborne Pathogen Standard if blood is present. Follow the rules of hand hygiene and the guidelines for glove use in Chapters 17 and 18.

See *Teamwork and Time Management: After the Exam.*

TEAMWORK AND TIME MANAGEMENT

After the Exam

Make sure the exam room is clean with supplies and equipment ready for the next exam. Otherwise you delay the person, the examiner, and the staff member assisting.

You may find an exam room that is not clean. Or exam equipment and supplies are not ready. Call for the nurse to see the problem before you proceed. The nurse can find out who last used the room or tray. The nurse can talk to the staff members involved.

FOCUS ON **PRIDE**

The Person, Family, and Yourself

Personal and Professional Responsibility

The person needs to feel safe and secure during the exam. The person should feel comfortable with the examiner and the assistant. Be professional and courteous. Provide care in a way that promotes dignity, self-esteem, and well-being.

Rights and Respect

The person has the right to privacy. Protect the person from exposure. Only the examiner and the assistant should see the person's body. The person must consent for others to be present. This includes family. Keep the person properly draped and screened. Expose only the body part being examined.

Independence and Social Interaction

Fears about the exam are common. Your interactions affect the person's mental comfort. Kindness and competence ease worries. To ease the person's fears:

- Greet the person. Introduce yourself by name and title. Use the examiner's name and title as well. For example: "Dr. Shaw will see you today."
- Talk with the person. Be pleasant. Listen with interest.
- Answer questions that you are able to answer. Note others for the examiner.
- Be prompt. Apologize for any delays. Ask if the person has needs while waiting.
- Be prepared. Have supplies and equipment ready.
- Make positive and honest comments. For example: "Dr. Shaw is kind and thorough."

Delegation and Teamwork

Good teamwork involves being helpful, prepared, and knowledgeable. Know where to find the supplies and equipment used for exams. When you need an item, you can get it quickly.

Plan ahead. Test equipment before each use. For example, check that the ophthalmoscope and otoscope lights work. If not, correct the issue.

Ethics and Laws

You must keep the person's information confidential. Talking about an exam with family, friends, or staff not involved in the person's care violates the *Health Insurance Portability and Accountability Act of 1996 (HIPAA)*. HIPAA protects the privacy and security of the person's health information (Chapter 5). Failure to follow HIPAA rules can result in fines, penalties, and criminal action.

FOCUS ON **PRIDE**: *Application*

Explain the importance of your role before, during, and after the physical exam. How do you prevent delays and promote comfort?

REVIEW QUESTIONS

Circle the BEST answer.

1 The otoscope is used to examine
   a Internal eye structures
   b The external ear and the eardrum
   c Reflexes
   d The vagina

2 When preparing for an exam, you should
   a Explain the purpose of the exam
   b Assume that the person knows what to do
   c Position and drape the person as directed
   d Obtain consent for the exam

3 You prepare a person for an exam. The person is at risk for falls. How will you notify the examiner that the person is ready?
   a Leave to get the examiner.
   b Stay with the person and use the call light.
   c Yell from the doorway.
   d Wait for the examiner to realize that you are ready.

4 Which part of an exam can you do?
   a Test reflexes.
   b Inspect the mouth, teeth, and throat.
   c Measure weight, height, and vital signs.
   d Examine the perineum and rectum.

5 A person is supine. The hips are flexed and externally rotated. The feet are supported in stirrups. The person is in the
   a Dorsal recumbent position
   b Knee-chest position
   c Semi-prone position
   d Lithotomy position

6 A female resident needs an exam. Which is *correct?*
   a Hand hygiene is practiced before and after the exam.
   b A male nursing assistant stays in the room to observe.
   c You may restrain the person for the exam if needed.
   d A family member is not allowed in the room.

Answers to Chapter 38 questions are on p. 903.

FOCUS ON **PRACTICE**

Problem Solving

During an exam, you must leave the room several times for supplies. What problems does this cause? How could this have been prevented?

OBJECTIVES

- Define the key terms and key abbreviations in this chapter.
- Explain why specimens are collected.
- Explain the rules for collecting specimens.
- Describe the different types of urine specimens.
- Describe 5 urine tests performed with reagent strips.
- Explain how to use reagent strips.
- Describe how to collect a stool specimen.

- Describe how to collect a sputum specimen.
- Describe the equipment used for blood glucose testing.
- Identify common skin puncture sites.
- Perform the procedures described in this chapter.
- Explain how to promote PRIDE in the person, the family, and yourself.

KEY TERMS

acetone See "ketone"
glucometer A device for measuring *(meter)* blood glucose *(gluco)*; glucose meter
glucosuria Sugar *(glucose)* in the urine *(uria)*
hematoma A swelling *(oma)* that contains blood *(hemat)*
hematuria Blood *(hemat)* in the urine *(uria)*
hemoptysis Bloody *(hemo)* sputum *(ptysis* means to spit)

ketone A substance appearing in urine from the rapid breakdown of fat for energy; acetone, ketone body
ketone body See "ketone"
melena A black, tarry stool
sputum Mucus from the respiratory system that is expectorated (expelled) through the mouth

KEY ABBREVIATIONS

APRN	Advanced practice registered nurse	mL	Milliliter
BM	Bowel movement	oz	Ounce
ID	Identification	PPE	Personal protective equipment
I&O	Intake and output	U/A; UA	Urinalysis

Specimens *(samples)* are collected and tested to prevent, detect, and treat disease. Some specimens are tested at the bedside. Most are tested in the laboratory. All laboratory specimens require *requisition slips* with identifying information and the test ordered. The specimen container is labeled following agency policy. To collect specimens, follow the rules in Box 39-1.

See *Teamwork and Time Management: Collecting and Testing Specimens.*

See *Promoting Safety and Comfort: Collecting and Testing Specimens.*

BOX 39-1	Collecting Specimens

- Follow agency policies and procedures to collect, label, and transport specimens correctly.
- Prevent infection (Chapters 17 and 18).
  - Practice medical asepsis.
  - Follow Standard Precautions and the Bloodborne Pathogen Standard. In nursing centers, follow Enhanced Barrier Precautions as required.
  - Wear personal protective equipment (PPE) as required for the task or by agency policy.
  - Follow the rules of hand hygiene and the guidelines for glove use.
- Use the correct container.
- Collect the specimen at the correct time.
- Do not contaminate the specimen.
  - Use a clean container for each specimen.
  - Do not touch the inside of the container or the inside of the lid.
  - Ask a female needing a urine specimen if she is having a menstrual period. Tell the nurse. Menstruating may cause blood to be in the urine specimen.
  - Ask the person not to have a bowel movement (BM) when collecting a urine specimen. Urine specimens must not contain stools.
  - Ask the person to void before collecting a stool specimen. Stool specimens must not contain urine.
  - Have the person put toilet paper in the toilet or in a disposable bag. Discard following agency policy. Urine and stool specimens must not contain toilet paper.
- Identify the person and label the specimen correctly.
  - Identify the person. Check the identification (ID) bracelet against the laboratory requisition slip or assignment sheet. Compare all information. Ask the person to state his or her first and last name and birthdate. (The person's room or bed number is *not* an acceptable identifier.)
  - Label the container in the person's presence. Provide clear, accurate information. Label the container—not the lid.
- Contain the specimen.
  - Secure the lid on the specimen container tightly.
  - Follow agency policies and procedures for using a plastic bag and *BIOHAZARD* labeling for transport (Fig. 39-1). Procedures in this chapter include placing the specimen in a *BIOHAZARD* bag. Do not let the container touch the outside of the bag. Seal the bag containing the specimen securely.
- Take the specimen and requisition slip to the laboratory or designated storage area.

TEAMWORK AND TIME MANAGEMENT
Collecting and Testing Specimens

Nursing centers have designated storage areas for specimens. Specimens are picked up at a certain time and transported to a laboratory. Have specimens collected and in the storage area by the pick-up time. If not collected in time, results are delayed. A new specimen may be needed. The delay can harm the person. Using more supplies and equipment costs more money.

PROMOTING SAFETY AND COMFORT
Collecting and Testing Specimens

Safety
Correct identification is very important when collecting and testing specimens. To identify the person, check the ID bracelet against all information on the requisition slip. The following identifying practices are also common.

- The person states or spells his or her first and last name.
- The person states his or her birthdate.
- The person identifies who ordered the test. For example, the person gives the name of the doctor or advanced practice registered nurse (APRN).

Blood and body fluids (including secretions and excretions) may contain microbes and blood. This includes urine, stool, and sputum specimens. Follow Standard Precautions and the Bloodborne Pathogen Standard when collecting, testing, and handling specimens. Follow the rules of hand hygiene and the guidelines for glove use in Chapters 17 and 18.

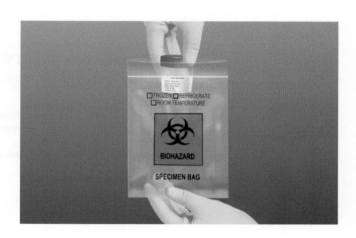

FIGURE 39-1 A specimen is placed in a plastic bag with a *BIOHAZARD* label. The specimen is labeled and securely sealed. The bag is then sealed and taken to the laboratory or storage area with the requisition slip. (From Melton Stein LN, Hollen CJ: *Concept-based clinical nursing skills: fundamental to advanced competencies,* ed 2, St Louis, 2024, Elsevier.)

URINE SPECIMENS

Urine specimens are collected for urine tests. Follow the rules in Box 39-1.

See *Delegation Guidelines: Urine Specimens*.
See *Promoting Safety and Comfort: Urine Specimens*.

The Random Urine Specimen

The random urine specimen is used for a routine urinalysis (U/A; UA). No special measures are needed. It is collected any time in a 24-hour period. Many people collect the specimen themselves. Weak and very ill persons need help.

See procedure: *Collecting a Random Urine Specimen*.

DELEGATION GUIDELINES

Urine Specimens

Collecting urine specimens is a routine nursing task. You need this information from the nurse and the care plan.
- Voiding device—bedpan, urinal, commode, or toilet with specimen pan (Fig. 39-2)
- The type of specimen needed
- What time to collect the specimen
- What special measures are needed
- If you need to test the specimen (p. 606)
- If measuring intake and output (I&O) is ordered (Chapter 32)

- What observations to report and record:
  - Problems obtaining the specimen
  - Color, clarity, and odor of urine
  - Blood in the urine
  - Particles in the urine
  - Complaints of pain, burning, urgency, difficulty voiding, or other problems
  - The time the specimen was collected
- When to report observations
- What patient or resident concerns to report at once

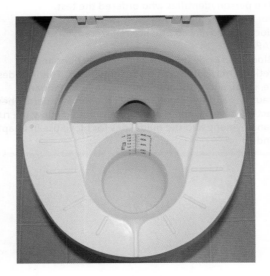

FIGURE 39-2 The specimen pan is at the front of the toilet on the toilet rim for a urine specimen. (NOTE: The toilet seat is lowered over the specimen pan for voiding.)

PROMOTING SAFETY AND COMFORT

Urine Specimens

Comfort
Clear specimen containers show urine. This may embarrass some people, including children. Cloudy urine specimen containers are common.

Collecting a Random Urine Specimen

QUALITY OF LIFE

- Knock before entering the person's room.
- Address the person by name.
- Introduce yourself by name and title.

- Explain the procedure before starting and during the procedure.
- Protect the person's rights during the procedure.
- Handle the person gently during the procedure.

PRE-PROCEDURE

1 Follow *Delegation Guidelines: Urine Specimens*. See *Promoting Safety and Comfort:*
   a *Collecting and Testing Specimens*, p. 597
   b *Urine Specimens*
2 Practice hand hygiene and get the following supplies.
   - Laboratory requisition slip
   - Specimen container
   - Voiding device (clean, un-used)—bedpan and cover (if used), urinal, commode, or specimen pan
   - Graduate to measure output (if needed)
   - Specimen label
   - Disposable bag (if needed)
   - Plastic bag with a *BIOHAZARD* label
   - Gloves

3 Arrange items in the person's room (bathroom). Open the plastic bag.
4 Practice hand hygiene.
5 Identify the person. Check the ID bracelet against the requisition slip. Compare all information. Also call the person by name. Ask the person to state his or her first and last name and birthdate.
6 Label the specimen container in the person's presence.
7 Provide for privacy.

PROCEDURE

8 Put on gloves.
9 Place the specimen pan on the toilet or commode container if used (see Fig. 39-2).
10 Ask the person to urinate into the voiding device. Have the person put toilet paper into the toilet. Or provide a disposable bag and follow agency policy for disposal. Toilet paper is not put in the bedpan or specimen pan.
11 Take the voiding device to the bathroom if a bedpan, urinal, or commode was used.
12 Pour about 120 mL (milliliters) (4 oz [ounces]) into the specimen container.
13 Secure the lid on the specimen container tightly. Put the container in the plastic bag. Do not let the container touch the outside of the bag.

14 Measure urine if I&O are ordered. Include the specimen amount.
15 Dispose of excess urine in the toilet. Avoid splashes. Rinse equipment. Pour the rinse into the toilet and flush. Follow agency procedures for cleaning and disinfection. Return equipment to its proper place.
16 Remove and discard the gloves. Practice hand hygiene. Put on clean gloves.
17 Seal the bag containing the specimen container.
18 Assist with hand hygiene. Remove and discard the gloves. Practice hand hygiene.

POST-PROCEDURE

19 Provide for comfort. (See the inside of the back cover.)
20 Make sure the bed is at a safe and comfortable level. Raise or lower bed rails. Follow the care plan.
21 Place the call light and other needed items within reach.
22 Follow the care plan and the person's preferences for privacy measures to maintain. Leaving the privacy curtain, window coverings, and door open or closed are examples.

23 Complete a safety check of the room. (See the inside of the back cover.)
24 Practice hand hygiene.
25 Take the specimen and requisition slip to the laboratory or storage area. Follow agency policies and procedures for labeling, containment, and transport.
26 Practice hand hygiene.
27 Report and record your care and observations.

The Midstream Specimen

The midstream specimen is also called a *clean-voided specimen* or *clean-catch specimen*. The perineal area is cleaned first to reduce the number of microbes in the urethral area. The person starts to void into a device. Then the person stops the urine stream and a sterile specimen container is positioned. The person voids into the container until the specimen is obtained.

Stopping and starting the urine stream is hard for many people. You may need to position and hold the specimen container after the person starts to void (Fig. 39-3).

See *Focus on Communication: The Midstream Specimen.*

See *Promoting Safety and Comfort: The Midstream Specimen.*

See procedure: *Collecting a Midstream Specimen.*

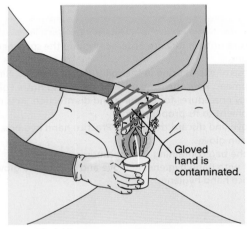

FIGURE 39-3 The labia are separated to collect a midstream specimen.

Gloved hand is contaminated.

FOCUS ON COMMUNICATION

The Midstream Specimen

Some persons can collect the midstream specimen without help. To explain the procedure, use words the person understands. Show the supplies and how to use them. Also, ask if the person has questions. For example:

> I need to collect a midstream urine specimen. This means I need urine from the middle of your urine stream. First, wipe well with this towelette (show the towelette) from the front to back. The specimen goes in this cup (show the specimen cup). Please do not touch the inside of the cup. Start urinating and then stop. Position the cup to catch urine and start urinating again. If you cannot stop the stream, position the cup during the middle of the stream. I need at least this much urine if possible (point to the measurement on the cup). Remove the cup when it is about that full. Finish urinating. Secure the lid on the cup. Please do not touch the inside of the lid. I will take the specimen when you are done.

Then ask if the person has questions. Make sure the person understands what to do. You can say: "Please tell me what you will do so I know that you understand."

PROMOTING SAFETY AND COMFORT

The Midstream Specimen

Safety

Some agencies require the use of sterile gloves to collect a midstream specimen. Follow agency policy. You must guard against contamination. Review "Surgical Asepsis" in Chapter 17.

Some urine specimen kits contain a collection cup with a transfer device and tubes (Fig. 39-4, *A*). Urine is transferred from the collection cup to a tube (Fig. 39-4, *B*). The tube is labeled and transported to the laboratory. The transfer device in the lid contains a "sharp." Discard the lid in a sharps container (Chapter 17). Follow agency policy to discard the remaining urine and collection cup.

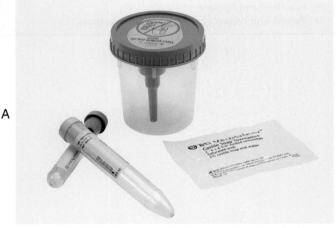

A

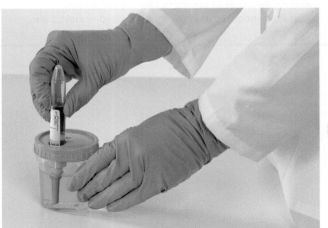

B

FIGURE 39-4 **A,** A urine specimen kit. This kit contains towelettes, a collection cup with a transfer device, and tubes with labels. **B,** Urine is transferred from the collection cup to a tube. (Courtesy and © Becton, Dickinson and Company.)

Collecting a Midstream Specimen

QUALITY OF LIFE

- Knock before entering the person's room.
- Address the person by name.
- Introduce yourself by name and title.

- Explain the procedure before starting and during the procedure.
- Protect the person's rights during the procedure.
- Handle the person gently during the procedure.

PRE-PROCEDURE

1 Follow *Delegation Guidelines: Urine Specimens*, p. 598. See *Promoting Safety and Comfort:*
   a *Collecting and Testing Specimens*, p. 597
   b *Urine Specimens*, p. 598
   c *The Midstream Specimen*
2 Practice hand hygiene and get the following supplies.
   - Laboratory requisition slip
   - Midstream specimen kit—specimen container, label, towelettes, sterile gloves
   - Voiding device—bedpan and cover (if used), urinal, commode, or specimen pan if needed
   - Graduate to measure output (if needed)
   - Supplies for perineal care (Chapter 24)
   - Plastic bag with a *BIOHAZARD* label
   - Sterile gloves (if not part of the specimen kit and required by agency policy)
   - Disposable gloves
   - Paper towels

3 Arrange items in the person's room (bathroom). Open the plastic bag.
4 Practice hand hygiene.
5 Identify the person. Check the ID bracelet against the requisition slip. Compare all information. Also call the person by name. Ask the person to state his or her first and last name and birthdate.
6 Provide for privacy.

PROCEDURE

7 Practice hand hygiene. Put on gloves.
8 Provide perineal care (Chapter 24). Follow agency policy for used linens. Remove and discard the gloves. Practice hand hygiene.
9 Open the specimen kit.
10 Put on gloves. Apply sterile gloves if required by agency policy.
11 Open the packet of towelettes.
12 Open the specimen container. Do not touch the inside of the container or lid. The inside is sterile. Set the lid down with the inside up.
13 *For a female*—Clean the perineal area with towelettes.
   a Spread the labia with your thumb and index finger. Use your non-dominant hand. (This hand is now contaminated. It must not touch anything sterile.)
   b Clean down the urethral area from front to back (top to bottom). Use a clean towelette for each stroke. Discard towelettes after use.
   c Keep the labia separated to collect the specimen (steps 15 through 18).
14 *For a male*—Clean the penis with towelettes.
   a Hold the penis with your non-dominant hand. (This hand is now contaminated. It must not touch anything sterile.)
   b Clean the penis starting at the meatus. (Retract the foreskin if the male is uncircumcised.) Clean in a circular motion. Start at the center and work outward. Discard towelettes after use.
   c Hold the penis (and keep the foreskin retracted in the uncircumcised male) until the specimen is collected (steps 15 through 18).
15 Have the person void into a device.

16 Pass the specimen container into the urine stream. Keep the labia separated (see Fig. 39-3) or the foreskin retracted.
17 Collect about 30 to 90 mL (1 to 3 oz) of urine. (Some agencies require 90 to 120 mL [3 to 4 oz]. Follow agency procedures for the amount to collect.)
18 Remove the specimen container. Set it on a paper towel.
19 Release the labia or penis. (Release the foreskin of the uncircumcised male.) Let the person finish voiding into the device.
20 Remove and discard soiled gloves. Practice hand hygiene. Put on clean gloves.
21 Secure the lid on the specimen container tightly. Touch only the outside of the container and lid. Wipe the outside of the container. Discard used paper towels.
22 Label the specimen container in the person's presence. Place the container in the plastic bag. The container must not touch the outside of the bag.
23 Provide toilet paper when the person is done voiding.
24 Take the voiding device to the bathroom if a bedpan, urinal, or commode was used.
25 Measure urine if I&O are ordered. Include the specimen amount.
26 Dispose of excess urine in the toilet. Avoid splashes. Rinse equipment. Pour the rinse into the toilet and flush. Follow agency procedures for cleaning and disinfection. Return equipment to its proper place.
27 Remove and discard the gloves. Practice hand hygiene. Put on clean gloves.
28 Seal the bag containing the specimen container.
29 Assist with hand hygiene. Remove and discard the gloves. Practice hand hygiene.

Continued

Collecting a Midstream Specimen—cont'd

POST-PROCEDURE

30 Provide for comfort. (See the inside of the back cover.)
31 Make sure the bed is at a safe and comfortable level. Raise or lower bed rails. Follow the care plan.
32 Place the call light and other needed items within reach.
33 Follow the care plan and the person's preferences for privacy measures to maintain. Leaving the privacy curtain, window coverings, and door open or closed are examples.

34 Complete a safety check of the room. (See the inside of the back cover.)
35 Practice hand hygiene.
36 Take the specimen and requisition slip to the laboratory or storage area. Follow agency policies and procedures for labeling, containment, and transport.
37 Practice hand hygiene.
38 Report and record your care and observations.

The 24-Hour Urine Specimen

All urine voided during 24 hours is collected for a 24-hour urine specimen. To prevent microbe growth, the urine is chilled on ice or refrigerated. A preservative may be added to the collection container.

The person voids to start the test with an empty bladder. Discard this voiding. Save *all voidings* for the next 24 hours. The person and staff must clearly understand the procedure and the test period. This test is re-started if:

- A voiding was not saved. (This includes if the person is incontinent.)
- Toilet paper was discarded into the specimen.
- The specimen contains stools.

See *Promoting Safety and Comfort: The 24-Hour Urine Specimen*.

See procedure: *Collecting a 24-Hour Urine Specimen*.

PROMOTING SAFETY AND COMFORT

The 24-Hour Urine Specimen

Safety

The urine container may include a preservative. Preservatives are hazardous. The person does not void directly into the container. Urine is poured into the container carefully to avoid splashes and splatters. Do not get the preservative or urine on your skin or in your eyes. If you do, flush your skin or eyes with a large amount of water. Tell the nurse what happened and check the safety data sheet (SDS) (Chapter 14). Also complete an incident report.

Keep the specimen chilled to prevent the growth of microbes as directed. A refrigerator or a basin with ice is used. Add ice to the basin as needed.

Assist the person with hand hygiene after every voiding. This prevents the spread of microbes.

Collecting a 24-Hour Urine Specimen

QUALITY OF LIFE

- Knock before entering the person's room.
- Address the person by name.
- Introduce yourself by name and title.

- Explain the procedure before starting and during the procedure.
- Protect the person's rights during the procedure.
- Handle the person gently during the procedure.

PRE-PROCEDURE

1 Follow *Delegation Guidelines: Urine Specimens*, p. 598. See *Promoting Safety and Comfort:*
   a *Collecting and Testing Specimens*, p. 597
   b *The 24-Hour Urine Specimen*
2 Practice hand hygiene and get the following supplies.
   - Laboratory requisition slip
   - Urine container for a 24-hour collection (Fig. 39-5)
   - Voiding device (clean, un-used)—bedpan and cover (if used), urinal, commode, or specimen pan
   - Graduate to measure output (if needed)
   - Specimen label
   - Preservative (if needed)
   - Two *24-HOUR URINE* labels
   - Funnel (if needed)
   - A basin with ice or an area for refrigeration as directed
   - Disposable bag as needed
   - *BIOHAZARD* label as required by agency policy
   - Gloves

3 Arrange items in the person's room (bathroom).
4 Practice hand hygiene.
5 Identify the person. Check the ID bracelet against the requisition slip. Compare all information. Also call the person by name. Ask the person to state his or her first and last name and birthdate.
6 Label the urine container in the person's presence (see Fig. 39-5). Place the labeled container in the bathroom.
7 Place one *24-HOUR URINE* label in the bathroom. Place the other near the bed.
8 Provide for privacy.

Collecting a 24-Hour Urine Specimen—cont'd

PROCEDURE

9 Put on gloves.

10 Ask the person to void. A toilet may be used for this first void (before the test begins). The person needs a voiding device for urine voided over the next 24 hours. Provide a device. Explain how to use it if needed. A specimen pan is on the front of the toilet or commode container (if used).

11 Measure urine if I&O are ordered. Discard (flush) the urine. Note the time. This starts the 24-hour period.

12 Follow agency procedures to clean and disinfect equipment. Return equipment to its proper place.

13 Remove and discard the gloves. Practice hand hygiene. Put on clean gloves.

14 Assist with hand hygiene.

15 Remove and discard the gloves. Practice hand hygiene.

16 Mark the start time on the urine container's label. Mark the time the test began and the time it is to end (24 hours later) on the room and bathroom labels.

17 Remind the person to:
  • Use the voiding device during the next 24 hours.
  • Not have a BM when voiding.
  • Put toilet paper in the toilet. Or provide a disposable bag. Follow agency policy for disposal.
  • Put on the call light after voiding.

18 Practice hand hygiene before leaving the room. Return to the room when the person signals for you. Knock before entering the room.

19 Do the following after every voiding during the test.
  a Practice hand hygiene. Put on clean gloves.
  b Measure urine if I&O are ordered.
  c Open the specimen container. Use the funnel or spout on the voiding device to pour urine into the container. Do not spill any urine. Tell the nurse if you spill or discard the urine. The test has to be re-started. Secure the lid on the specimen container.
  d Follow agency procedures to clean and disinfect equipment. Return equipment to its proper place.
  e Remove and discard the gloves. Practice hand hygiene. Put on clean gloves.
  f Assist with hand hygiene.
  g Remove and discard the gloves. Practice hand hygiene.
  h Follow the nurse's directions for storage of the container for the duration of the test (room temperature, on ice, or refrigerated).
  i Follow "Post-Procedure" steps (except for step 27).

20 Do the following at the end of the test.
  a Ask the person to void at the end of the 24-hour period.
  b Follow step 19 (a–g).
  c Remove the labels from the room and bathroom.
  d Note the end time on the urine container's label.

POST-PROCEDURE

21 Provide for comfort. (See the inside of the back cover.)

22 Make sure the bed is at a safe and comfortable level. Raise or lower bed rails. Follow the care plan.

23 Place the call light and other needed items within reach.

24 Follow the care plan and the person's preferences for privacy measures to maintain. Leaving the privacy curtain, window coverings, and door open or closed are examples.

25 Complete a safety check of the room. (See the inside of the back cover.)

26 Practice hand hygiene.

27 Take the specimen (labeled urine container) and requisition slip to the laboratory or storage area at the end of the test. Follow agency policies and procedures for labeling, containment, and transport.

28 Practice hand hygiene.

29 Report and record your care and observations.

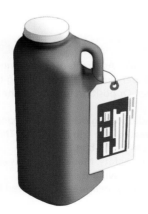

FIGURE 39-5 A 24-hour urine collection container and label. (From Melton Stein LN, Hollen CJ: *Concept-based clinical nursing skills: fundamental to advanced competencies,* ed 2, St Louis, 2024, Elsevier.)

Collecting a Urine Specimen From an Infant or Child

Sometimes urine specimens are needed from infants and children who are not toilet-trained. A collection bag ("wee bag") is applied over the urethra (Fig. 39-6). Follow the manufacturer's instructions for correct application. A parent or another staff member assists if the child is upset.

Voiding on request is hard for toilet-trained toddlers and young children. Potty chairs and specimen pans are useful. Remember to use terms the child understands. "Pee pee," "wee wee," "potty," and "tinkle" are examples. Or ask the parent what term the child uses and understands.

The nurse may have you give the child water or other fluids when a urine specimen is needed. Usually the child can void about 30 minutes after drinking fluids.

See procedure: *Collecting a Urine Specimen From an Infant or Child.*

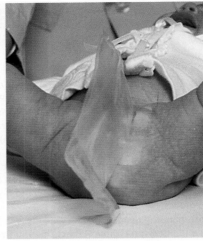

FIGURE 39-6 A urine collection bag applied to a baby's perineum.

Collecting a Urine Specimen From an Infant or Child

QUALITY OF LIFE

- Knock before entering the child's room.
- Address the child by name.
- Introduce yourself by name and title.
- Explain the procedure to the child and parents before starting and during the procedure.
- Protect the child's rights during the procedure.
- Handle the child gently during the procedure.

PRE-PROCEDURE

1 Follow *Delegation Guidelines: Urine Specimens*, p. 598. See *Promoting Safety and Comfort:*
  a *Collecting and Testing Specimens*, p. 597
  b *Urine Specimens*, p. 598
2 Practice hand hygiene and get the following supplies.
  • Laboratory requisition slip
  • Collection bag ("wee bag")
  • Plastic bag with a *BIOHAZARD* label
  • Specimen container
  • Scissors (if needed)
  • Items for perineal care as directed
  • Diapers
  • Gloves

3 Arrange items in the child's room.
4 Practice hand hygiene.
5 Identify the child. Check the ID bracelet against the requisition slip. Compare all information. Also call the child by name. Ask the parent to state the child's first and last name and the child's birthdate.
6 Provide for privacy.

PROCEDURE

7 Practice hand hygiene. Put on gloves.
8 Position the child on the back. Place a waterproof under-pad below the child if not already present.
9 Remove and discard the diaper.
10 Clean and dry the perineal and groin areas. Use towelettes; disposable wipes; or a wash basin, water, soap, washcloths, and towels as directed. The skin must be dried well for the adhesive on the bag to stick to the skin.
11 Remove and discard gloves if soiled. (Practice hand hygiene. Put on clean gloves.)
12 Flex the child's knees. Spread the legs.
13 Remove the adhesive backing from the collection bag. Apply the bag to the perineum (see Fig. 39-6).

14 Diaper the child. As directed, cut a slit in the bottom of a new diaper. Pull the collection bag through the slit in the diaper. Or position the bag to the side out 1 leg opening.
15 Remove and discard gloves. Practice hand hygiene.
16 Raise the head of the crib if allowed. This helps urine collect in the bottom of the bag.
17 Check for crib safety. Medical crib rails are raised and locked before leaving the bedside.
18 Maintain privacy measures as preferred by the child and parents.
19 Practice hand hygiene.

Collecting a Urine Specimen From an Infant or Child—cont'd

PROCEDURE—cont'd

20 Return to check the child often. Check the bag for urine. Do the following if the child has voided.
  a Provide for privacy.
  b Practice hand hygiene. Put on gloves.
  c Remove the diaper.
  d Remove the collection bag gently.
  e Follow agency procedures to contain the specimen.
    1) Method 1—Transfer the urine to the specimen container. Follow the manufacturer's instructions. Use the drainage tab if one is present.
    2) Method 2—Press the adhesive surfaces of the bag together. Make sure the seal is tight and there are no leaks. Place the sealed bag in the specimen container.
    3) Secure the cap on the specimen container tightly.
  f Clean the perineal area. Rinse and dry well.
  g Diaper the child.
  h Remove and discard the gloves. Practice hand hygiene.

21 Label the specimen container in the child's presence. Place it in the plastic bag. Seal the bag.

POST-PROCEDURE

22 Provide for comfort. (See the inside of the back cover.)
23 Check for crib safety. Medical crib rails are raised and locked before leaving the bedside.
24 Make sure the call light and other needed items are within reach for the child or parent.
25 Maintain privacy measures as preferred by the child and parents.

26 Complete a safety check of the room. (See the inside of the back cover.)
27 Practice hand hygiene.
28 Take the specimen and requisition slip to the laboratory or storage area. Follow agency policies and procedures for labeling, containment, and transport.
29 Practice hand hygiene.
30 Report and record your care and observations.

Urinary Catheter Specimens

A straight catheter (Chapter 28) may be needed to collect a specimen. A nurse inserts the catheter into the bladder and removes it after collecting the specimen. You may need to collect supplies or help position the person. Assist as the nurse directs.

A urine specimen can be collected from an indwelling catheter (Chapter 28). Urine in the drainage bag is not used. The port on the drainage tubing is used to collect the specimen. The nurse:

1 Clamps the drainage tubing so fresh urine can collect in the catheter.
2 Cleans the port.
3 Connects a syringe to the port (Fig. 39-7).
4 Aspirates (draws up) urine into the syringe.
5 Unclamps the drainage tubing.
  See *Delegation Guidelines: Urinary Catheter Specimens*, p 606.

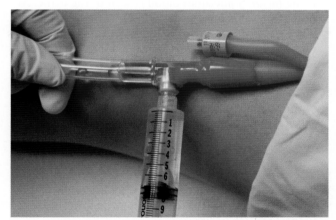

FIGURE 39-7 Collecting a specimen from a urinary catheter. A syringe is connected to the port on the drainage tubing. (From Perry AG, Potter PA, Ostendorf WR: *Nursing interventions & clinical skills,* ed 7, St Louis 2020, Elsevier.)

DELEGATION GUIDELINES
Urinary Catheter Specimens

Inserting a catheter is a nursing responsibility. With proper training, guidance, and assistance, some states and agencies let nursing assistants perform this sterile procedure. See Chapter 28.

In some agencies, collecting a specimen from an indwelling catheter is a delegated nursing task. Before collecting a urinary catheter specimen, make sure that:
- Your state allows you to perform the task.
- The task is in your job description (Chapter 3).
- You have the necessary education and training.
- The agency has determined that you are competent to perform the task safely.
- You know how to use the supplies and equipment.
- You review the procedure with the delegating nurse.
- The delegating nurse is available to answer questions and to guide and assist you as needed.

Testing Urine

The doctor or APRN orders the type and frequency of urine tests. Random or midstream urine specimens are needed as directed. Reagent strips (test strips) are used for various urine tests.

The nurse may have you do these simple tests.
- *Testing for pH*—Urine pH measures if urine is acidic or alkaline. Changes in normal pH (4.6 to 8.0) occur from illness, food, and drugs.
- *Testing for blood*—Injury and disease can cause hematuria. *Hematuria* means blood *(hemat)* in the urine *(uria)*. Sometimes blood is seen in the urine. At other times it is unseen *(occult)*.
- *Testing for glucose and ketones*—In diabetes, the pancreas does not secrete enough insulin (Chapter 51). The body needs insulin to use sugar for energy. If not used, sugar builds up in the blood. Some sugar appears in the urine. *Glucosuria* means sugar *(glucose)* in the urine *(uria)*. Diabetes may cause ketones in the urine. *Ketones (ketone bodies, acetone)* are substances appearing in urine from the rapid breakdown of fat for energy. The body uses fat for energy if it cannot use sugar.
- *Testing for infection*—The presence of certain white blood cells can signal a urinary tract infection.
- *Testing for protein*—Protein in the urine can signal kidney and other diseases.
  See *Teamwork and Time Management: Testing Urine.*
  See *Delegation Guidelines: Testing Urine.*
  See *Promoting Safety and Comfort: Testing Urine.*
  See procedure: *Testing Urine With Reagent Strips.*

TEAMWORK AND TIME MANAGEMENT
Testing Urine

In the past, urine testing was common for the management of diabetes. Urine was tested for glucose usually 4 times a day—30 minutes before meals and at bedtime. Test results were used for drug and diet decisions. Now, blood glucose testing (p. 614) is common.

When testing is needed at certain times, be prompt. Plan ahead to complete the test and report the result following the schedule.

DELEGATION GUIDELINES
Testing Urine

Testing urine is a nursing task that may be safely delegated to you. In some states and agencies testing urine with reagent strips is a routine nursing task. You need this information from the nurse and the care plan.
- What test is needed
- What equipment and reagent strips to use
- When to test urine
- If a random or midstream specimen is needed
- Instructions for the test ordered
- If the nurse will observe test results
- What observations to report and record:
  - The time you collected and tested the specimen
  - Test results
  - Problems obtaining the specimen
  - Color, clarity, and odor of urine
  - Blood or particles in the urine
  - Complaints of pain, burning, urgency, difficulty voiding, or other problems
- When to report test results and observations
- What patient or resident concerns to report at once

PROMOTING SAFETY AND COMFORT
Testing Urine

Safety
Accuracy is important. Promptly report results. Ordered drugs may depend on the results.

See Figure 39-8 for how to use reagent (test) strips. When using reagent (test) strips:
- Check the color of the strips. Do not use discolored strips.
- Check the expiration date on the bottle. Do not use the strips if the date has passed.
- Follow the manufacturer's instructions for an accurate result. Test results are used for diagnosis and treatment. A wrong result can cause serious harm.

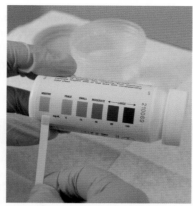

To use a reagent (test) strip:

• Do not touch the test area on the strip.
• Dip the strip into urine.
• Compare the strip with the color chart on the bottle.

FIGURE 39-8 Reagent (test) strips have sections that change color when reacting with urine.

Testing Urine With Reagent Strips

QUALITY OF LIFE

• Knock before entering the person's room.
• Address the person by name.
• Introduce yourself by name and title.

• Explain the procedure before starting and during the procedure.
• Protect the person's rights during the procedure.
• Handle the person gently during the procedure.

PRE-PROCEDURE

1 Follow *Delegation Guidelines: Testing Urine*. See *Promoting Safety and Comfort*:
   a *Collecting and Testing Specimens*, p. 597
   b *Testing Urine*
2 Practice hand hygiene and get the following supplies.
   • Reagent (test) strips for the ordered test
   • Equipment for the urine specimen (This procedure uses a random specimen. See procedure: *Collecting a Random Urine Specimen*, p. 599.)
   • Gloves

3 Arrange items in the person's room (bathroom).
4 Practice hand hygiene.
5 Identify the person. Check the ID bracelet against the assignment sheet. Use 2 identifiers (Chapter 14). Also call the person by name. Ask the person to state his or her first and last name and birthdate.
6 Provide for privacy.

PROCEDURE

7 Put on gloves.
8 Collect the urine specimen. (See procedure: *Collecting a Random Urine Specimen*, p. 599.)
9 Remove a strip from the bottle. Put the cap tightly on the bottle at once.
10 Dip the strip test area into the urine.
11 Remove the strip after the correct amount of time. See the manufacturer's instructions.
12 Tap the strip gently against the urine container. This removes excess urine.

13 Wait the required amount of time. See the manufacturer's instructions.
14 Compare the strip with the color chart on the bottle (see Fig. 39-8). Read the results.
15 Discard disposable items.
16 Dispose of urine in the toilet. Avoid splashes. Rinse equipment. Pour the rinse into the toilet and flush. Follow agency procedures for cleaning and disinfection. Return equipment to its proper place.
17 Remove and discard the gloves. Practice hand hygiene.

POST-PROCEDURE

18 Provide for comfort. (See the inside of the back cover.)
19 Make sure the bed is at a safe and comfortable level. Raise or lower bed rails. Follow the care plan.
20 Place the call light and other needed items within reach.
21 Follow the care plan and the person's preferences for privacy measures to maintain. Leaving the privacy curtain, window coverings, and door open or closed are examples.

22 Complete a safety check of the room. (See the inside of the back cover.)
23 Practice hand hygiene.
24 Report and record the test results and other observations.

Straining Urine

A stone *(calculus)* can develop in a kidney, a ureter, or the bladder. Stones *(calculi)* vary in size (Chapter 52). They can be as small as grains of sand, pearl-sized, or larger. Some stones are removed by medical or surgical procedures. Others pass through urine. When stones are present, all urine is strained. Passed stones are sent to the laboratory.

The person drinks 2000 to 3000 mL a day to help pass the stone. Expect the person to void in large amounts.

See procedure: *Straining Urine*.

Straining Urine

QUALITY OF LIFE

- Knock before entering the person's room.
- Address the person by name.
- Introduce yourself by name and title.
- Explain the procedure before starting and during the procedure.
- Protect the person's rights during the procedure.
- Handle the person gently during the procedure.

PRE-PROCEDURE

1 Follow *Delegation Guidelines: Urine Specimens*, p. 598. See *Promoting Safety and Comfort:*
   a *Collecting and Testing Specimens*, p. 597
   b *Urine Specimens*, p. 598
2 Practice hand hygiene and get the following supplies.
   - Laboratory requisition slip
   - Urine strainer
   - Specimen container
   - Specimen label
   - Voiding device (clean, un-used)—bedpan and cover (if used), urinal, commode, or specimen pan
   - Graduate to measure output (if needed)
   - 2 *STRAIN ALL URINE* labels
   - Plastic bag with a *BIOHAZARD* label
   - Gloves

3 Arrange items in the person's room (bathroom).
4 Practice hand hygiene.
5 Identify the person. Check the ID bracelet against the requisition slip. Compare all information. Also call the person by name. Ask the person to state his or her first and last name and birthdate.
6 Label the specimen container in the person's presence.
7 Provide for privacy.

PROCEDURE

8 Place 1 *STRAIN ALL URINE* label in the bathroom. Place the other near the bed.
9 Provide a voiding device and explain the procedure.
   a Show the person the voiding device. Explain its use if needed. Place the device in the room (bathroom) for use. A specimen pan is on the front of the toilet or commode container (if used). Remind the person to use the device for urinating.
   b Explain that all urine will be strained. Ask the person to put on the call light after each voiding.
10 Allow the person to void. Or return when the person has voided.
   a *If the person needs to void*—Continue to step 11 to strain the urine after voiding.
   b *If the person does not need to void*—Practice hand hygiene before leaving the room. Return to the room when the person signals. Knock before entering. Practice hand hygiene.
11 Put on gloves.

12 Place the strainer in the graduate.
13 Pour urine into the graduate. Urine passes through the strainer (Fig. 39-9).
14 Transfer any crystals, stones, or particles that appear in the strainer into the specimen container.
15 Secure the lid on the specimen container tightly. Place the container in the plastic bag. Do not let the container touch the outside of the bag.
16 Measure urine if I&O are ordered.
17 Dispose of urine in the toilet. Avoid splashes. Rinse equipment. Pour the rinse into the toilet and flush. Follow agency procedures for cleaning and disinfection. Return equipment to its proper place.
18 Remove and discard the gloves. Practice hand hygiene. Put on clean gloves.
19 Seal the bag containing the specimen container.
20 Assist with hand hygiene. Remove and discard the gloves. Practice hand hygiene.

POST-PROCEDURE

21 Provide for comfort. (See the inside of the back cover.)
22 Make sure the bed is at a safe and comfortable level. Raise or lower bed rails. Follow the care plan.
23 Place the call light and other needed items within reach.
24 Follow the care plan and the person's preferences for privacy measures to maintain. Leaving the privacy curtain, window coverings, and door open or closed are examples.

25 Complete a safety check of the room. (See the inside of the back cover.)
26 Practice hand hygiene.
27 Take the specimen and requisition slip to the laboratory or storage area. Follow agency policies and procedures for labeling, containment, and transport.
28 Practice hand hygiene.
29 Report and record your care and observations.

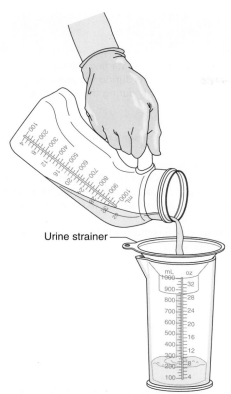

FIGURE 39-9 The strainer is placed in the graduate. Urine is poured through the strainer into the graduate.

STOOL SPECIMENS

Stools are studied for abnormal contents. Fat, microbes, worms, and blood are examples. Ulcers, colon cancer, and hemorrhoids are common causes of bleeding. Blood in stools can be:

- Visible. Bleeding from low in the bowels can cause red stools. Bleeding in the stomach or upper gastro-intestinal tract can cause black, tarry stools called *melena*.
- Unseen *(occult)*. *Occult* means hidden or not seen. Bleeding is in small amounts. Occult blood tests are used to screen for colon cancer and other digestive disorders. The procedure that follows includes an example of a test for occult blood. Occult blood test kits vary. Follow the manufacturer's instructions.

Urine must not contaminate the stool specimen. The person uses 1 device for voiding and another for a BM. Some tests require a warm stool. The specimen is taken at once to the laboratory or storage area. Follow the rules in Box 39-1.

See *Focus on Communication: Stool Specimens.*
See *Focus on Children and Older Persons: Stool Specimens.*
See *Delegation Guidelines: Stool Specimens.*
See *Promoting Safety and Comfort: Stool Specimens.*
See procedure: *Collecting and Testing a Stool Specimen*, p. 610.

FOCUS ON **COMMUNICATION**
Stool Specimens

Before you begin, explain what the person needs to do and what you will do. Show the equipment and supplies and how to use them. For example:

> I need to collect a specimen from a bowel movement. I'm going to place the specimen pan (show specimen pan) at the back of the toilet. Urinate into the toilet. Your bowel movement collects in the specimen pan. Please put toilet paper in the toilet, not in the specimen pan. After your bowel movement, put your call light on right away. I'll collect the specimen in this container (show the specimen container).

Then ask if the person has questions. If you do not know the answer, tell the nurse. Make sure the person understands what to do. You can say: "Please tell me what you will do so I know that you understand."

FOCUS ON **CHILDREN AND OLDER PERSONS**
Stool Specimens

Children
If the child wears a diaper, you can obtain stool from the diaper. You may need to scrape the diaper.

DELEGATION GUIDELINES
Stool Specimens

Collecting a stool specimen is a routine nursing task. Testing a stool specimen is a nursing task that may be safely delegated to you. Before collecting and testing a stool specimen, you need this information from the nurse.
- What time to collect and test the specimen
- What test is needed (if any)
- What equipment and special measures are needed
- Instructions for the test ordered
- If the nurse wants to observe the stool or test results
- What observations to report and record:
  - The time you collected and tested the specimen
  - Test results
  - Problems obtaining the specimen
  - Color, amount, consistency, and odor of stools
  - Complaints of pain or discomfort
- When to report observations
- What patient or resident concerns to report at once

PROMOTING SAFETY AND COMFORT
Stool Specimens

Safety
You must be accurate when testing stools. Follow the manufacturer's instructions for the test used. Promptly report the results to the nurse.

Comfort
Stools normally have an odor. A person may be embarrassed that you need a specimen. Complete the task quickly and carefully. Act in a professional manner.

Collecting and Testing a Stool Specimen

QUALITY OF LIFE

- Knock before entering the person's room.
- Address the person by name.
- Introduce yourself by name and title.

- Explain the procedure before starting and during the procedure.
- Protect the person's rights during the procedure.
- Handle the person gently during the procedure.

PRE-PROCEDURE

1 Follow *Delegation Guidelines: Stool Specimens*, p. 609. See *Promoting Safety and Comfort*:
   a *Collecting and Testing Specimens*, p. 597
   b *Stool Specimens*, p. 609
2 Practice hand hygiene and get the following supplies.
   - Laboratory requisition slip
   - Occult blood test kit (if needed)
   - Device to collect the BM (clean, un-used)—bedpan and cover (if used) or specimen pan
   - Device for voiding if the person will void—bedpan and cover (if used), commode, urinal, or specimen pan
   - Stool specimen container (Fig. 39-10)
   - Specimen label
   - Tongue blades (if needed)
   - Disposable bag
   - Plastic bag with a *BIOHAZARD* label
   - Toilet paper
   - Gloves

3 Arrange items in the person's room (bathroom). Open the plastic bag.
4 Practice hand hygiene.
5 Identify the person. Check the ID bracelet against the requisition slip. Compare all information. Also call the person by name. Ask the person to state his or her first and last name and birthdate.
6 Label the specimen container in the person's presence.
7 Provide for privacy.

PROCEDURE

8 Put on gloves.
9 Have the person void. Provide the voiding device if not using the bathroom. Empty the device into the toilet. Avoid splashes. Rinse the device. Pour the rinse into the toilet and flush. Follow agency procedures for cleaning and disinfection. Return the device to its proper place. (Change gloves and practice hand hygiene as needed.)
10 Put the specimen pan on the back of the toilet or commode if used (Fig. 39-11). Or provide the bedpan.
11 Ask the person not to put toilet paper into the bedpan, commode, or specimen pan. Have the person put toilet paper in the toilet. Or provide a disposable bag and follow agency policy for disposal.
12 Remove and discard the gloves. Practice hand hygiene.
13 *If the person can be left alone*:
   a Place the call light and toilet paper within reach. Ask the person to signal when done.
   b Maintain privacy measures.
   c Stay in the room or leave the room and close the door. Follow the care plan. Be respectful. Provide as much privacy as possible. (Practice hand hygiene before leaving the room.)
   d Return when the person signals. Or check on the person every 5 minutes. Knock before entering. Practice hand hygiene.
14 Put on gloves.
15 Assist the person off the toilet or commode (if used). Or remove the bedpan (if used). Assist with wiping and perineal care as needed.
16 Remove and discard soiled gloves. Practice hand hygiene. Put on clean gloves.
17 Note the color, amount, consistency, and odor of stools.

18 Collect the specimen.
   a Use the spoon attached to the lid to pick up several spoonfuls of stool. Or use a tongue blade to take about 2 tablespoons of stool to the specimen container (Fig. 39-12). Take the sample from:
      1) The middle of a formed stool
      2) Areas of pus, mucus, or blood and watery areas
      3) The middle and both ends of a hard stool
   b Secure the lid on the specimen container tightly.
   c Place the container in the plastic bag. Do not let the container touch the outside of the bag.
   d Wrap the tongue blade in toilet paper. Discard it in the disposable bag.
19 Test the specimen (if needed).
   a Open the test kit.
   b Use a tongue blade to obtain a small amount of stool.
   c Apply a thin smear of stool on *box A* on the test paper (Fig. 39-13, *A*).
   d Use another tongue blade to obtain stool from another part of the specimen.
   e Apply a thin smear of stool on *box B* on the test paper (Fig. 39-13, *B*).
   f Close the packet.
   g Wait 3 to 5 minutes or as required by the manufacturer.
   h Turn the test packet to the other side. Open the flap. Apply 2 drops of developer (from the kit) to both *A* and *B* boxes (Fig. 39-13, *C*). (Also apply 1 drop of developer to the card's quality control area. This checks that the card is functioning properly.) Follow the manufacturer's instructions.
   i Read the results within 60 seconds or as required by the manufacturer.
   j Note the color changes on your assignment sheet (Fig. 39-13, *D*).
   k Dispose of the test packet.
   l Wrap the tongue blades with toilet paper. Discard them in the disposable bag.

Collecting and Testing a Stool Specimen—cont'd

PROCEDURE—cont'd

20 Dispose of excess stool in the toilet. Avoid splashes. Rinse equipment. Pour the rinse into the toilet and flush. Follow agency procedures for cleaning and disinfection. Return equipment to its proper place.

21 Remove and discard the gloves. Practice hand hygiene. Put on clean gloves.
22 Seal the bag containing the specimen container. Assist with hand hygiene.
23 Remove and discard the gloves. Practice hand hygiene.

POST-PROCEDURE

24 Provide for comfort. (See the inside of the back cover.)
25 Make sure the bed is at a safe and comfortable level. Raise or lower bed rails. Follow the care plan.
26 Place the call light and other needed items within reach.
27 Follow the care plan and the person's preferences for privacy measures to maintain. Leaving the privacy curtain, window coverings, and door open or closed are examples.
28 Complete a safety check of the room. (See the inside of the back cover.)

29 Practice hand hygiene.
30 Take the specimen and requisition slip to the laboratory or storage area. Follow agency policies and procedures for labeling, containment, and transport.
31 Practice hand hygiene.
32 Report and record your care, observations, and the test results.

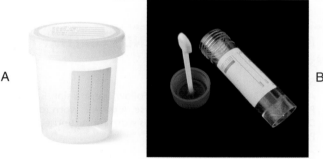

FIGURE 39-10 A, Stool specimen container. **B,** Stool specimen container with attached spoon. (A, © Fotofermer/Getty Images. B, From Healthlaw Medical Limited, Henso [Hangzhou] Co., Ltd. Hangzhou, China.)

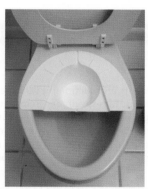

FIGURE 39-11 The specimen pan is placed at the back of the toilet for a stool specimen. (NOTE: The toilet seat is lowered over the specimen pan for the BM.)

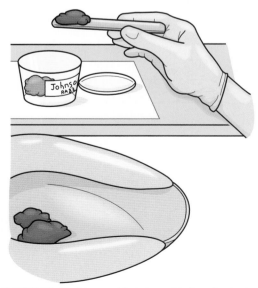

FIGURE 39-12 A tongue blade is used to transfer stool from the bedpan to the specimen container.

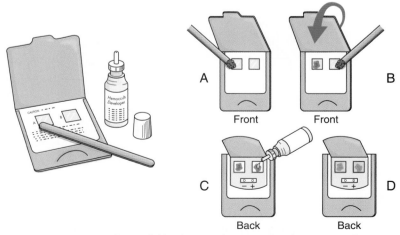

FIGURE 39-13 Testing for occult blood. **A,** Stool is smeared on *box A*. **B,** Stool is smeared on *box B* and then the flap is closed. **C,** Developer is applied to *boxes A* and *B* on the back side of the test packet. **D,** Color changes are noted.

SPUTUM SPECIMENS

Respiratory disorders cause the lungs, bronchi, and trachea to secrete mucus. Mucus from the respiratory system is called *sputum* when expectorated (expelled) through the mouth. Sputum specimens are studied for blood, microbes, and abnormal cells.

Sputum is not saliva. Saliva ("spit") is a thin, clear liquid produced by the salivary glands in the mouth. Sputum is coughed up from the bronchi and trachea. This can be painful and hard to do. Collecting a specimen is easier in the morning. Secretions collect in the trachea and bronchi during sleep. They are coughed up on awakening.

Follow the rules in Box 39-1. Also have the person rinse the mouth with water. Rinsing decreases saliva and removes food particles. Mouthwash is not used. It destroys some of the microbes in the mouth.

See *Focus on Children and Older Persons: Sputum Specimens*.
See *Delegation Guidelines: Sputum Specimens*.
See *Promoting Safety and Comfort: Sputum Specimens*.
See procedure: *Collecting a Sputum Specimen*.

FOCUS ON **CHILDREN AND OLDER PERSONS**

Sputum Specimens

Children
Breathing treatments and suctioning (Chapter 45) are often needed to obtain sputum specimens in infants and small children. The registered nurse (RN) or respiratory therapist (RT) gives the breathing treatment. The nurse suctions the trachea for the specimen. The infant or child is likely to be upset during suctioning. You may need to hold the child still.

Older Persons
Older persons may lack the strength to cough up sputum. Coughing is easier after *postural drainage*. It drains secretions by gravity. Gravity causes fluids to flow down. The person is positioned so a lung part is higher than the airway (Fig. 39-14). The nurse or respiratory therapist does postural drainage. Assist as directed.

DELEGATION GUIDELINES

Sputum Specimens

Collecting a sputum specimen is a routine nursing task. You need this information from the nurse.

- When to collect the specimen
- The amount needed—usually 1 to 2 teaspoons
- If the person uses the bathroom
- If the person can hold the sputum container
- If you need to wear a mask or respirator or other PPE (see *Promoting Safety and Comfort: Sputum Specimens*)
- What observations to report and record:
  - The time the specimen was collected
  - The amount collected
  - How easily the person raised the sputum
  - Sputum color—clear, white, yellow, green, brown, or red
  - Sputum odor—none or foul odor
  - Sputum consistency—thick, watery, or frothy (with bubbles or foam)
  - *Hemoptysis*—bloody *(hemo)* sputum *(ptysis* means to spit)
  - If the person could not produce sputum
  - Any other observations
- When to report observations
- What patient or resident concerns to report at once

PROMOTING SAFETY AND COMFORT

Sputum Specimens

Safety
Always use Standard Precautions. Follow Transmission-Based Precautions as directed by the nurse. A mask is worn for Droplet Precautions. A respirator is worn for Airborne Precautions. See Chapter 18.

Comfort
The procedure can embarrass the person. Coughing and expectorating sounds can disturb others. Also, sputum is not pleasant to look at. Privacy is important. Some sputum specimen containers are cloudy to hide the contents. Covering a clear container with a paper towel may be helpful.

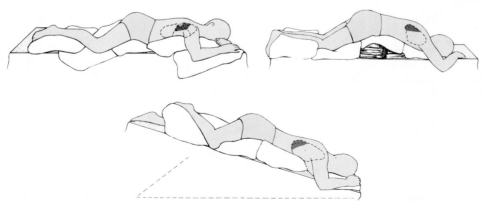

FIGURE 39-14 Some positions for postural drainage. (From Potter PA, Perry AG, Stockert PA, Hall AM: *Fundamentals of nursing*, ed 11, St Louis, 2023, Elsevier.)

Collecting a Sputum Specimen

QUALITY OF LIFE

- Knock before entering the person's room.
- Address the person by name.
- Introduce yourself by name and title.

- Explain the procedure before starting and during the procedure.
- Protect the person's rights during the procedure.
- Handle the person gently during the procedure.

PRE-PROCEDURE

1 Follow *Delegation Guidelines: Sputum Specimens.*
   See *Promoting Safety and Comfort:*
   a *Collecting and Testing Specimens*, p. 597
   b *Sputum Specimens*
2 Practice hand hygiene and get the following supplies.
   - Laboratory requisition slip
   - Sputum specimen container
   - Specimen label
   - Plastic bag with a *BIOHAZARD* label
   - Tissues
   - Gloves

3 Arrange items in the person's room (bathroom). Open the plastic bag.
4 Practice hand hygiene.
5 Identify the person. Check the ID bracelet against the requisition slip. Compare all information. Also call the person by name. Ask the person to state his or her first and last name and birthdate.
6 Label the specimen container in the person's presence.
7 Provide for privacy. If able, the person uses the bathroom for the procedure.

PROCEDURE

8 Put on gloves.
9 Have the person rinse the mouth with clear water.
10 Have the person hold the container. Only the outside is touched.
11 Have the person cover the mouth and nose with tissues when coughing. Follow agency policy for used tissues.
12 Have the person take 2 or 3 breaths and cough up the sputum.
13 Have the person expectorate (spit) directly into the container (Fig. 39-15). Sputum must not touch the outside of the container.

14 Collect 1 to 2 teaspoons of sputum.
15 Secure the lid on the specimen container tightly.
16 Place the container in the plastic bag. Do not let the container touch the outside of the bag.
17 Remove and discard gloves if soiled. Practice hand hygiene. Put on clean gloves.
18 Seal the bag containing the specimen container.
19 Assist with hand hygiene. Remove and discard the gloves. Practice hand hygiene.

POST-PROCEDURE

20 Provide for comfort. (See the inside of the back cover.)
21 Make sure the bed is at a safe and comfortable level. Raise or lower bed rails. Follow the care plan.
22 Place the call light and other needed items within reach.
23 Follow the care plan and the person's preferences for privacy measures to maintain. Leaving the privacy curtain, window coverings, and door open or closed are examples.

24 Complete a safety check of the room. (See the inside of the back cover.)
25 Practice hand hygiene.
26 Take the specimen and requisition slip to the laboratory or storage area. Follow agency policies and procedures for labeling, containment, and transport.
27 Practice hand hygiene.
28 Report and record your care and observations.

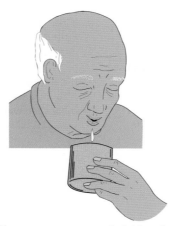

FIGURE 39-15 The person expectorates (spits) into the center of the specimen container.

BLOOD GLUCOSE TESTING

Blood glucose testing is used for persons with diabetes. The skin is punctured. A drop of blood is collected and tested. Measurements before meals and at bedtime are common. Results are used to regulate drugs and diet.

Blood Glucose Testing Equipment

To perform a blood glucose test, the following equipment and supplies are needed.

- *Gloves and antiseptic wipes.* Gloves are worn. The skin puncture site is cleaned with an antiseptic wipe. The puncture site is not touched after it is cleaned.
- *A sterile, disposable lancet in a lancing device.* A *lancet* is a short, pointed blade. It is used to puncture the skin to obtain the blood sample. The lancet is inside a lancing device. Usually a button on the device is pressed to activate the blade and puncture the skin. Retractable lancets protect staff from exposure to the blade. Discard the lancet in the sharps container after use (Chapter 17).
- *A glucometer* (Fig. 39-16). A *glucometer (glucose meter)* is a device for measuring *(meter)* blood glucose *(gluco).* The test result (a number) is displayed on the front of the device. Measurement time differs by the type of glucometer used. Around 5 seconds or less is common.
- *A bottle of reagent strips (test strips).* A strip is inserted into the glucometer. A drop of blood is applied to the reagent (test) strip. See Figure 39-16.
- *Gauze squares.* Pressure is applied with gauze squares over the puncture site until bleeding stops.

See *Teamwork and Time Management: Blood Glucose Testing Equipment.*

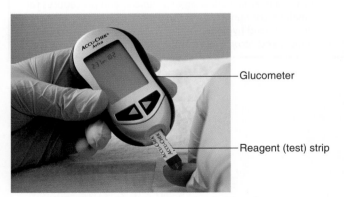

FIGURE 39-16 Blood glucose is tested with a glucometer.

Skin Puncture Sites

The side of a fingertip is the most common site for skin punctures (Fig. 39-17). Inspect the puncture site for trauma and skin breaks. Do not use swollen, bruised, cyanotic (bluish color), scarred, or calloused sites. Such areas have poor blood flow. A *callus* is a thick, hardened area on the skin. Calluses often form over frequently used areas, such as the tips of the thumbs and index fingers. Therefore thumbs and index fingers are not good skin puncture sites.

Use the side toward the tip of the middle or ring finger (see Fig. 39-17). Do not use the center, fleshy part of the fingertip. The site has many nerve endings making punctures painful. Explain that the person will feel a brief, sharp pinch.

See *Focus on Children and Older Persons: Skin Puncture Sites.*

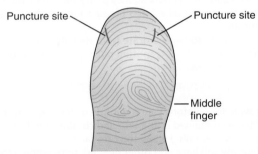

FIGURE 39-17 Sites for skin punctures on a fingertip.

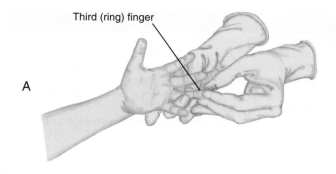

Third (ring) finger

A

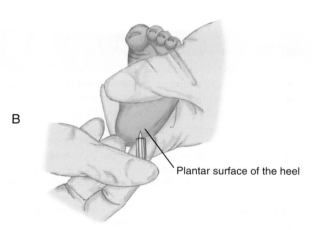

B

Plantar surface of the heel

FIGURE 39-18 A, The third finger (ring finger) is used for skin punctures in children. **B,** Heel site is used for skin punctures in infants. (From James SR, Nelson KA, Ashwill JW: *Nursing care of children: principles and practice,* ed 4, Philadelphia, 2013, Saunders.)

Measuring Blood Glucose

Some agencies allow nursing assistants to measure blood glucose. Others do not. If you perform blood glucose testing, you will learn to use your agency's equipment. Always follow the manufacturer's instructions and agency procedures. The procedure that follows is an example of how to measure blood glucose.

See *Teamwork and Time Management: Measuring Blood Glucose.*

See *Delegation Guidelines: Measuring Blood Glucose.*

See *Promoting Safety and Comfort: Measuring Blood Glucose.*

See procedure: *Measuring Blood Glucose,* p. 616.

TEAMWORK AND TIME MANAGEMENT
Measuring Blood Glucose

Perform blood glucose testing at times directed by the nurse and the care plan. Drugs are given at a certain time. The nurse needs the blood glucose results before giving the drugs.

DELEGATION GUIDELINES
Measuring Blood Glucose

In some agencies, blood glucose testing is a nursing task that may be delegated to you. If so, make sure that:
- Your state allows you to perform the task.
- The task is in your job description (Chapter 3).
- You have the necessary education and training.
- The agency has determined that you are competent to perform the task safely.
- You know how to use the supplies and equipment.
- You review the procedure with the delegating nurse.
- The delegating nurse is available to answer questions and to guide and assist you as needed.

If the above conditions are met, you need this information from the nurse and the care plan.
- What sites to avoid for a skin puncture
- When to collect and test the specimen—usually before meals and at bedtime
- If the person receives drugs that affect blood clotting (NOTE: If yes, it may take longer to stop bleeding. Apply pressure until bleeding stops.)
- What to report and record:
  - The time the specimen was collected
  - The blood glucose test result
  - The site used for the skin puncture
  - The amount of bleeding at the puncture site
  - Any signs of a *hematoma*—a swelling *(oma)* that contains blood *(hemat)*
  - How the person tolerated the procedure
  - Complaints of pain at the puncture site
  - Other observations or patient or resident complaints
- When to report observations and the test result
- What patient or resident concerns to report at once

PROMOTING SAFETY AND COMFORT
Measuring Blood Glucose

Safety
Accurate results are important. Inaccurate results can harm the person. Follow the rules in Box 39-2 (p. 616).

You must know how to use the equipment. Use only the reagent strips specified by the manufacturer. Otherwise you will get inaccurate results.

This procedure involves a risk of blood exposure and use of a lancet. Wear gloves. Discard the lancet in a sharps container. Follow the Bloodborne Pathogen Standard (Chapter 17).

Disinfect the glucometer before and after use. Follow the manufacturer's instructions for the disinfectant to use and how to use it.

BOX 39-2	Blood Glucose Testing

- Follow the manufacturer's instructions for the glucometer, lancing device, and disinfectant.
- Know how to use the equipment. Do not use equipment that you have not been trained to use. Request any necessary training.
- Make sure the glucometer was tested for accuracy. Check the testing log.
- Enter a code or user-ID if required by the glucometer. This is provided by the agency. Do not share your user-ID with others.

- Make sure you have the correct reagent (test) strips for the glucometer you are using. Scan the bar code on the bottle of reagent strips if needed. Or compare the code on the bottle of reagent strips to the code on the glucometer.
- Check the color of the reagent strips. Do not use discolored strips.
- Check the expiration date on the reagent strips. Do not use them if the date has passed.
- Report the result to the nurse at once.
- Record the result following agency policy.

Measuring Blood Glucose

QUALITY OF LIFE

- Knock before entering the person's room.
- Address the person by name.
- Introduce yourself by name and title.

- Explain the procedure before starting and during the procedure.
- Protect the person's rights during the procedure.
- Handle the person gently during the procedure.

PRE-PROCEDURE

1 Follow *Delegation Guidelines: Measuring Blood Glucose,* p. 615. See *Promoting Safety and Comfort:*
  a *Collecting and Testing Specimens,* p. 597
  b *Measuring Blood Glucose,* p. 615
2 Practice hand hygiene and get the following supplies.
  • Sterile lancet in a lancing device
  • Antiseptic wipes
  • Gloves
  • 2 × 2 gauze squares
  • Glucometer
  • Reagent (test) strips (Use the correct ones for the glucometer. Check the expiration date.)
  • Disinfectant
  • Paper towels
  • Warm washcloth (if needed)

3 Follow agency procedures to disinfect the glucometer before use. Follow the manufacturer's instructions for the disinfectant. (Wear gloves. Remove gloves and practice hand hygiene.)
4 Arrange items in the person's room. Place a barrier (paper towel) on the over-bed table if needed.
5 Practice hand hygiene.
6 Identify the person. Check the ID bracelet against the assignment sheet. Use 2 identifiers (Chapter 14). Also call the person by name. Ask the person to state his or her first and last name and birthdate.
7 Provide for privacy.
8 Raise the bed for body mechanics if needed. Lower the bed rail near you if needed.

PROCEDURE

9 Practice hand hygiene. Put on gloves.
10 Prepare the supplies.
  a Open the antiseptic wipes.
  b Prepare the glucometer. Follow the manufacturer's instructions and the prompts on the device.
    1) You may need to enter a user-ID and enter or scan the person's ID number (ID bracelet).
    2) Remove a test strip from the bottle. Close the cap tightly. Insert a test strip into the glucometer (Fig. 39-19, *A*). You may need to scan the bar code on the bottle of test strips. Or compare the code on the bottle of test strips to the code on the glucometer (Fig. 39-19, *B*).
  c Prepare the lancet. Follow the manufacturer's instructions for the lancing device.
11 Perform a skin puncture to obtain a drop of blood.
  a Inspect the person's fingers. Select a puncture site.
  b Do the following to increase blood flow to the puncture site.
    1) Warm the finger. Rub it gently or apply a warm washcloth.
    2) Massage the hand and finger toward the puncture site.
    3) Lower the finger below the person's waist.
  c Hold the finger with your thumb and index finger. Use your non-dominant hand. Hold the finger until step 12 (b).

  d Clean the site with an antiseptic wipe. *Do not touch the site after cleaning.*
  e Let the site dry.
  f Place the lancing device against the puncture site (Fig. 39-19, *C*).
  g Push the button on the device to puncture the skin. (Follow the manufacturer's instructions.)
  h Apply gentle pressure below the puncture site.
  i Let a large drop of blood form.
12 Collect and test the specimen. Follow the manufacturer's instructions and agency procedures for the glucometer used.
  a Touch the test strip to the drop of blood (Fig. 39-19, *D*). The glucometer will test the sample when enough blood is applied.
  b Apply pressure to the puncture site until bleeding stops. Use a gauze square. If able, let the person apply pressure to the site.
  c Read the result on the display (Fig. 39-19, *E*). Note the result on your note pad or assignment sheet. Tell the person the result.
  d Turn off the glucometer.
13 Discard the lancet in the sharps container.
14 Discard the gauze square and test strip. Follow agency policy.
15 Remove and discard the gloves. Practice hand hygiene.

Measuring Blood Glucose—cont'd

POST-PROCEDURE

16 Provide for comfort. (See the inside of the back cover.)
17 Lower the bed to a safe and comfortable level. Raise or lower bed rails. Follow the care plan.
18 Clean up and store supplies and equipment. (Wear gloves. Change gloves as needed.)
   a Discard disposable items.
   b Disinfect the glucometer. Follow agency procedures and the manufacturer's instructions.
   c Follow agency policy for any used linens.
   d Clean and dry the over-bed table as needed. Dry with paper towels. Discard paper towels. Position the over-bed table as the person prefers.
   e Remove and discard gloves. Practice hand hygiene.

19 Place the call light and other needed items within reach.
20 Follow the care plan and the person's preferences for privacy measures to maintain. Leaving the privacy curtain, window coverings, and door open or closed are examples.
21 Complete a safety check of the room. (See the inside of the back cover.)
22 Practice hand hygiene.
23 Return the glucometer to its proper place.
24 Report and record the test result and your care and observations (Fig. 39-20, p. 618).

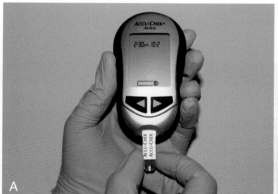
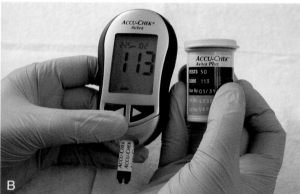
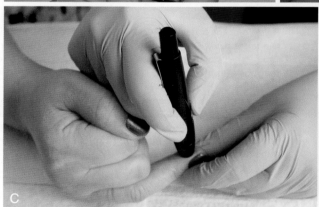
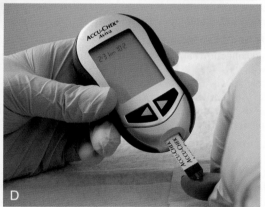
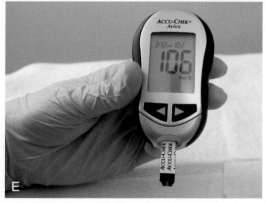

FIGURE 39-19 Measuring blood glucose. **A,** A reagent (test) strip is in the glucometer. **B,** The code on the bottle of reagent (test) strips is compared to the code on the glucometer. **C,** A lancet is used to puncture the skin. **D,** A drop of blood is applied to the reagent (test) strip. **E,** The result is displayed on the glucometer.

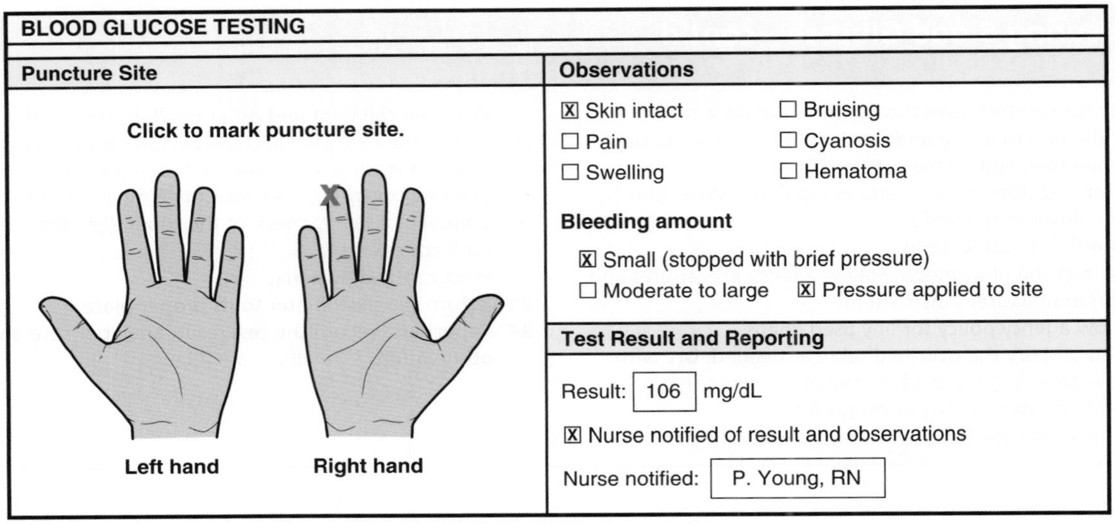

BLOOD GLUCOSE TESTING		
Puncture Site	**Observations**	
Click to mark puncture site. Left hand Right hand	☒ Skin intact ☐ Bruising ☐ Pain ☐ Cyanosis ☐ Swelling ☐ Hematoma **Bleeding amount** ☒ Small (stopped with brief pressure) ☐ Moderate to large ☒ Pressure applied to site	
	Test Result and Reporting	
	Result: [106] mg/dL ☒ Nurse notified of result and observations Nurse notified: [P. Young, RN]	

FIGURE 39-20 Charting sample.

FOCUS ON PRIDE

The Person, Family, and Yourself

Personal and Professional Responsibility

You must collect specimens on the right person. Otherwise, one or both persons could be harmed. Before collecting a specimen, carefully identify the person.

In some agencies, collection information is written on the specimen container. Collection date and time and the collector's name or initials are examples. Follow agency policy to properly collect and label specimens.

Rights and Respect

Specimen collection can be embarrassing. To respect the right to privacy:
- Politely ask visitors to leave the room.
- Close doors, privacy curtains, and window coverings.
- Leave the room if it is safe to do so. If you cannot leave, tell the person why.

Independence and Social Interaction

Some persons can collect their own specimens. Doing so promotes independence and reduces embarrassment.

Explain the procedure and show the person the container. Tell the person where you are placing the container. When ready to collect the specimen, the person knows where to find the container.

Delegation and Teamwork

Before taking a specimen to the laboratory, tell the nurse and your co-workers. Ask if other staff need specimens delivered. Doing so saves staff time. This also prevents having too many staff members off the unit at the same time. Return from the laboratory promptly.

Ethics and Laws

If you did not collect a specimen correctly, do not send it to the laboratory. Tell the nurse. Then collect the specimen at the next opportunity. Test results must be accurate for correct diagnosis and treatment. Take pride in honestly reporting mistakes.

FOCUS ON PRIDE: Application

What mistakes could occur in specimen collection? What can you do to prevent such mistakes? Explain why failing to report a mistake can be harmful.

REVIEW QUESTIONS

Circle the BEST answer.

1 Which specimen was collected *correctly*?
   a A stool specimen that contains urine
   b A urine specimen that contains toilet paper
   c A sputum specimen with a label and requisition slip
   d A urine specimen with a loose lid

2 A random urine specimen is collected
   a After sleep
   b Before meals
   c After meals
   d Any time

3 Perineal care is given before collecting a
   a Random urine specimen
   b Midstream urine specimen
   c 24-hour urine specimen
   d Stool specimen

4 To collect a midstream specimen on a female
   a Spread the labia to expose the urethral area
   b Clean the urethral area from back to front
   c Collect urine at the start of the urine stream
   d Collect about 10 mL of urine

5 A person is incontinent of urine 12 hours after the start of a 24-hour urine specimen. You should
   a Tell the nurse so the test can be re-started
   b Send the specimen collected over 12 hours to the laboratory
   c Not report the missed void so the 24-hour specimen is done on time
   d Ask the nurse to extend the collection time by 1 hour

6 Urine is tested for glucose
   a To measure the pH
   b To check for blood
   c To check for sugar
   d To check for infection

7 You are testing urine using reagent strips. Which is *correct*?
   a Obtain a 24-hour urine specimen for testing.
   b Touch the test area to make sure it is secure.
   c Use the reagent strips if the expiration date has passed.
   d Compare the strip with the color chart on the bottle.

8 You need to strain a person's urine. Straining is done to find
   a Blood
   b Stones
   c Ketones
   d Protein

9 A stool appears black and tarry. This is
   a Occult blood
   b Hematuria
   c Melena
   d Normal feces (stools)

10 A person has a BM in a bedpan. Part of the stool is red and watery. When collecting a sample, you should
   a Avoid the red, watery part
   b Collect from the red, watery part
   c Take the bedpan to the laboratory
   d Flush the stool and collect a different sample later

11 The best time to collect a sputum specimen is
   a On awakening
   b After meals
   c At bedtime
   d After oral hygiene

12 A sputum specimen is needed. Have the person
   a Use mouthwash
   b Rinse the mouth with clear water
   c Brush the teeth
   d Remove dentures

13 Which is the *best* site for a skin puncture?
   a At the center of the thumb
   b On a callus on the index finger
   c At the side toward the tip of the ring finger
   d On a swollen area of the little finger

14 Which is needed to measure blood glucose?
   a Glucometer
   b Sterile specimen container
   c Color-changing reagent strip
   d Sphygmomanometer

15 Which action when measuring blood glucose is *correct*?
   a Dispose of a used lancet in the wastebasket.
   b Only report an abnormal result.
   c Perform the test at a time convenient for you.
   d Check the expiration date on the reagent strips before use.

Answers to Chapter 39 questions are on p. 903.

FOCUS ON **PRACTICE**

Problem Solving

A midstream urine specimen is ordered. You give the patient the specimen cup and pack of towelettes and ask: "Do you know what to do?" The patient says: "Yes, I've done this before." You tell the patient to leave the specimen in the bathroom and signal for you when done.

You return and notice the towelettes are un-opened. What do you do? Should you send the specimen to the laboratory? How could this have been prevented?

The Person Having Surgery

OBJECTIVES

- Define the key terms and key abbreviations in this chapter.
- Describe the common fears and concerns of surgical patients.
- Describe pre-operative and post-operative care.
- List the signs and symptoms to report after surgery.

- Perform the procedures described in this chapter.
- Explain how to promote PRIDE in the person, the family, and yourself.

KEY TERMS

anesthesia The loss *(an)* of all sensation *(esthesia)*, especially pain, produced by a drug

antiseptic A substance applied to living tissue that prevents or stops the growth or action of microbes

elective surgery Surgery done by choice to improve life or well-being

embolus A blood clot (thrombus) that travels through the vascular system until it lodges in a blood vessel

emergency surgery Surgery done at once to save life or function

general anesthesia A treatment with certain drugs that produces a deep sleep and the absence of all sensation, especially pain

local anesthesia The loss of sensation, produced by a drug, in a small area

post-operative After *(post)* surgery; post-op

pre-operative Before *(pre)* surgery; pre-op

regional anesthesia The loss of sensation, produced by a drug, in a large area

sedation A state of quiet, calmness, or sleep produced by a drug

surgical site infection (SSI) An infection that occurs after surgery in the body part where the surgery took place

thrombus A blood clot

urgent surgery Surgery needed for health; it can be delayed for a few days

KEY ABBREVIATIONS

AE	Anti-embolism; anti-embolic	NPO	Nothing by mouth; *nil per os*
ASC	Ambulatory surgery center	OR	Operating room
CBC	Complete blood count	PACU	Post-anesthesia care unit
ECG; EKG	Electrocardiogram	post-op	Post-operative
ID	Identification	pre-op	Pre-operative
I&O	Intake and output	SCD	Sequential compression device
IV	Intravenous	SSI	Surgical site infection
NG	Naso-gastric	TED	Thrombo-embolic deterrent

There are many reasons for surgery. Surgery may be needed to:
- Remove, repair, or replace a diseased or injured body part.
- Remove a tumor.
- Make a diagnosis.
- Relieve symptoms.
- Restore or improve function or appearance.

Surgeries are done in hospitals or in ambulatory surgery centers. Hospital patients are admitted on the morning of surgery or 1 or 2 days before surgery. Some patients have surgery after receiving emergency room care. Called *in-patients*, surgical patients admitted to the hospital stay for 1 or more days after surgery. Most hospitals also offer ambulatory (same-day, outpatient) surgery services.

Ambulatory surgery centers (ASCs) are designed and equipped for certain surgical, diagnostic, or preventive procedures. Eye surgeries, colonoscopies to diagnose colon disorders, and pain management for back disorders are examples. Called *out-patients*, ASC patients go home in less than 23 hours. However, some ASCs offer overnight stays.

Surgeries are described as:

- *Elective surgery*—done by choice to improve life or well-being. It is not life-saving. Joint replacement surgery and cosmetic (plastic) surgery are examples. The surgery is scheduled in advance.
- *Urgent surgery*—needed for health. It can be delayed for a few days. Sometimes cancer surgery and coronary artery bypass surgery are delayed for a few days.
- *Emergency surgery*—done at once to save life or function. The need is sudden and not expected. Vehicle crashes, stabbings, and bullet wounds often require emergency surgery.

The person is prepared for what happens before, during, and after surgery. *Pre-operative* (*pre-op*) refers to before (*pre*) surgery. *Post-operative* (*post-op*) refers to after (*post*) surgery. Some people recover in nursing centers or rehabilitation centers. Some need home care.

PSYCHOLOGICAL CARE

Surgery causes many fears and concerns (Box 40-1). Past experiences affect feelings. Some persons have had surgery before. Others have not. Patients are affected when family and friends talk about their own surgeries. Some people do not share fears and concerns. They may cry, be quiet or withdrawn, or talk about other things. Some pace. Others are very cheerful.

Mental preparation is important. Respect the person's fears and concerns. Show warmth, sensitivity, and caring.

Your Role

You can assist in the person's psychological care before and after surgery.

- Listen. The person may talk about fears and concerns.
- Refer questions to the nurse.
- Explain the care you will give and its need.
- Follow communication rules (Chapters 7 and 8).
- Use verbal and nonverbal communication (Chapter 7).
- Provide care with skill and competence.
- Report signs of fear or anxiety (Chapter 53).
- Report a request to see a member of the clergy. See *Focus on Communication: Your Role.*

BOX 40-1	Surgery Fears and Concerns

Fear of

- Anesthesia and its effects (p. 626)
- Cancer
- Complications from surgery
- Disability
- Disfigurement and scarring
- Dying during or after surgery
- Exposure
- Not waking up after surgery
- Pain:
    - During surgery
    - After surgery
- Prolonged recovery
- Separation from family and friends
- Surgery on the wrong body part
- Tubes, needles, and other care equipment
- Waking up during surgery
- What happens after surgery:
    - More surgery
    - Treatments
    - Care

Concerns about

- Caring for children and other family members
- Finances:
    - Monthly bills
    - Loan payments
    - Mortgages
    - Hospital bills
    - Doctor bills
- House, lawn, and garden
- Pets
- Plants

FOCUS ON COMMUNICATION

Your Role

After surgery, the doctor talks to the patient and family about the results. Eager to know, they may ask you about reports. Refer their questions to the nurse. Never tell any results or diagnoses. You can say:

- "The doctor will talk to you about the surgery and the results. I'll tell the nurse that you're asking."
- "I'll get the nurse to answer your questions."

PRE-OPERATIVE CARE

The pre-operative (pre-op) period may be many days or a few minutes. If time allows, the person is prepared mentally and physically for anesthesia and surgery. The goal is to prevent complications before, during, and after surgery.

The nurse provides information. The nurse explains what to expect before, during, and after surgery.

- *Pre-op care*—includes tests and their purpose, skin preparation, personal care, and the purpose and effects of pre-op drugs.
- *Deep breathing, coughing, and incentive spirometry*—are practiced. Post-op, they are done every 1 to 2 hours when the person is awake. See Chapter 44.
- *Post-anesthesia care unit (PACU)*—commonly called the *recovery room*, this is where the person wakes up after surgery (Fig. 40-1). PACU care is explained.
- *Vital signs*—are taken often until they are stable. Equipment for monitoring vital signs electronically remains in place during and after surgery.
- *Food and fluids*—post-op, the person is NPO (nothing by mouth; *nil per os*) and has an intravenous (IV) site for IV therapy. Food and fluids are allowed when the person's condition is stable.
- *Turning and re-positioning*—are done at least every 1 to 2 hours post-op.
- *Early ambulation*—is done as soon as possible post-op.
- *Pain*—relates to the type and amount of pain to expect and how pain-relief drugs are given.
- *Equipment*—may involve a urinary catheter, naso-gastric (NG) tube, oxygen, wound suction, a cast, traction, or other equipment.
- *Position restrictions*—are common after some surgeries. For example, the hip is abducted after hip replacement surgery (Chapter 49).

See *Teamwork and Time Management: Pre-Operative Care.*
See *Focus on Children and Older Persons: Pre-Operative Care.*

Special Tests

Pre-op, the doctor evaluates the person's health status. These tests are common.
- Chest x-ray.
- Complete blood count (CBC).
- Urinalysis (U/A; UA).
- Electrocardiogram (ECG; EKG). See Figure 40-2.

Other tests depend on the person's condition and surgery. For expected blood loss, the person's blood is tested for blood type and compatible blood from a blood donor. This is called *type and crossmatch.*

The person is prepared for the tests as needed. Test results must be in the medical record before surgery.

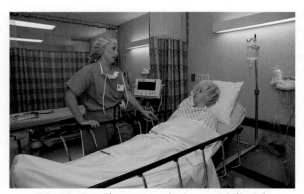
FIGURE 40-1 The post-anesthesia care unit (PACU).

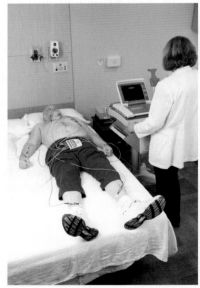
FIGURE 40-2 An electrocardiogram is performed.

Nutrition and Fluids

A light meal usually is allowed. Then the person is NPO for 6 to 12 hours before surgery. These measures reduce the risk of vomiting and aspiration during anesthesia and after surgery. An NPO sign is placed in the person's room. The water mug is removed.

Bowel Elimination

Bowel surgeries and procedures may require a *bowel prep*— cleansing the bowel of feces. Feces contain microbes. When the intestine is opened, feces can spill into the sterile abdominal cavity, causing a serious infection. The bowel prep helps prevent this contamination.

For the bowel prep, special fluids are ordered for the person to drink. Or enemas are ordered (Chapter 29).

Urinary Elimination

The person voids before the nurse gives pre-op drugs. If the person has a catheter, the drainage bag is emptied. The output is measured and recorded.

Catheters are commonly inserted in the OR. For pelvic and abdominal surgeries, the bladder must be empty. A full bladder is easily injured during surgery. Catheters also allow accurate output measurements during and after surgery.

Jewelry

Jewelry is easily lost or broken in the OR and PACU. Transfers to and from the OR, PACU, and the person's room also present safety risks. And jewelry can cause pressure injuries (Chapter 42). Therefore all jewelry is removed and stored or given to family for safe-keeping. This includes body-piercing jewelry. Record jewelry removal and storage according to agency policy.

The person may want to wear a wedding ring or religious item. Secure the item according to agency policy. Hand, arm, shoulder, and breast surgeries can cause swelling of the fingers on the affected side. Wedding rings are removed for such surgeries.

The Surgery Consent

The person's informed consent is needed for surgery. The patient and family are told about:

- The need for the surgery
- The surgery, risks, and possible complications
- Other treatment options
- The risks from not having surgery
- Who will do the surgery
- When the surgery will be done and how long it will take
- Expected length of recovery

Questions are answered. Misunderstandings are cleared up. A surgical consent is signed when the person understands the information. The doctor is responsible for securing the written consent. Often this is delegated to a nurse. *You do not obtain the person's written consent for surgery.*

Personal Care

Personal care before surgery may involve:

- *A complete bath, shower, or tub bath and shampoo.* A special soap or cleanser and shampoo are common. Their purpose is to reduce the number of microbes present. This lessens the risk of a wound infection. A patient gown and surgical cap are worn to the OR.
- *Make-up, nail polish, and non-natural nail removal.* The skin, lips, and nail beds are observed for color and circulation during and after surgery.
- *Hair care.* All hairpins, clips, combs, and other items are removed. So are wigs and hairpieces. A surgical cap keeps hair out of the face and operative site.
- *Oral hygiene.* Being NPO causes thirst and a dry mouth. Remind the person not to swallow any water during oral hygiene.
- *Dentures.* Provide denture care and store dentures following agency policy. Some people do not like to be without their dentures. Let them wear dentures as long as possible. This promotes dignity and self-esteem.
- *Adaptive (assistive) devices and prostheses.* Eyeglasses, contact lenses, hearing aids, artificial eyes, and artificial limbs are removed. Hearing aids may be worn if the surgeon needs to talk to or instruct the patient during surgery. Follow agency policy for storage and safe-keeping.
- *Other.* Often elastic stockings (p. 629) are put on before transport to the OR. So are sequential compression devices (p. 632).

See *Promoting Safety and Comfort: Personal Care.*

PROMOTING SAFETY AND COMFORT
Personal Care

Safety
Check for loose teeth when performing oral care. Loose teeth are common in children. Adults may have loose teeth from periodontal disease (Chapter 23). Report loose teeth to the nurse. The nurse notes this in the medical record and alerts the OR staff. A loose tooth can fall out during anesthesia. The person can aspirate the tooth.

The Pre-Operative Checklist

A pre-operative checklist is a list of what is to be completed before surgery (Fig. 40-3, p. 624). You may be delegated some tasks on the list. Promptly report when you complete each task and any observations. The checklist is completed before the nurse gives pre-op drugs.

PRE-OPERATIVE CHECKLIST

Username: T. Murphy, RN | Sign

Date: March 7 | Time: 07 ▼ 00 ▼

Medical Record	Yes	No
Surgical consent signed	X	☐
NPO since Date: March 6 Time: 22 ▼ 00 ▼	X	☐
Allergies verified Penicillin	X	☐
History and physical in medical record	X	☐
Advance directives in medical record	X	☐

Test results in medical record:

		Isolation precautions:
X CBC	X U/A	X None
X Type and crossmatch	X EKG	☐ Contact
X Urine pregnancy for females	X Chest x-ray	☐ Droplet
		☐ Airborne

Complete Before Surgery	Yes	No
Skin cleansing	X	☐
Patient gown and surgical cap applied	X	☐
Surgical side/site marked and verified	X	☐
IV inserted	X	☐
AE stockings/SCD on	X	☐
ID bracelet is on	X	☐
Voided or urinary catheter inserted	X	☐

Personal Belongings	In Place	Removed	N/A
Make-up, nail polish, non-natural nails	☐	X	☐
Hairpins, clips, combs, wig, hairpiece	☐	☐	X
Dentures (full, partial)	☐	X	☐
Eyeglasses, contact lenses	☐	X	☐
Hearing aid(s)	☐	☐	X
Prostheses (eye, limb)	☐	☐	X
Jewelry	☐	X	☐

Measurements

Vital Signs
Temperature 98.8 °F
Blood pressure 132/88 mm Hg
Pulse 68
Respirations 18
Pulse oximetry 98 %

Pain
Location Right hip
Intensity 6
Weight and Height
Weight 165 lbs
Height 5 ft 4 in

FIGURE 40-3 A sample pre-operative checklist.

Marking the Surgical Site. The surgeon has the person mark the surgical site before the surgery. Marking the site prevents surgery on the wrong part.

Site markings may be part of the pre-op checklist. The site is marked before pre-op drugs are given.

Skin Preparation

The incision is a portal of entry for microbes from the skin. A *surgical site infection (SSI)* is an infection that occurs after surgery in the body part where the surgery took place. A *skin prep* reduces the risk of SSI.

The area is cleaned with an antiseptic (Fig. 40-4). An *antiseptic* is a substance applied to living tissue that prevents or stops the growth or action of microbes. The incision and a large area around it are *prepped* (Fig. 40-5). The prep is done right before surgery.

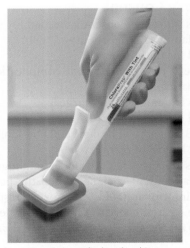

FIGURE 40-4 An antiseptic is applied to the skin to prevent infection. (Courtesy Becton, Dickinson and Company, Franklin Lakes, NJ.)

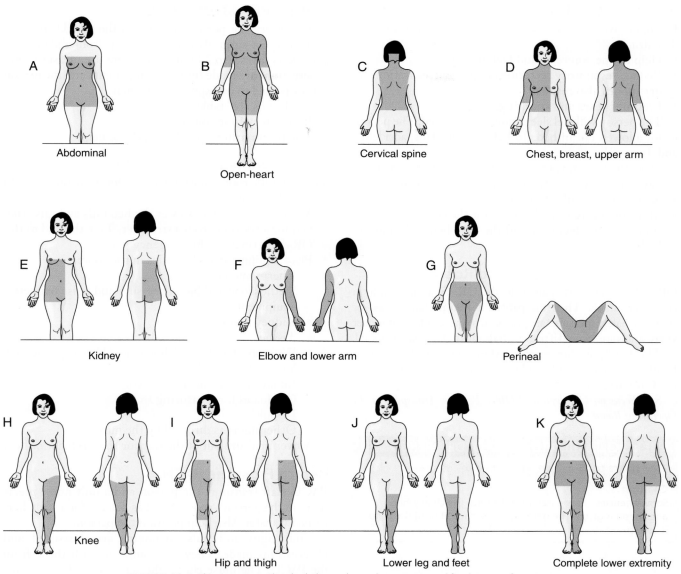

FIGURE 40-5 Skin prep sites. The *shaded area* shows the area prepped for the type of surgery.

Hair Removal. Hair is not removed from the surgical site unless it will interfere with surgery. If the surgeon orders hair removal, it is done before the antiseptic is applied. Electric clippers are used for hair removal (Fig. 40-6). Or a hair removal cream may be used. Shaving with a razor can cause small cuts in the skin. This increases the risk for SSI.

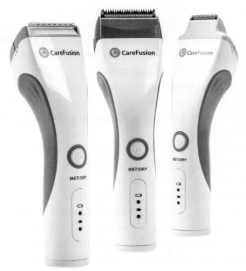

FIGURE 40-6 Surgical clippers. (Courtesy Becton, Dickinson and Company, Franklin Lakes, NJ.)

Pre-Operative Drugs

Pre-operative drugs are given before transport to the OR. The drugs:

- Help the person relax and feel drowsy.
- Reduce respiratory secretions to prevent aspiration. A dry mouth also results.
- Prevent nausea and vomiting.

The person will feel sleepy and light-headed. The person is not allowed out of bed. To help prevent falls, accidents, and damaged equipment:

- Have the person void before the drugs are given. Then have the person use the bedpan or urinal to void.
- Raise the bed rails after the drugs are given.
- Move furniture to make room for the stretcher if a transfer is needed. Clear off the over-bed table and the bedside stand.

Transport to the Operating Room

OR staff transport the patient to the OR. First, identification checks are made. Then the patient is transported by bed or stretcher. Safety measures are practiced to prevent falls. Stretcher safety straps are secured if present. Side rails or bed rails are raised.

The family is shown where they can wait. Sometimes family members are allowed to go with the patient as far as the OR entrance.

See *Focus on Children and Older Persons: Transport to the Operating Room.*

FOCUS ON CHILDREN AND OLDER PERSONS

Transport to the Operating Room

Children
Some agencies allow a parent to be with the child while anesthesia is given. The parent stays in the OR until the child is asleep.

SEDATION AND ANESTHESIA

Some procedures only require sedation. *Sedation* is a state of quiet, calmness, or sleep produced by a drug. Levels of sedation are minimal, moderate (conscious), and deep.

Anesthesia is the loss (*an*) of all sensation (*esthesia*), especially pain, produced by a drug.

- *General anesthesia* is a treatment with certain drugs that produces a deep sleep and the absence of all sensation, especially pain. Drugs are given IV or inhaled through a gas.
- *Regional anesthesia* is the loss of sensation, produced by a drug, in a large area. The person is awake. A drug is injected into a body part.
- *Local anesthesia* is the loss of sensation, produced by a drug, in a small area. A drug is injected at the site.

An *anesthesiologist* is a doctor specializing in giving sedation and anesthetics. An *anesthetist* is a registered nurse (RN) with advanced study in sedation and anesthetics.

POST-OPERATIVE CARE

After surgery the person is taken to the PACU to begin post-op (post-surgical) care. Recovery from sedation or anesthesia takes 1 to 2 hours. Vital signs are measured and observations are made often. For inpatient care, the person is transported to a hospital room when:

- Vital signs are stable.
- Respiratory function is good.
- The person can respond and call for help.

Preparing the Person's Room

The person's room must be ready for post-op care. To prepare the room:

- Make a surgical bed. Lower the bed rails and raise the bed for a transfer from a stretcher. Take the bed to the OR department if this is agency policy.
- Place equipment and supplies in the room.
  - Thermometer
  - Stethoscope and blood pressure and pulse oximetry equipment
  - Kidney basin
  - Tissues
  - Waterproof under-pad, linens, and blankets as needed
  - Vital signs flow sheet
  - Intake and output (I&O) record
  - Graduates for measuring I&O
  - IV pole
  - Other items as directed by the nurse
- Move furniture out of the way for the stretcher or bed.

Return From the PACU

PACU staff transport the person and a unit nurse meets them in the person's room. Assist as needed for a stretcher-to-bed transfer. Also help position the person.

Vital signs and pulse oximetry are measured and observations made. They are compared with those from the PACU. The nurse checks the surgical site for bleeding. Catheter, IV, and other tube placements and functions are checked. Bed rails are raised. The call light and other needed items are placed within the person's reach. Necessary care and treatments are given. Then the family can join the person.

Measurements and Observations

Your role in post-op care depends on the person's condition. Often you will measure vital signs and pulse oximetry and make post-op observations. These are usually done:

- Every 15 minutes until the person's condition is stable
- Then every 30 minutes for 1 to 2 hours
- Then every hour for 4 hours
- Then every 4 hours

The nurse tells you how often to check the person. Many serious complications can result from surgery (Box 40-2). Be alert for the signs and symptoms in Box 40-2. Report them at once.

BOX 40-2	**Post-Op Complications and Observations**

Complications

- Respiratory System
  - *Pneumonia*—inflammation and infection of lung tissue
  - *Atelectasis*—collapse of a portion of the lung
  - *Pulmonary embolism*—a blood clot from a vein that travels *(embolus)* in the bloodstream until it lodges in a lung
- Circulatory System
  - *Hypovolemia*—inadequate *(hypo)* amount *(vol)* of blood *(emia)*
  - *Hemorrhage*—the excessive loss *(rrhage)* of blood *(hemo)* in a short time
  - *Hypovolemic shock*—when organs and tissues do not get enough blood *(shock)* because of an inadequate *(hypo)* amount *(vol)* of blood *(emia)*
  - *Thrombophlebitis*—a blood clot *(thrombo)* causing inflammation *(itis)* of a vein *(phleb)*
  - *Thrombus*—a blood clot
  - *Embolus*—a blood clot that travels through the vascular system until it lodges in a blood vessel
- Urinary System
  - *Urinary retention*—urine collects *(retention)* in the bladder from being unable to void
  - *Urinary tract infection*—inflammation and infection of the urinary structures (bladder, ureters, urethra)
- Gastro-Intestinal System
  - Nausea
  - Vomiting
  - Constipation
  - Flatulence
  - *Post-operative ileus*—the absence of normal intestinal *(ileus)* function from the lack of peristalsis after surgery
- Integumentary System (Chapter 41)
  - Wound infection
  - *Hematoma*—a swelling *(oma)* that contains blood *(hemat)*
  - *Dehiscence*—the separation of wound layers
  - *Evisceration*—the separation of the wound along with the protrusion of abdominal organs

Observations to Report

- Abdominal: distention (swelling), pain, cramping
- Anxiety
- Bleeding: from the incision, drainage tubes, suction tubes, or other sites
- Blood pressure: increase or decrease
- Chest pain
- Choking
- Condition: any change in

Observations to Report—cont'd

- Confusion
- Cough: weak
- Discomfort in a leg
- Disorientation
- Drainage:
  - From wound (Chapter 41)
  - On or under dressings
  - On bed linens (including bottom linens and pillowcases)
  - Appearance from urinary catheter, NG tube, wound suction, and other tubes
- Hypoxia (Chapter 44)
- Intake and output (I&O)
- IV flow, flow rate: problem with
- Nausea
- Pain
- Pulse:
  - More than 100 beats per minute
  - Less than 60 beats per minute
  - Weak
  - Irregular
- Pulse oximetry measurement (Chapter 44)
- Respirations:
  - Shallow, slow breathing
  - Rapid
  - Gasping
  - Difficult *(dyspnea)*
  - Shortness of breath
  - Moist-sounding
  - Gurgling
- Restlessness
- Skin:
  - Moist or clammy
  - Pale *(pallor)*
  - *Cyanosis* (bluish color)
  - Cool
  - Warm or hot
- Sputum: clear, white, yellow, green, brown, or red; thick, watery, or frothy (with bubbles)
- Swelling in affected area
- Temperature: increase or decrease
- Thirst
- Urinary complaints: cannot void, burning, urgency, lower abdominal pain
- Urine: amount, character, and time of first voiding after surgery
- Vomiting

Positioning

The person is positioned for comfort and to prevent complications. There may be position restrictions after some surgeries. The person is usually positioned:

- To promote comfort
- For easy and comfortable breathing
- To prevent stress on the incision
- To prevent aspiration

When supine, the head of the bed is usually raised slightly. The person's head may be turned to the side.

The person is re-positioned at least every 1 to 2 hours. This prevents respiratory and circulatory complications. Turning may be painful. Provide support. Use smooth, gentle motions. Place pillows and positioning devices as the nurse directs (Chapters 19 and 35).

The nurse tells you when to re-position the person and the positions allowed. Usually you assist the nurse. The nurse may delegate these tasks when the person is stable and care is simple.

See *Focus on Children and Older Persons: Positioning.*

FOCUS ON **CHILDREN AND OLDER PERSONS**

Positioning

Older Persons

Many older persons have stiff and painful joints. Sore muscles, bones, and joints can occur from the OR table. Turn and re-position older persons slowly and gently.

Preventing Respiratory and Circulatory Complications

Coughing and deep-breathing exercises help prevent respiratory complications, including post-operative pneumonia (see Box 40-2). So does incentive spirometry. See Chapter 44.

Circulation must be stimulated for blood flow in the legs. If blood flow is sluggish, blood clots may form. A blood clot is called a *thrombus.* Blood clots (thrombi) can form in the deep leg veins in the lower legs or thighs (Fig. 40-7, *A*). Many people do not have signs or symptoms. Report the following at once.

- Swollen area of a leg.
- Pain or tenderness in a leg. This may be only when standing or walking.
- Warmth in the part of the leg that is swollen or painful.
- Red or discolored skin.

A blood clot can break loose and travel through the bloodstream. It then becomes an embolus. An *embolus* is a blood clot *(thrombus)* that travels through the vascular system until it lodges in a blood vessel (Fig. 40-7, *B*). An embolus from a vein lodges in the lungs *(pulmonary embolism)* and can cause severe respiratory problems and death. Report chest pain or shortness of breath at once.

Circulation is stimulated and thrombi prevented by:

- Leg exercises
- Ambulation as soon as possible
- Elastic stockings
- Elastic bandages (p. 631)
- Sequential compression devices (p. 632)
- No prolonged standing or sitting

See *Focus on Children and Older Persons: Preventing Respiratory and Circulatory Complications.*

See *Focus on Communication: Preventing Respiratory and Circulatory Complications.*

See *Promoting Safety and Comfort: Preventing Respiratory and Circulatory Complications.*

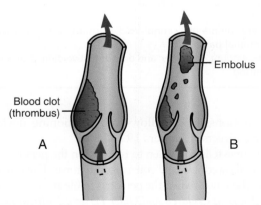

FIGURE 40-7 A, A blood clot is attached to the wall of a vein. The *arrows* show the direction of blood flow. **B,** Part of the thrombus breaks off and becomes an embolus. The embolus travels through the vascular system until it lodges in a distant vessel.

FOCUS ON CHILDREN AND OLDER PERSONS
Preventing Respiratory and Circulatory Complications

Older Persons
Older persons are at risk for respiratory complications. Respiratory muscles are weaker. The lungs are less elastic. The person has less strength for coughing. Coughing, deep breathing, and incentive spirometry are very important.

Older persons also are at risk for *thrombi* (blood clots) and *emboli* (dislodged blood clots). Blood is pumped through the body with less force. Circulation is already sluggish.

FOCUS ON COMMUNICATION
Preventing Respiratory and Circulatory Complications

The abbreviation "DVT" is often used in reference to thrombi. DVT stands for *deep vein thrombosis*—a blood clot in a vein deep in the body.

"TCDB" is often used for *turn, cough, and deep breathe.* Turning (re-positioning), coughing, and deep breathing are measures that help prevent complications after surgery.

At first, some terms and abbreviations will be unfamiliar. You must learn the common terms and abbreviations used in your work area. Ask the nurse if you do not know the meaning of a term or abbreviation.

PROMOTING SAFETY AND COMFORT
Preventing Respiratory and Circulatory Complications

Comfort
For coughing exercises, "splinting" the incision promotes comfort. To *splint* means to support or brace. To splint the incision, the person holds a pillow or the hands over the incision. See Chapter 44.

Leg Exercises. Leg exercises promote venous blood flow and help prevent thrombi. The nurse tells you when to do the exercises. They are done at least every 1 or 2 hours while the person is awake. Assist if the person is weak.

These exercises are usually done 5 times.

- Make circles with the toes. This rotates the ankles.
- Dorsiflex and plantar flex the ankles (Chapter 35).
- Flex and extend 1 knee and then the other (Fig. 40-8, *A*).
- Raise and lower the leg off the bed (Fig. 40-8, *B*).
  Repeat with the other leg.

After leg surgery, the surgeon may order other exercises and when to do them. Do not assist with leg exercises until the nurse tells you to.

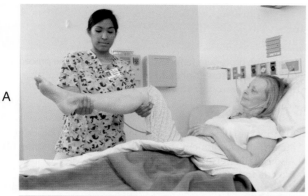

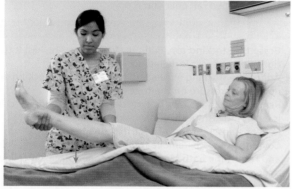

FIGURE 40-8 Leg exercises to stimulate circulation. **A,** The knee is flexed and then extended. **B,** The leg is raised and lowered.

Elastic Stockings. Elastic stockings put pressure on the veins. This promotes venous blood return to the heart. The stockings help prevent blood clots in leg veins. They also prevent leg swelling.

Persons at risk for thrombi include those who:
- Have had surgery.
- Have heart and circulatory disorders.
- Are on bed rest.
- Are older.
- Are pregnant.

Elastic stockings also are called AE stockings (AE means *anti-embolism* or *anti-embolic*). They also are called TED hose. (TED means *thrombo-embolic deterrent*. A *deterrent* prevents something from occurring.) AE stockings used after surgery are not used long-term. If a person needs stockings long-term, a *compression stocking* may be worn (Chapter 41). Compression stockings are available in different pressures (light to strong).

Stockings come in thigh-high and knee-high lengths and various sizes. The nurse measures the person for the correct size.

The person may have 2 pairs of stockings. Wash 1 pair while the other pair is worn. Wash them by hand with a mild soap. Hang them to dry.

See *Delegation Guidelines: Elastic Stockings.*
See *Promoting Safety and Comfort: Elastic Stockings.*
See procedure: *Applying Elastic Stockings*, p. 630.

DELEGATION GUIDELINES
Elastic Stockings

Applying elastic stockings is a routine nursing task. To apply elastic stockings, you need this information from the nurse and the care plan.
- What size to use—small, medium, large, extra-large, and so on
- What length to use—thigh-high or knee-high
- When to remove them and for how long—for bathing, some may be removed overnight
- What observations to report and record:
  - The size and length of stockings applied
  - When you applied the stockings
  - Skin color and temperature
  - Leg and foot swelling
  - Skin tears, wounds, or signs of skin breakdown
  - Complaints of pain, tingling, or numbness
  - When you removed the stockings and for how long
  - When you re-applied the stockings
  - When you washed the stockings
- When to report observations
- What patient or resident concerns to report at once

PROMOTING SAFETY AND COMFORT
Elastic Stockings

Safety
A toe opening on a stocking is used to check circulation, skin color, and skin temperature in the toes. Apply the stocking so the toe opening is over the top of the toes or under the toes. Follow the manufacturer's instructions.

Stockings must not have twists, creases, or wrinkles. Twists can affect circulation. So can stockings that roll up, bunch up, or have the toe opening wrapped around the toes. Creases and wrinkles can cause skin breakdown. Do not fold the top of the stocking down.

Loose stockings do not exert pressure on the veins. Stockings that are too tight can affect circulation. Tell the nurse if the stockings are too loose or too tight.

Comfort
Apply stockings before the person gets out of bed. Legs can swell from sitting or standing. Stockings are hard to put on swollen legs. The person is in bed while stockings are off. This prevents the legs from swelling.

Be sure the legs are dried well before applying stockings. Damp skin from water or lotion makes application hard. Powder may be applied as directed by the nurse.

The stocking is turned inside out down to the heel before application. Do not bunch up the stocking. When bunched, it is tight and difficult to unroll.

Gently handle and move the person's foot and leg. Do not force the joints (toes, foot, ankle, knee, and hip) beyond their range of motion or to the point of pain.

Applying Elastic Stockings

QUALITY OF LIFE

- Knock before entering the person's room.
- Address the person by name.
- Introduce yourself by name and title.

- Explain the procedure before starting and during the procedure.
- Protect the person's rights during the procedure.
- Handle the person gently during the procedure.

PRE-PROCEDURE

1 Follow *Delegation Guidelines: Elastic Stockings*, p. 629.
  See *Promoting Safety and Comfort: Elastic Stockings*, p. 629.
2 Practice hand hygiene and get the following supplies.
  - Elastic stockings in the correct size and length
  - Bath blanket (if needed)

3 Identify the person. Check the identification (ID) bracelet against the assignment sheet. Use 2 identifiers (Chapter 14). Also call the person by name.
4 Provide for privacy.
5 Raise the bed for body mechanics. Bed rails are up if used. Lower the bed rail near you if up.

PROCEDURE

6 Position the person supine.
7 Fan-fold top linens to the foot of the bed. Or fan-fold linens to the side, toward the other leg. If needed, use a bath blanket to cover the person.
8 Turn the stocking inside out down to the heel.
9 Slip the foot of the stocking over the toes, foot, and heel (Fig. 40-9, *A*). Properly position the heel pocket on the heel. The toe opening is over or under the toes. Follow the manufacturer's instructions.

10 Grasp the stocking top. Pull the stocking up the leg. It turns right side out as it is pulled up.
11 Adjust the stocking as needed. Make sure the stocking does not cause pressure on the toes.
12 Remove twists, creases, or wrinkles. Make sure the stocking is even, snug, smooth, and wrinkle-free (Fig. 40-9, *B*).
13 Repeat steps 8 through 12 for the other leg.
14 Cover the person. Remove the bath blanket (if used). Fold and return the bath blanket to its proper place. Or follow agency policy for used linens.

POST-PROCEDURE

15 Provide for comfort. (See the inside of the back cover.)
16 Lower the bed to a safe and comfortable level. Raise or lower bed rails. Follow the care plan.
17 Place the call light and other needed items within reach.
18 Follow the care plan and the person's preferences for privacy measures to maintain. Leaving the privacy curtain, window coverings, and door open or closed are examples.

19 Complete a safety check of the room. (See the inside of the back cover.)
20 Practice hand hygiene.
21 Report and record your care and observations.

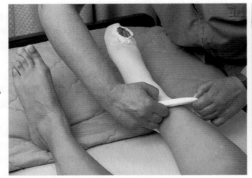 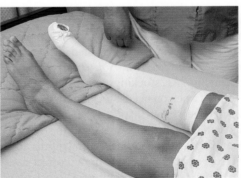

FIGURE 40-9 Applying elastic stockings. **A,** The stocking is slipped over the toes, foot, and heel. **B,** The stocking turns right side out as it is pulled up over the leg. The heel is positioned in the heel pocket of the stocking.

Elastic Bandages.

Elastic bandages have the same purposes as elastic stockings. They also provide support and reduce swelling from injuries. Another use is to hold dressings in place. They are applied to arms and legs. To apply bandages:

- Use the correct size—length and width.
- Position the person in good alignment.
- Face the person during the procedure.
- Start at the lower (*distal*) part of the extremity. Work upward to the top (*proximal*) part. See Figure 40-10.
- Expose the fingers or toes if possible. This allows circulation checks.
- Apply the bandage with firm, even pressure.
- Ask about comfort. Ask if the bandage feels too tight. Ask about pain, itching, and tingling or numbness.
- Check the color and temperature of the extremity every hour.
- Re-apply a loose or wrinkled bandage.
- Replace a moist or soiled bandage.
  See *Delegation Guidelines: Elastic Bandages*.
  See *Promoting Safety and Comfort: Elastic Bandages*.
  See procedure: *Applying an Elastic Bandage*.

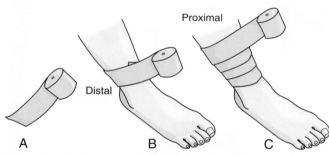

FIGURE 40-10 Applying an elastic bandage. **A,** The bandage roll is up. The loose end is at the bottom. **B,** The bandage is applied to the lower (*distal*) and smallest part with 2 circular turns. **C,** The bandage is applied with spiral turns in an upward (*proximal*) direction.

DELEGATION GUIDELINES

Elastic Bandages

Applying elastic bandages is a routine nursing task in some agencies. In others, it is a delegated nursing task. To apply elastic bandages, you need this information from the nurse and the care plan.

- Where to apply the bandage
- What width and length to use
- When to remove the bandage and for how long
- What observations to report and record:
  - The width and length applied
  - When you applied the bandage
  - Skin color and temperature
  - Swelling of the part
  - Skin tears, wounds, or signs of skin breakdown
  - Complaints of pain, itching, tingling, or numbness
  - A wet or soiled bandage
  - The amount and appearance of any drainage
  - When you removed the bandage and for how long
  - When you re-applied the bandage
- When to report observations
- What patient or resident concerns to report at once

PROMOTING SAFETY AND COMFORT

Elastic Bandages

Safety
Elastic bandages must be firm and snug but not tight. A tight bandage can affect circulation.

Manufacturers supply bandages with hook and loop, clip, tape, or Velcro closures. Metal or plastic clips can injure the skin if they are loose, fall off, or cause pressure. Check the clips often for correct placement.

Some agencies do not allow nursing assistants to apply elastic bandages. Know your agency's policy.

Comfort
A tight bandage can cause pain and discomfort. If the person complains of pain, tingling, or numbness, remove the bandage. Tell the nurse at once.

Applying an Elastic Bandage

QUALITY OF LIFE

- Knock before entering the person's room.
- Address the person by name.
- Introduce yourself by name and title.

- Explain the procedure before starting and during the procedure.
- Protect the person's rights during the procedure.
- Handle the person gently during the procedure.

PRE-PROCEDURE

1 Follow *Delegation Guidelines: Elastic Bandages*. See *Promoting Safety and Comfort: Elastic Bandages*.
2 Practice hand hygiene and get an elastic bandage with closures as directed by the nurse.

3 Identify the person. Check the ID bracelet against the assignment sheet. Use 2 identifiers (Chapter 14). Also call the person by name.
4 Provide for privacy.
5 Raise the bed for body mechanics. Bed rails are up if used. Lower the bed rail near you if up.

Continued

Applying an Elastic Bandage—cont'd

PROCEDURE

6. Help the person to a comfortable position in good alignment. Expose the part to bandage.
7. Make sure the area is clean and dry.
8. Hold the bandage with the roll up. The loose end is on the bottom (see Fig. 40-10, *A*).
9. Apply the bandage to the lower (*distal*) and smallest part of the wrist, foot, ankle, or knee (see Fig. 40-10, *B*).
10. Make 2 circular turns around the part.
11. Make over-lapping spiral turns in an upward (*proximal*) direction. Each turn over-laps ½ to ¾ (one-half to three-fourths) of the previous turn (see Fig. 40-10, *C*). Each over-lap is equal.

12. Apply the bandage smoothly with firm, even pressure. It is not tight.
13. End the bandage with 2 circular turns.
14. Secure the bandage with the manufacturer's closure. Clips are not under the body part.
15. Check the fingers or toes for coldness or *cyanosis* (bluish color). Ask about pain, itching, numbness, or tingling. Remove the bandage if any are noted. Report your observations.

POST-PROCEDURE

16. Provide for comfort. (See the inside of the back cover.)
17. Lower the bed to a safe and comfortable level. Raise or lower bed rails. Follow the care plan.
18. Place the call light and other needed items within reach.
19. Follow the care plan and the person's preferences for privacy measures to maintain. Leaving the privacy curtain, window coverings, and door open or closed are examples.

20. Complete a safety check of the room. (See the inside of the back cover.)
21. Practice hand hygiene.
22. Report and record your care and observations.

Sequential Compression Devices. *Sequential* means to be done in a sequence or pattern. *Compression* involves squeezing or pressing in. A *sequential compression device (SCD)* is a pump attached to sleeves (cuffs) that strap around the legs (Fig. 40-11). The pump inflates the sleeves with air 1 at a time. After 1 side deflates, the other inflates. This promotes venous blood flow to the heart by causing pressure on the veins.

SCDs are applied to both legs. The sleeves are made of cloth or plastic and are secured in place with Velcro following the manufacturer's instructions. Applied pre-op, SCDs also are worn post-op. Elastic stockings may be worn underneath.

Early Ambulation

Early ambulation prevents complications such as thrombi, pneumonia, atelectasis, constipation, and urinary tract infections. The person usually walks in the room or hallway the day of surgery. The person sits on the side of the bed first. Blood pressure and pulse are measured. If they are stable, the person is assisted out of bed.

The nurse tells you when the person can walk and how far to go. Distance increases as the person gains strength. Usually you assist the nurse the first time.

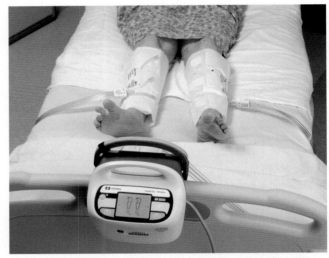

FIGURE 40-11 Sequential compression device. (From Stromberg HK: *deWit's Medical-surgical nursing: concepts and practice,* ed 4, St Louis, 2021, Elsevier.)

Wound Healing

The incision needs to heal. A dressing (bandage) may cover the incision for protection and to prevent infection. Your agency may let you do simple non-sterile dressing changes. See Chapter 41 for wound care.

Nutrition and Fluids

Post-op, the person has an IV. Continued IV therapy depends on the type of surgery and the person's condition. Anesthesia may cause nausea and vomiting. Diet progresses from NPO to clear liquids, to full liquids, to a regular diet or other special diet as the person requires. Frequent oral hygiene is important while NPO.

Some patients have NG tubes (Chapter 33). The NG tube may be attached to suction to keep the stomach empty. The person is NPO and has an IV.

Elimination

Anesthesia, surgery, and being NPO affect bowel and urinary elimination. Pain-relief drugs can cause constipation. Promote elimination as directed by the nurse and the care plan (Chapters 27 and 29). Fluid intake and a regular diet are needed for bowel elimination. Suppositories or enemas may be ordered for constipation.

Measure intake and output (I&O). The person must void within 6 to 8 hours after surgery. Report the time and amount of the first voiding. If the person does not void within 6 to 8 hours, a catheter may be needed. Some patients have a catheter after surgery. See Chapter 28.

Comfort and Rest

Pain is common after surgery. The degree of pain depends on:

* The extent of surgery.
* The incision site and size.
* If drainage tubes, casts, or other devices are present.
* Positioning during surgery. The position can cause discomfort.

Pain-relief drugs are ordered. The nurse uses the nursing process to promote comfort and rest. Many of the measures listed in Chapter 36 are part of the person's care plan.

Personal Hygiene

Personal hygiene is important for well-being. Wound drainage and skin prep solutions can irritate the skin and cause discomfort. NPO causes a dry mouth and breath odors. Moist, clammy skin from blood pressure changes or fever also cause discomfort.

Frequent oral hygiene, hair care, and a complete bed bath after surgery help refresh and renew the person. The gown and linens are changed when wet or soiled.

FOCUS ON **PRIDE**

The Person, Family, and Yourself

Personal and Professional Responsibility

What worries would you have about surgery—pain, loss of function, death, caring for your children and home, supporting your family? Imagine hours after being in an accident. You are told that your right leg was amputated.

Take time to listen to the person's fears and concerns. Avoid seeming rushed. Act professionally. Take pride in showing that you care.

Rights and Respect

The person has the right to accurate and complete information. You can answer questions about the care you give. If you do not know or are unsure of an answer, explain that you will ask the nurse.

Some questions are best answered by the nurse. For example: "How long will the surgery last?" or "What will be done for pain after surgery?" Even if you know the answer, say that you will ask the nurse to answer the question. Show good judgment. Only answer questions within the scope of your role.

Independence and Social Interaction

Some people prefer peace and quiet before and after surgery. Others want family and friends around. The support and conversation distracts from worries and pain. Each person is different. Ask what the person prefers. Tell the nurse. The nurse can talk with the family about the person's wishes and needs.

Delegation and Teamwork

You may be delegated parts of the person's post-op care. For example, you monitor vital signs. The patient and nurse rely on you. Complete post-op vital signs on time. Report abnormal values, sudden changes, and any concerns at once. Take pride in your role in post-op care. You can make a difference in the safety and quality of the person's care.

Ethics and Laws

When possible, the person signs the surgical consent. If unable, the person's spouse or nearest relative may be required to sign the consent. A parent or legal representative signs for a minor child. The legal representative signs for a person not mentally competent to sign.

FOCUS ON **PRIDE**: *Application*

Your attitude and conduct affect the person's surgical experience. You can either ease worries or increase stress. Explain how your behavior affects the person's outlook and comfort.

REVIEW QUESTIONS

Circle the BEST answer.

1 Which is true of elective surgery?
   a It is done at once.
   b The need is sudden and not expected.
   c It is scheduled at a later date.
   d General anesthesia is always used.

2 A person states: "I'm afraid of surgery." What should you do?
   a Call a member of the clergy.
   b Listen and provide care with skill and competence.
   c Change the subject.
   d Tell the family.

3 You assist with pre-op care by explaining
   a The reason for the surgery
   b The procedures you are doing
   c The risks and possible complications
   d What to expect during and after surgery

4 Which needs to be corrected before the person goes to surgery?
   a Nail polish, hair clips, and make-up are in place.
   b The person wears a patient gown.
   c Eyeglasses are removed.
   d Dentures are removed.

5 Before surgery, a person is
   a NPO
   b Allowed only water
   c Given breakfast
   d Given a tube feeding

6 A bowel prep is ordered to
   a Prevent bleeding
   b Relieve flatus
   c Prevent pain
   d Clean the intestines of feces

7 A skin prep is done to
   a Bathe the body completely
   b Sterilize the skin
   c Reduce the amount of microbes on the skin
   d Destroy non-pathogens and pathogens

8 After pre-op drugs are given, the patient
   a Must stay in bed
   b Can use the bathroom
   c Can use the commode to void
   d Can have sips of water

9 General anesthesia is
   a A specially educated nurse
   b A treatment causing deep sleep and absence of sensation
   c A treatment causing loss of sensation in a body part
   d A specially educated doctor

10 You are preparing a room for a post-op patient. Which should you expect?
   a The person will walk to the bed from a wheelchair.
   b Supplies for measuring I&O are not needed.
   c Supplies for skin preparation and hair removal are needed.
   d Equipment for measuring frequent vital signs is needed.

11 Which complication after surgery involves a blood clot in a leg?
   a Hemorrhage
   b Thrombus
   c Post-operative ileus
   d Dehiscence

12 Post-op, a person's position is changed at least
   a Every 2 hours
   b Every 3 hours
   c Every 4 hours
   d Every shift

13 Coughing and deep breathing after surgery prevent
   a Bleeding
   b A pulmonary embolus
   c Respiratory complications
   d Pain and discomfort

14 Leg exercises
   a Stimulate circulation and prevent thrombi
   b Are done only for leg surgery
   c Are done every 4 hours
   d Are not needed if elastic stockings are worn

15 Elastic stockings
   a Hold dressings in place
   b Slow blood flow
   c Prevent pressure injuries
   d Prevent blood clots

16 Elastic stockings are applied
   a When the person is standing
   b Before the person gets out of bed
   c After breakfast
   d For 30 minutes and then removed

17 The purpose of an elastic bandage is to
   a Prevent infection
   b Absorb drainage
   c Provide moisture for wound healing
   d Reduce swelling

18 When applying an elastic bandage
   a Position the part in good alignment
   b Cover the fingers or toes if possible
   c Apply it from the large to small part of the extremity
   d Apply it from the upper to lower part of the extremity

19 Which statement about walking after surgery is *correct*?
   a Walking is delayed as long as possible.
   b Ambulation occurs before vital signs are stable.
   c Early ambulation prevents complications.
   d The person walks without assistance at first.

20 Which is normal after surgery?
   a The blood pressure drops outside the normal range.
   b The person voids within 6 to 8 hours.
   c The pulse increases outside the normal range.
   d Skin is moist, clammy, and pale.

Answers to Chapter 40 questions are on p. 903.

FOCUS ON PRACTICE

Problem Solving

You are measuring a post-op patient's vital signs. The person is restless. The vital signs are similar to previous measurements. What do you do? Is there anything you need to report? If so, when?

Wound Care

OBJECTIVES

- Define the key terms and key abbreviations in this chapter.
- Identify different types of wounds and their causes.
- Describe skin tears and circulatory ulcers and the persons at risk.
- Explain how to help prevent skin tears and circulatory ulcers.
- Describe foot care for persons with diabetes.
- Describe the process and complications of wound healing.
- Describe what to observe about wounds.

- Explain the purposes of drains and wound dressings.
- Explain the rules for applying dressings.
- Explain the purpose of binders and compression garments and how to apply them.
- Describe care of the whole person when a wound is present.
- Perform the procedure described in this chapter.
- Explain how to promote PRIDE in the person, the family, and yourself.

KEY TERMS

abrasion A partial-thickness wound caused by the scraping away or rubbing of the skin from friction or trauma

arterial ulcer An open wound on the lower legs or feet caused by poor arterial blood flow; ischemic ulcer

avulsion A wound that occurs when skin or tissue is torn away

chronic wound A wound that does not heal easily and within about 3 months

circulatory ulcer An open sore on the lower legs or feet caused by decreased blood flow through the arteries or veins; vascular ulcer

diabetic foot ulcer An open wound on the foot caused by complications from diabetes

excoriation Damage to the epidermis (top skin layer) caused by scratching

incision A cut produced surgically by a sharp instrument; it creates an opening into an organ or body space

ischemic ulcer See "arterial ulcer"

laceration A wound with torn tissues and jagged edges caused by trauma

penetrating wound A wound caused by an object that breaks the skin and enters a body area, organ, or cavity

puncture wound A wound caused by piercing from a pointed object

purulent drainage Thick green, yellow, or brown drainage

sanguineous drainage Bloody (sanguis) drainage

serosanguineous drainage Thin, watery drainage (sero) that is blood-tinged (sanguineous)

serous drainage Clear, watery fluid (serum)

skin tear A break or rip in the outer layers of the skin; the epidermis (top skin layer) separates from the underlying tissues

stasis ulcer See "venous ulcer"

ulcer A shallow or deep crater-like sore of the skin or mucous membrane

vascular ulcer See "circulatory ulcer"

venous ulcer An open sore on the lower legs or feet caused by poor venous blood flow; stasis ulcer

wound Damage to the skin or mucous membrane

KEY ABBREVIATIONS

GI	Gastro-intestinal	ISTAP	International Skin Tear Advisory Panel
ID	Identification	PPE	Personal protective equipment

A *wound* occurs when there is damage to the skin or mucous membrane. Wounds commonly result from:
- Surgery.
- *Trauma*—an accident or violent act that injures the skin, mucous membranes, bones, and organs. Falls, vehicle crashes, gunshots, stabbings, bites, burns, and frostbite are examples.
- Unrelieved pressure or friction (Chapter 42).
- Decreased blood flow through the arteries or veins.
- Nerve damage.

Wounds are portals of entry for microbes. Infection is a major threat. Wound care includes preventing infection and further injury to the wound and nearby tissues. Blood loss and pain also are prevented.

The nurse uses the nursing process to keep the person's skin healthy. Some agencies have wound therapists or skin care teams to manage all skin problems. The team includes a nurse, physical therapist, and dietitian.

See *Promoting Safety and Comfort: Wound Care*, p. 636.

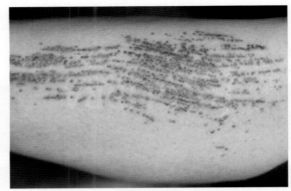

FIGURE 41-1 An abrasion. (From Lunn MM: *Essentials of medicolegal death investigation*, San Diego, 2017, Academic Press.)

TYPES OF WOUNDS

Wounds are closed or open. In a *closed wound*, the skin is intact (not broken). However, there is injury under the surface. Bruising is an example. In an *open wound*, the skin is broken (not intact).

Wounds vary in depth. In a *partial-thickness wound*, the epidermis and dermis of the skin are involved. In a *full-thickness wound*, the epidermis, dermis, and subcutaneous tissues are involved. Muscle and bone may also be involved.

The following are different types of open wounds.

- *Abrasion*—a partial-thickness wound caused by the scraping away or rubbing of the skin from friction or trauma (Fig. 41-1).
- *Avulsion*—a wound that occurs when skin or tissue is torn away. Skin tears are an example. See "Skin Tears."
- *Excoriation*—damage to the epidermis (top skin layer) caused by scratching (Fig. 41-2).
- *Incision*—a cut produced surgically by a sharp instrument. It creates an opening into an organ or body space (Fig. 41-3).
- *Laceration*—a wound with torn tissues and jagged edges caused by trauma (Fig. 41-4).
- *Penetrating wound*—a wound caused by an object that breaks the skin and enters a body area, organ, or cavity (Fig. 41-5). Gunshot wounds are examples.
- *Puncture wound*—a wound caused by piercing from a pointed object. A nail or a thin piece of metal, wood, or glass are examples. See Figure 41-6.
- *Ulcer*—a shallow or deep crater-like sore of the skin or mucous membrane (p. 638).

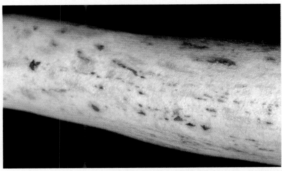

FIGURE 41-2 Excoriation. (From Marks JG, Miller JJ: *Lookingbill and Marks' principles of dermatology*, ed 6, London, 2019, Elsevier.)

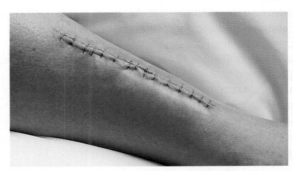

FIGURE 41-3 A surgical incision closed with staples. (From Perry AG, Potter PA, Ostendorf WR: *Nursing intervention and clinical skills*, ed 7, St Louis, 2020, Elsevier.)

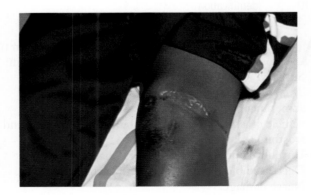

FIGURE 41-4 Laceration. (From Roberts JR, Custalow CB, Thomsen TW: *Roberts and Hedges' clinical procedures in emergency medicine and acute care*, ed 7, Philadelphia, 2019, Elsevier.)

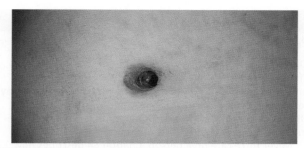

FIGURE 41-5 Penetrating wound. (From McCance KL, Huether SE: *Pathophysiology: the biologic basis for disease in adults and children,* ed 6, St Louis, 2010, Mosby.)

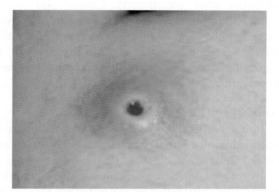

FIGURE 41-6 Puncture wound. (From Kordestani SS: *Atlas of wound healing: a tissue regeneration approach,* St Louis, 2019, Elsevier.)

Skin Tears

A *skin tear* is a break or rip in the outer layers of the skin. The epidermis (top skin layer) separates from the underlying tissues. The hands, arms, and lower legs are common sites for skin tears.

According to the International Skin Tear Advisory Panel (ISTAP), there are 3 types of skin tears.

- No skin loss (Fig. 41-7, *A*). The flap of skin can be placed back over the wound.
- Partial flap loss (Fig. 41-7, *B*). Part of the skin is lost. The remaining flap cannot be placed to cover the wound.
- Total flap loss (Fig. 41-7, *C*). The entire skin flap is lost. The wound is exposed.

Causes. Skin tears are caused by:

- Friction, shearing (Chapter 20), pulling, or pressure on the skin.
- Falls or bumping a hard surface. Beds, bed rails, chairs, wheelchair parts, walkers, and tables are dangers.
- Holding an arm or leg too tight.
- Removing tape or adhesives.
- Bathing, dressing, and other tasks.
- Pulling buttons and zippers across fragile skin.
- Jewelry—yours or the person's. Rings, watches, and bracelets are examples.
- Long or jagged fingernails (yours or the person's) and long or jagged toenails.

Skin tears are painful. They are portals of entry for microbes. Infection is a risk. Tell the nurse at once if you cause or find a skin tear. To prevent skin tears, follow the care plan and the measures in Box 41-1, p. 638.

A   B   C

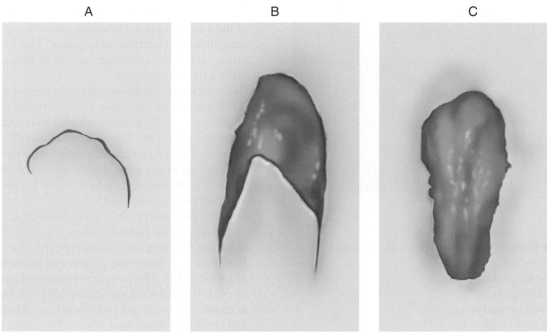

FIGURE 41-7 Skin tears. **A,** No skin loss. **B,** Partial flap loss. **C,** Total flap loss.

BOX 41-1	Preventing Skin Tears

- Follow the care plan and safety rules to:
  - Move, turn, position, or transfer the person.
    - Prevent shearing and friction.
    - Use an assist device to move and turn the person in bed.
    - Use pillows to support arms and legs.
  - Bathe the person.
  - Keep the skin moisturized and apply lotion.
  - Offer fluids.
- Keep your fingernails short and smoothly filed.
- Keep the person's fingernails short and smoothly filed. Report long, tough, or jagged toenails.
- Do not wear rings with large or raised stones. Do not wear bracelets.
- Check the person's rings and bracelets for broken, sharp, or jagged edges. If any are found, tell the nurse. The nurse will handle the matter.
- Be patient and calm when the person is confused, agitated, or resists care.
- Dress and undress the person carefully. The person wears soft clothes with long sleeves and long pants.
- Apply arm or leg protectors as ordered (Fig. 41-8).
- Provide a safe setting.
  - Pad bed rails and wheelchair arms, footplates, and leg supports.
  - Provide good lighting so the person can see. The person must avoid bumping into furniture, walls, and equipment.
  - Provide a safe setting for wandering (Chapter 54).
- Remove tape carefully. To remove tape, hold the skin down and gently pull the tape ends toward the wound.
- Do not apply adhesive tape (p. 644).

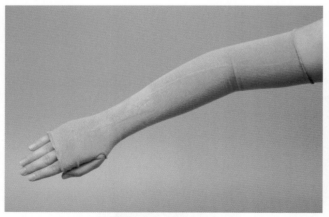

FIGURE 41-8 Skin protector.

Persons at Risk.
Persons at risk for skin tears:
- Need help moving.
- Have poor nutrition.
- Have poor hydration.
- Have altered mental awareness.
- Have thin and fragile skin.

See *Focus on Children and Older Persons: Persons at Risk (Skin Tears)*.

Prevention and Treatment. Careful and safe care helps prevent skin tears and further injury. Follow the measures in Box 41-1. Also follow the care plan and the nurse's directions. They may include dressings (p. 644) and elastic bandages (Chapter 40) to protect the skin and promote healing.

Circulatory Ulcers

Some diseases affect blood flow to and from the legs and feet, leading to circulatory ulcers. *Circulatory ulcers (vascular ulcers)* are open sores on the lower legs or feet. They are caused by decreased blood flow through the arteries or veins. Also called *leg and foot ulcers*, these wounds are hard to heal. Infection and gangrene can develop. *Gangrene* is a condition in which there is death of tissue.

Circulatory ulcers include:
- *Venous ulcers (stasis ulcers)*—open sores on the lower legs or feet caused by poor venous blood flow (Fig. 41-9, *A*). *Stasis* means stopped or slowed fluid flow. Leg veins do not return blood to the heart normally. Blood collects in the veins. The buildup of fluid and increased pressure prevent oxygen and nutrients from getting into tissues. The heels and inner part of the ankles are common sites. A dull, aching pain is common.
- *Arterial ulcers (ischemic ulcers)*—open wounds on the lower legs or feet caused by poor arterial blood flow (Fig. 41-9, *B*). *Ischemic* means reduced blood flow to a body part. Poor blood flow causes cell death and tissue damage. Arterial ulcers are found between the toes, on top of the toes, and on the outer side of the ankle. These wounds can be painful. Lowering the legs may help relieve pain.
- *Diabetic foot ulcers*—open wounds on the foot caused by complications from diabetes (Fig. 41-9, *C*). Diabetes (Chapter 51) can affect the nerves and blood vessels. With nerve damage, the person can lose sensation in a foot or leg. The person may not feel pain, heat, or cold. When blood vessels are affected, blood flow decreases. Tissues and cells do not get needed oxygen and nutrients. Sores heal poorly. Infection and tissue death (gangrene) are risks. Sometimes the affected part must be amputated.

A   B   C

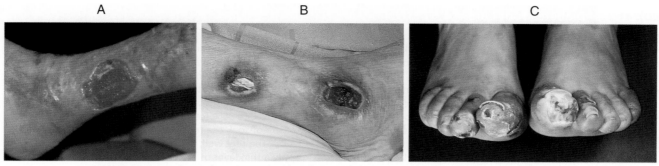

FIGURE 41-9 Circulatory ulcers. **A,** Venous ulcer. **B,** Arterial ulcers. **C,** Diabetic foot ulcers. (From Black JM, Hawks JH: *Medical-surgical nursing: clinical management for positive outcomes,* ed 8, St Louis, 2009, Saunders.)

Risk Factors. Risk factors for circulatory ulcers include:

- High blood pressure
- Diabetes
- Injury
- Narrowed arteries from aging
- Smoking
- History of blood clots (Chapter 40)
- Varicose veins (Fig. 41-10)
- Decreased mobility
- Obesity
- Surgery: leg, foot, bones, joints
- Advanced age
- *Phlebitis* (inflammation *[itis]* of a vein *[phleb]*)

Prevention and Treatment. Check the person's feet and legs daily. Report any sign of a problem at once. You must help prevent skin breakdown on the legs and feet. Follow the care plan to prevent and treat circulatory ulcers (Box 41-2). Diabetes foot care can prevent foot problems that cause diabetic foot ulcers (Box 41-3, p. 640). The doctor orders drugs and treatments as needed.

Persons at risk need professional foot care. You do not cut the toenails of persons with diseases affecting circulation.

See *Focus on Long-Term Care and Home Care: Prevention and Treatment*, p. 641.

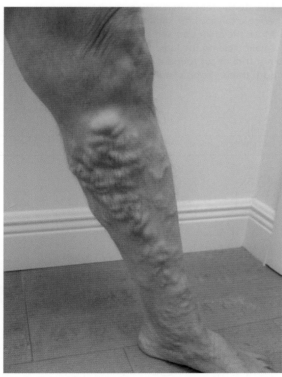

FIGURE 41-10 Varicose veins. Veins under the skin are dilated (wide) and bulging. (From Almeida JI: *Atlas of endovascular venous surgery,* ed 2, Philadelphia, 2019, Elsevier.)

BOX 41-2	Preventing Circulatory Ulcers

- Remind the person not to sit with the legs crossed.
- Re-position the person according to the care plan—at least every 2 hours.
- Do not use elastic or rubber band–type garters to hold socks or hose in place.
- Apply compression stockings or elastic bandages as directed to improve blood flow in the legs and prevent swelling. *Compression stockings* are available in different pressures (light to strong) and lengths (knee-high to thigh-high). *Elastic bandages* are available in different lengths and widths. Follow the rules for elastic stockings and elastic bandages in Chapter 40.
- Do not dress the person in tight clothes.
- Provide good skin care daily and as needed. Keep the feet clean and dry. Clean and dry between the toes.
- Report toenails in need of trimming and filing.
- Do not scrub or rub the skin during bathing and drying.
- Keep linens clean, dry, and wrinkle-free.
- Avoid injury to the legs and feet.
- Make sure shoes fit well.
- Keep pressure off the heels and other bony areas. Use pillows or other devices as directed.
- Check the person's legs and feet. Report skin breaks or changes in skin color.
- Do not massage over pressure points (Chapter 42). *Never rub or massage reddened areas.*
- Use protective devices as directed.
- Follow the care plan for walking and exercises.

BOX 41-3   Diabetes Foot Care

Common Problems

- *Corns and calluses* (Fig. 41-11, *A*). These are thick layers of skin caused by too much rubbing or pressure on the same spot. They occur over bony areas.
- *Blisters* (Fig. 41-11, *B*). These form when shoes rub on the same spot. Ill-fitting shoes and wearing shoes without socks are causes.
- *Ingrown toenails* (Fig. 41-11, *C*). An edge of a toenail grows into the skin. This occurs when the skin is cut while trimming toenails or from tight shoes.
- *Bunions* (Fig. 41-11, *D*). A *bunion* is a bump on the outside edge of the big toe. The big toe slants toward the small toes. Heredity is a factor. Shoes that fit poorly (too tight or narrow), high heels, and pointy shoes are causes.
- *Plantar warts* (Fig. 41-11, *E*). *Plantar* means sole. Plantar warts occur on the soles (bottoms) of the feet. Caused by a virus, plantar warts are painful.
- *Hammer toes* (Fig. 41-11, *F*). One or more toes are flexed. Diabetic nerve damage can weaken foot muscles. Because of deformed toes, the person has problems walking. Shoes do not fit well. Sores can develop on the tops of the toes and on the bottoms of the feet.
- *Dry and cracked skin* (Fig. 41-11, *G*). Dry skin can occur from nerve damage or poor blood flow in the legs and feet. The dry skin can crack, causing portals of entry for microbes. Infection can occur.
- *Athlete's foot* (Fig. 41-11, *H*). This is a fungus causing itching, burning, redness, and cracked skin between the toes and on the soles of the feet. The cracks are portals of entry for microbes.
- *Fungal infection of the toenails* (Fig. 41-11, *I*). The toenails become thick and hard to cut. They may be yellow, brown, or black. A nail may fall off.

Observations

- Check the feet daily for:
  - Cuts
  - Sores
  - Blisters
  - Redness
  - Calluses
  - Infected toenails
  - Ingrown toenails
  - Blood, pus, or watery drainage (p. 643)
  - Warm skin

Care Measures

- Wash the feet daily in warm water with mild soap.
  - Do not use hot water.
  - Test the water temperature with your elbow or use a water thermometer. Because burns are a risk, water temperature should be 90°F to 95°F (Fahrenheit) (32.2°C to 35°C [centigrade]).
  - Do not soak the feet in water. The skin could dry out.
  - Dry the feet well, especially between the toes.
- Apply a thin layer of talcum powder or cornstarch between the toes. This keeps the skin between the toes dry.
- Apply a thin layer of lotion, cream, or petroleum jelly on the tops and bottoms of the feet (not between the toes). Do so after washing and drying to keep the skin soft and smooth.
- Have the person wear closed-toed shoes and clean socks or stockings. This prevents blisters and sores.
  - Socks and stockings do not have holes or seams.
  - Lightly padded socks are best.
  - Tight socks or knee-high stockings are avoided.
  - Athletic and walking shoes are best. They have laces, Velcro, or buckles for easy adjustment.
  - Open-toed shoes, sandals, flip-flops, pointy shoes, and high-heels are not worn.
  - Vinyl and plastic shoes are not worn. They do not stretch and do not allow air movement inside the shoes.
- Check shoes for sharp edges or objects in the shoes. Make sure the lining is smooth.
- Do not allow the person to walk barefoot. The person could step on something and hurt the foot.
- Provide socks at night for cold feet.
- Promote blood flow to and from the feet. Have the person:
  - Elevate the feet when sitting.
  - Wiggle the toes for 5 minutes 2 or 3 times a day.
  - Move the ankles up and down and in and out.
  - Avoid crossing the legs.
- Do not trim or cut toenails or cut corns or calluses or try to smooth them. Professional foot care is needed.

Modified from National Institute of Diabetes and Digestive and Kidney Diseases: Diabetes and foot problems, January 2017.

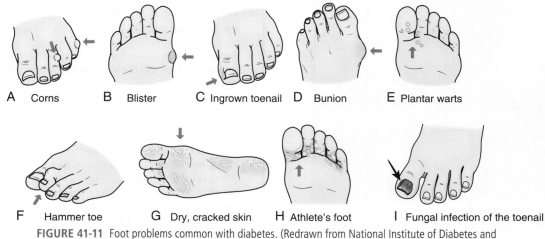

A Corns   B Blister   C Ingrown toenail   D Bunion   E Plantar warts

F Hammer toe   G Dry, cracked skin   H Athlete's foot   I Fungal infection of the toenail

FIGURE 41-11 Foot problems common with diabetes. (Redrawn from National Institute of Diabetes and Digestive and Kidney Diseases: *Prevent diabetes problems: keep your feet healthy*, Bethesda, 2014, U.S. Department of Health and Human Services.)

WOUND HEALING

The healing process has 3 phases.

- *Phase 1* (3 days). Bleeding stops. A scab forms, preventing microbes from entering the wound. An increased blood supply to the wound brings nutrients and healing substances. Signs and symptoms of inflammation appear—redness, swelling, heat or warmth, and pain. Loss of function may occur.
- *Phase 2* (days 3 to 21). Cells multiply to repair the wound. Some wounds do not heal in a timely manner. A *chronic wound* does not heal easily and within about 3 months.
- *Phase 3* (day 21 to 2 years). The scar gains strength. The red, raised scar becomes thin and pale.

Types of Wound Healing

Healing occurs in 3 ways (Fig. 41-12).

- *First (primary) intention.* The wound is closed. Sutures (stitches), staples, special glue, adhesive strips, or other wound closure devices are used to hold the wound edges together.
- *Second intention.* Contaminated and infected wounds (p. 642) are cleaned and dead tissue removed. Wound edges are not brought together. The wound gaps. Healing takes longer, leaving a larger scar. Infection is a great risk.
- *Third intention.* The wound is left open and closed later. It combines first and second intention. Infection and poor circulation are reasons for third intention.

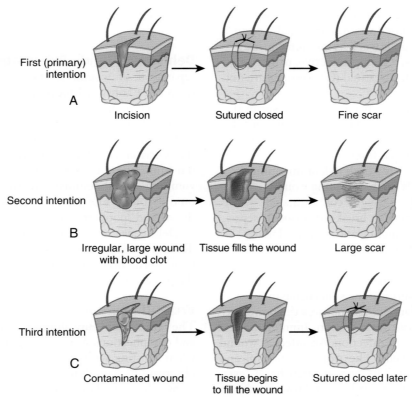

FIGURE 41-12 Wound healing. **A,** First (primary) intention. **B,** Second intention. **C,** Third intention. (Modified from Harding MM, Kwong J, Roberts D, et al: *Lewis's medical-surgical nursing: assessment and management of clinical problems,* ed 11, St Louis, 2020, Elsevier.)

Complications of Wound Healing

Many factors affect healing and the risk for complications. They include wound cause and type, age, health, nutrition, and life-style. Age, smoking, circulatory disease, and diabetes affect circulation. Some drugs prolong bleeding.

Good nutrition is needed. Protein is needed for tissue growth and repair.

Hemorrhage and Shock. *Hemorrhage* is the excessive loss *(rrhage)* of blood *(hemo)* in a short time (Chapter 58). *Shock* results when tissues and organs do not get enough blood (Chapter 58). Both are life-threatening.

- *Internal hemorrhage. Internal* means inside. You cannot see bleeding inside tissues and body cavities. A hematoma may form. A *hematoma* is a swelling *(oma)* that contains blood *(hemat)*. The area is swollen and reddish blue in color. Shock, vomiting blood, coughing up blood, and loss of consciousness signal internal hemorrhage.
- *External hemorrhage. External* means outside. You can see bleeding outside the body. Common signs are bloody drainage and dressings soaked with blood. Gravity causes fluid to flow down. Check under the body part for pooling of blood.

See Chapter 58 for the signs and symptoms of hemorrhage and shock. Hemorrhage and shock are emergencies. Alert the nurse at once. Assist as directed.

Infection. Contamination can occur during or after injury or surgery.

- *Clean wound*—is not infected. Microbes have not entered the wound. Closed wounds are usually clean. So are intentional wounds (such as incisions) made into sterile body areas. The reproductive, urinary, respiratory, and gastro-intestinal (GI) systems are not entered.
- *Clean-contaminated wound*—occurs from the surgical entry of the reproductive, urinary, respiratory, or GI system. Some or all parts of these systems are not sterile and contain normal flora.
- *Contaminated wound*—has a high risk of infection. Unintentional wounds (such as trauma wounds from vehicle crashes) are usually contaminated. Contamination occurs from breaks in surgical asepsis, spillage of intestinal contents, and trauma. Tissues may show signs of inflammation.
- *Infected wound (dirty wound)*—contains large amounts of microbes and shows signs of infection. Examples include old wounds, surgical incisions made into infected areas, and trauma that ruptures the bowel.

Wounds are at high risk for infection. Immune system changes increase the risk of infection. An infected wound appears inflamed (reddened). The wound is painful and tender. The area is warm. The person often has a fever. A bad odor and thick green, yellow, or brown drainage are signs of infection. See "Wound Drainage."

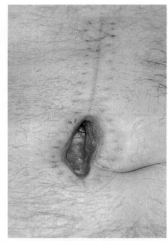

FIGURE 41-13 Wound dehiscence. (From Bale S, Jones V: *Wound care nursing: a patient-centered approach*, ed 2, St Louis, 2006, Mosby.)

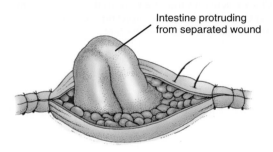

Intestine protruding from separated wound

FIGURE 41-14 Wound evisceration. (Modified from Ignatavicius DD, Workman ML: *Medical-surgical nursing: critical thinking for collaborative care*, ed 5, St Louis, 2006, Saunders.)

Dehiscence and Evisceration. *Dehiscence* is the separation of wound layers (Fig. 41-13). (*Dehiscence* is from the Latin word meaning to gap.) It may involve the skin layer or underlying tissues. Abdominal wounds are commonly affected.

Evisceration is the separation of the wound along with the protrusion of abdominal organs (Fig. 41-14). (*E* means out from. *Viscera* relates to the internal organs.) Coughing, vomiting, and abdominal distention (swelling) place stress on the wound. The person often describes the sensation of the wound "popping open."

Dehiscence and evisceration are surgical emergencies. Tell the nurse at once. The nurse covers the wound with large sterile dressings saturated with saline. Help prepare the person for surgery as directed.

Wound Appearance

The wound and any drainage are observed for healing and complications. See Box 41-4 for observations to make when assisting with wound care. Report and record your observations according to agency policy.

See *Focus on Long-Term Care and Home Care: Wound Appearance.*

- Wound site:
  - Surgery or trauma may involve multiple wounds.
- Wound size and depth are measured by the nurse in centimeters (cm). See Figure 41-15.
- Wound appearance:
  - Is the wound red and swollen?
  - Is the area around the wound warm to touch?
  - Are sutures, staples, or other closure devices intact or broken?
  - Are wound edges closed (*approximated*) or separated?
  - Did the wound break open?
- Drainage:
  - Is the drainage serous, sanguineous, serosanguineous, or purulent? (See "Wound Drainage.")
  - What is the amount of drainage?
- Odor:
  - Does the wound or drainage have an odor?
- Surrounding skin:
  - Is surrounding skin intact?
  - What is the color of surrounding skin?
  - Are surrounding tissues swollen?

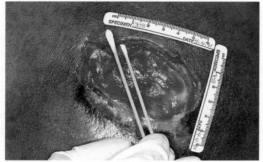

FIGURE 41-15 The size and depth of the wound are measured. (From Potter PA, Perry AG, Stockert PA, et al: *Fundamentals of nursing,* ed 8, St Louis, 2013, Mosby.)

FOCUS ON LONG-TERM CARE AND HOME CARE

Wound Appearance

Home Care

The nurse may use electronic images to assess the wound. Before you take photos or videos, make sure the person has signed the required consents. (The nurse obtains the consents.)

Make sure the date and time stamp features on your electronic device are working. Check that the date and time are correct.

Electronic images do not replace accurate observations. See Box 41-4.

Wound Drainage

During injury and wound healing, fluid and cells escape from tissues. The amount and kind of drainage depend on wound size and site, bleeding, and infection. Wound drainage is observed and measured.

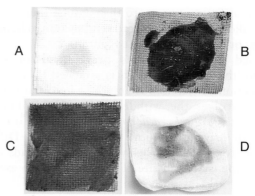

FIGURE 41-16 Wound drainage. **A,** Serous drainage. **B,** Sanguineous drainage. **C,** Serosanguineous drainage. **D,** Purulent drainage. (From Potter PA, Perry AG, Stockert PA, et al: *Fundamentals of nursing,* ed 11, St Louis, 2023, Elsevier.)

The following are different kinds of drainage (Fig. 41-16).

- *Serous drainage*—clear, watery fluid (*serum*). *Serous* comes from the word serum. Serum is the clear, thin, fluid portion of blood. Serum does not contain blood cells or platelets. Fluid in a blister is serous.
- *Sanguineous drainage*—bloody (*sanguis*) drainage. The Latin word *sanguis* means blood. Hemorrhage is suspected when large amounts are present. Bright drainage means fresh bleeding. Older bleeding is darker.
- *Serosanguineous drainage*—thin, watery drainage (*sero*) that is blood-tinged (*sanguineous*).
- *Purulent drainage*—thick green, yellow, or brown drainage.

Drainage must leave the wound for healing. Trapped drainage causes swelling of underlying tissues. The wound may heal at the skin level but underlying tissues do not close. Infection and complications can occur.

Drains. When large amounts of drainage are expected, the doctor inserts a drain. Drains allow an outlet for drainage to leave the wound.

An open drain such as a *Penrose drain (gravity drain)* is a rubber tube that drains onto a dressing (Fig. 41-17). The drain is open and uses gravity to drain fluids. Microbes entering the drain and wound are a risk.

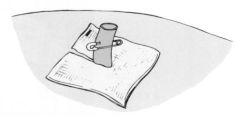

FIGURE 41-17 Penrose drain. A pin prevents the drain from slipping into the wound. (From Potter PA, Perry AG, Stockert PA, et al: *Fundamentals of nursing,* ed 9, St Louis, 2017, Elsevier.)

Sump drains contain more than 1 tube (lumen). Extra lumens allow openings for air to vent, suction to be applied, or fluids or drugs to be instilled (put in).

Closed drainage systems prevent microbes from entering the wound. A drain is attached to a reservoir with suction. A *reservoir* is an area where fluid collects. *Suction* involves the withdrawing of fluid. The term *evacuator* or *surgical evacuator* may be used. (To *evacuate* means to leave or remove from an area.) Different systems are available. The system used depends on the wound type, size, and site. The following are examples (Fig. 41-18).

- *Hemovac (3-spring) system.* This system is shaped like a cylinder. It compresses from top to bottom. A port (spout) on the top is opened to empty the contents. The device is pressed at the top and bottom and the port closed to create suction.
- *Jackson-Pratt (bulb) system.* This system is shaped like a bulb. A port (spout) at the top is opened to empty contents. The bulb is squeezed at the sides and the port closed to create suction.

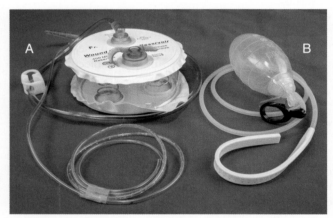

FIGURE 41-18 Closed drainage systems. **A,** Hemovac-type (3-spring) drain. **B,** Jackson-Pratt-type (bulb) drain (JP drain). (From Hollen CJ, Melton Stein LN: *Concept-based clinical nursing skills: fundamental to advanced competencies,* ed 2, St Louis, 2024, Elsevier.)

You may assist the nurse in observing wound drainage. For a closed drainage system, follow agency policy and the manufacturer's instructions.

DRESSINGS

Wound dressings have many functions. They:
- Protect wounds from injury and microbes.
- Absorb drainage.
- Remove dead tissue.
- Promote comfort.
- Cover unsightly wounds.
- Provide a moist environment for wound healing.
- Apply pressure (pressure dressings) to help control bleeding.

Dressing type and size depend on the type of wound, its size and site, and the amount of drainage (Fig. 41-19). Infection is a factor. The dressing's function and the frequency of dressing changes are other factors.

Some dressings have special agents for wound healing. If you assist with a dressing change, the nurse explains its use to you.

Securing Dressings

Dressings must be secured over wounds. Microbes can enter the wound and drainage can escape if the dressing is dislodged. Tape and Montgomery straps secure dressings. Binders (p. 648) hold dressings in place.

Tape. Adhesive, paper, plastic, cloth, and elastic tapes are common. Adhesive tape sticks well. However, adhesive problems include:
- It is hard to remove from the skin.
- It can irritate the skin.
- Skin tears or abrasions can occur when tape is removed.
- Adhesive tape allergies are common.

Paper, plastic, and cloth tapes usually do not cause allergic reactions. Elastic tape allows movement of the body part.

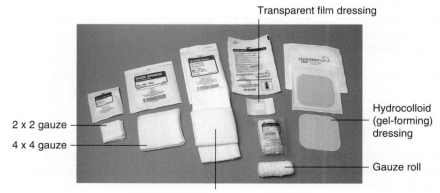

FIGURE 41-19 Types of dressings. (Modified from Williams P: *deWit's fundamental concepts and skills for nursing,* ed 6, St Louis, 2022, Elsevier.)

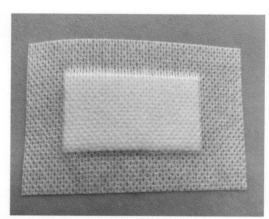

FIGURE 41-20 The tape extends beyond the sides of the dressing.

Tape comes in different widths—½-, ¾-, 1-, 2-, and 3-inch widths are common. Taping methods vary. Taping the top, middle, and bottom; taping the edges; and fully covering the dressing with tape are 3 methods. Tape should extend beyond the sides of the dressing (Fig. 41-20). *Do not apply tape to circle the entire body part. If swelling occurs, circulation to the part is impaired.*
See *Focus on Communication: Tape.*

FOCUS ON COMMUNICATION

Tape

Before applying tape, ask if the person has an allergy to tape. You can ask:
- "Do any types of tape irritate your skin?"
- "Do you have an allergy to tape?"

Montgomery Straps. Montgomery straps (Fig. 41-21) are used for large dressings and frequent dressing changes. A Montgomery strap has a tape strip and cloth tie. With the dressing in place, the tape strips are placed on both sides of the dressing. Then the straps are secured over the dressing.

The straps are undone for the dressing change. The tape strips stay in place. They are removed if soiled. Montgomery straps protect the skin from frequent tape application and removal.

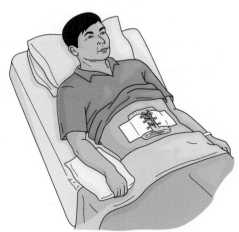

FIGURE 41-21 Montgomery straps.

Applying Dressings

A wound may not require a dressing and may be left "open to air." Or a transparent dressing covers the wound, which allows it to be seen for observations. Still other wounds require dressings that range from simple to complex. Some agencies allow nursing assistants to apply dry, non-sterile dressings to simple wounds. Follow the rules in Box 41-5.

See *Focus on Children and Older Persons: Applying Dressings.*
See *Teamwork and Time Management: Applying Dressings.*
See *Delegation Guidelines: Applying Dressings*, p. 646.
See *Promoting Safety and Comfort: Applying Dressings*, p. 646.
See procedure: *Applying a Dry, Non-Sterile Dressing*, p. 646.

BOX 41-5	Applying Dressings

- Let pain-relief drugs take effect, usually 30 minutes. The dressing change can cause discomfort. The nurse gives the drug and tells you how long to wait.
- Meet fluid and elimination needs before you begin.
- Collect equipment and supplies before you begin.
- Do not bend or reach over your work area.
- Control your nonverbal communication. Wound odors, appearance, and drainage may be unpleasant. Do not communicate your thoughts or reactions to the person.
- Remove soiled dressings so the person cannot see the soiled side. The drainage and its color may upset the person.
- Do not force the person to look at the wound. A wound can affect body image and self-esteem. The nurse helps the person deal with the wound.
- Remove tape by gently pulling the tape ends toward the wound.
- Remove dressings gently. They may stick to the wound, drain, or surrounding skin. If the dressing sticks, the nurse may have you wet the dressing with a saline solution. A wet dressing is easier to remove.
- Clean the wound with saline as directed by the nurse.
- Touch only the outer edges of new dressings as you would for a sterile field (Chapter 17).
- Report and record your observations. See *Delegation Guidelines: Applying Dressings*, p. 646.

FOCUS ON CHILDREN AND OLDER PERSONS

Applying Dressings

Children
Dressing changes may frighten children. Tape removal can be painful. Wound appearance can be frightening. A calm, cooperative child helps prevent contamination. A parent or caregiver may need to hold the child. Holding or playing with a toy can comfort the child.

TEAMWORK AND TIME MANAGEMENT

Applying Dressings

Collect all needed items before you start. Have extra dressings, tape, and other supplies on hand. Leave un-used items in the room for the next dressing change. Wound contamination can occur if you need to leave the room during the procedure.

DELEGATION GUIDELINES

Applying Dressings

Certain dressing changes can be delegated to nursing assistants in some agencies. When applying a dressing is delegated to you, make sure that:

- Your state allows you to perform the task.
- The task is in your job description (Chapter 3).
- You have the necessary education and training.
- The agency has determined that you are competent to perform the task safely.
- You know how to use the supplies and equipment.
- You review the procedure with the delegating nurse.
- The delegating nurse is available to answer questions and to guide and assist you as needed.

If the above conditions are met, you need this information from the nurse.

- When to change the dressing
- When a pain-relief drug will take effect
- What to do if the dressing sticks to the wound
- How to clean the wound
- What dressings to use
- How to secure the dressing—tape or Montgomery straps
- If tape is used, what kind and size to use
- How to apply tape over the dressing
- What observations to report and record:
  - Supplies used to dress the wound and secure the dressing
  - A red or swollen wound
  - An area around the wound that is warm to touch
  - If wound edges are closed or separated
  - A wound that has broken open *(dehiscence)*
  - Drainage appearance—clear; bloody; watery and blood-tinged; or thick and green, yellow, or brown
  - The amount of drainage and how to describe the amount—the size of a common object (quarter, dime) or guidelines for words such as small, moderate, and large
  - Wound or drainage odor
  - Intactness and color of surrounding tissues
  - Possible dressing contamination—urine, feces, other body fluids, dislodged dressing
  - Pain
  - Fever
- When to report observations
- What patient or resident concerns to report at once

PROMOTING SAFETY AND COMFORT

Applying Dressings

Safety

Tape removal can cause skin tears in persons with thin, fragile skin. Use extreme care to remove tape. Do not apply tape to irritated, injured, or non-intact skin. Tape can further damage the skin.

Dressings containing blood are biohazardous waste (Chapter 17). Follow the Bloodborne Pathogen Standard and agency policy to dispose of soiled dressings.

Comfort

Wounds and dressing changes can cause discomfort or pain. Allow time for a pain-relief drug to take effect before a dressing change. Gently apply and remove tape and dressings.

The person may not report discomfort from a dressing. You should ask:

- "Is the dressing comfortable?"
- "Does the tape cause pain or itching?"

Applying a Dry, Non-Sterile Dressing

QUALITY OF LIFE

- Knock before entering the person's room.
- Address the person by name.
- Introduce yourself by name and title.
- Explain the procedure before starting and during the procedure.
- Protect the person's rights during the procedure.
- Handle the person gently during the procedure.

PRE-PROCEDURE

1 Follow *Delegation Guidelines: Applying Dressings*. See *Promoting Safety and Comfort*:
  a *Wound Care*, p. 636
  b *Applying Dressings*
2 Practice hand hygiene and get the following supplies.
  - Gloves
  - PPE (personal protective equipment) as needed
  - Tape or Montgomery straps
  - Dressings as directed by the nurse
  - 4 × 4 gauze (see Fig. 41-19)
  - Saline solution as directed by the nurse
  - Cleaning solution as directed by the nurse
  - Adhesive remover (if needed)
  - Dressing set with scissors and forceps
  - Plastic bag with a *BIOHAZARD* label
  - Bath blanket
3 Arrange your work area. You should not have to reach over or turn your back on your work area.
4 Practice hand hygiene.
5 Identify the person. Check the identification (ID) bracelet against the assignment sheet. Use 2 identifiers (Chapter 14). Also call the person by name.
6 Provide for privacy.
7 Raise the bed for body mechanics. Bed rails are up if used. Lower the bed rail near you if up.

Applying a Dry, Non-Sterile Dressing—cont'd

PROCEDURE

8 Help the person to a comfortable position.
9 Cover the person with a bath blanket. Fan-fold top linens to the foot of the bed.
10 Expose the affected body part.
11 Make a cuff on the plastic bag. Place the bag within reach.
12 Practice hand hygiene.
13 Don needed PPE. Put on gloves.
14 Remove tape or undo Montgomery straps.
  a *Tape:* Hold the skin down. Gently pull the tape toward the wound. Apply adhesive remover during removal if needed. Follow the manufacturer's instructions.
  b *Montgomery straps:* Undo the straps. Fold the straps away from the wound.
15 Remove any adhesive from the skin. Follow the manufacturer's instructions for adhesive remover use. Clean away from the wound.
16 Remove dressings with a gloved hand or with forceps (Fig. 41-22). Start with the top dressing and remove each layer. Keep the soiled side away from the person's sight. Put dressings in the plastic bag. They must not touch the outside of the bag.

17 Remove the dressing over the wound very gently. It may stick to the wound or drain site. If directed by the nurse, moisten the dressing with saline if it sticks to the wound. Discard the dressing as in step 16.
18 Observe the wound, drain site, and wound drainage.
19 Remove the gloves. Put them in the bag. Practice hand hygiene.
20 Open the new dressings.
21 Put on clean gloves.
22 Clean the wound with saline or other solution as directed by the nurse. See Figure 41-23.
23 Apply dressings as directed by the nurse (Fig. 41-24, p. 648). Touch only the outer edges of the dressing. Do not touch the part that will have contact with the wound.
24 Secure the dressings. Use tape or Montgomery straps.
25 Remove the gloves. Put them in the bag.
26 Remove and discard PPE.
27 Practice hand hygiene.
28 Cover the person. Remove the bath blanket. Fold and return the bath blanket to its proper place. Or follow agency policy for used linens.

POST-PROCEDURE

29 Provide for comfort. (See the inside of the back cover.)
30 Lower the bed to a safe and comfortable level. Raise or lower bed rails. Follow the care plan.
31 Clean up and store supplies and equipment. (Wear gloves. Change gloves as needed.)
  a Discard used supplies in the bag. Tie the bag closed. Discard the bag following agency policy. Follow the Bloodborne Pathogen Standard.
  b Return equipment and supplies to their proper place. Leave extra dressings and tape in the room.
  c Clean and dry your work area. Dry with paper towels. Discard the paper towels.
  d Remove and discard gloves. Practice hand hygiene.

32 Place the call light and other needed items within reach.
33 Follow the care plan and the person's preferences for privacy measures to maintain. Leaving the privacy curtain, window coverings, and door open or closed are examples.
34 Complete a safety check of the room. (See the inside of the back cover.)
35 Practice hand hygiene.
36 Report and record your care and observations.

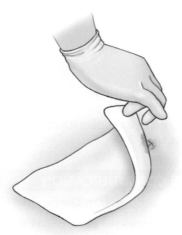

FIGURE 41-22 Removing a dressing. Keep the soiled side away from the person's sight.

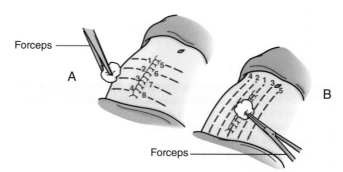

FIGURE 41-23 Cleaning a wound. **A,** Start at the wound and stroke out to the surrounding skin. Use new gauze for each stroke. **B,** Clean the wound from the top to the bottom. Start at the wound. Then clean the surrounding areas. Use new gauze for each stroke. (From Potter PA, Perry AG, Stockert PA, et al: *Fundamentals of nursing,* ed 11, St Louis, 2023, Elsevier.)

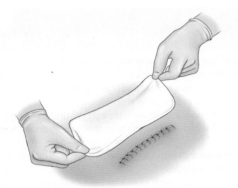

FIGURE 41-24 Applying a dressing. Wear clean gloves. Touch only the outer edges of the dressing. Do not touch the part that will contact the wound.

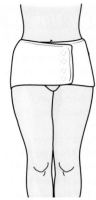

FIGURE 41-25 Abdominal binder. The top part is at the waist. The lower part is over the hips.

BINDERS AND COMPRESSION GARMENTS

Binders are wide bands of elastic fabric. They support wounds and hold dressings in place. They also prevent or reduce swelling, promote comfort, and prevent injury. These binders are common.

- *Abdominal binder*—provides abdominal support and holds dressings in place (Fig. 41-25). The top part is at the waist. The lower part is over the hips. Binders are secured in place with Velcro or with hook and loop closures.
- *Breast binder*—supports the breasts after surgery (Fig. 41-26). It is secured in place with Velcro or padded zippers.

Compression garments are made of a tight, stretchy fabric (Fig. 41-27). Common after plastic surgery, they help:

- Reduce swelling.
- Prevent fluid buildup at the surgical site.
- Hold the skin against the body.
- Achieve the desired shape.

Box 41-6 lists the rules for applying binders and compression garments.

See *Focus on Communication: Binders and Compression Garments*.

See *Promoting Safety and Comfort: Binders and Compression Garments*.

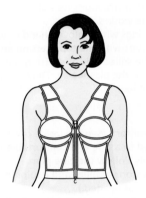

FIGURE 41-26 Breast binder.

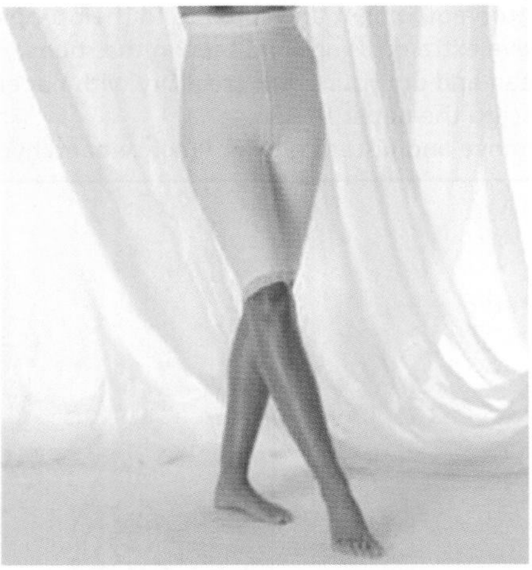

FIGURE 41-27 Compression garment. (Courtesy Rainey Compression Essentials, Atlanta, Ga.)

BOX 41-6   Binders and Compression Garments

- Follow the manufacturer's instructions.
- Position the person in good alignment.
- Apply the device for firm, even pressure over the area.
- Apply the device so it is snug. It must not interfere with breathing or circulation.
- Re-apply the device if it is out of position or causes discomfort.
- Change the device if moist or soiled. This prevents the growth of microbes.
- Tell the nurse at once if the person's breathing changes.
- Check the skin under and around the device. Tell the nurse at once if there is redness, irritation, or other signs of a skin problem.

FOCUS ON COMMUNICATION

Binders and Compression Garments

The person may not tell you about pain or discomfort. You need to ask:

- "Is the binder (garment) too tight or too loose?"
- "Does the binder (garment) cause pain?"
- "Do you feel pressure from the binder (garment)?" If yes: "Where? Please show me."

HEAT AND COLD APPLICATIONS

Heat and cold applications promote healing and comfort. They also reduce tissue swelling. See Chapter 43.

THE WHOLE PERSON

Wounds can have a minor or major effect on the person's life. The effect depends on the wound's cause, size, location, complexity, and complications. It also depends on the person's age and overall health. The wound is only part of the person's care. Nursing care must consider the *whole* person (Chapter 7).

Pain can affect breathing and moving. Turning, re-positioning, and walking may be painful. Be gentle. Let pain-relief drugs take effect before giving care.

Abdominal trauma and surgery can affect eating and elimination. Pain and odors from wound drainage can affect appetite. Follow the care plan to meet nutrition and elimination needs. Tell the nurse if the person wants certain foods or drinks.

Infection is always a threat. Follow the practices to prevent infection in Chapters 17 and 18. Carefully observe the wound for signs and symptoms of infection.

Delayed healing is a risk for persons who are older, are obese, or have poor nutrition. Protein is needed for tissue growth and repair. Poor circulation and diabetes also affect healing, increasing the risk of infection.

Worries and fears threaten a person's mental and emotional health. Scarring, disfigurement, delayed healing, and infection are common fears. So are fears about the wound "popping open." Worries about performing daily activities and work are common. Eye injuries can cause vision changes. Medical bills and ongoing care are other concerns.

Victims of violence may fear future attacks and worry about finding and convicting the attacker and about family safety. Victims of intimate partner, child, and elder abuse often hide the source of their injuries.

Wounds, dressings, drainage and drainage devices, and wound odors can be disturbing. Visitors may feel uncomfortable. Keep the wound covered and drainage containers out of sight if able. Promptly remove soiled dressings from the room. Use room deodorizers as directed.

Self-esteem is often affected when appearance changes. Clothing is useful in hiding some wounds. Other wounds are visible. Disfiguring wounds can affect body image and feelings of attraction.

The person may be sad and tearful or angry and hostile. Adjustment may require rehabilitation and counseling. Be gentle and kind, give thoughtful care, and practice good communication.

FOCUS ON **PRIDE**

The Person, Family, and Yourself

Personal and Professional Responsibility

As a nursing assistant, you have responsibilities for wound care. For example, if you are careless during a transfer, you can cause a skin tear. If you rush during a bath, you may not notice a wound between skin folds. If you do not apply shoes properly, a foot ulcer can develop.

How you provide care affects the person's health, safety, and quality of life. Take pride in working safely and carefully.

Rights and Respect

A person may have questions about the reasons for care. Avoid pat answers like: "It's to help you get better" or "The doctor (nurse) says you need it." The person has the right to be informed. Ask the nurse to explain reasons for care. Wait until questions are answered before performing the care measure.

Independence and Social Interaction

Body image involves thoughts and feelings about one's appearance. It relates to what a person believes others are thinking or saying about the person's appearance. Body image is a factor in a person's level of self-esteem.

Wounds can affect body image and self-esteem. Watch your reactions. Do not show disgust. Be professional. Talk about the person's wound as you need to. However, talk about other things as well. Remember, you are caring for a person. Your interactions make a difference.

Delegation and Teamwork

Wound care can be painful and tiring. To promote comfort and rest:

- Plan care with the nurse. Ask when pain-relief drugs will be given and will take effect. Allow rest periods before and after care.
- Be prepared. Leaving to get supplies causes delays. Care and procedures take longer than planned.
- Assist the nurse as instructed. You may need to position the person or raise a body part while the nurse changes a dressing. Teamwork reduces the amount of energy the person must use.

Ethics and Laws

Agency practices vary for charging supplies. Ethical practice involves honestly following agency rules. Not charging supplies correctly costs the nursing unit and agency money. Taking supplies home for your own use is unethical. This is stealing. Take pride in following agency rules and being an honest and reliable member of the nursing team.

FOCUS ON **PRIDE**: *Application*

Is body image the same for all persons? Is it the same throughout a person's life? Explain. How might a wound affect body image?

REVIEW QUESTIONS

Circle the BEST answer.

1 Which wound cause is *correct?*
   a Excoriation is caused by scratching.
   b An incision is caused by trauma.
   c A laceration is caused by a surgical instrument.
   d An abrasion is caused by poor blood flow.

2 Which can cause skin tears?
   a Keeping your nails trimmed and smooth
   b Dressing the person in soft clothing
   c Wearing rings
   d Padding wheelchair footplates

3 A person is at risk for circulatory ulcers. Which measure should you question?
   a Report toenails in need of trimming.
   b Hold socks in place with elastic garters.
   c Check the legs and feet carefully during skin care.
   d Re-position the person every hour.

4 Diabetic foot ulcers are caused by
   a Gangrene
   b Amputation
   c Infection
   d Nerve and blood vessel damage

5 A person has diabetes. When providing foot care
   a Dry well between the toes
   b Apply lotion between the toes
   c Trim the toenails
   d Use hot water

6 A person with diabetes wears socks with shoes to prevent
   a Corns
   b Bunions
   c Ingrown toenails
   d Blisters

7 A wound is separating. This is called
   a Primary intention
   b Third intention
   c Dehiscence
   d Evisceration

8 A patient has a surgical incision closed with staples. Which observation is *normal?*
   a The area around the wound is red, warm, and swollen.
   b The wound edges are closed (approximated).
   c The wound has a bad odor.
   d The wound has yellow drainage.

9 A person has clear, watery drainage from a wound. You describe this as
   a Serous drainage
   b Purulent drainage
   c Sanguineous drainage
   d Serosanguineous drainage

10 After surgery, a person has a wound dressing and a closed drainage system. Which is *true?*
   a The drainage system prevents fluids from leaving the wound.
   b The dressing protects the wound from injury and microbes.
   c The drainage system is not emptied.
   d The dressing is not changed.

11 To secure a dressing, apply tape
   a Around the entire body part
   b In an X pattern over the dressing
   c So it extends beyond the sides of the dressing
   d Loosely

12 What is the purpose of Montgomery straps?
   a To provide compression and prevent swelling
   b To lessen the frequency of dressing changes
   c To absorb more drainage
   d To prevent skin irritation from frequent dressing changes

13 The nurse needs help with a dressing change. Which shows good planning?
   a You leave the room to get supplies often.
   b You gather supplies while the person's pain-relief drug takes effect.
   c You set up supplies in an area that requires reaching over the wound.
   d You begin another patient's bed bath shortly before the nurse needs help.

14 Which action during a dressing change is *correct?*
   a Tape is removed by pulling it away from the wound.
   b Clean gloves are worn to apply the new dressing.
   c The same gauze is used for each stroke when cleaning the wound.
   d The part of the new dressing that will have contact with the wound is touched.

15 An abdominal binder is used to
   a Prevent blood clots
   b Absorb drainage
   c Provide support and hold dressings in place
   d Provide warmth

Answers to Chapter 41 questions are on p. 903.

FOCUS ON PRACTICE

Problem Solving

An older resident has thin, fragile skin. You notice a new skin tear on the person's arm. What do you do? How can you prevent skin tears?

Pressure Injuries

OBJECTIVES

- Define the key terms and key abbreviations in this chapter.
- Describe the causes and risk factors for pressure injuries.
- Identify the persons at risk for pressure injuries.
- Identify the sites for pressure injuries.
- Describe the stages of pressure injuries and the Kennedy terminal ulcer.

- Explain how to prevent pressure injuries.
- Identify the complications from pressure injuries.
- Explain how to promote PRIDE in the person, the family, and yourself.

KEY TERMS

avoidable pressure injury A pressure injury that develops from the improper use of the nursing process

bedfast Confined to bed

blanch To become white

bony prominence An area where the bone sticks out or projects from the flat surface of the body; pressure point

chairfast Confined to a chair

epidermal stripping Removing the epidermis (outer skin layer) as tape is removed from the skin

erythema Redness

eschar Thick, leathery dead tissue that may be loose or adhered to the skin; it is often black or brown

intact skin Skin that is not broken

pressure injury Localized damage to the skin and underlying soft tissue; the injury is usually over a bony prominence or related to a medical or other device and results from pressure or pressure in combination with shear

pressure point See "bony prominence"

shear When layers of the skin rub against each other; when the skin remains in place and underlying tissues move and stretch, tearing underlying capillaries and blood vessels and causing tissue damage

skin breakdown Changes or damage to intact skin

slough Dead tissue that is shed from the skin; it is usually light colored, soft, and moist; may be stringy at times

ulcer A shallow or deep crater-like sore of the skin or mucous membrane

unavoidable pressure injury A pressure injury that occurs despite efforts to prevent one through proper use of the nursing process

KEY ABBREVIATIONS

CMS	Centers for Medicare & Medicaid Services	**NPIAP**	National Pressure Injury Advisory Panel

Normal, healthy skin and tissues do not have damage or breaks (Fig. 42-1, p. 652). Pressure can damage the skin and tissues and cause severe wounds (Fig. 42-2, p. 652). Helping to prevent and treat wounds that occur from pressure is an important part of the nursing assistant's role.

TERMS AND CAUSES

The National Pressure Injury Advisory Panel (NPIAP) defines *pressure injury* as:

- Localized damage to the skin and underlying soft tissue.
- The injury is usually over a bony prominence or related to a medical or other device.
- The injury results from pressure or pressure in combination with shear.

Healthy Skin – Lightly Pigmented

A

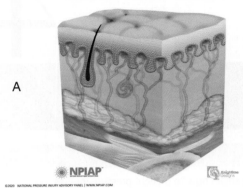

Healthy Skin – Darkly Pigmented

B

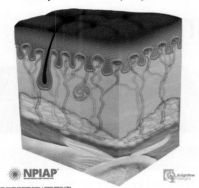

FIGURE 42-1 A, Healthy skin with light pigment. **B,** Healthy skin with dark pigment. (Note: *Pigment* gives color to the skin.) (Used with permission from the National Pressure Injury Advisory Panel [NPIAP]. Copyright 2020 NPIAP.)

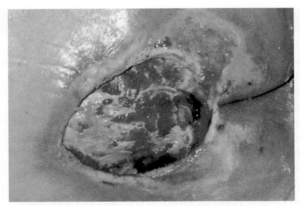

FIGURE 42-2 A pressure injury. (From Ostomy Wound Management, *Proceedings from the November National V.A.C.* ® 51[2A, supp]: 7S, Feb 2005, HMP Communications. Used with permission.)

A *bony prominence (pressure point)* is an area where the bone sticks out or projects from the flat surface of the body. The back of the head, shoulder blades, elbows, hips, spine, sacrum, knees, ankles, heels, and toes are bony prominences (Fig. 42-3).

Pressure injuries result from intense or prolonged pressure, shear, or both (Fig. 42-4). Pressure is a force that presses inward. Shear is a force that pulls across. *Shear* occurs when layers of the skin rub against each other. Or shear occurs when the skin remains in place and underlying tissues move and stretch, tearing underlying capillaries and blood vessels. Tissue damage occurs.

Possibly painful, a pressure injury may involve intact skin or an open ulcer.
- *Intact skin* is skin that is not broken.
- An *ulcer* is a shallow or deep crater-like sore of the skin or mucous membrane (see Fig. 42-2).

Some agencies and organizations use the term *pressure ulcer.* The term *bedsore* is commonly used by patients, residents, and families. Pressure injury, pressure ulcer, and bedsore essentially mean the same thing.

RISK FACTORS

Pressure and shearing are the major causes of pressure injuries (see Fig. 42-4). A common example of pressure is when the skin over a bony area is squeezed between hard surfaces (Fig. 42-5). The bone is 1 hard surface. The other is usually the mattress or seat of a chair. Unrelieved pressure squeezes tiny blood vessels. This prevents blood flow to the skin and underlying tissues. Oxygen and nutrients cannot get to the cells. Skin and tissues die. A common example of shear is when the person slides down in the bed or chair. Blood vessels and tissues are damaged. Blood flow to the area is reduced.

See Box 42-1 (p. 654) for pressure injury risk factors. Agencies must identify persons at risk for pressure injuries. The health team assesses the person's physical and mental health. A person's risk may increase during an illness, from condition changes, because of injury or surgery, or from medical devices. The person's care plan must include measures to reduce or remove risk factors. See "Persons at Risk" on p. 654.

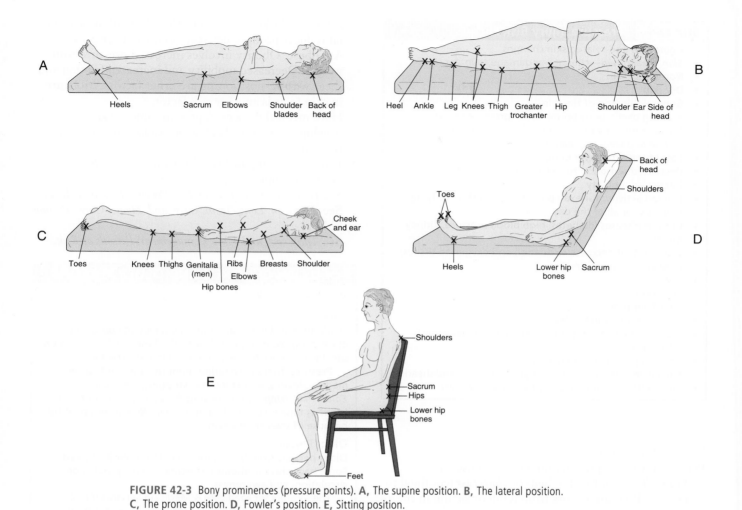

FIGURE 42-3 Bony prominences (pressure points). **A,** The supine position. **B,** The lateral position. **C,** The prone position. **D,** Fowler's position. **E,** Sitting position.

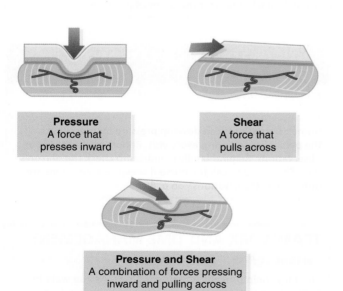

Pressure
A force that presses inward

Shear
A force that pulls across

Pressure and Shear
A combination of forces pressing inward and pulling across

FIGURE 42-4 The forces of pressure and shear. (Modified from Probst S: *Wound care nursing: a person-centered approach,* ed 3, St Louis, 2021, Elsevier.)

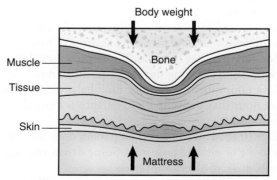

FIGURE 42-5 Tissue under pressure. The skin is squeezed between 2 hard surfaces—the bone and the mattress. (Redrawn from Agency for Healthcare Research and Quality: *Understanding your body: what are pressure ulcers?* Rockville, 2007, U.S. Department of Health and Human Services.)

BOX 42-1	Pressure Injury Risk Factors

- Aging and age-related skin changes
- *Skin breakdown*—changes or damage to intact skin
- Non-intact skin
- Dry skin
- General thinning of the skin
- Scarring over a bony prominence (pressure point)
- Pressure on bony prominences (pressure points)
- Fragile and weak capillaries
- Loss of the fatty layer under the skin
- Decreased sensation to touch, heat, and cold
- Decreased mobility
- Limited activity: for example, sitting in a chair or lying in bed most or all of the day
- Chronic diseases (diabetes, high blood pressure, kidney disease)
- Diseases that decrease circulation and oxygen to tissues; poor circulation to an area
- Fever
- Poor nutrition
- Poor hydration
- Incontinence: urinary, fecal
- Moisture in dark body areas: skin folds, under breasts, perineal area
- Poor fingernail and toenail care
- Friction (rubbing of 1 surface against another) and shearing
- *Edema* (the swelling of body tissues with water)

Persons at Risk

Persons at risk for pressure injuries are those who:

- Are *bedfast* (confined to bed) or *chairfast* (confined to a chair). Pressure occurs from lying or sitting in the same position too long.
- Need some or total help moving. For example, coma, paralysis, and hip fractures affect the ability to move.
- Are agitated, have muscle spasms, or have involuntary muscle movements. The movements cause rubbing (friction) against linens and other surfaces.
- Are incontinent. Urine and feces (stools) irritate the skin, leading to skin breakdown. They are also sources of moisture.
- Are exposed to moisture. Urine, feces (stools), wound drainage, sweat, and saliva are sources of moisture. Moisture irritates the skin. It also increases the risk of friction and shearing during re-positioning.
- Have poor nutrition or poor fluid balance. A balanced diet nourishes the skin. Fluid balance is needed for healthy skin.
- Have limited awareness. The person does not know to move or change positions. Some drugs and health problems can affect awareness.
- Have problems sensing pain or pressure. The person does not know to alert the staff to these symptoms of tissue damage.
- Have circulatory problems. Cells and tissues die when starved of oxygen and nutrients.

- Have weight loss or are very thin. Loss of muscle and fat reduces padding between bones and surfaces.
- Are obese. Obesity involves increased pressure from weight. Decreased mobility and increased friction and shear with re-positioning are other factors. Moisture in skin folds is another risk factor.
- Have medical devices. A pressure injury can develop where a medical device causes pressure on the skin.
- Have an existing or healed pressure injury. See "Pressure Injury Stages."

See *Focus on Children and Older Persons: Persons at Risk.*

See *Focus on Long-Term Care and Home Care: Persons at Risk.*

See *Teamwork and Time Management: Persons at Risk.*

FOCUS ON CHILDREN AND OLDER PERSONS
Persons at Risk

Children

Ill infants and children and those with mobility problems are at risk for pressure injuries. The back of the head is a common site. Incontinence (urinary and fecal) is also a risk factor.

Pressure, friction, shearing, poor nutrition, infection, medical devices, and epidermal stripping are causes. *Epidermal stripping* is removing the epidermis (outer skin layer) as tape is removed from the skin. Newborns are at risk because of their fragile skin.

Older Persons

Older persons have thin, fragile skin that is easily injured. Some have chronic diseases affecting mobility, nutrition, circulation, and awareness.

The Centers for Medicare & Medicaid Services (CMS) requires that nursing centers identify persons at risk for pressure injuries. A person can develop a pressure injury within 2 to 6 hours after the onset of pressure.

FOCUS ON LONG-TERM CARE AND HOME CARE
Persons at Risk

Home Care

Home care patients can develop pressure injuries. Check the person's skin during every visit. Report and record your observations. Remind family members to check the person's skin. They need to call the nurse if pressure injury signs are noted. See "Observations" on p. 658.

TEAMWORK AND TIME MANAGEMENT
Persons at Risk

You must help prevent pressure injuries. As you walk in hallways, look to see if a person has slid down in bed or in a chair. Do the same when people are in dining and lounge areas. Help re-position the person. Ask a co-worker to help you as needed. Report the re-positioning to the nurse.

PRESSURE INJURY SITES

Pressure injuries usually occur over bony prominences (pressure points). These areas bear the body's weight in certain positions (see Fig. 42-3). Pressure from body weight can reduce the blood supply to the skin. The sacrum and heels are common sites for pressure injuries.

Medical device–related pressure injuries can develop at sites where devices are used for diagnostic or treatment purposes. For example, eyeglasses can cause pressure and friction on the ears. Oxygen tubing (Chapter 44) can cause pressure on the nose, face, and ears. Pressure can occur on an ear from the mattress when in a side-lying position. Tubes, casts, braces, and other devices can cause pressure on the hands, arms, legs, and feet. Pressure can occur on the buttocks from bedpans.

Mucosal membrane pressure injuries are found in mucous membranes where a medical device is used. A urinary catheter can cause pressure and friction on the meatus. A feeding tube can cause pressure in the nose.

Pressure injuries can occur where skin has contact with skin. Common sites are between abdominal folds, the legs, the buttocks, the thighs, and under the breasts.

PRESSURE INJURY STAGES

Understanding the following terms will help you as you study the different pressure injury stages.

- *Erythema* means redness.
- *Blanch* means to become white.
  - *Blanchable*—When pressure is applied to the skin, blood is pressed away. This causes the skin to become white or pale (Fig. 42-6). When pressure is relieved, the skin returns to its normal color.
  - *Non-blanchable*—The skin does not become white or pale when pressure is applied and removed (see Fig. 42-6).
- *Slough* is dead tissue that is shed from the skin. It is usually light colored, soft, and moist. It may be stringy at times. See Figure 42-7.
- *Eschar* is thick, leathery dead tissue that may be loose or adhered to the skin. It is often black or brown. See Figure 42-8.

Pressure injuries range from reddened intact skin to tissue loss with bone exposure. For pressure injury stages, see Figure 42-9 (pp. 656–657).

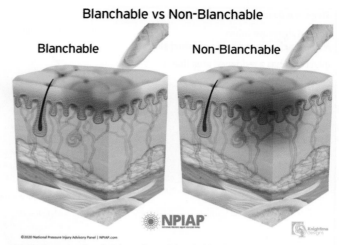

FIGURE 42-6 Blanchable and non-blanchable skin. (Used with permission from the National Pressure Injury Advisory Panel [NPIAP]. Copyright 2020 NPIAP.)

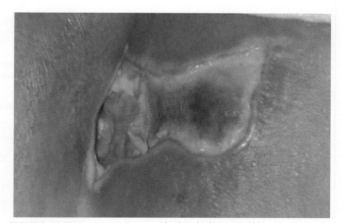

FIGURE 42-7 A pressure injury with slough. (From Braddom R: *Physical medicine and rehabilitation*, ed 4, Philadelphia, 2011, Elsevier Saunders, p 697.)

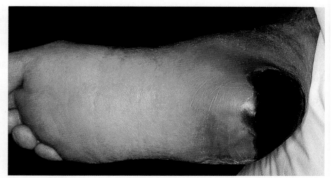

FIGURE 42-8 A pressure injury with eschar. (From Bolognia JL, Jorizzo JJ, Schaffer JV, et al: *Dermatology*, ed 3, Oxford, UK, 2012, Elsevier.)

Stage and Description	Drawing	Example

Stage 1 Pressure Injury

Non-blanchable erythema of intact skin

Intact skin has a reddened area that is non-blanchable.

Stage 1 Pressure Injury – Lightly Pigmented

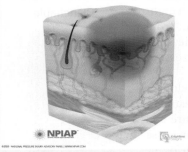

Stage 1 Pressure Injury – Darkly Pigmented

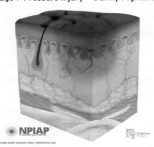

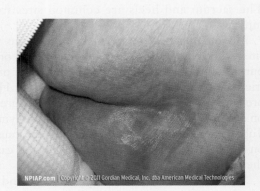

NOTE: *NPIAP defines a Stage 1 pressure injury as intact skin with a localized area of non-blanchable erythema, which may appear differently in darkly pigmented skin. Presence of blanchable erythema or changes in sensation, temperature, or firmness may precede visual changes. Color changes do not include purple or maroon discoloration; these may indicate deep tissue pressure injury.*

Stage 2 Pressure Injury

Partial-thickness skin loss with exposed dermis

The wound is pink or red and moist. It may involve a broken or intact blister. Fat and deeper tissues are not visible.

Stage 2 Pressure Injury

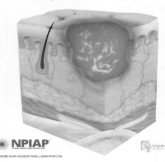

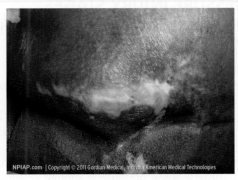

NOTE: *NPIAP defines a Stage 2 pressure injury as partial-thickness loss of skin with exposed dermis. The wound bed is viable, pink or red, moist, and may also present as an intact or ruptured serum-filled blister. Adipose (fat) is not visible and deeper tissues are not visible. Granulation tissue, slough and eschar are not present. These injuries commonly result from adverse microclimate and shear in the skin over the pelvis and shear in the heel. This stage should not be used to describe moisture associated skin damage (MASD) including incontinence associated dermatitis (IAD), intertriginous dermatitis (ITD), medical adhesive related skin injury (MARSI), or traumatic wounds (skin tears, burns, abrasions).*

Stage 3 Pressure Injury

Full-thickness skin loss

The skin is gone. Fat can be seen in the ulcer. Slough, eschar, or both may be present.

Stage 3 Pressure Injury

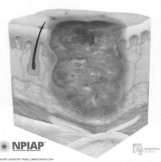

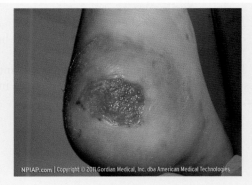

NOTE: *NPIAP defines a Stage 3 pressure injury as full-thickness loss of skin, in which adipose (fat) is visible in the ulcer and granulation tissue and epibole (rolled wound edges) are often present. Slough and/or eschar may be visible. The depth of tissue damage varies by anatomical location; areas of significant adiposity can develop deep wounds. Undermining and tunneling may occur. Fascia, muscle, tendon, ligament, cartilage and/or bone are not exposed. If slough or eschar obscures the extent of tissue loss this is an Unstageable Pressure Injury.*

FIGURE 42-9 Pressure injury stages. (Illustrations, photos, and definitions used with permission from the National Pressure Injury Advisory Panel [NPIAP], Copyright 2020 NPIAP.)

Stage and Description	Drawing	Example

Stage 4 Pressure Injury
Full-thickness skin and tissue loss

The skin is gone. Muscle, tendon, ligament, cartilage, or bone is exposed. Slough, eschar, or both may be present.

Stage 4 Pressure Injury

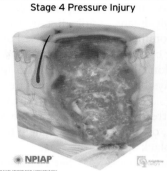

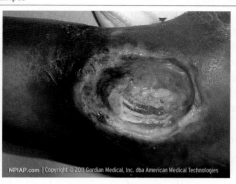

NOTE: *NPIAP defines a Stage 4 pressure injury as full-thickness skin and tissue loss with exposed or directly palpable fascia, muscle, tendon, ligament, cartilage or bone in the ulcer. Slough and/or eschar may be visible. Epibole (rolled edges), undermining and/or tunneling often occur. Depth varies by anatomical location. If slough or eschar obscures the extent of tissue loss this is an Unstageable Pressure Injury.*

Unstageable Pressure Injury
Obscured full-thickness skin and tissue loss

There is skin and tissue loss. The extent of tissue damage cannot be seen because of slough or eschar. (*Obscure* means to block from being seen.) When slough or eschar is removed, the injury can be seen.

Unstageable Pressure Injury
Slough and Eschar

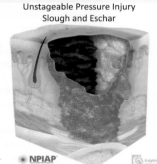

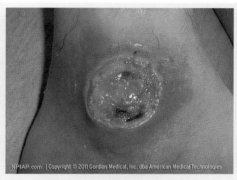

NOTE: *NPIAP defines an Unstageable Pressure Injury as full-thickness skin and tissue loss in which the extent of tissue damage within the ulcer cannot be confirmed because it is obscured by slough or eschar. If slough or eschar is removed, a Stage 3 or Stage 4 pressure injury will be revealed. Stable eschar (i.e. dry, adherent, intact without erythema or fluctuance) on the heel or ischemic limb should not be softened or removed.*

Deep Tissue Pressure Injury
Persistent non-blanchable deep red, maroon, or purple discoloration

Intact or non-intact skin is deep red, maroon, or purple and remains non-blanchable. The wound is dark or is a blood-filled blister.

Deep Tissue Pressure Injury

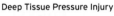

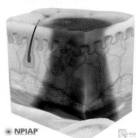

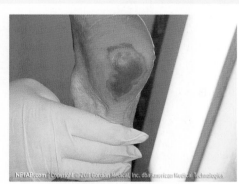

NOTE: *NPIAP defines a deep tissue pressure injury as intact or non-intact skin with localized area of persistent non-blanchable deep red, maroon, purple discoloration or epidermal separation revealing a dark wound bed or blood filled blister. Pain and temperature change often precede skin color changes. Discoloration may appear differently in darkly pigmented skin. This injury results from intense and/or prolonged pressure and shear forces at the bone-muscle interface. The wound may evolve rapidly to reveal the actual extent of tissue injury, or may resolve without tissue loss. If necrotic tissue, subcutaneous tissue, granulation tissue, fascia, muscle or other underlying structures are visible, this indicates a full thickness pressure injury (Unstageable, Stage 3 or Stage 4). Do not use DTPI to describe vascular, traumatic, neuropathic, or dermatologic conditions.*

FIGURE 42-9, cont'd

Kennedy Terminal Ulcer

Persons receiving end-of-life care (Chapter 59) are at risk for pressure injuries. Described by Karen Kennedy-Evans, the *Kennedy terminal ulcer* occurs over a bony prominence 2 to 3 days before death. The sacrum is the most common site. The cause is thought to be *skin failure*—the skin (along with other body organs) shuts down 10 to 14 days before death.

The onset is sudden. Shaped like a pear, butterfly, or horseshoe, the ulcer can be red, yellow, purple, or black (Fig. 42-10). At first it may look like a small black spot or a dried bowel movement. Within a few hours it can increase to the size of a quarter or larger. Usually Stage 2 with a blister at first, it rapidly progresses to Stage 3 or 4.

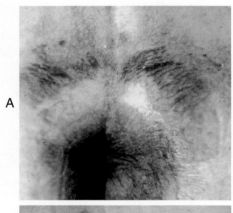

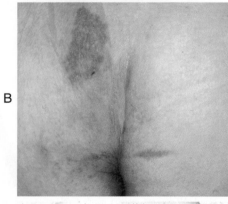

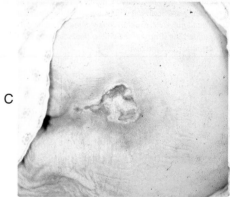

FIGURE 42-10 Kennedy terminal ulcer. **A** and **B,** First 4 to 8 hours. **C,** After 8 hours. (From Kennedy KL: *Understanding the Kennedy terminal ulcer,* Tucson, 2014.)

OBSERVATIONS

Inspect the skin every time you give care. This includes during or after transfers, re-positioning, bathing, and elimination procedures. Pay close attention to bony prominences. Also observe areas where skin has contact with skin. If needed, have help to lift the body part to look for skin changes. Check sites that have contact with medical devices.

Report areas of redness, skin color changes, blisters, or skin or tissue loss. The nurse needs to assess the site. If needed, help the nurse turn or position the person to assess the area.

See *Focus on Communication: Observations.*

FOCUS ON COMMUNICATION

Observations

When reporting observations, tell the nurse the site. Describe what you see as best as you can. For example, you can say:

- "I saw a reddened area on Mr. Smith's left heel. It was about the size of a quarter. The skin looked intact. Please look at it."
- "I noticed a red area with a blister on Ms. Clark's left buttock. I didn't see any drainage. Please look at it. I'll help you turn her."

PREVENTION AND TREATMENT

Preventing pressure injuries is much easier than trying to heal them. Unfortunately, some pressure injuries cannot be prevented. Called *unavoidable pressure injuries*, they occur despite efforts to prevent them through proper use of the nursing process. The Kennedy terminal ulcer is an example. An *avoidable pressure injury* develops from improper use of the nursing process.

Pressure injury prevention involves:

- Identifying persons at risk. The health team assesses the person's risk factors and skin condition.
- Prevention measures for those at risk. Good nursing care, cleanliness, and skin care are essential. Managing moisture, good nutrition and fluid balance, and relieving pressure also are key measures. Box 42-2 lists common measures used to prevent skin damage and pressure injuries. Always follow the person's care plan.

Some agencies use symbols or colored stickers as pressure injury alerts. Placed on the person's door or medical record, the alerts remind the staff that the person is at risk.

See *Focus on Surveys: Prevention and Treatment,* p. 660.

BOX 42-2	**Preventing Pressure Injuries**

Moving and Positioning
- Position the person according to the care plan. Use pillows for support as directed. The 30-degree lateral position is recommended (Fig. 42-11, p. 660).
- Do not position the person:
  - On a pressure injury
  - On a reddened area
  - On tubes or other medical devices
- Follow the person's re-positioning schedule (Fig. 42-12, p. 660). Re-position bedfast persons at least every 1 to 2 hours. Re-position chairfast persons at least every hour. Some persons are re-positioned every 15 minutes.
- Remind persons sitting in recliners, chairs, or wheelchairs to shift positions at least every 15 minutes.
- Do not leave a person on a bedpan longer than needed.
- Do not let the person sit on donut-shaped cushions.
- Prevent shearing and friction during moving and transfer procedures. Do not drag the person. Use assist devices as directed. See Chapters 20 and 21.
- Use slow, gradual turns and movements when re-positioning persons who are critically ill.
- Prevent shearing. Do not raise the head of the bed more than 30 degrees. Follow the care plan for:
  - When to raise the head of the bed
  - How far to raise the head of the bed
  - How long (in minutes) to raise the head of the bed
- Use pillows, foam wedges, or other devices to prevent bony areas from contact with other bony areas and firm surfaces. The ankles, knees, hips, and sacrum are examples.
- Keep the heels and ankles off of the bed. Use pillows or other devices as directed. Place the pillows or devices under the lower legs from mid-calf to the ankles.
- Use protective devices as directed (p. 660).
- Elevate the legs when the person is sitting in a recliner.
- Tilt the person's seat, if safely possible, when in a chair or wheelchair. Tilting prevents the person from sliding forward.
- Support the feet properly when the person is sitting upright in a chair or wheelchair. Use a footstool if the person's feet do not touch the floor when sitting in a chair. The body slides forward when the feet do not touch the floor. For the person in a wheelchair, position the feet on the footrests.

Skin Care
- Inspect the skin every time you give care. See "Observations." Report any concern at once.
- Follow the person's bathing schedule. Some persons do not need a bath or shower every day.
- Do not use hot water to bathe or clean the skin. Hot water can irritate the skin.
- Use a cleansing agent as directed. Some bar soaps can dry and irritate the skin.
- Provide good skin care.
  - The skin is clean and dry after bathing.
  - The skin is free of moisture from a bath or shower and from urine, feces (stools), perspiration, wound drainage, and other secretions.
  - Skin under the breasts, in the groin area, and under abdominal folds is clean and dry.

Skin Care—cont'd
- Prevent skin exposure to moisture.
  - Check persons who are at risk for moisture exposure often.
  - For persons who are incontinent of urine or feces (stools):
    - Follow measures to prevent incontinence.
    - Provide good skin care and change linens and garments at the time of soiling.
    - Use incontinence products as directed.
    - Apply an ointment or moisture barrier. Follow the care plan.
  - For persons who perspire heavily or have wound drainage, provide good skin care. Change linens and garments as needed.
- Apply moisturizer to dry areas—hands, elbows, hips, ankles, heels, and so on. The nurse tells you what to use and what areas need attention.
- Give a back massage when re-positioning the person. Do not massage bony areas.
- Do not massage over pressure points. *Never rub or massage reddened areas.*
- Keep linens clean, dry, and wrinkle-free.
- Make sure the bed or chair is free of objects. Crumbs, pins, pencils, pens, and coins are examples.
- Do not irritate the skin. Avoid scrubbing or vigorous rubbing when bathing or drying the person.
- Use pillows and blankets to prevent skin from being in contact with skin.
- Make sure clothes do not increase the risk for pressure injuries.
  - Avoid seams, buttons, or zippers that press against the skin.
  - Avoid tight clothes.
  - Keep clothes from bunching up or wrinkling.
- Make sure socks and shoes are in good repair. Socks should not have holes, wrinkles, or creases. Make sure there is nothing in the shoes before the person puts them on.
- Do not apply heat or cold (Chapter 43) directly on a pressure injury.
- See Chapter 41 for diabetes foot care.

Medical Devices
- Use the correct device in the correct size. Follow the care plan.
- Apply and secure the device correctly. Follow the manufacturer's directions.
- Move or re-position the device according to the care plan.
- Check the skin under a medical device for edema and signs of a pressure injury.
- Protect the skin under the device as directed by the nurse.
- Do not position the person on top of a medical device.
- Ask about the person's comfort. Tell the nurse if the device is causing discomfort or is too loose or too tight.

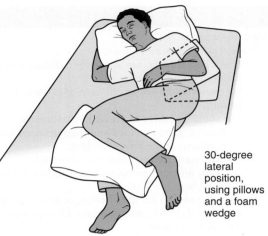
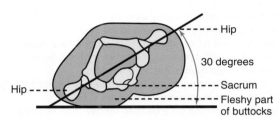

FIGURE 42-11 The 30-degree lateral position. Pillows are under the head, shoulder, and leg. This position inclines (lifts up) the hip to avoid pressure on the hip. The person does not lie on the hip as in the side-lying position.

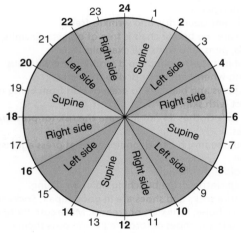

FIGURE 42-12 Turn clock. The clock shows the times to turn the person and to what position.

Protective Devices

Wound care products, drugs, treatments, dressings, and equipment are ordered to promote healing. Support surfaces relieve or reduce pressure. Such surfaces include foam, air, alternating air, gel, or water mattresses.

Protective devices are often used to prevent and treat skin breakdown and pressure injuries. These devices are common.

- *Bed cradle.* A bed cradle is a metal frame placed on the bed and over the person (Chapter 35). Top linens are brought over the cradle to prevent pressure on the legs, feet, and toes. Tuck and miter linens under the mattress bottom and sides. This protects against drafts and chilling.
- *Heel elevators.* These raise the heels and feet off of the bed (Fig. 42-13). They prevent pressure. Some also prevent footdrop (Chapter 35).
- *Elbow and heel protectors.* These devices are made of foam padding, pressure-relieving gel, sheepskin, or other cushioning materials. They fit the shape of elbows and heels (Fig. 42-14). Some are inside sleeves or mesh. Others are secured in place with straps. The devices promote comfort and reduce shear and friction.
- *Gel- or fluid-filled pads and cushions.* These devices have a pressure-relieving gel or fluid (Fig. 42-15). They are used for chairs and wheelchairs to prevent pressure. If the outer case is vinyl, the device may be placed in a fabric cover to protect the skin.
- *Special beds.* Some beds have air flowing through the mattresses. An *alternating pressure mattress* (Fig. 42-16) has many tubes that fill and release air at certain times. This changes where pressure is placed on the body. Some beds rotate from side to side. Alignment stays the same. Pressure points change as the bed rotates. They are useful for persons with spinal cord injuries. Follow the manufacturer's instructions and the nurse's directions for linens to use on special beds.
- *Other equipment.* Pillows, trochanter rolls, foot-boards, and other positioning devices may be used (Chapter 35). They maintain good alignment.

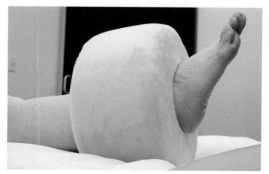

FIGURE 42-13 Heel elevator.

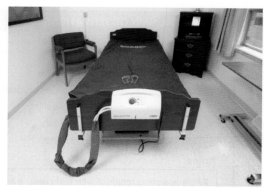

FIGURE 42-16 Alternating pressure mattress.

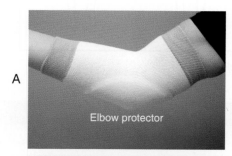

A

Elbow protector

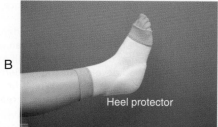

B

Heel protector

FIGURE 42-14 Elbow and heel protectors.

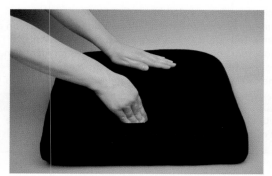

FIGURE 42-15 Gel cushion.

Dressings

A variety of dressings are available to treat pressure injuries. The dressing selected by the nursing team depends on the size, depth, and location of the pressure injury. Keeping the wound moist and the amount of drainage are other factors.

COMPLICATIONS

When skin is no longer intact, microbes contaminate and colonize the wound. *Contaminate* means that microbes are present. *Colonize* means that there is microbe replication (growth) but no tissue damage. There are no signs and symptoms of infection. When microbes increase in number and damage tissues, *infection* occurs. The person has signs and symptoms (Chapter 17). Wound healing is delayed. Pain increases. Infection is the most common complication of pressure injuries. Infection can spread to other parts of the body.

Osteomyelitis is a risk if the pressure injury is over a bony prominence. The risk is great if the wound is not healing. *Osteomyelitis* means inflammation *(itis)* of the bone *(osteo)* and bone marrow *(myel)*. Pain is severe. Treatment includes bed rest and antibiotics. Careful and gentle positioning is needed. Surgery may be done to remove dead bone and tissue.

Pain management is important. Pain may affect movement and activity. Immobility is a risk factor for pressure injuries. And it may delay healing of an existing pressure injury.

REPORTING AND RECORDING

Report and record any signs of skin breakdown or pressure injury at once. See Figure 42-17, p. 662. See "Wound Appearance" in Chapter 41.

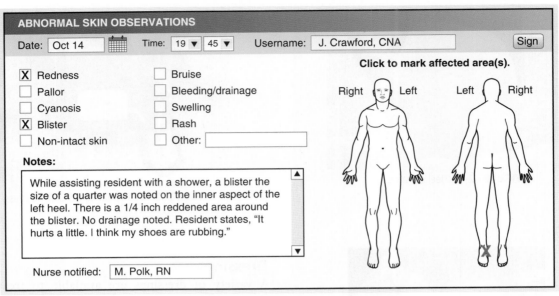

FIGURE 42-17 Charting sample.

FOCUS ON PRIDE

The Person, Family, and Yourself

Personal and Professional Responsibility

You have an important role in preventing and treating pressure injuries. Your attitude and quality of work affect the person. If you take your role seriously and believe you have a positive impact, the person benefits. If you are careless and lack concern for the person's well-being, harm can result.

You are an important part of the nursing team. Take pride in your role. Work to the best of your ability.

Rights and Respect

You have the right and responsibility to speak for patients and residents. This is called being an *advocate* (Chapter 2). You may be the first to notice a pressure injury. Reporting your observations can prevent further harm and result in prompt actions to promote healing. Take pride in being a voice for your patients and residents.

Independence and Social Interaction

Pressure injury healing can take a long time. As time passes, loneliness and depression can occur. Physical needs are great. Do not neglect mental and social needs. Be kind. Show compassion. Take time to listen. Give care in a way that improves quality of life.

Delegation and Teamwork

You must be thorough and accurate when completing, reporting, and recording care measures. The following example shows how poor communication, negligence, and false recording can cause harm.

A nursing assistant did not report placing a resident on the bedpan at 2250 (10:50 PM). The next shift began at 2300 (11:00 PM). Several hours later, the resident was still on the bedpan. A pressure injury had developed. The resident's care plan included re-positioning every 2 hours. While the chart showed that the person had been re-positioned, it really had not been done.

You must be careful and honest. Report and record when you complete a task. Give needed information to on-coming staff. Never report or record something you did not do. Also, do not report or record before completing a task.

Ethics and Laws

Agencies must have a plan to predict, prevent, and treat pressure injuries early. Assessments are done on admission and regularly. The agency must take action to address risks.

Know your agency's policies and procedures for identifying those at risk for pressure injuries. Follow the measures in Box 42-2 and the care plan to do your part to prevent pressure injuries.

FOCUS ON PRIDE: Application

Describe the physical, mental, and social effects a pressure injury can have. How can you help meet the person's needs?

REVIEW QUESTIONS

Circle the BEST answer.

1 A pressure injury is
   a An open wound
   b A localized injury to the skin and underlying tissue
   c A bony prominence
   d Dead tissue

2 Unrelieved pressure is a problem because it
   a Dilates (widens) blood vessels
   b Prevents pain sensation
   c Causes edema (swelling)
   d Prevents blood flow

3 A person is in Fowler's position. This places pressure on
 a The knees and ankles
 b The ribs and breasts
 c The cheek and ear
 d The sacrum and heels

4 Which contributes to the development of pressure injuries?
 a Shear
 b Slough
 c Eschar
 d Skin blanching

5 A person is bedfast (confined to bed). This person has
 a No risk of pressure injury
 b A low risk of pressure injury
 c An average risk of pressure injury
 d A high risk of pressure injury

6 Which is a risk factor for pressure injuries?
 a Balanced diet
 b Intact skin
 c Incontinence
 d Increased circulation

7 In a light-skinned person, a Stage 1 pressure injury has
 a A blister
 b A reddened area
 c Drainage
 d A bruise

8 Which is the most common site for a Kennedy terminal ulcer?
 a Back of the head
 b Hip
 c Sacrum
 d Heel

9 You are giving a bed bath. Why do you inspect the sacrum and heels?
 a The person cannot see these areas.
 b You are responsible for assessing the skin.
 c These are common sites for pressure injuries.
 d The skin is most fragile in these areas.

10 A person requires oxygen therapy. The person says the tubing rubs the ears. You should
 a Ask the nurse how to protect the skin under the tubing
 b Tape the tubing in place to prevent movement
 c Tell the person that pressure injuries cannot occur on the ears
 d Have the person remove the tubing if it feels uncomfortable

11 Which pressure injury prevention measure should you question?
 a Re-position the person every 2 hours.
 b Scrub the skin during bathing.
 c Apply lotion to dry areas.
 d Keep linens clean, dry, and wrinkle-free.

12 You should position the person
 a On an existing pressure injury
 b On a reddened area
 c On tubes or other medical devices
 d Using assist devices

13 What is the preferred position for preventing pressure injuries?
 a 30-degree lateral position
 b Fowler's position
 c Prone position
 d Supine position

14 A person in a chair should shift position at least every
 a 15 minutes
 b 30 minutes
 c Hour
 d 2 hours

15 You show you understand pressure injury prevention measures when you
 a Keep the head of the bed raised higher than 45 degrees
 b Inspect the person's skin every time you give care
 c Give a bath every day with bar soap and hot water
 d Rub bony areas firmly during a back massage

16 To prevent skin damage from moisture
 a Avoid using lotion on dry areas
 b Check incontinent persons every 4 hours
 c Dry under the breasts and in the groin area well
 d Change linens once daily for persons who perspire heavily

17 A person is sitting in a chair. The feet do not touch the floor. What should you do?
 a Have the person slide forward until the feet touch the floor.
 b Let the feet dangle.
 c Stack pillows under the person's feet.
 d Position the feet on a footstool.

18 Which keeps the heels and ankles off of the bed?
 a A bed cradle
 b Pillows
 c An alternating pressure mattress
 d Trochanter rolls

19 Which helps treat pressure injuries?
 a Donut-shaped cushions
 b Weight loss
 c Gel- or fluid-filled pads and cushions
 d Heat and cold applications

20 You see a reddened area on the person's skin. What should you do?
 a Rub the area.
 b Apply a moisturizer.
 c Apply a moisture barrier.
 d Tell the nurse.

21 You assist the nurse with pressure injuries by
 a Assessing pressure injury risk factors
 b Diagnosing pressure injury stages
 c Performing pressure injury prevention measures
 d Deciding how to treat pressure injuries

22 Pressure injury infection
 a Delays wound healing
 b Causes loss of sensation in the wound
 c Is not a common complication
 d Cannot spread infection to other body parts

Answers to Chapter 42 questions are on p. 903.

FOCUS ON **PRACTICE**

Problem Solving

A resident at risk for pressure injuries complains when awakened for care. You and a co-worker enter the room for re-positioning. The person is asleep. What will you do? What is the risk of waiting to re-position? How can you provide safe, quality care that avoids causing frustration?

OBJECTIVES

- Define the key terms and key abbreviations in this chapter.
- Explain the purpose, effects, and complications of heat and cold applications.
- Identify the persons at risk for complications from heat and cold applications.
- Describe the differences between moist and dry applications.

- Describe the rules for applying heat and cold.
- Identify when cooling and warming blankets are used.
- Perform the procedure described in this chapter.
- Explain how to promote PRIDE in the person, the family, and yourself.

KEY TERMS

compress A soft pad applied over a body area
constrict To narrow
cyanosis Bluish *(cyano)* color

dilate To expand or open wider
pack A commercial application for heat or cold therapy

KEY ABBREVIATIONS

C   Centigrade
F   Fahrenheit

ID   Identification

Heat and cold applications are applied to the skin. They are used to:
- Promote healing.
- Promote comfort.
- Reduce tissue swelling.

Heat and cold affect circulation (Fig. 43-1). Heat increases circulation—tissues receive more oxygen and nutrients. Cold decreases circulation—tissues receive less oxygen and nutrients. Severe injuries and changes in body function can occur. The risks are great.

See *Focus on Children and Older Persons: Heat and Cold Applications.*

See *Delegation Guidelines: Heat and Cold Applications.*

> ### FOCUS ON **CHILDREN AND OLDER PERSONS**
> #### *Heat and Cold Applications*
>
> **Children**
> Infants and young children have fragile skin. At risk for burns, they need careful attention. Always respond when a child cries. Crying can communicate pain.
>
> **Older Persons**
> Older persons often have fragile skin and changes in sensation. Persons with dementia may not be able to communicate about discomfort. They are at risk for complications.

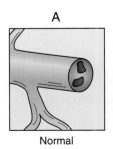
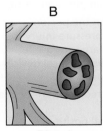
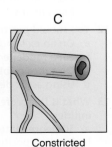

A   B   C

Normal   Dilated   Constricted

FIGURE 43-1 A, A blood vessel under normal conditions. **B,** Dilated (widened) blood vessel. **C,** Constricted (narrowed) blood vessel.

HEAT APPLICATIONS

Heat applications can be applied to almost any body part. They are used for musculo-skeletal injuries or problems (sprains, arthritis). Heat:
- Relieves pain.
- Relaxes muscles.
- Promotes healing.
- Reduces tissue swelling.
- Decreases joint stiffness.

When heat is applied to the skin, blood vessels in the area dilate. *Dilate* means to expand or open wider (see Fig. 43-1). Blood flow increases. Excess fluid is removed from the area faster. The skin is red and warm.

Complications of Heat

High temperatures can cause burns. Report pain, excess redness, and blisters at once. Also observe for pale skin. When heat is applied too long, blood vessels *constrict* (narrow) (see Fig. 43-1). Blood flow decreases. Tissues receive less oxygen. Tissue damage occurs. The skin is pale.

Older and fair-skinned persons have fragile skin that is easily burned. Persons with problems sensing heat and pain also are at risk. Nervous system damage, altered awareness, diabetes, and circulatory disorders can affect sensation. So can confusion and some drugs.

Metal implants pose risks with prolonged or high heat. Metal conducts heat. Deep tissues can be burned. Pacemakers (cardiac devices) and some joint replacements are made of metal. Certain applications may not be allowed over an implant area. Follow the doctors' orders and the nurse's instructions.

Heat is not applied right after an injury—within the first 24 to 48 hours. It is not applied to bleeding areas or to open wounds.

Heat is not applied to a pregnant woman's abdomen. The heat can affect fetal growth.

COLD APPLICATIONS

Cold applications are often used to treat sprains and fractures. Cold applications:
- Reduce pain.
- Prevent swelling.
- Decrease circulation and bleeding.
- Cool the body when fever is present.

Cold has the opposite effect of heat. When cold is applied to the skin, blood vessels constrict (see Fig. 43-1). Blood flow decreases.

Cold is useful right after an injury. Decreased blood flow reduces bleeding. Less fluid collects in the tissues. Cold helps reduce or relieve pain in the part.

Complications of Cold

Complications of cold applications include pain, burns, blisters, and poor circulation. Burns and blisters occur from intense cold. They also occur from dry cold in direct contact with the skin.

When cold is applied for a long time, blood vessels dilate. Blood flow increases. Prolonged application of cold has the same effect as heat applications.

Older and fair-skinned persons have fragile skin. They are at great risk for complications. So are persons with sensory impairments.

MOIST AND DRY APPLICATIONS

Applications are moist or dry.
- *Moist applications*—Water has contact with the skin.
- *Dry applications*—Water does not have contact with the skin.

Moist applications have greater and faster effects than dry applications. To prevent injury:
- Moist heat applications have lower (cooler) temperatures than dry heat applications.
- Moist cold applications have higher (warmer) temperatures than dry cold applications.

Dry applications stay at the desired temperature longer than moist applications. However, they do not penetrate as well as moist applications. Since higher or lower temperatures are needed for the desired effect, complications are still a risk.

Table 43-1 (pp. 666–667) describes different types of moist and dry heat and cold applications.

See *Focus on Long-Term Care and Home Care: Moist and Dry Applications*, p. 667.

TABLE 43-1	Types of Heat and Cold Applications	
Type	Description	Example
Hot or cold compress	• Moist heat or cold application, depending on the water temperature. • A *compress* is a soft pad applied over a body area. It is usually made of cloth. • The compress is placed in water, wrung out, applied to the area, and covered to maintain the desired temperature longer.	Plastic wrap / Compress / Towel
Hot soak	• Moist heat application. • A body part is in water. • Usually used for smaller parts—a hand, lower arm, foot, or lower leg. A tub is used for larger areas.	

Sitz bath	• Moist heat application.
	• A disposable sitz bath is used over a toilet seat. (*Sitz* means seat in German.)
	• The perineal and rectal areas are immersed in warm or hot water.
	• Common for hemorrhoids, after rectal or pelvic surgeries, and after childbirth. They are used to:
	  • Clean perineal and anal wounds
	  • Promote healing
	  • Relieve pain and soreness
	  • Increase circulation
	  • Stimulate voiding
		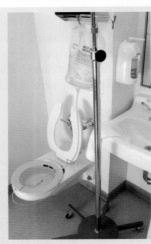

Aquathermia pad (Aqua-K, K-Pad)	• Dry heat application. • A therapy pad is connected to hoses on an electric heating unit. • The unit is filled with distilled water. (Distilled water has been purified.) Heated water is circulated through the hose to tubes inside the pad and back to the heating unit.	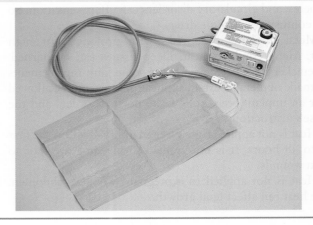

TABLE 43-1	Types of Heat and Cold Applications—cont'd	
Type	**Description**	**Example**
Hot or cold pack	• Moist or dry heat or cold application, depending on the type. • A *pack* is a commercial application for heat or cold therapy. • Some packs are disposable (single-use). Others are re-usable. • Packs are activated following the manufacturer's instructions. Striking, kneading, or squeezing the pack before use is common. • Re-usable cold packs are stored in the freezer. Follow agency policy and the manufacturer's instructions to clean a re-usable pack.	
Ice bag	• Dry cold application. • The bag is filled with crushed ice or ice chips and closed. • Bags, collars, gloves, and masks are different types.	

FOCUS ON LONG-TERM CARE AND HOME CARE

Moist and Dry Applications

Home Care

Heating pads have electrical coils made of wire. The coils present fire hazards if they break. Always make sure the heating pad is in good repair. Follow the manufacturer's instructions for use. Heating pad temperatures are easy to adjust. Burns are a great risk. Check the temperature often. Make sure the person has not changed the temperature.

Commercial cold packs are common in home settings. Some packs are designed for use as a heat or cold application. The pack is filled with a special fluid. For a cold application, the pack is kept in the freezer until needed. To use as a heating pack, follow the manufacturer's instructions. Cover the pack before application. A towel, dishcloth, or pillowcase may be used.

A bag of frozen peas or corn can serve as an ice bag. So can a plastic bag filled with ice. Close the bag securely to prevent leaks. Cover the bag of peas (corn) or plastic bag with a cloth before application.

APPLYING HEAT AND COLD

Protect the person from injury during heat and cold applications. Follow the rules in Box 43-1. See Table 43-2 for heat and cold temperature ranges.

See *Teamwork and Time Management: Applying Heat and Cold.*

See *Delegation Guidelines: Applying Heat and Cold.*
See *Promoting Safety and Comfort: Applying Heat and Cold.*
See procedure: *Applying Heat and Cold Applications.*

TABLE 43-2	Heat and Cold Temperature Ranges	
Temperature	Fahrenheit (F) Range	Centigrade (C) Range
Hot	99°F to 106°F	37°C to 41°C
Warm	93°F to 98°F	34°C to 37°C
Tepid	80°F to 92°F	26°C to 34°C
Cool	65°F to 79°F	18°C to 26°C
Cold	50°F to 64°F	10°C to 18°C

Modified from Perry AG, Potter PA, Ostendorf WR: Nursing interventions & clinical skills, ed 7, St Louis, 2020, Elsevier.

BOX 43-1	Applying Heat and Cold

- Know how to use the equipment. Follow the manufacturer's instructions for commercial devices.
- Measure the temperature of moist applications. Follow agency policy or use a water thermometer.
- Follow agency policies for safe temperature ranges. See Table 43-2.
- Do not apply *very hot* (above 106°F or 41.1°C) applications. Tissue damage can occur. A nurse applies *very hot* applications.
- Ask the nurse what temperature to use.
  - Heat—cooler temperatures for persons at risk.
  - Cold—warmer temperatures for persons at risk.
- Have the nurse show you the application site.
- Cover dry heat or cold applications before applying them. Use a flannel cover, towel, or other cover as directed.
- Provide for privacy. Properly screen and drape the person. Expose only the body part involved.
- Maintain comfort and body alignment during the procedure.
- Observe the skin every 5 minutes during the procedure. See *Delegation Guidelines: Applying Heat and Cold.*
- Do not let the person change the temperature of the application.
- Know how long to leave the application in place. Heat and cold are applied no longer than 15 to 20 minutes.
- Follow the rules for electrical safety when using electrical appliances for heat. See Chapter 14.
- Tell the person to notify you at once if:
  - The application feels too hot or too cold.
  - The person feels pain, numbness, or burning.
  - The person feels weak, faint, or drowsy.
- Place the call light within the person's reach.
- Complete a safety check before leaving the room. (See the inside of the back cover.)
- Follow agency procedures to clean and disinfect re-usable equipment after use. Discard disposable equipment.

TEAMWORK AND TIME MANAGEMENT
Applying Heat and Cold

After applying heat or cold, check the person and the application every 5 minutes. Plan your work so you can stay in or near the person's room. For example:
- Make the bed and straighten the person's unit.
- Provide care to the person's roommate if the person's care is assigned to you.
- Help the person complete the daily or weekly menu.
- Read cards and letters to the person, with the person's consent.
- Address envelopes and other correspondence for the person.
- Take time to visit with the person.

DELEGATION GUIDELINES
Applying Heat and Cold

To apply heat or cold, you need this information from the nurse and the care plan.
- What application to apply
- How to cover the application
- What temperature to use (see Table 43-2)
- The application site
- How long to leave the application in place
- What observations to report and record:
  - Complaints of pain or discomfort, numbness, or burning
  - Excess redness
  - Blisters
  - Pale, white, or gray skin
  - *Cyanosis*—bluish (cyano) color
  - Shivering
  - Rapid pulse, weakness, faintness, and drowsiness (sitz bath)
  - Time, site, and length of application
- When to report observations
- What patient or resident concerns to report at once

PROMOTING SAFETY AND COMFORT

Applying Heat and Cold

Safety

Sitz Bath

Blood flow increases to the perineum and rectum. Therefore less blood flows to other areas. Observe for signs of weakness, fainting, or fatigue. Also protect the person from injury, chills, and burns.

Aquathermia Pad

- Follow electrical safety measures (Chapter 14).
- Check the device for damage or flaws.
- Follow the manufacturer's instructions.
- Place the heating unit on an even, uncluttered surface.
- Check the hoses for kinks or bubbles. Water must flow freely.
- Place the pad in a flannel cover. The flannel absorbs perspiration at the application site. (Some agencies use towels or pillowcases.)
- Secure the pad in place with ties, tape, or rolled gauze. Do not use pins. They can puncture the pad and cause leaks.
- Do not place the pad under a body part. Heat cannot escape. Burns can result if heat cannot escape.
- Give the temperature setting key to the nurse. This prevents anyone from changing the temperature. The temperature is usually set at 105°F (40.5°C) with a key.

Commercial Hot and Cold Packs

Read warning labels. Follow the manufacturer's instructions. Cover the pack before application.

Medicated Patches and Ointments

Some persons have medicated patches or ointments applied to the skin. Do not apply heat over such areas.

Comfort

Cold applications can cause chills and shivering. Provide for warmth. Use bath blankets or other blankets as needed.

Keep the call light within reach. Check the person every 5 minutes.

Applying Heat and Cold Applications

QUALITY OF LIFE

- Knock before entering the person's room.
- Address the person by name.
- Introduce yourself by name and title.

- Explain the procedure before starting and during the procedure.
- Protect the person's rights during the procedure.
- Handle the person gently during the procedure.

PRE-PROCEDURE

1 Follow *Delegation Guidelines*:
 a   *Heat and Cold Applications*, p. 665
 b   *Applying Heat and Cold*
   See *Promoting Safety and Comfort: Applying Heat and Cold.*
2 Practice hand hygiene and get the following supplies.
  - *For a hot compress:*
    - Basin
    - Water thermometer
    - Small towel, washcloth, or gauze squares
    - Plastic wrap or aquathermia pad
    - Ties, tape, or rolled gauze
    - Bath towel
    - Waterproof under-pad
  - *For a hot soak:*
    - Water basin or arm or foot bath
    - Water thermometer
    - Waterproof under-pad
    - Bath blanket
    - Towel
  - *For a sitz bath:*
    - Disposable sitz bath
    - Water thermometer
    - 2 bath blankets, bath towels, and a clean gown
  - *For an aquathermia pad:*
    - Aquathermia pad and heating unit
    - Distilled water
    - Flannel cover or other cover as directed
    - Ties, tape, or rolled gauze (if needed)

  - *For a hot or cold pack:*
    - Commercial pack
    - Pack cover
    - Ties, tape, or rolled gauze (if needed)
  - *For an ice bag, ice collar, ice glove, or ice mask:*
    - Ice bag, collar, glove, or mask
    - Crushed ice
    - Flannel cover or other cover as directed (if needed)
    - Ties, tape, or rolled gauze (if needed)
    - Paper towels
    - Waterproof under-pad (if needed)
  - *For a cold compress:*
    - Large basin with ice
    - Small basin with cold water
    - Gauze squares, washcloths, or small towels
    - Waterproof under-pad
3 Arrange items in the person's room.
4 Practice hand hygiene.
5 Identify the person. Check the identification (ID) bracelet against the assignment sheet. Use 2 identifiers (Chapter 14). Also call the person by name.
6 Provide for privacy.

Applying Heat and Cold Applications—cont'd

7 Position the person for the procedure.
8 Place the waterproof under-pad under the body part (if needed).
9 *For a hot compress:*
   a Fill the basin ½ to ⅔ (one-half to two-thirds) full with hot water as directed. Measure water temperature.
   b Place the compress in the water and wring out.
   c Apply the compress over the area. Note the time.
   d Cover the compress as directed. Do 1 of the following.
      1) Apply plastic wrap and then a bath towel. Secure the towel in place with ties, tape, or rolled gauze.
      2) Apply an aquathermia pad.
10 *For a hot soak:*
   a Fill the container ½ (one-half) full with hot water. Measure water temperature.
   b Place the part into the water. Pad the edge of the container with a towel. Note the time.
   c Cover the person with a bath blanket for warmth.
11 *For a sitz bath:*
   a Place the sitz bath on the toilet seat.
   b Fill the sitz bath ⅔ (two-thirds) full with water. Measure water temperature.
   c Secure the gown above the waist.
   d Help the person sit on the sitz bath. Note the time.
   e Provide for warmth. Place a bath blanket around the shoulders. Place the other over the legs.
   f Stay with the person if the person is weak or unsteady.
12 *For an aquathermia pad:*
   a Fill the heating unit to the fill line with distilled water.
   b Open any hose clamps. Follow the manufacturer's instructions to fill the connecting hoses and pad with water and remove air. Be sure there are no kinks in the hoses or the pad.
   c Set the temperature as the nurse directs (usually 105°F [40.5°C]). Remove the key.
   d Place the pad in the cover.
   e Set the heating unit on the bedside stand. Keep the pad and connecting hoses level with the unit.
   f Plug in the unit. Let water warm to the desired temperature.
   g Apply the pad to the part. Note the time.
   h Secure the pad in place with ties, tape, or rolled gauze as needed.

13 *For a hot or cold pack:*
   a Squeeze, knead, or strike the pack as directed by the manufacturer.
   b Place the pack in the cover.
   c Apply the pack. Note the time.
   d Secure the pack in place with ties, tape, or rolled gauze as needed. Some packs are secured with Velcro straps.
14 *For an ice bag, collar, glove, or mask:*
   a Fill the device with water. Put in the stopper. Turn the device upside down to check for leaks.
   b Empty the device.
   c Fill the device ½ to ⅔ (one-half to two-thirds) full with crushed ice or ice chips.
   d Remove excess air. Bend, twist, or squeeze the device. Or press it against a firm surface.
   e Place the cap or stopper on securely.
   f Dry the device with paper towels.
   g Place the device in a cover if needed. Some are designed with a covering and can be applied directly to the skin.
   h Apply the device. Note the time.
   i Secure the device with ties, tape, or rolled gauze as needed.
15 *For a cold compress:*
   a Place the small basin with cold water into the large basin with ice.
   b Place the compress into the cold water.
   c Wring out the compress.
   d Apply the compress to the part. Note the time.
16 Place the call light and other needed items within reach. Maintain privacy measures as needed and as the person prefers.
17 Make sure the bed is at a safe and comfortable level. Raise or lower bed rails. Follow the care plan.
18 Do the following every 5 minutes.
   a Check the person for signs and symptoms of complications (see *Delegation Guidelines: Applying Heat and Cold*, p. 668). Remove the application if any occur. Tell the nurse at once.
   b Check the application for cooling (hot application) or warming (cold application).
19 Remove the application after 15 to 20 minutes.

20 Provide for comfort. (See the inside of the back cover.)
21 Make sure the bed is at a safe and comfortable level. Raise or lower bed rails. Follow the care plan.
22 Clean up and store supplies and equipment. (Wear gloves as needed.)
   a Discard disposable items.
   b Follow agency procedures to clean and disinfect re-usable equipment. Return supplies and equipment to their proper place.
   c Follow agency policy for used linens.
   d Clean and dry the over-bed table if used. Dry with paper towels. Discard paper towels. Position the over-bed table as the person prefers.
   e Remove and discard gloves. Practice hand hygiene.

23 Place the call light and other needed items within reach.
24 Follow the care plan and the person's preferences for privacy measures to maintain. Leaving the privacy curtain, window coverings, and door open or closed are examples.
25 Complete a safety check of the room. (See the inside of the back cover.)
26 Practice hand hygiene.
27 Report and record your care and observations.

COOLING AND WARMING BLANKETS

Cooling and warming blankets are used to cool or warm the body. Cooling is used for fever and heat-related illnesses. Warming is used for *hypothermia*—a very low *(hypo)* body temperature *(thermia)*. See Chapter 58 for cold- and heat-related illnesses.

Forced-air warming blankets circulate warm air to raise body temperature. Other blankets use warm or cool fluid to raise or lower body temperature. If your work area uses cooling or warming blankets, you will be trained in their use and in your role. Vital signs are measured often when in use. Continuous temperature monitoring measures body temperature at all times during treatment.

See *Focus on Children and Older Persons: Cooling and Warming Blankets.*

FOCUS ON CHILDREN AND OLDER PERSONS

Cooling and Warming Blankets

Children
Rapid temperature changes can occur in infants and children. Observe them closely. Measure temperature and other vital signs as the nurse directs. Report the following at once.
- The temperature measurement and other vital signs
- Changes in vital signs
- Changes in the child's condition

FOCUS ON **PRIDE**

The Person, Family, and Yourself

Personal and Professional Responsibility
Heat and cold are used for healing and comfort. You need to ask about the person's comfort. Also, the person may not know to report discomfort. The person may think an application that feels too cold (or hot) is normal. Or the person may think that numbness or burning is expected. You need to tell the person what to report (see Box 43-1).

Rights and Respect
Respect the right to privacy. Be sure the person is properly screened and covered. This will vary by application site, method, and personal preference. For example:
- A sitz bath is ordered. Ensure that the person is covered and no one enters the bathroom during the procedure.
- A resident receiving a hot soak to a foot wants the privacy curtain to remain pulled.
- A patient has an ice bag on 1 hand. So roommates can talk, the patient does not want the privacy curtain pulled during the application.

Independence and Social Interaction
Patients and residents can plan if they know what will happen. For example, a person wants to make a phone call before a hot compress. Or a person wants a hot soak done before visitors arrive. You promote independence when you involve the person in planning.

Delegation and Teamwork
Safety and comfort measures require time and planning. Heat and cold are usually applied for 15 to 20 minutes. The procedure involves:
- Meeting elimination needs before the procedure
- Positioning the person for comfort
- Placing needed items within reach—call light, water mug, reading material, electronic devices, phone, remotes, and other requested items
- Checking the person often
- Reporting and recording task completion and your observations

Ethics and Laws
Complications from heat and cold can be severe. Safety is a priority. Harm and legal action can result if you:
- Apply a heat or cold application without an order.
- Use the equipment without training.
- Apply an application that is too hot or too cold.
- Do not cover an application as directed.
- Neglect to check the person often.
- Leave the application on longer than directed.
- Fail to report complications to the nurse.
  Follow the rules in Box 43-1. Take pride in protecting the person from injury.

FOCUS ON **PRIDE**: *Application*
Providing comfort is an important part of every task. What special considerations are needed for heat and cold applications? How will you know if you have met the person's comfort needs?

REVIEW QUESTIONS

Circle the BEST answer.

1 Heat applications
   a Decrease blood flow
   b Constrict vessels before dilating them
   c Tighten muscles
   d Relieve pain

2 The *greatest* threat from heat applications is
   a Infection
   b Burns
   c Chilling
   d Skin tears

3 Who has the *greatest* risk for complications from heat applications?
   a An adult with dark skin
   b An older person with nerve damage
   c An adult with a wound
   d A pregnant woman

4 Which statement about moist and dry heat applications is *true?*
   a With moist applications, water has contact with the skin.
   b Moist heat has fewer effects than dry heat.
   c Dry heat penetrates deeper than moist heat.
   d Moist heat applications require higher temperatures than dry ones.

5 A warm application is usually
   a 80°F to 92°F
   b 93°F to 98°F
   c 99°F to 106°F
   d Above 106°F

6 A nurse asks you to apply a hot pack. Which should you question?
   a Check that the pack's temperature is at least 110°F (43.3°C).
   b Place the pack in a cover.
   c Secure the pack in place with ties.
   d Check the person for complications every 5 minutes.

7 Which statement about sitz baths is *true?*
   a Sitz baths last 25 to 30 minutes.
   b Weakness and fainting can occur.
   c The lower body is immersed in warm water.
   d Sitz baths decrease circulation to the perineum and rectum.

8 When using an aquathermia pad
   a Do not cover the pad
   b Place the pad under the person
   c Check for kinks in the hoses
   d Secure the pad in place with pins

9 Cold applications
   a Prevent swelling and decrease circulation
   b Dilate blood vessels
   c Prevent the spread of microbes
   d Increase bleeding

10 Which signals a complication of a cold application?
   a Cool skin
   b Cyanosis
   c Decreased swelling
   d Fever

11 You are applying a cold compress. You should
   a Use cooler temperatures for persons at risk
   b Observe the skin every 10 minutes
   c Re-apply the compress if the skin is bluish in color
   d Provide for warmth and privacy

12 Before applying an ice bag
   a Fill the bag with water and place it in the freezer
   b Measure the temperature of the ice
   c Check if the bag needs a cover
   d Explain that intense cold and numbness are normal

13 Moist cold compresses are left in place no longer than
   a 20 minutes
   b 30 minutes
   c 45 minutes
   d 60 minutes

14 A warming blanket is used for
   a Hypothermia
   b Heat-related illnesses
   c Cyanosis
   d Arthritis

Answers to Chapter 43 questions are on p. 903.

FOCUS ON **PRACTICE**

Problem Solving

You are to remove a hot pack. The person says: "My knee feels much better with that on. Can you leave it on longer?" What do you do? Is it safe or are there risks to leaving the application in place? Explain.

Oxygen Needs

- Define the key terms and key abbreviations in this chapter.
- Describe the factors affecting oxygen needs.
- Describe hypoxia and abnormal respirations.
- Identify the signs and symptoms of altered respiratory function.
- Describe pulse oximetry.

- Explain the measures to meet oxygen needs.
- Describe different devices used to give oxygen.
- Explain how to safely assist with oxygen therapy.
- Perform the procedures described in this chapter.
- Explain how to promote PRIDE in the person, the family, and yourself.

KEY TERMS

allergy A sensitivity to a substance that causes the body to react with signs and symptoms

apnea The lack or absence *(a)* of breathing *(pnea)*

atelectasis The collapse of a portion of a lung

Biot's respirations Rapid and deep respirations followed by 10 to 30 seconds of apnea

bradypnea Slow *(brady)* breathing *(pnea)*; respirations are fewer than 12 per minute

Cheyne-Stokes respirations Respirations gradually increase in rate and depth and then become shallow and slow; breathing may stop *(apnea)* for 10 to 20 seconds

cyanosis Bluish color *(cyano)* to the skin, lips, mucous membranes, and nail beds

dyspnea Difficult, labored, or painful *(dys)* breathing *(pnea)*

eupnea Normal *(eu)* breathing *(pnea)*

hemoptysis Bloody *(hemo)* sputum *(ptysis* means to spit)

hyperventilation Breathing *(ventilation)* is rapid *(hyper)* and deeper than normal

hypoventilation Breathing *(ventilation)* is slow *(hypo)*, shallow, and sometimes irregular

hypoxemia A reduced amount *(hypo)* of oxygen *(ox)* in the blood *(emia)*

hypoxia Cells do not have enough *(hypo)* oxygen *(oxia)*

Kussmaul respirations Very deep and rapid respirations

orthopnea Breathing *(pnea)* deeply and comfortably only when sitting *(ortho)*

orthopneic position Sitting up *(ortho)* and leaning over a table to breathe *(pneic)*

oxygen concentration The amount (percent [%]) of hemoglobin containing oxygen

pollutant A harmful chemical or substance in the air or water

pulse oximetry Measures *(metry)* the oxygen *(oxi)* concentration in arterial blood

respiratory arrest When breathing stops

respiratory depression Slow, weak respirations

sputum Mucus from the respiratory system that is expectorated (expelled) through the mouth

tachypnea Rapid *(tachy)* breathing *(pnea)*; respirations are more than 20 per minute

KEY ABBREVIATIONS

CO_2	Carbon dioxide	O_2	Oxygen
ID	Identification	RBC	Red blood cell
L/min	Liters per minute	SpO_2	Saturation of peripheral oxygen (oxygen concentration)

Oxygen is a gas. It has no taste, odor, or color. It is a basic need required for life. Death occurs within minutes if breathing stops. Brain and other organ damage can occur without enough oxygen. Illness, surgery, and injuries affect the amount of oxygen in the body.

To assist with oxygen needs, you need to be able to recognize altered respiratory function. You may help with tests, measurements, and measures to meet oxygen needs. You must also know your role in assisting with oxygen therapy.

See *Body Structure and Function Review: The Respiratory System*.

See *Delegation Guidelines: Oxygen Needs*.

BODY STRUCTURE AND FUNCTION REVIEW
The Respiratory System

Structure and Function

Every body cell needs oxygen. The respiratory system (Fig. 44-1) brings oxygen (O_2) into the lungs and removes carbon dioxide (CO_2). *Respiration* is the process of supplying the cells with O_2 and removing CO_2 from them. Respiration involves breathing in *(inhalation, inspiration)* and breathing out *(exhalation, expiration)*.

Air enters the body through the *mouth* and *nose*. Air passes through the *pharynx* (throat), *larynx* (voice box), and *trachea* (windpipe). The trachea divides at its lower end into the *right bronchus* and *left bronchus*. Each bronchus enters a *lung*. The bronchi divide many times into smaller branches *(bronchioles)*. The bronchioles further divide and end in tiny 1-celled air sacs *(alveoli)*. They are supplied by capillaries.

O_2 and CO_2 are exchanged between the alveoli and capillaries. Blood in the capillaries picks up O_2 from the alveoli. That blood is returned to the left side of the heart and pumped to the rest of the body. Alveoli pick up CO_2 from the capillaries for exhalation.

The lungs are separated from the abdominal cavity by a muscle called the *diaphragm*. The contraction and relaxation of the diaphragm allow air to enter and leave the lungs. A bony framework made up of the ribs, sternum, and vertebrae protects the lungs.

Changes With Aging

With age, respiratory muscles weaken. Some lung tissue is lost. Lung tissue becomes less elastic (more rigid). The chest is less able to expand and contract. Difficulty breathing and decreased strength for coughing and clearing the airway can occur. *Pneumonia* (inflammation and infection of the lungs) can develop. See Chapter 12 for more information.

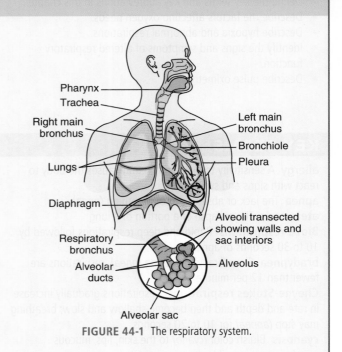

FIGURE 44-1 The respiratory system.

DELEGATION GUIDELINES
Oxygen Needs

Your state and agency determine the nursing assistant's role in assisting with oxygen needs. Some procedures and care measures in this chapter may be delegated nursing tasks. Before performing a delegated task, make sure that:
• Your state allows you to perform the task.
• The task is in your job description (Chapter 3).
• You have the necessary education and training.

• The agency has determined that you are competent to perform the task safely.
• You know how to use the supplies and equipment.
• You review the procedure with the delegating nurse.
• The delegating nurse is available to answer questions and to guide and assist you as needed.

FACTORS AFFECTING OXYGEN NEEDS

Any disease, injury, or surgery involving the respiratory or circulatory system affects the intake and use of O_2. Altered function of any system (for example, the nervous, musculo-skeletal, or urinary system) can also affect oxygen needs. Body systems depend on each other. Respiratory complications may result. Oxygen needs are affected by:

- *The circulatory system.* Narrowed vessels affect blood flow. Capillaries and cells must exchange O_2 and CO_2.
- *Red blood cell count.* Red blood cells (RBCs) contain hemoglobin. Hemoglobin picks up O_2 in the lungs and carries it to the cells. The bone marrow must produce enough RBCs. Blood loss also reduces the number of RBCs.
- *The nervous system.* Nervous system diseases and injuries can affect respiratory muscles. O_2 and CO_2 blood levels also affect brain function. When O_2 is lacking, respirations increase to bring in more oxygen. When CO_2 increases, respirations increase to rid the body of CO_2.
- *Aging.* See *Body Structure and Function Review: The Respiratory System.*
- *Exercise.* O_2 needs increase with exercise. Respiratory rate and depth increase to bring in O_2. Persons with heart and respiratory diseases may have enough oxygen at rest. However, even slight activity (exertion) can increase O_2 needs. Activity may be limited.
- *Fever.* O_2 needs increase. Respiratory rate and depth increase.
- *Pain.* O_2 needs increase, causing respirations to increase. Chest and abdominal injuries and surgeries often involve respiratory muscles. It hurts to breathe.
- *Drugs.* Some drugs depress the respiratory center in the brain. *Respiratory depression* means there are slow, weak respirations. *Respiratory arrest* is when breathing stops. Certain pain-relief drugs (opioids) can have these effects (Chapter 36). (Opioids may also be referred to as "narcotics.") Mis-use can cause respiratory depression and respiratory arrest. See "Opioid Overdose" in Chapter 58.
- *Smoking.* Smoking is a major risk factor for lung cancer, chronic bronchitis, emphysema, and coronary artery disease (Chapter 50).
- *Allergies.* An *allergy* is a sensitivity to a substance that causes the body to react with signs and symptoms. Runny nose, wheezing, and congestion are common. Mucous membranes in the upper airway swell. Severe swelling can close the airway. Shock and death are risks. Pollens, dust, foods, drugs, insect bites, powders, flowers, perfumes, sprays, animals, and cigarette smoke often cause allergies.
- *Pollutants.* A *pollutant* is a harmful chemical or substance in the air or water. Examples are dust, fumes, toxins, asbestos, coal dust, and sawdust. They damage the lungs.
- *Nutrition.* The body needs iron and vitamins (vitamin B_{12}, vitamin C, and folate) to produce RBCs.
- *Alcohol.* Alcohol depresses the brain. Excessive amounts reduce the cough reflex and increase the risk of aspiration. Obstructed airway and pneumonia are risks from aspiration.

ALTERED RESPIRATORY FUNCTION

Respiratory function involves 3 processes. Respiratory function is altered if even 1 process is affected.

- Air moves into and out of the lungs.
- Oxygen (O_2) and carbon dioxide (CO_2) are exchanged between the alveoli and capillaries.
- The blood carries O_2 to the cells and removes CO_2 from them.

Hypoxemia and hypoxia are risks. *Hypoxemia* is a reduced amount *(hypo)* of oxygen *(ox)* in the blood *(emia)*. It can lead to hypoxia. *Hypoxia* means that cells do not have enough *(hypo)* oxygen *(oxia)*. Cells cannot function properly. The brain is very sensitive to inadequate O_2. Restlessness, dizziness, and disorientation are early signs. Report the signs and symptoms of altered respiratory function in Box 44-1 at once.

Hypoxia threatens life. All organs need O_2 to function. Oxygen is given (p. 682). The cause of hypoxia is treated.

BOX 44-1 Altered Respiratory Function

- Restlessness
- Dizziness
- Disorientation and confusion
- Behavior and personality changes
- Trouble concentrating and following directions
- Anxiety and apprehension
- Fatigue
- Agitation
- Pulse rate: increased
- Respirations:
  - Increased rate and depth
  - Breathing pattern: abnormal (p. 676)
  - Shortness of breath or complaints of being "winded" or "short-winded"
  - Noisy, wheezing, wet-sounding, *stridor* (a loud, high-pitched sound from airway blockage)
- Sitting position—upright, leaning forward, hunched over a table
- *Cyanosis*—bluish color *(cyano)* to the skin, lips, mucous membranes, and nail beds
- Cough (note type, frequency, and time of day)
  - Dry and hacking
  - Harsh and barking
  - Productive (produces sputum) or non-productive
- *Sputum*—mucus from the respiratory system that is expectorated (expelled) through the mouth
  - Color—clear, white, yellow, green, brown, or red
  - Odor—none or foul odor
  - Consistency—thick, watery, or frothy (with bubbles or foam)
  - *Hemoptysis*—bloody *(hemo)* sputum *(ptysis* means to spit); note if the sputum is bright red, dark red, blood-tinged, or streaked with blood
- Chest pain (note location)
  - Constant or comes and goes
  - Person's description—sharp, dull, aching, pressure (Chapter 36)
  - What makes it worse—movement, activity, coughing, yawning, sneezing, sighing, deep breathing, position
- Vital signs: changes in

Abnormal Breathing Patterns

Adults normally breathe 12 to 20 times per minute. Infants and children have faster rates. Normal *(eu)* breathing *(pnea)* is called *eupnea*. Breaths are normally quiet, effortless, and regular. Both sides of the chest rise and fall equally. These breathing patterns are abnormal (Fig. 44-2):

- *Tachypnea*—rapid *(tachy)* breathing *(pnea)*. Respirations are more than 20 per minute. Fever, exercise, pain, pregnancy, and airway obstruction are among the causes.
- *Bradypnea*—slow *(brady)* breathing *(pnea)*. Respirations are fewer than 12 per minute. Drug overdose and nervous system disorders are causes.
- *Apnea*—the lack or absence *(a)* of breathing *(pnea)*. It occurs in cardiac arrest and respiratory arrest. Sleep apnea is another type of apnea (Chapter 50).
- *Hypoventilation*—breathing *(ventilation)* is slow *(hypo)*, shallow, and sometimes irregular. Lung disorders affecting the alveoli are causes. Pneumonia is an example. Other causes include obesity, airway obstruction, and drug side effects. Nervous system and musculo-skeletal disorders affecting the respiratory muscles also are causes.
- *Hyperventilation*—breathing *(ventilation)* is rapid *(hyper)* and deeper than normal. Causes include asthma, emphysema, infection, fever, nervous system disorders, hypoxia, anxiety, pain, and some drugs.
- *Dyspnea*—difficult, labored, or painful *(dys)* breathing *(pnea)*. Heart disease and anxiety are causes.
- *Cheyne-Stokes respirations*—respirations gradually increase in rate and depth and then become shallow and slow. Breathing may stop *(apnea)* for 10 to 20 seconds. Drug overdose, heart failure, renal failure, and brain disorders are causes. Cheyne-Stokes respirations are common when death is near.
- *Orthopnea*—breathing *(pnea)* deeply and comfortably only when sitting *(ortho)*. Causes are emphysema, asthma, pneumonia, angina, and other heart and respiratory disorders.
- *Biot's respirations*—rapid and deep respirations followed by 10 to 30 seconds of apnea. They occur with nervous system disorders.
- *Kussmaul respirations*—very deep and rapid respirations. They signal a serious and life-threatening complication of diabetes.

RESPIRATORY TESTS

Various tests may be ordered to detect lung changes. A chest x-ray is an example. You may be involved in pulse oximetry and the collection of sputum specimens (Chapter 39). Assist with other tests as directed by the nurse.

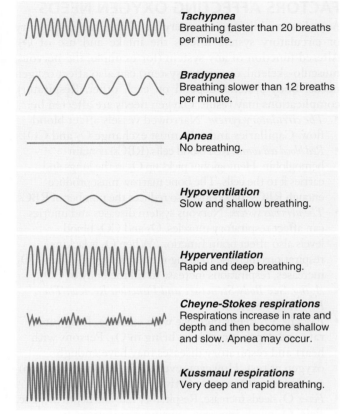

Tachypnea
Breathing faster than 20 breaths per minute.

Bradypnea
Breathing slower than 12 breaths per minute.

Apnea
No breathing.

Hypoventilation
Slow and shallow breathing.

Hyperventilation
Rapid and deep breathing.

Cheyne-Stokes respirations
Respirations increase in rate and depth and then become shallow and slow. Apnea may occur.

Kussmaul respirations
Very deep and rapid breathing.

FIGURE 44-2 Some abnormal breathing patterns.

Pulse Oximetry

Pulse oximetry measures *(metry)* the oxygen *(oxi)* concentration in arterial blood. *Oxygen concentration* is the amount (percent [%]) of hemoglobin containing O_2. An agency may use 1 of these terms.

- Pulse oximetry or pulse ox.
- O_2 saturation or O_2 sat.
- SpO_2 (saturation of peripheral oxygen). *Saturation* means to be filled. *Peripheral* relates to the surface. SpO_2 measures the amount of hemoglobin near the surface of the skin that is filled with oxygen.

The normal oxygen concentration range is between 95% and 100%. For example, if 97% of all hemoglobin carries O_2, tissues get enough oxygen. If only 90% contains O_2, tissues do not get enough oxygen. As low as 85% may be normal for persons with some chronic diseases.

A *pulse oximeter* is used to measure oxygen concentration. A sensor attaches to a finger, toe, earlobe, nose, or forehead (Fig. 44-3). Light beams on 1 side of the sensor pass through tissues. A detector on the other side measures the amount of light passing through the tissues. With this information, the oximeter measures the O_2 concentration.

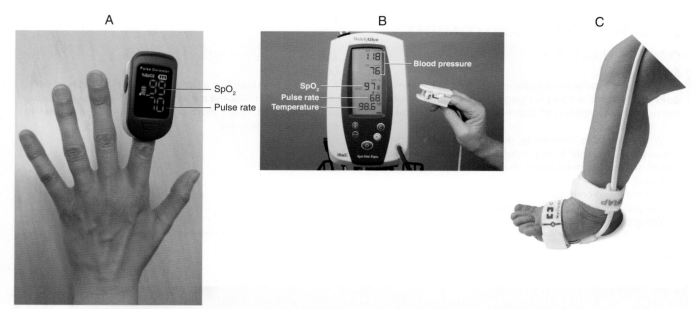

FIGURE 44-3 Pulse oximetry. **A,** A pulse oximetry sensor is attached to a finger. The device displays the O_2 concentration (SpO_2) and pulse. **B,** O_2 concentration (SpO_2) is often measured with vital signs. **C,** A pulse oximetry sensor for children. (C, From Covidien ©2015. All rights reserved. Used with permission of Covidien.)

Good blood flow to the site is needed. Avoid swollen sites and sites with skin breaks. Bright light, nail polish, non-natural nails, and movements affect measurements. For a good sensor site:

- Remove nail polish or use another site.
- Do not use finger sites with non-natural nails.
- Use the earlobe if there is finger movement from shivering, seizures, or tremors.
- Place a towel over the sensor to block bright lights if needed.
- Do not measure blood pressure on the side of a finger site at the same time. The cuff will affect blood flow and give an inaccurate measurement.

The pulse oximeter shows the pulse rate along with the oxygen concentration (see Fig. 44-3, *A*). Oxygen concentration is often measured along with vital signs (see Fig. 44-3, *B*). Report and record measurements according to agency policy.

See *Focus on Children and Older Persons: Pulse Oximetry.*
See *Delegation Guidelines: Pulse Oximetry.*
See *Promoting Safety and Comfort: Pulse Oximetry*, p. 678.
See procedure: *Using a Pulse Oximeter*, p. 678.

FOCUS ON **CHILDREN AND OLDER PERSONS**

Pulse Oximetry

Children
Different sensors may be used for children (see Fig. 44-3, *C*). The sensor is attached to the sole of the foot, palm of the hand, toe, or earlobe. If the child moves a lot, the earlobe is a better site.

DELEGATION GUIDELINES

Pulse Oximetry

In some agencies, pulse oximetry is a delegated nursing task. If so, the conditions in *Delegation Guidelines: Oxygen Needs* (p. 674) must be met. Pulse oximetry may be a routine nursing task in some agencies. Before the procedure, you need this information from the nurse and the care plan.

- Reason for the measurement: routine, continuous monitoring (p. 678), or condition change
- What site to use
- How to use the equipment
- What sensor to use
- What tape to use (if needed)
- The person's normal SpO_2 range
- Alarm limits for SpO_2 and pulse rate (if set)
- When to do the measurement
- What pulse site to use: apical or radial
- How often to check the site for continuous monitoring (usually at least every 2 hours)
- What observations to report and record:
  - The date and time
  - The SpO_2 and display pulse rate (see Fig. 44-3, *A*)
  - Apical or radial pulse rate
  - What the person was doing at the time
  - Oxygen flow rate and the device used (p. 684)
- When to report observations
- What patient or resident concerns to report at once:
  - An SpO_2 below the normal limit (usually 95%)
  - A pulse rate above or below the normal limit
  - The signs and symptoms listed in Box 44-1

PROMOTING SAFETY AND COMFORT

Pulse Oximetry

Safety

The person's condition can change quickly. Pulse oximetry does not lessen the need for good observation. Observe for signs and symptoms of altered respiratory function (see Box 44-1).

With continuous monitoring, pulse oximetry measurements are ongoing. A sensor is on the person at all times. Oximeter alarms are set. Tell the nurse if an alarm sounds. An alarm sounds if:

- O_2 concentration is low.
- The pulse rate is too fast or too slow.
- Other problems occur.

Comfort

A clip-on sensor feels like a clothespin. It should not hurt or cause discomfort. Ask the person to tell you at once if it causes pain, discomfort, or too much pressure. Change the sensor site as directed by the nurse.

Using a Pulse Oximeter

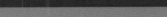

QUALITY OF LIFE

- Knock before entering the person's room.
- Address the person by name.
- Introduce yourself by name and title.

- Explain the procedure before starting and during the procedure.
- Protect the person's rights during the procedure.
- Handle the person gently during the procedure.

PRE-PROCEDURE

1 Follow *Delegation Guidelines:*
  a   *Oxygen Needs,* p. 674
  b   *Pulse Oximetry,* p. 677
  See *Promoting Safety and Comfort: Pulse Oximetry.*
2 Practice hand hygiene and get the following supplies.
  • Oximeter
  • Sensor (if not part of the device)
  • Tape (if needed)
  • Alcohol wipe

3 Arrange your work area.
4 Practice hand hygiene.
5 Identify the person. Check the identification (ID) bracelet against your assignment sheet. Use 2 identifiers (Chapter 14). Also call the person by name.
6 Provide for privacy.

PROCEDURE

7 Provide for comfort.
8 Select and clean the site. An alcohol wipe may be used. If needed, disinfect the sensor following the manufacturer's instructions. Discard the wipe. If measuring blood pressure, use 1 arm for blood pressure and a site on the other arm for pulse oximetry.
9 Clip or tape the sensor to the site. If needed, connect the sensor to the oximeter.
10 Turn on the oximeter.
11 *For continuous monitoring:*
  a   Set the high and low alarm limits for SpO_2 and pulse rate as directed by the nurse.
  b   Turn on audio and visual alarms.

12 Check the apical or radial pulse with the pulse on the display. The pulse rates should be about the same. Note both pulses on your assignment sheet.
13 Read the SpO_2 on the display. Note the value on the flow sheet and your assignment sheet.
14 Leave the sensor in place for continuous monitoring. Otherwise, turn off the device and remove the sensor.

POST-PROCEDURE

15 Provide for comfort. (See the inside of the back cover.)
16 Place the call light and other needed items within reach.
17 Follow the care plan and the person's preferences for privacy measures to maintain.
18 Complete a safety check of the room. (See the inside of the back cover.)

19 Practice hand hygiene.
20 Return the device to its proper place (unless monitoring is continuous). Follow agency policy for disinfection.
21 Report and record the SpO_2, the pulse rates, and your other observations.

MEETING OXYGEN NEEDS

Air must move deep into the lungs to alveoli where O_2 and CO_2 are exchanged. Disease, injury, and surgery can prevent air from reaching the alveoli. Pain, immobility, and some drugs interfere with deep breathing and coughing. Therefore secretions collect in the airway and lungs. Microbes can grow in the secretions. Infection is a threat.

Oxygen needs must be met. The following measures are common in care plans.

- Positioning
- Deep breathing and coughing
- Incentive spirometry (p. 681)

See *Focus on Communication: Meeting Oxygen Needs.*

Positioning

Breathing is usually easier in the semi-Fowler's and Fowler's positions. Persons with difficulty breathing often prefer the *orthopneic position*—sitting up (*ortho*) and leaning over a table to breathe (*pneic*). Place a pillow on the table to increase comfort (Fig. 44-4).

If the person must lie flat for a procedure, raise the head of the bed as soon as possible. Raise it at once if the person has difficulty breathing.

Frequent position changes are needed. Unless position limits were ordered, the person must not lie on 1 side for a long time. Secretions pool. The lungs cannot expand on that side. Position changes are needed at least every 2 hours. Follow the care plan.

Deep Breathing and Coughing

Deep breathing moves air into most parts of the lungs. Coughing removes mucus. Deep-breathing and coughing exercises are done after surgery or injury and during bed rest. The exercises are painful after surgery or injury. Breaking an incision open while coughing is a fear.

Deep breathing and coughing are usually done every 1 to 2 hours while awake. They help prevent pneumonia and atelectasis. *Atelectasis* is the collapse of a portion of a lung. It occurs when air cannot get to a part of the lung. Mucus blocking the airways and shallow breathing are some causes. Surgery, bed rest, lung diseases, and paralysis are risk factors.

See *Focus on Communication: Deep Breathing and Coughing.*

See *Focus on Children and Older Persons: Deep Breathing and Coughing.*

See *Delegation Guidelines: Deep Breathing and Coughing,* p. 680.

See *Promoting Safety and Comfort: Deep Breathing and Coughing,* p. 680.

See procedure: *Assisting with Deep-Breathing and Coughing Exercises,* p. 680.

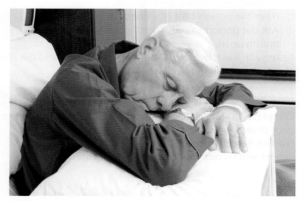

FIGURE 44-4 The person is in the orthopneic position. A pillow is on the over-bed table for comfort.

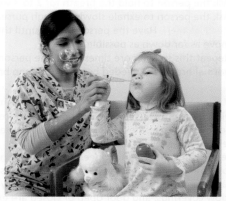

FIGURE 44-5 The child blows bubbles for a deep-breathing exercise.

DELEGATION GUIDELINES
Deep Breathing and Coughing

Assisting with deep-breathing and coughing exercises is a routine nursing task. To assist, you need this information from the nurse and the care plan.
- When to do them and how often
- How many deep breaths and coughs are needed
- What observations to report and record:
  - The number of deep breaths and coughs
  - How the person tolerated the procedure
- When to report observations
- What patient or resident concerns to report at once

PROMOTING SAFETY AND COMFORT
Deep Breathing and Coughing

Safety
Respiratory hygiene and cough etiquette are needed for a productive cough (Chapter 18). The person needs to:
- Cover the nose and mouth to cough or sneeze.
- Use tissues to contain respiratory secretions.
- Dispose of tissues in the nearest waste container after use.
- Wash the hands after coughing, sneezing, or contact with respiratory secretions.
  While the person is covering the nose and mouth, you need to splint a chest or abdominal incision with your hands or a pillow. See step 8 (b) in procedure: *Assisting With Deep-Breathing and Coughing Exercises*. Wear gloves to splint the incision.

Assisting With Deep-Breathing and Coughing Exercises

QUALITY OF LIFE
- Knock before entering the person's room.
- Address the person by name.
- Introduce yourself by name and title.
- Explain the procedure before starting and during the procedure.
- Protect the person's rights during the procedure.
- Handle the person gently during the procedure.

PRE-PROCEDURE
1 Follow *Delegation Guidelines: Deep Breathing and Coughing*. See *Promoting Safety and Comfort: Deep Breathing and Coughing*.
2 Practice hand hygiene and get gloves if needed.
3 Identify the person. Check the ID bracelet against the assignment sheet. Use 2 identifiers (Chapter 14). Also call the person by name.
4 Provide for privacy.
5 Raise the bed for body mechanics. Bed rails are up if used. Lower the bed rail near you if up.

PROCEDURE
6 Help the person to a comfortable sitting position.
  - Sitting on the side of the bed
  - Semi-Fowler's
  - Fowler's
7 *For deep breathing:*
  a Have the person place the hands over the rib cage (Fig. 44-6).
  b Have the person inhale through the nose and breathe as deeply as possible (Fig. 44-7).
  c Ask the person to hold the breath for 2 to 3 seconds.
  d Ask the person to exhale slowly through pursed lips (see Fig. 44-7). Have the person exhale until the ribs move as far down as possible.
  e Repeat this step 4 more times. Have the person take normal breaths as needed before each deep breath.
8 *For coughing:*
  a *If the person does not have a productive cough:*
    Have the person place both hands over the chest or abdominal incision. One hand is on top of the other (Fig. 44-8, *A*). Or the person holds a pillow or folded towel over the chest or abdominal incision (Fig. 44-8, *B*).
  b *If the person has a productive cough:*
    1) Have the person practice cough etiquette.
    2) Splint the chest or abdominal incision with your hands or a pillow. Wear gloves.
  c Have the person take in a deep breath as in step 7.
  d Ask the person to cough strongly 2 times with the mouth open.
9 Assist with hand hygiene. Wear gloves. Remove and discard gloves. Practice hand hygiene.

POST-PROCEDURE
10 Provide for comfort. (See the inside of the back cover.)
11 Lower the bed to a safe and comfortable level. Raise or lower bed rails. Follow the care plan.
12 Place the call light and other needed items within reach.
13 Follow the care plan and the person's preferences for privacy measures to maintain. Leaving the privacy curtain, window coverings, and door open or closed are examples.
14 Complete a safety check of the room. (See the inside of the back cover.)
15 Practice hand hygiene.
16 Report and record your care and observations (Fig. 44-9).

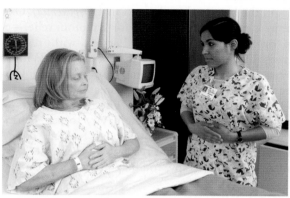

FIGURE 44-6 The hands are over the rib cage for deep breathing.

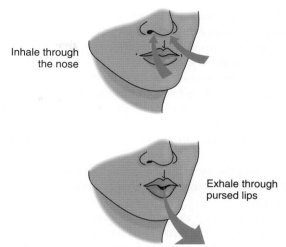

Inhale through the nose

Exhale through pursed lips

FIGURE 44-7 The person inhales through the nose and exhales through pursed lips during the deep-breathing exercise.

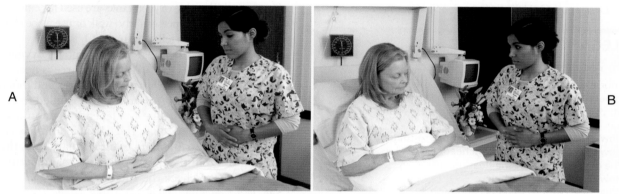

A

B

FIGURE 44-8 The incision is supported for the coughing exercise. **A,** The hands are over the incision. **B,** A pillow is held over the incision.

DATE: 04/19	TIME: 1530

OXYGEN NEEDS: CARE MEASURES

☒ Deep breathe   ☐ Turn
    ⑤ Times   ☒ Back
☒ Cough   ☐ Right side
    ② Times   ☐ Left side
☐ Incentive spirometry   ☐ Suction
    ☐ Times
    Volume ☐ mL

Assisted patient with deep-breathing and coughing exercises. Incision splinted with a pillow. Patient states: "It is getting easier." Denied pain or discomfort. Over-bed table with water mug and tissues in reach. Call light in reach.

Nurse notified: K. Somers, RN

FIGURE 44-9 Charting sample.

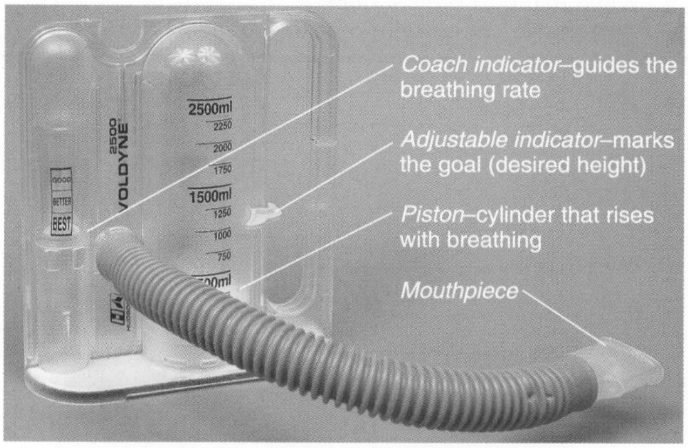

FIGURE 44-10 Parts of an incentive spirometer.

Coach indicator–guides the breathing rate

Adjustable indicator–marks the goal (desired height)

Piston–cylinder that rises with breathing

Mouthpiece

Incentive Spirometry

Incentive means to encourage. A *spirometer* is a machine that measures *(meter)* the amount (volume) of air inhaled with an inspiration *(spiro)* (Fig. 44-10). Incentive spirometry also is called *sustained maximal inspiration (SMI)*. *Sustained* means constant. *Maximal* means the most or the greatest. And *inspiration* is breathing in. The person inhales as deeply as possible and holds the breath for 3 to 5 seconds.

The goals are to improve lung function and prevent complications. Like yawning or sighing, breathing is long, slow, and deep. Air moves deep into the lungs. Secretions loosen. O_2 and CO_2 exchange occurs between the alveoli and capillaries.

The device is used as follows. The person:

1 Sits on the side of the bed, in Fowler's position, or in a chair.
2 Places the spirometer upright.
3 Exhales normally.
4 Seals the lips around the mouthpiece.
5 Takes a slow, deep breath until the piston rises to the desired height. A marker on the spirometer shows the desired height.
6 Holds the breath for 3 to 5 seconds to keep the piston floating.
7 Removes the mouthpiece and exhales slowly.
8 Rests for a few seconds and takes normal breaths.
9 Performs steps 3 through 8 at least 5 to 10 times. The doctor orders the number of breaths.
10 Coughs when needed or after the ordered number of breaths.
11 Repeats steps 1 through 10 every hour while awake.

See *Delegation Guidelines: Incentive Spirometry.*

DELEGATION GUIDELINES

Incentive Spirometry

The nurse teaches the person how to use the incentive spirometer. You may assist the person in using the device. To assist, you need this information from the nurse and the care plan.

- How often the person needs incentive spirometry
- How many breaths the person needs to take
- The desired height of the floating piston
- How to clean the mouthpiece
- What observations to report and record:
  - How many breaths the person took
  - The height of the floating piston
  - If the person coughed after the procedure
  - How the person tolerated the procedure
- When to report observations
- What patient or resident concerns to report at once

ASSISTING WITH OXYGEN THERAPY

Disease, injury, and surgery often affect breathing and oxygen needs. Oxygen therapy is ordered when the amount of O_2 in the blood is less than normal *(hypoxemia)*. Oxygen therapy is needed constantly or for symptom relief—chest pain or shortness of breath. Persons with respiratory diseases may have enough oxygen at rest. With mild exercise or activity, they become short of breath. Oxygen therapy helps relieve shortness of breath.

Oxygen is treated as a drug. The doctor orders when to give O_2, the amount, and the device to use. Harm can result from too much or not enough oxygen. *You do not give oxygen.* The nurse and respiratory therapist start and maintain oxygen therapy. You help provide safe care.

Oxygen Sources

Oxygen is supplied as follows.

- *Wall outlet.* O_2 is piped into each person's unit (Fig. 44-11).
- *Oxygen tank.* Portable oxygen tanks are used for emergencies, for transfers, and by persons who walk or use wheelchairs (Fig. 44-12). A gauge tells how much O_2 is left (Fig. 44-13).
- *Oxygen concentrator.* The machine removes oxygen from the air (Fig. 44-14). A power source is needed. An oxygen tank is needed for power failures and mobility.
- *Liquid oxygen system.* A portable unit is filled from a stationary unit (Fig. 44-15). Depending on unit size and the flow rate (p. 684), the portable unit has enough O_2 for about 8 to 20 hours of use. A dial shows the amount of O_2 in the unit. Follow the manufacturer's instructions to check the amount.

See *Focus on Long-Term Care and Home Care: Oxygen Sources.*

See *Teamwork and Time Management: Oxygen Sources,* p. 684.

See *Promoting Safety and Comfort: Oxygen Sources,* p. 684.

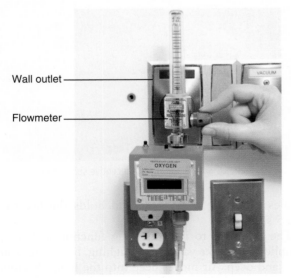

FIGURE 44-11 Wall oxygen outlet. The flowmeter is used to set the oxygen flow rate.

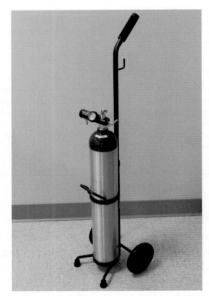

FIGURE 44-12 A portable oxygen tank.

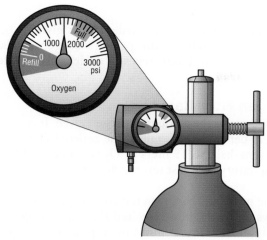

FIGURE 44-13 The gauge shows the amount of oxygen in the tank.

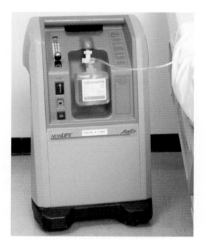

FIGURE 44-14 Oxygen concentrator.

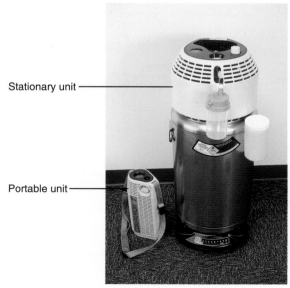

Stationary unit

Portable unit

FIGURE 44-15 A portable liquid oxygen unit and stationary unit. (Modified from Perry AG, Potter PA, Ostendorf WR, Laplante N: *Clinical nursing skills & techniques*, ed 10, St Louis, 2022, Elsevier.)

FOCUS ON **LONG-TERM CARE AND HOME CARE**

Oxygen Sources

Home Care

Oxygen tanks, oxygen concentrators, and liquid oxygen systems are used in home care. They are maintained by a medical supply company. The person (family) needs to have the company's name and phone number.

The patient and family must practice safety measures for using and storing oxygen. This includes measures to prevent fires. The nurse instructs them to:

- Practice fire prevention measures (Chapter 14) including:
  - Keeping a fire extinguisher in the room
  - Making sure smoke alarms are in working order
- Do not allow smoking in the room where oxygen is used.
  - Post *NO SMOKING* signs in the room and on the room door.
  - Remove smoking materials—cigarettes, cigars, pipes, electronic cigarettes, matches, lighters, and so on.
- Remove materials that can ignite, spark, or explode.
  - Personal products—nail polish remover, body oils, petroleum products (ointments), or products containing alcohol
  - Alcoholic beverages
  - Oils and greases
  - Lithium batteries
- Practice electrical safety (Chapter 14) including:
  - Using 3-pronged plugs.
  - Turning off electrical items before unplugging them.
  - Using electrical items that are in good repair. Examples include TVs, radios, music players, computers and other electronic devices, toys, and so on.
  - Avoiding the use of items that may spark. Such items include electric blankets, shavers, and heaters; hair dryers; wool and synthetic fabrics; and some toys.
- Store and use oxygen safely.
  - Keep oxygen sources and tubing at least 5 to 10 feet away from heat sources and open flames. Examples include:
    - Candles
    - Stoves, ovens, and cooktops
    - Heating ducts and pipes
    - Radiators
    - Space heaters—electrical and kerosene
    - Oil and kerosene lamps
  - Keep oxygen sources upright.
  - Keep oxygen sources in well-ventilated areas and away from the sun.
  - Do not drape or cover an oxygen source with clothing, blankets, or other materials.
  - Turn off oxygen when it is not in use.
  - Turn off oxygen if a fire occurs. Get the person and family out of the home. Call 911 to report a fire.

TEAMWORK AND TIME MANAGEMENT

Oxygen Sources

Oxygen tanks and liquid oxygen systems contain a certain amount of O_2. When the O_2 level is low, a new tank is needed or the liquid oxygen system is refilled. Check the O_2 level often. Report a low O_2 level at once.

PROMOTING SAFETY AND COMFORT

Oxygen Sources

Safety

Liquid oxygen is very cold. If touched, it can freeze the skin. Tampering with equipment is unsafe and could damage the equipment. Follow agency procedures and the manufacturer's instructions for liquid oxygen.

Many activities increase the need for O_2. These include moving in bed, transfer procedures, and walking. Do not remove the person's O_2. If needed, ask the nurse for longer tubing (extension tubing). Or ask the nurse to change to a portable oxygen tank.

Oxygen Devices

Different devices may be ordered for giving O_2. The type used depends on the person's oxygen needs. See Table 44-1 for different types of devices used to deliver oxygen.

Oxygen Flow Rates

The *flow rate* is the amount of oxygen given. It is measured in liters per minute (L/min). The ordered flow rate may be ½ (one-half) to 15 liters of O_2 per minute. The nurse or respiratory therapist sets the flow rate with a flowmeter (see Fig. 44-11).

The nurse and care plan tell you the person's flow rate. Always check the flow rate. Tell the nurse at once if it is too high or too low. A nurse or respiratory therapist will adjust the flow rate. Some states and agencies let nursing assistants adjust O_2 flow rates as directed. Know your agency's policy.

TABLE 44-1	Types of Oxygen Devices		
Device	**Description**	**Care Considerations**	**Example**
Nasal cannula	• Prongs are inserted into the nostrils. The prong openings face downward. • Tubing goes behind the ears and under the chin.	• Allows for eating and drinking. • Tight prongs can irritate the nose. • Pressure on the ears and cheekbones can occur. Pressure injuries are a risk.	Prong openings face downward
Simple face mask	• A mask covers the nose and mouth. • An elastic strap goes around the head to secure the device. • Small holes (vents) in the sides of the mask allow CO_2 to escape when exhaling. Vents also allow room air into the mask when inhaling.	• Talking and eating are hard to do with a mask. For eating, the nurse changes the mask to a cannula. • Moisture can build up under the mask. Keep the face clean and dry to prevent irritation. • Vomiting while wearing a mask can cause aspiration. • Pressure can occur where the mask and strap have contact with the skin. Pressure injuries are a risk.	Vents

TABLE 44-1	Types of Oxygen Devices—cont'd		
Device	Description	Care Considerations	Example
Partial-rebreather mask	• A bag is added to the simple face mask. • O_2, some exhaled air, and some room air are inhaled.	• See "Simple face mask." • The reservoir bag should not totally deflate (collapse) when inhaling.	Strap Adjustable nose clip Mask Vents O_2 tubing Reservoir bag
Non-rebreather mask	• The mask has a reservoir bag for O_2. • Exhaled air leaves through holes (vents) in the mask. Vent covers do not allow room air into the mask. • Only O_2 from the bag is inhaled. Exhaled air and room air are not inhaled.	• The reservoir bag must not totally deflate (collapse) when inhaling. Suffocation can occur if there is not enough air in the bag. • These masks are used for emergency situations. The person is closely monitored when in use.	Strap Adjustable nose clip Mask Vent cover O_2 tubing Reservoir bag
Venturi mask	• Precise amounts of O_2 are given. Color-coded adapters show the amount of O_2 given.	• See "Simple face mask."	

Continued

TABLE 44-1	Types of Oxygen Devices—cont'd		
Device	Description	Care Considerations	Example
Oxygen hood	• Used for infants, a plastic dome (hood) covers the infant's head. O_2 is delivered into the dome.	• The hood must be properly sized to prevent skin irritation on the neck (too small) and loss of O_2 (too big). • O_2 level, humidity, temperature, and noise level in the hood must be closely monitored.	

Safety

You assist the nurse with oxygen therapy. *You do not give oxygen. You do not remove or apply devices or adjust flow rates unless allowed by your state and agency.* You must give safe care. Follow the rules in Box 44-2. Also follow the rules for fire and the use of oxygen (Chapter 14).

Nursing assistant role limits regarding oxygen therapy differ by state and agency. Some do not allow nursing assistants to remove and replace oxygen devices during care. The nurse is responsible. Others allow removal and replacement of a nasal cannula for care such as cleaning the nostrils. Some allow nursing assistants to switch oxygen sources during transfer procedures without changing the flow rate. Others allow adjustment of the flow rate during activity as indicated on the person's care plan. All of the conditions in *Delegation Guidelines: Oxygen Needs* (p. 674) must be met. Follow the rules in your state and agency.

Oxygen Set-Up

Oxygen is a dry gas. If not humidified (made moist), O_2 dries the airway's mucous membranes. Distilled water is added to the humidifier (see Fig. 44-16). (Distilled water is water that has been purified with contaminants removed.) When added to the humidifier, distilled water creates water vapor. Oxygen picks up the water vapor as it flows into the system. Bubbling in the humidifier means water vapor is being produced. Low flow rates (up to 4 L/min) by cannula are usually not humidified.

BOX 44-2   Oxygen Safety

• Do not remove the oxygen device. Follow agency policy and your role limits on what to do when:
  • An oxygen device needs to be removed and replaced during care.
  • An oxygen source needs to be changed during care.
• Make sure the device is secure but not tight.
• Check areas where oxygen devices contact skin. Pressure injuries can develop where medical devices cause pressure on the skin. Report any sign of a pressure injury at once (Chapter 42). Check for irritation or skin changes:
  • Behind the ears
  • Under the nose (cannula)
  • Around the face (mask)
  • On the cheekbones
• Keep the face clean and dry when a mask is used.
• Do not shut off the O_2 flow unless there is a fire. *Turn off the O_2 flow if there is a fire. Remove the oxygen device.*
• Do not adjust the flow rate unless allowed by your state and agency.
• Tell the nurse at once if a:
  • Flow rate is too high or too low.
  • Humidifier is not bubbling (Fig. 44-16).
• Maintain an adequate water level in a humidifier.
• Secure tubing in place. Tape, clamp, or pin it to the person's garment following agency policy. Do not puncture the tubing.
• Make sure there are no kinks in the tubing.
• Make sure the person does not lie on any part of the tubing.
• Make sure an oxygen tank is secure in its holder.
• Report signs and symptoms of altered respiratory function or abnormal breathing patterns at once. See pp. 675–676.
• Follow the care plan for oral hygiene.
• Follow the care plan for hygiene and grooming. Do not use an electric shaver when oxygen is in use.
• Make sure the oxygen device is clean and free of mucus.
• Do not use petroleum products (ointments) near oxygen. For example, do not apply petroleum jelly to the nostrils or lips when a nasal cannula or mask is used. Burns can occur.
• See "Fire and Oxygen" in Chapter 14.

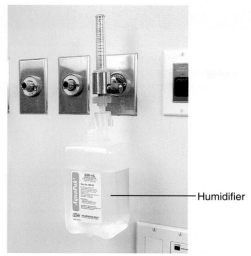

—Humidifier

FIGURE 44-16 Oxygen set-up with a humidifier.

You do not start oxygen therapy. You may be allowed to assist with set up. The procedure that follows is an example of how to set up for oxygen therapy with a humidifier.

See *Teamwork and Time Management: Oxygen Set-Up.*
See *Delegation Guidelines: Oxygen Set-Up.*
See *Promoting Safety and Comfort: Oxygen Set-Up.*
See procedure: *Setting Up Oxygen.*

TEAMWORK AND TIME MANAGEMENT
Oxygen Set-Up

As you walk past the room of any person receiving humidified O_2, always check the humidifier. Check for and tell the nurse if:
- There is no bubbling.
- The water level is low.

DELEGATION GUIDELINES
Oxygen Set-Up

Setting up oxygen is a nursing task that may be delegated to you in some agencies. The conditions in *Delegation Guidelines: Oxygen Needs* (p. 674) must be met. If setting up O_2 is delegated to you, you need this information from the nurse.
- The person's name and room and bed numbers
- What oxygen device to use
- If you need a humidifier

PROMOTING SAFETY AND COMFORT
Oxygen Set-Up

Safety
You do not give oxygen. Tell the nurse when the O_2 system is set up. The nurse turns on the O_2, sets the flow rate, and applies the O_2 device. *You do not adjust the flow rate unless allowed by your state and agency.*

Practice medical asepsis. Do not let the connecting tubing hang on the floor.

You must give safe care. Follow the rules in Box 44-2. Also follow the rules for fire and the use of oxygen (Chapter 14).

Setting Up Oxygen
QUALITY OF LIFE

- Knock before entering the person's room.
- Address the person by name.
- Introduce yourself by name and title.

- Explain the procedure before starting and during the procedure.
- Protect the person's rights during the procedure.
- Handle the person gently during the procedure.

PRE-PROCEDURE

1 Follow *Delegation Guidelines:*
  a *Oxygen Needs,* p. 674
  b *Oxygen Set-Up*
  See *Promoting Safety and Comfort: Oxygen Set-Up.*
2 Practice hand hygiene and get the following supplies.
  - Oxygen device with connecting tubing
  - Flowmeter
  - Humidifier (if ordered)
  - Distilled water (if using a humidifier)

3 Arrange your work area.
4 Practice hand hygiene.
5 Identify the person. Check the ID bracelet against the assignment sheet. Use 2 identifiers (Chapter 14). Also call the person by name.

Continued

Setting Up Oxygen—cont'd

PROCEDURE

6 Make sure the flowmeter is in the OFF position.
7 Attach the flowmeter to the wall outlet for oxygen.
8 Fill the humidifier with distilled water.
9 Attach the humidifier to the bottom of the flowmeter.
10 Attach the oxygen device and connecting tubing to the humidifier. *Do not set the flowmeter. Do not apply the O₂ device on the person.* Place the device and tubing in a clean place where the device will not fall to the floor.

11 Place the cap securely on the distilled water. Store the water according to agency policy.
12 Discard the packaging from the O_2 device and connecting tubing.

POST-PROCEDURE

13 Provide for comfort. (See the inside of the back cover.)
14 Place the call light and other needed items within reach.
15 Complete a safety check of the room. (See the inside of the back cover.)

16 Practice hand hygiene.
17 Tell the nurse when you are done. The nurse will:
   • Turn on the O_2 and set the flow rate.
   • Apply the O_2 device on the person.

FOCUS ON PRIDE

The Person, Family, and Yourself

Personal and Professional Responsibility

A person may say: "I'm not getting enough air." Yet the person seems to be breathing comfortably. You cannot feel what the person feels. Trust what the person tells you.

If the person uses oxygen therapy, you can check the oxygen set-up.
• Is the O_2 turned on and at the correct flow rate?
• Is there enough O_2 remaining in a portable oxygen tank or liquid oxygen unit?
• Is the tubing connected to the O_2 source?
• Are there any kinks in the tubing?
• Is the oxygen device (nasal cannula or mask) properly in place?

Do not dismiss what the person tells you. If you do not find a problem or you cannot correct the problem, tell the nurse at once.

Rights and Respect

People have the right to a safe setting. Smoking is not allowed where oxygen is used and stored. NO SMOKING signs are common in rooms and hallways. You may need to remind the person or visitors not to smoke. Be polite and respectful. Show the person where smoking is allowed.

Independence and Social Interaction

Needing long-term oxygen therapy changes a person's life. Portable oxygen sources increase independence. Small oxygen tanks and portable liquid oxygen units are examples. Such devices allow freedom and promote quality of life.

Delegation and Teamwork

Performing a task outside the limits of your role is wrong. Harm can result. You can lose your job and your ability to work as a nursing assistant. Take pride in following the limits of your role and providing safe care.

Ethics and Laws

The following case shows how harm resulted from unsafe use of oxygen by a certified nursing assistant (CNA) who was not supposed to handle oxygen.

A CNA took a group of residents outside to smoke. One resident, who used oxygen, was taken outside with her oxygen tank. Center policy stated that oxygen was to be used and handled only by nurses. The CNA tried to turn off the oxygen but she did not turn it off completely. The resident's cigarette set fire to the oxygen and caused severe facial burns.

The CNA lost her job. The state's board of nursing asked the CNA for a written response to complaints against her. The CNA did not respond.

The CNA's conduct provided grounds for disciplinary action. The CNA was charged with:
• *Committing an act that deceives, defrauds, or harms the public*
• *Conduct or practice that is or may be harmful to the health of a patient or the public*
• *Failing to follow policies and procedures designed to protect the patient or resident*
• *Neglecting or abusing a resident physically, verbally, emotionally, or financially*
• *Accepting care tasks that the CNA lacks the education or competence to perform*
• *Failing to cooperate with the board during an investigation by:*
  • *Not providing a complete, written explanation of the matter*
  • *Not completing and returning a board-issued questionnaire within 30 days*
The CNA's certificate was revoked.
(Arizona State Board of Nursing, 2010.)

FOCUS ON PRIDE: *Application*

What are the limits to your role when assisting with oxygen therapy? Why are such limits important? Explain the value of your role. How do you help the nurse and patient or resident?

REVIEW QUESTIONS

Circle the BEST answer.

1 Alcohol and opioids affect oxygen needs because they
 a Depress the brain
 b Are pollutants
 c Cause allergies
 d Cause infection

2 Hypoxia is
 a Not enough oxygen in the blood
 b The amount of hemoglobin that contains oxygen
 c Not enough oxygen in the cells
 d The lack of carbon dioxide

3 An early sign of altered respiratory function is
 a Cyanosis
 b Increased pulse
 c Restlessness
 d Dyspnea

4 A person breathes deeply and comfortably only while sitting. This is called
 a Apnea
 b Orthopnea
 c Bradypnea
 d Kussmaul respirations

5 Tachypnea means that respirations are
 a Slow
 b Rapid
 c Absent
 d Difficult or painful

6 Which should you report to the nurse at once?
 a A respiratory rate of 18 per minute
 b An SpO_2 of 97%
 c Bubbling in a humidifier
 d Dyspnea

7 A person's SpO_2 is 98%. Which is *true*?
 a The pulse oximeter is wrong.
 b The pulse is 98 beats per minute.
 c The measurement is within normal range.
 d The person has hypoxia.

8 A person has non-natural nails. Which is another pulse oximetry sensor site?
 a The wrist
 b The chest
 c The upper arm
 d An earlobe

9 You are assisting with deep breathing and coughing. You need to explain the procedure again if the person
 a Inhales through pursed lips
 b Sits in a comfortable position
 c Inhales deeply through the nose
 d Holds a pillow over an incision

10 A person has a productive cough. You remind the person to
 a Use an oxygen mask
 b Cover the nose and mouth when coughing
 c Cough and deep breathe twice daily
 d Inhale through the mouth

11 Which is useful for deep breathing?
 a Pulse oximeter
 b Incentive spirometer
 c Simple face mask
 d Partial-rebreather mask

12 Which oxygen device allows for eating?
 a Simple face mask
 b Partial-rebreather mask
 c Venturi mask
 d Nasal cannula

13 Oxygen flow rate is measured in
 a mm Hg
 b mL/h
 c L/min
 d SpO_2

14 When assisting with oxygen therapy, you can
 a Turn the oxygen on and off
 b Start the oxygen
 c Decide what device to use
 d Keep connecting tubing free of kinks

15 A person reports pressure on the ears from nasal cannula tubing. You should
 a Check for irritation and tell the nurse
 b Change the cannula to a mask
 c Remove the device
 d Explain that the pressure is normal

16 A person is receiving O_2. Which is *unsafe?*
 a Smoking materials are in the room.
 b Electrical items are turned off, then unplugged.
 c 3-pronged electrical items are used.
 d There is a fire extinguisher in the room.

17 A person is receiving O_2. Which should you question?
 a Provide oral hygiene.
 b Check that the flow rate is correct.
 c Turn off the O_2 for ambulation.
 d Secure tubing in place.

18 A person uses an oxygen concentrator with a humidifier. Which is expected?
 a The water level will move up and down as the person breathes.
 b The oxygen concentrator will be used for ambulation to the dining room.
 c Water will drip from the oxygen device.
 d There will be bubbling in the humidifier.

Answers to Chapter 44 questions are on p. 903.

FOCUS ON PRACTICE

Problem Solving

A person is receiving oxygen therapy by nasal cannula. The oxygen tubing will not reach from the wall oxygen outlet to the bathroom. The person removes the nasal cannula and walks to the bathroom. The person becomes short of breath and uses the call light in the bathroom to call for help. You respond. What will you do? How could this have been prevented?

CHAPTER 45

Respiratory Support and Therapies

OBJECTIVES

- Define the key terms and key abbreviations in this chapter.
- Explain how to assist in the care of persons with artificial airways.
- Describe the principles and safety measures for suctioning.
- Explain how to assist in the care of persons on mechanical ventilation.

- Explain how to assist in the care of persons with chest tubes.
- Describe devices used for sleep apnea.
- Explain how to promote PRIDE in the person, the family, and yourself.

KEY TERMS

hemothorax Blood *(hemo)* in the pleural space *(thorax)*
intubation Inserting an artificial airway
mechanical ventilation Using a machine to move air into and out of the lungs
patent Open and unblocked
pleural effusion The escape and collection of fluid *(effusion)* in the pleural space

pneumothorax Air *(pneumo)* in the pleural space *(thorax)*
suction The process of withdrawing or sucking up fluid *(secretions)*
tracheostomy A surgically created opening *(stomy)* in the neck into the trachea *(tracheo)*

KEY ABBREVIATIONS

BiPAP	Bilevel positive airway pressure	O_2	Oxygen
CO_2	Carbon dioxide	PPE	Personal protective equipment
CPAP	Continuous positive airway pressure	RT	Respiratory therapist
ET	Endotracheal		

Some persons have serious problems affecting the respiratory system. They need complex procedures and equipment. The nurse may ask you to assist in their care.

See *Body Structure and Function Review: The Respiratory System* (Chapter 44).

See *Promoting Safety and Comfort: Respiratory Support and Therapies*.

PROMOTING SAFETY AND COMFORT

Respiratory Support and Therapies

Safety

Respiratory secretions may contain microbes or blood. Follow Standard Precautions and the Bloodborne Pathogen Standard. Follow the rules of hand hygiene and the guidelines for glove use in Chapters 17 and 18. Wear other personal protective equipment (PPE) as directed. A mask or respirator with a face shield or goggles may be needed (Chapter 18).

In nursing centers, follow agency policies and procedures for using Enhanced Barrier Precautions when the person has an indwelling medical device. An artificial airway is an indwelling medical device. High-contact tasks and tasks involving the artificial airway require routine gown and glove use. See Chapter 18.

ARTIFICIAL AIRWAYS

Artificial airways keep the airway *patent* (open and unblocked). They are needed:

- When disease, injury, secretions, or aspiration obstructs (blocks) the airway
- For mechanical ventilation (p. 695)
- By some persons who are semi-conscious or unconscious
- During surgery and recovery from anesthesia

Intubation means inserting an artificial airway (Fig. 45-1). Airways are usually plastic and disposable.

- *Oro-pharyngeal airway*—inserted through the mouth and into the pharynx (see Fig. 45-1, *A*). The device prevents the tongue from blocking the airway. Use is temporary. A naso-pharyngeal airway is a similar device that is inserted through the nose. A nurse or respiratory therapist (RT) inserts the airway.
- *Endotracheal (ET) tube*—inserted through the mouth or nose into the trachea (see Fig. 45-1, *B*). A lighted scope is used to guide insertion by a doctor, specially trained nurse, or RT. The cuff on the tube is inflated to seal the airway. The seal prevents air leaks around the cuff. Airflow is directed to the lungs, not the upper airway. ET tubes are used short-term.
- *Tracheostomy tube*—inserted through a surgically created opening *(stomy)* into the trachea *(tracheo)* (see Fig. 45-1, *C*). Cuffed tracheostomy tubes are used in adults when mechanical ventilation (p. 695) is needed. Uncuffed tubes may be used long-term when the person can breathe without mechanical assistance. Doctors perform tracheostomies.

Vital signs and pulse oximetry are measured often. Observe for signs and symptoms of altered respiratory function (Chapter 44). If an airway comes out or is dislodged, tell the nurse at once.

Gagging and choking feelings are common. Imagine something in your mouth, nose, or throat. Comfort and reassure the person. Remind the person that the airway helps breathing. Use touch to show you care. Frequent oral hygiene is needed. Follow the care plan.

See *Focus on Communication: Artificial Airways.*

See *Promoting Safety and Comfort: Artificial Airways*, p. 692.

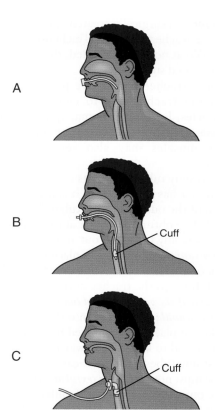

FIGURE 45-1 Artificial airways. **A,** Oro-pharyngeal airway. **B,** Endotracheal (ET) tube with cuff. **C,** Tracheostomy tube with cuff.

FOCUS ON **COMMUNICATION**

Artificial Airways

Usually, an artificial airway prevents speech because air cannot pass through the vocal cords. Some tracheostomy tubes allow speech. Follow the care plan for how to communicate when speech is affected. Paper and pencils, Magic Slates, and communication boards are some ways (Chapter 47). Hand signals, nodding the head, and hand squeezes are common for simple "yes" and "no" answers. Always keep the call light within reach.

Tracheostomies

A *tracheostomy* is a surgically created opening *(stomy)* in the
neck into the trachea *(tracheo)*. Tracheostomies are often
temporary. When no longer needed, the stoma is allowed
to heal or is closed surgically.

Sometimes tracheostomies are permanent. Removal
of part of the trachea due to cancer is one reason.
Airway injuries, long-term coma, spinal cord injuries,
and diseases causing weakness or paralysis of the
respiratory muscles may also require a permanent
tracheostomy.

A tracheostomy tube has 3 parts (Fig. 45-2).
- The *obturator* has a round end. It is used to guide
  insertion of the outer cannula (tube). Then it is
  removed. The obturator is kept at the bedside in case
  the tracheostomy tube falls out and needs insertion.
- The *outer cannula* is secured in place with ties around
  the neck or a Velcro collar. The outer cannula is not
  removed. It keeps the tracheostomy patent. *Call for the
  nurse at once if the outer cannula comes out.*
- The *inner cannula* is inserted into the outer cannula
  and locked in place. It is removed for cleaning and
  mucus removal to keep the airway patent. Most
  tracheostomy tubes have inner cannulas.

The tube must not come out *(extubation)*. If not secure, it
could come out with coughing or if pulled on. A loose tube
moves up and down, damaging the trachea. The tube must
remain patent. If able, the person coughs up secretions.
Otherwise, suctioning is needed. See "Suctioning." *Call
for the nurse at once if you note signs and symptoms of altered
respiratory function.*

Safety Measures. Nothing must enter the stoma.
Water and inhaled substances are examples. Otherwise, the
person can aspirate. These safety measures are needed.
- Dressings do not have loose gauze or lint.
- The stoma or tube is covered when outdoors. The
  person wears a stoma cover or shield, scarf, or shirt or
  blouse that covers the neck. The cover allows air to
  pass through for inhalation but prevents dust, insects,
  and other small particles from entering the stoma.
- The stoma is not covered with plastic, leather, or
  similar materials. Air cannot pass through such
  materials. Therefore air cannot be inhaled through
  the stoma and the person cannot breathe.
- Tub baths are taken. For showers, a shower guard is
  worn. A hand-held nozzle is used to direct water away
  from the stoma.
- The person is assisted with shampooing. Water must
  not enter the stoma.
- The stoma is covered when shaving.
- Swimming is not allowed. Water will enter the tube or
  stoma.
- Medical-alert jewelry is worn. The person carries a
  medical-alert ID (identification) card.

Assisting With Tracheostomy Care. Tracheostomy
care (trach care) is a nursing responsibility. The nurse may
ask you to assist. Trach care is done to prevent infection,
promote healing, and promote comfort. It also is done as
needed for excess secretions, soiled ties or collar, or soiled
or moist dressings. The nurse tells you when trach care is
needed and what supplies to collect. Assist as directed.

Trach care involves:
- Cleaning the inner cannula to remove mucus and
  keep the airway patent. A disposable inner cannula
  is discarded and a new one is inserted. Re-usable
  cannulas are cleaned with a small bottle brush or a
  pipe cleaner and a cleaning agent.
- Cleaning the stoma to prevent infection and skin
  breakdown.
- Applying clean ties or a Velcro collar. Clean ties are applied
  before removing the used ones. Hold the outer cannula in
  place until the nurse secures the new ties or collar. The ties
  or collar must be secure but not tight. For an adult, a finger
  should slide under the ties or collar (Fig. 45-3, *A*).

See *Focus on Children and Older Persons: Assisting With
Tracheostomy Care.*

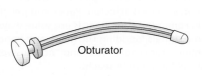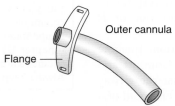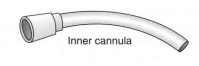

Obturator

Flange

Outer cannula

Inner cannula

FIGURE 45-2 Parts of a tracheostomy tube.

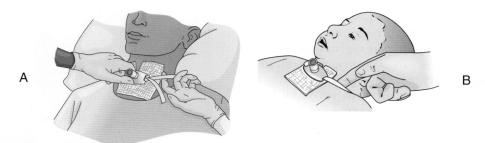

FIGURE 45-3 A, For an adult, a finger is inserted under the ties. **B,** For children, only a fingertip is inserted under the ties.

FOCUS ON CHILDREN AND OLDER PERSONS

Assisting With Tracheostomy Care

Children

Some children have congenital defects that are present at birth. (The Latin word *congenitus* means to be born with.) Tracheostomies are needed for some congenital defects affecting the neck and airway.

Some infections cause swelling of the airway structures. This obstructs air flow. So does foreign body aspiration. These problems may require emergency tracheostomies.

Tracheostomy ties must be secure but not tight. Only a fingertip should slide under the ties (Fig. 45-3, *B*). Ties are too loose if you can slide your whole finger under them.

Assist the nurse by holding the child still. Position the child's head as the nurse directs.

SUCTIONING

Secretions can collect in the airway. Retained secretions:

- Obstruct air flow into and out of the airway.
- Provide an environment for microbes.
- Interfere with oxygen (O_2) and carbon dioxide (CO_2) exchange.

Usually coughing removes secretions. Some persons cannot cough or the cough is too weak to remove secretions. They need suctioning.

Suction is the process of withdrawing or sucking up fluid (secretions). A tube connects to a suction source—wall outlet or portable suction machine—at 1 end and to a suction catheter at the other end. The catheter is inserted into the airway. Secretions are suctioned through the catheter.

The upper airway (nose, mouth, and pharynx) and lower airway (trachea and bronchi) can be suctioned. These routes are used to suction the airway.

- *Oro-pharyngeal.* A suction catheter is passed through the mouth (*oro*) into the pharynx (*pharyngeal*). A Yankauer suction catheter is used (Fig. 45-4). The Yankauer catheter is useful for removing thick secretions and vomit from the mouth and pharynx.
- *Naso-pharyngeal.* The suction catheter is passed through the nose (*naso*) into the pharynx (*pharyngeal*).
- *Lower airway.* The suction catheter is passed through an ET or tracheostomy tube (Fig. 45-5).

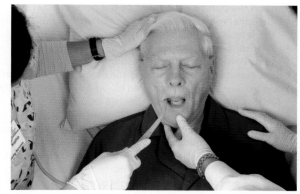

FIGURE 45-4 A Yankauer suction catheter is used to suction the mouth.

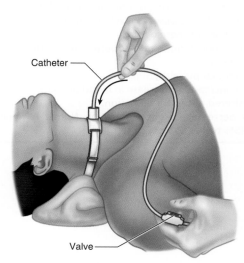

Catheter

Valve

FIGURE 45-5 A tracheostomy tube is suctioned. (From Potter PA, Perry AG, Stocker PA, Hall AM: *Fundamentals of nursing,* ed 11, St Louis, 2023, Elsevier.)

Oxygen levels drop during naso-pharyngeal and lower airway suctioning. To prevent complications, the nurse or RT performs hyperoxygenation before and after the procedure. To *hyperoxygenate* means to give extra *(hyper)* oxygen. This is done with a mechanical ventilator or manually with an Ambu bag (Fig. 45-6) (Chapter 58). During the procedure, suction is applied for only 5 to 10 seconds for an adult. The person is monitored closely, given more oxygen, and suctioned again if needed and if tolerating the procedure well.

To assist the nurse with suctioning, follow the safety measures in Box 45-1.

See *Focus on Children and Older Persons: Suctioning.*
See *Delegation Guidelines: Suctioning.*
See *Promoting Safety and Comfort: Suctioning.*

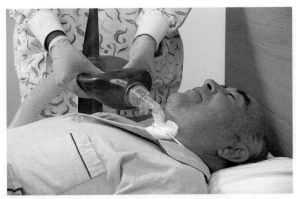

FIGURE 45-6 An Ambu bag used for oxygenation. The device is squeezed with 2 hands.

BOX 45-1	Assisting With Suctioning

- Review the procedure with the nurse. Know what you are expected and allowed to do.
- Report coughing and the signs and symptoms of altered respiratory function (Chapter 44). Suctioning is done as needed, not on a schedule.
- Position the person as directed by the nurse.
  - Oro-pharyngeal suctioning—semi-Fowler's position or the lateral position
  - Naso-pharyngeal or lower airway suctioning—semi-Fowler's or Fowler's position
- Follow Standard Precautions and the Bloodborne Pathogen Standard. Secretions may contain blood and are potentially infectious. Wear gloves and other PPE as directed.
- Follow sterile technique (Chapter 17) when assisting the nurse or RT with naso-pharyngeal or lower airway suctioning. This helps prevent microbes from entering the airway.
- Collect and keep suction catheter supplies and equipment at the bedside as directed by the nurse. They are ready when the person needs suctioning. Collect the correct catheter type and size. If too large, it can injure the airway.
- Check the pulse, respirations, and pulse oximeter measurements before, during, and after the procedure as directed. Also observe level of consciousness. Tell the nurse if any of these occur:
  - A change in pulse rate or pulse rate less than 60 beats per minute.
  - Irregular pulse rhythm.
  - An increase or decrease in blood pressure.
  - Altered respiratory function.
  - A decrease in oxygen saturation. Normal range is 95% to 100%. See Chapter 44.

FOCUS ON CHILDREN AND OLDER PERSONS

Suctioning

Children

Suctioning may frighten children. They need clear, simple explanations about the procedure. You may need to control the child's head and arm movements.

DELEGATION GUIDELINES

Suctioning

Suctioning is a nursing responsibility or that of an RT. Some states and agencies allow nursing assistants to perform oro-pharyngeal suctioning. If delegated to you, make sure that:

- Your state allows you to perform the task.
- The task is in your job description (Chapter 3).
- You have the necessary education and training.
- The agency has determined that you are competent to perform the task safely.
- You know how to use the supplies and equipment.
- You review the procedure with the delegating nurse.
- The delegating nurse is available to answer questions and to guide and assist you as needed.

If the above conditions are met, you need the following information from the nurse and the care plan.

- What suction catheter and tubing to use
- What suction source to use—wall suction or portable suction
- What suction pressure to use
- How to position the person—semi-Fowler's with the head to the side or lateral position
- What to use to clear (rinse) the suction catheter and tubing
- Where to store the suction catheter when not in use
- What observations to report and record:
  - The amount, color, and consistency of secretions
  - Signs and symptoms of altered respiratory function (Chapter 44)
  - How the person tolerated the procedure
- When to report observations
- What patient or resident concerns to report at once (see Box 45-1)

Suctioning

Safety

Oro-pharyngeal suctioning is to be performed carefully. Trauma to tissues in the mouth and stimulation of the gag reflex are risks.

Naso-pharyngeal and lower airway suctioning can have serious complications. The nurse or RT performs these procedures. Altered respiratory function and life-threatening problems can occur from the respiratory, cardiovascular, and nervous systems. Cardiac arrest is a risk. Airway injuries, bleeding, and infection are possible.

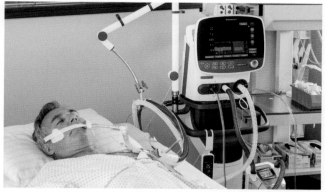

FIGURE 45-7 A mechanical ventilator. (© Hamilton Medical.)

MECHANICAL VENTILATION

Mechanical ventilation is using a machine to move air into and out of the lungs (Fig. 45-7). An ET or tracheostomy tube is needed.

Problems that interfere with breathing or normal oxygen levels include:

- Weak muscle effort, obstructed airway, and damaged lung tissue
- Nervous system diseases and injuries affecting the respiratory center in the brain
- Nerve damage interfering with messages between the lungs and the brain
- Drug overdose depressing the brain

Ventilator alarms sound when something is wrong. One alarm means the person is disconnected from the ventilator and can die from the lack of oxygen. The nurse shows you how to reconnect the ET or tracheostomy tube. When any alarm sounds, check if the tube is attached to the ventilator. If not, re-attach it to the ventilator. Call for the nurse at once when an alarm sounds. Do not re-set alarms.

Persons needing mechanical ventilation are often very ill. Other problems and injuries are common. Some persons are disoriented, confused, or fearful. The machine, fear of dying, and needing the machine life-long are concerns. Some are relieved to get enough oxygen. Mechanical ventilation can be painful for those with chest injuries or chest surgery. Tubes and hoses restrict movement, causing more discomfort.

The nurse may have you assist with the person's care. See Box 45-2.

See *Focus on Long-Term Care and Home Care: Mechanical Ventilation*, p. 696.

BOX 45-2   Assisting With Mechanical Ventilation

- Keep the call light and other needed items within reach.
- Answer call lights promptly. The person depends on others for basic needs.
- Make sure hoses and connecting tubes have slack. They must not pull on the artificial airway.
- Explain who you are and what you are going to do. Do this each time you enter the room.
- Give the day, date, and time every time you give care.
- Report signs of altered respiratory function or discomfort at once.
- Do not change machine settings or re-set alarms.
- Follow the care plan for communication. The person cannot talk. Use agreed-upon hand or eye signals for "yes" and "no." Everyone must use the same signals. Some persons can use the communication aids described in Chapter 7. Ask questions with simple answers. It may be hard to write long responses.
- Be professional. Watch what you say and do. This includes when the person is not conscious. Do not say or do anything that could upset the person.
- Use touch to comfort and reassure the person. Also tell the person about the weather, pleasant news events, and gifts and cards.
- Meet basic needs. Follow the care plan.
- Tell the person when you are leaving the room and when you will return.
- Complete a safety check before leaving the room. (See the inside of the back cover.)

CHEST TUBES

Air, blood, or fluid can collect in the pleural space (sac or cavity). This occurs when the chest is entered because of injury or surgery.

- *Pneumothorax* is air *(pneumo)* in the pleural space *(thorax).*
- *Hemothorax* is blood *(hemo)* in the pleural space *(thorax).*
- *Pleural effusion* is the escape and collection of fluid *(effusion)* in the pleural space.

Pressure from air, blood, or fluid in the pleural space collapses the lung. Air cannot reach affected alveoli for O_2 and CO_2 exchange. Altered respiratory function results. Pressure on the heart affects the heart's ability to pump blood.

The doctor inserts chest tubes to remove the air, blood, or fluid (Fig. 45-8). The sterile procedure is done in surgery, the emergency room, or at the bedside. A nurse assists.

Chest tubes attach to a drainage system. A water seal mechanism prevents air from entering the chest cavity. Figure 45-9 shows the different chambers in a 3-chambered drainage system:

- The tube from the patient connects to the first chamber. Drainage collects in this chamber.
- The second chamber is a water seal. This prevents air from returning to the person.
- The third chamber is used for suction control. See Box 45-3 for care of the person with chest tubes.

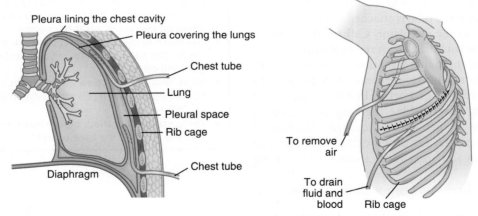

FIGURE 45-8 Chest tubes inserted into the pleural space. (Modified from Harding MM: *Lewis's medical-surgical nursing: assessment and management of clinical problems,* ed 11, St Louis, 2020, Elsevier.)

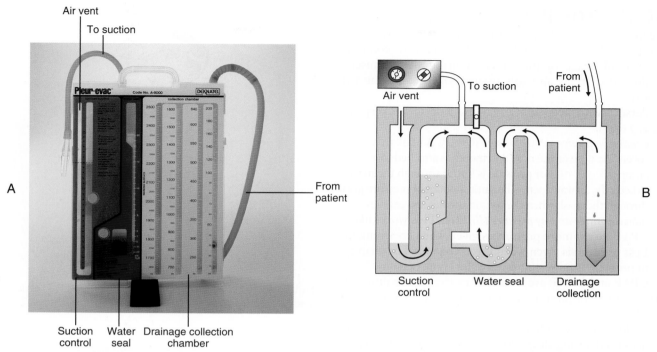

FIGURE 45-9 A, Chest tube drainage system. **B,** The system has 3 chambers—a drainage collection chamber, a water seal chamber, and a chamber for suction control. (From Ignatavicius DD, Workman ML, Rebar CR, Heimgartner NM: *Medical-surgical nursing: concepts for interprofessional collaborative care,* ed 10, St Louis, 2021, Elsevier.)

BOX 45-3	Assisting With Chest Tubes

- Keep the drainage system below the chest.
- Report the following at once:
  - Vital signs and pulse oximetry measurements. The nurse tells you when to take them.
  - Signs and symptoms of altered respiratory function. See Chapter 44.
  - Complaints of pain or difficulty breathing.
  - Changes in chest drainage. This includes increases in drainage or the appearance of bright red drainage.
  - If bubbling in the drainage system increases, decreases, or stops. The nurse shows you what is expected.
  - If any part of the drainage system is loose or disconnected. Follow agency policy for placing the end of a disconnected tube in a container of sterile water until help arrives.

- Keep connecting tubing straight or coiled on the bed as directed. Allow enough slack so the chest tubes are not dislodged when the person moves. Prevent the tubing from hanging in loops. Drainage collects in loops.
- Prevent tubing kinks. Kinks obstruct the chest tube. Air, blood, or fluid collects in the pleural space.
- Assist with recording chest drainage according to agency policy.
- Turn and position the person as directed. Be careful and gentle to prevent the chest tubes from dislodging.
- Assist with deep-breathing and coughing exercises and incentive spirometry as directed. See Chapter 44.
- Call for help at once if a chest tube comes out. Cover the insertion site with sterile gauze or other dressing according to agency policy. Stay with the person. Follow the nurse's directions.
- Complete a safety check before leaving the room. (See the inside of the back cover.)

DEVICES FOR SLEEP APNEA

Sleep apnea is a sleep disorder that causes pauses in breathing during sleep (Chapter 50). The most common cause is blockage of the airway. During sleep, muscles in the throat relax and soft tissues collapse, closing the airway.

Persons with sleep apnea may use a device to keep the airway open.

- *Continuous positive airway pressure (CPAP).* A mask that covers the nose or the nose and mouth is attached to a pump (Fig. 45-10). Air pressure is forced through the mask to keep the airway open. The same amount of pressure goes through the mask when the person inhales and exhales.
- *Bilevel positive airway pressure (BiPAP).* This works like a CPAP except more pressure is given when breathing in. Less pressure is given when breathing out. The change in pressure is more comfortable for some persons.

CPAP and BiPAP are also used to treat other disorders affecting the respiratory system. A nurse or RT manages the device.

Follow agency policy for your role in assisting with devices used during sleep. Pressure injuries are a risk where the mask contacts the skin (Chapter 42).

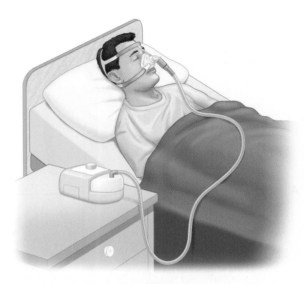

FIGURE 45-10 A continuous positive airway pressure (CPAP) device used for sleep apnea.

FOCUS ON **PRIDE**

The Person, Family, and Yourself

P ersonal and Professional Responsibility

Observing the person and reporting concerns are important parts of your role. Tell the nurse at once if you suspect a problem. Delay can cause harm or death. Take pride in safely assisting with respiratory support and therapies.

R ights and Respect

Persons requiring respiratory support may be comatose or sedated. However, the person may hear and understand. Show dignity and respect when providing care.

- Tell the person when he or she will be moved or touched.
- Explain what the person will feel and where it will be felt.
- Talk to the person. Tell about pleasant things.
- Focus on the person. Do not ignore the person or talk with co-workers about personal matters.
- Use touch to show you care.

I ndependence and Social Interaction

Mechanical ventilation brings fears and worries for the family. Quality time with the person can bring the family peace and ease stress. To provide social support, you can:

- Encourage the family to talk to the person. If the person cannot respond, explain that he or she may hear and understand.
- Allow private time.
- Promote the use of touch. Provide chairs so the family can sit by the person to hold a hand, stroke the hair, and so on.
- Allow family involvement in care measures. Brushing hair, applying lotion, and giving nail care are examples.

D elegation and Teamwork

Some team members have 1 focus of care. For example, the RT provides respiratory treatments and therapies. Develop a good working relationship with the RT. Politely offer to help as needed. The RT is a good source for respiratory issues. Ask questions and thank the RT for answering them.

E thics and Laws

Many respiratory support measures and therapies in this chapter are outside the scope of your role. Serious problems can occur from the wrong care. Know your limits. Assist with care measures as directed. Remember your legal and ethical responsibilities. You have the right to refuse a function or task that is beyond your legal scope, preparation, skill level, and job description.

FOCUS ON **PRIDE**: *Application*

Imagine if a family member required mechanical ventilation. What concerns and fears would you have? Describe the quality of care you would expect. How will you apply these qualities in your interactions with the person and family?

REVIEW QUESTIONS

Circle the BEST answer.

1 A person has a tracheostomy. Which is *true*?
   a The person must not cough.
   b The obturator is kept at the nurses' station.
   c The tube must remain patent.
   d The nurse removes the outer cannula for cleaning.

2 A person with an ET tube vomits. Which is *true*?
   a The ET tube needs to be replaced.
   b The person cannot be suctioned.
   c Aspiration is a risk.
   d The ET tube needs to be removed.

3 A person with a tracheostomy *cannot*
   a Swim
   b Shave
   c Shower with a hand-held nozzle
   d Shampoo

4 The nurse is changing tracheostomy ties. You must
   a Remove the inner cannula
   b Clean the stoma
   c Remove the dressing
   d Hold the outer cannula in place

5 You cannot slide a finger under the tracheostomy ties. This means that the ties
   a Are secured correctly
   b Are too tight
   c Are too loose
   d Need to be replaced

6 Which signals the need for suctioning?
   a A pulse rate of 90 beats per minute
   b Signs and symptoms of altered respiratory function
   c It has been 2 hours since the last suctioning
   d Being unable to speak

7 Suctioning the lower airway requires
   a Sterile technique
   b Mechanical ventilation
   c A Yankauer catheter
   d Chest tubes

8 Your role in suctioning involves
   a Selecting the type of suction catheter
   b Hyperoxygenating the lungs
   c Deciding when to suction the airway
   d Keeping needed supplies at the bedside

9 You note the following while assisting with suctioning. Which should you report at once?
   a A pulse rate of 82 beats per minute
   b A regular heart rhythm
   c Oxygen saturation of 90%
   d Thick secretions

10 A person has an ET tube with mechanical ventilation. Which is *true*?
   a The ET tube must stay attached to the ventilator.
   b You should remove slack from hoses and tubing.
   c The person cannot respond or sense touch.
   d You can re-set alarms on the ventilator.

11 A ventilator alarm sounds. What should you do?
   a Re-set the alarm.
   b Check if the airway is attached to the machine.
   c Do nothing.
   d Ask the person what is wrong.

12 A person has a pneumothorax. This is
   a Fluid in the pleural space
   b Blood in the pleural space
   c Air in the pleural space
   d Secretions in the pleural space

13 Assisting with chest tube care involves
   a Avoiding deep breathing and coughing
   b Making sure tubing is not kinked
   c Keeping the drainage system at chest level
   d Hanging tubing in loops

14 A CPAP is used
   a To collect chest tube drainage
   b For sleep apnea
   c To suction the airway
   d For portable oxygen therapy

Answers to Chapter 45 questions are on p. 903.

FOCUS ON **PRACTICE**

Problem Solving

The nurse suctioned a patient's tracheostomy tube 2 hours ago. Now the person's breathing is noisy and wet-sounding. Coughing has a harsh sound. Is this normal? What do you do? How often is suctioning done?

OBJECTIVES

- Define the key terms and key abbreviations in this chapter.
- Identify the goals of rehabilitation.
- Describe common rehabilitation therapies.
- Describe how rehabilitation involves the whole person.
- Explain the importance of preventing complications.
- Identify complication prevention measures.

- Identify the common reactions to rehabilitation.
- Explain your role in rehabilitation and restorative care.
- List the common rehabilitation programs and services.
- Explain how to promote PRIDE in the person, the family, and yourself.

KEY TERMS

activities of daily living (ADL) The activities usually done during a normal day in a person's life
disability Any lost, absent, or impaired physical or mental function
prosthesis An artificial replacement for a missing body part
rehabilitation The process of restoring a person's highest possible level of physical, psychological, social, and economic function

restorative aide A nursing assistant with special training in restorative nursing and rehabilitation skills
restorative nursing care Nursing care that helps persons regain health and strength for safe and independent living

KEY ABBREVIATIONS

ADL	Activities of daily living	ROM	Range-of-motion

Disease, injury, and surgery can affect body function. So can birth injuries and birth defects (Chapter 55). Often more than 1 function is lost.

A *disability* is any lost, absent, or impaired physical or mental function. Causes are acute or chronic (Box 46-1).

- An *acute problem* has a short course with complete recovery. A fracture (broken bone) is an example.
- A *chronic problem* has a long course. The problem is controlled—not cured—with treatment. Arthritis and paralysis are chronic health problems.

Disabilities can affect eating, speaking, bathing, dressing, walking, work ability, and other functions. The focus of rehabilitation is to restore function or adapt to lost function. Quality of life is promoted.

BOX 46-1	Common Problems Requiring Rehabilitation

- Amputation
- Birth defects
- Brain tumor
- Burns
- Cancer
- Chronic obstructive pulmonary disease
- Fractures
- Head injury
- Intellectual and developmental disabilities (Chapter 55)
- Joint replacement surgery
- Myocardial infarction (heart attack)
- Spinal cord injury or tumor
- Stroke
- Substance use disorder—drug, alcohol
- Wound healing

REHABILITATION

Rehabilitation is the process of restoring a person's highest possible level of physical, psychological, social, and economic function. The goals of rehabilitation are to:

* Prevent or reduce the degree of disability.
* Improve abilities for the highest level of independence. Self-care or returning to work may be a goal. If improved function is not possible, the goal is to prevent further loss of function for the best possible quality of life.
* Help the person adjust to the disability.

Many factors affect recovery. The degree of disability affects how much function is possible. Age and other health problems *(comorbidities)* contribute. For example, heart and respiratory disorders can limit activity level, and diabetes can slow healing. Finances, social support, and motivation are other factors.

Rehabilitation is delivered in different settings. Hospitals and sub-acute and long-term care settings provide rehabilitation services. Out-patient rehabilitation and home care are other options.

See *Focus on Long-Term Care and Home Care: Rehabilitation.*

See *Focus on Children and Older Persons: Rehabilitation.*

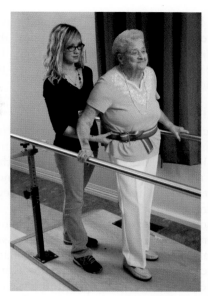

FIGURE 46-1 The person is assisted with walking in physical therapy.

Common Rehabilitation Therapies

Rehabilitation therapies are managed by health care professionals including physical, occupational, speech-language, and respiratory therapists (Chapter 1). Common therapies are:

* *Physical therapy*—focuses on movement and mobility. Exercises and the use of adaptive (assistive) devices help to maintain or improve mobility and function. A physical therapist (PT) plans and directs the person's care (Fig. 46-1).
* *Occupational therapy*—focuses on skills needed for daily living and work. Exercises and adaptations in the person's setting or technique are common. So is the use of adaptive (assistive) devices. An occupational therapist (OT) plans and directs care.
* *Speech-language therapy*—focuses on communication and swallowing. A speech-language pathologist (speech therapist) plans and directs care.
* *Respiratory therapy*—focuses on breathing and respiratory system function. A respiratory therapist (RT) plans and directs care.

RESTORATIVE NURSING

Restorative nursing supports progress made in a rehabilitation therapy program. *Restorative nursing care* is nursing care that helps persons regain health and strength for safe and independent living. The nursing staff delivers care.

Restorative nursing measures promote:

* Healing
* Self-care
* Elimination
* Positioning
* Mobility
* Communication
* Cognitive function

Restorative nursing may begin after a rehabilitation program ends. Or it occurs at the same time. Nursing care

---

FOCUS ON LONG-TERM CARE AND HOME CARE

Rehabilitation

Long-Term Care

Short-term rehabilitation in a long-term care setting is common. The person receives care and therapy until able to return home.

Others have disabilities that are progressive. (The disability gets worse in time.) As function declines, goals and the amount of assistance needed change. However, goals should still promote:

* Maintaining the highest level of function
* Preventing unnecessary decline in function

FOCUS ON CHILDREN AND OLDER PERSONS

Rehabilitation

Older Persons

Rehabilitation may take longer in older persons than in other age-groups. Changes from aging affect healing, mobility, vision, hearing, and other functions. Chronic health problems can slow recovery. Older persons are at risk for injuries. Because fast-paced rehabilitation may be hard, programs for older persons usually are slower-paced.

is aimed at helping the person practice and retain learned skills. For example, a person needs physical therapy for rehabilitation after joint replacement surgery. Outside of therapy, the nursing care plan includes measures to promote mobility and prevent complications.

Restorative Aides

Some agencies have restorative aides. A *restorative aide* is a nursing assistant with special training in restorative nursing and rehabilitation skills. These aides assist the nursing and health teams. Required training varies among states. If there are no state requirements, the agency provides needed training.

The various care measures learned throughout this book are common parts of a restorative aide's role. Assisting with moving, transfers, hygiene, grooming, elimination, feeding, and exercise and activity are examples. Communicating with the person and assisting with the use of adaptive (assistive) devices are others.

Goals will differ depending on the person's needs and abilities. While assisting with care, the restorative aide must understand the goals in the person's care plan to promote independent function.

THE WHOLE PERSON

Health problems and disabilities affect the whole person. Physical, psychological, social, and economic effects occur. The health and nursing teams help the person learn to adjust to changes. Abilities—what the person can do—are stressed.

Physical Aspects

Physical aspects of rehabilitation and restorative nursing involve the prevention of further complications and the promotion of body function and self-care.

Preventing Complications. Complications delay recovery and can cause declines in function. Prevention measures must begin when the person first seeks care for illness, injury, or surgery. Table 46-1 summarizes common complications and prevention measures that are important to your role.

Elimination. Some persons need bladder training (Chapter 27). The method depends on the person's problems, abilities, and needs. Some need bowel training (Chapter 29). Bowel control and regular elimination are goals.

TABLE 46-1	Preventing Complications
Complication	**Prevention Measures**
Muscle atrophy and contractures (Chapter 35)	• Range-of-motion (ROM) exercises • Exercise, activity, and ambulation • Proper use of positioning devices
Pressure injuries (Chapter 42)	• Proper positioning and frequent re-positioning • Proper use of protective devices • Good skin care, hygiene, and incontinence care • Good nutrition and fluid balance
Infection (Chapters 17 and 18)	• Good hand hygiene • Practicing medical asepsis • Following Standard Precautions, Transmission-Based Precautions, and Enhanced Barrier Precautions
Blood clots (Chapter 40)	• Leg exercises • Elastic stockings, elastic bandages, or sequential compression devices • Ambulation
Altered respiratory function (Chapter 44)	• Deep-breathing and coughing exercises • Incentive spirometry • Exercise and activity
Urinary problems—urinary incontinence, urinary retention, urinary tract infection (Chapter 27)	• Promoting normal urinary elimination • Following voiding routines and habits • Following the person's bladder training program if ordered
Bowel problems—constipation, fecal impaction, fecal incontinence (Chapter 29)	• Good nutrition and fluid balance (including increased fiber intake and adequate fluid intake) • Exercise, activity, and ambulation • Promoting normal bowel elimination • Following the person's bowel training program if ordered
Falls (Chapter 15)	• Meeting basic needs • Keeping the call light in reach and responding promptly • Frequent observation • Reminding the person to ask for help to get up • Using a transfer/gait belt and needed walking aids • Performing a safety check before leaving the room

Self-Care. Self-care is a major goal. *Activities of daily living (ADL)* are the activities usually done during a normal day in a person's life. ADL include bathing, oral hygiene, dressing, eating, elimination, and mobility. The health team evaluates the person's ADL abilities and the need for adaptive (assistive) devices. Devices are often changed, made, or bought for the person's needs (Fig. 46-2).

- Eating devices include plate guards and silverware with curved handles or cuffs (straps) (Chapter 31). Some devices attach to splints (see Fig. 46-2, *F*). Special cups with handles, lids, and cut-outs are common.
- Elevated (raised) toilet seats and shower chairs (benches) are common in bathrooms.
- Electric toothbrushes have back-and-forth brushing motions for oral hygiene. Other devices for hygiene, grooming, and changing garments promote independence. See Chapters 24, 25, and 26.
- Various devices are useful for cooking, writing, phone calls, and other tasks. Some are shown in Figure 46-2. See *Focus on Surveys: Self-Care.*

FOCUS ON SURVEYS

Self-Care

Surveyors focus on rehabilitation goals. The ability to perform self-care is an example. Surveyors try to determine if:

- Care measures address the person's needs and rehabilitation goals. For example, is a needed bath mitt available? Does the person use the mitt to bathe?
- The staff follow the care plan. For example, do staff allow and encourage residents to bathe themselves to the extent possible?

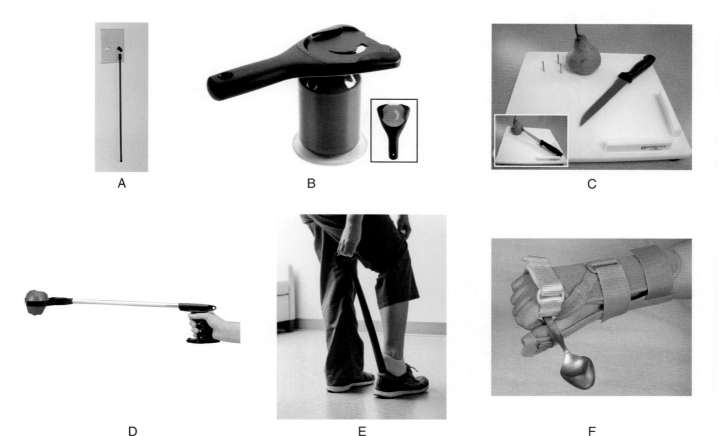

A

B

C

D

E

F

FIGURE 46-2 A, Light switch extender. **B,** Jar opener. **C,** Cutting board. **D,** Reacher. **E,** Shoehorn. **F,** Eating device attached to a splint. (A and C, Courtesy Parsons ADL, Inc. Tottenham, Ontario. B, Courtesy OXO International, Inc., New York, NY. D, Image provided by Performance Health. E, From Perry AG, Potter PA, Ostendorf WR, Laplante N: *Clinical nursing skills and techniques*, ed 10, St. Louis, 2021, Mosby.)

Mobility. The person may need to learn how to move in bed. Or the person may need crutches or a walker, cane, orthotic device, or brace (Chapter 35). Some people need wheelchairs. If possible, they learn wheelchair transfers. Such transfers include to and from the bed, toilet, bathtub, sofa, and chair and in and out of vehicles (Figs. 46-3, 46-4, and 46-5).

An amputation also affects mobility. A *prosthesis* is an artificial replacement for a missing body part. The person learns how to use the artificial arm or leg (Chapter 49). The goal is for the device to be like the missing body part in function and appearance.

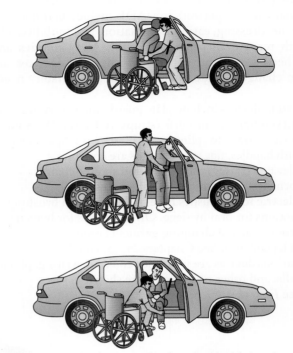

FIGURE 46-5 The person transfers from the wheelchair to the car.

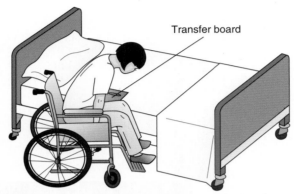

FIGURE 46-3 The person uses a transfer board (sliding board) to transfer from a wheelchair to bed.

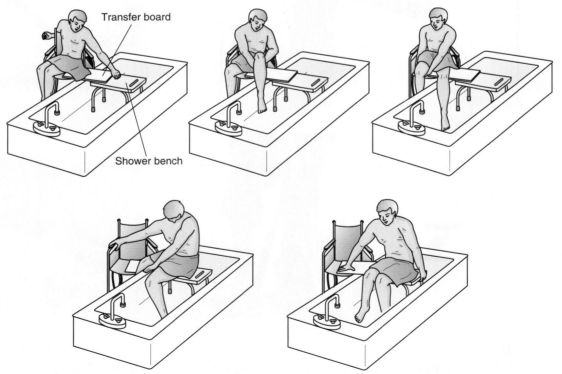

FIGURE 46-4 A wheelchair to tub transfer. A transfer board (sliding board) and shower bench are used.

Nutrition. Difficulty swallowing *(dysphagia)* may occur after a stroke. The person may need a dysphagia diet (Chapter 31). If possible, the person learns exercises to improve swallowing. Persons who cannot swallow need enteral nutrition (Chapter 33).

Mechanical Ventilation. Some persons needing mechanical ventilation (Chapter 45) are weaned from the ventilator. That is, the person learns to breathe without the machine. The process may take many weeks. Other persons learn to live with life-long mechanical ventilation.

Communication

Aphasia (Chapter 47) may occur from a stroke. *Aphasia* is the total or partial loss *(a)* of the ability to use or understand language *(phasia)*. It results from damage to parts of the brain responsible for language and speech. Speech therapy and communication devices are helpful (Chapters 7 and 47).

See *Focus on Communication: Communication*.

FOCUS ON COMMUNICATION

Communication

Persons with speech disorders may need other communication methods. Pictures, reading, writing, facial expressions, and gestures are examples. All health team members and the family use the same method with the person. Changing methods can cause confusion and delay progress.

Psychological and Social Aspects

Functional changes affect the person mentally and socially. Self-esteem, family and work roles, and relationships may change. Appearance is often affected. Feelings of being unwhole, useless, unattractive, or undesirable can occur. Some persons become depressed or angry.

Some persons deny the disability. Others expect that therapy will quickly correct the problem. Some think therapy time alone is enough to make progress. The nurse and therapist help the person with expectations, goals, and a plan of care.

A good attitude and motivation are important. Maintaining these can be hard for the person. Progress may be slow. Learning a new task is a reminder of the disability. The fear of losing independence brings many worries. The person may need help coping. Report these signs.

- Expressing feelings like hopelessness, uselessness, or worry
- Anger directed at others
- Expressing a negative self-image
- Dependence (relying on others for care)
- Depression (Chapter 53)

Allow persons to express their feelings. Listen patiently. Remind persons of their progress. Give support, reassurance, and encouragement. Focus on abilities and strengths. Psychological and social needs are part of the care plan. Spiritual support helps some persons.

See *Focus on Communication: Psychological and Social Aspects*.

FOCUS ON COMMUNICATION

Psychological and Social Aspects

Emotional needs are great during rehabilitation. Good communication and support provide encouragement.

- Listen to the person.
- Show concern, not pity.
- Focus on what the person can do. Point out even slight progress.
- Be polite but firm. Do not let the person control you.
- Do not shout at or insult the person. Such behaviors are abuse and mistreatment.
- Do not argue with the person.
- Tell the nurse about problems. The person may need other support measures.

Economic Aspects

Some persons return to their jobs. Those who cannot do so are assessed for work skills, work history, interests, and talents. A job skill may be restored or a new one learned. The goal is gainful employment. Help is given finding a job.

THE PERSON'S SETTING

The setting must be safe and meet the person's needs (Chapter 13). Needed changes are made. For example, the over-bed table, bedside stand, call light, and other needed items are moved to a person's strong (unaffected) side. If unable to use the call light, another communication aid is used. The rehabilitation team helps the person and family plan for needed changes at home.

See *Focus on Long-Term Care and Home Care: The Person's Setting*.

FOCUS ON LONG-TERM CARE AND HOME CARE

The Person's Setting

Home Care

The rehabilitation team assesses the person's home setting. For safety and care needs, some persons require personal attendants 24 hours a day. Changes or repairs in the home are made as needed. For example:

- Grab bars (safety bars) are installed in the bathroom.
- A hand-held shower nozzle is installed. A shower chair is purchased.
- Door knobs are changed to lever handles.
- Hand rails are installed in stairways and by outside steps.
- Night-lights are placed in bedrooms and bathrooms.
- An electric lift chair is purchased for the person to use.
- Chairs are placed where the person can sit with ease.

THE REHABILITATION TEAM

Rehabilitation is a team effort. The person is the key team member. The person, family, doctor, and nursing and health teams set goals and plan care. The focus is to regain function and independence.

The team meets often to discuss the person's progress. The rehabilitation plan is changed as needed. The person and family attend the meetings when possible. Families provide support and encouragement. Often they help with home care.

Your Role

You help promote the person's independence. Preventing decline in function also is a goal. The many procedures, care measures, and rules in this book apply. Safety, communication, legal, and ethical aspects apply. So do the measures in Box 46-2.

See *Focus on Communication: Your Role.*

FOCUS ON COMMUNICATION

Your Role

The nurse or therapist teaches the person and family about measures to gain function and independence. If the person or family needs more teaching, tell the nurse.

You may need to guide and direct the person during care. Listen to how the nurse or therapist guides and directs the person. Use those words. Hearing the same thing helps the person learn and remember what to do.

REHABILITATION PROGRAMS

Common rehabilitation programs include:
- *Cardiac rehabilitation*—for heart disorders
- *Brain injury rehabilitation*—for nervous system disorders including traumatic brain injury
- *Spinal cord rehabilitation*—for spinal cord injuries
- *Stroke rehabilitation*—after a stroke
- *Respiratory rehabilitation*—for respiratory system disorders such as chronic obstructive pulmonary disease, after lung surgery, for respiratory complications from other health problems, and for mechanical ventilation
- *Orthopedic rehabilitation*—for fractures, joint replacement surgery, and other musculo-skeletal problems
- *Amputee rehabilitation*—for amputation of a limb
- *Hearing, speech, and vision rehabilitation*—for persons who are hard of hearing or deaf, have speech problems, are blind, or have severe vision problems
- *Drug and alcohol treatment*—for persons addicted to drugs or alcohol
- *Behavioral health treatment*—for those with mental health disorders
- *Rehabilitation for complex medical and surgical conditions*—wound care, diabetes, and burns are examples

See *Focus on Children and Older Persons: Rehabilitation Programs.*

See *Focus on Long-Term Care and Home Care: Rehabilitation Programs.*

BOX 46-2 Assisting With Rehabilitation Needs

Physical Needs
- Follow the care plan and the nurse's instructions.
- Follow the person's daily routine.
- Provide for safety.
- Report early signs and symptoms of complications. See Table 46-1 for complications.
- Keep the person in good alignment.
- Turn and re-position the person as directed.
- Use safe transfer methods.
- Practice measures to prevent pressure injuries.
- Perform ROM exercises as instructed.
- Remember that muscles will atrophy if not used. Contractures can also develop.
- Provide needed adaptive (assistive) devices.
- Know how to use and apply needed devices. For splints, orthotic devices, and prostheses:
  - Have the nurse or therapist show you how to apply the device. Do not guess. Practice application with supervision before doing so alone.
  - Check skin that has contact with the device for signs of pressure (Chapter 42). Report concerns.
  - Provide good skin care to areas that have contact with the device. Skin should be clean and dry before application.

Psychological and Social Needs
- Protect the person's rights. Privacy and personal choice are very important.
- Encourage performing ADL to the extent possible.
- Allow time to complete tasks. Do not rush the person.
- Give praise for even a little progress.
- Provide emotional support and reassurance.
- Try to understand and appreciate the person's situation, feelings, and concerns.
- Do not pity the person or give sympathy.
- Provide for spiritual needs.
- Practice the methods developed by the rehabilitation team. You will better assist the person.
- Practice the task that the person must do. This helps you guide and direct the person.
- Stress what the person can do. Focus on abilities and strengths, not on disabilities and weaknesses.
- Have a hopeful outlook.

FOCUS ON **CHILDREN AND OLDER PERSONS**

Rehabilitation Programs

Children

Federal laws require that schools provide needed therapies. In-school therapy is required to meet the child's learning needs.

FOCUS ON **LONG-TERM CARE AND HOME CARE**

Rehabilitation Programs

Long-Term Care

Nursing centers must provide rehabilitation services required by a person's care plan. If not provided by center staff, the service is obtained from another source. For example, a person's care plan includes speech therapy. The center does not have a speech therapist. The service is obtained from another agency.

QUALITY OF LIFE

Successful rehabilitation improves quality of life. A hopeful and winning outlook is needed. The more the person can do alone, the better the person's quality of life. See *Focus on PRIDE: The Person, Family, and Yourself* for ways to promote independence.

To promote quality of life:

* Protect the right to privacy.
* Encourage personal choice.
* Protect the right to be free from abuse and mistreatment.
* Encourage activities.
* Provide a safe setting.
* Show patience, understanding, and sensitivity.

FOCUS ON **PRIDE**

The Person, Family, and Yourself

Personal and Professional Responsibility

Often nursing assistants are promoted to restorative aide positions. Professional behaviors are highly valued for promotions. Patience, kindness, and good communication skills are needed. Staff with a positive attitude, good work ethics, and excellent job performance are considered first.

Becoming a restorative aide allows you to advance as a nursing assistant. Seek out learning opportunities and practice positive work habits. Take pride in continuing to learn, improve, and grow as a nursing assistant.

Rights and Respect

Rehabilitation is challenging for the person, the family, and the nursing staff. No matter how difficult the situation, the person's rights are always protected. See Chapter 2.

Losing patience can cause frustration. Unkind remarks and actions toward the person are not allowed. Protect the person from abuse and mistreatment. Treat the person with dignity and respect.

Independence and Social Interaction

Quality of life improves the more the person can do independently. To promote independence:

* Stress the person's abilities and strengths.
* Let the person choose activities of interest.
* Remain patient. Do not rush the person.
* Promote self-care. Know what the person can do. Resist the urge to do those things for the person.
* Provide limited help if the person needs only some help.
* Offer encouragement and support.
* Have the person use adaptive (assistive) devices as needed.
* Encourage personal choice. Personal choice allows control.

Delegation and Teamwork

Disability affects the whole person. The person may be overwhelmed, sad, angry, or discouraged. Such feelings can be hard to control. Outbursts may occur.

The person does not choose loss of function. If the person's emotional responses upset you, think how the person must feel. You must:

* Show patience, understanding, sensitivity, and respect.
* Be calm and act in a professional manner.
* Control your words and actions.

The nurse can suggest ways to help you control or express your feelings. You may need to assist with other persons for a while. Take pride in being a part of a strong, supportive team.

Ethics and Laws

The person may not want to practice rehabilitation procedures or methods. The person may want you to give care instead. To make progress, the person needs to follow the rehabilitation plan. Report any problems to the nurse.

FOCUS ON **PRIDE**: *Application*

Do you know someone with a disability? How does the disability affect the whole person? How does it affect the person's family?

REVIEW QUESTIONS

Circle the BEST answer.

1 Which statement about rehabilitation is *true*?
   a Only chronic problems require rehabilitation.
   b Rehabilitation for older persons is usually fast-paced.
   c You do not need to know how to use the person's adaptive (assistive) devices.
   d Personal preferences are considered in the rehabilitation plan.

2 What is the focus of rehabilitation and restorative nursing care?
   a Depending on others to meet basic needs
   b Recovering quickly from injury or illness
   c Restoring and maintaining function
   d Accepting loss of function with a positive attitude

3 Complications following illness, injury, or surgery
   a Cannot be prevented
   b Are minor
   c Are only a concern if signs and symptoms are present
   d Delay recovery and rehabilitation

4 You are helping a person dress. The person is supposed to practice using a shoehorn to put on shoes. Which comment is *best*?
   a "If I put your shoes on you, we will finish faster."
   b "You are doing well. Let me know if you need help tying."
   c "It is so sad that you cannot put your shoes on anymore."
   d "You should be able to do this without the shoehorn."

5 A person has weakness on the right side. ADL are
   a Done by the person to the extent possible
   b Done by you
   c Delayed until the right side can be used
   d Done by a therapist

6 Which shows you understand the psychological effects of rehabilitation?
   a You laugh when the person makes mistakes.
   b You talk about the person's weaknesses more than strengths.
   c You convey hopefulness and talk about what the person can do.
   d You argue with the person about the best way to do a task.

7 To provide emotional support during rehabilitation
   a Remind residents of their limits
   b Give sympathy and show pity
   c Talk about your feelings
   d Listen and give praise

8 A person is not allowed food until exercises are done. This is abuse and mistreatment.
   a True
   b False

9 During therapy, a person wants music played. You should
   a Explain that music is not allowed
   b Choose some music
   c Ask the person to choose some music
   d Ask a therapist to choose some music

10 A person's right side is weak. You move the call light to the left side. You promote quality of life by
   a Encouraging self-care
   b Allowing personal choice
   c Providing for safety
   d Taking part in activities

Answers to Chapter 46 questions are on p. 903.

FOCUS ON PRACTICE

Problem Solving

A person's care plan includes long-handled devices for dressing and bathing. During the bath, you provide a long-handled sponge. The person says: "I don't feel like using that today. Will you wash my feet for me?" What will you say and do? How will your response affect the person's progress?

Hearing, Speech, and Vision Problems

OBJECTIVES

- Define the key terms and key abbreviations in this chapter.
- Describe the common ear, speech, and eye disorders.
- Describe how to communicate with persons who have hearing loss.
- Explain the purpose of a hearing aid.
- Describe how to care for hearing aids.

- Explain how to communicate with persons who have speech disorders.
- Explain how to assist persons who are visually impaired or blind.
- Explain how to protect an ocular prosthesis from loss or damage.
- Perform the procedure described in this chapter.
- Explain how to promote PRIDE in the person, the family, and yourself.

KEY TERMS

aphasia The total or partial loss *(a)* of the ability to use or understand language *(phasia)*

blindness The absence of sight

braille A touch reading and writing system that uses raised dots for each letter of the alphabet; the first 10 letters also represent the numbers 0 through 9

Broca's aphasia See "expressive aphasia"

cerumen Earwax

deafness Hearing loss in which it is impossible for the person to understand speech through hearing alone

expressive aphasia Difficulty expressing or sending out thoughts through speech or writing; Broca's aphasia

global aphasia Difficulty expressing or sending out thoughts and difficulty understanding language; mixed aphasia

hearing loss Not being able to hear the range of sounds associated with normal hearing

low vision Impaired vision that cannot be corrected with eyeglasses, contact lenses, drugs, or surgery; vision changes interfere with every-day activities

mixed aphasia See "global aphasia"

presbycusis Decreased hearing ability due to aging; age-related hearing loss

presbyopia The gradual loss of the ability to focus on close-up objects that occurs with aging

receptive aphasia Difficulty understanding language; Wernicke's aphasia

tinnitus A ringing, roaring, hissing, or buzzing sound in the ears or head

vertigo Dizziness

Wernicke's aphasia See "receptive aphasia"

KEY ABBREVIATIONS

ADA	Americans with Disabilities Act of 1990
AMD	Age-related macular degeneration

ASL	American Sign Language

Hearing, speech, and vision are important for self-care, work, most activities, and safety and security needs. Hearing, speech, and vision disorders occur in all age-groups. Common causes are birth defects, injuries, infections, diseases, and aging.

HEARING DISORDERS

The ear functions in hearing and balance. Hearing is needed for clear speech, responding to others, safety, and awareness of surroundings.

See *Body Structure and Function Review: The Ear*, p. 710.

BODY STRUCTURE AND FUNCTION REVIEW
The Ear

Structure and Function
A sense organ, the ear (Fig. 47-1) functions in hearing and balance. It has 3 parts: the *external ear, middle ear,* and *inner ear.*

Sound waves are guided through the external ear (outer part) into the *auditory canal.* Glands in the auditory canal secrete a waxy substance called *cerumen.* The auditory canal extends about 1 inch into the *eardrum.* The eardrum *(tympanic membrane)* separates the external and middle ear.

The middle ear contains the *eustachian tube* and 3 small bones called *ossicles.* The eustachian tube connects the middle ear and the throat. Air enters the eustachian tube so there is equal pressure on both sides of the eardrum. The ossicles amplify sound received from the eardrum and transmit the sound to the inner ear. The 3 ossicles are:
- The *malleus*—looks like a hammer.
- The *incus*—looks like an anvil.
- The *stapes*—is shaped like a stirrup.

The inner ear consists of *semicircular canals* and the *cochlea.* The cochlea looks like a snail shell. It contains fluid that carries sound waves from the middle ear to the *acoustic nerve.* The acoustic nerve then carries messages to the brain.

The 3 semicircular canals are involved with balance. They sense the head's position and changes in position. They send messages to the brain.

Changes With Aging
Presbycusis (age-related hearing loss) is decreased hearing ability due to aging. Changes in hearing occur gradually. Changes in the inner ear and acoustic nerve are part of the cause. High-pitched sounds especially become hard to hear. Age-related hearing loss is common.

Earwax can harden and thicken with age. It can become lodged (impacted) in the ear and affect hearing.

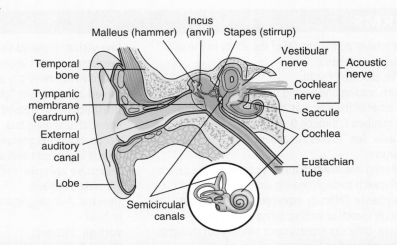

FIGURE 47-1 The ear.

Otitis Media
Otitis media is an infection *(itis)* of the middle *(media)* ear *(ot)*. It often begins with sore throats, colds, the flu, allergies, or other respiratory infections that spread to the middle ear. Viruses and bacteria are causes.

Otitis media is acute or chronic. Chronic otitis media can damage the structures needed for hearing. Permanent hearing loss can occur.

Fluid builds up in the ear. Pain (earache), hearing loss, fever, and tinnitus occur. *Tinnitus* is a ringing, roaring, hissing, or buzzing sound in the ears or head. An untreated infection can spread to nearby structures in the head. Antibiotics, pain-relief drugs, and drugs to relieve congestion are often used for treatment.

See *Focus on Children and Older Persons: Otitis Media.*

FOCUS ON CHILDREN AND OLDER PERSONS
Otitis Media

Children
Otitis media is common in infants and children. Infants cannot tell you about an earache. The child may:
- Have ear pain or an earache.
- Have a fever.
- Tug or pull at the ears.
- Roll the head back.
- Cry more than usual.
- Be fussy and irritable.
- Have fluid draining from the ear.
- Sleep poorly.
- Be dizzy or have problems with balance.
- Have trouble hearing.
- Not respond to quiet sounds.

Older Persons
Otitis media can occur in adults. They may have some of the same signs and symptoms as children. Persons with dementia may show behavior changes.

Meniere's Disease

Meniere's disease involves the inner ear. Fluid buildup in the inner ear causes swelling and pressure. Usually 1 ear is affected. Symptoms are sudden. They include:

- *Vertigo*—dizziness
- Tinnitus
- Hearing loss
- Feeling of fullness or pressure in the ear

An attack usually involves vertigo, tinnitus, and hearing loss. Vertigo causes whirling and spinning sensations. The dizziness causes severe nausea and vomiting. An episode can last 20 minutes or 2 to 24 hours.

Drugs and a low-salt diet may decrease fluid in the ear. Smoking, caffeine, and alcohol are avoided. Safety is needed during vertigo.

- Have the person lie down.
- Prevent falls. Assist with walking and use bed rails according to the care plan.
- Have the person keep the head still and focus on an object that does not move. The person avoids turning the head. Do not move around while talking with the person.
- Avoid sudden movements. The person moves slowly.
- Prevent flashing lights (such as from TV) and bright lights.

Hearing Loss

Hearing loss is not being able to hear the range of sounds associated with normal hearing. Losses are mild to deafness. *Deafness* is hearing loss in which it is impossible for the person to understand speech through hearing alone.

Causes include damage to the outer, middle, or inner ear or to the acoustic nerve. See Box 47-1 for the risk factors and signs and symptoms of hearing loss.

Temporary hearing loss can occur from earwax *(cerumen)*. Hearing improves after the earwax is removed.

See *Focus on Communication: Hearing Loss.*
See *Promoting Safety and Comfort: Hearing Loss.*

FOCUS ON COMMUNICATION

Hearing Loss

The National Association of the Deaf (NAD) uses the terms *deaf* and *hard of hearing* to describe persons with hearing loss. Do not use the terms *deaf and dumb, deaf-mute,* or *hearing-impaired.* Such terms may offend persons who are hard of hearing.

PROMOTING SAFETY AND COMFORT

Hearing Loss

Safety
Do not try to remove earwax. This is done by a doctor or a nurse. Do not insert anything, including cotton swabs, into the ear.

Effects on the Person. A person may deny hearing loss or not notice gradual hearing loss. Others may see changes in the person's behavior or attitude but not suspect hearing loss.

Psychological and social changes may occur. People may shun social events to avoid embarrassment because of giving wrong answers or responses. Or they try to control conversations. They may feel lonely, bored, and left out. Only parts of conversations are heard. They think others are talking about them or are talking softly on purpose. Straining and working hard to hear can cause fatigue, frustration, and irritability.

Hearing is needed for clear speech. Pronouncing words and voice volume depend on hearing yourself. Hearing loss may result in slurred speech or pronouncing words wrong. Some people have monotone speech or drop word endings. It may be hard to understand the person. Do not assume or pretend that you understand. Serious problems can result. See "Speech Disorders" on p. 715.

See *Focus on Children and Older Persons: Effects on the Person,* p. 712.

BOX 47-1	Hearing Loss

Risk Factors

- Aging—ear structures change
- Loud noise:
  - A short blast (explosion, gunshot)
  - Occupational exposure (farming, factory work)
  - Recreational exposure (loud music including with earbuds, motorcycle, airplane)
- Heredity—greater risk for ear damage or changes from aging
- Some drugs—antibiotics, chemotherapy
- Some illnesses—ear infection, stroke, tumor
- Trauma—head injury

Signs and Symptoms

- Problems:
  - Hearing on the phone
  - Hearing with background noise or in noisy areas
  - Following conversations when 2 or more people are speaking
  - Understanding women and children
- Straining to understand a conversation
- Hearing voices as mumbled or slurred
- Misunderstanding what others say
- Answering questions or responding inappropriately
- Asking others to repeat themselves
- Speaking too loudly
- Leaning forward to hear
- Turning and cupping the better ear toward the speaker
- Turning up the TV, radio, music, or other sound sources so loud that others complain

FOCUS ON CHILDREN AND OLDER PERSONS

Effects on the Person

Children

Hearing problems may be present at birth or develop as the child grows. Hearing is needed for speech and language development. Children learn to talk by imitating sounds and voices.

Medical attention is needed if a child does not hear well or speak clearly. See Box 47-2. Items checked "No" may signal hearing loss or a communication problem. Report concerns about a child's hearing to the nurse.

Communication. Persons with hearing loss may wear hearing aids (p. 714) or lip-read (speech-read). They watch facial expressions, gestures, and body language. American Sign Language (ASL) uses signs made with the hands and other movements such as facial expressions, gestures, and postures (Figs. 47-2 and 47-3). (Different sign languages are used in different countries. For example, British Sign Language is different from ASL.)

Some people have *hearing dogs.* The dog alerts the person to sounds. Phones, doorbells, smoke alarms, alarm clocks, babies' cries, sirens, and on-coming cars are examples.

See Box 47-3 (p. 714) for measures to promote hearing and communication.

BOX 47-2   Hearing Checklist for Children

Items marked "No" may signal hearing loss or a communication problem.

Birth to 3 Months
- Reacts to loud sounds.
- Calms down or smiles when spoken to.
- Recognizes your voice and calms down if crying.
- When feeding, starts or stops sucking in response to sound.
- Coos and makes pleasure sounds.
- Has a special way of crying for different needs.
- Smiles when he or she sees you.

4 to 6 Months
- Follows sounds with his or her eyes.
- Responds to changes in the tone of your voice.
- Notices toys that make sounds.
- Pays attention to music.
- Babbles in a speech-like way and uses many different sounds, including sounds that begin with *p, b,* and *m.*
- Laughs.
- Babbles when excited or unhappy.
- Makes gurgling sounds when alone or playing with you.

7 Months to 1 Year
- Enjoys playing peek-a-boo and pat-a-cake.
- Turns and looks in the direction of sounds.
- Listens when spoken to.
- Understands words for common items such as "cup," "shoe," or "juice."
- Responds to requests ("Come here.").
- Babbles using long and short groups of sounds ("tata," "upup," "bibibi").
- Babbles to get and keep attention.
- Communicates using gestures such as waving or holding up arms.
- Imitates different speech sounds.
- Has 1 or 2 words ("Hi," "dog," "Dada," or "Mama") by first birthday.

1 to 2 Years
- Knows a few parts of the body and can point to them when asked.
- Follows simple commands ("Roll the ball.") and understands simple questions ("Where's your shoe?").
- Enjoys simple stories, songs, and rhymes.

1 to 2 Years—cont'd
- Points to pictures, when named, in books.
- Acquires new words on a regular basis.
- Uses some 1- or 2-word questions ("Where kitty?" or "Go bye-bye?").
- Puts 2 words together ("More cookie.").
- Uses many different consonant sounds at the beginning of words.

2 to 3 Years
- Has a word for almost everything.
- Uses 2- or 3-word phrases to talk about and ask for things.
- Uses *k, g, f, t, d,* and *n* sounds.
- Speaks in a way that is understood by family members and friends.
- Names objects to ask for them or to direct attention to them.

3 to 4 Years
- Hears you when you call from another room.
- Hears the TV or radio at the same sound level as other family members.
- Answers simple "Who?" "What?" "Where?" and "Why?" questions.
- Talks about activities at day care, pre-school, or friends' homes.
- Uses sentences with 4 or more words.
- Speaks easily without repeating syllables or words.

4 to 5 Years
- Pays attention to a short story and answers simple questions about it.
- Hears and understands most of what is said at home and in school.
- Uses sentences that give many details.
- Tells stories that stay on topic.
- Communicates easily with other children and adults.
- Says most sounds correctly except for a few (*l, s, r, v, z, ch, sh,* and *th*).
- Uses rhyming words.
- Names some letters and numbers.
- Uses adult grammar.

Modified from National Institute on Deafness and Other Communication Disorders: Your baby's hearing and communicative development checklist, *NIH Publication No. 10-4040, Bethesda, Md, updated March 6, 2017, National Institutes of Health.*

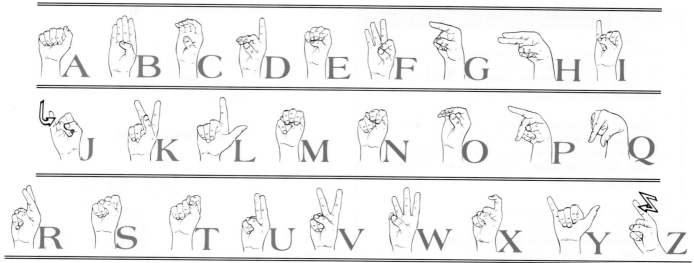

FIGURE 47-2 Manual alphabet. (Courtesy National Association of the Deaf, Silver Spring, Md.)

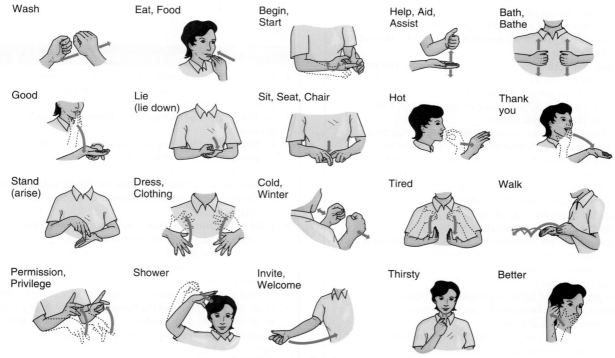

FIGURE 47-3 American Sign Language examples.

BOX 47-3 Measures to Promote Hearing

The Setting

- Reduce or eliminate background noises. Turn off radios, music players, TVs, fans, and so on.
- Provide a quiet place to talk. Avoid areas with loud sound.
- Have the person sit where able to hear best.

The Person

- Make sure the person's hearing aid is turned on, working, and properly placed in or behind the ear.
- Have the person wear needed eyeglasses or contact lenses. The person needs to see your face to lip-read (speech-read).

You

- Gain attention. Alert the person to your presence. Raise an arm or hand or lightly touch the person's hand, arm, or shoulder. Do not startle or approach the person from behind.
- Position yourself at the person's level. Sit if the person is sitting. Stand if the person is standing.
- Face the person when speaking. Do not turn or walk away while you are talking. Do not talk from the doorway or another room.
- Have light shine on your face. Shadows and glares affect the ability to see your face clearly.
- Maintain eye contact with the person.
- Speak clearly, distinctly, and at a normal rate. Do not talk too fast or too slow.
- Speak in a normal tone of voice. Do not shout or mumble.
- State the person's name before starting a conversation. This gains the person's attention and focus.
- Adjust the pitch of your voice as needed. Ask if the person can hear you better.
  - If no hearing aid, lower the pitch. Higher-pitched voices can be harder to hear than lower-pitched voices.
  - If a hearing aid is worn, raise the pitch slightly.
- Do not cover your mouth, smoke, eat, or chew gum while talking. Mouth movements are affected.
- Keep your hands away from your face.
- Stand or sit on the side of the better ear.
- State the topic of conversation first.
- Say when you are changing the subject. State the new topic.
- Use short sentences and simple words.
- Pause between sentences. Ensure understanding before speaking again.
- Use gestures and facial expressions as useful clues.
- Write out important names, words, numbers, addresses, appointments, and so on.
- Re-phrase if the person does not seem to understand. Do not repeat the same words again and again.
- Keep conversations and discussions short. This avoids tiring the person.
- Be alert to messages sent by your facial expressions, gestures, and body language.
- Be alert to the person's nonverbal communication. For example, watch for puzzled looks and expressions of anger, frustration, excitement, fatigue, and so on.

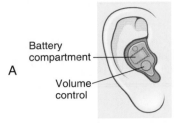

In-the-ear hearing aid

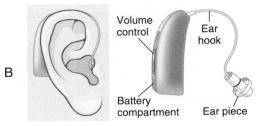

Behind-the-ear hearing aid

FIGURE 47-4 Hearing aids. **A,** An in-the-ear hearing aid. **B,** A behind-the-ear hearing aid. (From Chabner D-E: *The language of medicine*, ed 12, St Louis, 2021, Elsevier.)

BOX 47-4 Hearing Aids: Care Measures

- Hold and handle hearing aids gently. This includes when removing, inserting, or cleaning the device and when inserting batteries.
- Do the following if a hearing aid does not seem to work properly.
  - Check if the hearing aid is *on.* The device has an *on* and *off* switch or function.
  - Check the battery position.
  - Insert a new battery if needed. Use the correct battery size.
  - Clean the hearing aid. Follow the manufacturer's instructions.
- Hold the hearing aid over a soft cloth or soft surface to change the battery or to clean the device.
- Clean the hearing aid according to the manufacturer's instructions. Wiping with a soft, dry cloth is a common cleaning method.
- Do not expose the hearing aid to heat or extreme cold.
- Have the person remove the hearing aid before using a hair dryer, hair spray, spray perfumes, shaving lotions, or powders.
- Protect the hearing aid from water. The person does not wear a hearing aid during a bath or shower or when shampooing the hair.
- Check meal trays and bed linens for hearing aids. The person may have removed the hearing aid and set it aside.
- Remove and turn off the hearing aid at bedtime. This saves battery life. Remove the battery if the person prefers.
- Place the hearing aid in its storage case when not worn. Place the storage case in the top drawer of the bedside stand.

Hearing Aids. *Hearing aids* make sounds louder. They do not correct, restore, or cure hearing problems. The person hears better because the device makes sounds louder. Background noise and speech are louder. Some types can reduce background noise. The measures in Box 47-3 apply.

Two common types of hearing aids are in-the-ear and behind-the-ear (Fig. 47-4). Hearing aids are costly. Protect them from damage. The care measures in Box 47-4 are general. Follow the manufacturer's instructions and the nurse's directions for how to insert, remove, and care for the person's hearing aid.

Other Hearing Devices and Services. Other devices and services can help the person with hearing loss.

- *Phone amplifying devices.* Special phone receivers make sounds louder. Some phones work with hearing aids.
- *Telecommunications Relay Services (TRS).* These services allow persons with hearing loss or speech disorders to communicate by telephone. The *Americans with Disabilities Act (ADA) of 1990* requires access to such services. There are different types of TRS available. All involve a communications assistant (CA) or use of technology to relay messages between callers (Fig. 47-5). Confidentiality of all conversations is maintained. In the United States, dial 711 to access TRS. Emergency 911 services are accessible by dialing 911 directly.
- *Internet services and equipment.* The *Twenty-First Century Communications and Video Accessibility Act* requires that persons with disabilities be able to access and use Internet services and equipment.
- *TV and radio listening systems.* These are used with or without hearing aids. The person does not have to turn the volume up high.
- Smoke alarms with strobe lights.
- Doorbells that can be heard throughout the house.

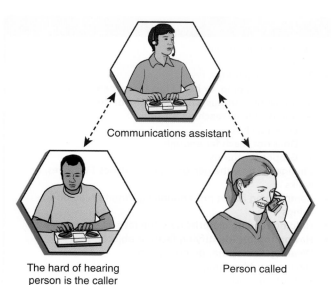

Communications assistant

The hard of hearing person is the caller

Person called

FIGURE 47-5 Telecommunications Relay Services (TRS) allow persons with hearing loss or speech disorders to communicate by telephone. With the system shown, a teletypewriter (text telephone; TTY) and communications assistant (CA) are used to relay typed and spoken messages between callers.

SPEECH DISORDERS

Speech disorders affect oral communication. Hearing loss, developmental disabilities (Chapter 55), and brain injury are common causes. These problems are common.

- *Aphasia.* See "Aphasia" on p. 716.
- *Apraxia of speech. Apraxia* means not (*a*) to act, do, or perform (*praxia*). The brain is unable to direct the movements needed for normal sound production. The person understands and knows what to say. However, the person cannot use speech muscles to make words for understandable speech.
- *Dysarthria. Dysarthria* means difficult or poor (*dys*) speech (*arthria*). The muscles used for speech are weak. Slurred, soft, slow, or hoarse speech can occur.

To communicate with a person with a speech disorder, practice the measures in Box 47-5.

A speech-language pathologist can help the person:

- Use remaining abilities.
- Restore or improve language abilities to the extent possible.
- Learn communication methods.
- Strengthen speech muscles.

BOX 47-5	Communicating With Persons With Speech Disorders

The Person
- Have the person repeat or re-phrase statements as needed.
- Have the person write down key words or the message.
- Have the person point, gesture, or draw key words.
- Have the person use picture boards (Chapter 7) as needed.

You
- Follow the care plan for a consistent approach.
- Provide a calm, quiet setting. Turn off the TV, radio, music, and other distractions.
- Include the person in conversations.
- Listen and give the person your full attention.
- Use short, simple sentences.
- Repeat yourself as needed.
- Repeat what the person has said. Ask if you understood correctly.
- Write down key words as needed.
- Speak in a normal tone. Do not talk in a babyish or child-like way.
- Ask questions to which you know the answers. This helps you learn how the person speaks.
- Allow the person enough time to talk.
- Determine the topic being discussed. This helps you understand main points.
- Watch lip movements.
- Watch facial expressions, gestures, and body language. They give clues about what is being said.
- Do not correct the person's speech.
- Be patient and kind. Emotional needs are great. Frustration, depression, and anger can occur.

Improvement depends on many factors. They include the cause, amount, and area of brain or nerve damage; age; health; and willingness and ability to learn.

Aphasia

Aphasia is the total or partial loss *(a)* of the ability to use or understand language *(phasia)*. Parts of the brain responsible for language are damaged. Stroke, head injury, brain infections, dementia, and brain tumors are common causes.

Expressive aphasia (Broca's aphasia) relates to difficulty expressing or sending out thoughts through speech or writing. The person knows what to say but has problems speaking or writing. The person can usually understand others. The person may:

- Omit small words such as "is," "and," "of," and "the."
- Speak in 1-word or short sentences (fewer than 4 words). For example, the person says "2 cup table" to mean "There are 2 cups on the table."
- Put words in the wrong order. The person may say "room bath" for "bathroom."
- Think one thing but say another. For example, the person wants food but asks for a book.
- Call people the wrong names.
- Make up words.
- Produce sounds and no words.

Receptive aphasia (Wernicke's aphasia) is difficulty understanding language. The person has trouble understanding what is said or written. The person may speak using long sentences with no meaning. The person says unnecessary words and uses made-up words. The person is often unaware of mistakes.

Some people have both expressive and receptive aphasia. *Global aphasia (mixed aphasia)* involves difficulty expressing or sending out thoughts and difficulty understanding language. The person has problems speaking and understanding language.

EYE DISORDERS

Vision problems range from mild loss to complete blindness. *Blindness* is the absence of sight. Vision loss is sudden or gradual. One or both eyes are affected. See Box 47-6 for the signs and symptoms of vision problems.

See *Body Structure and Function Review: The Eye.*

BOX 47-6	**Vision Problems: Signs and Symptoms**

The Person Reports:

- Hazy, blurred, cloudy, or double vision
- Pain or discomfort by or in the eye: sudden or recurring
- Flashes of light
- Halos, rainbows, or rings around lights
- Spots or "floaters"
- Sensitivity or pain to light or glares
- Headaches
- Pain or pressure on the forehead or behind the eyes
- Sudden change or loss of vision in an eye
- Burning, itching, or redness in an eye
- Drainage from an eye
- Tearing
- Seeing a dark "curtain" come down over the eye
- Problems seeing at night
- An eye injury
- A swollen eye

You Observe the Person:

- Squinting
- Bumping into things
- Shuffling, tripping, or being hesitant when walking
- Being overly cautious when going up or down stairs
- Having problems reaching for things:
  - Over-reaches
  - Does not reach far enough
  - Gropes for things
- Changes in how the person reads, watches TV, drives, or walks
- Complaining about not enough lighting to read or do things
- Holding reading material near the face or at an angle
- Having trouble identifying faces or objects
- Wearing clothes that do not match
- Having trouble eating:
  - Cutting food
  - Getting food on a fork or spoon
  - Spilling or dropping food
  - Pouring liquids
- Having problems seeing at night

BODY STRUCTURE AND FUNCTION REVIEW
The Eye

Structure and Function

Receptors for vision are in the eyes (Fig. 47-6). Bones of the skull, eyelids and eyelashes, and tears protect the eyes from injury. The eye has 3 layers.

- The *sclera,* the white of the eye, is the outer layer. It is made of tough connective tissue. The *conjunctiva* is a mucous membrane that lines the eyelids and the front of the sclera.
- The *choroid* is the second layer. Blood vessels, the *ciliary muscle,* and the *iris* make up the choroid. The iris gives the eye its color. The opening in the middle of the iris is the *pupil.* Pupil size varies with the amount of light entering the eye. The pupil *constricts* (narrows) in bright light. It *dilates* (widens) in dim or dark places.
- The *retina* is the inner layer. It has receptors for vision and the nerve fibers of the *optic nerve.* The *macula* is near the center of the retina. The area contains cells that are sensitive to light, color, and the fine detail needed for central vision.

Light enters the eye through the *cornea*—the transparent part of the outer layer that lies over the eye. Light rays pass to the *lens,* which lies behind the pupil. The light is then reflected to the retina. Light is carried to the brain by the optic nerve.

The *aqueous chamber* separates the cornea from the lens. The chamber is filled with a fluid called *aqueous humor.* The fluid helps the cornea keep its shape and position. The *vitreous humor* is behind the lens. It is a gelatin-like substance that supports the retina and maintains the eye's shape.

Changes With Aging

Vision changes occur with age. *Presbyopia* is the gradual loss of the ability to focus on close-up objects that occurs with aging. It is caused by changes in the eye's lens. The pupils become less responsive to light with age. Decreased vision at night or in dark areas can occur. Older persons may also have problems seeing green and blue colors.

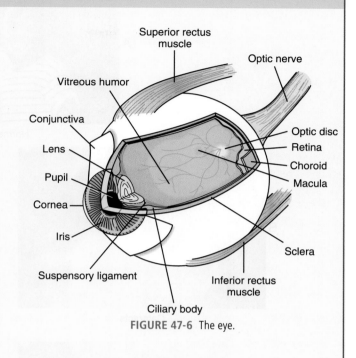

FIGURE 47-6 The eye.

Cataracts

A cataract is clouding of the lens (Fig. 47-7). The normal lens is clear. *Cataract* comes from the Greek word for waterfall. Trying to see is like looking through a waterfall. Cataracts can occur in 1 or both eyes. Signs and symptoms include:

- Cloudy, blurry, or dimmed vision. Colors seem faded and brownish. Blues and purples are hard to see. See Figure 47-8, *A* and *B* (p. 718).
- Sensitivity to light and glares.
- Poor vision at night.
- Halos around lights.
- Double vision in the affected eye.

Risk Factors. Most cataracts are caused by aging. A family history, diabetes, smoking, excessive alcohol use, and prolonged exposure to sunlight are risk factors. So are high blood pressure, obesity, and eye injuries and surgeries.

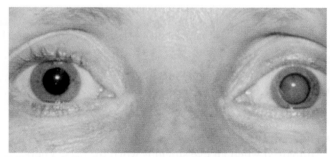

FIGURE 47-7 The right eye is normal. The left eye has a cataract. (From Swartz MH: *Textbook of physical diagnosis,* ed 8, Philadelphia, 2021, Elsevier.)

Treatment. Surgery is the only treatment. Surgery is done when the cataract affects daily activities. The lens is replaced with a plastic lens. Vision improves after surgery.

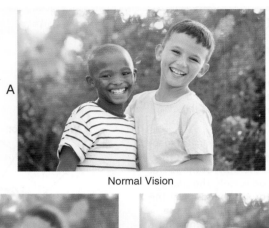

Normal Vision

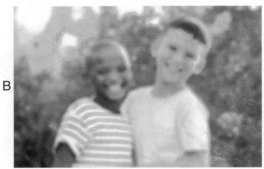

Cataracts

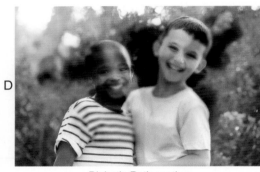

Age-Related Macular Degeneration

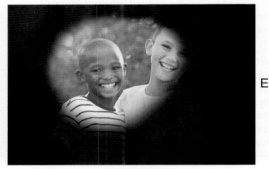

Diabetic Retinopathy

Glaucoma

FIGURE 47-8 Vision loss with eye disorders. **A,** Normal vision. **B,** Vision loss from cataracts. **C,** Vision loss from macular degeneration. **D,** Vision loss from diabetic retinopathy. **E,** Vision loss from glaucoma. (From National Eye Institute, National Institutes of Health.)

Post-operative care includes:
- Have the person wear ordered eyeglasses or eye shield as directed. If ordered, the shield is worn for sleep, including naps.
- Follow measures for persons who are blind or visually impaired when an eye shield is worn (p. 721). There may be vision loss in the other eye.
- Remind the person not to rub or press the affected eye.
- Do not bump the eye.
- Place the over-bed table and bedside stand on the un-operative side.
- Place the call light and needed items within reach.
- Report eye drainage or complaints of pain at once.
- Remind the person not to bend, stoop, or lift heavy things. Avoid coughing, sneezing, and vomiting if possible.

Age-Related Macular Degeneration

Age-related macular degeneration (AMD) damages the macula in the center of the retina. AMD causes blurring of central vision. *Central vision* is what you see "straight-ahead." It is needed to read, write, drive, cook, and see faces and for fine detail. Over time, blind spots (blank spots) occur in the center of vision (see Fig. 47-8, *A* and *C*). Onset is gradual and painless.

Risk Factors. AMD is common in people age 50 and older. Besides age, risk factors include:
- Smoking.
- Race. Whites are at greater risk than any other group.
- Family history.

Treatment. For advanced AMD, no treatment can prevent vision loss. Eye injections and laser treatments may stop or slow the disease progress. It may save what is left of central vision.

The following can reduce the risk of AMD.
- Eating a healthy diet high in green, leafy vegetables and fish
- Not smoking
- Maintaining normal blood pressure and cholesterol levels
- Regular exercise

Diabetic Retinopathy

In diabetic retinopathy, blood vessels in the retina are damaged. A complication of diabetes, it is a leading cause of blindness. Usually both eyes are affected.

Vision blurs and the person may see dark "floating" spots or streaks (see Fig. 47-8, *A* and *D*). Often there are no early warning signs.

Risk Factors. Everyone with diabetes (Chapter 51) is at risk for diabetic retinopathy. The risk increases the longer the person has diabetes. Good management of diabetes can help lower risk.

Treatment. The person needs to control diabetes, blood pressure, and cholesterol. Eye injections, laser treatments, or eye surgery may be used to prevent worsening vision.

Glaucoma

With glaucoma, fluid builds up in the eye, causing pressure on the optic nerve. The optic nerve is damaged. Vision loss with eventual blindness occurs.

Glaucoma can affect 1 or both eyes. Onset is usually gradual. Peripheral vision (side vision) is lost. The person sees through a tunnel (see Fig. 47-8, *A* and *E*), has blurred vision, and sees halos around lights.

Glaucoma of sudden onset is less common. Severe eye pain, nausea, vomiting, and sudden blurring of vision occur. With sudden onset, emergency care is needed to prevent blindness.

Risk Factors. Glaucoma is a leading cause of vision loss in the United States. Persons at risk include:
- African Americans over 40 years of age
- Everyone over 60 years of age, especially Mexican Americans
- Those with a family history of the disease

Treatment. Glaucoma has no cure. Prior damage cannot be reversed. Drugs, laser treatments, or surgery may be used to control glaucoma and prevent further damage to the optic nerve.

Low Vision

Low vision is impaired vision that cannot be corrected with eyeglasses, contact lenses, drugs, or surgery. Vision changes interfere with every-day activities. While wearing eyeglasses or contact lenses, the person still has vision problems that affect activities like reading, driving, recognizing faces, and seeing a TV or computer screen clearly.

Causes. Eye injuries and the eye disorders already described are common causes of low vision. Birth defects and brain injuries are other causes. The vision problem depends on the cause. There may be:
- Central vision loss—affecting the center of the person's vision
- Peripheral vision loss—affecting side vision
- Problems seeing at night or in low light
- Problems telling colors apart
- Blurred vision

Living With Low Vision. The person learns to use visual and adaptive (assistive) devices. Examples include:
- Prescription reading glasses
- Large-print reading materials
- Hand-held, stand (mounted), or video magnifiers
- Electronic reading machines
- Computers with large print and speech systems
- Phones, clocks, and watches with large numbers and that talk
- Lighting that can be adjusted
- Motion lights that turn on when the person enters a room

Changes in the home are made as needed for safety. See "Meeting Needs" on p. 720 for specific caregiving measures. The person may need help with transportation from family or friends. Continuing work, hobbies, and social activities promote quality of life.

Impaired Vision and Blindness

Some people are totally blind. Others sense some light but have no usable vision. Others have some usable vision but cannot read newsprint. A person who is legally blind sees at 20 feet what a person with normal vision sees at 200 feet. See Box 47-6 for the signs and symptoms of vision problems.

Loss of sight is serious. Adjustments can be hard and long. Rehabilitation programs help the person adjust to the vision loss and learn to be independent. The goal is to be as active as possible and have quality of life.

Braille. *Braille* is a touch reading and writing system that uses raised dots for each letter of the alphabet (Fig. 47-9). The first 10 letters also represent the numbers 0 through 9. Braille is read by moving the hands from left to right along each line of braille (Fig. 47-10).

Special devices allow computer access—keyboards, displays, and printers. A "braille display" lets the person read the information. Braille printers produce printouts in braille.

Mobility. Persons who are blind or visually impaired learn to move about independently using a long cane or a guide dog. Both are used world-wide.

- Long canes are white or silver-gray with red tips. Do not interfere with the arm holding the cane. The person stores the cane when not in use. If you store the cane, ask the person where to place it.
- A guide dog sees for a person. The dog responds to the master's commands. Commands are disobeyed to avoid danger. For example, the guide dog disobeys a command to cross the street if a car is coming. Do not pet, feed, or distract a guide dog. Such actions can place the person in danger.

Meeting Needs. The person's care plan includes measures to meet the person's needs. Safety measures are included. Follow the practices in Box 47-7 according to the care plan.

See *Focus on Long-Term Care and Home Care: Meeting Needs.*

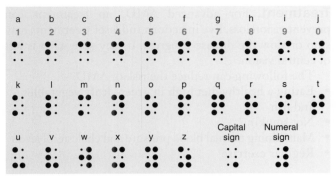

FIGURE 47-9 Braille.

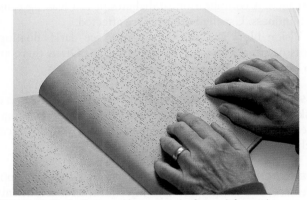

FIGURE 47-10 Braille is read by moving the fingers left to right across the braille lines.

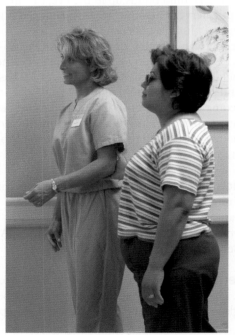

FIGURE 47-11 The blind person walks slightly behind the nursing assistant and touches the nursing assistant's arm lightly.

BOX 47-7 Caring for Persons Who Are Blind or Visually Impaired

The Setting

- Report worn or loose carpeting and other flooring. Also report throw rugs, plastic runners, and furniture with wheels.
- Keep furniture, equipment, electrical cords, and other items out of areas where the person will walk.
- Keep chairs pushed in under the table or desk.
- Keep room doors fully open or fully closed.
- Keep drawers and cabinet, cupboard, and closet doors fully closed.
- Report burnt-out light bulbs.
- Provide preferred lighting. Tell the person if lights are on or off.
- Adjust window coverings to prevent glares. Sunny days and bright, snowy days cause glares.
- Keep the call light and TV, light, and other controls within reach.
- Use night-lights in the person's room, bathroom, and hallway.
- Practice safety measures to prevent falls (Chapter 15).
- Orient the person to the room. Describe the layout. Include the location and purpose of furniture and equipment.
- Let the person touch and find furniture and equipment.
- Do not re-arrange furniture and equipment.
- Use colors and contrast. Solid, bright colors (red, orange, yellow) are best. Avoid pastels, patterns, prints, designs, and stripes. Light against dark provides contrast. For example, use a white plate with a dark placemat.
- Provide the same meal-time setting. Arrange things in the same way for each meal.
  - Have the person sit in good light.
  - Arrange the place setting.
    - The knife and spoon are to the right of the plate or as the person prefers.
    - The fork and napkin are to the left of the plate or as the person prefers.
    - The glass or cup is to the right of the plate if the person is right-handed. It is to the left of the plate if left-handed.
  - Arrange dishes, seasonings, and condiments in a straight line or in a semi-circle just beyond the place setting.
  - Explain the location of food and beverages. Use the face of a clock (Chapter 31). Or guide the person's hand to each item on the tray or place setting.
  - Cut meat, open containers, and perform other tasks as needed.
- Complete a safety check before leaving the room. (See the inside of the back cover.)

The Person

- Have the person wear comfortable shoes that fit correctly.
- Have the person use hand and stair railings and grab (safety) bars.
- Assist with walking as needed. Offer to guide and help the person. Respect the person's answer. If help is accepted:
  - Offer your arm. State which arm is offered. Tap the back of your hand against the person's hand.
  - Have the person hold on to your arm just above the elbow (Fig. 47-11). Do not grab the person's arm.
  - Walk at a normal pace. Walk 1 step ahead of the person. Stand next to the person at the top and bottom of stairs and when crossing streets.
  - Never push, pull, or guide the person in front of you.
  - Pause to change direction, step up, or step down.
  - Warn of stairs, elevators, escalators, doors, turns, furniture, and other obstructions. State if steps are up or down.
  - Have the person hold on to a railing, the wall, or a strong surface if you need to step away. Tell the person that you are leaving and what to hold on to.

The Person—cont'd

- Guide the person to a seat by placing your guiding arm on the seat. The person moves a hand down your arm to the seat.
- Let the person do as much as possible. Do not do things that the person can do.
- Provide visual and adaptive (assistive) devices. Follow the care plan.

You

- Identify yourself when you enter the room. Give your name, title, and reason for being there. Do not touch the person before the person is aware of your presence.
- Ask how much the person can see. Do not assume the person is totally blind or has some vision.
- Identify others. Say where each person is and what the person is doing.
- Offer to help. Simply say: "May I help you?" Respect the person's answer.
- Leave the person's belongings where you found them. Do not move or re-arrange things. If you must move things, tell the person what you moved and where.

Communication

- Face the person when speaking. Speak slowly and clearly.
- Use a normal tone of voice. Do not shout or speak loudly.
- Address the person by name. This shows that you are directing a comment or question to the person.
- Speak directly to the person. Do not talk just to others who are present.
- Feel free to use words such as "see," "look," "read," or "watch TV." You can use "blind" and "visually impaired." However, it is respectful to refer to the person first. You also can use colors, sizes, shapes, patterns, designs, and so on.
- Describe people, places, and things thoroughly. Do not leave out a detail because you do not think it is important.
- Warn of dangers. Give a calm and clear warning. You can say "wait" first. Then describe the danger. For example: "Wait, there is ice on the sidewalk."
- Greet the person by name when the person enters a room. This alerts the person to your presence. Say who you are. Also identify others in the room.
- Listen to the person. Give verbal cues that you are listening. Say: "yes," "okay," "I see," "tell me more," "I don't understand," and so on.
- Answer questions. Provide specific and descriptive responses.
- Give step-by-step explanations as you give care. Say when the procedure is over.
- Give specific directions.
  - Say "right behind you," "on your left," or "in front of you." Avoid phrases like "over here" or "over there."
  - Tell the distance. For example: "three steps in front of you" or "at the end of the hallway by the nurses' station."
  - Give landmarks if possible. Sounds and scents can serve as "landmarks." "By the kitchen" is an example.
- Tell the person when you are leaving the room or the area. If appropriate, state where you are going. For example: "I'm going to go into your bathroom now."
- Tell the person when you are ending a conversation. For example: "Thank you for sharing stories about your children."

Corrective Lenses

Eyeglasses and contact lenses correct many vision problems.

- *Eyeglasses.* Eyeglasses are worn for reading, for seeing at a distance, or for all activities. Eyeglass lenses are hardened glass or plastic. Clean them daily and as needed. Wash glass lenses with warm water. Dry them with a lens cloth or cotton cloth. Plastic lenses scratch easily. Use special cleaning solutions and cloths.
- *Contact lenses.* Contact lenses fit on the eye. There are hard and soft contacts. Contact lenses are usually only worn while awake. Some can be worn day and night for up to 30 days. Contacts are removed, cleaned, and stored according to the manufacturer's instructions. Depending on the type, they are discarded daily, weekly, or monthly. Report and record the following:
- Eye redness or irritation
- Eye drainage
- Eye pain or discomfort
- Blurred vision

See *Delegation Guidelines: Corrective Lenses.*
See *Promoting Safety and Comfort: Corrective Lenses.*
See procedure: *Caring for Eyeglasses.*

Caring for Eyeglasses

QUALITY OF LIFE

- Knock before entering the person's room.
- Address the person by name.
- Introduce yourself by name and title.
- Explain the procedure before starting and during the procedure.
- Protect the person's rights during the procedure.
- Handle the person gently during the procedure.

PRE-PROCEDURE

1 Follow *Delegation Guidelines: Corrective Lenses.* See *Promoting Safety and Comfort: Corrective Lenses.*

2 Practice hand hygiene and get the following supplies.
   - Eyeglass case
   - Cleaning solution or warm water
   - Lens cloth or cotton cloth

PROCEDURE

3 Remove the eyeglasses.
   a Hold the frames in front of the ears (Fig. 47-12, *A*).
   b Lift the frames from the ears. Bring the eyeglasses down away from the face (Fig. 47-12, *B*).
4 Clean the lenses with a cleaning solution or warm water. Clean in a circular motion. Dry the lenses with the cloth.
5 *For the person not wearing eyeglasses:*
   a Open the eyeglass case.
   b Fold the glasses. Put them in the case. Do not touch the clean lenses.
   c Place the case in the top drawer of the bedside stand.

6 *For the person wearing eyeglasses:*
   a Hold the frames at each side. Place them over the ears.
   b Adjust the eyeglasses so the nose-piece rests on the nose.
   c Return the case to the top drawer of the bedside stand.

POST-PROCEDURE

7 Provide for comfort. (See the inside of the back cover.)
8 Return the cleaning solution and cloth to their proper place. Discard a disposable cloth. Or follow agency policy for used linens.
9 Place the call light and other needed items within reach.
10 Complete a safety check of the room. (See the inside of the back cover.)
11 Practice hand hygiene.
12 Report and record your care and observations.

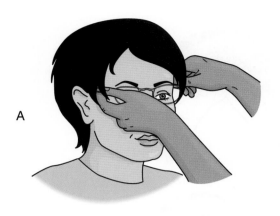 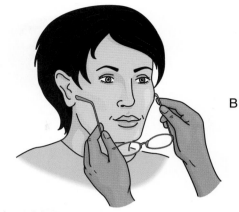

FIGURE 47-12 Removing eyeglasses. **A,** Hold the frames in front of the ears. **B,** Lift the frames from the ears. Bring the glasses down away from the face.

Ocular Prostheses

Injury or disease may require removing an eyeball. The person is fitted with an ocular (eye) prosthesis. This artificial eye does not provide vision. It matches the other eye in color and shape. The other eye may have normal, some, or no vision.

Worn all the time, even for sleep, the prosthesis usually needs little care. The prosthesis is briefly removed for cleaning and then re-inserted. Cleaning frequency varies. It is done regularly—every 3 weeks is common—and when irritation and excessive tearing occur.

To clean an ocular prosthesis:

1 Collect a kidney basin, denture cup, or other container as directed by the nurse. Line the container with a soft cloth or 4 × 4 gauze. This prevents scratches and damage.
2 Line the sink or work area with a towel.
3 Practice hand hygiene. Apply gloves.
4 Have the person put the eye in the container.
5 Wash the artificial eye, using your fingertips, with mild soap and warm water or saline as directed. Baby shampoo is often recommended. Do not use alcohol, chemicals, or antibacterial soap. Do not use a cloth.
6 Rinse well.
7 Air dry if directed. If directed, dry gently with a soft, lint-free cloth. Do not use a cloth that will leave fibers on the eye.
8 Line a container with a new soft cloth or 4 × 4 gauze.
9 Place the eye in the container. Remove gloves and practice hand hygiene.
10 Have the person insert the prosthesis.
    See *Promoting Safety and Comfort: Ocular Prostheses.*

PROMOTING SAFETY AND COMFORT
Ocular Prostheses

Safety
See Figure 47-13 (p. 724) for how an ocular prosthesis is removed and inserted. When handling an ocular prosthesis, you must prevent chips, scratches, and other damage. It must not fall on the floor or other hard surface. Always hold the eye over a towel or other soft surface. The prosthesis is the person's property. Protect it from loss or damage.

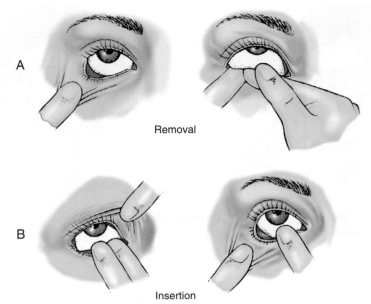

A

Removal

B

Insertion

FIGURE 47-13 Removing and inserting an ocular prosthesis. **A,** Removal. The lower eyelid is pulled down. The prosthesis is removed. **B,** Insertion. The upper eyelid is pulled up. The prosthesis is inserted. The lower eyelid is pulled down to set the prosthesis in place. (Modified from Monahan FD, Drake DT, Neighbors M, editors: *Medical-surgical nursing: foundations for clinical practice*, ed 2, Philadelphia, 1998, Saunders.)

FOCUS ON PRIDE

The Person, Family, and Yourself

P ersonal and Professional Responsibility

Hearing aids, contact lenses, eyeglasses, and ocular prostheses are costly to repair or replace. Protect devices from loss or damage. If a device is lost or damaged, tell the nurse. Take pride in being responsible and honest.

R ights and Respect

Many persons with hearing, speech, and vision problems have overcome great challenges. They take pride in how they have adapted. They deserve to be treated with dignity and respect. Do not pity the person. Treat the person like an adult, not like a child. Focus on the person's abilities, not disabilities.

Always refer to the person first. Then state the disability if needed. For example, a nurse says: "Please take Mrs. Jones a warm blanket. She is blind, so remember to knock and introduce yourself before entering the room. She will place the blanket as she prefers."

I ndependence and Social Interaction

Adjusting to a hearing, speech, or vision problem is often long and hard. Take time to listen. Be patient, understanding, and sensitive to the person's needs and feelings. Allow the person to be in control to the extent possible. This helps promote independence to improve quality of life.

D elegation and Teamwork

Hearing loss requires changes in communication. Communication measures are part of the care plan. A consistent approach is needed. The health team uses the same methods to communicate with the person. Follow the care plan.

E thics and Laws

The *Americans with Disabilities Act (ADA) of 1990* protects the rights of persons with disabilities. It includes persons with limited hearing, speech, and vision. The ADA covers rights such as employment, access to services and places, and the use of communication devices.

To comply with the ADA, agencies often provide:
- Braille on signs for areas with public access. Lobbies, restrooms, elevators, and cafeterias are examples.
- Communication devices for hearing or speech problems. For example, a device with a keyboard and screen is connected to a phone line. The device is used instead of a phone.
- Sign language interpreters.
- Information in large print and braille.

Ask about your agency's resources. Offer to help. If not sure how to help, ask the nurse. Take pride in helping others.

FOCUS ON PRIDE: *Application*

Hearing, speech, and vision problems do not affect intelligence. Some behaviors insult the person. Treating the person like a child and talking to others but not the person are examples. What are other examples? Identify ways to show dignity and respect.

REVIEW QUESTIONS

Circle the BEST answer.

1 Care of the person with Meniere's disease includes
   a Wearing a hearing aid
   b Preventing falls from vertigo
   c Speech therapy
   d Treating infection

2 Which is a sign of hearing loss?
   a An adult tugs or pulls at the ears.
   b A 5-month-old babbles and makes gurgling sounds.
   c An adult asks others to repeat themselves.
   d A 10-month-old uses gestures to communicate.

3 When talking to a person with hearing loss
   a Shout
   b Change the subject if the person does not seem to understand
   c Avoid using gestures and facial expressions
   d Use short sentences and simple words

4 A hearing aid
   a Corrects a hearing problem
   b Makes sounds louder
   c Makes speech clearer
   d Removes background noise

5 A hearing aid does not seem to be working. Your *first* action is to
   a See if it is turned on
   b Wash it with soap and water
   c Have it repaired
   d Remove the batteries

6 A person wears hearing aids. Which care measure is *correct*?
   a Leave the hearing aids in while showering.
   b Leave the hearing aids in while styling hair with a hair dryer and hair spray.
   c Hold the hearing aids over a sink when cleaning them.
   d Store the hearing aids in their case when not worn.

7 A person has aphasia. You know that
   a The person cannot hear
   b Swallowing is affected
   c The person has a language disorder
   d The person cannot speak

8 A person with receptive aphasia
   a Has trouble understanding speech and writing
   b Is aware of mistakes in speech
   c Speaks in phrases or short sentences
   d Has trouble hearing sounds

9 A person has a speech disorder. You should
   a Correct the person's speech
   b Discourage the writing of words
   c Leave the TV on while talking
   d Ask the person to repeat as needed

10 A person with a cataract
    a Has cloudy, blurry, or dim vision
    b Loses central vision
    c Has eye pain
    d Is blind

11 A person had cataract surgery. Which would you question?
    a Remind the person not to bend or lift heavy objects.
    b Let the person rub the eye.
    c Place the over-bed table on the un-operative side.
    d Leave an eye shield on during naps.

12 A person has AMD. Which is *true?*
    a There is a blind spot in the center of vision.
    b Lost vision can be restored with surgery.
    c Peripheral (side) vision is lost.
    d Vision is blurry with spots.

13 With low vision
    a There is no usable vision
    b Surgery can correct vision loss
    c Visual and adaptive devices are needed
    d Every-day activities are not affected

14 Braille involves
    a A long cane for walking
    b Raised dots arranged for letters of the alphabet
    c A guide dog
    d Corrective lenses

15 Which are dangers for persons who are blind or visually impaired?
    a Closed drawers
    b Doors that are fully open
    c Equipment in hallways
    d Night-lights

16 A person is blind. At meal times,
    a Provide a consistent setting
    b Feed the person even if the person can eat independently
    c Use plates, napkins, and placemats with designs
    d Provide the same foods every day

17 A person is visually impaired. You should
    a Move furniture to provide variety
    b Avoid words such as "see" and "look"
    c Assume that the person has no sight
    d Explain procedures step-by-step

18 A person is blind. To give directions you can say
    a "Over there"
    b "Right here"
    c "Across the room"
    d "On your left"

19 When eyeglasses are not worn they should be
    a Soaked in a cleaning solution
    b Taken to the nurses' station
    c Put in the eyeglass case
    d Placed in the bathroom

20 To care for an ocular prosthesis
    a Clean the prosthesis with alcohol
    b Wash the prosthesis with mild soap and warm water
    c Soak the prosthesis in a cleaning solution overnight
    d Scrub the prosthesis with a brush

Answers to Chapter 47 questions are on p. 903.

FOCUS ON **PRACTICE**

Problem Solving

A resident asks for help completing the weekly menu. You are to read each option and mark the choices. Hard of hearing, the resident struggles to hear you. You repeat the meal options many times. What will you do? How can you promote hearing and communication?

OBJECTIVES

- Define the key terms and key abbreviations in this chapter.
- Explain the differences between benign tumors and cancer.
- Identify cancer risk factors and signs and symptoms.
- Describe common cancer treatments and side effects.
- Describe the needs of persons with cancer.
- Explain how immune system disorders affect the body.
- Identify different autoimmune disorders.
- Describe human immunodeficiency virus (HIV) infection and acquired immunodeficiency syndrome (AIDS).

- Explain how to assist in the care of persons with AIDS.
- Identify different skin disorders.
- Describe the causes, signs and symptoms, and treatments of shingles and cellulitis.
- Explain how to promote PRIDE in the person, the family, and yourself.

KEY TERMS

benign tumor A tumor that does not spread to other body parts
biopsy A procedure in which a piece of tissue is removed for testing
cancer See "malignant tumor"
malignant tumor A tumor that invades and destroys nearby tissues and can spread to other body parts; cancer

metastasis The spread of cancer to other body parts
mole A brown, tan, or black spot on the skin that is flat or raised and round or oval
stomatitis Inflammation *(itis)* of the mouth *(stomat)*
tumor A new growth of abnormal cells that is benign or malignant

KEY ABBREVIATIONS

AIDS	Acquired immunodeficiency syndrome	STD; STI	Sexually transmitted disease; sexually transmitted infection
CDC	Centers for Disease Control and Prevention	TB	Tuberculosis
HIV	Human immunodeficiency virus		

You will care for persons with health problems. This chapter will help you better understand cancer and some immune system problems and skin disorders. Learning about disorders gives meaning to the required care. The nurse gives you more information as needed.

CANCER

Cells reproduce for tissue growth and repair. Cells divide in an orderly way. Sometimes cell division and growth are out of control. A mass or clump of cells develops. This new growth of abnormal cells is called a *tumor*. Tumors are benign or malignant (Fig. 48-1).

Benign tumors do not spread to other body parts (see Fig. 48-1, *A*). They can grow to a large size but rarely threaten life. They usually do not grow back when removed.

Malignant tumors (cancer) invade and destroy nearby tissues. They can spread to other body parts (see Fig. 48-1, *B*). They may be life-threatening. Sometimes they grow back after removal.

Metastasis is the spread of cancer to other body parts (Fig. 48-2). If not treated and controlled, cancer cells break off the tumor and travel to other body parts. New tumors grow at those sites.

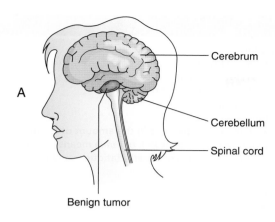

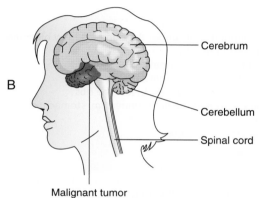

FIGURE 48-1 Tumors. **A,** A benign tumor grows within a local area. **B,** A malignant tumor invades other tissues.

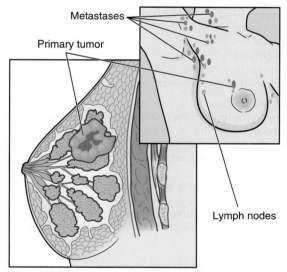

FIGURE 48-2 A tumor in the breast has metastasized to the lymph nodes.

A biopsy is often needed to diagnose cancer. A *biopsy* is a procedure in which a piece of tissue is removed for testing. The tissue sample is removed with a needle, using a scope, or with surgery. Sometimes the entire tumor and tissue around the tumor are removed. The sample is examined for cancer.

Risk Factors

Cancer is the second leading cause of death in the United States. The National Cancer Institute describes these risk factors.

- *Age.* Advancing age is the most important risk factor. However, cancer can occur at any age.
- *Tobacco.* This includes using tobacco (smoking, snuff, and chewing tobacco) and being around tobacco (second-hand smoke). This risk can be avoided.
- *Radiation.* Sources are sun light, x-rays, and radon gas that forms in the soil and some rocks.
- *Infections.* Certain viruses and bacteria increase the risk of cancers—cervix, penis, vagina, anus, nose and throat, lung, liver, lymphoma, leukemia, Kaposi's sarcoma (associated with acquired immunodeficiency syndrome [AIDS], p. 733), and stomach.
- *Immuno-suppressive drugs.* Such drugs are often used for organ transplant patients to prevent rejection of the transplant. They lower the body's ability to stop cancer from forming.
- *Alcohol.* Alcohol is linked to the increased risk of cancers of the mouth, throat, esophagus, larynx, liver, and breast.
- *Hormones.* The female hormones estrogen and progesterone are known to increase the risk of breast and uterine cancers.
- *Diet and obesity.* A healthy diet, physical activity, and a healthy weight may reduce the risk of some cancers. Obesity is linked to post-menopausal breast cancer and cancers of the colon, rectum, uterus, esophagus, kidney, pancreas, and gallbladder.
- *Environment.* Air pollution, second-hand smoke, and asbestos are linked to lung cancer. Drinking water with large amounts of arsenic is linked to skin, bladder, and lung cancers.

Cancer Signs and Symptoms

Cancer can occur almost anywhere. Box 48-1 (pp. 728-729) lists some signs and symptoms of common types of cancer. Cancer may not cause pain. Waiting for pain as a symptom can delay diagnosis and treatment. If detected early, cancer may be better treated and controlled.

See *Focus on Children and Older Persons: Cancer Signs and Symptoms,* p. 729.

BOX 48-1   Cancer: Signs and Symptoms

Brain Tumor
- Headache—morning headache, headache that goes away after vomiting
- Seizures
- Vision, hearing, and speech problems
- Loss of appetite
- Frequent nausea and vomiting
- Changes in personality, mood, ability to focus, or behavior
- Loss of balance and trouble walking
- Weakness
- Unusual sleepiness, change in activity level

Pancreatic Cancer
- *Jaundice*—yellowish skin and eyes
- Light-colored stools
- Dark urine
- Pain in the upper or middle abdomen and back
- Weight loss
- Loss of appetite
- Fatigue

Uterine Cancer
- Unusual vaginal bleeding or discharge
- Vaginal bleeding after menopause
- *Dysuria*—painful or difficult urination
- Pain during sex
- Pelvic pain

Cervical Cancer
- Vaginal bleeding after sex
- Vaginal bleeding after menopause
- Unusual vaginal bleeding or discharge
- Pelvic pain
- Pain during sex

Breast Cancer
- Lump or thickening in or near the breast or underarm
- Change in the size or shape of the breast
- Dimple or puckering in the breast skin, dimples that look like the skin of an orange
- Nipple turned inward into the breast
- Fluid (other than breast-milk) from the nipple, especially if bloody
- Scaly, red, or swollen skin on the breast, nipple, or areola (the dark area of skin around the nipple)

Bladder Cancer
- Blood in the urine (urine looks rusty or bright red)
- Urinary frequency
- Dysuria
- Feeling the need to void even when the bladder is not full
- *Nocturia*—frequent urination at night

Colon Cancer
- Change in bowel habits
- Blood in the stool (bright red or very dark)
- Diarrhea, constipation, feeling that the bowel does not empty completely
- Stools that are narrower than usual
- Frequent gas pains, bloating, fullness, cramping
- Weight loss
- Fatigue
- Vomiting

Kidney Cancer
- Blood in the urine
- Lump in the abdomen
- Pain in the side that does not go away
- Loss of appetite
- Weight loss
- Signs of *anemia* (a decrease in the amount of healthy red blood cells; *an* means lack of, *emia* means blood condition)—shortness of breath, fatigue, rapid pulse, dizziness, pale skin

Leukemia
- Weakness
- Fatigue
- Fever or night sweats
- Easy bruising or bleeding
- Flat, pinpoint spots under the skin caused by bleeding
- Shortness of breath
- Weight loss, loss of appetite
- Pain in the bones or stomach
- Pain or feeling of fullness below the ribs
- Painless lumps in the neck, underarm, stomach, or groin
- Having many infections

Lung Cancer
- Chest discomfort or pain
- Cough that does not go away or worsens over time
- Trouble breathing, wheezing
- Blood in sputum
- Hoarseness
- Loss of appetite
- Weight loss
- Fatigue
- Dysphagia
- Swelling in the face, neck veins, or both

Lymphoma
- Swelling in the lymph nodes in the neck, underarm, groin, or stomach
- Fever
- Night sweats
- Fatigue
- Weight loss
- Skin rash or itchy skin
- Pain in the chest, abdomen, or bones

Mouth and Lip Cancer
- Sore on the lip or in the mouth that does not heal
- Lump or thickening on the lips, gums, or in the mouth
- A white or red patch on the gums, tongue, or lining of the mouth
- Lip or mouth bleeding, pain, or numbness
- Voice change
- Loose teeth or dentures that no longer fit well
- Trouble chewing, swallowing, or moving the tongue or jaw
- Jaw swelling
- Sore throat or feeling that something is caught in the throat

| **BOX 48-1** | **Cancer: Signs and Symptoms—cont'd** |

Melanoma
- Change in the size, shape, or color of a *mole* (a brown, tan, or black spot on the skin that is flat or raised and round or oval) (Fig. 48-3)
- Mole with irregular edges
- Mole with more than 1 color
- Uneven mole shape—1 half does not match the other half
- Mole that itches, oozes, bleeds, or has an ulcer (Chapter 41)
- New moles growing near an existing mole
- Skin color changes

Skin Cancer
- A sore that does not heal
- Skin that is raised, smooth, shiny, and pearly
- Skin that is firm and looks like a scar (may be white, yellow, or waxy)
- Raised and red or reddish-brown skin
- Scaling, bleeding, or crusty areas

Prostate Cancer
- Trouble starting the urine flow
- Frequent urination, especially at night
- Urinary retention
- Weak urine stream
- Urine stream that starts and stops
- Pain in the back, hips, or pelvis
- Signs of anemia—shortness of breath, fatigue, rapid pulse, dizziness, pale skin

Thyroid Cancer
- A lump (nodule) in the neck
- Dyspnea
- Dysphagia, pain with swallowing
- Hoarseness

Modified From National Cancer Institute:
- Adult central nervous system tumors treatment (PDQ®)–patient version, updated January 5, 2024.
- Pancreatic cancer treatment (PDQ®)–patient version, updated February 28, 2024.
- Endometrial cancer treatment (PDQ®)–patient version, updated November 13, 2020.
- Cervical cancer symptoms, updated October 13, 2022.
- Breast cancer treatment (PDQ®)–patient version, updated February 26, 2024.
- Bladder cancer symptoms, updated February 16, 2023.
- Colon cancer treatment (PDQ®)–patient version, updated April 6, 2022.
- Renal cell cancer treatment (PDQ®)–patient version, updated July 21, 2023.
- Adult acute lymphoblastic leukemia treatment (PDQ®)–patient version, updated November 17, 2023.
- Non–small cell lung cancer treatment (PDQ®)–patient version, updated October 11, 2023.
- Non-Hodgkin lymphoma treatment (PDQ®)–patient version, updated November 16, 2023.
- Lip and oral cavity cancer treatment (adult) (PDQ®)–patient version, updated October 14, 2021.
- Melanoma treatment (PDQ®)–patient version, updated June 30, 2023.
- Skin cancer treatment (PDQ®)–patient version, updated May 15, 2023.
- Prostate cancer treatment (PDQ®)–patient version, updated February 16, 2023.
- Thyroid cancer treatment (adult) (PDQ®)–patient version, updated July 21, 2023.

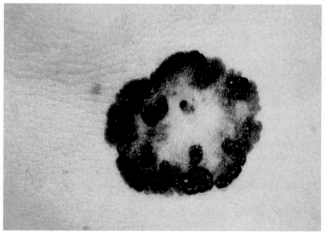

FIGURE 48-3 Melanoma. (From Centers for Disease Control and Prevention, Department of Health and Human Services/Carl Washington, MD, Emory University School of Medicine; Mona Saraiya, MD, MPH.)

FOCUS ON CHILDREN AND OLDER PERSONS

Cancer Signs and Symptoms

Children
The most common childhood cancers are:
- Leukemia—a cancer of the blood and bone marrow. The bone marrow is a spongy substance found inside bones. Blood cells are made in the bone marrow. Leukemia is the most common form of childhood cancer.
- Brain and spinal cord tumors.
- Lymphomas—tumors of the lymph tissues.

Early signs and symptoms are often similar to common illnesses and injuries. Fever, fatigue, swollen glands, weight loss, bruising, and tender joints or bones are examples. Children should see a doctor when signs and symptoms are severe or do not go away.

Treatment

Treatment depends on the tumor type, its site and size, and if it has spread. The treatment goal may be to:
- Cure the cancer. Remove cancer from the body and kill cancer cells.
- Control the disease. Help the person live longer.
- Reduce symptoms from the cancer and its treatments.

Some cancers respond to 1 type of treatment. Others require 2 or more types. Cancer treatments also damage healthy cells and tissues. Side effects depend on the type and extent of the treatment.

Surgery. Surgery removes tumors. It is done to cure or control cancer or to relieve pain. See Chapter 40 for care of the person having surgery.

Radiation Therapy. Radiation therapy *(radiotherapy)* kills cancer cells. X-ray beams are aimed at the tumor. Sometimes radioactive material is implanted in or near the tumor. Radiation therapy:

- Destroys certain tumors.
- Shrinks a tumor before surgery.
- Destroys cancer cells that remain after surgery.
- Controls tumor growth to prevent or relieve pain.

Cancer cells and normal cells receive radiation. Healthy cells are damaged. Skin changes occur at the treatment site—dryness, itching, swelling, peeling, redness, blistering, and hair loss. Special skin care measures are ordered.

Fatigue is common. Extra rest is needed. Other side effects depend on the part of the body being treated. Discomfort, nausea, vomiting, diarrhea, and loss of appetite *(anorexia)* are common. Radiation to the head and neck can cause dry mouth, mouth pain or swelling, and *dysphagia* (difficulty swallowing).

See *Promoting Safety and Comfort: Radiation Therapy.*

PROMOTING SAFETY AND COMFORT

Radiation Therapy

Safety

Radiation implants (seeds, ribbons, capsules) are placed near the tumor. Therefore the person's body gives off radiation. Practice these safety measures.

- Tell the nurse if you are or may be pregnant or are younger than 18. The nurse needs to change your assignment.
- Follow agency policy for wearing a badge or device to measure radiation exposure.
- Talk to the person from the doorway if you do not need to enter the room. Radiation exposure decreases with distance.
- Follow agency policies for wearing personal protective equipment (PPE) including a gown, gloves, and shoe coverings. Don items before entering the person's room.
- Minimize your time in the room and near the person. Follow limits for time in the person's room and for the distance between you and the person.
- Leave trash, linens, and food trays in the room. These items will be removed by staff trained to do so. Disposable items are used as much as possible.
- Remove and discard PPE before leaving the room.
- Wash your hands after leaving the room.

Comfort

The person has a private room to protect others from radiation exposure. A visitor may be limited to 30 minutes or less a day. Visitors may stand at the doorway rather than enter the room. Children under 18 years of age and pregnant women are not allowed to visit.

Therefore the person may feel sad, lonely, and depressed. Assure the person that care needs will be met. Treat the person with caring, kindness, and dignity.

Chemotherapy. Chemotherapy involves drugs that kill cancer cells. It is used to:

- Cure the cancer.
- Shrink a tumor before surgery.
- Slow the growth of the cancer.
- Prevent the cancer from spreading.
- Kill cells that break off of the tumor to prevent metastasis.
- Relieve symptoms caused by the cancer.

Chemotherapy affects the whole body. Cancer cells and normal cells are affected. Side effects depend on the drug used.

- Fatigue.
- Hair loss *(alopecia).*
- Gastro-intestinal irritation. Poor appetite, nausea, vomiting, and diarrhea can occur. *Stomatitis,* an inflammation *(itis)* of the mouth *(stomat),* may occur.
- Decreased blood cell production (red blood cells, white blood cells, platelets). The person may be weak and tired. Infection and bleeding are risks.
- Changes in thinking and memory.
- Emotional changes.

Chemotherapy is often given in cycles. A period of treatment is followed by a rest period. The rest period allows the body to recover and build healthy new cells before the next treatment.

The drug usually stays in the person's body for 3 to 7 days. It is excreted through body fluids—urine, feces (stools), vomit, tears, saliva, semen, and vaginal secretions. Safety measures are listed in Box 48-2.

BOX 48-2   Safety During Chemotherapy

General Safety

- Wear gloves for any contact with the person's body fluids (including secretions and excretions). Wash your hands after removing and discarding the gloves.
- Wash the hands or any body part or area that has contact with the person's body fluids. Do so at once. Use soap and water. This applies to you, the person, and others.

Elimination and Vomiting

- Wear gloves to handle bedpans, urinals, or kidney basins.
- Empty and rinse bedpans, urinals, and kidney basins after use. Follow agency policies and procedures for disinfection. In home settings, such items should be washed at least once a day with soap and water.
- Flush after the person uses the toilet or you empty a bedpan, urinal, or kidney basin. Put the lid down first to avoid splashing. Flush twice if young children or pets will have contact with the toilet.
- Wear gloves when handling used diapers, incontinence products, waterproof under-pads, and ostomy pouches.
- Double-bag diapers, incontinence products, waterproof under-pads, and ostomy pouches. Follow agency policy.
- Place ostomy waste in a tied plastic bag or a Ziploc bag. Then place the bag in another plastic bag. Discard following agency policy.

Laundry

- Follow agency policy for soiled linens and clothing. In the home setting:
  - Wash soiled linens as soon as possible. If unable to wash right away, place them in a plastic bag. Discard the plastic bag in the trash after washing the items.
  - Wash soiled items separately from other linens or garments.
  - Wash soiled items twice.

Modified from UPMC: Patient education: safe handling of chemotherapy waste material, Pittsburgh, Pa, Reviewed February 2023, UPMC.

Hormone Therapy. Some cancers need hormones to grow. Hormone therapy involves drugs or surgery to remove hormone sources from the body. For example, to treat breast cancer, drugs are given to block hormones from the ovaries or the ovaries are removed. For prostate cancer, drugs are given to block hormones from the testicles or the testicles are removed.

Side effects include hot flashes, fatigue, nausea, and loss of sexual desire. Men may have weakened bones, diarrhea, and enlarged and tender breasts. Women may have vaginal dryness, menstrual changes (if pre-menopausal), and mood changes. Fertility is affected in men and women. Men may experience erectile dysfunction (impotence) (Chapter 12).

Immunotherapy. Immunotherapy helps the immune system fight the cancer. Side effects include flu-like symptoms—fever, chills, weakness, dizziness, nausea and vomiting, muscle or joint aches, fatigue, headache, dyspnea, and blood pressure changes. Pain, swelling, redness, itching, and rash may occur.

Other Therapies. Other therapies include:

- *Targeted therapy.* There are differences in how cancer cells grow, divide, and spread. Targeted drugs focus on these differences to treat cancer. Most healthy cells are not harmed. Targeted therapy may be used alone or with surgery, chemotherapy, or radiation.
- *Stem cell transplants.* High doses of chemotherapy or radiation therapy can kill cancer cells and blood cells (red blood cells, white blood cells, and platelets). With a stem cell transplant, the person is given blood-forming stem cells. A stem cell is an immature cell from which new cell types develop. New blood cells develop from the stem cells.
- *Complementary and alternative medicine (CAM). Complementary medicine* is used with standard cancer treatments. *Alternative medicine* is used instead of standard cancer treatments. CAM includes massage therapy, herbal products, vitamins, special diets, spiritual healing, aromatherapy, and acupuncture. Aromatherapy involves the use of fragrant oils to improve symptoms. Acupuncture involves inserting small needles at certain points in the skin to control pain and other symptoms.

The Person's Needs

Persons with cancer have many needs. They include:

- Pain relief or control. Tell the nurse if the person reports pain or if there are signs of pain. Provide comfort measures. See Chapter 36.
- Rest and exercise. Follow the care plan for the person's specific needs. The person may tire easily.
- Fluids and nutrition. Follow the person's ordered diet. Small portions and more frequent meals may be needed for nausea or poor appetite. Soft foods or a dysphagia diet may be needed for chewing or swallowing problems.

- Preventing skin breakdown. Give good skin care and monitor for skin changes. Follow the care plan for skin care measures if irritation is present.
- Preventing infection. Chemotherapy, especially, can weaken the person's immune system. (*Immunocompromised* refers to a person who has a weakened immune system.) Practice good hand hygiene and the other infection prevention measures in Chapter 17. Rest, good nutrition, exercise as able, and stress reduction are important measures for immune system health. The person avoids contact with others who may have an infection.
- Oral care. Treatments, nausea, and vomiting can cause a bad taste in the mouth, dry mouth, and irritation in the mouth (stomatitis). Follow the care plan to promote comfort. Use a soft toothbrush or sponge swabs gently. Do not use a mouthwash that contains alcohol.
- Preventing bowel problems. Constipation can occur from pain-relief drugs. Some cancer treatments cause diarrhea. Promote normal bowel elimination. See Chapter 29.
- Dealing with treatment side effects. Report weakness, fatigue, nausea, vomiting, bowel changes, appetite changes, weight loss, skin changes, signs of infection, or pain. Report blood in the urine or feces (stool). Report irritation, sores, or bleeding in the mouth. Ask the nurse for specific side effects to report.
- Psychological, social, spiritual, and sexual needs. Cancer affects the whole person.

Psychological and social needs are great. Anger, fear, and depression are common. Some surgeries are disfiguring. The person may feel unwhole, unattractive, or unclean. The person and family need support.

Spiritual needs are important. A spiritual leader may provide comfort. To many people, spiritual needs are just as important as physical needs.

Cancer treatment may affect sexual function. This depends on the cancer type and treatment method. Fatigue, pain, hormone changes, surgery in the pelvic area, and drug side effects are some factors. Changes may be temporary or long-term. Connection and intimacy are important. The health team helps the person manage and cope with changes.

Persons dying of cancer often receive hospice care (Chapters 1 and 59). Support is given to the person and family.

See *Focus on Communication: The Person's Needs.*

FOCUS ON COMMUNICATION

The Person's Needs

Knowing what to say to a person with cancer can be hard. Talk as you would with any other person. Avoid comments like "I'm sure you will be fine" or "It will be okay."

Often the person needs to talk and share thoughts, feelings, or experiences. Listen patiently and with interest. Being there when needed is important. You may not have to say anything. Just listen. Others prefer quiet. Be sensitive to the person's individual needs.

IMMUNE SYSTEM DISORDERS

Immune system disorders occur from problems with the immune response. The response may be inappropriate, too strong, or lacking.

See *Body Structure and Function Review: The Immune System*.

BODY STRUCTURE AND FUNCTION REVIEW

The Immune System

Structure and Function

The immune system protects the body from microbes, cancer cells, and other harmful substances. The system defends against threats inside and outside the body.

Immunity is protection against a disease or condition. *Specific immunity* is the body's reaction to a certain threat. *Non-specific immunity* is the body's reaction to anything it does not recognize as a normal body substance. Special cells and substances function to protect the body.

- *Antibodies and antigens.* Antibodies are normal body substances that recognize other substances. Antigens cause an immune response. Antibodies recognize and bind with unwanted antigens. This leads to the destruction of unwanted substances and the production of more antibodies.
- *Phagocytes.* White blood cells that digest and destroy microbes and other unwanted substances.
- *Lymphocytes.* White blood cells that produce antibodies. Lymphocyte production increases as the body responds to an unwanted substance. *B lymphocytes (B cells)* and *T lymphocytes (T cells)* are different types. B cells cause antibody production. Some T cells kill infected cells and tumor cells. Others stop the immune response when the antigens have been destroyed.

Changes With Aging

Older persons have fewer numbers of certain immune cells. The immune response slows. There is increased risk for infection. Usual signs of infection are lessened or absent (Chapter 12). Healing slows. The ability to detect and correct cell defects (problems) declines. There is increased risk of cancer.

Autoimmune Disorders

Autoimmune disorders occur when the immune system attacks the body's own *(auto)* healthy cells, tissues, or organs. The body parts affected depend on the type of disorder (Fig. 48-4).

Common autoimmune disorders include:

- *Celiac disease.* The person cannot tolerate gluten—a substance in wheat, rye, and barley. When gluten is ingested, the immune system responds and damages the lining of the small intestines. Over time, the damage prevents nutrient absorption. Diarrhea, fatigue, weight loss, bloating, and anemia occur. Poor nutrition and serious complications can result. A gluten-free diet is needed (Chapter 30).

Body Parts That Can Be Affected by Autoimmune Diseases

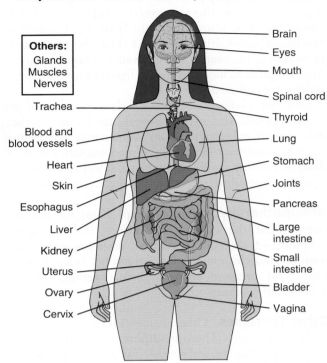

FIGURE 48-4 Body parts affected by autoimmune disorders. (Redrawn from Office on Women's Health, U.S. Department of Health and Human Services: *Autoimmune diseases,* updated April 1, 2019.)

- *Lupus.* This disease can damage the joints, skin, kidneys, heart, lungs, and other body parts. A rash across the nose and cheeks is common. See Figure 48-5.
- *Multiple sclerosis* (Chapter 49). The immune system attacks the protective coating around nerves. Damage affects the brain and spinal cord.
- *Rheumatoid arthritis* (Chapter 49). The immune system attacks the lining of the joints.
- *Inflammatory bowel disease* (Chapter 51). This disorder causes chronic inflammation of the digestive tract.
- *Type 1 diabetes* (Chapter 51). The immune system attacks the cells that make insulin (a hormone that regulates blood glucose [sugar] levels). Unable to make insulin, too much glucose remains in the blood.
- Thyroid disorders (Chapter 51):
  - *Graves' disease* causes *hyperthyroidism* (too much thyroid hormone production).
  - *Hashimoto's disease* causes *hypothyroidism* (not enough thyroid hormone production).

Most autoimmune disorders are chronic. Treatment depends on the disorder and the tissues and organs affected. Treatment is aimed at:

- Relieving symptoms
- Replacing needed hormones
- Suppressing the immune system

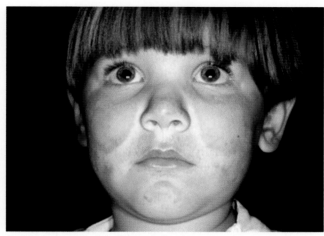

FIGURE 48-5 Called the "butterfly" rash, the rash from lupus is across the nose and cheeks. (From Kliegman RM et al: *Nelson textbook of pediatrics,* ed 21, Philadelphia, 2020, Elsevier.)

HIV/AIDS

The *human immunodeficiency virus (HIV)* attacks the immune system. It destroys the body's ability to fight infections and disease.

HIV is spread through certain body fluids—blood, semen, vaginal fluids, rectal fluids, and breast-milk (from mother to baby). HIV is not spread by air, water, saliva, tears, sweat, insects, pets, casual contact (shaking hands, hugging, dancing, sharing dishes), closed mouth or social kissing, or toilet seats.

HIV is transmitted *mainly* by:

- Having sex with someone who has HIV.
  - Anal sex
  - Vaginal sex
  - Multiple sex partners
- Sharing needles, syringes, rinse water, or other equipment used to prepare injection drugs.

While less common, HIV-infected mothers can transmit HIV to babies during pregnancy, birth, or breast-feeding. The Centers for Disease Control and Prevention (CDC) reports that while HIV *may* be spread by the following methods, the risk is low.

- Being stuck with an HIV-contaminated needle or other sharp object in the workplace.
- Receiving blood transfusions, blood products, or organ or tissue transplants contaminated with HIV. This is *very* unlikely. Donated blood, blood products, organs, and tissues are thoroughly tested in the United States.
- Eating food pre-chewed by an HIV-infected person if the food mixes with blood.
- Being bitten and skin broken by an HIV-infected person.
- Oral sex. Risk increases when there are mouth or genital sores, bleeding gums, or another sexually transmitted disease (infection) present.
- Touch is only risky if there is contact between broken skin, wounds, or mucous membranes and HIV-infected blood or body fluids.
- Deep, open-mouth kissing if blood is exchanged when the person with HIV has sores or bleeding gums.

BOX 48-3   HIV: Stages and Signs and Symptoms

Acute Infection
- May occur within 2 to 4 weeks after HIV infection.
- Risk of transmitting HIV to others is high.
- Flu-like symptoms often described as the "worst flu ever."
  - Fever
  - Chills
  - Rash
  - Night sweats
  - Muscle aches
  - Sore throat
  - Fatigue
  - Swollen lymph nodes
  - Mouth ulcers
- Symptoms may last a few days to several weeks.

Clinical Latency Stage (Chronic HIV Infection)
- *Latency* means present and developing but not obvious or visible.
- The HIV virus is still active and reproducing, but at very low levels. (*Viral load* is the amount of HIV in the blood.)
- The person may have no HIV-related symptoms or only mild ones.
- HIV can still be spread to others even if there are no symptoms. Persons with HIV need to have their viral load checked regularly to know their risk of spreading HIV.
- This stage can last 10 years or longer. Some people progress to the next stage faster.

AIDS
- The immune system is badly damaged.
- The person is at risk for infections, illnesses, and cancers. (Known as *opportunistic infections,* these health problems occur more often and are more severe due to the person's damaged immune system.) They include pneumonia, tuberculosis (TB), fungal infections, Kaposi's sarcoma (a type of cancer), and nervous system disorders.
- Viral load may be high. Risk of transmitting HIV to others may be high.
- Signs and symptoms:
  - Rapid weight loss
  - Recurring fever
  - Night sweats
  - Fatigue: extreme and unexplained
  - Swollen lymph glands: underarms, groin, neck
  - Diarrhea lasting more than a week
  - Sores: mouth, anus, genitals
  - Pneumonia
  - Red, brown, pink, or purple blotches: on or under the skin; inside the mouth, nose, or eyelids
  - Memory loss
  - Depression

Modified from HIV.gov: Symptoms of HIV, updated June 15, 2022 and Centers for Disease Control and Prevention: About HIV, reviewed June 30, 2022.

If untreated, HIV infection progresses in stages. Acquired immunodeficiency syndrome (AIDS) is the final and most severe stage. Box 48-3 lists the stages and signs and symptoms of HIV infection and AIDS.

Drugs are used to treat HIV symptoms. They also reduce complications and the risk of spreading HIV. Treatment can slow or prevent progression to AIDS and prolong life. AIDS has no vaccine and no cure at present. Without treatment, persons with AIDS live for about 3 years. Common care measures for persons with AIDS are listed in Box 48-4.

HIV Testing. The CDC recommends HIV testing at least once for everyone ages 13 to 64. Pregnant women and those planning to become pregnant should be tested as early as possible. A person with HIV will test positive (HIV-positive). If HIV is not present, the person tests negative (HIV-negative).

BOX 48-4   Caring for the Person With AIDS

- Follow Standard Precautions and the Bloodborne Pathogen Standard. HIV is a bloodborne pathogen (Chapter 17).
- Provide daily hygiene. Avoid irritating soaps.
- Follow the care plan for oral hygiene. A toothbrush with soft bristles is best.
- Provide oral fluids as ordered.
- Measure and record intake and output.
- Measure weight daily.
- Encourage deep-breathing and coughing exercises as ordered.
- Prevent pressure injuries.
- Assist with range-of-motion exercises and ambulating as ordered.
- Encourage self-care. The person may use adaptive (assistive) devices (walker, commode, eating devices).
- Encourage the person to be as active as possible.
- Change linens and garments when damp or wet.
- Listen and provide emotional support.
- Report changes to the nurse:
  - Fever
  - Cough
  - Appetite changes
  - Swallowing problems
  - Weight loss
  - Diarrhea
  - Fatigue
  - Night sweats
  - Skin changes
  - Signs of pressure injury (Chapter 42)
  - Mouth pain, mouth sores, white patches in the mouth
  - Sores in the perineal area
  - Confusion or behavior changes
  - Depression

According to the CDC, testing should be done once a year if the person:
- Is a man who has had sex with another man
- Has had sex with an HIV-positive partner
- Has had more than 1 partner since the last HIV test
- Has shared needles or equipment used for injection drugs
- Has exchanged sex or drugs for money
- Has another sexually transmitted disease (infection) (STD; STI) (Chapter 52), hepatitis (Chapter 51), or TB (Chapter 50)
- Has had sex with anyone who has done anything listed above
- Does not know the sexual history of a sexual partner

HIV Prevention. The CDC recommends the following measures to prevent HIV infection.
- Choosing less risky sexual behaviors. Oral sex is less risky than anal or vaginal sex. Sexual activities that do not involve contact with body fluids (semen, vaginal fluid, blood) do not transmit HIV.
- Using condoms consistently and correctly.
- Reducing the number of sexual partners or choosing not to have sex. The greater the number of partners, the greater the risk of a partner with HIV.
- Taking pre-exposure prophylaxis (PrEP) drugs. (*Prophylaxis* means prevention measures.) Such drugs are indicated for persons who are HIV-negative and at risk for getting HIV from sex or use of injection drugs.
- Seeing a doctor within 3 days after possible exposure to HIV. The doctor may order post-exposure prophylaxis (PEP).
- Testing and treatment for other STDs (STIs).
- Encouraging HIV-positive partners to get and continue treatment. HIV treatment reduces the amount of HIV in the blood and prevents transmission to others.

SKIN DISORDERS

There are many types of skin disorders. Alopecia, hirsutism, dandruff, lice, and scabies are discussed in Chapter 25. See Chapter 41 for skin tears and wounds related to circulatory problems. Pressure injuries are discussed in Chapter 42. Burns are discussed in Chapter 58.

See *Body Structure and Function Review: The Integumentary System*.

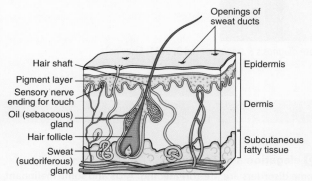
Shingles

Shingles (herpes zoster) is caused by the same virus that causes chicken pox. The virus lies dormant in nerve tissue. (*Dormant* means to be inactive.) The virus can become active years later.

At first there is pain, itching, or tingling of the skin. Then the person has a painful rash of fluid-filled blisters. This usually occurs on 1 side of the face or body (Fig. 48-7).

Persons who have had chicken pox are at risk. So are persons with weakened immune systems from HIV

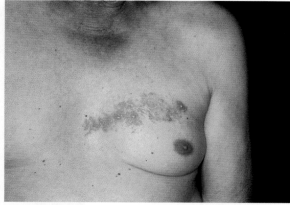

FIGURE 48-7 Shingles. (Courtesy Department of Dermatology, School of Medicine, University of Utah, Salt Lake City, Utah.)

infection, certain cancers and cancer treatments, immuno-suppressive drugs, and stress. The risk of getting shingles increases with age.

Anti-viral drugs and pain-relief drugs are used. For many healthy people, the rash is gone in 2 to 4 weeks. Pain can last for months or years after the rash heals. A vaccine is available to prevent shingles. The CDC recommends that persons age 50 and older be vaccinated against shingles.

Fluid from the blisters can spread the virus to persons who have not had chicken pox or the chicken pox vaccine. The blisters usually develop a crust (scab) within 7 to 10 days. Shingles lesions are infectious until they crust over. The person needs to cover the rash, avoid touching or scratching the rash, and practice hand hygiene often.

Avoid contact with an infected person if you:

- Have never had chicken pox or the vaccine to prevent chicken pox.
- Are pregnant and have not had chicken pox or the vaccine to prevent chicken pox.
- Have a weakened immune system.

Cellulitis

Cellulitis is an infection of the skin and underlying tissue. It is usually caused by a break in the skin that allows bacteria to enter. The skin is red, swollen, warm, and painful (Fig. 48-8, p. 736). Cellulitis can occur anywhere on the body. It occurs most often on a foot or leg.

Factors that increase the risk of cellulitis include:

- Having an injury, wound, or other skin condition
- Having a weakened immune system
- Chronic swelling of a body part
- A history of cellulitis
- Diabetes
- Being overweight

Good hand hygiene and wound care can prevent cellulitis. Cellulitis is treated with antibiotics. The affected area is elevated if possible. If untreated, the infection can spread to other areas of the body. Persons with diabetes are at risk for severe complications, including amputation. For persons with diabetes, the feet need to be checked daily for changes in the skin (Chapter 41).

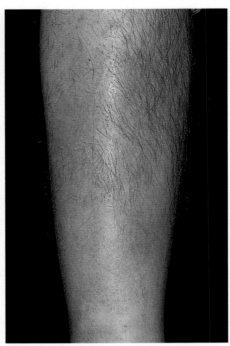

FIGURE 48-8 Cellulitis. (From Habif TP et al: *Skin disease diagnosis & treatment*, ed 3, 2011, Elsevier.)

FOCUS ON **PRIDE**

The Person, Family, and Yourself

Personal and Professional Responsibility

Oncology is the study of cancer. Oncology staff are experienced with the care and needs of persons with cancer. Staff need to be kind, caring, patient, and compassionate. Good communication skills are needed to provide quality care and to work well with the team.

Rights and Respect

The person and family have many reactions to illness—fear, anger, worry, guilt. Families respond in different ways. Family bonds are stronger when the family relies on each other during stress. A helpful and supportive family benefits the person's quality of life.

   Promote pride in the family. Show respect. Compliment their efforts. Encourage the family's help and support.

Independence and Social Interaction

A *stigma* relates to negative attitudes and beliefs about someone or something. *Discrimination* involves the behaviors that result from such attitudes and beliefs. The CDC lists some examples of HIV stigma and discrimination.
- Believing that only certain groups of people get HIV
- Making judgments about persons who take measures to prevent HIV transmission
- Thinking that HIV is deserved because of life choices
- Refusing to care for or have casual contact with a person with HIV
- Socially isolating persons who are HIV positive
- Using labels that insult persons with HIV
   Stigmas and discrimination harm mental health and well-being. Treat all persons with dignity and respect.

Delegation and Teamwork

Some disorders are life-threatening. AIDS and some malignant tumors are examples. Caring for dying persons is a challenge. You may have emotions and responses similar to the family. Share your feelings with the nursing team. Listen when others need to talk. See Chapter 59 for end-of-life care.

Ethics and Laws

Oncology staff often care for a person many times. Staff get to know the person's likes, dislikes, and preferences. Staff learn about the person's family, school or work, hobbies, and so on. Interest in the person adds to quality of care.

   Maintaining professional boundaries can be hard when caring for persons you see often and get to know well. However, you must protect the person's privacy and rights. Watch your behavior closely to avoid crossing boundaries (Chapter 5).

FOCUS ON **PRIDE**: *Application*

Many of the disorders in this chapter are life-changing. Choose 1 disorder in this chapter. Discuss the impact on the person and others.

REVIEW QUESTIONS

Circle the BEST answer.

1 A person has cancer. You know that
   a The tumor will not threaten life
   b The tumor can spread to other body parts
   c The tumor is benign
   d The cancer can be cured with surgery

2 Metastasis means that
   a Cancer cells have been killed
   b A benign tumor has grown larger
   c A malignant tumor has spread to other body parts
   d Healthy cells have been damaged by cancer treatments

3 Who has the greatest risk of cancer?
   a The person who smokes
   b The person who is physically active
   c The person who limits time in the sun
   d The person who is 43 years old

4 Your friend has severe fatigue and weight loss for no known reason. The person says, "I don't have pain, so it isn't cancer." Which reply is *best*?
   a "It's probably something else."
   b "Cancer may not cause pain. Have you told your doctor?"
   c "You are right. I'm sure you are fine."
   d "Wait a few weeks and see if you feel better."

5 A patient had surgery to remove a tumor. Which is appropriate for this patient?
   a You report signs of pain to the nurse right away.
   b You tell the person to expect hair loss.
   c You refuse tasks involving body fluids to protect yourself.
   d You avoid getting close to the person.

6 A patient has a radiation implant. You need to
   a Remove trash and linens from the room as usual
   b Give a pregnant visitor a gown to wear before a visit
   c Use re-usable items as much as possible
   d Limit your time in the room

7 Common side effects of chemotherapy include
   a Numbness and weakness on 1 side of the body
   b Chest pain and dyspnea
   c Fatigue, hair loss, and nausea
   d Fever and night sweats

8 A person receiving chemotherapy becomes sad when talking about treatment side effects. You should
   a Change the subject
   b Talk about how other patients respond to treatment
   c Tell the person: "It will be okay"
   d Listen

9 A person has stomatitis from receiving cancer treatment. Which shows you understand the person's oral care needs?
   a You do not give oral care if the person has a dry mouth.
   b You use sponge swabs gently.
   c You use a mouthwash containing alcohol for mouth sores.
   d You use a toothbrush with firm bristles.

10 In an autoimmune disorder, the immune system
   a Is weakened
   b Does not respond at all
   c Attacks the body's own healthy cells, tissues, and organs
   d Produces abnormal cells that spread to other body parts

11 A person with celiac disease requires
   a Hormone therapy
   b A diet without gluten
   c Immunotherapy
   d Antibiotics

12 HIV is spread through
   a Blood and certain body fluids
   b Coughing and sneezing
   c Using public phones and restrooms
   d Hugging or dancing with an infected person

13 Which poses the *lowest* risk for HIV transmission?
   a Sex with an infected person
   b Needle-sharing
   c Sharing dishes with an infected person
   d Being born to an infected mother

14 Which statement about HIV and AIDS is *true*?
   a HIV treatment does not lower the risk of transmission.
   b HIV is only spread when symptoms are present.
   c The person with AIDS is at risk for infections and cancers.
   d HIV treatment cannot slow progression to AIDS.

15 HIV can be prevented by
   a Taking immuno-suppressive drugs
   b Getting an HIV vaccine
   c Using antibiotics
   d Avoiding risky sexual behaviors

16 A person with shingles needs to
   a Keep the rash covered until lesions crust over
   b Avoid contact with persons who have had chicken pox
   c Gently scratch areas of the rash that itch
   d Avoid pain-relief drugs

17 A person has shingles. You know that
   a Healing occurs in 3 to 5 days
   b Itching and pain are common
   c Lesions are not infectious
   d Antibiotics are used for treatment

18 Which statement about cellulitis is *true*?
   a Cellulitis is inflammation of the mouth that occurs with cancer treatment.
   b The infection cannot spread to other body areas.
   c Persons with diabetes are at risk for severe complications.
   d Cellulitis cannot be prevented.

Answers to Chapter 48 questions are on p. 903.

FOCUS ON **PRACTICE**

Problem Solving

You work for a home health agency. You have 2 visits today. One is a patient with AIDS. The other is a patient receiving chemotherapy for cancer. You have a cough and fever. Do you go to work or call to say you cannot work? Explain the reason for your decision.

Nervous System and Musculo-Skeletal Disorders

OBJECTIVES

- Define the key terms and key abbreviations in this chapter.
- Describe different nervous system disorders and the care required—stroke, Parkinson's disease, multiple sclerosis (MS), amyotrophic lateral sclerosis (ALS), traumatic brain injury, and spinal cord injury.
- Describe different musculo-skeletal disorders and the care required—arthritis, osteoporosis, and fractures.

- Explain how to assist in the care of persons after joint replacement surgery.
- Explain how to assist in the care of persons in casts, in traction, and with hip fractures.
- Describe the effects of amputation.
- Explain how to promote PRIDE in the person, the family, and yourself.

KEY TERMS

amputation The removal of all or part of an extremity

arthritis Joint (arthr) inflammation (itis)

arthroplasty The surgical replacement (plasty) of a joint (arthro)

closed fracture The bone is broken but the skin is intact; simple fracture

compound fracture See "open fracture"

fracture A broken bone

gangrene A condition in which there is death of tissue

hemiparesis Partial paralysis (paresis) on 1 side (hemi) of the body

hemiplegia Paralysis (plegia) on 1 side (hemi) of the body

open fracture The broken bone has pierced the skin; compound fracture

paralysis Loss of muscle function

paraplegia Paralysis in the legs and lower trunk

paresis Weak or impaired muscle function without complete paralysis; partial paralysis

quadriplegia Paralysis in the arms, legs, and trunk; tetraplegia

simple fracture See "closed fracture"

tetraplegia See "quadriplegia"

KEY ABBREVIATIONS

AD	Autonomic dysreflexia	MS	Multiple sclerosis
ADL	Activities of daily living	RA	Rheumatoid arthritis
ALS	Amyotrophic lateral sclerosis	ROM	Range-of-motion
CVA	Cerebrovascular accident	TBI	Traumatic brain injury
JA	Juvenile arthritis	TIA	Transient ischemic attack

This chapter will help you understand some disorders of the nervous and musculo-skeletal systems. Learning about disorders gives meaning to the required care. The nurse gives you more information as needed.

NERVOUS SYSTEM DISORDERS

Nervous system disorders can affect mental and physical function. They can affect the ability to speak, understand, feel, see, hear, touch, think, control bowels and bladder, and move. Some problems are short-term. Others are long-term.

See *Body Structure and Function Review: The Nervous System.*

BODY STRUCTURE AND FUNCTION REVIEW

The Nervous System

Structure and Function

The nervous system controls, directs, and coordinates body functions. It has 2 main divisions—the central nervous system (CNS) and the peripheral nervous system (PNS). The CNS consists of the brain and spinal cord (Fig. 49-1). The PNS involves the nerves throughout the body (Fig. 49-2).

Neurons (nerve cells) are the specialized cells in the nervous system that conduct (send and receive) signals (impulses). *Neurotransmitters* are chemicals that allow signals to pass between nerve cells. Nerve cells can also transmit signals to muscles and glands. *Nerves* are groupings (bundles) of nerve cells. Some nerves have a protective covering called a *myelin sheath*. The myelin insulates the nerve fiber and increases the rate of impulse conduction.

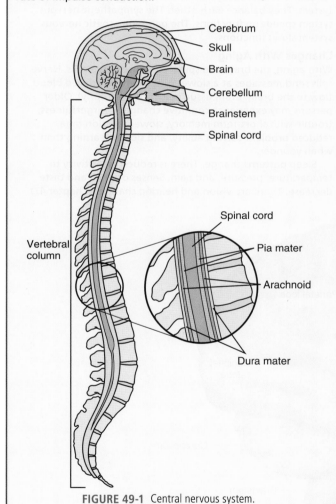

FIGURE 49-1 Central nervous system.

Cerebrum
Skull
Brain
Cerebellum
Brainstem
Spinal cord
Vertebral column
Spinal cord
Pia mater
Arachnoid
Dura mater

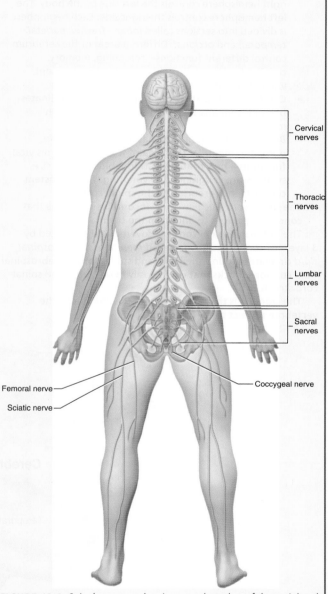

FIGURE 49-2 Spinal nerves and major nerve branches of the peripheral nervous system. (Modified from Solomon EP: *Introduction to human anatomy and physiology*, ed 4, St Louis, 2016, Saunders.)

Cervical nerves
Thoracic nerves
Lumbar nerves
Sacral nerves
Coccygeal nerve
Femoral nerve
Sciatic nerve

Continued

BODY STRUCTURE AND FUNCTION REVIEW—cont'd

The Nervous System

The Central Nervous System

Major structures in the central nervous system (CNS) include:

- The *brain* (Fig. 49-3). The 3 main parts of the brain are the:
  - *Cerebrum.* This is the largest part of the brain. It is divided into 2 hemispheres—*right* and *left hemispheres.* The right hemisphere controls the left side of the body. The left hemisphere controls the right side. Each hemisphere is divided into sections called *lobes—frontal, parietal, temporal,* and *occipital.* Different areas of the cerebrum control different functions—reasoning, memory, consciousness, speech, voluntary muscle movement, vision, hearing, sensation, and other activities.
  - *Cerebellum.* This structure regulates and coordinates body movements including balance and smooth movements.
  - *Brainstem.* The brainstem has 3 parts—*midbrain, pons,* and *medulla.* This area of the brain controls vital functions—heart rate, breathing, blood vessel size, swallowing, coughing, and vomiting. The brainstem connects the cerebrum to the spinal cord.
- The *spinal cord* (see Fig. 49-1). It contains pathways that conduct messages to and from the brain.

The brain and spinal cord are covered and protected by 3 layers of connective tissue called *meninges. Cerebrospinal fluid* circulates around the brain and spinal cord. Cerebrospinal fluid cushions shocks that could easily injure brain and spinal cord structures.

The cranium is the bone that protects the brain. The vertebrae protect the spinal cord. See Figure 49-1.

The Peripheral Nervous System

The peripheral nervous system (PNS) has 12 pairs of *cranial nerves* and 31 pairs of *spinal nerves.* The cranial nerves conduct impulses between the brain and the head, neck, chest, and abdomen. They conduct impulses for smell, vision, hearing, taste, pain, touch, temperature, and pressure. They also conduct impulses for voluntary and involuntary muscles. Spinal nerves (see Fig. 49-2) carry impulses from the skin, extremities, and internal structures not supplied by the cranial nerves.

Some peripheral nerves form the *autonomic nervous system.* This system controls involuntary muscles and certain body functions—heartbeat, blood pressure, intestinal contractions, and glandular secretions.

The autonomic nervous system is divided into the *sympathetic nervous system* and the *parasympathetic nervous system.* They balance each other. The sympathetic nervous system speeds up functions. The parasympathetic nervous system slows functions.

Changes With Aging

With aging, the brain and spinal cord lose nerve cells. Nerve cells send messages at a slower rate. There is reduced blood flow to the brain. Brain tissue may shrink *(atrophy).* Older persons may experience cognitive changes—forgetfulness, trouble with short-term memory, slower reaction time, reduced problem-solving ability, and slower learning than when younger.

Sleep patterns change. There is reduced sensitivity to temperature, pressure, and pain. Senses of smell and taste decrease. There are vision and hearing changes (Chapter 47).

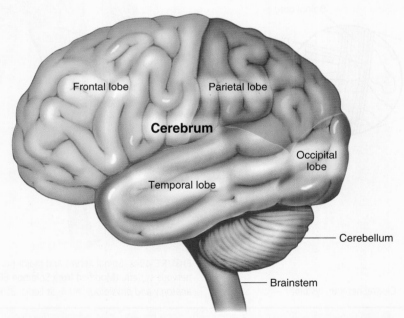

FIGURE 49-3 Major structures and lobes of the brain. (Modified from Bell F, Patton KT, Williamson P, Thompson T: *The human body in health & disease,* ed 8, St Louis, 2024, Elsevier.)

Stroke

Stroke (*brain attack* or *cerebrovascular accident [CVA]*) occurs when 1 of these happens.

- A blood vessel in the brain bursts and bleeds into the brain (cerebral hemorrhage).
- A blood clot blocks a blood vessel in the brain. Blood flow stops.

Brain cells in the affected area do not get enough oxygen and nutrients. Brain damage occurs. Functions controlled by that part of the brain are lost (Fig. 49-4).

Stroke is a leading cause of disability and death in the United States. The person needs emergency care (Chapter 58).

Risk Factors.
Risk factors include:

- High blood pressure
- Smoking or second-hand smoke
- Heart disease
- Diabetes
- High cholesterol
- Transient ischemic attack (TIA) (see "Signs and Symptoms")
- Age 55 and older
- Being over-weight
- Lack of physical activity
- Family history of stroke, heart disease, or TIAs
- Substance use disorder (Chapter 53)
- Biological sex—men are at higher risk than women
- Race—African Americans have a higher risk than other races
- Hormones—use of birth control pills

Signs and Symptoms.
Stroke occurs suddenly. See Box 49-1 for the major signs and symptoms. Nausea and vomiting, seizures, or loss of consciousness may occur.

When signs and symptoms only last a few minutes, this is called a *transient ischemic attack (TIA)*. (*Transient* means temporary or short term. *Ischemic* means reduced blood flow to a body part.) During a TIA, blood supply to the brain is interrupted for a short time. A TIA may occur before a stroke.

All stroke-like symptoms signal the need for emergency care. Blood flow to the brain must be restored as soon as possible.

BOX 49-1	Stroke: Signs and Symptoms

- Sudden numbness or weakness of the face, arm, or leg; especially on 1 side of the body
- Sudden confusion, trouble speaking, or trouble understanding speech
- Sudden trouble seeing in 1 or both eyes
- Sudden trouble walking, dizziness, or loss of balance or coordination
- Sudden, severe headache with no known cause

From National Institute of Neurological Disorders and Stroke: Know stroke. Know the signs. Act in time. *Bethesda, Md, reviewed December 18, 2023, National Institutes of Health.*

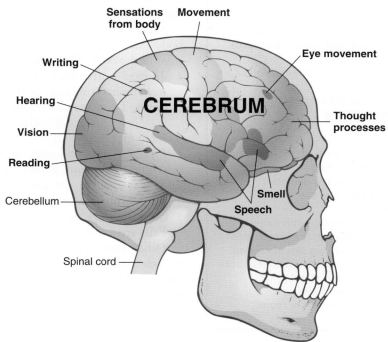

FIGURE 49-4 Functions lost from a stroke depend on the area of brain damage. (From Chabner DE: *The language of medicine,* ed 12, St Louis, 2021, Elsevier.)

Effects on the Person. If the person survives, some brain damage is likely. Effects of stroke can include:

- Weakness or inability to move parts of the body.
  - *Hemiparesis*—partial paralysis (*paresis*) on 1 side (*hemi*) of the body. *Paresis* is weak or impaired muscle function without complete paralysis.
  - *Hemiplegia*—paralysis (*plegia*) on 1 side (*hemi*) of the body. *Paralysis* is loss of muscle function.
- Changing emotions. The person cries easily or has mood swings sometimes for no known reason.
- Difficulty swallowing (*dysphagia*).
- Aphasia or slowed or slurred speech (Chapter 47).
- Changes in sight, touch (sensation), movement, and thought.
- Impaired memory.
- Urinary frequency, urgency, or incontinence.
- Loss of bowel control or constipation.
- Depression and frustration.
- Behavior changes.

The person may forget about or ignore the weaker side. This is called *neglect*. It is from the loss of vision or movement and feeling on that side. Sometimes thinking is affected. The person may not recognize or know how to use common items. Activities of daily living (ADL) and other tasks are hard to do. The person may forget what to do and how to do it. If the person does know, the body may not respond.

Rehabilitation starts at once. The person may depend in part or totally on others for care. The goal is to regain the highest possible level of function (Box 49-2).

See *Focus on Long-Term Care and Home Care: Effects on the Person (Stroke)*.

FOCUS ON LONG-TERM CARE AND HOME CARE

Effects on the Person (Stroke)

Long-Term Care

Some persons return home after rehabilitation. For others, long-term care is often permanent. Many measures listed in Box 49-2 are part of the person's care.

Home Care

Many stroke survivors return home. Family assistance and home health care are often needed. Many measures in Box 49-2 continue. The health team recommends home changes to help the person function.

BOX 49-2   Stroke Care Measures

- Position the person in the side-lying position to prevent aspiration.
- Keep the bed in semi-Fowler's position.
- Approach the person from the strong (unaffected) side. The person may have loss of vision on the affected side.
- Turn and re-position the person at least every 2 hours.
- Use assist devices to move, turn, re-position, and transfer the person.
- Encourage incentive spirometry and deep breathing and coughing.
- Prevent contractures. Assist with range-of-motion (ROM) exercises.
- Prevent pressure injuries.
- Meet food and fluid needs. A dysphagia diet with thickened liquids and modified food texture is common (Chapter 31).
- Apply elastic stockings as directed to prevent *thrombi* (blood clots) in the legs.
- Meet elimination needs. Follow the care plan for:
  - Catheter care or bladder training
  - Bowel training
- Practice safety precautions.
  - Keep the call light and other needed items within reach on the strong (unaffected) side.
  - Check the person often. Follow the care plan.
  - Use bed rails according to the care plan.
  - Prevent falls and other injuries.
- Encourage as much self-care as possible. This includes turning, positioning, and transferring. The person uses adaptive (assistive) devices and walking aids as needed.
- Do not rush the person. Movements are slower after a stroke.
- Follow established communication methods.
- Give support, encouragement, and praise.
- Complete a safety check before leaving the room. (See the inside of the back cover.)

Parkinson's Disease

Parkinson's disease is a progressive disorder affecting movement. It occurs when nerve cells in the brain do not produce enough of a chemical (neurotransmitter) called *dopamine*. Dopamine is needed for smooth, purposeful movement. Persons over the age of 60 are at higher risk.

Signs and symptoms are mild at first on 1 side of the body (Fig. 49-5). They worsen over time and affect both sides of the body. The main signs are:

- *Tremors*—often start in the hand. Pill-rolling movements (rubbing the thumb and index finger) may occur. There may be trembling in the hands, arms, legs, jaw, and face. Shaking has a rhythmic back-and-forth motion.
- *Rigid, stiff muscles*—occur in the arms, legs, neck, and trunk. (The trunk [torso] is the chest and abdomen.)
- *Slow movement*—the person develops short, shuffling steps. Simple tasks are hard to do.
- *Stooped posture and impaired balance*—it is hard to walk. Falls are a risk.

Other signs and symptoms develop over time. They include swallowing and chewing problems, constipation, sleep problems, depression, and emotional changes (fear, insecurity). Memory loss and slow thinking can occur. The person may have slow, monotone, and soft speech. A fixed stare and trouble blinking and smiling can occur.

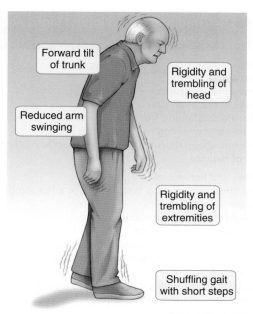

FIGURE 49-5 Signs of Parkinson's disease. (From Patton KT, Thibodeau GA: *The human body in health & disease*, ed 7, St Louis, 2018, Elsevier.)

With no cure, drugs are ordered to control the disease. Exercise and physical therapy help improve strength, posture, balance, and mobility. Therapy is needed for speech and swallowing problems. The person may need help with eating and self-care. Normal elimination is a goal. Safety measures are needed to prevent falls and injuries.

Multiple Sclerosis

Multiple means many. *Sclerosis* means hardening or scarring. Multiple sclerosis (MS) is an autoimmune disorder (Chapter 48) that damages the myelin covering nerve fibers. In MS, the immune system attacks myelin in the brain and spinal cord, causing scarring and damage. Nerve impulses between the body and brain are not sent in a normal way. Functions are impaired or lost.

Symptoms usually start between the ages of 20 and 40. MS occurs more often in women than in men. The risk increases if a family member has MS. Signs and symptoms of MS vary widely depending on the severity and the areas affected. They may include:

- Blurred or double vision; blindness in 1 eye
- Muscle weakness in the arms and legs
- Problems with coordination, balance, and walking *(ataxia)*
- Tingling, prickling, or numb sensations
- Partial or complete paralysis
- Pain
- Speech problems
- Tremors
- Dizziness
- Concentration, attention, memory, and judgment problems
- Depression
- Bladder problems
- Problems with sexual function
- Hearing loss
- Fatigue

MS can present in many ways. For example:
- Symptoms appear for a while then seem to go away. The person is in *remission*. Later, symptoms flare up again *(relapse)*.
- More symptoms appear. The person's condition worsens.
- There are remissions and relapses at first. Eventually symptoms become worse. More symptoms occur with each flare-up. The person's condition declines.

MS has no cure. Some drugs can slow the disease and help control symptoms. Persons with MS are kept as active and as independent as possible. The care plan reflects changing needs. Skin care, hygiene, and ROM exercises are important. So are turning, positioning, and deep breathing and coughing. Elimination needs are met. Injuries and complications from bed rest are prevented.

See *Focus on Long-Term Care and Home Care: Multiple Sclerosis*.

FOCUS ON **LONG-TERM CARE AND HOME CARE**

Multiple Sclerosis

Home Care
The person may need help with housekeeping to avoid fatigue. As mobility decreases, the person depends more on others. Occupational and physical therapists are often involved in the person's care.

Amyotrophic Lateral Sclerosis

Amyotrophic lateral sclerosis (ALS) affects the nerve cells in the brain and spinal cord that control voluntary muscles. Muscles in the arms and legs and those used for chewing and talking are voluntary. Commonly called *Lou Gehrig's disease*, it is rapidly progressive and fatal. (Lou Gehrig was a New York Yankees baseball player who died of the disease.)

ALS usually strikes persons between 55 and 75 years of age. Most die 3 to 5 years after onset.

Affected nerve cells in the brain and spinal cord stop sending messages to the voluntary muscles. Muscles weaken, waste away *(atrophy)*, and twitch. Over time, the brain cannot start or control voluntary movements. The person cannot move the arms, legs, and body. Muscles for speaking, chewing and swallowing, and breathing also are affected. Eventually respiratory muscles fail. The person needs a ventilator to breathe (Chapter 45).

The disease usually does not affect the mind, intelligence, or memory. However, some persons develop dementia. Sight, smell, taste, hearing, and touch are not affected. Usually bowel and bladder functions remain intact.

ALS has no cure. Some drugs can slow the disease and improve symptoms. However, damage cannot be reversed. The person is kept active and independent to the extent possible. The care plan reflects changing needs.

Persons with ALS may need:

- Physical, occupational, speech-language, and respiratory therapies
- ROM exercises
- Mobility aids—braces, walker, wheelchair
- Comfort and pain-relief measures
- Communication methods
- Dysphagia diet or feeding tube
- Respiratory support—suctioning, mechanical ventilation
- Safety measures to prevent falls and injuries
- Psychological and social support
- Hospice care

Head Injuries

Head injuries result from trauma to the scalp, skull, or brain. Injuries range from a minor bump to a serious, life-threatening brain injury. Falls, vehicle accidents, violence (assaults, gunshots), and sports injuries are common causes.

Head injuries are open or closed. Bleeding may occur.

- Closed—the skull did not break but the brain is injured.
- Open (penetrating)—an object broke the skull and entered the brain.

Symptoms may develop at the time of the injury. Or they can take several hours or days to develop. Symptoms are from bleeding or swelling inside the skull.

Most head injuries need emergency care. See Chapter 58.

Traumatic Brain Injury. Traumatic brain injury (TBI) occurs from violent injury to the brain—a bump, blow, jolt, or an object entering the brain. Common causes include:

- *Falls.* Older persons and children are at risk for falling out of bed, slipping in the shower or bathtub, falling down steps, and falling from ladders.
- *Vehicle accidents.* Cars, motorcycles, and bikes are often involved. Persons who were walking or jogging have been injured.
- *Violence.* Gunshots, intimate partner violence (Chapter 5), and child abuse can result in TBI.
- *Sports.* Many sports increase the risk of TBI—football, soccer, boxing, baseball, hockey, lacrosse, skateboarding, and other high-impact sports.
- *Explosive blasts and combat injuries.* TBI can occur from penetrating injuries, blows to the head, and falls. Military personnel are at risk.

Brain tissue is bruised or torn. Bleeding is in the brain or in nearby tissues. Spinal cord injuries are likely.

Men, infants and children, young adults, and older persons are at risk for TBI. Death can occur at the time of injury or later. See Box 49-3 for the signs and symptoms of TBI.

BOX 49-3	Traumatic Brain Injury: Signs and Symptoms

Physical
- Headache
- Convulsions, seizures
- Unequal eye pupil size, large pupil
- Clear fluids draining from the nose or ears
- Nausea and vomiting
- New neurological problem—slurred speech, weakness, loss of balance

Cognitive and Behavioral
- Loss of consciousness: a few seconds to a few minutes or longer
- Altered level of consciousness
- Confusion, disorientation
- Problems with memory, concentration, or decision-making
- Problems sleeping, sleeping more than usual, cannot be awakened
- Frustration, irritability, mood changes (agitation, combativeness, unusual behavior)
- Anxiety, depression
- Drowsiness, lack of energy or motivation

Perception and Sensation
- Dizziness, loss of balance or coordination
- Blurred vision, double vision
- Hearing problems, ringing in the ears
- Bad taste in the mouth
- Sensitivity to light or sound

Modified from National Institute of Neurological Disorders and Stroke: Traumatic brain injury, last reviewed November 28, 2023, National Institutes of Health.

If the person survives, some permanent damage is likely. Disabilities depend on the severity and site of injury. They include:

- Cognitive problems—thinking, memory, reasoning
- Sensory problems—sight, hearing, touch, taste, smell
- Communication problems—expressing or understanding language
- Emotional problems—depression, anxiety, personality changes, aggressive behavior, acting out, socially inappropriate behavior
- Changes in level of consciousness:
  - Stupor—The person is unresponsive but can be briefly aroused by a strong stimulus (such as pain).
  - Coma—The person is unconscious, does not respond, is unaware, and cannot be aroused.
  - Vegetative state (Fig. 49-6)—The person is unconscious and unaware of surroundings. The person has sleep-wake cycles and may open the eyes, make sounds, or move.
  - Brain death (see Fig. 49-6)—Despite complete loss of brain function, the heart continues to beat. Reflex activity, movement, and spontaneous respirations are absent.

Healthy control

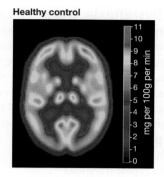

Vegetative state   **Brain death**

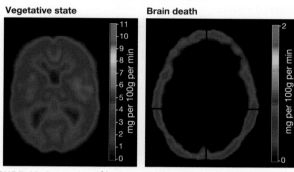

FIGURE 49-6 Imaging of brains with altered levels of consciousness. (Images courtesy *Nature Reviews Neuroscience*, McMillan Publishers Limited, 2014.)

Emergency care involves drugs and surgery to limit brain damage. Rehabilitation is required. Physical, occupational, speech-language, and mental health therapies depend on the person's needs. Nursing care depends on the person's needs and abilities.

See *Focus on Children and Older Persons: Traumatic Brain Injury.*

FOCUS ON **CHILDREN AND OLDER PERSONS**

Traumatic Brain Injury

Children
Birth injuries are a major cause of head injuries in newborns. As children grow older, vehicle accidents, wheel-related sports (bikes, scooters, skates, skateboards), and falls are major causes of TBI.

Falls are a great danger for infants and toddlers. Falling down stairs and from windows are common accidents. Specific safety practices to prevent injuries and falls are discussed in Chapters 14, 15, and 56 and Appendix D.

The National Institute of Neurological Disorders and Stroke lists these signs of TBI in infants and children.
• A change in eating or nursing habits
• Persistent crying or irritability
• Inability to be consoled (comforted)
• Change in ability to pay attention
• Loss of interest in favorite toys or activities
• Change in sleep habits
• Sad or depressed mood
• Loss of a skill (such as toilet training)
• Loss of balance or unsteady walking
• Vomiting
• Seizures

Spinal Cord Injury

Spinal cord injury usually results from a sudden, traumatic blow to the spine. Common causes are vehicle accidents, falls, violence (knife and gunshot wounds), and sports injuries. Cancer and other diseases can also cause injury. Young adult men have the highest risk.

Serious damage to the nervous system can occur. The trauma fractures or dislocates vertebrae in the spine. Spinal cord tissue is torn or bruised. Problems depend on the amount of damage to the spinal cord and the level of injury. Paresis or paralysis can result. Sensation and body functions are also affected. The higher the level of injury, the more functions lost (Fig. 49-7).
• Lumbar injuries—occur in the low back. Sensory (feeling) and muscle function (movement) in the legs is lost. The person has paraplegia. *Paraplegia* is paralysis in the legs and lower trunk. (*Para* means beyond; *plegia* means paralysis.)
• Thoracic injuries—occur in the middle and upper back. Sensory and muscle function below the chest is lost. The person has paraplegia.
• Cervical injuries—occur at the neck. Sensory and muscle function of the arms, legs, and trunk (torso) is lost. Paralysis in the arms, legs, and trunk is called *quadriplegia* or *tetraplegia*. (*Quad* and *tetra* mean 4. *Plegia* means paralysis.)

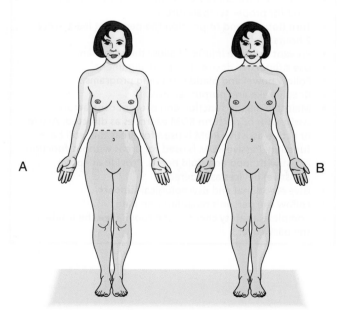

FIGURE 49-7 The *shaded areas* show the area of paralysis. **A,** Paraplegia. **B,** Quadriplegia (tetraplegia).

Damage to the spinal cord may be incomplete or complete.
- Incomplete—Some sensory and muscle function below the level of the injury remains.
- Complete—No sensory or muscle function below the level of the injury remains.

The person with a spinal cord injury has 1 or more of these signs and symptoms.
- Severe back, neck, or head pain or pressure
- Loss of movement
- Loss of sensation—heat, cold, touch
- Bladder and bowel incontinence
- Problems with balance and walking
- Breathing problems
- Twisted or odd position of the neck or back
- Spasms

Emergency care is needed. Cervical traction with a special bed may be needed (p. 752). The spine is kept straight at all times. See Box 49-4 for care measures for paralysis. Emotional needs are great. Reactions to paralysis and loss of function are often severe.

If the person lives, rehabilitation is needed. The person learns to function at the highest possible level with adaptive (assistive) and other devices. Some persons live independently at home or with home care. Others need long-term care or assisted-living settings.

BOX 49-4 Paralysis: Care Measures

- Practice safety measures to prevent falls. Use bed rails as directed.
- Keep the bed in a low position. Follow the care plan.
- Keep the call light and other needed items within reach. If unable to use the call light, check the person often.
- Prevent burns. Check bath water, heat applications, and food for proper temperature.
- Turn (logroll) and re-position the person at least every 2 hours.
- Prevent pressure injuries. Follow the care plan.
- Use supportive devices for good alignment.
- Follow bowel and bladder training programs.
- Keep intake and output records.
- Maintain muscle function and prevent contractures. Assist with or perform ROM exercises as directed. Active or active-assistive ROM is used for areas that still have function. Passive ROM is used for areas without function.
- Assist with food and fluid needs. Provide adaptive (assistive) devices as ordered.
- Give emotional and psychological support.
- Follow the person's rehabilitation plan.
- Complete a safety check of the room. (See the inside of the back cover.)

Autonomic Dysreflexia (AD). This syndrome can occur with spinal cord injuries above the mid-thoracic (middle back) level. The autonomic nervous system over-reacts to a stimulus *(reflexia)*. A full bladder, constipation, fecal impaction, and skin disorders are some triggers. With AD, there is sudden onset of excessively high blood pressure. Stroke, seizures, heart attack, and death are risks. AD is life-threatening. Report any of the following at once.
- High blood pressure
- Headache: throbbing or pounding
- Pulse: slow or rapid; irregular
- Blurred vision
- Muscle spasms, especially the jaw
- Heavy sweating
- "Goose bumps" and flushed (red) skin above the level of the spinal cord injury
- Nasal congestion
- Anxiety
- Dizziness
- Fainting
- Bowel or bladder problems

To treat AD, the head of the bed is raised or the person sits upright if allowed. Tight clothing is removed. And the cause is treated. See Box 49-5.

BOX 49-5 Autonomic Dysreflexia

- Monitor urinary output.
- Follow measures for catheter care. Do not let the drainage bag get too full.
- Prevent urinary tract infections.
- Promote bowel elimination. Prevent constipation and fecal impaction.
- Prevent skin injuries—skin tears, pressure injuries, cuts, bruises, burns, and so on.
- Check the feet for ingrown toenails, blisters, pressure injuries, and so on.
- Have the person wear loose and comfortable clothing.
- Remove wrinkles from clothing and linens.
- Re-position the person at least every 2 hours. Avoid prolonged pressure from the bed or chair.
- Report pain and menstrual cramps.

MUSCULO-SKELETAL DISORDERS

Musculo-skeletal disorders affect movement. Injury and aging are common causes. Daily living, social activities, and quality of life are affected.

See *Body Structure and Function Review: The Musculo-Skeletal System*.

BODY STRUCTURE AND FUNCTION REVIEW

The Musculo-Skeletal System

Structure and Function

Bones

Bones are hard, rigid structures.

- *Long bones* bear the body's weight. Leg bones are long bones.
- *Short bones* allow skill and ease in movement. Bones in the wrists, fingers, ankles, and toes are short bones.
- *Flat bones* protect the organs. They include the ribs, skull, pelvic bones, and shoulder blades.
- *Irregular bones* are the vertebrae in the spinal column. They allow various degrees of movement and flexibility.

Joints

A *joint* is the point at which 2 or more bones meet (Fig. 49-8). Joints allow movement.

- *Ball-and-socket joint* allows movement in all directions. The rounded end of 1 bone fits into the hollow end of another bone.
- *Hinge joint* allows movement in 1 direction.
- *Pivot joint* allows turning from side to side.

Cartilage is connective tissue at the end of the long bones. It cushions the joint so that the bone ends do not rub together. The *synovial membrane* lines the joints. It secretes *synovial fluid*. Synovial fluid acts as a lubricant so the joint can move smoothly. Bones are held together at the joint by strong bands of connective tissue called *ligaments*.

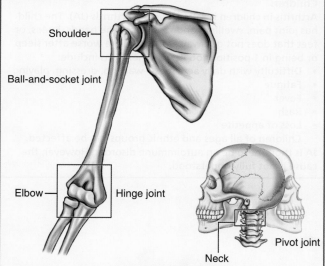

FIGURE 49-8 Types of joints. (Modified from Herlihy B: *The human body in health and illness,* ed 7, St Louis, 2022, Elsevier.)

Muscles

Muscles function in the movement of body parts and the maintenance of posture. Strong, tough connective tissues called *tendons* connect muscles to bones. When muscles *contract* (shorten), tendons at each end of the muscle cause the bone to move. (The body also contains involuntary muscles and cardiac muscle with specific functions. See Chapter 10.)

Changes With Aging

With age, bone mass decreases. Bones become weaker and more brittle. They can break easily. The vertebrae shorten. There is a gradual loss of height. Joints can become stiff and painful. Muscles may shrink (atrophy). Muscle strength, tone, and contractility decrease. Mobility is often affected.

Arthritis

Arthritis means joint *(arthr)* inflammation *(itis)*. Affected joints have swelling, stiffness, and reduced range of motion. The joints are hard to move.

The 2 main types of arthritis are:

- *Osteoarthritis.* Cartilage at the ends of bones is damaged and wears away, causing the bones to rub together. The hands, knees, hips, and spine are often affected (Fig. 49-9).
- *Rheumatoid arthritis (RA).* RA is an autoimmune disorder (Chapter 48) that attacks the lining of the joint. RA causes inflammation and painful swelling. Many joints are affected at the same time. The wrists, hands, and knees are commonly affected. RA can also affect the neck, shoulders, elbows, hips, ankles, and feet. RA occurs on both sides of the body. For example, both the right and left wrists are affected. RA can cause fever and fatigue and affect other tissues and organs. The lungs, heart, and eyes are examples.

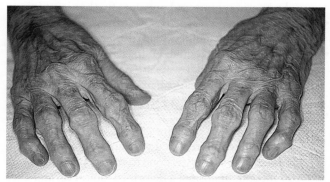

FIGURE 49-9 Osteoarthritis in the finger joints. (From Swartz MH: *Textbook of physical diagnosis: history and examination,* ed 8, Philadelphia, 2021, Elsevier.)

Risk Factors. Arthritis risk factors include:

- *Aging.* The risk increases with age.
- *Being over-weight.* Stress is placed on the weight-bearing joints—hips and knees. Stress also is placed on the spine.
- *Biological sex.* Arthritis is more common in women.
- *Joint injury.* A previous joint injury or over-use of a joint may develop into osteoarthritis.
- *Family history.* Arthritis tends to run in families.

Treatment. Osteoarthritis and RA have no cure. Treatments are similar.

- *Pain control.* Drugs decrease swelling and inflammation and relieve pain.
- *Heat and cold.* Heat relieves pain, increases blood flow, and reduces stiffness. Heat applications, a warm bath or shower, and water therapy in a heated pool are helpful. Cold applied for 20 minutes is useful after joint use and for severe pain. Cold slows circulation to reduce swelling. Nerve endings are numbed, which dulls the pain. See Chapter 43.
- *Exercise.* Exercise helps joint flexibility. It helps with weight control and promotes fitness. The person is taught needed exercises. Walking, biking, swimming, and water aerobics have a low risk of joint stress or injury.
- *Rest and joint care.* Good body mechanics, posture, and regular rest protect the joints. Relaxation methods are helpful.
- *Adaptive (assistive) devices.* Canes and walkers provide support. Splints support weak joints and promote alignment. Devices for hands and wrists are useful.
- *Weight control.* Weight loss reduces stress on weight-bearing joints and prevents further joint injury.
- *Healthy life-style.* The focus is on fitness, exercise, rest, managing stress, and good nutrition.
- *Safety.* Falls are prevented. Help is given with ADL as needed. Elevated toilet seats are helpful when hips and knees are affected. So are chairs with higher seats and armrests.
- *Joint replacement surgery. Arthroplasty* is the surgical replacement *(plasty)* of a joint *(arthro)*. The damaged joint is removed and replaced with an artificial joint *(prosthesis)*. The surgery is done to relieve pain, restore joint function, or correct a deformed joint. Hip and knee replacements are common (Fig. 49-10). Ankle, foot, shoulder, elbow, and finger joints also can be replaced. See Box 49-6 for care measures following a hip or knee replacement. After a hip replacement, the person is taught precautions to protect the hip (see Fig. 49-11). See *Focus on Children and Older Persons: Arthritis.*

BOX 49-6	Care After Joint Replacement: Hip or Knee

- Incentive spirometry and deep-breathing and coughing exercises to prevent respiratory complications.
- Elastic stockings to prevent *thrombi* (blood clots) in the legs.
- Physical therapy exercises to restore movement and return to normal activity. For knee replacement, sometimes a machine is used to slowly move the knee while in bed (continuous passive motion [CPM]).
- Assistance with walking and a walking aid—cane, walker, or crutches.
- Measures to protect the hip as shown in Figure 49-11.
- Food and fluids for tissue healing and to restore strength.
- Safety measures to prevent falls.
- Measures to prevent infection. Wound, urinary tract, and skin infections must be prevented.
- Measures to prevent pressure injuries.
- Assist devices for moving, turning, re-positioning, and transfers.
- Long-handled devices for reaching things.

FOCUS ON **CHILDREN AND OLDER PERSONS**

Arthritis

Children

Arthritis in children is called juvenile arthritis (JA). The child has joint pain, swelling, and stiffness in the hands, knees, or feet that does not go away. Symptoms are worse after sleep or being in 1 position too long. Other signs include:
- Difficulty with daily activities—walking, dressing, playing
- Fatigue
- Fever
- Rash
- Loss of appetite

Children of all ages and ethnic groups can be affected. JA is thought to be an autoimmune disorder. However, the cause is not fully understood.

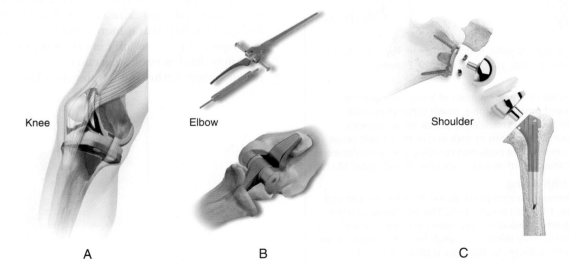

FIGURE 49-10 A, Knee replacement prosthesis. **B,** Elbow replacement prosthesis. **C,** Shoulder replacement prosthesis. (Courtesy Zimmer, Inc., A Bristol-Meyers Squibb Company, Warsaw, Ind.)

Do   Do Not

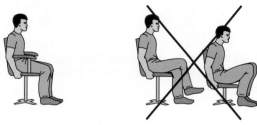

Do not cross your operated leg past the mid-line of the body or turn your kneecap in toward your body.

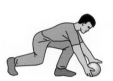

Do not sit in low chairs or cross your legs.

To sit: Use a high chair with arms or add pillows to elevate the seat.

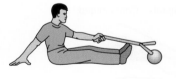 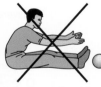

Avoid flexing your hips past 90 degrees.

To bend: Keep the operative leg behind you or as instructed by your therapist.

To reach: Use long-handled grabbers or as your therapist advises.

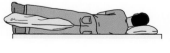 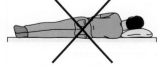

Use an elevated toilet.

Sleep with a pillow between the legs.

FIGURE 49-11 Measures to protect the hip after hip replacement surgery. (Modified from Monahan FD et al: *Phipps' medical-surgical nursing: health and illness perspectives,* ed 8, St Louis, 2007, Mosby.)

Osteoporosis

With osteoporosis, the bone *(osteo)* becomes porous and brittle *(porosis)*. Bones are fragile and break easily. Fractures (broken bones) can occur during normal daily activities. Spine, hip, and wrist fractures are common. (See "Fractures" on p. 750.)

Risk factors include:
- Aging.
- Biological sex. Women are at higher risk because of the loss of estrogen after menopause.
- Being thin and small.
- A family history of osteoporosis.
- A diet low in calcium and vitamin D.
- Tobacco and alcohol use.
- Eating disorders (Chapter 53).
- Bed rest, immobility, and lack of exercise. Bones must bear weight for strength and to form properly.

A broken bone is often the first sign of osteoporosis. Changes in the spine cause sloped shoulders, curving of the back, loss of height, back pain, and a hunched (bent over) posture (Fig. 49-12).

Prevention is important. Calcium and vitamin supplements may be ordered to prevent bone loss and build new bone. Estrogen is ordered for some women. Other preventive measures include:
- Exercising weight-bearing joints—walking, jogging, stair climbing, weight-lifting, dancing, and so on
- Eating foods that contain calcium and vitamin D
- No smoking and limiting alcohol
- Good posture and body mechanics
- Safety measures to prevent falls and accidents
- Safe moving, transferring, turning, and positioning procedures

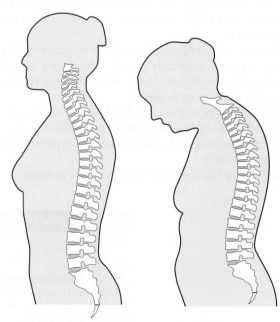

FIGURE 49-12 Osteoporosis in the spine. (Modified from Office of Women's Health: *Osteoporosis,* page updated May 20, 2019, U.S. Department of Health & Human Services.)

Fractures

A *fracture* is a broken bone. Depending on the type of fracture, tissues around the fracture—muscles, blood vessels, nerves, and tendons—may be injured. Fractures are open or closed (Fig. 49-13).

- *Open fracture (compound fracture)*—the broken bone has pierced the skin.
- *Closed fracture (simple fracture)*—the bone is broken but the skin is intact.

Different types of fractures can occur depending on how the bone breaks or the cause (Fig. 49-14). Some are more severe than others. For example, in a *stress (hairline) fracture,* only a small crack is present. In a *comminuted fracture,* the bone is shattered or broken into 3 or more pieces.

Falls, accidents, sports injuries, bone tumors, and osteoporosis are some causes. Signs and symptoms of a fracture are:

- Pain
- Swelling and tenderness
- Problems moving the part
- Deformity (the part looks out of place)
- Bruising and skin color changes at the fracture site
- Bleeding (internal or external)
- Numbness and tingling

For healing, bone ends are brought into and held in normal position. This is called *reduction and fixation.*

- Reduction—the bone is moved back into place.
  - Closed reduction—the bone is not exposed.
  - Open reduction—the bone is surgically exposed and moved into alignment.
- Fixation—the bone is held (fixed) in place (Fig. 49-15).
  - External fixation—Pins, screws, or wires are set into the bone outside the skin (see Fig. 49-15, *A*). The device is removed after healing or when the person is healthy enough for internal fixation of the fracture.
  - Internal fixation—Nails, rods, pins, screws, plates, or wires are surgically placed. The device is under the skin (see Fig. 49-15, *B*). After healing, the device is left in place or removed.

Casts and traction also are used. Devices such as splints, slings, and walking boots are common. Healing can take 6 to 8 weeks or longer depending on age, type of fracture, and general health.

See *Focus on Children and Older Persons: Fractures.*

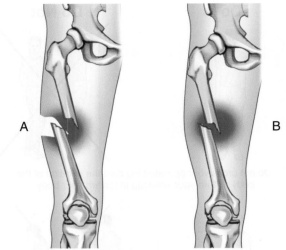

FIGURE 49-13 A, Open fracture. **B,** Closed fracture. (From Patton KT, Thibodeau GA: *The human body in health & disease,* ed 7, St Louis, 2018, Elsevier.)

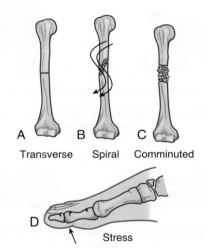

FIGURE 49-14 Examples of different types of fractures. **A,** Transverse—straight across. **B,** Spiral—fracture that occurs from twisting. **C,** Comminuted—shattered or broken in 3 or more pieces. **D,** Stress—a small crack. (From Harding MM et al: *Lewis's medical-surgical nursing: assessment and management of clinical problems,* ed 12, St Louis, 2023, Elsevier.)

FOCUS ON CHILDREN AND OLDER PERSONS

Fractures

Children
Falls and accidents involving motor vehicles, bikes, skateboards, and roller blades are common causes of fractures in children. Fractures may signal child abuse in infants and children.

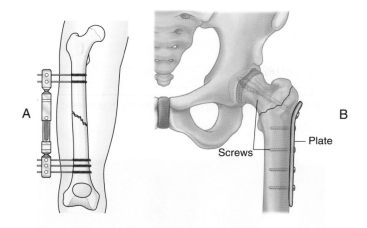

FIGURE 49-15 A, External fixation. **B,** Internal fixation. (A, From Mackenzie SP, White TO: *McRae's orthopaedic trauma and emergency management,* ed 4, St Louis, 2024, Elsevier. B, From Silvestri AE, Silvestri LA: *Saunders comprehensive review for the NCLEX-RN® examination,* ed 9, St Louis, Elsevier.)

Casts. Casts are made to fit the affected body part. They are made of fiberglass or plaster. First, a stockinette and padding are applied to protect the skin. Then, wet plaster or fiberglass strips or rolls are wrapped around the part.

Fiberglass casts dry quickly. A plaster cast dries in 24 to 48 hours. When wet, it is gray and cool and has a musty smell. It is odorless, white, and shiny when dry. The nurse may ask you to assist with care. See Box 49-7 for cast care. See Figure 49-16 (p. 752) for examples of casts.

BOX 49-7	Cast Care

The Cast

- Do not cover the cast with blankets, plastic, or other material. A cast gives off heat as it dries. Covers prevent the escape of heat. Burns can occur if heat cannot escape.
- Promote drying of the cast. All cast surfaces need exposure to air. Follow the nurse's directions to:
  - Turn the person. The person is turned at least every 2 hours.
  - Use a fan to move air over the cast.
- Maintain the shape of the cast.
  - Do not place a wet cast on a hard surface. It flattens the cast.
  - Use pillows to support the entire length of the cast (Fig. 49-17, p. 752).
  - Support the wet cast with your palms to turn and position the person (Fig. 49-18, p. 752). Fingertips can dent the cast, causing pressure areas and skin breakdown.
  - Report rough cast edges. The nurse may cushion the cast edges.
  - Keep the cast dry. A wet cast loses its shape. For casts near the perineal area, the nurse may apply a waterproof material after the cast dries.
- Do not remove the stockinette or padding around the cast edges.

Positioning

- Position the person as directed.
- Elevate a casted arm or leg on pillows to reduce swelling.
- Have enough help to turn and re-position the person. Plaster casts are heavy and awkward. Balance is lost easily.

Safety

- Follow the care plan for elimination needs. A fracture pan may be needed.
- Do not let the person insert things into the cast (pencils, back scratchers, and so on). Itching under the cast causes an intense desire to scratch. Items used to scratch can damage the skin, wrinkle the stockinette or padding, or be lost into the cast. Skin breakdown, pressure injury, and infection are risks.
- Do not put powder inside the cast.
- Do not let the person wear rings on the fingers or toes. The fingers or toes may swell or be swollen.
- Complete a safety check before leaving the room. (See the inside of the back cover.)

Reporting and Recording

- Report these signs and symptoms at once.
  - *Pain*—pressure injury, poor circulation, nerve damage
  - *Swelling and a tight cast*—reduced blood flow to the part
  - *Pale skin*—reduced blood flow to the part
  - *Cyanosis* (bluish skin color)—reduced blood flow to the part
  - *Odor*—infection
  - *Inability to move the fingers or toes*—pressure on a nerve
  - *Numbness*—pressure on a nerve, reduced blood flow to the part
  - *Temperature changes*—cool skin means poor circulation; hot skin means inflammation
  - *Drainage on or under the cast*—infection or bleeding
  - *Chills, fever, nausea, and vomiting*—infection

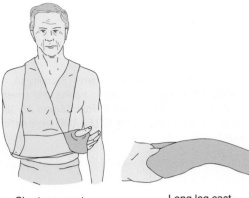

Short arm cast   Long leg cast

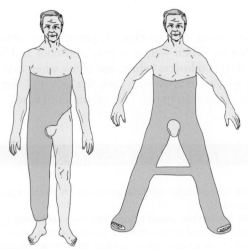

Single hip spica   Double hip spica

FIGURE 49-16 Examples of casts.

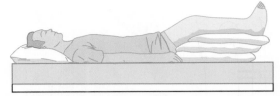

FIGURE 49-17 Pillows support the entire length of the wet cast.

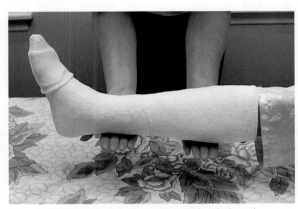

FIGURE 49-18 The cast is supported with the palms.

Traction. With traction, a steady pull from 2 directions keeps the bone in place. Weights, ropes, and pulleys are used (Fig. 49-19). Traction is applied to the neck, arms, legs, or pelvis.

For *skeletal traction*, wires or pins are inserted through the bone (see Fig. 49-19, *A*). For *cervical traction*, tongs are applied to the skull (Fig. 49-20). Weights are attached to the device. With *skin traction*, a boot, splint, or wraps are used. Weights are attached (see Fig. 49-19, *B*).

The person is at risk for complications from immobility (Chapter 35). To assist with the person's care, see Box 49-8.

BOX 49-8	Traction Care

- Keep the person in good alignment.
- Do not remove the traction.
- Keep the weights off of the floor. Weights must hang freely from the traction set-up (see Fig. 49-19).
- Do not add or remove weights.
- Check for frayed ropes. Report fraying at once.
- Perform ROM exercises for uninvolved joints as directed.
- Position the person as directed. Usually only the supine position is allowed. Slight turning may be allowed.
- Provide the fracture pan for elimination.
- Give skin care as directed.
- Put bottom linens on the bed from the top down. The person uses a trapeze to raise the body off of the bed (see Fig. 49-19).
- Check pin, nail, wire, or tong sites for redness, drainage, and odor. Report observations at once.
- Observe for the signs and symptoms listed for cast care (see Box 49-7). Report them at once.
- Complete a safety check before leaving the room. (See the inside of the back cover.)

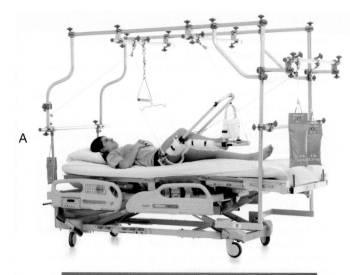

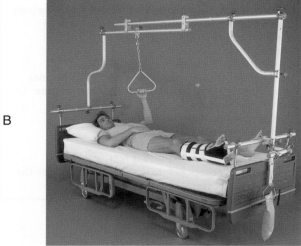

FIGURE 49-19 Traction set-up. Note the weights, pulleys, and ropes. A trapeze is used to raise the upper body off the bed. **A,** Skeletal traction. **B,** Skin traction. (A, Courtesy Zimmer, Inc. B, Courtesy Zimmer Biomet.)

Hip Fractures. Fractures of the hip are common in older persons. In addition to aging, risk factors include:

- Biological sex. Hip fractures are more common in older women. (Women are at higher risk for osteoporosis.)
- Osteoporosis. See p. 749.
- Drugs. Some drugs can weaken bones or have dizziness as a side effect.
- Nutrition. Calcium and vitamin D are needed for healthy bones.
- Inactivity. Weight-bearing exercise and activities are needed to strengthen bones.
- Smoking and alcohol use. These can cause bone loss.

Falls are the most common cause of hip fractures. However, fractures have occurred upon standing or twisting. Signs and symptoms include:

- Being unable to move after falling
- Severe hip or groin pain
- Shorter leg on the injured side
- Turning the leg inward or outward on the injured side
- Not being able to stand on the injured side
- Swollen and bruised area around the hip

Hip fractures require surgical repair or a hip replacement (Fig. 49-21). Adduction, internal rotation, external rotation, and severe hip flexion are avoided after surgery. Post-operative problems present life-threatening risks. They include pneumonia, urinary tract infections, and *thrombi* (blood clots) in the leg veins or lungs. Pressure injuries, constipation, and confusion are other problems. Box 49-9 (p. 754) describes the required care.

Rehabilitation is usually needed. Physical therapy and occupational therapy are common. Adaptive (assistive) devices are used for dressing and bathing. A walker is usually needed at first.

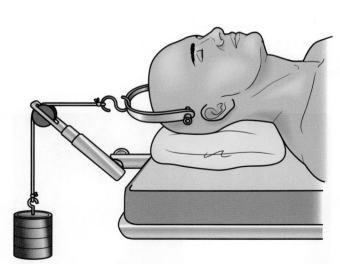

FIGURE 49-20 Cervical traction for spinal cord injury. (From Linton A, Matteson M: *Medical-surgical nursing,* ed 8, St Louis, 2022, Saunders.)

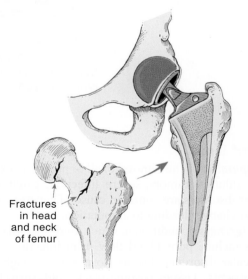

Fractures in head and neck of femur

FIGURE 49-21 Hip fracture repaired with a prosthesis. (Modified from Cooper K, Gosnell K: *Adult health nursing,* ed 8, St Louis, 2019, Elsevier.)

BOX 49-9	Hip Fracture Care

- Give good skin care. Skin breakdown can be rapid.
- Prevent pressure injuries.
- Prevent wound, skin, and urinary tract infections.
- Encourage incentive spirometry and deep-breathing and coughing exercises as directed.
- Report pain.
- Turn and position the person as directed. Usually the person is not positioned on the operative side.
- Prevent external rotation of the hip. Use trochanter rolls, pillows, or sandbags.
- Keep the leg abducted. Use pillows (Fig. 49-22) or a hip abduction wedge (abductor splint) in bed (Chapter 35).
- Do not exercise the affected leg. The physical therapist helps the person with rehabilitation exercises.
- Provide a straight-back chair with armrests. The person needs a high, firm seat.
- Place the chair on the unaffected side for transfers. The physical therapist teaches the person how to sit and stand while recovering.
- Use assist devices to move, turn, re-position, and transfer the person.
- Elevate the leg following the care plan. The leg is not elevated when the person sits in a chair. (The knee is kept lower than the hip while seated. Elevation puts strain on the hip.)
- Apply elastic stockings as directed to prevent *thrombi* (blood clots) in the legs.
- Do not let the person stand on the operated leg until allowed by the doctor.

- Assist with walking according to the care plan. Use of a walking aid (crutches, walker, cane) is expected. Know the person's weight-bearing restrictions (limitations) on the operated leg.
  - *Non-weight bearing (NWB)*—No weight is to be placed on the operative side.
  - *Toe-touch (touch-down) weight bearing*—The toes or foot on the operative side may lightly touch the floor for balance only. However, weight is not placed on the leg.
  - *Partial weight bearing*—Some body weight can be placed on the operative leg.
  - *Weight bearing as tolerated*—Weight is applied as it is comfortable to do so. If pain occurs, less weight is applied.
  - *Full weight bearing*—No restrictions (limitations). The person can put full body weight on the leg.
- Follow measures to protect the hip. (The measures from Fig. 49-11 apply.) The person:
  - Does not cross the affected leg past the mid-line of the body.
  - Does not turn the kneecap on the affected side in toward the body.
  - Does not sit in low chairs.
  - Does not cross the legs.
  - Does not flex the hips past 90 degrees. (This includes bending over at the waist and sitting with the knee higher than the hip.)
  - Uses long-handled devices for reaching.
  - Uses an elevated toilet seat.
  - Sleeps with a pillow between the legs.
- Practice safety measures to prevent falls.
- Complete a safety check before leaving the room. (See the inside of the back cover.)

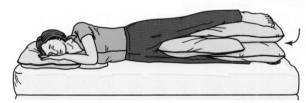

FIGURE 49-22 Pillows are used to keep the hip in abduction. (From Monahan FD et al: *Phipps' medical-surgical nursing: health and illness perspectives,* ed 8, St Louis, 2007, Mosby.)

Loss of Limb

An *amputation* is the removal of all or part of an extremity. Severe injuries, tumors, severe infection, gangrene, and vascular disorders are common causes. Diabetes can cause vascular changes leading to amputation.

Gangrene is a condition in which there is death of tissue. Causes include poor blood flow from infection, injuries, or vascular disorders. Tissues do not get enough oxygen and nutrients. Tissues become black, cold, shriveled, and die (Fig. 49-23). Surgery is needed to remove dead tissue. Gangrene can cause death.

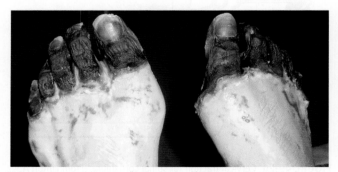

FIGURE 49-23 Gangrene. (From Centers for Disease Control and Prevention/Christina Nelson, MD, MPH, 2012.)

Much support is needed. The amputation affects the person's life—body image, appearance, daily activities, moving about, work, and so on. Fear, shock, anger, denial, and depression are common emotions.

A *prosthesis* is an artificial replacement for a missing body part (Fig. 49-24). For a proper fit, the stump is shaped into a cone (Fig. 49-25). Exercises are done to strengthen other limbs. Occupational and physical therapists help the person learn to use the prosthesis. Have the nurse or therapist show you how to assist the person with applying the device. Do not guess. Practice application with supervision before doing so alone.

The person may feel that the limb is still there. Aching, tingling, and itching are common sensations. Or the person reports pain in the amputated part *(phantom pain)* (Chapter 36). This is a normal reaction. It may occur for a short time or for many years.

Because of other health problems, many older persons cannot use a leg prosthesis. They need to use wheelchairs. After amputation, most older persons need long-term care or home care.

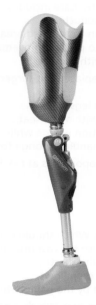

FIGURE 49-24 Above-the-knee prosthesis. (Courtesy Otto Bock Health Care, Minneapolis, Minn.)

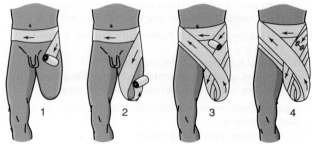

FIGURE 49-25 A mid-thigh amputation is bandaged to shape the stump. (From Monahan FD et al: *Phipps' medical-surgical nursing: health and illness perspectives,* ed 8, St Louis, 2007, Mosby.)

FOCUS ON **PRIDE**

The Person, Family, and Yourself

P ersonal and Professional Responsibility

Think about the life changes that occur with the disorders in this chapter. Consider how you will interact with and care for persons experiencing them. There is a big difference between a nursing assistant who wants to make a difference and one who is just doing a job. When you genuinely care, you can make a difference in the person's life. Consistently show that you care.

R ights and Respect

Feeling alone in a struggle can worsen mental and emotional effects. Having a support system is important. The person's family and caregivers need support and encouragement. Treat them with dignity, kindness, and respect.

I ndependence and Social Interaction

The disorders in this chapter affect independence. Many require rehabilitation (Chapter 46). To promote independence:
- Focus on the person's abilities, not disabilities.
- Encourage as much self-care as possible.
- Allow personal choice.
- Praise the person's progress.

D elegation and Teamwork

Rehabilitation therapies are commonly needed for many disorders in this chapter (Chapter 46). Physical, occupational, and speech-language therapies are examples. The therapists are valuable members of the health team. They may remind you of ways to promote independence with a person. Listen to their directions. Ask for help if you have questions or need to be shown how to do something. Give good effort in trying the requested methods.

E thics and Laws

Emotional lability refers to rapid changes in mood that cannot be controlled. Laughing, crying, and angry outbursts are examples. Stroke and head injuries can cause such sudden expressions without a reason for them. The person has no control over the behavior.

Your conduct must be professional. Mocking, insulting, yelling back, and use of force are examples of abuse. Show patience and self-control in your responses.

FOCUS ON **PRIDE**: *Application*

Some disorders in this chapter have sudden effects. Others have progressive effects. Explain why both are life-changing. Describe the challenges of a disorder with long-term effects.

REVIEW QUESTIONS

Circle the BEST answer.

1 A stroke also is called
   a A cerebrovascular accident
   b Aphasia
   c Hemiplegia
   d A transient ischemic attack

2 Sudden weakness on 1 side of the body and trouble speaking and walking are signs of
   a A hip fracture
   b Stroke
   c Multiple sclerosis
   d Parkinson's disease

3 A person had a stroke. Which should you question?
   a Give thickened liquids for dysphagia.
   b Perform ROM exercises.
   c Turn and re-position the person every 2 hours.
   d Place needed items on the weak (affected) side.

4 Which statement about Parkinson's disease is *true?*
   a There is a cure.
   b Mental function is affected first.
   c Tremors, slow movements, and a shuffling gait occur.
   d Paralysis occurs but mental function is intact.

5 A person with multiple sclerosis is in remission. This means that symptoms
   a Have gone away for a while
   b Are worsening
   c Will not return
   d Are being treated

6 Amyotrophic lateral sclerosis affects nerve cells that control
   a Involuntary muscles
   b Voluntary muscles
   c Memory
   d Bowel and bladder function

7 A person has amyotrophic lateral sclerosis. Which can you perform?
   a Range-of-motion exercises
   b Tracheostomy suctioning
   c Feeding tube insertion
   d Fall risk assessment

8 Persons with head or spinal cord injuries require
   a Rehabilitation
   b Drugs to cure paralysis
   c A prosthesis
   d Chemotherapy

9 Which carries the *lowest* risk for traumatic brain injury?
   a Falling in the bathroom
   b Motorcycle accident
   c Transferring with a mechanical lift
   d Child abuse

10 A person has quadriplegia from a spinal cord injury. Care includes
   a Active ROM exercises to the arms and legs
   b Pressure injury prevention
   c Removing the call light from the room
   d Using a long-handled device for reaching

11 After spinal cord injury, autonomic dysreflexia is usually triggered by
   a Sweating
   b High blood pressure
   c A full bladder
   d A slow pulse

12 Arthritis affects
   a The joints
   b Bone mass
   c Voluntary muscles
   d Involuntary muscles

13 A person has arthritis. Care includes
   a Keeping joints abducted
   b Applying traction to affected areas
   c Wearing a cast to prevent movement
   d Rest balanced with exercise

14 A person had hip replacement surgery. Which should you question?
   a Do not cross the legs.
   b Provide a chair with a low seat.
   c Use a hip abduction wedge while in bed.
   d Provide a long-handled sponge for bathing the feet.

15 A person with osteoporosis is at risk for
   a Fractures
   b An amputation
   c Phantom pain
   d Paralysis

16 A cast needs to dry. Which should you question?
   a Turn the person so the cast dries evenly.
   b Cover the cast with plastic.
   c Elevate the cast on pillows.
   d Support the cast by the palms when lifting.

17 A person has an arm cast. Which is normal?
   a Numbness and inability to move the fingers
   b Chills and nausea
   c Cool skin and cyanosis
   d Pulse rate of 76 and a respiratory rate of 18

18 A person is in traction. Care includes
   a Avoiding ROM exercises for uninvolved joints
   b Keeping the weights on the floor
   c Removing the weights if the person is uncomfortable
   d Using a fracture pan for elimination

19 A person had surgery for a hip fracture. Which do you expect during recovery?
   a The person will use a walker or other walking aid.
   b The person will not have weight-bearing restrictions.
   c You will teach the person rehabilitation exercises.
   d You will position the person on the operative side with the legs together.

20 A person needs help applying a prosthesis. You are not sure how to assist the person in applying it correctly. You should
   a Act confident and guess how to apply it
   b Convince the person not to wear it
   c Ask the nurse or therapist to help you
   d Tell the person to apply it without help

Answers to Chapter 49 questions are on p. 903.

FOCUS ON PRACTICE

Problem Solving

After a stroke a person has hemiplegia, aphasia, and dysphagia. How will you modify the care measures listed below? Apply learning from this and other chapters.
- Transferring from the bed to the wheelchair
- Changing garments
- Assisting with food and fluids
- Explaining a procedure
- Performing a safety check of the room

Cardiovascular, Respiratory, and Lymphatic Disorders

OBJECTIVES

- Define the key terms and key abbreviations in this chapter.
- Describe congenital heart defects.
- Identify the causes and effects of anemia.
- Identify cardiovascular disorder risk factors and complications.
- Describe the care required for hypertension, coronary artery disease, angina, myocardial infarction, heart failure, and dysrhythmias.

- Describe chronic obstructive pulmonary disease, asthma, and sleep apnea.
- Describe different infectious respiratory disorders and the care required—influenza, pneumonia, and tuberculosis.
- Describe different lymphatic disorders—lymphedema and lymphoma.
- Explain how to promote PRIDE in the person, the family, and yourself.

KEY TERMS

anemia A decrease in the amount of healthy red blood cells (*an* means lack of; *emia* means blood condition)
apnea The lack or absence *(a)* of breathing *(pnea)*
arrhythmia See "dysrhythmia"
congenital To be born with
dysrhythmia An abnormal *(dys)* heart rhythm *(rhythmia)*; arrhythmia

hypertension High blood pressure
lymphedema A buildup of lymph in the tissues causing edema (swelling)
pneumonia Inflammation and infection of lung tissue
sleep apnea Pauses *(a)* in breathing *(pnea)* that occur during sleep

KEY ABBREVIATIONS

BiPAP	Bilevel positive airway pressure		**IV**	Intravenous
CAD	Coronary artery disease		**MI**	Myocardial infarction
CDC	Centers for Disease Control and Prevention		**mm Hg**	Millimeters of mercury
CHF	Congestive heart failure		**O₂**	Oxygen
CO₂	Carbon dioxide		**RBC**	Red blood cell
COPD	Chronic obstructive pulmonary disease		**TB**	Tuberculosis
CPAP	Continuous positive airway pressure		**WBC**	White blood cell
ICD	Implantable cardioverter defibrillator			

Cardiovascular and respiratory system disorders are leading causes of death in the United States. Many people have these disorders. Disorders also occur in the lymphatic system. Understanding these disorders gives meaning to the care you provide.

CARDIOVASCULAR DISORDERS

The circulatory (cardiovascular) system delivers blood to the body's cells. Problems occur in the heart or blood vessels. See Chapter 40 for blood clots (thrombi and emboli). See Chapter 41 for circulatory ulcers.

See *Body Structure and Function Review: The Circulatory System*, pp. 758-759.

See *Focus on Children and Older Persons: Cardiovascular Disorders*, p. 759.

BODY STRUCTURE AND FUNCTION REVIEW

The Circulatory System

Structure and Function

The circulatory system (cardiovascular system) is made up of the *blood, heart,* and *blood vessels*. The heart and blood vessels make up a continuous circuit that circulates (moves) blood through the system. Blood moves from the heart, to the lungs, back to the heart, to the rest of the body, and back to the heart to repeat the circuit.

The Blood

The blood consists of *blood cells* and *plasma*. Plasma is mostly water. It carries blood cells—red blood cells, white blood cells, and platelets. Plasma also carries substances (nutrients, hormones, and chemicals) that cells need to function.

Red blood cells (RBCs) are called *erythrocytes*. Hemoglobin in the RBCs transports oxygen (O_2) and carbon dioxide (CO_2). Hemoglobin picks up O_2 as RBCs circulate through the lungs. As blood circulates through the body, O_2 is given to cells. Cells release CO_2 (a waste product). It is picked up by the hemoglobin and transported back to the lungs to be removed from the body.

Blood also contains *white blood cells (WBCs)* and *platelets (thrombocytes)*. WBCs are called *leukocytes*. They protect the body against infection. Platelets are needed for blood clotting.

The Heart

The heart is a muscle. It pumps blood through the blood vessels to the tissues and cells. The heart has 4 chambers (Fig. 50-1).

- Upper chambers receive blood and are called *atria*. The *right atrium* receives blood from body tissues. The *left atrium* receives blood from the lungs.
- Lower chambers are called *ventricles*. Ventricles pump blood. The *right ventricle* pumps blood to the lungs for O_2. The *left ventricle* pumps blood to all parts of the body.

Valves are between the atria and ventricles (see Fig. 50-1). The valves allow blood flow in 1 direction. They prevent blood from flowing back into the atria from the ventricles. The *tricuspid valve* is between the right atrium and the right ventricle. The *mitral valve (bicuspid valve)* is between the left atrium and the left ventricle.

Heart action has 2 phases.

- *Diastole* is the resting phase. Heart chambers fill with blood.
- *Systole* is the working phase. The heart contracts. Blood is pumped through the blood vessels when the heart contracts.

The heart has its own electrical system that stimulates the heart to contract. The electrical signal begins in the *sinoatrial (SA) node* (see Fig. 50-1). The SA node sets the pace of the heart. It stimulates the heart to beat at 60 to 100 beats per minute. The electrical signal spreads through the heart, causing the heart to contract.

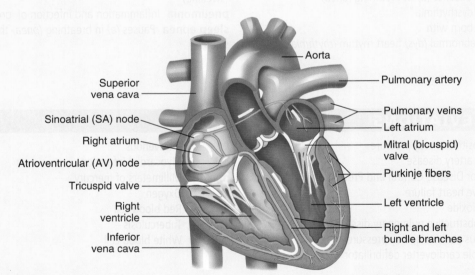

FIGURE 50-1 Structures of the heart. Chambers and major vessels that carry blood full of O_2 are shown in red. Chambers and major vessels that carry blood low in O_2 are shown in blue. Valves are white. The heart's electrical system is yellow. (Modified from Patton KT, Thibodeau GA: *The human body in health & disease,* ed 6, St Louis, 2014, Mosby.)

BODY STRUCTURE AND FUNCTION REVIEW—cont'd

The Circulatory System

The Blood Vessels

Blood flows to body tissues and cells through the blood vessels (Fig. 50-2). There are 3 groups of blood vessels: *arteries, capillaries,* and *veins.*

Arteries carry blood away from the heart. Arterial blood is rich in O_2. The *aorta* is the largest artery (see Figs. 50-1 and 50-2). It receives blood directly from the left ventricle. The aorta branches into other smaller arteries that carry blood to all parts of the body. The smallest arteries (arterioles) connect to capillaries.

Capillaries are very tiny blood vessels. Nutrients, O_2, and other substances pass from capillaries into the cells. The capillaries pick up waste products (including CO_2) from the cells. Capillaries connect to small veins (venules).

Veins return blood with waste products to the heart. Venous blood has little O_2 and a lot of CO_2. The many veins branch together as they near the heart to form 2 main veins—the *inferior vena cava* and the *superior vena cava* (see Figs. 50-1 and 50-2). Both empty into the right atrium.

Changes With Aging

Changes in the circulatory system can occur with aging. Heart walls thicken, and the heart may enlarge slightly. Heart valves thicken and become stiff. The heart pumps with less force. The rate may slow or abnormal rhythms may occur.

Arteries narrow and become stiffer. It is harder to pump blood through them. Less blood flows through narrowed arteries. The number of RBCs decreases. Such changes cause fatigue.

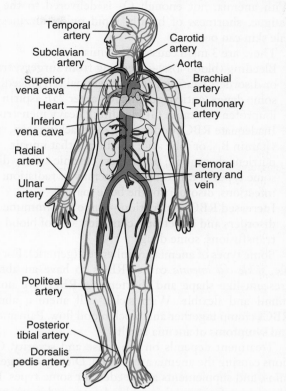

Temporal artery
Carotid artery
Subclavian artery
Aorta
Superior vena cava
Brachial artery
Heart
Pulmonary artery
Inferior vena cava
Radial artery
Femoral artery and vein
Ulnar artery
Popliteal artery
Posterior tibial artery
Dorsalis pedis artery

FIGURE 50-2 Arterial and venous systems. Arterial system is red. Venous system is blue.

FOCUS ON CHILDREN AND OLDER PERSONS

Cardiovascular Disorders

Children

Some babies have congenital heart defects. *Congenital* means to be born with. Defects occur during pregnancy as the baby's heart develops. The defect can involve the heart walls, heart valves, or the blood vessels near the heart. Blood flow is affected. The flow can slow down, go in the wrong direction or place, or be blocked.

Usually the cause is unknown. Risk factors include:

- Family history. A family history of defects may increase the risk.
- Environment. Smoking during pregnancy and second-hand smoke increase risk. So does taking certain drugs early in pregnancy. Drinking alcohol during pregnancy also increases the risk.
- Some medical conditions during pregnancy. Diabetes and a viral infection with rubella (German measles) are examples.

The common signs of congenital heart defects are:

- *Cyanosis* (bluish tint to the skin, lips, and fingernails)
- Fatigue
- Heart murmurs (heart sounds other than "lub-dub" during an apical pulse)
- Poor circulation
- Fast breathing

Heart defects are found during pregnancy or when the child is very young. Some are not diagnosed until the child is older. Treatment may involve:

- Drugs.
- Correcting the defect with a catheter procedure. A catheter is inserted into a blood vessel and then into the heart.
- Surgery.
- A heart transplant.

With successful treatment, many children with heart defects grow into healthy adults. Some need life-long treatment.

Anemia

Anemia is a decrease in the amount of healthy red blood cells (RBCs) (*an* means lack of; *emia* means blood condition). With anemia, not enough O_2 is delivered to the body. Fatigue, shortness of breath, rapid pulse, dizziness, and pale skin can occur.

There are 3 main causes of anemia.

- Bleeding (blood loss)—bleeding from surgery, trauma, or disorders causing gastro-intestinal (GI) bleeding; some drugs (anticoagulants [Chapter 25]; aspirin and ibuprofen can cause GI bleeding); heavy menstruation
- Inadequate RBC production—diet lacking iron, vitamin B_{12}, or folic acid; conditions that impair nutrient absorption; pregnancy; chronic kidney disease; some types of cancer; chemotherapy or radiation; some infections; disorders of the bone marrow
- Increased RBC destruction—some autoimmune disorders and infections; complications of blood transfusions; some drugs

Some types of anemia are inherited (genetic). For example, *sickle cell anemia* causes RBCs to have an abnormal crescent-like shape and shorter life. RBCs are normally round and flexible. With sickle cell anemia, abnormal RBCs clump together and block blood flow. Pain and signs and symptoms of anemia result.

Treatment depends on the cause and severity. Conditions causing the anemia are treated. Dietary changes, vitamins, and supplements are needed for some types. Drugs, blood transfusions (giving blood from a donor), or stem cell transplants (Chapter 48) may be needed. Some persons require oxygen therapy (Chapter 44).

Hypertension

With every heartbeat, blood is pumped into arteries. Blood pressure is the force of blood pressing against artery walls. Pressure is higher when the heart beats *(systole)*. Pressure is lower when the heart rests *(diastole)*.

Hypertension means high blood pressure. Blood pressure is high when:

- The systolic pressure is 140 mm Hg (millimeters of mercury) or higher.
- The diastolic pressure is 90 mm Hg or higher.

When risk factors are present (Box 50-1), a systolic pressure between 130 and 139 mm Hg or a diastolic pressure between 80 and 89 mm Hg may signal hypertension. Report abnormal blood pressures at once.

Hypertension often does not cause symptoms. Measuring blood pressure regularly is important. Over time, hypertension causes the heart to work harder, leading to other disorders. Heart attack (p. 762), heart failure (p. 763), stroke (Chapter 49), and kidney failure (Chapter 52) are examples.

Life-style changes can lower blood pressure. A diet low in fat and salt, a healthy weight, and regular exercise are needed. No smoking is allowed. Alcohol and caffeine are limited. Managing stress and sleeping well also lower blood pressure. Certain drugs lower blood pressure.

BOX 50-1	Cardiovascular Disorders: Risk Factors

Factors You *Cannot* Control
- Age and biological sex—45 years or older for men; 55 years or older for women (risk increases for women after menopause)
- Family history—tends to run in families; early onset in a close family member increases the risk

Factors You *Can* Control
- Being over-weight
- Stress
- Smoking and tobacco use
- Poor diet—high in fat, salt, sugar, and cholesterol
- Excessive alcohol use
- Lack of exercise
- Not getting enough sleep
- High blood pressure
- Unhealthy blood cholesterol levels
- Diabetes

Modified from National Heart, Lung, and Blood Institute: *Understand your risk for heart disease*, National Institutes of Health, updated March 24, 2022.

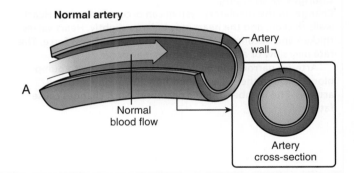

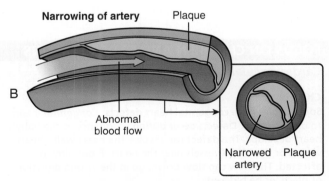

FIGURE 50-3 A, Normal artery. **B,** Plaque on the artery wall in atherosclerosis.

Coronary Artery Disease

The *coronary arteries* supply the heart muscle with blood. In coronary artery disease (CAD) (coronary heart disease, heart disease), the coronary arteries become hardened and narrow. One or all are affected. The heart muscle gets less blood and O_2.

The most common cause is atherosclerosis (Fig. 50-3). Plaque—made up of cholesterol, fat, and other substances—collects on artery walls. The narrowed arteries block some or all blood flow. Blood clots can form along the plaque and block blood flow.

Major complications of CAD are angina, heart attack, heart failure, irregular heartbeats, and sudden death. The more risk factors present (see Box 50-1), the greater the chance of CAD and its complications.

Treatment goals are to:

- Relieve symptoms (see "Angina")
- Slow or stop atherosclerosis
- Lower the risk of blood clots
- Widen or bypass clogged arteries
- Prevent complications

CAD requires life-style changes (see "Hypertension").

Drugs may be given to:

- Lower cholesterol
- Lower blood pressure
- Prevent blood clots
- Decrease the heart's workload and relieve symptoms
- Delay medical and surgical procedures that open or bypass diseased arteries (Fig. 50-4)

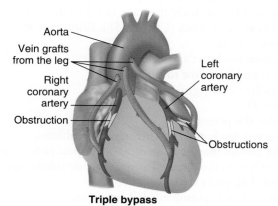

Triple bypass

FIGURE 50-4 Coronary artery bypass surgery. Arteries or veins from other parts of the body are used to bypass (go around) narrowed coronary arteries. (Modified from Patton KT, Thibodeau GA: *The human body in health & disease,* ed 7, St Louis, 2018, Elsevier.)

Cardiac Rehabilitation. CAD complications may require cardiac rehabilitation (cardiac rehab). The cardiac rehab team includes doctors (the person's doctor, a heart specialist, a heart surgeon), nurses, exercise specialists, physical and occupational therapists, dietitians, and mental health professionals.

Cardiac rehab programs include:

- Exercise. Exercise begins slowly. At first, the heart is monitored during exercise. Activity increases over time. Exercise outside of rehab is encouraged. Walking and yard work are examples.
- Healthy eating. The person learns how to make healthy food choices. Diet planning for health problems such as diabetes, obesity, hypertension, and high cholesterol is included.
- Education. The person learns ways to stay healthy. Quitting smoking and managing other health problems are examples.
- Support. The rehab team provides support for life-style changes. Some persons need help coping with anxiety and depression (Chapter 53).

Angina

Angina is chest pain from reduced blood flow to part of the heart muscle *(myocardium)*. (*Angina* comes from the Latin word *angor* that means strangling.) It occurs when the heart needs more O$_2$. Normally blood flow to the heart increases when O$_2$ needs increase. Exertion, a heavy meal, stress, and excitement increase the heart's need for O$_2$. So does smoking and very hot or cold temperatures. In CAD, narrowed vessels prevent increased blood flow.

Chest pain is described as tightness, pressure, squeezing, or burning in the chest. Pain can occur in the shoulders, arms, neck, jaw, or back (Fig. 50-5). The person may also have nausea, fatigue, dyspnea, sweating, light-headedness, and weakness.

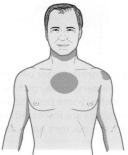
- Chest
- Left shoulder and down both arms
- Neck

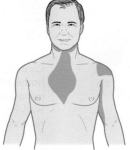
- Chest radiating to neck and jaw
- Left shoulder and down left arm

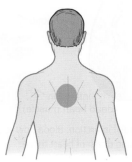
- Back

FIGURE 50-5 *Shaded areas* show common locations and patterns of angina. (Modified from Harding M et al: *Lewis's medical-surgical nursing: assessment and management of clinical problems,* ed 11, St Louis, 2020, Elsevier.)

Rest often relieves symptoms in a few minutes. Persons with angina need to know:

- The usual pattern of their symptoms. This includes the causes, usual description and duration of the pain, and if rest or drugs relieve pain.
- What drugs to use and how to use them. *Nitroglycerin* dissolved under the tongue is common.
- How to control angina. Avoiding triggers like physical exertion, stress, and large meals are examples.
- The limits of physical activity. The person should stop activity before symptoms occur. For example, a person usually has angina walking up a flight of stairs. The person should stop half-way and rest before continuing.
- When to get emergency care. Pain that is severe, lasts longer than a few minutes, or is not relieved by rest or drugs may signal a heart attack. Emergency care is needed.

See "Coronary Artery Disease" for the treatment of angina. Increased blood flow to the heart lowers the risk of heart attack and death.

Myocardial Infarction

Myocardial refers to the heart muscle. *Infarction* means tissue death. With myocardial infarction (MI) part of the heart muscle dies from sudden blockage of blood flow in a coronary artery. A thrombus (blood clot) in an artery with atherosclerosis blocks blood flow (Fig. 50-6).

MI also is called:

- Heart attack
- Acute myocardial infarction (AMI)
- Acute coronary syndrome (ACS)

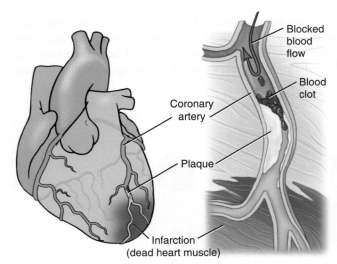

FIGURE 50-6 Myocardial infarction. Blood flow to part of the heart muscle is blocked, causing death of heart tissue.

BOX 50-2	Myocardial Infarction: Signs and Symptoms

- Chest pain, heaviness, or discomfort in the center or left side of the chest (this is the most common symptom)
- Upper body discomfort—pain in 1 or both arms, the back, shoulders, neck, jaw, or upper stomach
- *Dyspnea* (difficulty breathing)—with rest or during mild physical activity (this is more common in older adults)
- Breaking out in a sweat for no reason
- Unexplained fatigue—feeling unusually tired for no reason, sometimes for days (this is more common in women)
- Nausea and vomiting
- Light-headedness or sudden dizziness
- Rapid or irregular pulse

Modified from National Heart, Lung, and Blood Institute: Heart attack: symptoms, National Institutes of Health, updated March 24, 2022.

CAD, angina, and previous MI are risk factors. See Box 50-2 for signs and symptoms. Symptoms may start slowly and be mild. Or they are sudden and severe.

MI is an emergency (Chapter 58). Efforts are made to:

- Relieve pain.
- Reduce the heart's workload.
- Restore blood flow to the heart.
- Stabilize vital signs.
- Give O$_2$.
- Calm the person.
- Prevent death and life-threatening problems.

The person may need medical or surgical procedures to open or bypass the diseased artery. Cardiac rehabilitation is needed. The goals are to:

- Recover and resume normal activities.
- Prevent another MI.
- Prevent complications such as heart failure or sudden cardiac arrest (sudden cardiac death) (Chapter 58).

See *Focus on Long-Term Care and Home Care: Myocardial Infarction.*

FOCUS ON LONG-TERM CARE AND HOME CARE

Myocardial Infarction

Home Care

Cardiac rehabilitation continues for persons who return home after an MI. The person may go to a gym, health club, or hospital fitness center. Some persons like indoor malls for walking. Normal activities are increased slowly. The person returns to work with the doctor's approval.

Heart Failure

Heart failure or congestive heart failure (CHF) occurs when the weakened heart cannot pump normally. Blood backs up. Tissue congestion occurs. Heart failure is caused by conditions that damage or over-work the heart muscle (Box 50-3).

Heart failure can affect 1 or both sides of the heart.

- Left side—When the left side of the heart cannot pump normally, blood backs up into the lungs. Respiratory congestion occurs.
- Right side—When the right side of the heart cannot pump normally, blood backs up into the venous system. Swelling occurs *(edema)*.
- Both left side and right side—Signs and symptoms occur from the effects of poor circulation on other organs. See Box 50-3.

Pulmonary edema (fluid in the lungs) can result from heart failure. It is an emergency. The person can die.

The goals of treatment are to:

- Treat the cause of heart failure.
- Reduce symptoms.
- Prevent worsening heart failure.
- Improve quality of life.
- Prolong life.

BOX 50-3 | **Heart Failure**

Common Causes
- Coronary artery disease
- Heart attack
- Hypertension
- Dysrhythmia (abnormal heart rhythm)
- Cardiomyopathy (enlarged, thick, or rigid heart muscle)
- Damaged heart valves
- Congenital heart defects
- Chronic conditions: diabetes, HIV, thyroid problems, kidney disease, serious lung diseases

Signs and Symptoms
- Dyspnea: worse with exertion or lying down
- Sputum: white, pink, blood-tinged, foamy
- Cough
- Lung sounds: gurgling, wheezing
- Concentration problems, decreased alertness
- Reduced ability to exercise
- Fatigue and weakness
- *Nocturia* (frequent urination at night)
- Nausea
- Decreased appetite
- Swelling: feet, ankles, legs, abdomen, neck veins
- Rapid weight gain
- Rapid or irregular pulse

Drugs are used to strengthen the heart, decrease strain on the heart, and reduce fluid buildup. A sodium-controlled diet is ordered. Oxygen is given. Semi-Fowler's position is preferred for breathing. The person must reduce CAD risk factors. If acutely ill, the person needs hospital care.

You assist with these aspects of the person's care.

- Promoting rest and activity as ordered
- Measuring intake and output (I&O)
- Measuring weight daily
- Reporting signs of fluid overload (Chapter 32) including weight change (gain) as directed—usually 2 pounds in 1 day is significant
- Measuring vital signs and pulse oximetry
- Restricting fluids as ordered
- Promoting a low-sodium, low-fat, and low-cholesterol diet
- Providing good skin care and preventing pressure injuries
- Assisting with range-of-motion (ROM) and other exercises
- Assisting with transfers and ambulation
- Assisting with self-care activities
- Maintaining good alignment and elevating swollen extremities as directed
- Applying elastic stockings

Many older persons have heart failure. Skin breakdown is a risk. Tissue swelling, poor circulation, and fragile skin increase the risk of pressure injuries. Good skin care and regular position changes are needed.

Dysrhythmias

A *dysrhythmia (arrhythmia)* is an abnormal *(dys)* heart rhythm *(rhythmia)*. The rhythm may be too fast, too slow, or irregular. Dysrhythmias are caused by changes in the heart's electrical system. Changes may result from hypertension, CAD, MI, or heart failure. Weakening and changes in the heart muscle are other causes. So are substance use disorders (Chapter 53), excess caffeine intake, smoking, stress, and thyroid problems. Some drugs can cause dysrhythmias.

The person may notice the change in the pulse—slow, irregular, skipped beats, pounding, racing. Feeling dizzy or light-headed, chest pain, sweating, and dyspnea are other symptoms. The person may faint (Chapter 58). Some dysrhythmias are minor. Others are life-threatening.

Treatment depends on the type of dysrhythmia. Drugs may be given. A procedure may be needed.

- *Defibrillation* (Chapter 58) or *cardioversion*—an electrical shock is given to stop an abnormal rhythm.
- *Ablation*—areas of tissue in the heart sending abnormal electrical signals are destroyed.

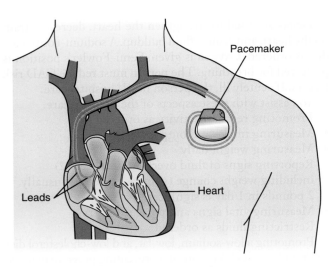

FIGURE 50-7 Pacemaker.

Some abnormal rhythms are treated with a pacemaker (Fig. 50-7). This device monitors and regulates the heart's rhythm. The device is inserted under the skin near the heart. One or more wires (leads) are placed in the heart muscle and connected to the pacemaker. The pacemaker sends signals through the leads to stimulate the heart to beat normally.

For life-threatening dysrhythmias, an implantable cardioverter defibrillator (ICD) may be placed. The ICD delivers a shock when the heart is in a life-threatening rhythm. The goal is to restore a regular heart rhythm. Some devices are both a pacemaker and an ICD.

See *Focus on Long-Term Care and Home Care: Dysrhythmias*.

RESPIRATORY DISORDERS

The respiratory system brings O_2 into the lungs and removes CO_2 from the body. Respiratory disorders interfere with this function and threaten life.

See *Body Structure and Function Review: The Respiratory System*.

BODY STRUCTURE AND FUNCTION REVIEW

The Respiratory System

Structure and Function
Oxygen is needed to live. The respiratory system (Fig. 50-8) brings O_2 into the lungs and removes CO_2. *Respiration* is the process of supplying the cells with O_2 and removing CO_2 from them. Respiration involves breathing in (*inhalation, inspiration*) and breathing out (*exhalation, expiration*).

Air enters the body through the *nose*. Then air passes into the *pharynx* (throat), the *larynx* (voice box), and the *trachea* (windpipe). The trachea divides into the *right bronchus* and the *left bronchus*. Each bronchus enters a *lung*. The bronchi divide many times into smaller branches (*bronchioles*). They end up in tiny one-celled air sacs called *alveoli*.

The alveoli and capillaries exchange O_2 and CO_2. Blood in the capillaries picks up O_2 from the alveoli. Then the blood is returned to the left side of the heart and pumped to the rest of the body. Alveoli pick up CO_2 from the capillaries for exhalation.

Each lung is divided into lobes. The right lung has 3 lobes; the left lung has 2. The lungs are separated from the abdominal cavity by a muscle called the *diaphragm*. A bony framework made up of the ribs, sternum, and vertebrae protects the lungs.

Changes With Aging
With age, respiratory muscles weaken. Some lung tissue is lost. Lung tissue becomes less elastic (more rigid). The chest is less able to expand and contract. Difficulty breathing and decreased strength for coughing and clearing the airway can occur.

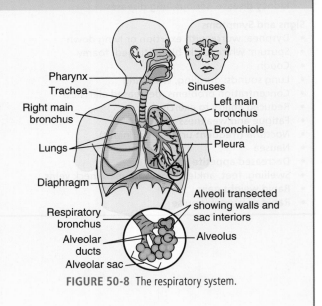

FIGURE 50-8 The respiratory system.

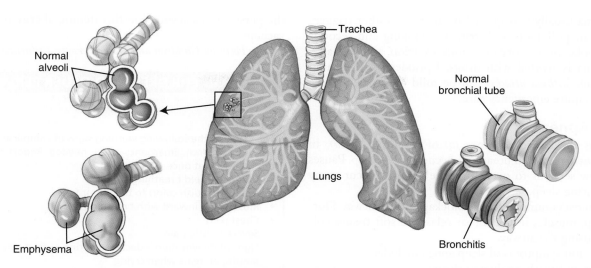

FIGURE 50-9 COPD. Emphysema damages the inner walls of alveoli. Chronic bronchitis causes inflammation and mucus in the airways. (Modified from Brooks ML, Brooks DL: *Exploring medical language: a student-directed approach,* ed 11, St Louis, 2022, Elsevier.)

Chronic Obstructive Pulmonary Disease

Chronic obstructive pulmonary disease (COPD) involves 2 disorders—emphysema and chronic bronchitis (Fig. 50-9). These disorders interfere with O_2 and CO_2 exchange in the lungs. They obstruct (block) airflow. Lung function is gradually lost.

Most people with COPD have both emphysema and chronic bronchitis. The severity of each varies for each person.

Cigarette smoking is the greatest risk factor. Pipe, cigar, and other smoking tobaccos are also risk factors. So is exposure to second-hand smoke. Not smoking is the best way to prevent COPD. COPD has no cure. Air pollution and industrial dusts are other risk factors.

COPD affects the airways and alveoli. Less air gets into the lungs; less air leaves the lungs. These changes occur.
- The airways and alveoli (air sacs) become less elastic. They are like old rubber bands.
- The walls between many alveoli are destroyed.
- Airway walls become thick, inflamed, and swollen.
- The airways secrete more mucus than usual. Excess mucus clogs the airways.

Emphysema. In emphysema, the alveoli are damaged (see Fig. 50-9). Alveoli lose their shape and become less elastic. They do not expand and shrink normally. As a result, air is trapped and not exhaled. Over time, more alveoli are involved. O_2 and CO_2 exchange cannot occur in affected alveoli. As more air is trapped in the lungs, the person develops a *barrel chest* (Fig. 50-10).

The person has shortness of breath and a cough. At first, shortness of breath occurs with exertion. Over time, it occurs at rest. Fatigue is common. The body does not get enough O_2. Breathing is easier when sitting upright and slightly forward (Chapter 44).

The person must stop smoking. Respiratory therapy, breathing exercises, oxygen, and drug therapy are ordered.

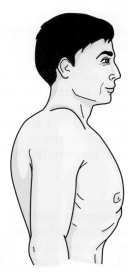

FIGURE 50-10 Barrel chest from emphysema.

Chronic Bronchitis. *Bronchitis* means inflammation (*itis*) of the bronchi (*bronch*). With chronic bronchitis, airways are narrowed from inflammation and mucus (see Fig. 50-9).

The main symptom is an on-going cough or a cough that produces a lot of mucus (*smoker's cough*). The person has difficulty breathing and tires easily. The body cannot get enough O_2. Wheezing and chest tightness can occur.

The person must stop smoking. Oxygen therapy and breathing exercises are common. Drugs are given to open the airways. Respiratory tract infections are prevented. If one occurs, prompt treatment is needed.

Asthma

With asthma, the airway becomes inflamed and narrow. Extra mucus is produced. Coughing, wheezing, chest tightness, and shortness of breath can occur.

Asthma usually is triggered by allergies. Other triggers include air pollutants and irritants, smoking and second-hand smoke, respiratory infections, exertion, and cold air.

Asthma is treated with drugs. Episodes of worsening symptoms *(asthma attacks)* can be mild or severe. Severe attacks require emergency care.

Sleep Apnea

Apnea is the lack or absence *(a)* of breathing *(pnea)*. In *sleep apnea*, pauses in breathing occur during sleep. Pauses last a few seconds to over a minute and can occur many times during sleep.

The most common cause is blockage of the airway. During sleep, muscles in the throat relax and soft tissues collapse, closing the airway.

Signs and symptoms of sleep apnea include:
* Pauses in breathing during sleep
* Loud snoring
* Waking during sleep with a gasp or shortness of breath
* Difficulty staying asleep
* Day-time sleepiness
* Headache in the morning
* Dry mouth or sore throat after sleeping
* Problems with attention
* Irritability

Life-style changes may help. A healthy diet, exercise, weight loss, no smoking, limiting alcohol before sleep, and having healthy sleep habits are examples. For more severe sleep apnea, surgery or use of a positive airway pressure device (continuous positive airway pressure [CPAP] or bilevel positive airway pressure [BiPAP]) may be needed (Chapter 45).

Influenza

Influenza *(flu)* is a respiratory infection caused by viruses. In the United States, "flu season" occurs in the fall and winter months. During these months—usually ranging from October through March—flu activity is highest. Children and older persons are at great risk.

Coughing and sneezing spread flu viruses. The virus is also spread when a person touches a contaminated surface or object and then touches the mouth, eyes, or nose. Standard Precautions and Droplet Precautions are needed (Chapter 18).

Signs and symptoms of flu begin rapidly and include fatigue, headache, muscle or body aches, chills, and a fever. (A fever is not always present.) Chest discomfort and cough are common and can be severe. The person may have a runny nose, stuffy nose, or sore throat.

Treatment involves fluids and rest. Drugs are ordered for symptom relief and to shorten the flu episode. Pneumonia, ear and sinus infections, and worsening of chronic health problems (heart failure, asthma, diabetes) are complications.

The flu vaccine is the best prevention. The Centers for Disease Control and Prevention (CDC) recommends the flu vaccine for all persons 6 months old and older unless the person has a severe, life-threatening allergy to the flu vaccine.

See *Focus on Children and Older Persons: Influenza.*

FOCUS ON **CHILDREN AND OLDER PERSONS**

Influenza

Children
The CDC lists the following warning signs of complications of the flu in children. Emergency care is needed. Report any of the following at once.
* *Dyspnea*, rapid breathing
* *Cyanosis* (bluish color) to the lips or face
* Ribs pulling inward with breathing
* Chest pain
* Severe muscle pain
* Signs of dehydration—decreased urine output, dry mouth, no tears when crying
* Not being alert or interacting when awake
* Seizures
* Any fever in children younger than 12 weeks; high fever (above 104°F) not controlled with fever-reducing drugs in older children
* Fever or cough that improves but then returns or worsens
* Worsening chronic health condition

Older Persons
Older persons may not have the usual flu signs and symptoms. The following may signal flu in older persons:
* Changes in mental status or behavior
* Worsening of other health problems
* A body temperature below the normal range
* Fatigue
* Decreased appetite and fluid intake

Pneumonia

Pneumonia means inflammation and infection of lung tissue. (*Pneumo* means lungs.) Affected tissues fill with fluid. O_2 and CO_2 exchange is affected. Bacteria, viruses, and other microbes are causes. Depending on the setting and cause, these descriptions may be used:
* *Community-acquired pneumonia*—pneumonia that develops outside of a health care setting.
* *Healthcare-associated pneumonia*—pneumonia that develops while receiving care in a health care setting (hospital, long-term care center, and so on).
* *Ventilator-associated pneumonia*—pneumonia that develops from being on a mechanical ventilator (Chapter 45).

Risk factors and the signs and symptoms of pneumonia are listed in Box 50-4. Onset may be sudden. The person is very ill.

Drugs are ordered for infection and pain. Fluid intake is increased for fever and to thin secretions. Thin secretions are easier to cough up. Intravenous (IV) therapy and oxygen may be needed. Semi-Fowler's position eases breathing. Rest and mouth care are important. Standard Precautions are followed. Transmission-Based Precautions depend on the cause. Frequent linen changes are needed because of fever.

See *Focus on Children and Older Persons: Pneumonia.*

BOX 50-4	Pneumonia

Risk Factors
- Age—2 years or younger, 65 years or older
- Smoking
- Excessive alcohol use
- Poor nutrition
- Trouble coughing
- Dysphagia
- Decreased mobility
- Sedative use (drugs for anxiety or sleep)
- Recent cold or the flu
- Some chronic diseases—asthma, COPD, diabetes, cardiovascular disorders
- Weakened immune system from HIV/AIDS, organ transplant, chemotherapy
- Hospital care (especially if on a ventilator)

Signs and Symptoms
- Fever
- Chills
- Cough—productive (with mucus) or dry (without mucus)
- Chest pain with breathing or coughing
- Dyspnea
- Headache
- Fatigue

FOCUS ON CHILDREN AND OLDER PERSONS

Pneumonia

Children
Pneumonia occurs in children of all ages. It is more common in infants and toddlers.

Older Persons
Changes from aging, diseases, and decreased mobility increase the risk of pneumonia in older persons. Decreased mobility after surgery is a risk factor. Aspiration pneumonia is common. Dysphagia, decreased cough and gag reflexes, and nervous system disorders are risk factors. So are substances that depress the brain—narcotics, sedatives, alcohol, and drugs for anesthesia. For older adults, pneumonia can be life-threatening.

Older persons may not have the usual signs and symptoms. Older persons may have lower-than-normal body temperature. Confusion or changes in mental awareness can occur.

Tuberculosis

Tuberculosis (TB) is a bacterial infection in the lungs. It also can occur in the kidneys, spine, and brain. If not treated, the person can die.

TB is spread by airborne droplets with coughing, sneezing, speaking, singing, or laughing. Nearby persons can inhale the bacteria. Those with close, frequent contact with an infected person are at risk. TB is more likely to occur in close, crowded areas. Age (very young or very old), poor nutrition, and human immunodeficiency virus (HIV) infection are other risk factors.

TB can be present in the body but not cause signs and symptoms (latent TB). *Latent* means present but not active. An active infection may not occur for many years. Only persons with an active infection can spread the disease to others.

Chest x-rays and TB testing can detect the disease. Signs and symptoms are fatigue, loss of appetite, weight loss, fever, chills, and night sweats. The person has a bad cough that lasts 3 weeks or longer. Sputum may contain blood. Chest pain occurs.

Drugs for TB are given. Standard Precautions and Airborne Precautions are needed, including wearing a respirator (Chapter 18). The person must cover the mouth and nose with tissues when sneezing, coughing, or producing sputum. Tissues are discarded in a no-touch waste container. Hand-washing after contact with sputum is essential.

See *Focus on Children and Older Persons: Tuberculosis*.
See *Focus on Long-Term Care and Home Care: Tuberculosis*.

FOCUS ON CHILDREN AND OLDER PERSONS

Tuberculosis

Older Persons
With aging, persons infected long ago can develop active TB from declining general health. Other older people with extended contact with those infected can become infected. Nursing center residents are examples.

FOCUS ON LONG-TERM CARE AND HOME CARE

Tuberculosis

Long-Term Care
According to the CDC, persons with suspected or confirmed TB should not be treated in long-term care settings. Such settings include skilled nursing facilities and hospices. Persons with suspected or confirmed TB can be treated in long-term care settings if:
- Administrative and environmental controls are in place.
- The agency has a respiratory-protection program.

Cough-inducing procedures are not done unless needed infection control measures are in place. Or such procedures are done outside.

Standard Precautions and Airborne Precautions are followed. See Chapter 18. The person wears a mask during transport to other areas, in waiting areas, and when others are present.

Home Care
The nurse teaches the person and household members about taking drugs, respiratory hygiene and cough etiquette, and the need for medical care. The person may have to stay at home until TB tests are negative or the person is no longer infectious.

Wear a respirator (Chapter 18) to enter the home of a person with suspected or confirmed TB. Also wear a respirator to transport the person in a vehicle. The person wears a mask during transport to other areas, in waiting areas, and when others are present.

Cough-inducing procedures are not done unless needed infection control measures are in place. Or such procedures are done outdoors.

LYMPHATIC DISORDERS

The lymphatic system drains extra fluid from the tissues, helps fight infection, and absorbs and transports fats. Lymphatic disorders affect these functions.

See *Body Structure and Function Review: The Lymphatic System.*

BODY STRUCTURE AND FUNCTION REVIEW
The Lymphatic System

Structure and Function

The lymphatic (lymph) system transports lymph throughout the body (Fig. 50-11). *Lymph* is a clear, thin, watery fluid that contains WBCs, proteins, and fats. (Water, proteins, and other substances normally leak out of the capillaries into surrounding tissues.)

The lymphatic system:

- Collects extra lymph from the tissues and returns it to the blood. Otherwise, the tissues swell.
- Defends the body against infection by producing lymphocytes (a type of WBC).
- Absorbs fats from the intestines and transports them to the blood.

Lymph is transported by *lymphatic vessels. Lymph nodes* are bean-shaped structures that filter bacteria, cancer cells, and damaged cells from the lymph. This prevents such substances from circulating throughout the body. Lymph nodes are found in the neck, underarm, groin area, chest, abdomen, and pelvis. Normally, lymph nodes are not felt. They swell when producing more lymphocytes to fight infection.

See Figure 50-11 for the location of the *thymus (thymus gland).* Certain lymphocytes—T lymphocytes (T cells)—develop in the thymus. Such lymphocytes are important for immune system function.

The *tonsils* are in the back of the throat. *Adenoids* are behind the nose. These structures trap microbes in the mouth and nose to help prevent infection.

The *spleen* is the largest structure in the lymphatic system. The spleen:

- Filters and removes bacteria and other substances.
- Destroys old RBCs.
- Saves the iron found in hemoglobin when RBCs are destroyed.
- Stores blood. When needed, the blood is returned to the circulatory system.

Changes With Aging

With age, thymus gland tissue is slowly replaced by fat and connective tissue. By age 80, the thymus is usually gone.

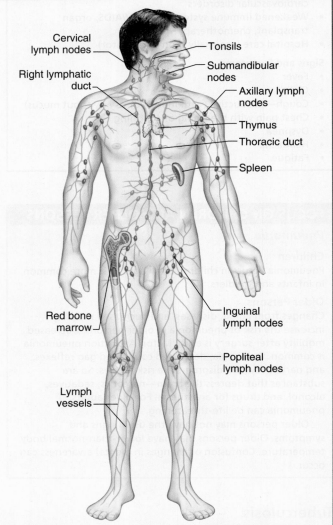

FIGURE 50-11 The lymphatic system. The bean-shaped structures shown in green are lymph nodes. (Modified from Patton KT, Thibodeau GA: *The human body in health and disease,* ed 7, St Louis, 2018, Elsevier.)

Lymphedema

Lymphedema is a buildup of lymph in the tissues causing edema (swelling). It occurs with blockage or damage to the lymph system. Causes include:

- Cancer
- Infection
- Surgical removal of lymph nodes
- Scar tissue from radiation therapy or surgery
- Absent or abnormal lymph nodes present at birth

Lymphedema usually affects an arm or leg (Fig. 50-12). Other body parts can be involved. The person may have a tight or heavy feeling and have trouble moving the body part. Thickening of the skin, pain, itching or burning, and hair loss are also common. Daily activities are often affected.

Damage to the lymph system cannot be reversed. Care measures can prevent lymphedema or keep it from getting worse (Box 50-5). Treatment may include careful exercise, good skin care, fluid balance, and massage therapy. Pressure garments (compression sleeves, lymphedema sleeves or stockings) may be used. The garment applies a certain amount of pressure to the arm or leg to move fluid and prevent fluid buildup. The goals are to control swelling, decrease pain, improve movement and use of the body part, and allow daily activities.

See *Promoting Safety and Comfort: Lymphedema.*

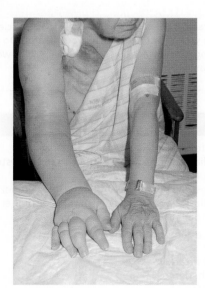

FIGURE 50-12 Lymphedema. (From Swartz MH: *Textbook of physical diagnosis: history and examination*, ed 8, Philadelphia, 2021, Elsevier.)

BOX 50-5	**Lymphedema: Care Measures**

Preventing Infection

- Monitor for signs of skin infection. Report redness, pain, swelling, heat, red streaks below the skin, or fever.
- Apply lotion to keep the skin moist.
- Report small cuts or breaks in the skin. Treatment with an antibacterial ointment is needed.
- Avoid needle-sticks on the affected arm or leg. This includes blood glucose testing (Chapter 39).
- Do not use a hand with lymphedema to test water temperature. Burns are a risk from decreased sensation.
- Report long or jagged toenails. A nurse or doctor (podiatrist) performs toenail care. Nails are cut straight across to prevent ingrown nails and infections.
- Keep the feet clean, dry, and protected. Cotton socks and shoes are worn.
- The person:
  - Wears gloves for gardening and cooking.
  - Wears sunscreen and clothing for sun protection when outside.

Promoting Fluid Flow

- Do not use a blood pressure cuff on an arm with or at risk for lymphedema.
- Do not use elastic bandages or stockings with tight bands.
- Apply compression garments as directed.
- Position the affected arm or leg higher than heart level if possible.
- Do not apply heat to the affected arm or leg.
- The person:
  - Does not sit with the legs crossed.
  - Changes sitting position at least every 30 minutes.
  - Wears clothes without tight bands or elastic. If jewelry is worn, it is loose.
  - Does not carry bags on an arm with lymphedema.
  - Does not swing the affected arm or leg quickly in circles.
  - Does not let the arm or leg hang down.

Modified from National Cancer Institute: Lymphedema (PDQ®)—patient version, *updated March 6, 2024, National Institutes of Health.*

PROMOTING SAFETY AND COMFORT

Lymphedema

Safety

In persons at risk, actions that block fluid flow or increase fluid buildup can cause lymphedema or make it worse. Never apply a blood pressure cuff to an arm with or at risk for lymphedema. For example, lymph nodes are often removed during breast cancer surgery. Do not use the arm on the surgery side to check blood pressure.

If not sure which arm to use, ask the nurse. Also, ask if the person has an arm that must not be used.

Comfort

Lymphedema can be painful and affect movement. Handle the person gently. Tell the person before you move the body part. Ask the person to tell you if pain is felt. Stop movements that cause pain.

Lymphoma

Lymphoma is cancer involving cells in the immune system (lymphocytes). Lymphocytes are a type of WBC that protects the body from infection. They are found in lymph nodes and other lymph tissues.

In cancer, an abnormal cell divides and makes more abnormal cells (Chapter 48). Lymphoma begins with an abnormal lymphocyte. Abnormal lymphocytes cannot protect the body.

There are 2 main types of lymphoma—Hodgkin lymphoma and non-Hodgkin lymphoma. They differ in the types of cells involved, how they spread, and how they respond to treatment.

Signs and symptoms of lymphoma include:
- Painless swelling in the lymph nodes in the neck, underarm, groin, or stomach
- Fever
- Night sweats
- Fatigue
- Weight loss
- Skin rash or itchy skin
- Pain in the chest, abdomen, or bones

Treatment may include chemotherapy, radiation, or other cancer treatments (Chapter 48). Psychological, social, and spiritual support are needed.

FOCUS ON PRIDE

The Person, Family, and Yourself

Personal and Professional Responsibility

Apply the information in this chapter to your own life. Are there life-style factors that put you at risk for a cardiovascular or respiratory disorder? A healthy life-style benefits you personally and professionally. You must be healthy and strong to care for others.

Rights and Respect

Some choices are unhealthy. For example, a person with COPD continues to smoke. Or a person with CAD chooses not to exercise or make diet changes. The health team teaches the person the risks and encourages healthy changes. They cannot force changes. However, they must be sure the person understands the risks.

While aware of the risks, some persons choose not to make life-style changes. You may not agree with the person's decision, but you must treat the person with dignity and respect. Personal choice is part of quality of life.

Independence and Social Interaction

Infections like the flu, pneumonia, and TB can spread to others. Transmission-Based Precautions may be needed. If family and friends avoid visiting, loneliness can result.

Social and emotional needs are important. As you give care, talk with the person. Show interest in the conversation. Be polite and kind. Tell the nurse about any concerns.

Delegation and Teamwork

A person's condition can change quickly. A person with angina may have an MI. Hypertension may lead to a stroke. A person may have a severe asthma attack.

Sudden condition changes require the nurse's attention. Assist as directed. You may need to help other patients or residents while the nurse gives care. Help willingly. The entire nursing team must give "extra effort" during an emergency.

Ethics and Laws

Some agencies use color-coded wristbands to promote safety and prevent harm (Chapter 14). They communicate alerts or warnings. "Limb alert" or "forbidden extremity" wristbands communicate that an arm must not be used for blood pressures, intravenous infusions, or blood draws. These are useful for lymphedema.

Know what wristbands are used in your agency. Check for wristbands when providing care. Take pride in using such safety measures to prevent harm.

FOCUS ON PRIDE: Application

List the risk factors for cardiovascular disorders. Circle those that apply to you. Which factors can you change? Do you plan to make changes to lower your risk? Explain. What would help you make changes?

REVIEW QUESTIONS

Circle the BEST answer.

1 A patient is being treated for anemia. Which would you expect?
   a Shortness of breath and fatigue with activity
   b Productive cough and fever
   c Pauses in breathing during sleep
   d Swelling and trouble moving the affected arm or leg

2 A person with a congenital heart defect
   a Needs heart surgery
   b Has damaged heart valves
   c Has blocked coronary arteries
   d Was born with the defect

3 In hypertension
   a The diastolic pressure is higher than the systolic pressure
   b The systolic pressure is 140 mm Hg or higher
   c The diastolic pressure is 70 mm Hg or higher
   d Chest pain is a common symptom

4 Which is a complication of hypertension?
   a COPD
   b Heart attack
   c Lymphedema
   d Anemia

5 Which life-style practice *increases* the risk of high blood pressure?
  a Regular exercise
  b A low-sodium diet
  c Smoking
  d Sleeping at least 7 hours per night

6 Cardiac rehabilitation involves
  a Exercise
  b Surgery
  c Catheter procedures
  d A vaccine

7 A person with angina has pain that is severe and not relieved by rest or drugs. This
  a Is normal angina pain
  b Signals hypertension
  c Signals heart failure
  d Signals a heart attack

8 A person reports sudden, squeezing pain in the center of the chest. You should
  a Report the pain if it is not relieved in 15 minutes
  b Report the pain at once
  c Give the person a nitroglycerin tablet
  d Give the person oxygen

9 You are measuring a daily weight on a person with heart failure. The person gained 4 pounds since yesterday. This is
  a Expected and you do not need to report it
  b Not accurate so you should record yesterday's weight
  c A significant change and you need to report it
  d A minor change and you do not need to record it

10 A person has heart failure. Which should you question?
  a Encourage fluids.
  b Measure intake and output.
  c Restrict sodium.
  d Perform range-of-motion exercises.

11 A person has a dysrhythmia. The nurse asks you to check an apical pulse for 1 minute. Why?
  a The wrists cannot be used to feel for a pulse.
  b The radial pulse will be too weak to feel.
  c The person will not have pulses at other pulse sites.
  d The pulse is likely to be slow, fast, or irregular.

12 The most common cause of COPD is
  a Smoking
  b Allergies
  c Being over-weight
  d A high-sodium diet

13 A person has emphysema. Which is *true?*
  a The person has an infection.
  b Breathing is usually easier lying down.
  c The person has dyspnea and a cough.
  d A pacemaker is used for treatment.

14 Which is *least* likely to help the person with sleep apnea?
  a Weight loss
  b Quitting smoking
  c Drinking alcohol before sleep
  d CPAP

15 The flu virus is spread by
  a Coughing and sneezing
  b Contaminated food
  c Blood
  d Needle sharing

16 Which position eases breathing in the person with pneumonia?
  a Supine
  b Semi-Fowler's
  c Prone
  d Trendelenburg's

17 Which statement about pneumonia in older persons is *true?*
  a Older persons have a low risk of pneumonia.
  b Older persons may not have the usual signs and symptoms.
  c Having dysphagia lowers the risk of pneumonia.
  d Pneumonia is not life-threatening in older persons.

18 Care of a person with tuberculosis (TB) involves
  a Airborne Precautions including wearing a respirator
  b Elastic stockings and fluid restriction
  c Special precautions for handling urine and feces (stools)
  d Bed rest and dietary changes

19 A person with tuberculosis (TB) coughs on your hand. You should
  a Watch for signs of latent TB
  b Get a TB vaccine
  c Ask the nurse about being treated
  d Wash your hands

20 A person has lymphedema in the left arm. Which should you question?
  a Apply lotion to the skin.
  b Elevate the left arm on pillows.
  c Use the right arm for blood pressure.
  d Apply a hot compress to the left arm.

Answers to Chapter 50 questions are on p. 903.

Answers to Chapter 50 questions are on p. 903.

FOCUS ON **PRACTICE**

Problem Solving

An 82-year-old resident is tired and does not want to eat breakfast. The person is confused. This is not normal behavior. When should you report these changes? Why is it important to monitor for such changes in older persons?

OBJECTIVES

- Define the key terms and key abbreviations in this chapter.
- Describe gastro-esophageal reflux disease, gastritis and peptic ulcers, diverticular disease, inflammatory bowel disease, hemorrhoids, and gallstones.
- Explain the safety and comfort measures to perform when vomiting occurs.

- Describe hepatitis and cirrhosis and the care required.
- Describe diabetes and the care required.
- Describe hypothyroidism and hyperthyroidism.
- Explain how to promote PRIDE in the person, the family, and yourself.

KEY TERMS

acid reflux See "heartburn"
emesis See "vomitus"
heartburn A burning sensation in the chest or throat; acid reflux
hyperglycemia High *(hyper)* sugar *(glyc)* in the blood *(emia)*

hypoglycemia Low *(hypo)* sugar *(glyc)* in the blood *(emia)*
jaundice Yellowish color of the skin or whites of the eyes
vomitus Food and fluids expelled from the stomach through the mouth; emesis

KEY ABBREVIATIONS

BMs	Bowel movements	IBD	Inflammatory bowel disease
C. diff	*Clostridioides difficile*	I&O	Intake and output
GERD	Gastro-esophageal reflux disease	TH	Thyroid hormone
GI	Gastro-intestinal		

Problems can develop in any part of the digestive system. This includes the accessory organs of digestion—liver, gallbladder, and pancreas. The pancreas also is part of the endocrine system. This chapter describes some common disorders of the digestive and endocrine systems.

DIGESTIVE DISORDERS

The digestive system breaks down food into nutrients for the body to absorb. Solid wastes are eliminated. Disorders affect digestive system structures and function. See Chapter 29 for diarrhea, constipation, flatulence, fecal incontinence, and ostomy care.

- *Diarrhea* is the frequent passage of liquid stools. (Contagious infections with *Clostridioides difficile* [*C. diff*] and norovirus are discussed in Chapter 29. *C. diff* causes *colitis*—inflammation of the colon. Norovirus causes *gastroenteritis*—inflammation of the stomach and intestines.)
- *Constipation* is the passage of hard, dry stool.
- *Flatulence* is the excessive formation of gas or air in the stomach and intestines.
- *Fecal incontinence* is the inability to control the passage of feces and gas through the anus.
- *Ostomy* involves a surgically created opening that connects an internal organ to the body's surface.
  See *Body Structure and Function Review: The Digestive System.*

BODY STRUCTURE AND FUNCTION REVIEW
The Digestive System

Structure and Function

The digestive system *(gastro-intestinal [GI] system)* extends from the mouth to the anus (Fig. 51-1). Digestion begins in the *mouth (oral cavity)* as food is chewed and mixed with saliva. Swallowed food moves into the *esophagus* and to the *stomach.* Movement of food through the GI tract occurs because of *peristalsis*—alternating contraction and relaxation of muscles.

The stomach is a muscular, pouch-like sac. The mucous membrane lining the stomach contains glands that secrete *gastric juices.* Food is mixed and churned with the gastric juices to form a semi-liquid substance called *chyme.* Peristalsis pushes chyme from the stomach into the small intestine.

The first part of the *small intestine* is the *duodenum.* More digestive juices are added to the chyme. One is called *bile*—a greenish liquid made in the *liver.* Bile is stored in the *gallbladder.* Juices from the *pancreas* and small intestine are added to the chyme. Digestive juices chemically break down food into nutrients for absorption. Peristalsis moves the chyme through the 2 other parts of the small intestine: the *jejunum* and the *ileum.* Most nutrient absorption takes place in the small intestine.

Undigested chyme passes from the small intestine into the *large intestine (large bowel* or *colon).* The colon absorbs most of the water from the chyme. The remaining semi-solid material is called *feces.* Feces contain a small amount of water, solid wastes, and some mucus and germs. These are the waste products of digestion. Feces pass through the colon into the *rectum* by peristalsis. Feces pass out of the body through the *anus.*

Changes With Aging

With age, secretion of saliva and digestive juices decreases. Some foods are difficult to chew, swallow, and digest. Peristalsis decreases and can cause flatulence (gas) and constipation.

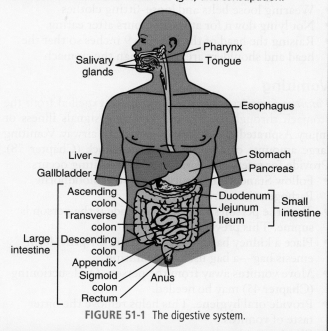

FIGURE 51-1 The digestive system.

Gastro-Esophageal Reflux Disease

Gastro-esophageal reflux disease (GERD) occurs when a muscle at the end of the esophagus does not close properly. Stomach *(gastro)* contents flow back up *(reflux)* into the esophagus *(esophageal).* Stomach contents contain acid that can irritate and inflame the esophagus lining. This is called *esophagitis*—inflammation *(itis)* of the esophagus.

Heartburn is the most common symptom. *Heartburn (acid reflux)* is a burning sensation in the chest or throat. The person may taste stomach fluid in the back of the mouth. Besides heartburn, other signs and symptoms of GERD include:

- Pain in the chest or upper abdomen
- Hoarseness or sore throat
- *Dysphagia* (difficult or painful swallowing)
- Dry cough
- Bad breath
- Nausea and vomiting

Risk factors include being over-weight, alcohol or coffee use, pregnancy, and smoking. Hiatal hernia is a risk factor. *Hernias* occur when part of an organ protrudes or projects through an opening in a muscle wall. With *hiatal hernia,* the upper part of the stomach is above the diaphragm (Fig. 51-2). Large meals, eating late at night, and lying down after eating can cause gastric reflux. So can chocolate, alcohol, caffeine drinks, fried and fatty foods, spicy foods, and acidic foods (such as citrus fruits and tomatoes).

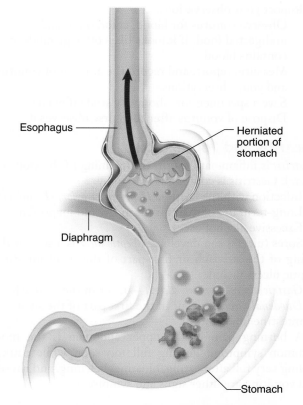

FIGURE 51-2 Hiatal hernia. (Modified from Patton KT, Thibodeau GA: *The human body in health & disease,* ed 7, St Louis, 2018, Elsevier.)

The doctor may order drugs to prevent stomach acid production or to promote stomach emptying. Surgery may be needed. Life-style changes include:

- No smoking or drinking alcohol
- Losing weight
- Eating small meals and eating slowly
- Avoiding foods and drinks that cause reflux
- Wearing loose belts and loose-fitting clothes
- Not lying down for at least 3 hours after eating
- Raising the head of the bed 6 to 9 inches so that the head and shoulders are higher than the stomach

Vomiting

Vomitus (emesis) is the food and fluids expelled from the stomach through the mouth. Vomiting signals illness or injury. Aspirated vomitus can obstruct the airway. Vomiting large amounts of blood can lead to shock (Chapter 58). Provide for safety and comfort when vomiting occurs.

- Follow Standard Precautions and the Bloodborne Pathogen Standard.
- Turn the person's head well to 1 side if the person is supine. This prevents aspiration.
- Place a kidney basin under the chin. Or provide an emesis bag—a bag used for vomiting.
- Move vomitus away from the person. Oral suctioning (Chapter 45) may be needed.
- Provide oral hygiene. This helps remove the bitter taste of vomitus.
- Eliminate odors.
- Provide comfort measures.
- Report your observations.
  - Observe vomitus for blood, color, odor, and undigested food. If it looks like coffee grounds, it contains blood.
  - Measure, report, and record the amount of vomitus and your observations.
  - Save a specimen for laboratory study if needed.
  - Dispose of vomitus after the nurse observes it.

Gastritis and Peptic Ulcers

Gastritis is inflammation *(itis)* of the lining of the stomach *(gastr)*. Gastritis is commonly caused by:

- Infection with the bacteria *Helicobacter pylori (H. pylori)*
- Long-term use of drugs like aspirin and ibuprofen
- Excessive alcohol use

Sores (ulcers) can develop. A *peptic ulcer* is a sore in the lining of the stomach or first part of the small intestine. Peptic ulcers include:

- *Gastric ulcers (stomach ulcers)*—occur in the stomach
- *Duodenal ulcers*—occur in the first part of the small intestine (duodenum)

A burning pain in the upper abdomen is the most common symptom. Feeling full too soon while eating, feeling very full after eating, bloating, belching, and nausea and vomiting are other signs and symptoms.

Treatment involves drugs to heal the ulcer and manage the underlying cause. Without treatment, peptic ulcers can worsen and lead to complications. Bleeding in the stomach or intestines and anemia (Chapter 50) can occur. Vomitus that contains blood, black stools, and bloody stools indicate bleeding. Report signs of bleeding at once. Ulcers can also cause holes (perforations) in the stomach wall and lead to a serious infection of the abdominal cavity *(peritonitis)*. (The *peritoneum* is the membrane that lines the abdominal cavity.)

An *upper GI endoscopy* is a procedure using a scope to examine *(scopy)* inside *(endo)* the upper GI tract. The procedure is also called an "EGD" for the parts of the upper GI system examined—esophagus, stomach (gastr [o]), duodenum. It may be done for diagnosis or to treat complications. Surgery may be required for complications.

Diverticular Disease

Small pouches can develop in the colon. The pouches bulge outward through weak spots in the colon wall (Fig. 51-3). A pouch is called a *diverticulum*. (*Diverticulare* means to turn inside out). *Diverticulosis* is the condition of having these pouches. (*Osis* means condition of.) The pouches can become infected or inflamed—*diverticulitis*. (*Itis* means inflammation.)

Diverticular disease becomes more common with aging. Obesity, smoking, lack of exercise, low-fiber diet, a diet high in animal fat, and some drugs are risk factors.

When feces enter the pouches, they can become inflamed and infected. The person has abdominal pain and tenderness in the lower left abdomen. Fever, nausea and vomiting, bloating, and constipation or diarrhea can occur.

Diet changes are ordered. Sometimes antibiotics and probiotics are ordered. *Probiotics*—found in dietary supplements and some foods—are live bacteria normally found in the colon. Surgery is done for severe disease, obstruction, and ruptured pouches. The diseased part of the bowel is removed. A colostomy may be needed (Chapter 29).

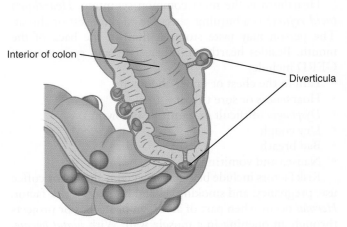

FIGURE 51-3 Diverticulosis. (From Harding MM, et al: *Lewis's medical-surgical nursing: assessment and management of clinical problems*, ed 11, St Louis, 2020, Elsevier.)

Inflammatory Bowel Disease

Inflammatory bowel disease (IBD) involves chronic inflammation of the GI tract. IBD often occurs before 30 years of age. Risk factors include a family history of IBD and cigarette smoking. The 2 types of IBD are shown in Figure 51-4.

- *Crohn's disease.* Inflammation commonly affects the small intestine and the beginning of the large intestine. However, any part of the GI tract from the mouth to the anus can be affected.
- *Ulcerative colitis.* The lining of the large intestine and rectum is inflamed and has ulcers.

Signs and symptoms include:
- Persistent diarrhea
- Abdominal pain and cramping
- Fever
- Rectal bleeding and bloody stools (common with ulcerative colitis)
- Fatigue
- Weight loss

Complications include blockage *(bowel obstruction)*, abnormal passages in the body *(fistulas)*, infected areas *(abscesses)*, tears in the anus *(anal fissures)*, ulcers in the GI tract, poor nutrition, and dehydration. Persons with IBD may be at higher risk for colon cancer.

Treatment involves diet changes and drug therapy for inflammation, infection, diarrhea, pain, and nutrition. Surgery may be needed to remove damaged parts of the small intestine or colon. A colostomy or ileostomy (Chapter 29) may be necessary.

Hemorrhoids

Hemorrhoids are swollen veins in the lower rectum or anus. Hemorrhoids may be internal (inside the rectum) or external (under the skin around the anus). Hemorrhoids are very common. Persons more likely to have them are those who:
- Are older—over age 50
- Are pregnant
- Strain during bowel movements
- Have a low-fiber diet
- Have chronic diarrhea or constipation
- Sit for a long time on the toilet
- Often lift heavy objects

Hemorrhoids can cause pain and bleeding from the rectum after a bowel movement. A high-fiber diet, drinking enough water, and not straining during bowel movements can help. Drugs to soften stools and creams, ointments, or suppositories may be used.

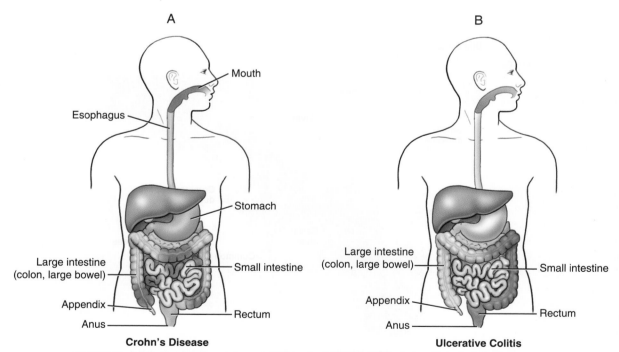

FIGURE 51-4 Inflammatory bowel disease. (Affected areas are shown in dark red.) **A,** Crohn's disease. Damaged areas appear in patches. **B,** Ulcerative colitis. The rectum and colon are damaged. (Modified from Centers for Disease Control and Prevention: *Inflammatory bowel disease (IBD): What is it?*, May 18, 2018.)

Gallstones

Bile is a liquid made in the liver. It is stored in the gallbladder until needed to digest fat. Gallstones form when the bile hardens into stone-like pieces (Fig. 51-5).

Ducts (tubes) carry bile from the liver through the gallbladder and to the small intestine. Gallstones can lodge in any duct (Fig. 51-6). Bile flow is blocked. The gallbladder and ducts become inflamed. The liver and pancreas may be involved. Severe infections or damage can cause death.

Gallstones can be as small as a grain of sand or as big as a golf ball. A person may have 1 large stone or several that vary in size. Persons at risk include those who are:

- Women—especially women who:
  - Are pregnant
  - Use hormone replacement therapy
  - Take birth control pills
- Older persons—the risk increases with aging
- Known to have a family history of gallstones
- American Indians or Mexican Americans
- Over-weight or obese or have had fast weight loss
- Have diabetes (p. 779) or cirrhosis (p. 778)

A "gallbladder attack" or "gallstone attack" usually occurs in the evening or at night after having a heavy meal. Signs and symptoms include nausea, vomiting, and pain in the upper right abdomen, back, or right shoulder. Removal of the gallbladder is common.

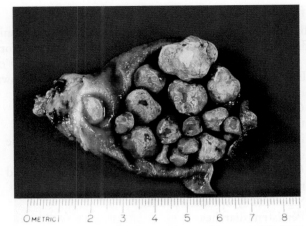

FIGURE 51-5 Inflamed gallbladder with gallstones. (From Williamson P, et al: *The human body in health and disease*, ed 8, St Louis, 2024, Elsevier.)

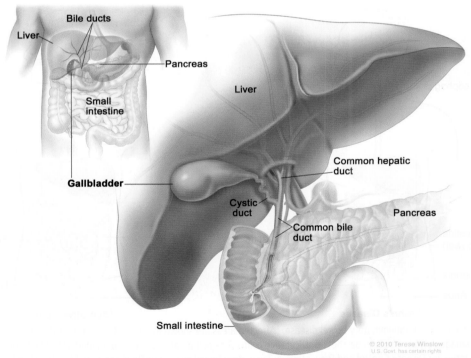

FIGURE 51-6 The gallbladder and ducts that carry bile from the liver to the gallbladder and to the small intestine. (© 2010 Terese Winslow LLC, U.S. Govt. has certain rights.)

Hepatitis

Hepatitis is inflammation *(itis)* and infection of the liver *(hepat)* caused by a virus. See Box 51-1 for signs and symptoms. Some people have no symptoms. There are 5 major types of hepatitis. See Box 51-1 for the methods of transmission for each type.

- *Hepatitis A* is caused by the hepatitis A virus (HAV). It is spread through contact with feces (stools) from an infected person. Handle bedpans, toilets, commodes, incontinence products, and rectal thermometers carefully. The hepatitis A vaccine protects against the disease.
- *Hepatitis B* is caused by the hepatitis B virus (HBV). It is spread through contact with infected blood or body fluids. The hepatitis B vaccine protects against the disease.
- *Hepatitis C* is caused by the hepatitis C virus (HCV). It is spread through contact with infected blood. A person may have no symptoms but can spread the disease. Serious liver disease and damage may appear years later. While there is no vaccine for hepatitis C, it can usually be cured with treatment.
- *Hepatitis D* is caused by the hepatitis D virus (HDV). It is spread through contact with infected blood or body fluids. It only infects persons who have hepatitis B. Vaccination for hepatitis B protects against hepatitis D.
- *Hepatitis E* is caused by the hepatitis E virus (HEV). There are different types. This disease is not common in developed countries.

Hepatitis A and E are usually acute (short-term) conditions. Hepatitis B, C, and D can become chronic (long-term). The person needs rest, fluids, and a healthy diet. Alcohol and drugs that may cause more liver damage are not used. Some types can be treated with antiviral drugs. Early diagnosis and treatment can prevent complications of chronic hepatitis—cirrhosis, liver cancer, and liver failure.

See *Promoting Safety and Comfort: Hepatitis*, p. 778.

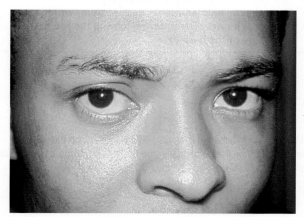

FIGURE 51-7 Jaundice. (Photo courtesy the DCD/Dr. Thomas F. Sellers.)

BOX 51-1	Hepatitis

Signs and Symptoms

- *Jaundice*—yellowish color of the skin or whites of the eyes (Fig. 51-7)
- Fatigue
- Pain: abdominal, joint
- Appetite: loss of
- Nausea and vomiting
- Diarrhea (hepatitis A)
- Bowel movements (BMs): light, clay-colored
- Urine: dark
- Fever
- Itching: severe
- Weight loss

Transmission

Hepatitis A

Spread through contact with an infected person's feces (stools) by:

- Eating food prepared by the infected person with poor hand-washing after a BM
- Drinking untreated water
- Eating food washed in untreated water
- Placing a finger or object that is contaminated with the infected person's feces (stools) into the mouth
- Close personal contact with an infected person—sex, providing care

Hepatitis B

Spread through contact with an infected person's blood, semen, or other body fluids by:

- Being born to an infected mother
- Having unprotected sex with an infected person
- Sharing drug needles or materials with an infected person
- Getting an accidental stick with a needle that was used on an infected person
- Being tattooed or pierced with tools not cleaned properly after use on an infected person
- Having contact with blood or open sores of an infected person
- Using an infected person's razor, toothbrush, or nail clippers

Hepatitis C

Spread through contact with an infected person's blood (see Hepatitis B)

Hepatitis D

Spread through an infected person's blood or body fluids by:

- Sharing drug needles or materials with an infected person
- Having unprotected sex with an infected person
- Getting an accidental stick with a needle that was used on an infected person

Hepatitis E

Different types are spread by:

- Drinking water contaminated with feces (stools) of an infected person
- Eating raw or under-cooked pork, venison, wild boar, or shellfish

---

Modified from National Institute of Diabetes and Digestive and Kidney Diseases: What is viral hepatitis?, *May 2017;* Hepatitis A, *September 2019;* Hepatitis B, *June 2020;* Hepatitis C, *March 2020;* Hepatitis D, *May 2017; and* Hepatitis E, *June 2017; National Institutes of Health.*

PROMOTING SAFETY AND COMFORT

Hepatitis

Safety

The viruses that cause hepatitis can be transmitted (see Box 51-1). Protect yourself and others. Follow the rules of hand hygiene and the guidelines for glove use in Chapters 17 and 18. Follow Standard Precautions and the Bloodborne Pathogen Standard. Transmission-Based Precautions are ordered as necessary.

Alcohol-based hand sanitizer may not be as effective against the hepatitis A virus as washing with soap and water. Good hand hygiene is important. Hand-washing after elimination, after handling diapers or incontinence products, and before preparing or eating food are essential. Assist the person with hand-washing as needed.

Having one's own personal care items (toothbrush, razor, nail clippers, and so on) is important. Sharing personal care items with an infected person can spread infections.

Cirrhosis

Cirrhosis is a liver condition caused by chronic liver damage (Fig. 51-8). (*Cirrho* means yellow-orange. *Osis* means condition.) Healthy liver tissue is replaced with scar tissue. Some blood flow through the liver is blocked. Normal liver functions are affected:

- Fighting infection
- Processing, storing, and delivering nutrients to the body
- Cleaning the blood of toxins, fats, cholesterol, and drugs
- Making proteins for blood clotting
- Producing bile for fat digestion

Alcohol use disorder (Chapter 53), chronic hepatitis B and C, and extra fat in the liver are common causes. Obesity is becoming a common cause. The person may not have signs or symptoms until the liver is badly damaged. See Box 51-2 for signs and symptoms that can occur as cirrhosis progresses.

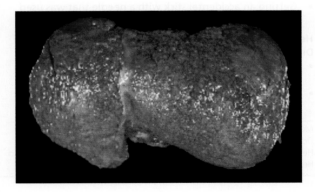

BOX 51-2   Cirrhosis

Signs and Symptoms

- Weakness and fatigue
- Loss of appetite and weight loss
- Nausea and vomiting
- Pain or discomfort in the right upper abdomen
- *Ascites*—abdominal bloating from fluid buildup in the abdomen (Fig. 51-9)
- *Edema* (swelling) in the feet and legs
- Itching (severe)
- Spider-like blood vessels on the skin
- Jaundice
- Bruising and bleeding easily
- Dark urine
- *Encephalopathy*—mental changes that occur from the buildup of toxins in the brain—confusion, memory loss, trouble thinking, personality changes
- Sleep problems

General Care

- Follow the care plan to prevent complications from bed rest—pneumonia, blood clots, pressure injuries.
- Provide good skin care and prevent itching.
  - Follow the care plan for what cleanser to use.
  - Apply lotion to the skin.
  - Discourage the scratching of itchy skin.
- Provide mouth care before meals and every 2 hours.
- Follow diet and fluid restriction orders.
- Turn the person at least every 2 hours or as noted on the care plan.
- Promote comfort and the ability to breathe.
  - Semi-Fowler's or Fowler's position
  - Pillows under the arms for support
  - Coughing and deep-breathing exercises
- Assist with ambulation and activities of daily living (ADL) as needed.

Measurements and Observations

- Observe vomitus, urine, and BMs for blood.
- Observe for signs of decreased mental function—confusion, memory loss, behavior changes, and so on.
- Measure vital signs every 2 to 4 hours.
- Measure intake and output (I&O).
- Measure weight daily.

Safety

- Use bed rails according to the care plan.
- Keep the call light and other needed items within reach.
- Complete a safety check before leaving the room. (See the inside of the back cover.)

FIGURE 51-8 A damaged liver has nodules (bumps) on the surface. (The surface of the liver is normally smooth.) (From Shiland BJ: *Mastering healthcare terminology*, ed 7, St Louis, 2023, Elsevier.)

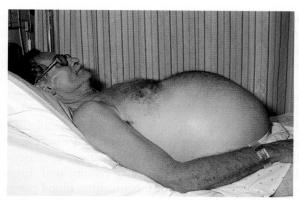

FIGURE 51-9 Fluid in the membrane lining the abdominal cavity *(ascites)*. (From Swartz MH: *Textbook of physical diagnosis*, ed 8, Philadelphia, 2021, Elsevier.)

Cirrhosis has many serious complications. Blocked blood flow in the liver increases blood pressure in the large vein that brings blood from the GI tract to the liver *(portal hypertension)*. Enlarged veins *(varices)* in the esophagus, stomach, or intestines can burst and cause GI bleeding. Infections, gallstones, and mental changes can occur. Liver cancer is a risk. Liver failure (end-stage liver disease) can occur—the liver stops working.

Treatment is aimed at treating the cause to keep the cirrhosis from getting worse. Complications are treated. A low-sodium diet is needed for edema and ascites. Diuretic drugs (water pills) are ordered to remove fluid. Sometimes a procedure is performed to drain excess fluid from the abdomen. Antibiotics are ordered for infection. The person must avoid alcohol and may need a liver transplant.

The measures listed in Box 51-2 may be part of the person's care plan.

ENDOCRINE DISORDERS

The endocrine system is made up of glands that secrete hormones. Disorders occur from too much or too little secretion of hormones or from an inadequate response to the hormone. The disorders discussed in this chapter involve the pancreas and thyroid gland.

See *Body Structure and Function Review: The Endocrine System (Pancreas and Thyroid Gland)*.

BODY STRUCTURE AND FUNCTION REVIEW

The Endocrine System (Pancreas and Thyroid Gland)

Structure and Function

The *endocrine glands* (Fig. 51-10) secrete chemical substances called *hormones* into the bloodstream. Hormones regulate the activities of other organs and glands in the body.

The *pancreas* is in the abdomen behind the stomach. It secretes *insulin*. Insulin regulates the amount of sugar in the blood available for use by the cells. Insulin is needed for sugar to enter the cells. Without insulin, excess sugar builds up in the blood.

The *thyroid gland* is in the neck. It secretes *thyroid hormone (TH)*. TH regulates metabolism—how the body uses nutrients to provide energy and maintain body functions. Body processes, movement, and weight are affected by too little or too much TH.

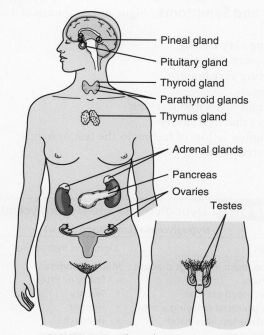

FIGURE 51-10 The endocrine system.

Changes With Aging

Insulin and TH usually remain stable with age. They may decrease slightly. With age, the body may become less sensitive to insulin. Insulin is not used as well.

Diabetes

In diabetes, the body cannot produce or use insulin properly. Without any or enough insulin, sugar builds up in the blood. Blood glucose (sugar) is high. Cells do not have enough sugar for energy and cannot function.

Types of Diabetes. A family history of the disease is a common risk factor for the 3 types of diabetes.

- *Type 1 diabetes.* Occurs most often in children and young adults but can develop at any age. The pancreas makes no insulin. Too much glucose stays in the blood. Onset is rapid.
- *Type 2 diabetes.* This is the most common type. It occurs most often in middle and older adulthood. It can develop during childhood. In type 2 diabetes, the body does not make enough insulin or use insulin well. Risk factors include being age 45 or older, having a family history of diabetes, being over-weight or obese, and being physically inactive.
- *Gestational diabetes.* This type develops during pregnancy. This type usually goes away after the baby is born. However, the mother is at risk for type 2 diabetes later in life.

Signs and Symptoms. Signs and symptoms of diabetes are:

- Being very thirsty
- Frequent urination
- Feeling very hungry
- Fatigue
- Weight loss without trying
- Sores that heal slowly
- Tingling or loss of feeling in the feet or hands
- Blurred vision

Complications. Diabetes must be controlled to prevent complications. High blood glucose levels can cause serious health problems. Heart disease, stroke, kidney disease, eye problems, dental problems, and nerve damage (*neuropathy*) are examples. With nerve problems, the person may lose sensation in the feet. Foot problems can occur (Chapter 41).

Treatment. Type 1 diabetes is treated with daily insulin therapy, healthy eating (Chapter 30), and exercise. Type 2 diabetes is treated with healthy eating, exercise, and weight loss if needed. Type 2 may require oral drugs or insulin. Types 1 and 2 involve controlling blood pressure, cholesterol, and the risk factors for coronary artery disease.

Good foot care is needed. Corns, blisters, calluses, and other foot problems can lead to an infection and amputation. See Chapters 25 and 41.

Blood sugar level can fall too low or go too high.

- *Hypoglycemia* means low (*hypo*) sugar (*glyc*) in the blood (*emia*).
- *Hyperglycemia* means high (*hyper*) sugar (*glyc*) in the blood (*emia*).

Blood glucose is monitored as often as ordered (Chapter 39). For example, type 1 testing may be done 4 to 10 times a day. For type 2, testing can range from daily to 4 times a day—before meals and at bedtime.

See Table 51-1 for the causes, signs, and symptoms of hypoglycemia and hyperglycemia. Both can lead to death if not corrected. Call for the nurse at once.

TABLE 51-1	Hypoglycemia and Hyperglycemia		
Hypoglycemia (Low Blood Sugar)		**Hyperglycemia (High Blood Sugar)**	
Causes	Signs and Symptoms	Causes	Signs and Symptoms
• Too much insulin or diabetic drugs • Increased exercise • Skipping or delaying a meal • Eating too little food • Vomiting • Drinking alcohol	**Mild to Moderate** • Shaky or jittery • Sweaty • Hunger • Headache • Blurred vision • Sleepy or tired • Dizzy or being light-headed • Confused or disoriented • Skin: pale • Uncoordinated movements • Irritable or nervous • Arguing or being combative • Behavior or personality changes • Trouble concentrating • Weakness • Pulse: rapid or irregular **Severe** • Cannot eat or drink • Seizures or convulsions • Unconsciousness	• Not enough insulin or diabetic drugs • Too little exercise • Eating too much food • Emotional stress • Infection or sickness • Undiagnosed diabetes	**Early** • Frequent urination • Increased thirst • Blurred vision • Being tired • Headache **Late** • Breath that smells fruity • Weakness • Dry mouth • Shortness of breath • Nausea and vomiting • Confusion • Abdominal pain • Coma

Thyroid Disorders

Hypothyroidism (under-active thyroid) is when the thyroid gland does not produce enough *(hypo)* thyroid hormone (TH). Body processes slow. When hypothyroidism is caused by an autoimmune problem (Chapter 48), it is called *Hashimoto's disease*. It can also be caused by inflammation of the thyroid. Radiation treatment of the thyroid, surgical removal of all or part of the thyroid, and some drugs cause hypothyroidism.

Hyperthyroidism (over-active thyroid) is when the thyroid gland produces too much *(hyper)* TH. When hyperthyroidism is caused by an autoimmune disorder (Chapter 48), it is called *Graves' disease*. Inflammation of the thyroid, excessive iodine intake, and having growths (nodules) within the thyroid are other causes.

Table 51-2 describes some signs and symptoms of hypothyroidism and hyperthyroidism. A *goiter* is swelling in the neck caused by an enlarged thyroid gland. It may occur with either condition.

Treatment includes measures to return TH levels to normal. Hypothyroidism is treated with a thyroid hormone drug. Drugs or surgery may be needed for hyperthyroidism.

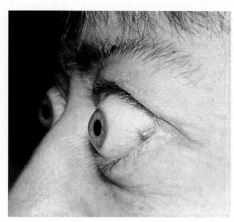

FIGURE 51-11 Bulging of the eyes can occur with hyperthyroidism. (From Goldman L, Cooney K: *Goldman-Cecil medicine,* ed 27, St Louis, 2024, Elsevier.)

TABLE 51-2	Signs and Symptoms: Thyroid Disorders
Hypothyroidism	**Hyperthyroidism**
Weight gain	Weight loss despite increased appetite
Trouble tolerating cold	Trouble tolerating heat, sweating
Slow pulse	Fast pulse
Constipation	Frequent bowel movements
Muscle and joint pain	Muscle weakness, shaky hands
Fatigue	Fatigue
Depression	Nervousness, irritability, trouble sleeping
Dry skin, dry and thinning hair	Bulging eyes (Fig. 51-11)

Modified from National Institute of Diabetes and Digestive and Kidney Diseases: Hypothyroidism (underactive thyroid), *March 2021;* Hyperthyroidism (overactive thyroid), *August 2021; National Institutes of Health.*

FOCUS ON **PRIDE**

The Person, Family, and Yourself

Personal and Professional Responsibility

Understanding health problems allows you to safely assist with care. You may want to know more about a health problem. Or a person may have a disorder you did not learn about in your training. Ask the nurse for more information. You can also look up the problem in a medical dictionary or on the Internet. Take pride in learning more.

Rights and Respect

The Bloodborne Pathogen Standard protects workers from bloodborne pathogens (Chapter 17). Health care workers are at risk for accidental needle-stick injuries. One infection prevention measure in the Standard is hepatitis B vaccination. The hepatitis B vaccine protects against hepatitis B. You will be offered the vaccine. You have the right to refuse. You must sign a document saying you refuse. You can have the vaccine at a later time.

Independence and Social Interaction

Many digestive and endocrine disorders require diet changes. Dietary practices are cultural and personal. The person may feel loss of control over an important part of life. The person and family need education, support, and encouragement.

Delegation and Teamwork

Complications are worsening problems that can occur with a disorder. You have an important role in observing for signs and symptoms of complications. Report concerns at once. Value your role as part of the nursing team.

Ethics and Laws

Some problems need attention right away. Care delays can cause harm. For example, a person who is vomiting uses the call light to signal for help. Minutes pass before anyone responds. The person aspirates. Vomitus obstructs the airway. The person dies.

Prompt responses are needed. Otherwise negligence, neglect, and other legal problems can result (Chapter 5).

FOCUS ON **PRIDE**: *Application*

Identify a complication of a disorder in this chapter. What might signal that the complication is occurring? What will you do if you are unsure what to watch for?

REVIEW QUESTIONS

Circle the BEST answer.

1 A person has gastro-esophageal reflux disease. Which should you question?
  a Loose clothing
  b Supine position after meals
  c Small meals
  d No smoking or alcohol

2 A person with gastro-esophageal reflux disease has these food choices. Which is *best* for the person?
  a Baked chicken
  b Pasta with tomato sauce
  c Fried ravioli
  d Chicken wings with hot sauce

3 A person is vomiting. You should
  a Position the person supine
  b Leave to get the nurse
  c Do nothing
  d Turn the person's head to the side

4 Vomiting is dangerous because of
  a Aspiration
  b Diverticular disease
  c Ascites
  d Jaundice

5 A person with peptic ulcer disease vomits. It looks like coffee grounds. This signals
  a Healing of the ulcer
  b Gallstones
  c Bleeding
  d Hemorrhoids

6 A person has diverticular disease. How will you assist with care?
  a Giving antibiotics
  b Promoting normal bowel elimination
  c Dietary teaching and planning
  d Assessing risk factors

7 Crohn's disease and ulcerative colitis can cause
  a Flank pain and dysuria
  b Jaundice and itching
  c Diarrhea and bloody stools
  d Ascites and edema

8 Which helps prevent hemorrhoids?
  a Sitting on the toilet for long periods
  b Straining during bowel movements
  c A low-fiber diet
  d Drinking water

9 Gallbladder attacks usually occur
  a On awakening
  b During a fast
  c After a heavy meal
  d When the person is lying down

10 Which is a sign of gallstones?
  a Extreme thirst
  b Abdominal pain
  c Black, tarry stools
  d Hoarseness and a choking sensation

11 Hepatitis is inflammation of the
  a Liver
  b Gallbladder
  c Pancreas
  d Stomach

12 Which is spread by food or water contaminated with feces from an infected person?
  a Hepatitis A
  b Hepatitis B
  c Hepatitis C
  d Hepatitis D

13 A vaccine is available to protect against
  a Inflammatory bowel disease
  b Hepatitis B
  c Hepatitis C
  d Diabetes

14 Which is a common cause of cirrhosis?
  a Thyroid disease
  b Alcohol use disorder
  c Gastritis
  d GERD

15 A person has cirrhosis. Which should you question?
  a Measure I&O.
  b Weigh the person daily.
  c Observe the stools and vomitus for blood.
  d Encourage fluids.

16 Which may signal diabetes?
  a Decreased urine output and dark urine
  b Edema and weight gain
  c Being very hungry and thirsty
  d Jaundice and a swollen abdomen

17 Why is good foot care important for persons with diabetes?
  a Foot pain is common with diabetes.
  b Persons with diabetes cannot wear footwear.
  c Blood glucose testing is usually done through the feet.
  d Foot problems can lead to infection and amputation.

18 A person with diabetes is vomiting after a meal. The person is at risk for
  a Hypoglycemia
  b Hyperglycemia
  c Jaundice
  d Bleeding

19 With type 2 diabetes, blood glucose
  a Does not need to be monitored
  b Is low if the disorder is not treated
  c Is often tested before meals and at bedtime
  d Returns to normal after pregnancy

20 Hypothyroidism can cause
  a Weight loss
  b A slow pulse
  c Trouble tolerating heat
  d Frequent bowel movements

Answers to Chapter 51 questions are on p. 904.

FOCUS ON PRACTICE

Problem Solving

A resident with diabetes is confused, weak, and shaky after an exercise activity. What do you do? What might these signs and symptoms indicate? How does understanding the person's health problems help you give better care?

Urinary and Reproductive Disorders

OBJECTIVES

- Define the key terms and key abbreviations in this chapter.
- Describe urinary tract infections and the care required.
- Describe prostate enlargement and the care required.
- Describe urinary diversions and the care required.
- Describe renal calculi and the care required.
- Describe chronic kidney disease and the care required.

- Describe vaginitis, sexually transmitted diseases (infections), and pelvic inflammatory disease.
- Describe pelvic organ prolapse.
- Explain how to promote PRIDE in the person, the family, and yourself.

KEY TERMS

dialysis The process of removing waste products from the blood
dysuria Difficult or painful *(dys)* urination *(uria)*
hematuria Blood *(hemat)* in the urine *(uria)*
oliguria Scant amount *(olig)* of urine *(uria)*
pyuria Pus *(py)* in the urine *(uria)*

urinary diversion A surgically created pathway for urine to leave the body
urostomy A surgically created opening *(stomy)* that connects to the urinary tract *(uro)*

KEY ABBREVIATIONS

AIDS	Acquired immunodeficiency syndrome		**PID**	Pelvic inflammatory disease
BPH	Benign prostatic hyperplasia		**STD**	Sexually transmitted disease
CKD	Chronic kidney disease		**STI**	Sexually transmitted infection
HIV	Human immunodeficiency virus		**TURP**	Transurethral resection of the prostate
HPV	Human papilloma viruses		**UTI**	Urinary tract infection
mL	Milliliter			

Urinary and reproductive disorders are common. Understanding the disorders gives meaning to the required care.

URINARY SYSTEM DISORDERS

Disorders can occur in urinary system structures—kidneys, ureters, bladder, and urethra. Men can develop prostate problems.

See *Body Structure and Function Review: The Urinary System*, p. 784.

BODY STRUCTURE AND FUNCTION REVIEW

The Urinary System

Structure and Function

The urinary system includes the kidneys, ureters, the bladder, and the urethra (Fig. 52-1). Its functions include:

- Removing waste products from the blood.
- Maintaining water balance.
- Maintaining electrolyte balance. *Electrolytes* are substances that dissolve in water—sodium, potassium, calcium, and magnesium.
- Maintaining acid-base balance (Chapter 10).

The 2 *kidneys* lie in the upper abdomen against the back muscles on each side of the spine. Blood is filtered by the kidneys. Each kidney has over a million tiny *nephrons*—the basic working units of the kidney. Most of the water and other needed substances are re-absorbed by the body. The rest of the fluid and the waste products form *urine*. The kidneys also produce hormones that help control blood pressure, stimulate red blood cell production, and maintain bone strength.

A *ureter* is attached to each kidney. Urine flows from the kidneys through the ureters to the bladder. Urine is stored in the bladder. The *urethra* connects the bladder to the outside of the body. Men have a gland called the *prostate gland* that lies just below the bladder and surrounds the urethra. Urine passes from the body through the *meatus* at the end of the urethra. Urine is a clear, yellowish liquid. Normal urine output for an adult is about 1500 mL (milliliters) per day.

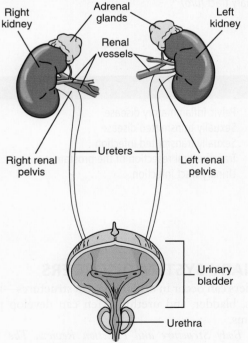

FIGURE 52-1 The urinary system.

Changes With Aging

In older persons, there is reduced blood supply to the kidneys, and the kidneys *atrophy* (shrink). Kidney function decreases. Bladder muscles weaken, and the tissues are less able to stretch. The bladder may hold less urine and not empty completely. Changes increase the risk for urinary system problems—infection, frequency, urgency, incontinence, night-time urination. In men, the prostate gland enlarges.

Urinary Tract Infections

A urinary tract infection (UTI) is an infection in any part of the urinary system. UTIs most often involve the lower urinary tract (bladder and urethra). Microbes can enter the system through the urethra. Urological exams, intercourse, poor perineal hygiene, immobility, and poor fluid intake are common causes. Persons with urinary catheters are at high risk (Chapter 28). UTI is a common healthcare-associated infection (Chapter 17). The infection can spread to other urinary structures.

Women are at high risk. Microbes can easily enter the female urethra and travel a short distance to the bladder. Prostate gland secretions help protect men from UTIs. However, an enlarged prostate increases the risk of UTI.

See Box 52-1 for signs and symptoms and the 2 types of UTIs. UTIs are treated with antibiotics. Fluids, especially water, are encouraged to flush bacteria from the urinary tract. Normal elimination is promoted. The person should urinate when the urge is felt. For prevention and treatment, proper perineal care and catheter care are needed.

BOX 52-1	**Urinary Tract Infections**

Signs and Symptoms

- Urinary frequency
- Urgency
- Burning on urination
- *Oliguria*—scant amount *(olig)* of urine *(uria)*
- *Dysuria*—difficult or painful *(dys)* urination *(uria)*
- *Hematuria*—blood *(hemat)* in the urine *(uria)*
- *Pyuria*—pus *(py)* in the urine *(uria)*
- Cloudy urine
- Urine that appears red, pink, or dark
- Fever
- Fatigue
- Weakness
- Pressure in the lower abdomen
- Urine odor
- Pelvic pain—women
- Rectal pain—men

Types of Urinary Tract Infections

- *Cystitis* (bladder infection)—a bladder *(cyst)* infection *(itis)* caused by bacteria. Specific symptoms:
  - Pelvic pressure
  - Lower abdominal discomfort
  - Frequent, painful urination
  - Hematuria
- *Pyelonephritis* (kidney infection)—inflammation *(itis)* of the kidney *(nephr)*. (*Pyelo* relates to the renal pelvis [see Fig. 52-1]). Specific symptoms:
  - Flank pain—pain in the back between the ribs and the hip (Fig. 52-2)
  - High fever
  - Nausea and vomiting
  - Shaking and chills

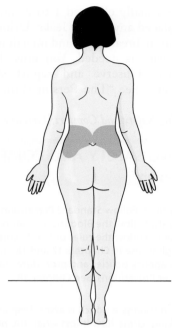

FIGURE 52-2 *Shading* shows the flank area.

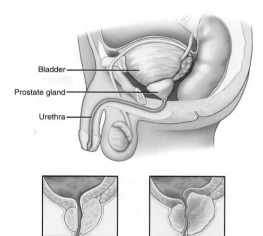

Bladder

Prostate gland

Urethra

Normal prostate   Enlarged prostate

FIGURE 52-3 Enlarged prostate. The prostate presses against the urethra. Urine flow is obstructed.

Prostate Enlargement

The prostate is a walnut-shaped gland in men. It lies just below the bladder (Fig. 52-3). The prostate surrounds the urethra. The prostate grows larger (enlarges) as the man grows older. This is called benign prostatic hyperplasia (BPH). *Benign* means non-malignant. *Hyper* means excessive. *Plasia* means formation or development. Benign prostatic hypertrophy is another name for enlarged prostate. (*Trophy* means growth.)

BPH is common in older men. The enlarged prostate presses against the urethra, obstructing urine flow (see Fig. 52-3). The following are signs and symptoms of BPH.

- Urinary frequency—voiding 8 or more times a day
- Urgency—cannot delay voiding
- Trouble starting a stream
- Weak or "stop and start" urine stream
- Dribbling after voiding
- Frequent voiding during sleep *(nocturia)*
- Urinary retention—the bladder does not empty; urine remains in the bladder
- Urinary incontinence
- Pain during urination *(dysuria)*
- Urine has an unusual color or smell

For mild BPH, drugs can shrink the prostate or stop its growth. Procedures or surgery may be needed to remove tissue or widen the urethra. A transurethral resection of the prostate (TURP) is a common surgical procedure used to treat BPH. The surgery uses a scope inserted through *(trans)* the urethra *(urethral)* to remove prostate tissue. *Resection* involves removing tissue. A catheter is in place after the procedure. Some bleeding

and blood clots in the urine are normal at first. The catheter is usually removed in 1 to 3 days. The person's care plan may include:

- No straining or sudden movements
- Drinking a least 8 cups of water daily
- No straining to have a bowel movement
- A balanced diet to prevent constipation
- No heavy lifting

Urinary Diversion

Cancer and bladder injuries are common reasons for blocked urine flow or surgical removal of the bladder. Urine must be re-routed from the body. A *urinary diversion* is a surgically created pathway for urine to leave the body.

Often an ostomy is involved. A *urostomy* is a surgically created opening *(stomy)* that connects to the urinary tract *(uro)*. The 2 main types of urostomies are:

- *Ileal conduit.* A small section of the small intestine *(ileal)* is used as a passageway *(conduit)* for urine. The ureters are connected to the piece of intestine. The intestine is brought out onto the body's surface to create a stoma (Fig. 52-4, p. 786).
- *Cutaneous ureterostomy.* A *ureter* is brought through the abdominal wall and a stoma *(ostomy)* is created on the skin *(cutaneous)*. This type may involve 1 or 2 ureters and stomas (Fig. 52-5, p. 786).

Urine drains constantly from the stoma into a pouch applied over the stoma (Fig. 52-6, p. 786). Pouches are emptied when becoming ⅓ (one-third) to ½ (one-half) full. Pouches become heavy as they fill with urine. For sleep, the person can attach drainage tubing to the pouch for urine to flow to a bigger urine collection device. A heavy pouch can loosen the seal between the pouch and the skin. Urine can leak onto the skin.

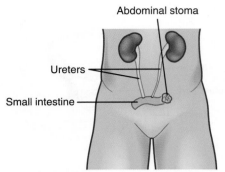

FIGURE 52-4 Ileal conduit. (Modified from Harding MM, et al: *Lewis's medical-surgical nursing: assessment and management of clinical problems,* ed 11, St Louis, 2020, Elsevier.)

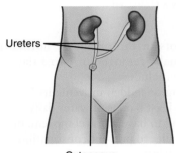

FIGURE 52-5 Cutaneous ureterostomy. The left ureter is connected to the right ureter. One stoma is needed. (Modified from Harding MM, et al: *Lewis's medical-surgical nursing: assessment and management of clinical problems,* ed 11, St Louis, 2020, Elsevier.)

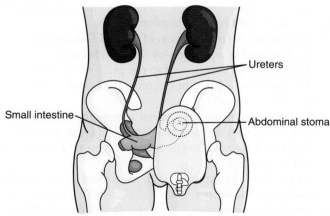

FIGURE 52-6 Ileal conduit with a urostomy pouch.

Pouches are usually changed 1 to 2 times per week. A pouch is replaced any time it leaks. Urine on the skin can cause irritation, breakdown, and infection.

Good skin care is needed. You must help prevent skin breakdown. Observe and report skin changes around the stoma. See "The Person With an Ostomy" in Chapter 29.

See *Promoting Safety and Comfort: Urinary Diversion.*

PROMOTING SAFETY AND COMFORT
Urinary Diversion

Safety
Urine is a body fluid. Follow Standard Precautions if contact with urine is likely. Follow the Bloodborne Pathogen Standard if blood is present. Follow the rules of hand hygiene and the guidelines for glove use in Chapters 17 and 18. In nursing centers, follow agency policies and procedures for using Enhanced Barrier Precautions. See Chapter 18.

Comfort
The best time to change a pouch is after sleep and before eating or drinking. Urine flow is less when the person has not had anything to eat or drink for 2 to 3 hours.
   The stoma does not have sensation. Touching the stoma does not cause pain or discomfort.

Kidney Stones

Kidney stones *(renal calculi)* are hard, pebble-like materials that develop in 1 or both kidneys (Fig. 52-7). They vary in size—from a grain of sand to pea-sized. Larger stones can develop. Stones may be smooth or jagged. They are usually yellow or brown.

Men are at higher risk than women. A family history of kidney stones increases the risk. So does having kidney stones before. Not drinking enough liquids is another risk factor.

Signs and symptoms include:
- Severe, sharp pain in the back, side, lower abdomen, or groin (Fig. 52-8)
- *Dysuria*—difficult or painful *(dys)* urination *(uria)*
- Urinary frequency and urgency
- Inability to urinate or can only urinate a small amount
- *Hematuria*—blood *(hemat)* in the urine *(uria)*
- Cloudy urine
- Foul-smelling urine
- Nausea and vomiting
- Fever and chills

Drugs are given for pain relief. The person needs to drink 2000 to 3000 mL a day. Fluids help flush stones out through the urine. All urine is strained (Chapter 39). Medical or surgical removal of the stone may be necessary. Diet changes may prevent stones.

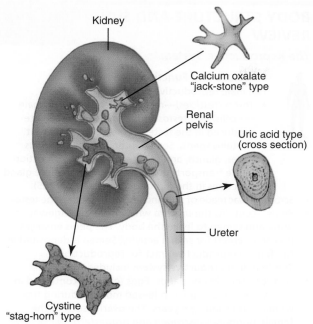

FIGURE 52-7 Kidney stones. Stones vary in shape and size. (Modified from Nix S: *Williams' basic nutrition & diet therapy*, ed 16, St Louis, 2022, Elsevier.)

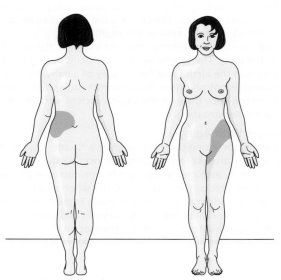

FIGURE 52-8 Shaded areas show where the pain from a left kidney stone is located.

BOX 52-2	Chronic Kidney Disease

Signs and Symptoms

- Appetite—loss of
- Chest pain (related to fluid build-up)
- Concentration: problems with
- *Edema*—swelling in the feet, ankles, or legs (less often in the hands or face)
- Fatigue
- Headaches
- Muscle cramps
- Nausea and vomiting
- Numbness
- Shortness of breath (related to fluid build-up)
- Skin—dry, itching
- Sleep problems
- Thirst: excessive
- Urinary output: decreased
- Weight loss

Care Measures

- Diet planning (Chapter 30)
  - Lowering sodium
  - Lowering phosphorus and potassium in advanced CKD
  - Choosing certain types and amounts of protein
- Fluid restriction
- Measuring blood pressure in the supine, sitting, and standing positions
- Measuring daily weight
- Measuring and recording intake and output (I&O)
- Turning and re-positioning at least every 2 hours
- Measures to prevent pressure injuries
- Range-of-motion (ROM) exercises
- Measures to prevent itching (bath oils, lotions, creams)
- Measures to prevent injury and bleeding
- Frequent oral hygiene
- Measures to prevent infection
- Deep-breathing and coughing exercises
- Measures to prevent diarrhea or constipation
- Measures to meet emotional needs
- Measures to promote rest

Signs and symptoms modified from National Institute of Diabetes and Digestive and Kidney Diseases: What is chronic kidney disease?, *June 2017, National Institutes of Health.*

Chronic Kidney Disease

In chronic kidney disease (CKD), the kidneys are damaged and do not function normally. Waste products are not removed from the blood. Fluid is retained. Diabetes and hypertension are common causes of CKD.

Blood and urine tests are used to check kidney function. Early CKD may not have signs or symptoms. As CKD advances, signs and symptoms occur (Box 52-2). Anemia, high blood pressure, and heart disease can develop (Chapter 50). Bone disease (weak and brittle bones) and poor nutrition (malnutrition) can also occur.

CKD can worsen over time and may lead to kidney failure (end-stage renal disease; ESRD). ESRD requires a kidney transplant or dialysis. *Dialysis* is the process of removing waste products from the blood.

- *Hemodialysis* filters blood (*hemo*) through a machine that works as an artificial kidney (Fig. 52-9, p. 788).
- *Peritoneal dialysis* uses the lining of the abdominal cavity (*peritoneal membrane*) to remove waste and fluid from the blood (Fig. 52-10, p. 788).

Dietary changes are needed. See "The Renal Diet" in Chapter 30. The person's care plan may include the measures in Box 52-2.

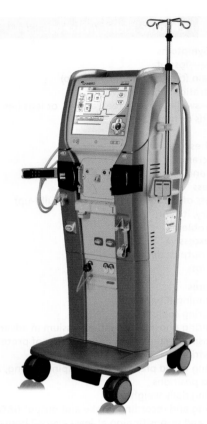

FIGURE 52-9 Dialysis machine. (Image courtesy Baxter International Inc.)

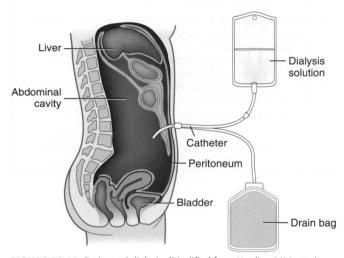

Liver

Abdominal cavity

Dialysis solution

Catheter

Peritoneum

Bladder

Drain bag

FIGURE 52-10 Peritoneal dialysis. (Modified from Harding MM, et al: *Lewis's medical-surgical nursing: assessment and management of clinical problems*, ed 11, St Louis, 2020, Elsevier.)

REPRODUCTIVE DISORDERS

The reproductive system includes organs and hormone-producing glands. Aging, infection, injury, some chronic illnesses, and surgeries can affect reproductive structures and functions. Problems can occur with menstruation and fertility (ability to reproduce). Altered sexual function related to aging is discussed in Chapter 12. This chapter describes different infections that affect the reproductive system.

See *Body Structure and Function Review: The Reproductive System*.

BODY STRUCTURE AND FUNCTION REVIEW

The Reproductive System

Structure and Function

The male reproductive system includes the:
- *Testes (testicles)*—male sex glands. *Sperm* (male sex cells) and *testosterone* (male hormone) are produced in the testes. *Semen* is the fluid that contains sperm. See Chapter 10 for the various tubes, glands, and other structures that function in the transportation of sperm. The prostate gland functions in the reproductive system (p. 785).
- *Scrotum*—sac made of skin and muscle that holds the testes.
- *Penis*—contains the *urethra* which is the passageway for urine and semen to leave the body. The penis enlarges (becomes erect) for sexual activity. Semen is deposited in the female reproductive tract for reproduction.

The female reproductive system includes the:
- *Ovaries*—female sex glands. Eggs *(ova)* are contained in the ovaries. One ovum is released monthly during the woman's reproductive years. The ovaries secrete the female hormones *(estrogen* and *progesterone).*
- *Fallopian tubes*—passageways for ova from each ovary to the uterus. There are 2 fallopian tubes.
- *Uterus*—a hollow, muscular organ where a fertilized cell implants, grows into a fetus (unborn baby), and is nourished during pregnancy. The tissue lining the uterus is the *endometrium.* The *cervix* is the lower, narrow part of the uterus that leads to the vagina.
- *Vagina*—the passageway from the uterus to the outside of the body. The vagina receives the penis during sex. It serves as the birth canal for delivery of a baby. When a woman is not pregnant, the endometrium is discharged from the body through the vagina each month. This is called *menstruation.*

Changes With Aging

In men, testosterone decreases slightly with age. Erections take longer, are less forceful, and are lost quickly.

In women, estrogen and progesterone decrease with age. *Menopause* occurs. This is when menstruation stops. The woman can no longer become pregnant. Female structures atrophy. There is thinning of vaginal walls and vaginal dryness. See Chapter 12 for more information.

Vaginitis

Vaginitis is inflammation or infection of the vagina. The most common types and causes are:
- Bacterial vaginosis. This occurs from an imbalance in the normal bacterial flora in the vagina.
- *Candida* infection. *Candida* is a yeast (a type of fungus) often present in the vagina. Overgrowth can cause an infection *(vaginal candidiasis).*
- Trichomoniasis. This is sexually transmitted. It is caused by a parasite. (A *parasite* is an organism that lives in or on a host to get nourishment from the host.) See "Sexually Transmitted Diseases."
- Irritation from products. Some women are sensitive or allergic to soaps, detergents, or other products. There is no infection, but inflammation occurs.

Vaginal burning, itching, pain, discharge, and a bad odor are signs and symptoms. Treatment depends on the cause. Report discomfort, discharge, or odor to the nurse. Even women who are not sexually active can have vaginitis.

Sexually Transmitted Diseases

Sexually transmitted diseases (STDs) are passed from person to person through sexual contact. They are also known as sexually transmitted infections (STIs). Common infection sites are the genitals, rectum, mouth, and throat.

STDs/STIs can be caused by bacteria, parasites, or viruses. The most common STDs/STIs are described in Box 52-3. Signs and symptoms vary depending on the cause. A person may not have signs and symptoms and still spread infection. Vaginal, anal, and oral sex can transmit STDs/STIs. Needle sharing (injection drug use) can spread HIV and other bloodborne infections.

Correct use of latex condoms reduces the risk of becoming infected or spreading STDs/STIs. Not having vaginal, anal, or oral sex is the best way to avoid infection.

In health care settings, Standard Precautions and the Bloodborne Pathogen Standard are followed.

STDs/STIs caused by bacteria or parasites can be cured. Those caused by a virus cannot be cured. However, treatment can reduce symptoms and the risk of transmission to others.

See *Focus on Children and Older Persons: Sexually Transmitted Diseases*, p. 790.

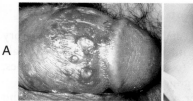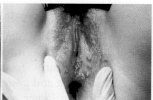

FIGURE 52-11 Herpes. **A,** Sores on the penis. **B,** Sores on the female perineum. (Courtesy United States Public Health Service, Washington, DC.)

BOX 52-3	Sexually Transmitted Diseases/Sexually Transmitted Infections

- **Chlamydia**—a bacterial infection, both men and women can become infected. Babies can become infected during childbirth.
  - Men—may have discharge from the penis and burning with urination. Testicular pain and swelling are less common, but they can occur.
  - Women—may have abnormal vaginal discharge with a strong odor and burning with urination. Abdominal pain, painful sex, nausea, and fever can occur if the infection spreads.
  - Both men and women—infection of the rectum can cause rectal pain, discharge, and bleeding.
- **Genital herpes**—caused by the herpes simplex virus. Sores can appear on the genital or rectal area, buttocks, and thighs (Fig. 52-11). The virus can spread when sores are not present. Babies can become infected during childbirth.
  - "Outbreaks" occur causing signs and symptoms. Sores (blisters) usually occur where the virus entered the body. The blisters become painful and break before healing.
  - The virus stays in the body for life. Repeated outbreaks are common. Treatment can lessen symptoms, decrease outbreaks, and lower the risk of transmission to others.
- **Gonorrhea**—a bacterial infection that can infect the genital area, mouth, or anus. Babies can become infected during childbirth. There may be no symptoms or:
  - Men—pain with urination and discharge from the penis. If untreated, prostate or testicle problems can develop.
  - Women—early symptoms may be mild. Bleeding between menstrual periods, pain with urination, and vaginal discharge are later signs. If untreated, pregnancy and fertility problems can develop.

- **HIV/AIDS**—caused by the human immunodeficiency virus (HIV), the immune system is harmed. The person is at risk for infections and certain cancers. AIDS (acquired immunodeficiency syndrome) is the final stage of HIV infection. See Chapter 48 for the stages and signs and symptoms of HIV infection and AIDS. HIV transmission occurs most by unprotected sex with an infected person and by needle-sharing with injection drug users. See Chapter 48 for less common methods of transmission including contact with an infected person's blood and from mother to baby during pregnancy, birth, or breast-feeding.
- **Human papilloma viruses (HPV)**—a group of viruses that cause warts on the genitals. Some types cause cancer if the infection persists and causes cell changes. Vaccines can protect against diseases caused by some types of HPV.
- **Syphilis**—a bacterial infection that infects the genital areas, lips, mouth, or anus in men and women. Babies can become infected during pregnancy.
  - A single, small, painless sore usually develops at first. If untreated, a rash that does not itch may occur on the hands and feet. Symptoms may come and go for many years.
  - During the late stages, syphilis can cause serious health problems and even death.
- **Trichomoniasis**—caused by a parasite.
  - Men—usually do not have symptoms. However, they can have itching or irritation inside the penis, burning with urination or after ejaculation, and discharge from the penis.
  - Women—develop vaginitis. Signs and symptoms include a yellow-green or gray vaginal discharge; discomfort during sex; vaginal odor; dysuria; and genital itching, burning, and soreness

Modified from MedlinePlus: Sexually transmitted diseases, Bethesda, Md, February 17, 2023, U.S. National Library of Medicine including content from Centers for Disease Control and Prevention: Chlamydia—CDC basic fact sheet, *April 12, 2022;* Genital herpes—CDC basic fact sheet, *January 3, 2022;* Gonorrhea—CDC basic fact sheet, *August 22, 2022;* Syphilis—CDC basic fact sheet, *February 10, 2022;* Trichomoniasis—CDC basic fact sheet, *April 25, 2022; and U.S. Food & Drug Administration (from the FDA Office of Women's Health):* HPV (human papillomavirus), *November 1, 2023.*

Pelvic Inflammatory Disease

In females, STDs/STIs can lead to pelvic inflammatory disease (PID). PID is infection of the upper female reproductive structures (cervix, uterus, fallopian tubes, ovaries). Chlamydia and gonorrhea are common causes.

Abdominal pain, fever, vaginal discharge, pain during sex, and dysuria are some signs and symptoms. PID is treated with antibiotics. Without treatment, PID can cause infertility and other serious complications.

PELVIC ORGAN PROLAPSE

Normally, muscles and tissues support the organs in the pelvic area. In females, these include the uterus, bladder, and rectum. As muscles and tissues become weak or damaged, 1 or more organs can drop (prolapse) into or out of the vagina.

- A *cystocele* occurs when the bladder bulges into the vaginal wall. This is the most common type.
- A *rectocele* occurs when the rectum bulges into the vaginal wall.
- *Uterine prolapse* occurs when the uterus drops into the vagina.

Childbirth, aging, hormonal changes of menopause, family history, and long-term pressure on the abdomen (obesity, chronic cough, straining during bowel movements) increase the risk of pelvic organ prolapse. Pelvic pain and pressure occur. The person may feel or see a bulge within or coming out of the vaginal opening. Discomfort during sex, urinary incontinence, and problems having bowel movements can occur.

Surgery performed through the vagina or abdomen may be done if the prolapse impairs quality of life. Non-surgical treatments include pelvic floor muscle exercises (Chapter 27) or use of a pessary. A *pessary* is a removable device that is used to support prolapsed organs. The device is inserted into the vagina. There are different shapes and sizes. It should not cause discomfort. The person may remove the device weekly for cleaning. Report problems to the nurse.

REVIEW QUESTIONS

Circle the BEST answer.

1   A person has cystitis. This is a
   a   Kidney infection
   b   Kidney stone
   c   Sexually transmitted disease (infection)
   d   Bladder infection

2   BPH causes urinary problems because
   a   An enlarged prostate presses against the urethra
   b   Stones in the kidneys block urine flow
   c   Kidney damage reduces urine output
   d   Cancer cells damage the bladder

3   After a TURP, which measure should you question?
   a   No sudden movements
   b   No oral fluids
   c   No heavy lifting
   d   No straining to have a bowel movement

4   A person with a urostomy
   a   Has a new pathway for urine to exit the body
   b   Needs dialysis
   c   Had surgery for an enlarged prostate
   d   Has pyuria

5   A person has kidney stones. Which do you expect to do?
   a   Assist with transport to dialysis.
   b   Restrict fluids.
   c   Strain all urine.
   d   Explain that nothing can be done for the pain.

6   With chronic kidney disease
   a   Excess waste products are removed from the blood
   b   The body retains fluid and waste products
   c   Urinary diversion is needed
   d   Kidney function returns after dialysis

7   Chronic kidney disease care includes
   a   A diet high in sodium and potassium
   b   Encouraging fluids
   c   Measuring weight daily
   d   Straining the urine

8   An older female resident reports burning and itching in the vaginal area. You should
   a   Only report the concern if a discharge is present
   b   Explain that there is no concern if she is not sexually active
   c   Refuse to perform perineal care
   d   Report the symptoms to the nurse

9   A person makes the following statements about STDs/STIs. Which shows the person needs more teaching from the nurse?
   a   "Using condoms correctly reduces my risk of infection."
   b   "I can get an infection from oral sex."
   c   "Infections are only spread when there are symptoms."
   d   "Some infections can be cured. Others cannot."

10   A woman with a cystocele uses a pessary. You know that the device
   a   Is used to support the prolapsed bladder
   b   Is surgically placed and permanent
   c   Needs removed before a bowel movement
   d   Needs cleaned during perineal care

Answers to Chapter 52 questions are on p. 904.

FOCUS ON PRACTICE

Problem Solving

A patient has a urinary catheter. Does this affect UTI risk? Describe the care measures for perineal care and catheter care that help lower the risk of UTI. Use what you have learned from this and other chapters.

OBJECTIVES

- Define the key terms and key abbreviations in this chapter.
- Explain mental health and the effects of mental health disorders.
- Identify the risk factors and warning signs of mental health disorders.
- Describe anxiety disorders and the defense mechanisms used to relieve anxiety.
- Describe psychotic disorders and schizophrenia.
- Describe mood disorders.

- Describe personality disorders.
- Describe substance use disorder and addiction.
- Describe 3 eating disorders.
- Describe suicide and the persons at risk.
- Describe the care required by persons with mental health disorders.
- Explain how to promote PRIDE in the person, the family, and yourself.

KEY TERMS

addiction A chronic disease involving substance-seeking behaviors and use that is compulsive and hard to control despite the harmful effects

anxiety A feeling of worry, nervousness, or fear about an event or situation

compulsion An over-whelming urge to repeat certain rituals, acts, or behaviors

coping Strategies to manage stress and reduce negative emotions caused by stress

defense mechanism An unconscious reaction that blocks unpleasant or threatening feelings

delusion A false belief

delusion of grandeur An exaggerated belief about one's importance, fame, wealth, power, or talents

delusion of persecution A false belief that one is being mistreated, abused, or harassed

detoxification The process of removing a toxic substance from the body

drug addiction A strong urge or craving to use a substance; the person cannot stop using it; tolerance develops

flashback Reliving a trauma over and over in thoughts during the day and in nightmares during sleep

hallucination Seeing, hearing, smelling, feeling, or tasting something that is not real

mental health Involves a person's emotional, psychological, and social well-being

mental health disorder A serious illness that can affect a person's thinking, mood, behavior, function, and ability to relate to others; psychiatric disorder

obsession A frequent, upsetting, and unwanted thought, idea, or image

panic An intense and sudden feeling of fear, anxiety, or dread

personality The set of attitudes, values, behaviors, and traits of a person

phobia An intense fear of something that has little or no real danger

psychiatric disorder See "mental health disorder"

psychosis A condition that affects the mind and causes a loss of contact with reality

stress The response or change in the body caused by any emotional, psychological, physical, social, or economic factor

stressor The event or factor that causes stress

suicidal ideation Thinking about, considering, or planning suicide

suicide To end one's life on purpose

suicide contagion Exposure to suicide or suicidal behaviors within one's family, one's peer group, or through media reports of suicide

tolerance Needing more of a drug for the same effect

withdrawal syndrome The physical and mental response after stopping or severely reducing the use of a substance that was used regularly

KEY ABBREVIATIONS

AUD	Alcohol use disorder		GAD	Generalized anxiety disorder
BPD	Borderline personality disorder		OCD	Obsessive-compulsive disorder
CBT	Cognitive behavioral therapy		PTSD	Post-traumatic stress disorder
CDC	Centers for Disease Control and Prevention		SUD	Substance use disorder

Mental health involves a person's emotional, psychological, and social well-being. Important from childhood through old age, mental health affects how a person:

- Thinks.
- Feels.
- Relates to others.
- Makes choices.
- Acts when coping with life.
- Handles stress. *Stress* is the response or change in the body caused by any emotional, psychological, physical, social, or economic factor.

Mental health disorders (psychiatric disorders) are serious illnesses that can affect a person's thinking, mood, behavior, function, and ability to relate to others. Risk factors and early warning signs are listed in Box 53-1. Mental health disorders are common. They may be occasional or long-term. Many persons recover completely.

ANXIETY DISORDERS

Anxiety is a feeling of worry, nervousness, or fear about an event or situation. Some anxiety is normal. It is a normal reaction to stress. Anxiety disorders happen when anxiety cannot be controlled and interferes with every-day activities, work, school, and relationships. The anxiety does not go away and can get worse over time. See Box 53-2 for signs and symptoms.

Anxiety level depends on the stressor. A *stressor* is the event or factor that causes stress. It can be physical, emotional, social, or economic. Past experiences and the number of stressors affect how a person reacts.

Coping and defense mechanisms may help relieve anxiety.

- *Coping* involves strategies to manage stress and reduce negative emotions caused by stress. Unhealthy coping includes over-eating, drinking alcohol, smoking, and fighting. Healthy coping includes discussing the problem, exercising, listening to music, and having time alone or being with others who are helpful.
- *Defense mechanisms* are unconscious reactions that block unpleasant or threatening feelings (Box 53-3, p. 794). (In this context, *unconscious* involves being outside of the person's awareness.) Some use of defense mechanisms is normal. In mental health disorders, they are used poorly.

Anxiety disorders often occur with other mental health disorders. Depression (p. 796), eating disorders (p. 799), and substance use disorder (p. 797) are examples. Anxiety may be linked to health problems. Heart disease, diabetes, thyroid problems, and respiratory disorders are examples.

BOX 53-1 Mental Health Disorders

Risk Factors

- Genetics and family history. Mental health disorders tend to run in families.
- Life experiences. Stress or history of abuse are examples.
- Chemical imbalances in the brain.
- Traumatic brain injury.
- Fetal exposure to viruses or toxic chemicals.
- Use of alcohol or recreational drugs.
- Serious health problems.
- Having few friends and feeling lonely or isolated.

Early Warning Signs

- Eating or sleeping too much or too little
- Pulling away from people or usual activities
- Having low or no energy
- Feeling numb or like nothing matters
- Having unexplained aches and pains
- Feeling helpless or hopeless
- Smoking, drinking, or using drugs more than usual
- Feeling unusually confused, forgetful, on edge, angry, upset, worried, or scared
- Yelling or fighting with family and friends
- Having severe mood swings that cause relationship problems
- Having persistent thoughts and memories
- Hearing voices or believing things that are not true
- Thinking of harming oneself or others
- Being unable to perform daily tasks

Modified from Substance Abuse and Mental Health Services Administration: What is mental health, Washington, D.C., updated April 24, 2023, U.S. Department of Health & Human Services and MedlinePlus: Mental disorders, Washington, D.C., page updated March 16, 2023, U.S. Department of Health & Human Services.

BOX 53-2 Anxiety: Signs and Symptoms

- Weakness
- Breathing problems: shortness of breath, smothering or choking sensations
- Rapid heart rate; pounding heartbeat
- Nausea
- Abdominal pain
- Hot flashes (women)
- Dizziness
- Chest pain
- Nightmares
- Restlessness
- Fatigue
- Difficulty concentrating
- Irritability
- Muscle tension
- Sleep problems
- Sweating
- Trembling or shaking
- Tingling or numb hands

BOX 53-3	Defense Mechanisms

Compensation. *Compensate* means to make up for, replace, or substitute. A weakness is replaced with a strength.
  EXAMPLE: Not good in sports, a child develops another talent.
Conversion. *Convert* means to change. An emotion is changed into a physical symptom.
  EXAMPLE: Not wanting to read out loud in school, a child complains of a headache.
Denial. *Deny* means refusing to accept or believe something that is true. The person refuses to accept unpleasant or threatening things.
  EXAMPLE: A person ignores pain and refuses to see a doctor.
Displacement. *Displace* means to move or take the place of. Behaviors or emotions are moved from one person, place, or thing to a safe person, place, or thing.
  EXAMPLE: Angry at your boss, you yell at a friend.
Identification. *Identify* means to relate to or associate with. A person assumes the ideas, behaviors, or traits of another person.
  EXAMPLE: Fearing rejection, a person acts differently around peers.
Projection. *Project* means to blame another. Unacceptable behaviors, thoughts, or emotions are attributed to someone else.
  EXAMPLE: Not understanding a lesson, a student thinks: "The teacher does not understand it enough to teach it well."

Rationalization. *Rational* means sensible, reasonable, or logical. An acceptable reason—not the real reason—is given for behaviors or actions.
  EXAMPLE: A student did not study and failed a test. The student thinks: "I failed because I wasn't feeling well."
Reaction formation. A person acts in a way opposite to how the person truly feels.
  EXAMPLE: A worker does not like the boss. The worker gives the boss a gift.
Regression. *Regress* means to move back or to retreat. The person retreats or moves back to an earlier time or condition.
  EXAMPLE: A 3-year-old wants a baby bottle when a new baby arrives.
Repression. *Repress* means to hold down or keep back. Unpleasant or painful thoughts or experiences are kept from the conscious mind. They cannot be recalled or remembered.
  EXAMPLE: A child was sexually abused. Now 33 years old, there is no memory of the event.

Generalized Anxiety Disorder

The person with generalized anxiety disorder (GAD) has extreme anxiety, fear, or worry. GAD occurs on most days for at least 6 months. The person has worry and concern about many things. Health, work, social situations, and every-day life are examples. Serious problems in such areas can result.

Panic Disorder

Panic is an intense and sudden feeling of fear, anxiety, or dread. The person with panic disorder has sudden, recurring periods of panic when there is no real danger. *Panic attacks* can be unexpected or brought on by a trigger—fear of an object or situation. The person cannot function. Signs and symptoms of anxiety are severe (see Box 53-2).

Panic attacks can occur at any time and can last several minutes or longer. The person may try to avoid places where panic attacks have occurred.

Call for the nurse if the person has severe signs and symptoms of anxiety. During a panic attack, these actions can help.
- Help the person to a quiet area.
- Stay with the person and remain calm.
- Speak in short, simple sentences. Give reminders of the person's safety.
- Talk the person through deep-breathing exercises (Chapter 44) or other relaxation methods (Chapter 36). Follow the person's care plan.
See *Focus on Communication: Panic Disorder.*

FOCUS ON COMMUNICATION

Panic Disorder

A calm and focused approach can help reduce stress in a stressful situation. Pay attention to your voice tone, posture, and facial expressions. Help the person focus and relax. This is an example.

You are safe. I am with you. The nurse is coming. Let's focus on taking slow breaths. Breathe in through your nose. (Wait and allow the person to follow the instruction. Do the action with the person. Make eye contact. Give positive feedback.) *Good job. Now breathe out through your mouth.*

Phobias

A *phobia* is an intense fear of something that has little or no real danger. Common phobias are fear of:
- Being in an open, crowded, or public place (*agoraphobia—agora* means marketplace)
- Water (*aquaphobia—aqua* means water)
- Being in or trapped in an enclosed or narrow space (*claustrophobia—claustro* means closing)
- The slightest uncleanliness (*mysophobia—myso* means anything that is disgusting)
- Night or darkness (*nyctophobia—nycto* means night or darkness)
- Strangers (*xenophobia—xeno* means strange)

The person avoids what is feared. When faced with the fear, the person has high anxiety and cannot function.

Obsessive-Compulsive Disorder

Obsessive-compulsive disorder (OCD) occurs when a person has recurring thoughts, behaviors, or both that cannot be controlled.

- An *obsession* is a frequent, upsetting, and unwanted thought, idea, or image. Microbes, dirt, fear of losing things, violent thoughts, or sexual acts are common obsessive thoughts.
- A *compulsion* is the over-whelming urge to repeat certain rituals, acts, or behaviors. The compulsion is done in response to obsessive thoughts and the resulting anxiety. Hand-washing, counting, checking on things, cleaning, hoarding, and doing things in a certain order are examples.

OCD behaviors can take a long time, are very distressing, and affect daily life.

Post-Traumatic Stress Disorder

Post-traumatic stress disorder (PTSD) occurs in some people after a terrifying, traumatic, scary, or dangerous event. There was harm or threat of harm. PTSD can develop at any age after:

- Being harmed or after a loved one was harmed
- Seeing a harmful event happen to a loved one or stranger
- The sudden, unexpected death of a loved one
- Traumatic events
  - War, terrorist attack, bombing
  - Abuse, mugging, rape, torture
  - Kidnapping, being held captive
  - Crashes—vehicle, train, plane
  - Natural disaster—flood, tornado, hurricane, earthquake

Signs and symptoms may begin within 3 months or years after the event (Box 53-4). Flashbacks are common. A *flashback* is reliving a trauma over and over in thoughts during the day and in nightmares during sleep. Every-day things can trigger them—words, objects, situations, thoughts, or reminders of the event. During a flashback, the trauma seems to be happening all over again. The person has symptoms of PTSD.

Some people recover within 6 months. For others, PTSD is a chronic condition. Depression, substance use disorder, and other anxiety disorders may occur with PTSD.

See *Focus on Children and Older Persons: Post-Traumatic Stress Disorder.*

FOCUS ON CHILDREN AND OLDER PERSONS

Post-Traumatic Stress Disorder

Children
Older children and teenagers may have symptoms similar to adults. They also may show disruptive, disrespectful, or destructive behaviors. There may be feelings of guilt for not preventing injury or death. They may have thoughts of revenge.

Children less than 6 years old will have different signs and symptoms than adults.
- Wetting the bed after being toilet-trained
- Not being able to talk
- Acting out the traumatic event during play
- Having frightening dreams
- Being unusually clingy with a parent or other adult

| BOX 53-4 | Post-Traumatic Stress Disorder: Signs and Symptoms |

- Flashbacks
- Nightmares or bad dreams
- Frightening thoughts
- Experiencing physical effects of stress (see Box 53-2)
- Avoiding places, events, or things that are reminders of the trauma
- Avoiding thoughts or feelings related to the trauma
- Being easily startled or frightened
- Feeling tense, on guard, or "on edge"
- Trouble concentrating
- Sleep problems
- Angry outbursts
- Risky, reckless, or destructive behavior
- Problems remembering key parts of the trauma
- Negative thoughts about oneself or the world
- Ongoing negative emotions—blame, fear, anger, guilt, shame
- Loss of interest in enjoyed activities
- Social isolation
- Difficulty feeling positive emotions—happiness, satisfaction

Modified from National Institute of Mental Health: Post-traumatic stress disorder, National Institutes of Health, last reviewed May 2023.

PSYCHOTIC DISORDERS

Psychosis describes a condition that affects the mind and causes a loss of contact with reality. Psychotic disorders cause abnormal thinking and perceptions. (To *perceive* means to become aware of something through the mind or the senses—sight, hearing, touch, smell, and taste.) In a psychotic state, the person has lost touch with what is real.

Two main symptoms of psychosis are:
- *Delusions*—false beliefs.
- *Hallucinations*—seeing, hearing, smelling, feeling, or tasting something that is not real. Hearing voices is a common hallucination. "Voices" may comment on the person's behavior or order the person to do things, warn of danger, or talk to other voices.

Schizophrenia is one disorder that causes psychosis. Other causes include sleep deprivation, alcohol and some drugs, brain tumors, brain infections, and stroke.

See *Focus on Communication: Psychotic Disorders.*

FOCUS ON COMMUNICATION

Psychotic Disorders

Delusions and hallucinations can frighten a person. Good communication is important.
- Speak slowly and calmly.
- Do not pretend to experience what the person does. Help the person focus on reality.
- Do not try to convince the person that the experience is not real. To the person, it is real.

For example, a person hears voices. You can say: "I don't hear the voices. But I believe you do. Try to listen to my voice and not the other voices."

Schizophrenia

Schizophrenia is a serious brain illness affecting how a person thinks, feels, and behaves. *Schizophrenia* means split *(schizo)* mind *(phrenia)*. Age of onset is usually between 16 and 30. Schizophrenia in children is rare. Gradual changes in mood, thinking, and social function begin before the first episode of psychosis. Signs and symptoms (Box 53-5) make it hard to perform daily tasks.

BOX 53-5	Schizophrenia: Signs and Symptoms

- Hallucinations
- Delusions
  - *Delusions of grandeur*—exaggerated beliefs about one's importance, fame, wealth, power, or talents
  - *Delusions of persecution*—false beliefs that one is being mistreated, abused, or harassed
- Abnormal thinking and speech
  - Trouble organizing or logically connecting thoughts
  - Stopping speech in the middle of a thought
  - Making up words that have no meaning
- Abnormal body movements
  - Repeating motions over and over
  - Sitting for long periods without moving, speaking, or responding
- Emotional and behavioral problems
  - No facial expression (flat affect), dull voice
  - Trouble being happy or showing emotions
  - Loss of motivation and interest in daily activities
  - Trouble planning and staying with an activity
  - Socially withdrawn
- Cognitive problems
  - Trouble paying attention, understanding, or remembering
  - Trouble making decisions

People with schizophrenia do not tend to be violent. However, if a person becomes violent, it is often directed at oneself. Some persons with schizophrenia attempt suicide (p. 800).

MOOD DISORDERS

Mood disorders are also called affective disorders. (*Affect* relates to feelings, emotions, and mood.) Feeling sad, irritable, or in a bad mood from time to time is normal. Mood disorders can cause feelings of constant sadness, loss of interest in life, and extremes in feeling happy and sad. Bipolar disorder and depression are 2 types.

Bipolar Disorder

Bipolar means 2 *(bi)* poles or ends *(polar)*. The person with bipolar disorder has severe extremes in mood, energy, and function. There are emotional highs or "ups" *(mania)* and emotional lows or "downs" *(depression)*. Therefore the disorder is sometimes called manic-depressive disorder.

The disorder runs in families. It usually develops during the late teens or early adulthood. Signs and symptoms range from mild to severe (Table 53-1). Mood changes are called "episodes."

If not treated, bipolar disorder can cause problems with relationships, school, or work. Some persons are suicidal. Life-long management is needed.

Depression

Depression (major depressive disorder, clinical depression) is a mood disorder that affects feeling, thinking, and daily activities. See "Depressive Episode" in Table 53-1 for signs and symptoms. The person has prolonged feelings of sadness, loss, anger, or frustration that affect daily life. Work, study, sleep, eating, and other activities are affected.

TABLE 53-1	Bipolar Disorder: Signs and Symptoms	
Manic Episode		**Depressive Episode**
• Feeling very up, high, happy, or very irritable or touchy		• Feeling very down, sad, or anxious
• Feeling jumpy, wired, or more active than usual		• Feeling slowed down or restless
• Decreased need for sleep		• Trouble falling asleep, waking up too early, or sleeping too much
• Talking fast about many different things ("flight of ideas")		• Talking very slowly, feeling that one has nothing to say, or forgetting a lot
• Racing thoughts		• Problems concentrating or making decisions
• Thinking one can do many things at once without getting tired		• Feeling unable to do simple things
• Excessive appetite for food, drinking, sex, or other pleasurable activities		• Lack of interest in almost all activities
• Feeling unusually important, talented, or powerful		• Feeling hopeless or worthless or thinking about death or suicide

Modified from National Institute of Mental Health: Bipolar disorder, U.S. Department of Health and Human Services, last reviewed February 2024.

Depression is thought to be caused by a combination of factors. Persons with a family history are at higher risk. Major life changes, trauma, and stress are other risk factors. Depression can occur with other illnesses. Diabetes, cancer, heart disease, stroke, and Parkinson's disease are examples. Depression can make an illness worse. Or an illness can make depression worse. Some drugs have the side effect of depression.

Depression in Older Persons.
Depression occurs in older persons. However, it is not a normal part of aging. Older persons have many losses—death of family and friends, loss of body functions, loss of independence. See Box 53-6 for the signs and symptoms of depression in older persons.

Depression in older persons is often overlooked or a wrong diagnosis is made. Instead of depression, the person is thought to have a cognitive disorder (Chapter 54). Therefore the depression goes untreated.

BOX 53-6	Depression in Older Persons: Warning Signs

- Changes in mood, energy level, or appetite
- Feeling "flat" or trouble feeling good emotions
- Problems sleeping or sleeping too much
- Problems concentrating
- Feeling restless, worried, or "on edge"
- Angry, irritable, or aggressive behaviors
- On-going headaches, gastro-intestinal problems, or pain
- Need for alcohol or drugs
- Feeling sad or hopeless
- Suicidal thoughts
- High-risk activities
- Obsessive thinking or compulsive behavior
- Thoughts or behaviors that interfere with work, family, or social activities
- Unusual thinking or behaviors that are concerning to others

Modified from National Institute of Mental Health: Older adults and mental health, last reviewed May 2023.

PERSONALITY DISORDERS

Personality is the set of attitudes, values, behaviors, and traits of a person. Personality development starts at birth. Genes, growth and development (Chapter 11), environment, parenting, and social experiences influence personality. Normally, people can form relationships and cope with normal stresses.

Personality disorders involve long-term patterns of thoughts and behaviors that can:
- Interfere with daily life.
- Cause problems at school or work.
- Cause problems in relationships.

There are many types of personality disorders. Two examples are described in this chapter.

Antisocial Personality Disorder
A person has a long-term pattern of manipulating, exploiting, or violating the rights and safety of others. Behavior is often criminal. Setting fires and animal cruelty during childhood are often seen. The person may
- Act witty and charming
- Flatter and manipulate others for personal gain or pleasure
- Break the law repeatedly—lying, stealing, fighting
- Have no regard for the safety of self and others
- Have problems with substance use
- Show no guilt or remorse (regret, sorrow)
- Be angry or arrogant often

Borderline Personality Disorder
In borderline personality disorder (BPD), the person has a long-term pattern of unstable moods, behaviors, and emotions. Relationship problems and impulsive actions often result. (To be *impulsive* means to be reckless or act in haste without considering the consequences.) Genes and family and social factors may be causes. Childhood abandonment, abuse, and family problems are risk factors.

Signs and symptoms of BPD include:
- Changing interests and values rapidly
- Viewing things in terms of extremes—all good or all bad
- Shifting and changing feelings about other people—liking a person one day but not the next
- Having an intense fear of being abandoned
- Being unable to stand being alone
- Feeling empty and bored
- Inappropriate anger
- Impulsive substance use or sexual relationships
- Self-injury such as wrist cutting or overdosing (p. 799)
- Suicide attempts or suicide (p. 800)

SUBSTANCE USE DISORDER
Substance use disorder (SUD) is when the use of alcohol or another substance (a drug) leads to health issues or problems at work, school, or home. *Addiction* (p. 799) is often used to describe the most severe form of SUD.

The exact cause is unknown. Influencing factors include genetics, how the substance affects the person, changes in the brain, peer pressure, anxiety, depression, and stress. The person with SUD may have other mental health problems.

Legal substances (such as alcohol) and illegal substances (such as heroin) are used. Legal drugs are approved for use in the United States. Illegal drugs are not approved for use. Legal drugs may be bought or obtained illegally. Commonly used substances include:

- *Opioids (narcotics).* Opioids are pain-relief drugs (Chapter 36).
- *Stimulants.* These drugs stimulate the brain and nervous system.
- *Depressants.* Such drugs depress the nervous system, causing drowsiness and reduced anxiety. Alcohol is a depressant.

- *Hallucinogens.* These drugs cause sensations and images (hallucinations) that are not real. LSD is an example.
- *Marijuana (cannabis).* This drug affects the brain, causing a "high." Mood changes are common. Legal in some states, medical use includes treating rare forms of seizures, nausea from cancer therapy, and loss of appetite from HIV/AIDS.

Signs and symptoms of SUD are listed in Box 53-7. See *Focus on Children and Older Persons: Substance Use Disorder.*

BOX 53-7	Substance Use Disorder: Signs and Symptoms

Behavior Changes
- Missing school or work; decreased school or work performance
- Getting into trouble—fights, violence, accidents, car crashes, illegal activities
- Using a substance in hazardous situations—driving, using a machine
- Secretive or suspicious behaviors; hiding substance use
- Appetite: changes in
- Sleep pattern: changes in
- Personality and attitude: changes in
- Mood swings
- Irritability
- Angry outbursts
- Hyperactivity
- Agitation
- Giddiness
- Motivation: lacking
- Fearful, anxious, or paranoid behaviors for no reason

Physical Changes
- Eyes: bloodshot, abnormal pupil size
- Weight: loss or gain
- Appearance: decline in
- Smells: body, breath, clothing
- Tremors
- Speech: slurred
- Coordination: impaired

Social Changes
- Sudden change in friends, hangouts, or hobbies
- Legal problems related to substance use
- Unexplained need for money
- Financial problems
- Continued substance use despite harmful effects on health, work, or family

Modified from Substance Abuse and Mental Health Services Administration: Mental health and substance use co-occurring disorders, *updated April 24, 2023.*

FOCUS ON CHILDREN AND OLDER PERSONS

Substance Use Disorder

Children
According to the Centers for Disease Control and Prevention (CDC), alcohol is the most commonly used and abused substance among teenagers. As a consequence, under-age drinking is more likely to result in:
- School problems—absences, failing grades
- Social problems—fighting, not taking part in activities
- Legal problems—driving arrests, hurting someone while drunk
- Physical problems—hang-overs, illness
- Unwanted, unplanned, unprotected sexual activity
- Disrupted growth and sexual development
- Physical and sexual violence
- Risk for suicide and homicide
- Alcohol-related car crashes
- Alcohol-related injuries—burns, falls, drowning
- Memory problems
- Mis-use of other substances
- Changes in brain development with life-long effects
- Death from alcohol poisoning

Older Persons
Aging can lead to physical and social changes that may increase the risk of substance use. Some older adults use substances to cope with life changes such as retirement, grief and loss, health

problems, or a change in living situation. Sometimes the effects of substance use are mistaken for other health problems. When this happens, SUD can be overlooked.

Older adults often have more prescription drugs than other age-groups. This can lead to accidental mis-use of drugs. A person may forget to take a drug, take a drug too often, or take the wrong amount.

Alcohol is the most used substance among older adults. Drinking too much alcohol over a long time can:
- Cause health problems. Certain types of cancer, liver damage, immune system disorders, and brain damage are examples.
- Worsen some health problems. Osteoporosis, diabetes, high blood pressure, stroke, memory loss, and mood disorders are examples.
- Make it hard to diagnose and treat some health problems. For example, body changes from alcohol use can dull the pain that signals a heart attack.
- Cause confusion and forgetfulness. These may be mistaken as signs of Alzheimer's disease (Chapter 54).

Changes from aging can affect how the body handles alcohol. Alcohol use increases the risk for falls, fractures, vehicle crashes, and other injuries. Mixing alcohol with some prescribed drugs is harmful.

Addiction

Addiction is a chronic disease involving substance-seeking behaviors and use that is compulsive and hard to control despite the harmful effects. See Box 53-8 for signs of addiction.

In *drug addiction,* there is a strong urge or craving to use the substance. The person cannot stop using the drug. Tolerance develops. *Tolerance* is needing more of a drug for the same effect.

In alcohol use disorder (AUD), there is impaired ability to stop or control alcohol use despite harmful effects. AUD is sometimes referred to as alcohol abuse, alcohol dependence, alcohol addiction, or alcoholism. The more signs present (see Box 53-8), the more severe the AUD.

Persons with addiction cannot stop taking the substance without treatment. Treatment for SUD is a long-term process. The person may *relapse*—use the substance again after stopping. Treatment may involve:

- Emergency treatment. An overdose is life-threatening. See "Complications." Treatment depends on the substance used.
- Detoxification (detox). A *toxin* is a harmful substance that can cause death or serious illness. *Detoxification* is the process of removing a toxic substance from the body.
- Drug therapy. A drug with a similar action on the body is slowly given to reduce withdrawal effects.
- Counseling. See "Care and Treatment" on p. 801.

Complications

Complications of SUD include:

- Sudden death. This can occur from one use of the substance.
- Stroke.
- Lung disease.
- Cancer. Cancers of the mouth and throat, esophagus, larynx, liver, and breast are linked to alcohol.
- Infection. HIV/AIDS and hepatitis B and C are risks from shared needles (Chapters 48 and 51).
- Job loss.
- Depression.
- Memory and concentration problems.
- Problems with police and legal issues.
- Relationship problems.
- Unsafe sexual practices. Unwanted pregnancy, sexually transmitted disease (infection), HIV/AIDS, or hepatitis can result.
- Suicide.

Overdose occurs when too much of a substance is taken. The dose (amount) is toxic and can be fatal. Signs of an overdose are listed in Box 53-9. Emergency care is needed (Chapter 58). Opioid mis-use and overdose are a growing concern in the United States. Emergency care for opioid overdose is discussed in Chapter 58.

BOX 53-8 Signs of Addiction

- The substance is taken in larger amounts. Or it is taken for longer than intended.
- The person tries to cut down or stop using the substance but is unable.
- The person craves or has a strong urge for the substance.
- Dangerous activities occur during or after substance use.
- Much time is spent using the substance or recovering from its effects. Or the person spends much time trying to obtain the substance. This interferes with family, work, school, or interests. Substance use continues despite problems.
- The person continues to use the substance even when it causes depression or anxiety or worsens other health problems.
- Substance use causes impaired memory *(blackouts).*
- The person has tolerance to the substance.
  - The substance has less and less effect on the person.
  - More of the substance is needed for the same effect.
- The person has withdrawal symptoms. *Withdraw* means to stop, remove, or take away. *Withdrawal syndrome* is the physical and mental response after stopping or severely reducing the use of a substance that was used regularly. The body may respond with restlessness, shakiness, insomnia, nausea, sweating, rapid pulse, feeling unwell, hallucinations, or seizures.

Modified from National Institute on Alcohol Abuse and Alcoholism: Understanding alcohol use disorder, National Institutes of Health, updated January 2024.

BOX 53-9 Signs of Overdose

- "Pinpoint pupils"—small (constricted) eye pupils
- Losing consciousness or falling asleep
- Abnormal breathing—slow, weak, or no breathing
- Choking or gurgling sounds
- Limp body—without strength or movement
- Cold, clammy (moist) skin
- Discolored skin (especially in the lips and nails)

Modified from Centers for Disease Control and Prevention: Stop overdose: stigma reduction, last reviewed July 25, 2023.

EATING DISORDERS

An eating disorder involves a severe disturbance in eating behavior with thoughts and emotions related to eating. Eating disorders often develop during the teen years or in young adulthood. However, they can develop during childhood or later in life. The person may have other mental health disorders.

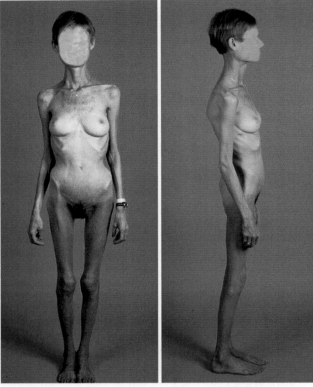

FIGURE 53-1 A person with anorexia nervosa. (Courtesy George D. Comerci, MD, Tucson.)

Eating disorders include:

- *Anorexia nervosa. Anorexia* means no *(a)* appetite *(orexis). Nervosa* relates to nerves or emotions. The person has an intense fear of gaining weight. A fat body image is felt despite being quite thin (Fig. 53-1). Eating very small amounts, exercising excessively, forcing vomiting, and using laxatives (drugs to promote bowel movements) are common. Serious health problems can result. Death is a risk from cardiac arrest or suicide.

- *Bulimia nervosa.* Binge-eating occurs—eating large amounts of food. Over-eating is followed by forced vomiting and intense exercise. Enema and laxative use rid the body of food. Diuretic mis-use may occur. (Diuretics cause the kidneys to produce large amounts of urine. Weight loss occurs with the fluid loss.)

- *Binge-eating disorder.* The person often eats large amounts of food. Eating is out of control. Binge-eating is not followed by purging, fasting, or exercise. Often the person is over-weight or obese. High blood pressure, heart disease, diabetes, and joint pain can occur.

SUICIDE

Suicide means to end one's life on purpose. Violence is directed at oneself. The action results in death. If the person survives, it is called a *suicide attempt*.

BOX 53-10	Suicide

Risk Factors
- Prior suicide attempt
- Depression or other mental health disorders
- Substance use disorder
- Chronic pain
- Family history of a mental health disorder, substance use disorder, or suicide
- Family violence (including physical or sexual abuse)
- Having guns or other firearms in the home
- Being in prison or jail recently
- Exposure to the suicidal behavior of others (family, peers, media figures)

Warning Signs
- Talking or thinking about death
- Talking about wanting to die or to kill oneself
- Talking about feeling empty, hopeless, or having no reason to live
- Talking about feeling trapped or having no solutions
- Talking about being a burden to others
- Talking about guilt or shame
- Posting suicidal messages on social media sites
- Planning or looking for a way to kill oneself—searching on-line, saving pills, obtaining lethal items (guns, ropes, knives)
- Feeling unbearable pain—physical, emotional
- Withdrawing from family and friends
- Saying good-bye to family and friends
- Giving away important belongings
- Putting legal affairs in order—will, advance directive
- Taking risks that could lead to death, such as reckless driving
- Having extreme mood swings—a sudden change from very sad to very calm or happy
- Using alcohol or drugs often
- Acting anxious or agitated
- Changing eating or sleeping habits
- Showing rage or talking about revenge

Modified from National Institute of Mental Health: Frequently asked questions about suicide, NIH publication No. 23-MH-6389, Bethesda, Md, National Institutes of Health, 2023.

Suicide is a leading cause of death in the United States. Risk factors and warning signs are listed in Box 53-10. *Suicidal ideation* refers to thinking about, considering, or planning suicide. *If a person mentions or talks about suicide, take the person seriously. Call for the nurse at once. Do not leave the person alone.*

Agencies treating persons with mental health disorders must identify persons at risk for suicide. They must:
- Identify specific factors or features that increase or decrease the risk for suicide.
- Meet the person's immediate safety needs.
- Provide the most appropriate setting to treat the person.
- Provide crisis information to the person and family. A crisis "hotline" phone number is an example.

See *Focus on Communication: Suicide.*
See *Focus on Children and Older Persons: Suicide.*

FOCUS ON COMMUNICATION

Suicide

A person thinking about suicide may say:
- "I just don't want to live anymore."
- "I wish I was dead."
- "I wish I had never been born."
- "Everyone would be better off without me."

A person may ask you not to tell anyone about the suicidal thoughts. Protecting personal information is important. But the person's safety is the priority. Never promise that you will not tell anyone. *Call for the nurse at once if a person talks about suicide.*

FOCUS ON **CHILDREN AND OLDER PERSONS**

Suicide

Children

The CDC reports that in 2021, suicide was the second leading cause of death among 10- to 14-year-olds. Besides the risk factors and warning signs listed in Box 53-10, others include:
- Having problems at school—lower grades, lacking interest in school, refusing to go to school, bullying
- Writings or drawings about death or suicide

Older Persons

Older adults are at risk for suicide. The CDC reports that persons age 85 and older have the highest rates of suicide. Many older persons suffer from depression (p. 797). Depression can severely affect an older person's heath. It can worsen conditions such as heart disease, diabetes, and stroke. Especially when untreated, depression can lead to suicide.

Depression in older persons is treatable. Noticing and reporting the warning signs (see Box 53-6) can prevent depression from being overlooked and untreated.

Suicide Contagion

Suicide contagion is exposure to suicide or suicidal behaviors within one's family, one's peer group, or through media reports of suicide. The exposure has led to suicides and suicidal behaviors in persons at risk. Adolescents and young adults are at risk for suicide contagion.

Following suicide exposure, those close to the victim need evaluation by a mental health professional. They include family, friends, peers, and co-workers. Persons at risk for suicide need mental health services.

CARE AND TREATMENT

Treatment of mental health disorders involves therapy, prescription drugs, or both. Counseling and psychotherapy (talk therapy) help a person identify and change troubling emotions, thoughts, and behaviors. There are different therapy types. Cognitive behavioral therapy (CBT) is a common method used. CBT teaches new ways to think, behave, and respond to situations.

The care plan reflects the needs of the total person. This includes physical, safety and security, and emotional needs.

Communication is important. Be alert to nonverbal communication—the person's and your own. The person may respond to stress with anxiety, panic, anger, or violence. Protect yourself. Once you are safe, the health team can protect the person and others. To protect yourself:
- Call for help. Do not try to resolve an unsafe situation on your own.
- Keep a safe distance between you and the person.
- Be aware of your setting. Do not let the person block your exit.

See *Focus on Communication: Care and Treatment.*
See *Promoting Safety and Comfort: Care and Treatment*, p. 802.

FOCUS ON **COMMUNICATION**

Care and Treatment

Nonverbal communication involves eye contact, tone of voice, facial expressions, body movements, and posture. Persons with depression often have little eye contact, poor posture, and speak softly. Some do not say much at all. Facial expressions may not change. Some persons cry.

Persons with anxiety may be restless, unable to sit still, and talk fast. Eye contact may be prolonged and intense. Others have poor eye contact. The eyes may dart about. Be alert to nonverbal cues. Report what you observe.

Your nonverbal communication is important. When interacting with persons with mental health disorders:
- Face the person.
- Maintain an appropriate level of eye contact.
- Position yourself near the person but not too close. Do not invade the person's space.
- Crouch, sit, or stand at the person's level if safe to do so.
- Show interest and concern through your posture and facial expressions.
- Speak calmly.

PROMOTING SAFETY AND COMFORT

Care and Treatment

Safety

Mental health disorders can be very distressing for the person. Chapter 7 discusses how behaviors communicate needs and how to manage difficult behavior. Chapter 14 describes measures to promote safety in situations that are or may become violent.

To *de-escalate* is to safely lower the intensity of a situation. Measures that help calm the person are performed. You must remember to stay calm. Your own behavior can raise or lower the intensity of the situation. Be aware of your verbal and non-verbal communication.

- *Position and body language.* Be at the same level as the person (sitting or standing). Face the person. Maintain a safe distance between you and the person. Maintain a relaxed stance. Keep the hands at the front of the body in a relaxed manner—not raised defensively (unless required for protection), on the hips, or with arms crossed. Do not shake a finger or point. Refrain from the use of touch—it will likely be considered a threat.

- *Facial expressions.* Maintain an attentive, caring expression. Use some eye contact, but do not glare or stare intensely.
- *Speech.* Use a moderate, calm volume. Resist being defensive and arguing. Listen and respond in a way that communicates that you want to help.

Follow the care plan for specific measures to de-escalate. Meeting needs, re-direction (distraction), and relaxation techniques are helpful. The nursing team needs to understand and manage the person's triggers. (*Triggers* are things that provoke the reaction. The setting, unmet needs, a conversation, a thought, or an emotion are some.)

Know your limits. Calmly get help if your efforts to de-escalate are not working.

FOCUS ON PRIDE

The Person, Family, and Yourself

Personal and Professional Responsibility

Just as a person does not choose to have a physical illness, a person does not choose a mental health disorder. How you view the disorder affects how you treat the person. Treat the person with kindness, respect, and compassion. Provide quality care.

Rights and Respect

Agencies have strict rules to protect the person's rights to privacy and confidentiality (Chapter 2). Do not talk about the person with your family or friends. Never give information to someone not involved in the person's care. This includes the person's family. Direct questions to the nurse. Follow agency policies. Take pride in protecting the person's rights.

Independence and Social Interaction

Social support is important in treating mental health disorders. Family and friends provide support and a sense of worth and belonging. *Support groups* connect people who share common problems. People can share experiences and coping strategies. Groups may be in-person or on-line.

Delegation and Teamwork

Some situations are urgent. If someone calls for help, respond at once. Assist as the nurse directs. Take pride in working as a team.

Ethics and Laws

Sometimes a person's speech or behaviors may seem strange or odd to you. You must show professional and ethical conduct. Never laugh at or insult a person. Do not joke with others about a person. Treat the person with dignity and respect.

FOCUS ON PRIDE: *Application*

Why are persons with mental health disorders at risk for violations of their rights? How must the health team protect the person's rights?

REVIEW QUESTIONS

Circle the BEST answer.

1 Stress is
   a A way to cope with or adjust to every-day living
   b A response or change in the body caused by some factor
   c A mental health disorder
   d An unwanted thought or idea

2 A young adult reports feeling hopeless and without energy. The person has lost interest in usual activities and has trouble doing daily tasks. These are
   a Normal for this stage of life
   b Personality qualities that will not change
   c Signs of a mental health disorder
   d Normal coping mechanisms

3 Which is a healthy coping strategy?
   a Exercising
   b Eating a lot
   c Drinking alcohol
   d Smoking cigarettes

4 These statements are about defense mechanisms. Which is *true?*
   a Using them signals a mental health disorder.
   b They can help relieve anxiety.
   c They prevent mental health disorders.
   d Persons with mental health disorders use them well.

5 A person with panic disorder becomes anxious in a noisy room. Which response is *best?*
 a Ignore the person's reaction.
 b Tell the person that there is no reason to feel anxious.
 c Give the person something to read as a distraction.
 d Help the person to a quiet area.

6 A phobia is
 a The event that causes stress
 b A false belief
 c An intense fear of something
 d A ritual

7 A person cleans and cleans in response to anxious thoughts. This behavior is
 a A delusion
 b A hallucination
 c A compulsion
 d Panic

8 Flashbacks with PTSD can cause the person to
 a Relive the trauma in thoughts and during sleep
 b Forget the past
 c Regress to an earlier time
 d Have emotional highs and lows

9 A person with schizophrenia has delusions and hallucinations. This means that the person has
 a False beliefs and perceptions
 b Enhanced sensations and awareness
 c Anger and aggression
 d Impulsive and inappropriate behavior

10 A person has psychosis causing delusions of persecution. The person says the food is poisoned. Which response is *best?*
 a "Your food is fine. Eat it."
 b "That is all you are getting to eat today."
 c "You seem worried. How can I help?"
 d "They fired the person who was poisoning the food."

11 Bipolar disorder means that the person
 a Is very suspicious
 b Has anxiety
 c Is very unhappy and feels unwanted
 d Has severe extremes in mood

12 Which is a sign of depression in older persons?
 a Hallucinations
 b Appetite changes
 c Memory loss
 d Slurred speech

13 In antisocial personality disorder, the person
 a Lacks regard for the rights and safety of others
 b Has a sad, anxious, or empty mood
 c Withdraws from people and interests
 d Is paranoid and avoids social situations

14 Which statement about substance use disorder is *true?*
 a Legal substances cannot cause addiction.
 b Substance use causes problems at work, home, or school.
 c Complications of substance use disorder are minor.
 d There is no treatment for substance use disorder.

15 Which statement shows *correct* understanding of addiction?
 a "People with addictions do not know the substance is harmful."
 b "Stopping addiction just requires self-control."
 c "Addiction is a chronic disease and is treatable."
 d "If relapse occurs, addiction is permanent."

16 A person has withdrawal syndrome. This means that
 a The person has a physical and mental response when the drug is not taken
 b The person needs higher doses of the drug
 c The effect is reduced with the same amount of drug
 d The person has a relapse after treatment

17 A person uses opioid drugs. Constricted pupils, slow breathing, clammy skin, and loss of consciousness
 a Are normal effects
 b Indicate tolerance and the person needs more of the drug
 c Indicate overdose and the person needs to sleep
 d Indicate overdose and the person needs emergency care

18 Binge-eating followed by forced vomiting occurs in
 a Anorexia nervosa
 b Binge-eating disorder
 c Bulimia nervosa
 d Borderline personality disorder

19 A 14-year-old talks about suicide. You know that suicide
 a Is uncommon in this age-group
 b Does not occur in this age-group
 c Is more common in young persons than in those age 85 and older
 d Is a leading cause of death in this age-group

20 A person talks about suicide. What should you do?
 a Call for the nurse.
 b Identify factors that increase the risk of suicide.
 c Ask what method the person plans to use.
 d Restrain the person.

21 A patient's family member asks what to say when the person talks about suicide. You should
 a Give advice
 b Direct the question to the nurse
 c Suggest a local support group
 d Call a crisis hotline

22 Which can help de-escalate a person showing agitated and aggressive behavior?
 a Use touch to show care and concern.
 b Loudly tell the person to calm down.
 c Threaten to restrain the person.
 d Listen calmly and respond in a way that shows you want to help.

Answers to Chapter 53 questions are on p. 904.

FOCUS ON PRACTICE

Problem Solving

A person with panic disorder becomes restless in a group setting. The person feels short of breath and hot and says: "My heart is pounding. I need to leave." What might be the cause? What will you do?

Confusion and Dementia

- Define the key terms and key abbreviations in this chapter.
- Describe confusion and its causes.
- List the measures that help confused persons.
- Explain the difference between delirium and dementia.
- Describe the signs, symptoms, and behavior and function changes that can occur with Alzheimer's disease (AD).

- Explain the care required by persons with AD and other dementias.
- Describe the effects of AD on the family.
- Explain validation therapy.
- Explain how to promote PRIDE in the person, the family, and yourself.

KEY TERMS

cognitive function Involves memory, thinking, reasoning, ability to understand, judgment, and behavior

confusion A state of being disoriented to person, time, place, situation, or identity

delirium A state of sudden, severe confusion and rapid changes in brain function

delusion A false belief

dementia The loss of cognitive function that interferes with daily life and activities

elopement When a patient or resident leaves the agency without staff knowledge

hallucination Seeing, hearing, smelling, feeling, or tasting something that is not real

paranoia A disorder *(para)* of the mind *(noia)*; false beliefs (delusions) and suspicion about a person or situation

sundowning Signs, symptoms, and behaviors of dementia increase during hours of darkness

KEY ABBREVIATIONS

AD	Alzheimer's disease	CMS	Centers for Medicare & Medicaid Services
ADL	Activities of daily living	NIA	National Institute on Aging

Changes in the brain and nervous system occur with certain diseases and with age. See Box 54-1. Cognitive function may be affected. (*Cognitive* relates to knowledge.) *Cognitive function* involves memory, thinking, reasoning, ability to understand, judgment, and behavior. Changes in function affect quality of life.

BOX 54-1	Nervous System Changes From Aging

- Nerve cells are lost.
- Nerve conduction slows.
- Reflexes, responses, and reaction times are slower.
- Vision, hearing, taste, smell, and touch decrease.
- Sensitivity to pain decreases.
- Blood flow to the brain is reduced.
- Sleep patterns change.
- Memory is shorter; forgetfulness occurs.
- Dizziness can occur.

CONFUSION

Confusion is a state of being disoriented to person, time, place, situation, or identity. *Disoriented* means to be apart from *(dis)* one's awareness *(oriented)*. Memory and the ability to make good judgments are lost. Daily activities may be affected. A person may not know people, the time, or the place. Behavior changes are common—anger, restlessness, depression, irritability.

Disease, brain injury, infections, fever, alcohol or drug use, and drug side effects are some causes of confusion. Hypoxia (Chapter 44), hypoglycemia (Chapter 51), sleep problems (Chapter 36), and seizures (Chapter 58) are other causes. Poor nutrition and fluid and electrolyte imbalances (Chapters 30 and 32) can cause confusion.

Depending on the cause, onset may be fast or slow. Report sudden onset of confusion at once. Confusion may be temporary or permanent. Treatment is aimed at the cause. Some measures help improve function (Box 54-2). You must meet the person's basic needs.

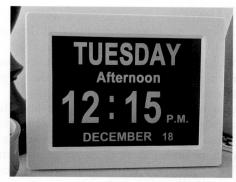

FIGURE 54-1 A large clock can help persons who are confused.

Delirium

Delirium is a state of sudden, severe confusion and rapid changes in brain function. Usually temporary and reversible, it can occur with physical or mental illness. Surgery, drug side effects, severe lack of sleep, electrolyte imbalances, and substance use disorder or withdrawal (Chapter 53) are some causes. Infections such as urinary tract infections (Chapter 52) and pneumonia (Chapter 50) can cause delirium.

Onset is usually fast—within hours or a few days. Signs and symptoms (Box 54-3) may come and go during the day and worsen at night. Depending on the cause, delirium lasts for hours or a week or more. It may take several weeks for normal mental function to return.

Delirium signals illness. It is an emergency. The cause must be found and treated.

See *Focus on Children and Older Persons: Delirium*.

BOX 54-2	**Confusion: Care Measures**

- Follow the care plan.
- Provide for safety.
- Face the person. Speak clearly.
- Call the person by name each time you have contact.
- State your name. Show your name tag.
- Give the date and time each morning. Repeat as needed during the day or evening.
- Explain what you are going to do and why.
- Give clear, simple directions and answers to questions.
- Break tasks into small steps.
- Ask clear and simple questions. Allow time to respond.
- Make sure the person can see a calendar and clock (Fig. 54-1). Remind the person of holidays, birthdays, and other events.
- Have the person wear needed eyeglasses and hearing aids.
- Use touch to communicate as appropriate for the person (Chapter 7).
- Place familiar objects and photos within view.
- Provide newspapers, magazines, TV, radio, phone, and any other personal electronic devices. Read to the person if appropriate.
- Discuss current events that are not upsetting.
- Maintain the day-night cycle.
  - Open window coverings during the day. Close them at night.
  - Use night-lights in rooms, bathrooms, hallways, and other areas at night.
  - Have the person wear day-time clothes during the day.
- Provide a calm, relaxed, and peaceful setting. Prevent loud noises, rushing, and crowded hallways and dining rooms.
- Follow the person's routine. Meals, bathing, exercise, TV, bedtime, and other activities have a schedule. This promotes a sense of order and what to expect.
- Do not re-arrange furniture or the person's belongings.
- Encourage the person to take part in self-care.

BOX 54-3	**Delirium: Signs and Symptoms**

- Alertness: changes in (usually more alert in the morning and less alert at night)
- Sensation and perception: changes in
- Awareness and level of consciousness: changes in
- Movement: very active or slow moving
- Drowsiness, changes in sleep patterns
- Confusion about time or place
- Thinking: disorganized
- Memory: decreased short-term memory and recall (cannot remember events since the delirium began)
- Concentration: problems with
- Speech: does not make sense
- Incontinence
- Emotional or personality changes: agitation, anger, depression, euphoria (extremely happy), irritability

Modified from MedlinePlus: Delirium, Bethesda, Md, reviewed November 9, 2021, U.S. National Library of Medicine, National Institutes of Health.

FOCUS ON **CHILDREN AND OLDER PERSONS**

Delirium

Older Persons
Older persons in a hospital or long-term care setting are at risk for delirium. Do not assume the nurse knows about a problem. Report the signs and symptoms in Box 54-3 or a change in the person's normal behavior at once.

DEMENTIA

Dementia is the loss of cognitive function that interferes with daily life and activities. (*De* means from. *Mentia* means mind.) Changes in personality, mood, behavior, and communication are common. Dementia is a group of symptoms, not a specific disease.

Dementia is caused by damage to brain cells. Some conditions cause thinking and memory problems that can be reversed when the cause is treated. Head injury and blood clots, tumors, or infections in the brain are some treatable causes. Thyroid problems, certain vitamin deficiencies, drug side effects, and substance use disorder are other examples.

Permanent dementias result from changes in the brain (Box 54-4). There is no cure. Function declines over time.

Dementia is not a normal part of aging. The risk increases with age. Persons over 65 and those with a family history of dementia are at higher risk.

Early warning signs include:
- Memory loss (losing things, forgetting names)
- Problems with common tasks (dressing, cooking, driving)
- Problems with language and communication; forgetting simple words
- Getting lost in familiar places
- Misplacing things and putting things in odd places (for example, putting a watch in the oven)
- Personality, mood, and behavior changes
- Poor or decreased judgment (for example, going out in the snow without shoes)

See *Focus on Children and Older Persons: Dementia.*

Mild Cognitive Impairment

Mild cognitive impairment (MCI) causes slight changes in memory or thinking. For example, the person loses things often, forgets important events or appointments, or forgets which words to use. Changes are greater than those with normal aging. The person can do normal activities and care for oneself. The person is at risk for dementia.

ALZHEIMER'S DISEASE

Alzheimer's disease (AD) is the most common type of permanent dementia. Many nerve cells (neurons) are damaged and die. Connections between nerve cells are lost. Over time, the brain shrinks from nerve cell death and tissue loss (Fig. 54-2). Two abnormal structures are thought to cause damage.
- *Plaques*—protein pieces (called *beta-amyloid*) build up in the spaces between nerve cells.
- *Tangles*—twisted protein fibers (called *tau*) build up inside nerve cells.

With aging, most people develop some plaques and tangles. In AD, plaque and tangle development is severe. The parts of the brain responsible for memory, language, and thinking are affected before other areas.

AD onset is gradual. Most persons with AD are age 65 and older. However, it can occur in younger persons.

AD is progressive. Symptoms gradually get worse over time. Currently, there is no cure. The goals of treatment are to slow the progression of symptoms and improve quality of life. Persons with AD can live for 4 to 8 years or longer.

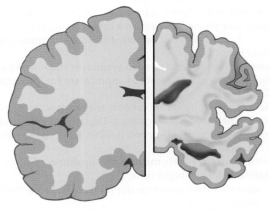

Healthy brain   Severe AD

FIGURE 54-2 Nerve cell death and tissue loss shrink the brain in the person with AD. (Redrawn from National Institute on Aging: *Alzheimer's disease fact sheet,* National Institutes of Health, U.S. Department of Health and Human Services, content reviewed April 5, 2023.)

Risk Factors

The greatest risk factor for AD is increasing age. The risk increases after age 65. About one-third (⅓) of people age 85 and older have AD. A family history of AD increases the person's risk. More persons with AD are women because women live longer than men.

BOX 54-4	Types of Permanent Dementia

- Alzheimer's disease—most common type. See "Alzheimer's Disease."
- Vascular dementia—stroke or other blood vessel problems damage vessels that supply blood to the brain.
- Lewy body dementia—abnormal protein deposits in the brain (Lewy bodies) affect chemicals in the brain. (Dementia that can occur with Parkinson's disease [Chapter 49] is a type of Lewy body dementia.)
- Fronto-temporal disorders—nerve cells in certain areas of the brain (front and sides) break down.
- Mixed dementia—2 or more types of dementia occur together.

FOCUS ON **CHILDREN AND OLDER PERSONS**

Dementia

Older Persons
Depression is a common mental health disorder in older persons. Confusion and attention problems from depression may be mistaken for dementia. Dementia, depression, aging, and some drug side effects have similar signs and symptoms. See "Depression in Older Persons" in Chapter 53.

The National Institute on Aging (NIA) recommends the following to maintain cognitive health.

- Get regular exercise.
- Eat a healthy diet.
- Spend time with family and friends.
- Keep the mind active.
- Control type 2 diabetes (Chapter 51).
- Maintain healthy blood pressure (Chapter 50) and cholesterol levels (Chapter 30).
- Maintain a healthy weight.
- Do not smoke.
- Get help for depression (Chapter 53).
- Avoid excess alcohol intake.
- Get enough sleep.

Signs of AD

Memory problems are usually one of the first signs of AD. According to the Alzheimer's Association, the most common early sign is difficulty remembering newly learned information. Over time, there is a slow decline in memory, thinking, and reasoning.

Box 54-5 lists early signs and symptoms of AD. AD is not a normal part of aging. See Box 54-6 for the differences between AD and normal age-related changes.

BOX 54-5 Alzheimer's Disease: Early Signs and Symptoms

Memory Loss That Disrupts Daily Life
- Forgets newly learned information
- Forgets important dates or events
- Asks the same questions over and over
- Relies more on memory aids—reminder notes, electronic devices
- Relies on family members for things usually handled alone

Problems With Planning or Problem Solving
- Has trouble making a plan or working with numbers
- Has problems following a recipe
- Has trouble keeping track of monthly bills
- Difficulty concentrating
- Takes longer to do things than before

Problems Completing Familiar Tasks
- Has a hard time with tasks in the home, at work, or with recreation
- Has problems driving to familiar places
- Has trouble organizing a grocery list
- Forgets the rules to a favorite game

Confusion With Time or Place
- Loses track of dates, seasons, and passing of time
- Has trouble understanding something that is not happening right away
- Forgets the current location
- Forgets the method of arrival (how the person got to the current location)

Problems With Vision and Spatial Relationships
- Balance problems
- Difficulty reading
- Difficulty judging distance
- Has problems with color or contrast
- Has trouble driving

Problems With Speaking or Writing
- Has trouble following or joining a conversation
- Stops in the middle of a conversation and does not know how to continue
- Repeats things
- Has trouble finding the right word
- Calls things by the wrong name—calling a "watch" a "hand-clock" is an example

Misplacing Items and Being Unable to Find Them
- Puts things in strange places
- Loses things and is unable to retrace steps to find them
- Accuses others of stealing

Decreased or Poor Judgment
- Changes in judgment or decision making
- Poor judgment with money—giving away large amounts is an example
- Pays less attention to hygiene and grooming

Withdrawal From Work or Social Activities
- No longer does hobbies, social activities, work projects, or sports
- Has trouble keeping up with a favorite sports team
- Has trouble remembering how to do a hobby
- Avoids being social

Mood and Personality Changes
- Is confused
- Is depressed
- Is suspicious, afraid, or anxious
- Is easily upset at home, at work, with friends, or outside of the usual setting

Modified from Alzheimer's Association: 10 early signs and symptoms of Alzheimer's and dementia, 2024.

BOX 54-6 Alzheimer's Disease and Normal Aging

Signs of AD
- Poor judgment and decision making.
- Cannot manage a budget.
- Loses track of the date or season.
- Problems having a conversation.
- Misplaces things. Cannot retrace steps to find them.

Normal Age-Related Changes
- Makes a bad decision once in a while.
- Misses a monthly payment.
- Forgets which day it is but remembers later.
- Sometimes forgets which word to use.
- Loses things from time to time.

Modified from Alzheimer's Association: 10 early signs and symptoms of Alzheimer's and dementia, 2024.

Stages of AD

Signs and symptoms become more severe as AD progresses. The disease ends in death. AD is described in 3 stages. See Figure 54-3 and Box 54-7.

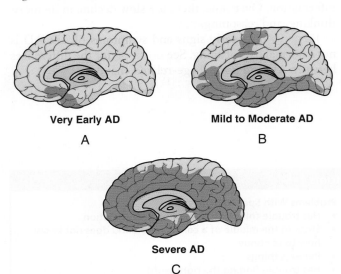

FIGURE 54-3 A, Very early AD. **B,** Mild to moderate AD. **C,** Severe AD. (NOTE: Blue shading shows the areas of the brain affected.) (Redrawn from National Institute on Aging: *Alzheimer's disease: unraveling the mystery,* Bethesda, Md, September 2008, National Institutes of Health.)

Behavior and Function Changes

AD changes how a person behaves and acts. Besides the signs and symptoms in Boxes 54-5 and 54-7, these common behaviors and changes of AD are described in the following pages.

- Wandering and getting lost
- Sundowning
- Hallucinations
- Delusions
- Paranoia
- Catastrophic reactions
- Agitation and aggression
- Communication changes
- Screaming
- Repetitive behaviors
- Rummaging and hiding things
- Changes in intimacy and sexuality

Behaviors communicate needs (Chapter 7). With dementia, communication skills decline (p. 811). It is important for caregivers to be attentive to the person's needs and to remember that behaviors are often attempts to communicate needs.

BOX 54-7	Alzheimer's Disease: Stages

Mild AD
- Memory loss that disrupts daily life
- Poor judgment causing bad decisions
- Loss of spontaneity and initiative
- Losing track of dates or knowing the current location
- Taking longer to do daily tasks
- Repeating questions
- Forgetting recently learned information
- Problems handling money and paying bills
- Trouble with planning and problem solving
- Wandering and getting lost
- Losing things or misplacing them in odd places
- Difficulty completing tasks—bathing is an example
- Mood and personality changes
- Anxiety or aggression

Moderate AD
- Increased memory loss and confusion
- Withdrawal from social activities
- Cannot learn new things
- Problems with language, reading, writing, and working with numbers
- Trouble with thoughts and thinking logically
- Shortened attention span
- Problems coping with new situations
- Change in sleep patterns—sleeping more during the day, restlessness at night
- Problems with familiar tasks that have multiple steps—getting dressed is an example
- Problems recognizing family and friends
- Hallucinations, delusions, and paranoia
- Impulsive behavior—undressing at inappropriate times or places and using vulgar language are examples
- Emotional outbursts
- Restlessness, agitation, anxiety, tearfulness
- Wandering—especially in the late afternoon or evening
- Repetitive statements or movements, occasional muscle twitches

Severe AD
- Depends on others for care
- In bed most or all of the time
- Cannot communicate
- No awareness of recent experiences or surroundings
- Weight loss with little interest in eating
- Seizures
- General physical decline—dental problems, skin problems, foot problems
- Difficulty swallowing (a common cause of death is pneumonia from aspiration)
- Groaning, moaning, or grunting
- Increased sleeping
- Loss of bowel and bladder control

Modified from National Institute on Aging: What are the signs of Alzheimer's disease?, content reviewed October 18, 2022, National Institutes of Health.

Besides brain changes, the following can affect behavior.

- Health problems—illness, pain, infection, drugs, lack of sleep, constipation, hunger, thirst, poor vision or hearing, alcohol use, too much caffeine
- Emotions—sadness, fear, feeling overwhelmed, stress, anxiety
- Changes in routine
- A caregiver's approach—rushed, impatient, critical, unfamiliar
- Problems in the person's setting:
  - A strange setting. The person does not know the setting well.
  - Too much noise or distraction (TV, music, people talking at once) can cause confusion and frustration.
  - Not understanding signs. For example, the person may think that a *WET FLOOR* sign is an instruction to wet the floor.
- Mirrors. The person may think that a mirror image is another person in the room.

Triggers are things that provoke a reaction. The factors listed above are some. Identifying and managing triggers are important in dementia care. The setting and situation are adapted to remove triggers if possible.

See *Promoting Safety and Comfort: Behavior and Function Changes.*

PROMOTING SAFETY AND COMFORT

Behavior and Function Changes

Safety
Some behaviors are caused by illness, injury, or drugs—not AD. Without treatment, life may be threatened. Always report changes in behavior.

Wandering and Getting Lost. Persons with AD are often not oriented to person, time, and place. They may wander off and not find their way back. Wandering is by foot, car, bike, or other means. They may be with you one moment and gone the next.

Judgment is poor. They cannot tell what is safe or dangerous. Life-threatening accidents are great risks. They can walk into traffic or a nearby river, lake, ocean, or forest. If not properly dressed, heat or cold exposure is a risk.

Wandering may have no cause. Or the person is looking for something or someone—the bathroom, the bedroom, a child, or a partner. Pain, drug side effects, stress, restlessness, too much stimulation, and anxiety are other causes. A wandering pattern may reflect a life-long routine—leaving work, getting children from school, and so on. Sometimes finding the cause prevents wandering.

See *Teamwork and Time Management: Wandering and Getting Lost.*

See *Focus on Long-Term Care and Home Care: Wandering and Getting Lost*, p. 810.

TEAMWORK AND TIME MANAGEMENT

Wandering and Getting Lost

Patients and residents may try to wander to another nursing unit or out of the agency. Leaving the agency without staff knowledge is called *elopement*. Serious injury and death have resulted. State and federal guidelines to prevent elopement are followed. The agency's emergency plan includes elopement prevention and response measures (Chapter 14).

All staff must be alert to persons who wander. Staff must monitor for exit-seeking behaviors—expressing a desire to leave, staying close to doors, pacing to and from exits, trying to open doors or windows. Tell other staff that a person wanders. You cannot be with the person all the time. All staff can help monitor the person. Help other staff in the same way.

Wandering is allowed in safe areas (Fig. 54-4). Unsafe areas within the agency include kitchens, shower rooms, and utility rooms. If you see a person wandering into an unsafe area, gently guide the person to a safe place (Fig. 54-5). Tell the nurse.

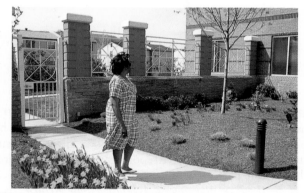

FIGURE 54-4 An enclosed garden allows persons with AD to wander in a safe setting.

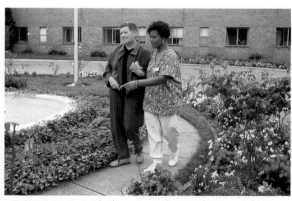

FIGURE 54-5 Guide the person who wanders to a safe area.

FOCUS ON LONG-TERM CARE AND HOME CARE

Wandering and Getting Lost

Home Care

A person who wanders should not be left alone. The following may prevent wandering from home.

- Keep doors locked. A keyed deadbolt or locks in places the person is not likely to look (Fig. 54-6) may be used. Door knob covers are another option. The device turns instead of the door knob. In case of emergency, a caregiver must be present to help the person exit.
- Place *STOP*, *DO NOT ENTER*, or *CLOSED* signs on doors.
- Place a poster, curtain, or brightly colored streamers across the door. Or wallpaper the door to match the walls. The person does not focus on the exit.
- Install safety devices on windows to limit how much windows open.
- Use a door chime that sounds when a door is opened.
- Secure the yard with a fence and a locked gate.
- Keep shoes, keys, suitcases, coats, hats, and other items used when leaving the home out of sight.

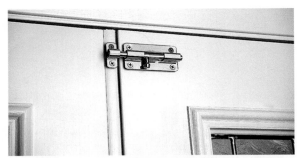

FIGURE 54-6 A slide lock is at the top of a door.

MedicAlert® + Alzheimer's Association Safe Return®. Some states have safety alert systems for older persons who are missing. Called "Silver Alert" or "Code Silver" in some states, such programs involve reporting and alert procedures to help locate persons with dementia who are lost.

MedicAlert® + Alzheimer's Association Safe Return® is a nationwide 24-hour emergency service for persons who wander or have a medical emergency. The purpose is to find and safely return persons who wander and become lost. A small fee is charged.

A family member provides required information and a photo. The person receives an ID (wallet card and bracelet or necklace). If reported missing, the person's information is sent to the police. When the person is found, someone calls the toll-free number on the ID. *MedicAlert® + Alzheimer's Association Safe Return®* then calls the family member or caregiver. The person is returned home.

Sundowning. With *sundowning*, signs, symptoms, and behaviors of dementia increase during hours of darkness. As daylight ends and darkness starts, confusion and restlessness increase. So do anxiety, agitation, and other symptoms. Behavior is worse after sundown. It may continue during the night.

Brain changes affecting the sleep-wake cycle may cause sundowning. Other possible causes include fatigue, hunger or thirst, depression, pain, and boredom. Confusion and fear can occur when poor lighting and shadows cause the person to see things that are not there.

Hallucinations and Delusions. A *hallucination* is seeing, hearing, smelling, feeling, or tasting something that is not real. Affected persons see animals, insects, or people that are not present. Some hear voices. They may feel bugs crawling or feel that they are being touched.

Poor vision or hearing may be a cause. The person should wear needed eyeglasses and hearing aids. Other causes include infection, pain, and drugs.

Delusions are false beliefs. To the person, the beliefs are real. People with AD may think they are another person. Some believe they are in jail, are being killed, or are being attacked. A person may believe the caregiver is someone else. Many other false beliefs can occur.

Paranoia. *Paranoia* is a disorder (*para*) of the mind (*noia*). The person has false beliefs (delusions) and suspicion about a person or situation. Paranoia is a type of delusion. The person believes others are mean, lying, not fair, or intend harm. The person may be suspicious, fearful, or jealous.

Paranoia may worsen as memory loss gets worse. For example, the person thinks misplaced items have been stolen. Or the person no longer recognizes a caregiver. The person does not trust the caregiver.

The person may express loss through paranoia. Reasons for the loss do not make sense. Therefore the person blames or accuses others.

See *Promoting Safety and Comfort: Paranoia.*

PROMOTING SAFETY AND COMFORT

Paranoia

Safety

Behaviors may not mean paranoia. Fears of harm, strangers, stealing, mistreatment, and so on may be real. Some people abuse vulnerable adults (Chapter 5). This includes sexual and financial abuse.

Abuse may be by phone, mail, e-mail, or in person. The abuser may be a friend or family member. Financial abuse occurs when money or belongings are stolen. Financial abuse can include:

- Forging checks or cashing checks without permission
- Taking retirement and Social Security benefits
- Using the person's credit cards or bank accounts
- Changing names on wills, bank accounts, insurance policies, or titles to homes or cars
- "Scams" such as identity theft, phone prizes, and threats
- Borrowing money and not paying it back
- Giving away or selling the person's property without permission
- Forcing the person to sign over property
  Protect the person from harm, abuse, and mistreatment.
Report the following at once.
- What the person is saying
- The person seems afraid or worried about money
- Missing items
- The person's behaviors
- Signs and symptoms of problems
- Visitors or family members acting strangely

Catastrophic Reactions. *Catastrophic reactions* are extreme responses to normal events or things. The person reacts as if there is a disaster or tragedy. The person may scream, cry, or be agitated or combative (ready to fight). These reactions are common from too many stimuli. Eating, music or TV playing, and being asked questions all at once can overwhelm the person.

Agitation and Aggression. When agitated, the person is restless or worried and cannot settle down. The person may pace, move about, or not sleep. Agitation may lead to aggression. The person may yell, scream, swear, hit, pinch, grab, or try to hurt someone. Common causes are:

- Pain or discomfort.
- Anxiety, depression, or stress.
- Loneliness.
- Drug interactions.
- Fatigue.
- Too many stimuli. Too much noise or too many people in the room are examples.
- Hunger or thirst.
- Elimination needs, constipation, or incontinence.
- Feeling lost or abandoned.
- A feeling of loss. Missing driving or caring for children are examples.
- Care measures (bathing, dressing) that upset or frighten the person.
- Feeling pressured to do something that is now hard or impossible. Remembering an event or person are examples.
- Change in routine, caregiver, or setting.
- Caregivers. A caregiver may rush the person or be impatient. Or mixed verbal and nonverbal messages are sent. For example, a caregiver talks too fast or too loud. Consider how your behaviors affect the person. You can ask yourself:
  - Am I being calm and respectful?
  - Are there any distractions that need removed?
  - Am I at the person's level (seated, standing)?
  - Am I making eye contact?
  - Am I being patient and waiting for a response before giving the next step?
  - Have I praised the person's effort?
  - Am I focusing on the person more than the task?

Communication Changes. Communication skills gradually decline. The person has trouble expressing thoughts and emotions. Communication changes include:

- Struggling to find the right word
- Problems understanding the meaning of words
- Attention problems during conversations
- Losing one's train of thought when talking
- Problems blocking background noises—radio, TV, music, phones, others talking, and so on
- Frustration with communication problems
- Being sensitive to touch, tone, and voice volume

As the person loses the ability to talk clearly, other communication methods may be used. Facial expressions and gestures are examples. In time, the person cannot understand others and communicate verbally.

See *Caring About Culture: Communication Changes.*
See *Focus on Communication: Communication Changes.*

✿ CARING ABOUT CULTURE
Communication Changes

For some, English is a second language. For example, the first language learned is Spanish, Italian, French, Russian, Chinese, or Japanese. With AD, the person may forget or no longer understand English. The person uses and understands only the first language learned.

FOCUS ON COMMUNICATION
Communication Changes

To promote communication with the person with AD, see Box 54-8 (p. 812). Avoid:

- *Giving orders.* For example: "Sit down and eat" is bossy. It does not show respect. Instead say: "Let me help you sit down."
- *Wanting the truth.* For example, do not say: "Don't you remember?" or "What day is it?" Instead say: "Today is Friday."
- *Correcting errors.* For example, do not say: "I just told you it's time to get dressed. You already had breakfast." Instead say: "Let me help you get dressed."
- *Pointing out errors.* Instead of saying: "You missed a button," say: "Let's try it this way."
- *Giving many choices.* For example: "What would you like for dinner?" involves many choices. Instead, limit choices. Say: "Do you want potatoes or rice?"
- *Asking open-ended questions.* For example, do not say: "How do you feel?" Instead, ask "yes" or "no" questions. You can say: "Are you tired?"

Screaming. At first, persons with AD have problems finding the right words. As AD progresses, they speak in short sentences or just words. Often speech is not understandable.

Screaming to communicate is common in persons who are very confused and have poor communication skills. They may scream a word or a name. Or they just make screaming sounds.

Possible causes include hearing and vision problems, pain or discomfort, fear, and fatigue. Too much or not enough stimulation is another cause. A person may react to a caregiver or family member by screaming. The following measures and those in Box 54-8 may be helpful.

- Provide a calm, quiet setting.
- Play soft music.
- Have the person wear hearing aids and eyeglasses.
- Have a family member or favorite caregiver comfort and calm the person.
- Use touch to calm the person.

BOX 54-8	Dementia Care: Communication

- Treat the person with dignity and respect.
- Approach the person in a calm, quiet manner.
- Approach the person from the front—not from the back. This avoids startling the person. Stand if the person is standing. Sit if the person is sitting. (Politely ask to sit if the person is able to reply.)
- Make eye contact to get the person's attention. Maintain an appropriate level of eye contact.
- Have the person's attention before you start speaking.
- Identify yourself and other people by name.
- Call the person by name.
- Avoid pronouns (he, she, them, it, and so on). For example, instead of saying: "They are here," say: "Jon and Stacy are here."
- Follow the rules and measures to promote communication (Chapter 7).
- Do not talk about the person as if the person is not there.
- Control distractions and noise. TV, radio, and music are examples.
- Speak in a calm, gentle voice. Be patient.
- Be aware of your body language. Smile and avoid frowning, grimacing, or other negative actions. Standing with the arms folded tightly signals tension or anger.
- Use gestures or cues. Point to objects. Show the motion you want the person to do.
- Watch the person's facial expressions and gestures. Expressions may show sadness, anger, or frustration. Pulling at under-garments may signal incontinence or elimination needs.
- Comfort the person with touch as appropriate for the person. For example, hold the person's hand while you talk.
- Speak slowly. Use simple words and short sentences.
- Do not "baby talk" or use a "baby voice."
- Ask or say 1 thing at a time. Present 1 idea, statement, or question at a time.
- Give simple, step-by-step instructions.
- Explain all procedures and activities.
- Repeat instructions as needed. Allow time to respond or react.
- Avoid interruptions. If you must leave the room, start from the beginning.
- Ask simple questions with simple answers. Do not ask complex questions.
- Let the person speak. Do not interrupt or rush the person.
- Give the person time to respond. If there is no response, try giving the direction again with a cue. You may need to show the item to use, show the motion to do, or gently guide the person's body part (arm, hand) through the motion.
- Try other words if the person does not seem to understand.
- Provide the word if the person is struggling to communicate a thought.
- Do not criticize, correct, interrupt, argue, or try to reason with the person.
- Give consistent responses.
- Practice the measures in Chapter 47:
  - To promote hearing
  - To communicate with speech-impaired persons
  - For blind and visually impaired persons

Repetitive Behaviors. *Repetitive* means to do over and over. (The term *perseveration* may also be used for repetitive behaviors.) The person repeats the same motions, words, or questions over and over. For example, the same napkin is folded over and over. Or the person says the same words or asks the same question over and over. Such behaviors are not harmful. However, they can annoy caregivers and the family.

Rummaging and Hiding Things. To *rummage* means to search for things by moving things around, turning things over, or looking through something such as a drawer or closet. The behavior may have no meaning. Or the person is looking for a certain item but cannot tell you what or why.

The person may hide things, throw things away, or lose things. Eyeglasses, hearing aids, and dentures must stay with the person. Always make sure these items are safe. Money, jewelry, and other important items usually are sent home with the family.

Changes in Intimacy and Sexuality. *Intimacy* is a special bond between people who love and respect each other. It includes the way people talk and act toward each other. *Sexuality* includes the way partners physically express feelings for each other. The person with dementia may:
- Depend on and cling to a partner.
- Not remember life with a partner.
- Not remember feelings for a partner.
- Express affection for another person.
- Have side effects from drugs that affect sexual interest.
- Have memory loss, brain changes, or depression that affects sexual interest.
- Have inappropriate sexual behaviors. Sexual behaviors are labeled inappropriate because of how and when they occur—wrong person, wrong place, or wrong time. (Also known as *disinhibition*, the person lacks the ability to control inappropriate behavior.)

Healthy persons do not undress or expose themselves in front of others. They do not masturbate or engage in sexual acts in public. They know their sexual partners. Persons with dementia may mistake someone else for a sexual partner. The person kisses and hugs the other person.

Appropriate affection is encouraged. The nurse encourages the person's partner to show affection with the couple's usual practices. Hand-holding, hugging, kissing, touching, and dancing are examples. Distraction and privacy measures may be helpful when actions occur with the wrong person or in public (undressing, masturbating). For example, a resident is distracted with an activity or guided to the resident's room.

Some behaviors are not sexual. Touching, scratching, and rubbing the genitals can signal infection, pain, or discomfort in the urinary or reproductive systems. Poor hygiene and incontinence are other causes. Good hygiene prevents itching. Clean the person promptly and thoroughly after elimination. Do not let the person stay wet or soiled.

CARE OF PERSONS WITH AD AND OTHER DEMENTIAS

The person may be cared for at home until symptoms become severe. Adult day care may help. Often assisted living or nursing center care is required. Other illnesses may require hospital care. The person may need hospice care as death nears (Chapter 59). You may care for persons with AD or other dementias in such settings. The person and family need your support and understanding.

People with dementia do not choose the signs and symptoms of the disease. They cannot control what is happening to them. *The disease is responsible, not the person.*

Remember, often the person's behavior is an attempt to communicate needs. See "Meeting Basic Needs" on p. 814.

You must treat persons with dementia with dignity and respect. They have the same rights as everyone else. The care plan addresses the person's specific needs related to behavior changes. See Box 54-9 for examples. See Box 54-8 for measures to promote communication.

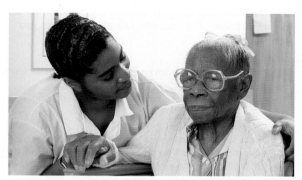

FIGURE 54-7 Gentle touch can be calming for some persons.

BOX 54-9	Dementia Care: Behavior Changes

Wandering
- Follow agency policy for locking doors and windows. Some doors lock automatically. Staff use an identification badge or enter a code into an electronic key pad for entry and exit.
- Keep door alarms and electronic doors turned on. Respond to alarms at once.
- Follow agency policy for fire exits. Everyone must be able to leave the building for a fire.
- Have the person wear an ID bracelet or *MedicAlert®* + *Alzheimer's Association Safe Return®* ID at all times. Follow agency policies and procedures for electronic bands or bracelets used to prevent elopement.
- Know when the person is more likely to wander.
- Follow the care plan for daily routine, activities, and exercise. Meet food, fluid, and elimination needs.
- Involve the person in activities—folding napkins, dusting a table, sorting socks, rolling yarn, sweeping, sanding blocks of wood, or watering plants.
- Do not use restraints. They tend to increase confusion and disorientation. See Chapter 16.
- Do not argue with the person who wants to leave. The person will not understand.
- Go with the person who insists on going outside. Provide proper clothing. Direct the person to a safe area (p. 809). Guide the person inside after a few minutes.
- Allow wandering in enclosed and safe areas.

Sundowning
- Complete treatments and activities early in the day.
- Encourage exercise and activity early in the day.
- Avoid too many activities in a day.
- Allow for rest during the day if needed. If a nap is needed, it should be short and not late in the day.
- Keep the person on a schedule. Waking up, meal times, and bedtime should involve a set routine.
- Avoid caffeine (coffee, tea, colas, chocolate), sweets, and alcohol late in the day.

Sundowning—cont'd
- Provide a calm, quiet setting late in the day.
- Do not restrain the person.
- Meet nutrition and elimination needs. Unmet needs can increase restlessness.
- Use night-lights at night.
- Do not try to reason with the person. The person will not understand.
- Do not ask the person to explain the problem. Communication changes impair understanding and speech.
- Promote sleep at night. See p. 815.

Hallucinations and Delusions
- Have the person wear eyeglasses and hearing aids as needed.
- Do not argue with the person. The person will not understand.
- Reassure the person. Say that you will keep the person safe.
- Distract the person with an item or activity. Or take the person to another room or for a walk.
- Turn off TV or movies when violent and disturbing programs are on. The person may believe the story is real.
- Provide comfort if the person seems afraid. Gentle touch may calm and reassure some persons (Fig. 54-7).
- Eliminate noises that can be misinterpreted. TV, radio, music, furnaces, and air conditioners are examples.
- Check lighting. Eliminate glares, shadows, or reflections.
- Cover or remove mirrors. The person could misinterpret the reflection.
- Remove anything that could be used to hurt the self or others.
- Report behavior changes. They may signal a physical illness.

Continued

BOX 54-9	Dementia Care: Behavior Changes—cont'd

Paranoia
- Do not react if the person blames you for something.
- Do not argue with the person.
- Give reminders of the person's safety.
- Use touch correctly. Know how the person responds to touch. Touch can comfort some people. Others do not like being touched.
- Search for missing things to distract the person. Talk about what you found. For example, talk about a photo you found.

Catastrophic Reactions
- Approach the person from the front. Do not startle from behind or the side.
- Be calm. Do not appear rushed. Give the person time to calm down.
- Use touch correctly. See "Paranoia."
- Explain in simple terms what you want the person to do. For example: "It's time for bed. I'll help you into bed."
- Do not argue with the person.
- Follow the person's daily routine, including naps and bedtime.
- Distract the person with an item or activity.

Agitation and Aggression
- Look at how your behaviors affect the person.
- Provide a calm, quiet setting.
- Follow the care plan and a set routine for activities of daily living (ADL). Meet basic needs.
- Observe for early signs of agitation and aggression. Try to remove the cause before the agitation or aggression worsens.
- Do not ignore the problem. Try to find the cause.
- Allow personal choice to the extent possible.
- Try to distract the person. A snack or activity may help.
- Reassure the person.
  - Speak calmly.
  - Listen to concerns.
  - Try to show that you understand the person's anger or fears.
- Keep personal items within the person's sight. Photos and treasures are examples.
- Reduce glares, noise, and clutter.
- Limit the number of people in the room.
- Use touch correctly. See "Paranoia."
- Provide soothing music.
- Read to the person with a gentle voice.
- Try taking the person for a walk.
- Provide quiet times.

Agitation and Aggression—cont'd
- Limit the amount of caffeine (coffee, tea, colas, chocolate) and sweets.
- See Chapter 7 for managing difficult behavior, including anger and aggression.
- See Chapter 14 for workplace violence.

Repetitive Behaviors
- Allow harmless acts. Holding a purse, folding napkins, caring for a doll, and petting a stuffed animal are examples.
- Look for a reason for the repetition. The action may have meaning if it occurs around certain people, in certain places, or at certain times.
- Know when repetitive behaviors are likely. For example, a person constantly calls for a nurse at bedtime.
- Consider how the person may be feeling. Think about the emotion instead of reacting to the behavior.
- Engage the person in a pleasant activity. Boredom may be the cause.
- Take the person for a walk.
- Turn the action into an activity. For example, a person has repetitive hand motions. You provide a pile of washcloths and ask the person to help fold laundry.
- Use a calm voice and gentle touch. Be patient.
- Do not argue with the person.
- Answer questions. You may have to answer the same question many times.
- Follow the care plan for memory aids when the person asks the same questions over and over. Clocks, calendars, and photos are examples.

Rummaging and Hiding Things
- Keep harmful items and products out of sight and reach.
- Remove spoiled items from refrigerators and cabinets. The person may look for food and eat whatever is found.
- Guide the person away from other patient or resident rooms.
- Keep wastebaskets covered or out of sight. The person may rummage through a wastebasket or throw things away.
- Check wastebaskets, linens, and food trays. Look for items thrown away or hidden.
- Keep bathroom doors closed and toilet seats down. The person cannot flush things down the toilet.
- Allow rummaging in a safe place. The agency may have a drawer, closet, bag, box, basket, or chest with safe items.

Meeting Basic Needs

Over time, the person depends on others more and more for care. Safety, hygiene, food and fluids, elimination, and activity needs must be met. So must comfort and sleep needs. Good skin care and alignment prevent skin breakdown and contractures. The agency's safety plan and the person's care plan will include many of the measures listed in Box 54-10.

The person can have other health problems and injuries. The person may not be aware of or able to communicate about pain, fever, constipation, incontinence, or other problems. Carefully observe the person. Report any change in usual behavior.

Infection is a risk. Infection can occur from poor hygiene. This includes poor skin care, oral hygiene, and perineal care after elimination. Inactivity and immobility can cause pneumonia and pressure injuries. Dysphagia can cause aspiration and pneumonia.

See *Teamwork and Time Management: Meeting Basic Needs*, p. 817.

See *Focus on Surveys: Meeting Basic Needs*, p. 817.

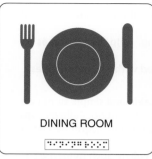 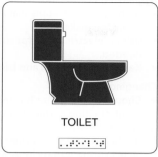

FIGURE 54-8 Signs give cues to persons with dementia.

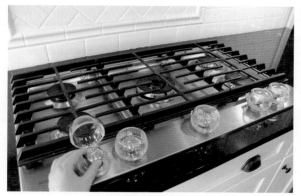

FIGURE 54-9 Safety covers are on stove knobs.

BOX 54-10	Dementia Care: Meeting Basic Needs

Environment
- Follow set routines. Avoid changing roommates or rooms.
- Place picture signs by room doors, bathrooms, dining rooms, and other areas (Fig. 54-8).
- Keep personal items where the person can see and reach them.
- Stay within the person's sight to the extent possible.
- Place memory aids (large clocks and calendars) where the person can see them.
- Keep noise levels low.
- Play music and show movies from the person's past.

Safety
- Reassure the person that you are there to help.
- Remove harmful, sharp, and breakable items from the area. This includes knives, scissors, glasses, dishes, razors, and tools.
- Provide plastic eating and drinking utensils. They help prevent breakage and cuts.
- Practice electrical safety measures (Chapter 14). Also remove electric appliances from the bathroom. Hair dryers, curling irons, make-up mirrors, and electric shavers are examples.
- Provide safe storage for:
  - Personal care items (shampoo, deodorant, lotion, and so on)
  - Cleaners and drugs
  - Dangerous equipment and tools
  - Cigarettes, cigars, pipes, matches, and other smoking materials
  - Car keys
- Keep childproof caps on drug containers and cleaners.
- Remove knobs from stoves or place safety covers on the knobs (Fig. 54-9).
- Remove dangerous appliances, power tools, and firearms and weapons from the home.
- Supervise the person who smokes.
- Practice safety measures to prevent:
  - Falls (Chapter 15)
  - Fires (Chapter 14)
  - Burns (Chapter 14)
  - Poisoning (Chapter 14)
- Lock doors to kitchens, utility rooms, and housekeeping closets. Keep them locked.

Meals
- Maintain a routine. Have meals at usual times. Serve food in a familiar place and in a consistent way.
- Serve favorite foods.
- Respect personal, cultural, and religious food preferences.
- Use the meal as a time for social interaction. Use a kind and pleasant tone of voice.
- Play music during the meal.
- Be patient. Give the person time to eat.
- Provide finger foods.
- Avoid coffee, tea, and cola. The caffeine can increase restlessness, confusion, and agitation.
- Cut food and pour liquids as needed.
- Tell the nurse about changes in eating habits and appetite.
- Watch for signs of dysphagia (Chapter 31) and dehydration (Chapter 32).

Sleep
- Develop a regular bedtime. Bedtime should be the same each evening.
- Perform activities that use more energy early in the day.
- Provide a quiet, peaceful mood in the evening—dimmed lights, low noise level, and soft music.
- Follow bedtime rituals.
- Use night-lights in rooms, hallways, bathrooms, and other areas. They help the person see and prevent accidents and disorientation.
- Limit caffeine.
- Limit naps during the day.
- Follow the person's exercise plan. Play music to the exercise.
- Reduce noises.

Oral Care
- Allow the person to do as much as possible.
- Explain what to do 1 step at a time. For example: "Pick up the toothpaste. Take off the cap. Squeeze the toothpaste on the toothbrush. Put the toothbrush in your mouth. Brush."
- Show the person how to brush the teeth step-by-step.
- Help the person clean dentures.
- Try a long-handled, angled, or electric toothbrush.

Continued

BOX 54-10	Dementia Care: Meeting Basic Needs—cont'd

Bathing

- Follow the care plan for how often to give a bath or shower. Bathing 2 to 3 times a week is enough. A partial bath is done on other days.
- Follow the person's habits and routines.
  - Use the person's preferred bathing method—tub bath, shower. Follow the care plan. Some persons may need complete bed baths.
  - Perform the bath at the same time—in the morning, before bed.
- Practice safety measures. See Chapter 24.
  - Do not leave the person alone in the bath or shower.
  - Check for a comfortable water temperature.
  - Use a hand-held shower head.
  - Use a bath mat and grab (safety) bars.
  - Use a sturdy shower chair.
  - Do not use bath oils. They make the tub slippery and may increase the risk of urinary tract infection.
- Expect that bathing will be a difficult task. Plan ahead to calm the person. Before the bath:
  - Gather supplies—soap, washcloths, towels, shampoo, and so on.
  - Make sure the bathroom is warm and well lit.
  - Play soft music if this relaxes the person.
  - Be matter-of-fact. Say: "It is time for a bath now." Try the bath when the person is calm. Never use force.
  - Provide privacy.
- Promote comfort and independence. During the bath or shower:
  - Be gentle and respectful.
  - Tell the person what you will do step-by-step.
  - Do not rush the person.
  - Allow the person to do as much as possible. This shows dignity and helps the person feel in control.
  - Give the person a washcloth to hold.
  - Put a towel over the shoulders or lap. The person feels less exposed. Clean under the towel with a washcloth.
  - Talk to the person about something else. Talk about something the person enjoys. This may distract the person.
- Dry the skin well after bathing to prevent a rash or infection. Dry well between skin folds.

Hygiene and Grooming

- Provide good skin care.
- Provide incontinence care as needed. Apply a barrier cream or moisturizer (cream, lotion, paste) as directed by the nurse and care plan.

Hygiene and Grooming—cont'd

- Help the person apply make-up if this is a routine. Do not apply eye make-up.
- Use an electric razor for shaving. Help the person as needed.
- Keep the nails clean and trimmed without rough edges.

Changing Garments

- Choose clothing that is comfortable and simple to put on. Front-opening garments are easy to put on. Pullover tops are harder. And the person may become frightened when the head is inside a garment.
- Select clothing that closes with Velcro. Such items are easy to put on and take off. Buttons, zippers, snaps, and other closures can frustrate the person.
- Apply slip-on shoes that will not slide off or shoes with Velcro straps.
- Offer simple clothing choices (Fig. 54-10). Let the person choose between 2 shirts or 2 blouses, 2 pants or 2 slacks, and so on.
- Lay clothing out in the order it will be put on. Hand the person 1 item at a time. Tell or show the person what to do. Do not rush.

Other Basic Needs

- Follow a daily routine. This helps the person know when certain things will happen.
- Promote urinary and bowel elimination and prevent incontinence.
- Promote exercise and activity during the day. This helps reduce wandering and sundowning behaviors. The person may also sleep better.
- Provide a quiet, restful setting. Soft music is better than loud TV programs.
- Have equipment ready for any procedure. This lessens the time for care measures.
- Observe for signs and symptoms of health problems (Chapter 8). Common health problems include:
  - Dental problems (Chapter 23)
  - Incontinence (Chapters 27 and 29)
  - Constipation and diarrhea (Chapter 29)
  - Dehydration (Chapter 32)
  - Flu and pneumonia (Chapter 50)
  - Fever—may signal infection, dehydration, heat-related illness (Chapter 58), or constipation
- Prevent infection.

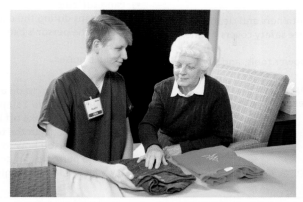

FIGURE 54-10 The person is offered simple clothing choices.

Secured Units

Many nursing centers have secure memory care units (Chapter 1). Entrances and exits are locked. Residents cannot wander away. They have a safe setting to move about. Some persons have behaviors that disrupt or threaten others. They need a secured unit.

According to the Centers for Medicare & Medicaid Services (CMS), persons on a secured unit must be protected from involuntary seclusion (Chapter 5). The agency must identify the reason for placement on the unit. The reason must *not* be:

- For staff convenience or discipline.
- Based on a diagnosis alone. Placement is made on an individual basis.
- By request of the family or the person's representative without a medical reason.

The person's medical record must include:

- The reason for placement on the unit.
- How the resident or resident's representative was involved in the decision.
- If the secured unit is the least restrictive approach to protect the person.
- The person's reaction to placement on the unit.
- On-going review and revision of the care plan as needed. For example, are interventions meeting the resident's needs? Is a secured unit still needed?

At some point, the secured unit is no longer needed. For example, a person's condition progresses to severe AD (see Box 54-7). The person cannot sit or walk. Wandering is not a concern. The person is transferred to another unit.

Activities

Persons with dementia need to feel useful, worthwhile, and active. This promotes self-esteem. Therapies and activities focus on strengths and past successes. For example:

- A person who used to cook helps clean fruit.
- Once a good dancer, activities are planned so the person can dance.
- A person who likes to clean helps with dusting.

Supervised activities meet the person's needs and cognitive abilities. Activities are based on what the person enjoys and can do. Some people like crafts, exercise, gardening, and listening and moving to music. Others like sing-alongs, board games, and reminiscing. (*Reminiscence* or *to reminisce* means to talk about or recall past events.) Some like to string beads, fold towels, or roll dough. Massage, music, and aromatherapy can be comforting and relaxing.

Sometimes activities are used for re-direction (distraction). The person is calmly encouraged to do an enjoyed activity. In all activities, *enjoyment* is what matters. Achievement (doing the activity well) is not the goal.

The Family

The person may live at home or with a partner, children, or other family members. Or someone stays with the person. Home care may help for a while. Adult day care and assisted living are options (Chapters 1 and 57). Nursing center care is needed when:

- The family cannot meet the person's needs.
- The person no longer knows the caregiver.
- Family members have health problems.
- The person's behavior presents dangers to self and others.

Doctor's visits, drugs, home care, and assisted living are costly. So is nursing center care. The person's medical care can drain finances.

Home care and nursing center care are stressful. The family has physical, emotional, social, and financial stresses. Adult children are in the *sandwich generation*. Their own children need attention while an ill parent needs care. Caring for 2 families is stressful. Often adult children have jobs too.

Caregivers can suffer from anger, anxiety, guilt, depression, and sleep problems. Some cannot concentrate or are irritable. Health problems can develop. They need to focus on their own health. They need a healthy diet, exercise, and plenty of rest. Asking family and friends for help is hard for some people.

Caregivers need support and encouragement. The NIA suggests how family members can take care of themselves. See Box 54-11 (p. 818). AD support groups are sponsored by hospitals, nursing centers, and the Alzheimer's Association. The Alzheimer's Association has chapters across the country. Support groups offer encouragement and advice. Members share feelings, anger, frustration, guilt, and other emotions. They also share coping and caregiving ideas.

BOX 54-11	Family Caregivers: Taking Care of Yourself

- Ask for help when you need it. Asking for something specific may be useful. For example:
  - "Can you make Mom's dinner Sunday night?"
  - "Can you stay with Dad from 2 to 4 Monday afternoon?"
- Join a support group.
- Take breaks every day.
- Spend time with friends.
- Maintain hobbies and interests.
- Eat healthy foods and exercise often.
- See a doctor regularly.
- Keep health, legal, and financial information current.
- Remember that these feelings are normal—being sad, lonely, frustrated, confused, angry. Say to yourself:
  - "I'm doing the best I can."
  - "What I'm doing would be hard for anyone."
  - "I'm not perfect and that's okay."
  - "I can't control some things."
  - "I need to do what works for right now."
  - "Even when I do everything I can, there will still be problems. They are caused by the illness, not by what I do."
  - "I will enjoy our peaceful times together."
  - "I will get counseling if caregiving becomes too much."
- Do not neglect your own mental, emotional, and social needs. You may need to talk to a mental health professional, counselor, or social worker.
- Do not neglect your own spiritual needs (Chapter 7).
- Understand that you may feel powerless and hopeless about what is happening.
- Understand that you may feel a sense of loss and sadness.
- Understand why you are caring for a person with AD. Was the choice made out of love, loyalty, duty or obligation, money concerns, fear, or another reason?
- Let yourself feel "uplifts." Examples include good feelings about the person, support from caring people, and time for your interests.

Modified from National Institute on Aging: Alzheimer's caregiving: caring for yourself, Bethesda, Md, content reviewed May 17, 2017, National Institutes of Health.

The family often feels hopeless. No matter what is done, dementia gets worse. Much time, money, energy, and emotion are needed to care for the person. Anger and resentment may result. Guilt feelings are common. The family knows that the person did not choose the disease and its signs, symptoms, and behaviors. Sometimes behaviors are embarrassing. The family may be upset and angry that the loved one cannot show love or affection.

The family is an important part of the health team. They help plan care when possible. The nurse and support group help the family learn how to provide a safe home setting and give needed care. They learn how to bathe, feed, dress, and give oral care.

In nursing centers, some family members take part in unit activities. For many persons, family members provide comfort. They also need support and understanding from the health team.

See *Focus on Long-Term Care and Home Care: The Family.*

See *Focus on Long-Term Care and Home Care: The Family.*

FOCUS ON LONG-TERM CARE AND HOME CARE

The Family

Home Care

Home care is an option for many families. They may need help with meeting the person's needs—preparing meals, bathing, elimination, and so on. Someone needs to supervise the person while family members work, do errands, and have alone time. The amount and kind of care depend on the person's needs and the family's ability to provide care.

Validation Therapy

Validation therapy is a way to communicate with persons with dementia. *Validate* means to show that a person's feelings and needs are fair (valid) and have meaning. Behaviors signal the need to express feelings and needs—safety, security, comfort, love and belonging, feeling useful, and so on. Caregivers help the person express feelings and needs verbally or nonverbally. With validation, the person's reality (what the person thinks is real and true) is accepted. The person is treated with dignity and self-worth.

Validation therapy is based on these principles.

- All behavior has meaning.
- A person may have unresolved issues and emotions from the past.
- A person's mind may return to the past to resolve issues and emotions.
- Caregivers need to listen and provide empathy.
- Attempts are not made to correct thoughts or bring the person back to reality (reality orientation). For example:
  - A person talks about waiting for the bus to go to work. The caregiver does not say: "You don't work anymore." Instead, the caregiver says: "Tell me about your work."
  - A resident says she is at the train station waiting for her husband. Killed in a war, her husband never came home. The caregiver does not remind the resident of what happened. Instead, the caregiver asks the resident about her husband.
  - A patient was 3 years old when his father died. He holds a ball constantly. He calls for his father and repeats "play ball, play ball." The caregiver does not remind the patient that his father is not alive. Instead, the caregiver says: "Tell me about playing ball."

Validation therapy is useful for some persons. If used in your agency, you will be trained to use validation therapy correctly.

FOCUS ON **PRIDE**

The Person, Family, and Yourself

Personal and Professional Responsibility

Everyone has different talents, abilities, and interests. Persons with dementia are no different. Understanding the person's past, hobbies, talents, family, and work helps you give better care.

Learn about the person. Engage the person in activities once enjoyed. Treat each person as unique with a history, interests, strengths, and needs.

Rights and Respect

The person has the right to privacy and confidentiality. Protect the person from exposure. Only those involved in the person's care are present during care. The person is allowed to visit in private. Do not share information about the person with others.

The person has the right to keep and use personal items. A pillow, blanket, or sweater may have meaning. The person may not know why or recognize the item. Still, it is important and provides comfort. Keep personal items safe. Protect property from loss or damage.

Independence and Social Interaction

Maintaining routines can help persons with dementia remain independent longer. For example, a person uses the bathroom, washes hands, brushes teeth, brushes hair, and dresses in the morning. The person is more independent when ADL are done in this order. Changing the order causes confusion.

Break down tasks into simple steps. Patiently tell the person each step. Repeat directions as needed. Allow extra time for each task. Resist the urge to take over. Let the person do what is safely possible.

Delegation and Teamwork

Persons with dementia may respond better to certain staff or caregivers. This can vary by day or time of day. Do not be offended if someone else provides care. The team works together to meet the person's needs.

Sometimes the person resists care from everyone. Convincing the person to allow care is often useless. Use a calm and caring approach. Try giving care at a different time. Never use force.

Ethics and Laws

Persons with dementia may not be able to control their words and actions. However, you must control your reactions. The following is a real example of a poor response to the person's behavior.

While a licensed nursing assistant (LNA) was feeding a resident with AD, the resident threw the tray on the floor. The LNA called the resident a degrading name and swore at her.

The Board of Nursing concluded that the LNA abused and improperly cared for the resident. The unprofessional conduct violated the Administrative Rules of the Board of Nursing because of:

- *Abusing or neglecting a patient*
- *Performing unsafe or unacceptable patient care*
- *Failing to conform to acceptable standards of practice*
- *Engaging in conduct likely to harm the public*

The nursing assistant's license was reprimanded. **(Author note: A *reprimand* means that the Board considered the conduct to be improper. However, the Board did not limit the LNA's ability to work as an LNA.)**

(State of Vermont Board of Nursing, 2000.)

Patience and kindness are important qualities when caring for persons with dementia. If you find yourself feeling impatient or frustrated, tell the nurse. You may need an assignment change. Never act out against the person. You cannot yell at the person or be rough. The person must be protected from verbal and physical abuse and mistreatment.

FOCUS ON **PRIDE**: *Application*

You can practice explaining tasks step-by-step. This will help build confidence in working with persons with dementia. Choose a task. Break the task into simple steps. Explain it to another student or family member step-by-step. Have the person perform the task as you explain it.

REVIEW QUESTIONS

Circle the BEST answer.

1 A person is confused during recovery from surgery. The confusion is likely to be
   a Permanent
   b Temporary
   c Caused by dementia
   d Caused by a brain injury

2 A person is confused. Which should you question?
   a Restrain in bed at night.
   b Give clear, simple directions.
   c Provide a calm, consistent setting.
   d Open drapes during the day.

3 A person has AD. Which is *true?*
   a AD is a normal part of aging.
   b Diet and drugs can cure the disease.
   c AD and delirium are the same.
   d AD ends in death.

4 During the final stage of AD, the person is likely to
   a Wander and become lost
   b Follow simple commands
   c Need total assistance with ADL
   d Repeat questions over and over

Continued

5 Which is common in persons with AD?
   a Paralysis
   b Dyspnea
   c Vision loss
   d Sleep disturbances

6 A person has AD. To communicate, you should
   a Give orders
   b Limit choices
   c Correct mistakes
   d Ask open-ended questions

7 Which can be helpful when giving care and communicating with a person with dementia?
   a Stand if the person is seated.
   b Use gestures and cues.
   c Speak loudly and quickly.
   d Avoid calling the person by name.

8 A person with AD is screaming. You know that this
   a Is a way to communicate
   b Signals aggression
   c Is caused by a delusion
   d Signals attention-seeking behavior

9 Which statement about sundowning is *true*?
   a AD behaviors improve at night.
   b Encouraging activity late in the day can help.
   c Being tired or hungry can increase restlessness.
   d Dim lighting or darkness is calming.

10 A person with AD has delusions. Which should you question?
    a Distract the person with an activity.
    b Tell the person you will provide protection.
    c Tell the person the beliefs are not real.
    d Use touch to calm the person.

11 Which can cause delusions in persons with AD?
    a Mirrors
    b Eyeglasses
    c Hearing aids
    d Night-lights

12 A person with AD keeps telling you that someone is stealing things. What should you do?
    a Nothing. The person has paranoia.
    b Tell the nurse. Someone could be abusing the person.
    c Tell the person not to worry.
    d Send other items home with the family.

13 A person with AD is at risk for elopement. Which should you question?
    a Make sure door alarms are turned on.
    b Make sure an ID bracelet is worn.
    c Assist with exercise as ordered.
    d Remind the person not to wander.

14 A person with AD keeps moving an empty cup back and forth across the table. Which response is *best*?
    a Take the cup away.
    b Ask the person to stop.
    c Allow the person to continue.
    d Fill the cup with coffee.

15 Which can help with rummaging?
    a Keep the person's room locked.
    b Provide safe places to rummage.
    c Ask the person to explain the behavior.
    d Hide items the person looks for.

16 A person with AD is upset. Which is a *correct* response?
    a Try to reason with the person.
    b Ask what is bothering the person.
    c Ignore the problem.
    d Provide reassurance and try to find the cause.

17 Which is *unsafe* for persons with AD?
    a Utility rooms are locked.
    b Cleaners and drugs are locked up.
    c The person keeps smoking materials.
    d Sharp objects are removed from the setting.

18 A person with moderate AD is more restless than usual. The person screams when voiding. You know that this
    a Is normal for this stage
    b May signal pain or infection
    c Is a sign that AD is progressing
    d Is a treatment side effect

19 You are preparing to give oral care to a person with moderate AD. Which will you do?
    a Give step-by-step directions.
    b Brush the teeth yourself if the person resists.
    c Help the person to the bathroom before gathering supplies.
    d Play loud music to distract the person.

20 You need to help a person with AD change clothes. You should
    a Ask the person to get clothes from the closet and signal for you when ready
    b Dress the person quickly to prevent agitation
    c Avoid showing the person what to do
    d Offer 2 clothing options that are comfortable and easy to put on

21 You are caring for a person with AD. You should avoid
    a Trying to bring the person back to reality
    b Offering support to the family
    c Following a set routine
    d Removing distractions

22 Validation therapy involves
    a Support groups and counseling for persons with severe AD
    b Drugs to treat AD
    c Helping the person with AD express needs and feelings
    d Orienting the person with AD to reality

Answers to Chapter 54 questions are on p. 904.

FOCUS ON **PRACTICE**

Problem Solving

A person has moderate AD. While preparing for a bath, the person becomes upset and repeats: "Go away" over and over. How will you respond? How might you meet hygiene needs?

Intellectual and Developmental Disabilities

OBJECTIVES

- Define the key terms and key abbreviations in this chapter.
- Explain how intellectual and developmental disabilities affect the person and family across the life-span.
- Explain when intellectual and developmental disabilities occur and their causes.

- Identify the types of support and services available to persons with intellectual and developmental disabilities.
- Describe the intellectual and developmental disabilities presented in this chapter.
- Explain how to promote PRIDE in the person, the family, and yourself.

KEY TERMS

birth defect A problem that develops during pregnancy, often during the first 3 months; it may involve a body structure or function

developmental disability A life-long condition that begins during the developmental period and impairs physical or intellectual function or both

disability Any lost, absent, or impaired physical or mental function

inherited That which is passed down from parents to children

intellectual disability A life-long condition that begins during the developmental period and limits intellectual function and adaptive behavior

spastic Uncontrolled contractions of skeletal muscles

KEY ABBREVIATIONS

ADA	Americans With Disabilities Act of 1990	FASDs	Fetal alcohol spectrum disorders
ADHD	Attention-deficit/hyperactivity disorder	Fragile X	Fragile X syndrome
ASD	Autism spectrum disorder	IDD	Intellectual and developmental disability
CP	Cerebral palsy	IQ	Intelligence quotient
DS	Down syndrome	SB	Spina bifida
FAS	Fetal alcohol syndrome		

A *disability* is any lost, absent, or impaired physical or mental function. Disabilities can begin before birth or during childhood and affect physical function, mental function, or both. This chapter describes some common causes of life-long intellectual and developmental disabilities and the support and services required to meet the person's needs.

DEVELOPMENTAL DISABILITIES

A *developmental disability* is a life-long condition that begins during the developmental period and impairs physical or intellectual function or both. ("Developmental period" refers to the time before adulthood.) Screening during childhood monitors progress in growth and development. (See Chapter 11.) Trained specialists perform developmental evaluations when there are delays and areas of concern.

According to the *Developmental Disabilities Assistance and Bill of Rights Act of 2000*, a developmental disability occurs before the age of 22. The person has limited functioning in at least 3 of these areas.

- Self-care
- Communication—receiving and expressing language
- Learning
- Mobility
- Self-direction
- Ability to live independently
- Ability to financially support oneself

Early intervention can help young children learn important skills. Depending on the child's needs, therapies and services can help the child with speech, mobility, learning, and interaction with others. The person usually requires support and assistance long-term.

Intellectual Disabilities

An intellectual disability (ID) is a type of developmental disability. An *intellectual disability* is a life-long condition that begins during the developmental period and limits intellectual function and adaptive behavior. *Intellectual function* includes skills such as learning, reasoning, and problem solving. *Adaptive behavior* involves social and life skills needed for daily living (Box 55-1).

The Arc is a national organization focusing on people with intellectual and related disabilities. The Arc describes an intellectual disability as:

- An IQ score of about 70 or below. (*IQ* means intelligence quotient.) Learning ability is less than normal. The person learns at a slower pace.
- A significant limitation in at least 1 adaptive behavior. See Box 55-1.
- Onset before age 18.

IQ scores and adaptive behavior are measured using standardized tests given by trained professionals.

Intellectual disabilities can be mild to severe. Persons mildly affected have delays in learning in school. As adults, they can function in society with some support. For example, they need help finding a job. Support is not needed every day. Others need much support every day at home and at work. Still others need constant support in all areas.

See *Focus on Communication: Intellectual Disabilities*.

FOCUS ON **COMMUNICATION**

Intellectual Disabilities

Mental retardation was once a common term for intellectual disabilities. However, the term is offensive and out-dated. *Intellectual disability* is the preferred term.

Signed in 2010, *Rosa's Law* replaced *mental retardation* with *intellectual disability* in federal health, education, and labor laws. The law was inspired by Rosa Marcellino, a person with Down syndrome. Rosa was 9 years old when the law was signed. The change promoted respect, value, and dignity for persons with intellectual disabilities.

Do not use "mental retardation" or "mentally retarded." Refer to the person. Then state the disability as an "intellectual disability" if needed.

BOX 55-1 Adaptive Behaviors

- Communication—receiving and expressing language
- Reading
- Writing
- Money concepts and managing money
- Social skills—interpersonal skills, responsibility, not being tricked by others, following rules, obeying laws
- Activities of daily living—eating, dressing, mobility, elimination, preparing meals, taking needed drugs, using the phone, using transportation, housekeeping, job skills, and maintaining a safe setting

Modified from The Arc: Introduction to intellectual disabilities, Washington, DC.

IDDs

"Intellectual and developmental disabilities" (IDDs) refers to the many conditions that can cause life-long mental or physical disabilities or both. IDDs begin before, during, or after birth or during childhood. IDDs can be mild to severe. Some causes and warning signs are listed in Box 55-2.

Some IDDs involve birth defects. A *birth defect* is a problem that develops during pregnancy, often during the first 3 months. It may involve a body structure or function. Birth defects may affect how the body looks, functions, or both.

BOX 55-2 Intellectual and Developmental Disabilities: Causes and Warning Signs

Causes
- Genetics
  - Genes inherited from 1 or both parents. *Inherited means to be passed down from parents to children.*
  - Problems when genes combine during fertilization.
- Fetal exposure to certain substances. Alcohol, drugs, and certain environmental toxins (such as lead) are examples.
- Malnutrition during pregnancy.
- Infections during pregnancy. German measles is an example.
- Problems during childbirth.
  - Lack of oxygen to the brain
  - Head injury during birth
- Premature birth.

Causes—cont'd
- Problems after birth.
  - Infections
  - Head injuries
  - Near drowning
  - Exposure to environmental toxins (lead and mercury are examples)
  - Poisoning
  - Malnutrition

Warning Signs
- Delays in sitting up, crawling, or walking
- Delays in talking or having difficulty speaking
- Trouble remembering things
- Trouble understanding the rules of social behavior
- Trouble "seeing" or "understanding" the outcomes of actions
- Trouble solving problems

"Causes" modified from The Arc of the United States: Causes and prevention of intellectual disabilities, Silver Spring, Md, revised March 1, 2011. "Warning Signs" modified from Eunice Kennedy Shriver National Institute of Child Health and Human Development: What are the signs of intellectual and developmental disabilities (IDDs)? Bethesda, Md, last reviewed November 9, 2021.

Children with IDDs become adults. *Independence to the extent possible* is the goal. This includes having a job and living in the community. Many need life-long help, support, and special services.

- Personal services:
  - Self-care
  - Adaptive (assistive) devices for eating, dressing, bathing, mobility, and other needs
  - Health care including drug therapy or surgery
  - Home and vehicle needs
  - Therapies: physical, occupational, speech and language, respiratory, recreation, and other
  - Hearing and vision aids
- Housing—family, independent living, group homes, or long-term care centers
- Education:
  - An individualized education program (IEP)—free program offered to public school children needing special education services; the program outlines the individual goals and support services needed for the child to succeed in school
  - Job training
- Finances and employment
- Protection of their rights:
  - The *Americans With Disabilities Act of 1990 (ADA)*—civil rights (equal opportunities—employment; access to goods and services; participation in state and local government programs, services, and activities)
  - The *Individuals with Disabilities Education Act (IDEA)*—educational rights
  - The *Developmental Disabilities Assistance and Bill of Rights Act of 2000*—involvement in shaping policies and services that affect persons with developmental disabilities; includes advocacy and protection

An IDD affects the family throughout life. Both the child and parents grow older. It can be hard to provide care and financial support. A parent may become ill, injured, or disabled or may die. Still, the person needs care.

See *Focus on Long-Term Care and Home Care: IDDs.*

FOCUS ON LONG-TERM CARE AND HOME CARE

IDDs

Long-Term Care

Changes from aging (Chapter 12) may occur earlier when IDDs are severe. Some adults with IDDs need nursing center care. They are further protected by the *Omnibus Budget Reconciliation Act of 1987 (OBRA)*. OBRA requires that centers provide age-appropriate activities. Staff must have special training to meet care needs.

Some severely disabled children live in agencies for persons with developmental disabilities.

Sexuality

Forming relationships, making choices about sexuality, and family planning are part of a person's well-being. The person's needs and desires are to be respected.

The Arc's beliefs about sexuality include the right to:
- Develop friendships and emotional and sexual relationships. This involves the right to:
  - Love and be loved.
  - Choose to begin and end a relationship.
- Dignity and respect.
- Privacy and confidentiality.
- Freely choose associations (groups to belong to).
- Education to promote informed decision-making. Information about reproduction, marriage and family, abstinence, safe sex, sexual orientation, sexually transmitted diseases (infections), and abuse are included.
- Be protected from sexual harassment and abuses—physical, sexual, emotional.
- Personal choice in sexual expression.
- Decide about having and raising children.
- Make birth control decisions.
- Have control over one's own body.
- Protection from sterilization because of the disability. *Sterilization* means to remove or block sex organs so the person cannot have children.

DOWN SYNDROME

Down syndrome (DS) is named for the doctor who identified the syndrome. DS is a genetic cause of mild to moderate intellectual disabilities. It is caused by an error in cell division that causes a full or partial extra chromosome (chromosome 21) to be present.

The child with DS has certain features caused by the extra chromosome (Fig. 55-1, p. 824).
- A flattened face, especially the bridge of the nose
- Almond-shaped eyes that slant upward
- Short neck
- Small ears
- A tongue that tends to stick out of the mouth
- Small hands and feet
- Small pinky fingers that may curve toward the thumb
- Shorter-than-average height
- Poor muscle tone

Developmental delays may occur in childhood. There may be delays in motor skills (moving and walking), language (speech) development, learning, and social skills (play).

Persons with DS may be more likely to have heart defects, thyroid problems, sleep apnea, hearing and vision problems, ear infections, and obesity. Some persons have gastro-intestinal problems such as constipation and gastro-esophageal reflux disease. Children are monitored for conditions that are more common in persons with DS.

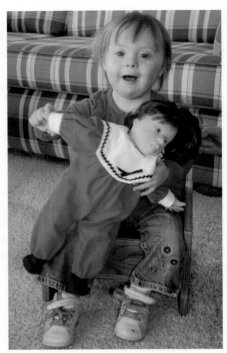

FIGURE 55-1 A child with Down syndrome. (From Hockenberry MJ, Wilson D, Rodgers CC: *Wong's nursing care of infants and children,* ed 11, St Louis, 2019, Elsevier.)

Adults with DS have a higher risk of developing Alzheimer's disease (Chapter 54).

Persons with DS need the support and services listed on p. 823. Therapies help the person learn self-care skills. Many persons with DS live to age 60 or older.

See *Focus on Communication: Down Syndrome.*

FOCUS ON COMMUNICATION

Down Syndrome

The National Down Syndrome Society identifies these as respectful ways to refer to persons with Down syndrome.
- Always refer to the person first.
- Instead of saying "a Down syndrome child," say "a child with Down syndrome."
- Avoid describing the condition as "Down's" or saying "Down's child." (Down syndrome without "apostrophe s" is preferred.)
- Do not say the person is "afflicted by" or "suffers from" Down syndrome. The person "has" the condition.

FRAGILE X SYNDROME

Fragile X syndrome (Fragile X) is the most common form of inherited IDD. There is a change in the gene that makes a protein needed for brain development. The body makes little or none of the protein.

Girls usually have milder symptoms than boys do. Fragile X has no cure. The following signs and symptoms are treated with educational, speech, behavioral, physical, and drug therapies.
- *Learning.* Learning disabilities range from mild to severe.
- *Physical.* Physical features become more apparent with age. The person may have a long and narrow face, large ears, and a prominent jaw and forehead. Poor muscle tone, flat feet, and flexible finger joints are other signs.
- *Social and emotional.* Behavior problems are common. Attention problems, being very active (hyperactive), poor eye contact, anxiety, and shyness are some. The person may flap or bite the hands.
- *Speech and language.* Boys may have more severe delays than girls.

ADHD

Attention-deficit/hyperactivity disorder (ADHD) is a common developmental disorder that begins in childhood. ADHD causes:
- Attention problems—trouble focusing, being organized, and staying on task.
- Hyperactivity—excessive movement, activity, and talking.
- Impulsivity—acting in the moment without thinking through the outcome and having trouble with self-control.

Symptoms interfere with different areas of life—home, school, friendships. As the person ages, ADHD can affect school and work performance, relationships, and daily life.

Causes and risk factors are not fully understood. Differences in brain structure and function are present in persons with ADHD.

Treatment includes behavioral and drug therapies. A healthy life-style including regular exercise, a healthy diet, and adequate sleep is important. Parents need to develop effective methods of discipline for inappropriate behavior. Instead of harsh forms (yelling, scolding, spanking), giving clear directions and consequences (time-out, removal of a privilege) are more effective. The following strategies may help manage ADHD.
- Have a routine and organizational methods in place.
- Remove distractions.
- Limit choices to few options when many choices are overwhelming.
- Give clear, specific, step-by-step directions. Have the person's attention before giving the direction.
- Do not rush the person.
- Set realistic goals and give positive reinforcement (praise) or other rewards for the person's efforts.
- Know the person's strengths and create opportunities for success.

BOX 55-3 | **Autism Spectrum Disorder: Signs and Symptoms**

Social Communication and Interaction Skills
- Avoids eye contact or does not keep eye contact.
- Does not respond to own name by 9 months of age.
- Does not show facial expressions (happy, sad, angry, surprised) by 9 months of age.
- Does not play simple, interactive games like pat-a-cake by 12 months of age.
- Uses few or no gestures by 12 months of age. Not waving good-bye is an example.
- Does not share interests with others by 15 months of age. Showing a parent a liked object is an example.
- Does not point to show interest in an item by 18 months of age.
- Does not notice when others are hurt or upset by 2 years of age.
- Does not notice other children and join them to play by 3 years of age.
- Does not engage in pretend play by 4 years of age.
- Does not sing, dance, or act for a parent by 5 years of age.

Restricted or Repetitive Behaviors or Interests
- Lines up toys or other objects. Gets upset when the order is changed.
- Repeats words or phrases over and over (*echolalia—echo* means to repeat; *lalia* means disorder of speech).
- Plays with toys the same way every time.
- Is focused on parts of objects. For example, focuses on wheels.
- Gets upset by small changes.
- Has narrow (obsessive) interests.
- Must follow certain routines.
- Rocks, spins in circles, or flaps the hands.
- Has unusual reactions to the way things sound, smell, taste, look, or feel.

Other
- Delayed language skills.
- Delayed movement skills.
- Delayed learning.
- Is hyperactive (very active).
- Acts without thinking (impulsive).
- Has a short attention span.
- Has unusual eating and sleeping habits.
- Has unusual mood or emotional reactions.
- Has anxiety or excessive worry.
- Lacks fear or has more fear than expected.

Modified from Centers for Disease Control and Prevention: Signs and symptoms of autism spectrum disorder, Atlanta, Ga, January 25, 2024.

AUTISM SPECTRUM DISORDER

Autism spectrum disorder (ASD) is a developmental disorder that begins in early childhood. Persons with ASD may have a wide range of symptoms affecting communication, behavior, social interaction, and learning. Examples are listed in Box 55-3. Symptoms usually appear before the age of 3.

The cause of ASD is unknown. Genetics and environment are factors. Early diagnosis and treatment are important. ASD treatment involves a variety of life-long therapies depending on the person's changing needs. Examples include behavior, speech, language, and communication therapies; physical, occupational, and recreational therapies; diet therapy; and drug therapy.

A daily routine is helpful for persons with ASD. A change in routine can be very upsetting. As adults, some persons with ASD work and live independently. Others need family support and community services. Some live in group homes or residential facilities.

Other disorders may occur with ASD. Fragile X syndrome and seizure disorders are examples.

CEREBRAL PALSY

Cerebral palsy (CP) is a group of disorders affecting the ability to move and maintain balance and posture. Areas of the brain (*cerebral*) that control movement and posture do not develop correctly or are damaged. *Palsy* means weakness or problems using the muscles.

BOX 55-4 | **Cerebral Palsy: Early Signs**

Younger Than 6 Months of Age
- Head falls back when picked up while lying on the back.
- Feels stiff.
- Feels floppy.
- Seems to over-extend the back and neck when held.
- Legs get stiff and cross or scissor when picked up.

Older Than 6 Months of Age
- Does not roll over in either direction.
- Cannot bring the hands together.
- Has difficulty bringing the hands to the mouth.
- Reaches out with 1 hand while keeping the other fisted.

Older Than 10 Months of Age
- Crawls in a lop-sided manner. Pushes off with 1 hand and leg; drags the other hand and leg.
- Scoots on buttocks or hops on knees.
- Does not crawl on all fours.

Modified from Centers for Disease Control and Prevention: About cerebral palsy, Atlanta, Ga, May 14, 2024.

Damage can occur before, during, or after birth. A movement disorder, CP causes problems controlling the muscles. Delays in reaching motor (movement) milestones may signal CP (Box 55-4). Signs and symptoms vary and range from mild to severe.

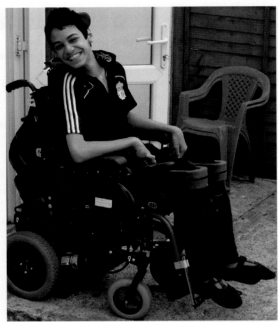

FIGURE 55-2 A person with cerebral palsy. (From Lissauer T, Carroll W: *Illustrated textbook of paediatrics*, ed 6, Oxford, 2022, Elsevier.)

There are different types of CP. Spastic CP is the most common type. *Spastic* means uncontrolled contractions of skeletal muscles. The person has increased muscle tone, causing stiff muscles and awkward movements. Different body parts may be involved—legs; 1 side of the body; both arms and legs, the trunk, and face. Posture, balance, and movement are affected. The person may be able to walk with adaptive (assistive) devices or not be able to walk at all (Fig. 55-2). When the arms are affected, there are problems with eating, writing, dressing, and other activities of daily living.

The person may have other health problems.

- Seizure disorders
- Intellectual disabilities
- Delayed growth and development
- Spinal deformities and arthritis
- Impaired vision
- Hearing problems
- Speech and language disorders
- Drooling
- Incontinence
- Pain or difficulty feeling sensations
- Learning problems
- Infections and long-term illnesses—heart and lung diseases, pneumonia
- Contractures
- Malnutrition
- Dental problems
- Inactivity

CP has no cure. Treatment may involve drugs, surgery, and various therapies—physical, occupational, speech and language, recreational. Various orthotic devices, walking aids, wheelchairs, and adaptive (assistive) devices may be needed.

SPINA BIFIDA

Spina bifida (SB) is a defect in the spine (vertebrae). (*Spina* means backbone. *Bifid* means split in 2 parts.) The spine and membranes that protect the spinal cord do not form and close properly. An opening occurs along the spine. The defect occurs during the first month of pregnancy. (SB is a type of neural tube defect. In the fetus, the brain and spine develop from the neural tube. Having enough folic acid [a vitamin] during pregnancy can help prevent neural tube defects.)

SB can cause mild to severe physical and intellectual disabilities. Severity depends on the size and location of the spinal opening and if the spinal cord and nerves are affected. The most common types of SB include:

- *Spina bifida occulta. Occult* means hidden. There is a small gap in the spine but no "sac" (protrusion) along the back. The spinal cord and nerves are not damaged. The person has a dimple or tuft of hair on the back (Fig. 55-3). This is the most common and mildest form of SB. Often there are no symptoms. Foot weakness and bowel and bladder problems can occur.
- *Meningocele. Meninges* are the membranes that cover and protect the brain and spinal cord. *Cele* means hernia or swelling. With a meningocele, a sac comes through a gap (opening) in the spine (Fig. 55-4, *A* and Fig. 55-5). The sac contains meninges and spinal fluid. The spinal cord and nerve tissue do not enter the sac. Usually there is little to no nerve damage. Minor disabilities can occur. Surgery corrects the defect.
- *Myelomeningocele (or meningomyelocele).* This is the most severe type. Like a meningocele, there is a sac coming through an opening in the spine. However, with a myelomeningocele, the sac contains part of the spinal cord along with meninges and spinal fluid (Fig. 55-4, *B*). (*Myelo* means spinal cord.) Nerve damage occurs. Loss of function occurs below the level of damage. Leg paralysis and lack of sensation are common. So is the lack of bowel and bladder control. Hydrocephalus can occur. (See "Hydrocephalus.") The defect is closed with surgery.

Children with severe forms of SB are at risk for bladder, bowel, and mobility problems. Skin breakdown, depression, and social and sexual issues are other risks. Some children have learning problems.

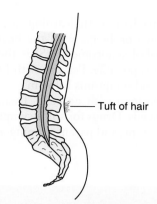

FIGURE 55-3 Spina bifida occulta.

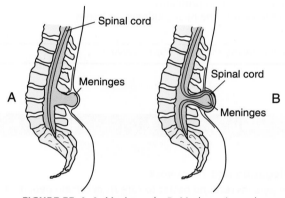

FIGURE 55-4 A, Meningocele. B, Myelomeningocele.

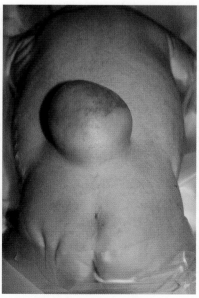

FIGURE 55-5 Meningocele. (From Swaiman KF et al: *Swaiman's pediatric neurology, principles and practice,* ed 6, Philadelphia, 2017, Elsevier.)

HYDROCEPHALUS

With hydrocephalus, cerebrospinal fluid collects in and around the brain. (*Hydro* means water. *Cephalo* means head.) The head enlarges (Fig. 55-6). Pressure inside the head increases. Intellectual disabilities and neurological damage occur without treatment. Vision problems, seizures, and learning disabilities can occur.

If untreated, hydrocephalus usually causes death. Treatment involves a shunt placed in the brain. It allows cerebrospinal fluid to drain from the brain. The shunt is a long, flexible tube. It goes from the brain into a body cavity to drain (Fig. 55-7). The shunt must remain open (*patent*). If blocked, the cerebrospinal fluid cannot drain from the brain.

Hydrocephalus can be present at birth. Genetic problems and problems with fetal development are causes. Hydrocephalus also can occur at any age after birth. Injury, stroke, infections, tumors, and bleeding in the brain are causes.

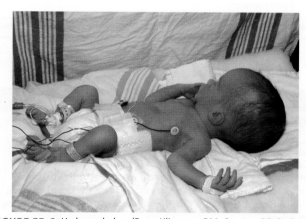

FIGURE 55-6 Hydrocephalus. (From Kliegman RM, Stanton BF, St Geme JW III, Schor NF: *Nelson textbook of pediatrics,* ed 21, Philadelphia, 2020, Elsevier.)

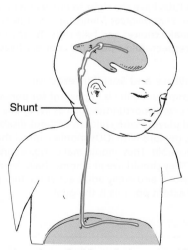

FIGURE 55-7 A shunt drains fluid from the brain. (Modified from Hockenberry MJ, Wilson D, Rodgers CC: *Wong's nursing care of infants and children,* ed 11, St Louis, 2019, Elsevier.)

FETAL ALCOHOL SPECTRUM DISORDERS

Drinking alcohol during pregnancy can cause a group of conditions called fetal alcohol spectrum disorders (FASDs). Children born with FASD have a mix of problems—medical, behavioral, educational (learning), and social. Signs and symptoms are listed in Box 55-5.

Types of FASD depend on the signs and symptoms present. For example, a person might have an intellectual disability and problems with learning and behavior. Or a person may have problems with the heart, kidneys, or bones. Fetal alcohol syndrome (FAS) is the most serious type. Fetal death is possible. Persons with FAS may have a mix of the signs and symptoms listed in Box 55-5.

FASDs are life-long with no cure. Treatment depends on the person's needs. Drugs for some symptoms, behavior and education therapy, and parent training are common.

BOX 55-5   Fetal Alcohol Spectrum Disorders: Signs and Symptoms

- Atypical facial features such as a smooth ridge between the nose and upper lip
- Small head size
- Shorter-than-average height
- Low body weight
- Poor coordination
- Hyperactive behavior
- Attention problems
- Poor memory
- Learning disabilities and difficulty in school (especially with math)
- Speech and language delays
- Intellectual disabilities
- Poor reasoning and judgment skills
- Sleep and sucking problems as a baby
- Vision or hearing problems
- Problems with the heart, kidneys, or bones

Modified from Centers for Disease Control and Prevention: About fetal alcohol spectrum disorders (FASDs), Atlanta, Ga, May 15, 2024.

FOCUS ON PRIDE

The Person, Family, and Yourself

P ersonal and Professional Responsibility

Caring for persons with IDDs is a joy and a challenge. The person may struggle with speech, learning, mobility, or self-care. Care needs can be great. Despite these challenges, the person often has a positive outlook on life and brings joy to others.

Do not allow challenges to affect your attitude. Instead, let your attitude overcome the challenges. Take pride in your decision to have a positive attitude.

R ights and Respect

Persons with IDDs have the right to enjoy and maintain a good quality of life. That involves friendships, health and safety, and the right to make choices and take risks. Treat the person with dignity and respect. Allow personal choice. Always provide quality care.

I ndependence and Social Interaction

Inclusion in community life is important for persons with IDDs. The Arc supports opportunities such as living in a family home, learning, and playing with children without disabilities.

As adults, persons with IDDs should control their lives as much as possible. They should make choices and act for themselves. They should live in a home, have friends, do meaningful work, and enjoy adult activities. Independence to the greatest extent possible is the goal.

D elegation and Teamwork

Some persons respond better to care from certain people at certain times. For example, you are patient and kind but a person refuses to eat. Another staff member is able to get the person to eat.

Do not be offended if the person responds to someone else. It does not mean you have done something wrong. And it does not mean the person does not like you.

Do not be discouraged. Also, be willing to learn. Ask the staff member if there is a different method to try. Or ask if there are preferences you should know about. Thank the person for helping.

E thics and Laws

Persons with IDDs must be protected from abuse, mistreatment, and neglect (Chapters 2 and 5). They may have limited communication skills. Or they may fear what will happen if they tell. Changes in mood or behavior, frequent injuries, poor hygiene, weight loss, and anxiety around a caregiver are signs of abuse. See Chapter 5 for others. Tell the nurse right away if you suspect abuse. Take pride in protecting the person's safety and well-being.

FOCUS ON PRIDE: Application

What factors affect quality of life? Are these the same for persons with IDDs? How do family members, caregivers, friends, and others affect the person's quality of life and self-worth?

REVIEW QUESTIONS

Circle the BEST answer.

1 Which statement about developmental disabilities is *true?*
   a Being able to live independently is not possible.
   b Early intervention can help the person learn important skills.
   c Support and services are usually only needed during childhood.
   d The person does not have the same rights as others.

2 A person with an intellectual disability has limitations in adaptive behavior. This means that the person
   a Has trouble with social and life skills needed for daily living
   b Is unable to learn or problem solve
   c Will not be able to form relationships
   d Cannot make independent choices

3 A person has an IQ score below 70. Which is expected?
   a The person cannot learn.
   b The person will not be able to learn until adulthood.
   c The person will learn at a slower pace.
   d The person cannot attend public school.

4 Intellectual and developmental disabilities (IDDs)
   a Begin before, during, or after birth or in childhood
   b Begin in adulthood
   c Do not affect a person in adulthood
   d Cause death before adolescence

5 Which is a common goal for a person with a mild IDD?
   a Curing the condition
   b Coping with life without a partner or a family
   c Managing life without job skills
   d Independence to the extent possible

6 Down syndrome involves
   a Muscle weakness and paralysis
   b Excess fluid and pressure in the brain
   c Spinal defects and nerve damage
   d Physical feature changes and intellectual disabilities

7 Fragile X syndrome is
   a The result of brain injury
   b Caused by alcohol use during pregnancy
   c Inherited from parents
   d Caused by an infection

8 A person with ADHD is impulsive and has trouble focusing. Which approach is *best* to manage the condition?
   a Harsh discipline
   b Behavioral therapy
   c Avoiding public settings
   d Ignoring the behavior

9 Autism spectrum disorder affects
   a Physical features
   b Mobility
   c Bowel and bladder control
   d Social and communication skills

10 Which statement about cerebral palsy is *true?*
   a CP affects posture, balance, and movement.
   b Children with CP have distinct facial features.
   c Drugs and therapies can cure CP.
   d CP is a genetic disorder.

11 With spina bifida there is
   a An extra chromosome that affects facial features
   b A defect in the spine that may cause nerve damage
   c Abnormal brain development causing behavioral symptoms
   d Birth trauma causing developmental delays

12 The person with spina bifida may have
   a Bowel and bladder problems
   b A short attention span
   c Hearing and vision problems
   d Speech and language problems

13 Hydrocephalus often occurs with
   a Down syndrome
   b Cerebral palsy
   c Spina bifida
   d Autism

14 Hydrocephalus is treated with
   a Braces and crutches
   b A shunt
   c Drugs
   d Social services

15 Alcohol use during pregnancy is
   a Safe in moderation
   b Safe in early pregnancy
   c Safe in late pregnancy
   d Harmful to the developing fetus

Answers to Chapter 55 questions are on p. 904.

FOCUS ON **PRACTICE**

Problem Solving

A child with ADHD has trouble focusing and following directions. Is this behavior expected? What strategies might help your interactions with the child?

OBJECTIVES

- Define the key terms and key abbreviations in this chapter.
- Describe how to meet the safety and security needs of infants and children.
- Identify the signs and symptoms of illness in infants.
- Explain how to help mothers with breast-feeding.
- Describe 3 forms of baby formulas.
- Explain how to bottle-feed babies.
- Explain how to burp a baby.
- Describe how to give cord care.

- Describe the purposes of circumcision, needed observations, and the required care.
- Explain how to bathe infants.
- Explain why infants are weighed.
- Describe the care needed by mothers after childbirth.
- Perform the procedures described in this chapter.
- Explain how to promote PRIDE in the person, the family, and yourself.

KEY TERMS

breast-feeding Feeding a baby milk from the mother's breasts; nursing

circumcision The surgical removal of foreskin from the penis

episiotomy Incision *(otomy)* into the perineum

lochia The vaginal discharge that occurs after childbirth

meconium A newborn's first bowel movement; it is a dark green to black, tarry bowel movement

nursing See "breast-feeding"

postpartum After *(post)* childbirth *(partum)*

prenatal care The health care a woman receives while pregnant

umbilical cord The structure that connects the mother and fetus (unborn baby); it carries blood, oxygen, and nutrients from the mother to the fetus

KEY ABBREVIATIONS

BM	Bowel movement	ID	Identification
C	Centigrade	SIDS	Sudden infant death syndrome
CPSC	Consumer Product Safety Commission	SUID	Sudden unexpected infant death
C-section	Cesarean section		
F	Fahrenheit		

Mothers and newborns usually have short hospital stays. Some need home care after discharge because of:
- Complications before or after childbirth
- Health problems
- Needing help with other young children
- A multiple birth (twins, triplets, and so on)
- Needing help with meals and housekeeping

Babies depend on others for basic needs—physical, safety and security, and love and belonging. A review of growth and development will help you care for babies (Chapter 11).

See *Promoting Safety and Comfort: Caring for Mothers and Babies.*

PROMOTING SAFETY AND COMFORT

Caring for Mothers and Babies

Safety
Some care measures in this chapter involve exposing and touching a baby's private areas—the perineum and rectum. Sexual abuse has occurred in health care settings. Perform such care measures with a parent present. Always act in a professional manner.

Contact with urine or feces (stools) is likely when assisting with diaper changing and bathing. Follow Standard Precautions. Follow the Bloodborne Pathogen Standard if blood is present. Follow the rules of hand hygiene and the guidelines for glove use in Chapters 17 and 18.

SAFETY AND SECURITY

Babies cannot protect themselves. They need to feel safe and secure. They feel secure when warm and when wrapped and held snugly. Babies cry to communicate. They cry when soiled, hungry, hot or cold, tired, uncomfortable, or in pain. To promote safety and security, respond to their cries—feed them, change diapers as needed, comfort them, talk to them, and so on.

Follow the infant safety measures in Box 56-1. Follow the measures in Chapters 14 and 15 to protect children from burns, poisoning, choking and suffocation, and falls. Also see Appendix D, p. 909.

See *Focus on Long-Term Care and Home Care: Safety and Security*, p. 832.

BOX 56-1 **Infant Safety**

General Safety
- Keep the baby warm. Check windows for drafts. Close windows securely.
- Keep your fingernails short. Do not wear non-natural nails. Long nails can scratch the baby.
- Do not wear rings or bracelets. Jewelry can scratch the baby.
- Respond to the baby's crying. Babies communicate by crying. Responding to their cries helps them feel safe and secure.
- Keep 1 hand on a child lying in a crib or on a scale, bed, table, or other surface or furniture (Fig. 56-1).
- Keep pins and small objects out of the baby's reach.
- Do not shake powder directly over the baby. The powder can get into the baby's eyes and lungs. Shake some on your hand away from the baby.
- Do not tie a pacifier around the baby's neck.

Holding a Baby
- Use both hands to lift a newborn. Use 1 hand to support the head and upper back. Use your other hand to support the legs. Do not lift a newborn by the arms.
- Hold the baby securely. Use the cradle hold, football hold, or shoulder hold (Fig. 56-2, p. 832).
- Support the baby's head and neck when lifting or holding the baby. Neck support is necessary for the first 3 months after birth.
- Handle the baby with gentle, smooth movements. Avoid sudden or jerking movements. Do not startle the baby.
- Hold and cuddle infants. It is comforting and helps them learn to feel love and security.

Crib and Furniture Safety
- Make sure the crib is within hearing distance of the caregivers.
- Do not put a pillow, quilts, bumper pads, or soft toys in the crib. They can cause suffocation.
- Place infants on a firm surface to sleep. Do not lay an infant on soft bedding products. This includes fluffy, plush products such as sheepskin, quilts, comforters, pillows, and toys. Soft products can cause suffocation.
- Report crib or furniture problems at once. Loose nuts, bolts, screws or bent or broken parts are examples.
- See "Crib Safety" on p. 833.
- See Appendix D (p. 909) for nursery equipment safety. Nursery equipment must be safe and in good repair.

Sleep
- Remove bibs and necklaces before sleep.
- Lay babies on their backs for sleep. *Do not lay babies on their stomachs for sleep. This can interfere with chest expansion and breathing. The baby can suffocate.* Infants can lie on their sides and stomachs when awake and supervised.
- Make sure there is no soft bedding under the baby.
- Maintain a comfortable temperature. Babies must not get too hot during sleep. Do not use clothing that may cover the infant's head or cause over-heating.

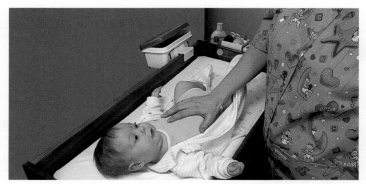

FIGURE 56-1 Keep 1 hand on a child lying on a raised surface.

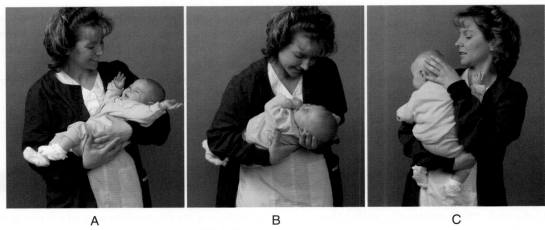

A   B   C

FIGURE 56-2 Holding a baby. **A,** The cradle hold. **B,** The football hold. **C,** The shoulder hold.

FOCUS ON LONG-TERM CARE AND HOME CARE

Safety and Security

Home Care

Injuries in the home are preventable. Safety measures can protect infants and children from harm.

- Supervise infants and children at all times.
- Use childproof locks or door knob covers leading to non-childproof areas (Fig. 56-3). Older children may try to open doors.
- Use safety gates at the top and bottom of stairs.
- Do not let children climb on furniture. Also prevent furniture from tipping.
- Remove or pad furniture with sharp or rough edges.
- Check that the crib meets federal safety standards.
- Store harmful items where children cannot reach them. Keep items in locked storage areas.
- Keep child-resistant caps on drugs and other harmful substances.
- Keep cords and strings out of reach and away from cribs and playpens.
- Use outlet safety covers or outlet plugs on electrical outlets (Chapter 14). A choking hazard, use outlet plugs with caution. The plug must not be easily removed by children.
- Keep the hot water heater temperature below 120°F (Fahrenheit) (48°C [centigrade]) to prevent burns.

- Supervise children in or near water. Prevent children from entering areas that contain water.
- Follow safety measures for car seats.
  - Use a federally approved car seat. Choose a seat based on the child's age and size (Fig. 56-4).
  - Follow the car seat manufacturer's weight and height limits. The child should use the car seat for as long as possible—until weight or height limits are outgrown.
  - Use the seat correctly. Follow the manufacturer's instructions for how to install.
  - Keep the seat rear-facing for as long as possible. See Figure 56-4.
- Check that the child's clothing is safe and fits well. Drawstrings, ribbons, and cords are hazards. Loose clothing, long clothing, and items around the neck are dangerous.
- Check that all toys are age-appropriate and are not damaged.
- Keep small items away from children. Make sure the child cannot fit items in the mouth.
- Follow the safety measures in Appendix D, p. 909.

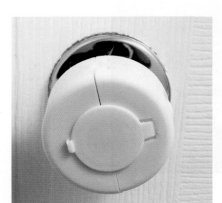

FIGURE 56-3 Door knob cover. The device turns instead of the door knob.

Using the correct car seat or booster seat can be a lifesaver: make sure your child is always buckled in an age- and size-appropriate car seat or booster seat.

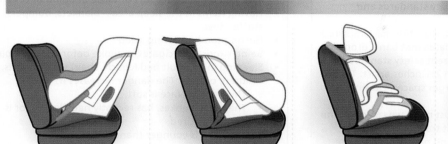

REAR-FACING CAR SEAT	**FORWARD-FACING CAR SEAT**	**BOOSTER SEAT**	**SEAT BELT**
Birth until age 2-4	**After outgrowing rear-facing seat until at least age 5**	**After outgrowing forward-facing seat and until seat belts fit properly**	**Once seat belts fit properly without a booster seat**
Buckle children in a rear-facing car seat until they reach the maximum weight or height limit of their car seat. Keep children rear-facing as long as possible.	When children outgrow their rear-facing car seat, they should be buckled in a forward-facing car seat until they reach the maximum weight or height limit of their car seat.	Once children outgrow their forward-facing seat, they should be buckled in a booster seat until seat belts fit properly. Proper seat belt fit usually occurs when children are 4 feet 9 inches tall and age 9-12.	Children no longer need to use a booster seat once seat belts fit them properly. Seat belts fit properly when the lap belt lays across the upper thighs (not the stomach) and the shoulder belt lays across the chest (not the neck).

Keep children ages 12 and under properly buckled in the back seat. Never place a rear-facing car seat in front of an active air bag.

*Recommended age ranges for each seat type vary to account for differences in child growth and height/weight limits of car seats and booster seats. Use the car seat or booster seat owner's manual to check installation and the seat height and weight limits, and proper seat use.

Child safety seat recommendations: American Academy of Pediatrics.
Graphic design: adapted from National Highway Traffic Safety Administration.

FIGURE 56-4 Car seat guidelines. (From Centers for Disease Control and Prevention, Department of Health and Human Services.)

Crib Safety

Cribs and crib linens present safety hazards. They can strangle and suffocate the baby. Mattresses, linens, and bumper pads pose many dangers. For safety:

- The sleep surface is firm, flat, and level.
- The mattress fits tightly.
- The mattress is covered with a fitted crib sheet that fits snugly.
- Sheets for larger beds are not used.
- Sheets are not used if they are frayed, worn, or have loose threads or stitching.
- Bumper pads are not used. In 2021, the *Safe Sleep for Babies Act* prohibited the manufacture and sale of crib bumpers.
- Blankets or pillows are not placed between the mattress and fitted crib sheet.
- Pillows, blankets, comforters, quilts, sheepskin, sleep positioners, and pillow-like stuffed toys and other soft products are not placed in the crib.
- Plastic trash bags, dry-cleaning bags, or plastic packaging materials are not used to protect the mattress. The plastic can cling to the baby's face, nose, and mouth. This prevents breathing and causes suffocation.

Report any hazard to the nurse.

See *Focus on Long-Term Care and Home Care: Crib Safety*, p. 834.

FOCUS ON LONG-TERM CARE AND HOME CARE

Crib Safety

Home Care

Cribs must meet federal safety standards. The American Academy of Pediatrics lists these safety standards and guidelines.

- Cribs with drop-side rails are not used. Cribs manufactured since June 2011 meet safety standards that ban a drop-side rail. Older cribs may not meet current safety standards.
- Crib slats (bars) are no more than 2⅜ inches apart. The baby's head can get caught in larger spaces, causing suffocation and death.
- Head-boards and foot-boards must not have cut-outs. The baby's head, arms, or legs can get trapped in cut-outs.
- Corner posts are flush with the end panels. Or they are very tall (as on a canopy bed). Clothing and ribbons can catch on corner posts and strangle a baby.
- Screws, bolts, nuts, plastic parts, and other hardware are original from the manufacturer and in place. Loose, missing, or replacement parts from a hardware store can cause the crib to collapse. This can trap and suffocate the baby.
- There are no rough edges or sharp points on metal parts. There are no cracks or splinters in wood.
- The mattress is the same size as the crib. There are no gaps to trap body parts. No more than 2 fingers should fit between the mattress and the sides or ends of the crib.
- Plastic wrapping from a new mattress is removed and destroyed. Plastic wrapping can suffocate a child.
- The crib is away from windows. Strangulation can occur from cords on window coverings. The Consumer Product Safety Commission (CPSC) recommends cordless window coverings.
- The following guide is used for when to lower the mattress and change beds.
  - *Before the baby can sit:* Lower the mattress so the baby cannot fall out by leaning against a side or pulling over a side.
  - *Before the child can stand:* Lower the mattress to the lowest position.
  - *When the child is 35 inches tall or when the height of the side rail is about nipple-level:* Use a different bed. Falls occur most often when a child tries to climb out of the crib.

Check the crib after assembly and then weekly for loose joints, missing or broken parts, or sharp edges. Do not use the crib if parts are missing or broken.

Sudden Unexpected Infant Death

Sudden unexpected infant death (SUID) is any sudden and unexpected death in an infant younger than 1 year old. The death may be explained or unexplained. The most common causes of SUID are:

- *Sudden infant death syndrome (SIDS)*—the sudden, unexplained death of an infant younger than 1 year old. It usually occurs during sleep.
- Accidental suffocation or strangulation in bed.
- Unknown causes.

Crib and sleep safety help prevent sudden infant death. See Box 56-2 and Figure 56-5.

BOX 56-2	Sudden Infant Death Syndrome: Sleep Safety

SIDS **Risk Factors**

- Sleeping on the stomach.
- Sleeping on soft surfaces—adult mattress, couch, chair.
- Sleeping on or under soft or loose bedding or coverings.
- Having items in the sleep area—blankets, bumpers, stuffed toys.
- Getting too hot during sleep.
- Being exposed to cigarette smoke before or after birth.
- Sleeping in an adult bed (couch, chair) with parents, other children, or pets. The danger increases if:
  - The sleep surface is soft.
  - The adult smokes, has recently had alcohol, or is drowsy or tired.
  - The baby is younger than 4 months old.
  - The baby was born early or at a low birth weight.
  - The sleep area includes unsafe items—pillows, blanket, and so on.

Safety Measures

- Lay babies on their backs to sleep—for naps and at night.
- Use a firm, flat, level sleep surface.
  - Use a crib that meets CPSC safety standards.
  - Use a tight-fitting mattress covered by a fitted sheet.
- Do not use any other bedding or soft items in the sleep area—soft objects, toys, crib bumpers, loose bedding. See "Crib Safety."
- Place babies to sleep in the same room as the parents but not in the same bed. Do so for at least the first 6 months. It is best to do so for the first year.
- Do not smoke or allow smoking around babies or in their setting—home, car, and so on.
- Offer a pacifier for sleep.
  - Do not attach the pacifier to anything that could cause suffocation, choking, or strangulation. Strings, clothing, stuffed toys, and blankets are examples.
  - Wait until babies breast-feed well before using a pacifier. For formula-fed babies, a pacifier can be offered at any time. Do not force the baby to use one.
- Do not let babies get too hot during sleep. Dress babies in clothes suitable for the room's temperature. A wearable blanket may be used. Do not use a loose blanket or over-bundle the baby. Watch for signs of over-heating—sweating, the chest feels hot to the touch. Do not cover the face or head.
- Do not use products that claim to reduce SIDS risk—wedges, positioning devices, heart and breathing monitors.
- Provide supervised time on the stomach (tummy time) when babies are awake.

Modified from Eunice Kennedy Shriver National Institute of Child Health and Human Development: What are the known risk factors? *and* Ways to reduce baby's risk, *National Institutes of Health, U.S. Department of Health and Human Services.*

WHAT DOES A SAFE SLEEP ENVIRONMENT LOOK LIKE?

The following image shows a safe sleep environment for baby.

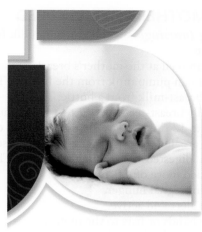

Room share: Give babies their own sleep space in your room, separate from your bed.

Use a firm, flat, and level sleep surface, covered only by a fitted sheet*.

Remove everything from baby's sleep area, except a fitted sheet to cover the mattress. No objects, toys, or other items.

Use a wearable blanket to keep baby warm without blankets in the sleep area.

Make sure baby's head and face stay uncovered during sleep.

Place babies on their backs to sleep, for naps and at night.

Couches and armchairs are not safe for baby to sleep on alone, with people, or with pets.

Keep baby's surroundings smoke/vape free.

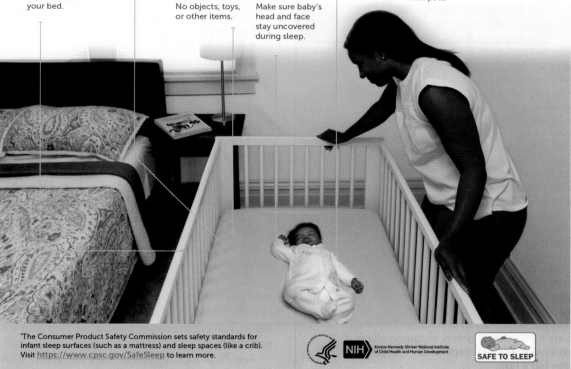

*The Consumer Product Safety Commission sets safety standards for infant sleep surfaces (such as a mattress) and sleep spaces (like a crib). Visit https://www.cpsc.gov/SafeSleep to learn more.

FIGURE 56-5 A safe sleep setting can reduce SIDS risk. (From Eunice Kennedy Shriver National Institute of Child Health and Human Development: *Safe sleep environment for baby*, U.S. Department of Health and Human Services.)

Regular wellness visits are important for infant and child health. Vaccines and breast-feeding protect against sudden infant death.

The mother's health during pregnancy affects the baby's risk. Women should receive regular prenatal care. *Prenatal care* is the health care a woman receives while pregnant. Mothers must avoid smoking, alcohol, and illegal drug use during pregnancy and after childbirth.

SIGNS AND SYMPTOMS OF ILLNESS

Babies can become ill quickly. Signs and symptoms may be sudden. You must be very alert. Report any of the signs and symptoms in Box 56-3 at once. Be alert to any change in the baby's behavior—sleep pattern, cry, appetite, or activity.

Tell the nurse when a sign or symptom began. You may need to measure the baby's temperature, pulse, and respirations (Chapter 34). The nurse tells you what temperature site to use—tympanic, rectal, temporal artery, or axillary. Apical pulses are taken on infants and young children.

BOX 56-3	Illness in Babies: Signs and Symptoms

- The baby has *jaundice*—a yellowish color to the skin and whites of the eyes.
- The baby looks sick.
- The baby has redness or drainage around the cord stump or circumcision (p. 845).
- The baby has a fever (Chapter 34).
- The baby is limp and slow to respond.
- The baby is hard to wake up.
- The baby is less active than usual.
- The baby cries all the time or does not stop crying.
- The baby screams for a long time.
- The baby is flushed, pale, or perspiring.
- The baby has noisy, rapid, difficult, or slow respirations.
- The baby is coughing or sneezing.
- The baby has reddened or irritated eyes.
- The baby turns the head to 1 side or puts a hand to 1 ear (signs of an earache).
- The baby is feeding poorly or has skipped feedings.
- The baby has vomited most of the feeding or vomits between feedings.
- The baby has watery stools or hard, formed stools.
- Stools are light-colored, green, or foul-smelling.
- The baby has fewer wet diapers.
- The baby has a rash.

HELPING MOTHERS BREAST-FEED

Breast-feeding (nursing) is feeding a baby milk from the mother's breasts.

- The baby can feed at the mother's breast.
- The mother can pump milk from the breasts. The baby is fed breast-milk from a bottle.

Babies usually breast-feed every 2 to 3 hours during the first month (8 to 12 times a day). They are fed on demand. That is, they are fed when hungry, not on a schedule. Breast-milk is digested faster than formula. Therefore nursing is needed more often.

The following signal hunger.

- Being more alert and active
- Putting the hands or fists to the mouth
- Making sucking motions with the mouth
- Turning the head to look for the breast (rooting reflex)
- Crying (may be a late sign)

Babies nurse for a short time the first few days. These early feedings are important. The mother makes a rich, thick, yellowish milk called *colostrum*. Colostrum protects the baby from infection and helps the gastro-intestinal system grow and function. By day 3 to 5, mature milk is formed. Nursing time takes longer—about 15 to 20 minutes at each breast. The rate varies for each baby. With time, feedings often are shorter and less frequent.

A feeding ends when:

- The baby's sucking slows.
- The baby pulls away from the breast.
- The baby is no longer interested in feeding.

Weight, elimination, and behavior are monitored. Babies are getting enough milk if they:

- Gain weight steadily after the first week of age.
- Pass enough clear or pale urine (p. 842). Urine is not deep yellow or orange.
- Have enough bowel movements (p. 842).
- Have short sleeping periods and wakeful, alert periods.
- Are satisfied and content after feedings.

Nurses help new mothers learn to breast-feed and about breast care. Tell the nurse if the mother or baby is having problems nursing.

Mothers may need help getting ready to nurse. They may need help with hand-washing and positioning. Provide for privacy and make sure the call light is within reach before leaving the room. Follow the care plan and the measures in Box 56-4.

See *Focus on Long-Term Care and Home Care: Helping Mothers Breast-Feed*, p. 838.

BOX 56-4	Assisting With Breast-Feeding

- Practice hand hygiene and Standard Precautions.
- Place milk, juice, or water near the mother. Most mothers become thirsty while breast-feeding.
- Help the mother wash the hands before breast-feeding.
- Help the mother to a comfortable position. The cradle position, side-lying position, and football hold are the basic positions for breast-feeding (Fig. 56-6).
- Change the baby's diaper if necessary. Bring the baby to the mother.
- Provide for privacy. Close doors and window coverings. A baby blanket or nursing cover can be used if desired.
- Make sure the mother holds the baby close to the breast.
- Have the mother use the nipple to stroke the baby's cheek or lower lip. This stimulates the *rooting reflex* (Chapter 11). The baby turns the head toward the breast and starts to suck.
- Make sure the baby's nose is not blocked by the mother's breast. One nostril must be clear for breathing. If the nose seems blocked, have the mother do 1 of the following.
  - Re-position the baby. The mother can raise the baby's hips or move the baby's head back slightly.
  - Use the thumb to keep breast tissue away from the baby's nose (Fig. 56-7, p. 838).
- Encourage nursing from both breasts at each feeding. If the last feeding ended at the right breast, the next feeding is started at the right breast. The mother can use a ribbon or diaper pin on a bra strap as a reminder of which breast to start with.

- Remind the mother how to remove the baby from the breast. To break the suction between the baby and the breast, the mother can insert a finger into a corner of the baby's mouth (Fig. 56-8, p. 838).
- Help the mother burp the baby (p. 841). The baby is burped after nursing at 1 breast. Then the baby is burped after nursing at the other breast.
- Remind the mother to air-dry the nipples after a feeding.
- Change the baby's diaper after the feeding.
- Lay the baby in the crib if the baby has fallen asleep. *Lay the baby on the back. Do not lay the baby on the stomach.*
- Help the mother prevent dry and cracked nipples. Follow the nurse's directions and the care plan.
  - Milk is left on the nipple after a feeding. The milk is allowed to air-dry.
  - The mother applies prescribed ointment or cream after each feeding if the nipples are cracked. If directed, remind the mother to wash the breasts with water before a feeding to remove the ointment or cream.
  - A clean washcloth and warm water are used to gently wash the breasts and nipples. Soap is not used.
  - Nipples are air-dried to help prevent cracking and soreness.
- Help the mother straighten clothing after the feeding if necessary.
- Encourage the mother to wear a nursing bra day and night. The bra supports the breasts and promotes comfort.
- Encourage the mother to place nursing pads in the bra. The pads absorb leaking milk.

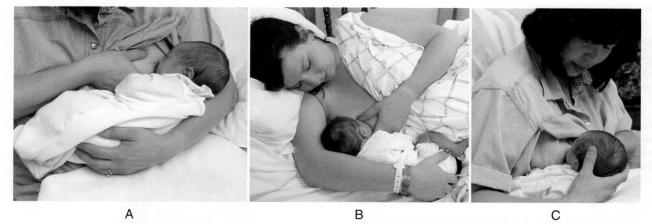

A   B   C

FIGURE 56-6 Basic breast-feeding positions. **A,** Cradle position. **B,** Side-lying position. **C,** Football hold. (From James SR, Nelson KA, Ashwill JW: *Nursing care of children: principles and practice*, ed 4, St Louis, 2013, Saunders.)

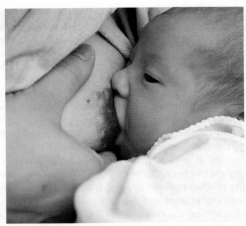

FIGURE 56-7 The mother supports the breast with 1 hand. The thumb is on top of the breast to keep breast tissue away from the baby's nose. (From James SR, Nelson KA, Ashwill JW: *Nursing care of children: principles and practice*, ed 4, St Louis, 2013, Saunders.)

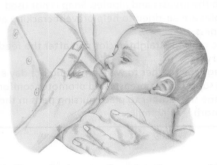

FIGURE 56-8 The mother inserts a finger into the corner of the baby's mouth to remove the baby from the breast. (From James SR, Ashwill JW, Droske SC: *Nursing care of children: principles and practice*, ed 2, Philadelphia, 2002, Saunders.)

BOTTLE-FEEDING BABIES

Babies who are not breast-fed use formula. The doctor prescribes the formula. It provides the nutrients the infant needs.

Formula comes in 3 forms.
- *Ready-to-feed.* Ready to use, it is poured from the container into a baby bottle (Fig. 56-9). The container may have more than 1 feeding. Refrigerate after opening. Use the contents within 48 hours.
- *Powdered.* Container directions tell how much powder and water to use.
- *Liquid concentrate.* Container directions tell you how much liquid and water to use.

Bottles are prepared 1 at a time or in batches for the whole day. To prepare a bottle:
- Practice hand hygiene.
- Use water from a safe water source as directed by the nurse.
  - Bottled water.
  - Tap water. State and local health departments determine tap water safety.
  - Boiled tap water. Bring cold tap water to a boil for 1 minute. Cool to room temperature for no more than 30 minutes.
- Follow the container directions carefully. Measure exact amounts.
- Pour the correct amount of water and formula into the bottle.
- Gently shake or swirl the bottle to mix.
- Check the temperature by placing drops on the inside of your wrist. The formula should feel warm, not hot.
- Cap extra bottles (Fig. 56-10). Store them in the refrigerator. Use stored bottles within 24 hours.

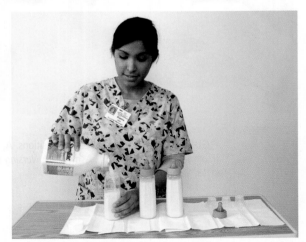

FIGURE 56-9 Ready-to-feed formula is poured from the container into the bottle.

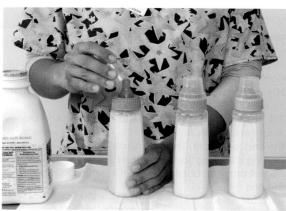

FIGURE 56-10 Bottles are capped for storage in the refrigerator.

Cleaning Baby Bottles

Protect the baby from infection. Baby bottles, caps, nipples, and other items must be clean. Disposable equipment is often used in hospitals. Reusable equipment is common in homes. It is carefully washed in hot, soapy water or in a dishwasher. Complete rinsing is needed to remove all soap. Some bottles have plastic liners that are discarded after 1 use.

See *Delegation Guidelines: Cleaning Baby Bottles.*
See *Promoting Safety and Comfort: Cleaning Baby Bottles.*
See procedure: *Cleaning Baby Bottles.*

Cleaning Baby Bottles

PRE-PROCEDURE

1 Follow *Delegation Guidelines: Cleaning Baby Bottles.* See *Promoting Safety and Comfort: Cleaning Baby Bottles.*
2 Practice hand hygiene and get the following supplies.
- Bottles, nipples, caps, and any other bottle parts (rings, valves, and so on)
- Wash basin—clean, used only for washing baby-feeding items
- Bottle brush—clean, used only for washing baby-feeding items (use a brush that will not scratch or damage items)
- Dishwashing soap
- Other items used to prepare formula
- Towel
- Gloves (if needed)

PROCEDURE

3 Follow agency policy for glove use. Apply gloves if needed.
4 Take apart the bottles. Separate the parts of each bottle—bottle, nipple, cap, and any other parts.
5 Rinse the bottles, nipples, caps, and other bottle parts in warm or cold running water.
6 Place the items in the basin.
7 Fill the basin with hot water. Add dishwashing soap.
8 Wash the bottles, nipples, caps, and other bottle parts. Wash any other items used to prepare formula.
9 Clean inside baby bottles with the bottle brush (Fig. 56-11, p. 840).
10 Squeeze hot, soapy water through the nipples (Fig. 56-12, p. 840).
11 Rinse all items thoroughly. Squeeze water through the nipples to remove soap.
12 Lay a clean towel on the counter. Or use a drying rack as directed.
13 Stand bottles upside down to drain. Place nipples, caps, and other items on the towel or on the drying rack. Let the items air-dry.
14 Rinse the basin and bottle brush well. Let them air-dry after use.
15 Remove and discard gloves if worn. Practice hand hygiene.
16 Follow agency policies and procedures to sanitize or sterilize items.

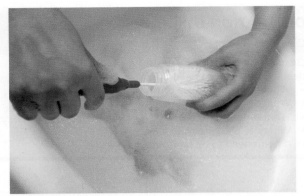

FIGURE 56-11 A bottle brush is used to clean inside a baby bottle.

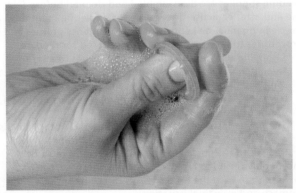

FIGURE 56-12 Water is squeezed through the nipple during washing and rinsing.

BOX 56-5	Bottle-Feeding Babies

- Warm a refrigerated bottle. The formula should feel warm to the inside of your wrist (Fig. 56-13).
- Assume a comfortable position for the feeding.
- Hold the baby close to you. Relax and snuggle the baby.
- Stroke the baby's cheek or lip with the nipple. The baby's head will turn to the nipple.
- Tilt the bottle so that the neck of the bottle and the nipple are always full (Fig. 56-14). Otherwise some air is in the neck or nipple. The baby sucks air into the stomach, causing cramping and discomfort.
- Do not prop the bottle and lay the baby down for the feeding (Fig. 56-15).
- Burp the newborn after every ½ to 1 ounce of formula. (Measurements are marked on the bottle.) Older babies are burped less often—after every 2 to 3 ounces. Also burp the baby at the end of the feeding.
- Do not leave the baby alone with a bottle.
- Do not force the baby to finish the bottle.
- Discard remaining formula. Do not save or reheat it for another feeding.
- Wash the bottle, cap, nipple, and any other bottle parts after the feeding (see procedure: *Cleaning Baby Bottles*).

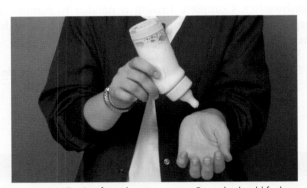

FIGURE 56-13 Testing formula temperature. Formula should feel warm on the inside of your wrist.

Feeding the Baby

Formula-fed babies usually want to be fed every 2 to 4 hours. They are fed on demand. The amount of formula taken increases as they grow older. The nurse or the mother tells you how much formula a baby needs at each feeding. Babies usually take as much formula as they need. The baby stops sucking and turns away from the bottle when satisfied.

Most babies do not like cold formula out of the refrigerator. To warm a bottle, hold the bottle under warm running tap water or in a container of warm water. Turn the bottle to warm the formula evenly.

The formula should feel warm. To test the temperature, sprinkle a few drops on the inside of your wrist. Allow the formula to cool if it is hot. The guidelines in Box 56-5 will help you bottle-feed babies.

Solid foods are given around 6 months. Usually baby rice or oatmeal cereal is the first solid food given. The cereal is mixed with breast-milk or formula to a thin consistency. Other solid foods are added as the baby grows. The nurse tells you what foods the baby can have.

See *Promoting Safety and Comfort: Feeding the Baby*.

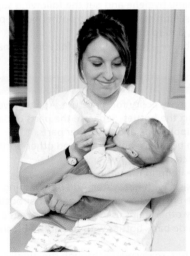

FIGURE 56-14 The bottle is tilted so that formula fills the bottle neck and nipple.

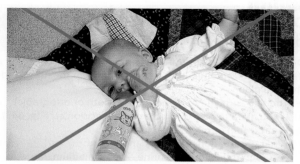

FIGURE 56-15 Do NOT prop the bottle to feed the baby.

PROMOTING SAFETY AND COMFORT

Feeding the Baby

Safety

Do not set the bottle out to warm at room temperature. This takes too long and allows the growth of microbes. Do not heat formula in microwave ovens. The formula can heat unevenly and burn the baby's mouth.

BURPING THE BABY

Babies take in air during feedings. Air in the stomach and intestines causes cramping and discomfort. This can lead to vomiting. Burping helps to get rid of the air. Most babies burp mid-way and after a feeding.

To burp a baby, gently pat or rub the baby's back with circular motions. Figure 56-16 shows how to position the baby for burping.

- *Over the shoulder.* First place a clean towel or rag (burp rag, burp cloth) over your shoulder. This protects your clothing if the baby "spits up." Then hold the infant over your shoulder.
- *On your lap.* Support the baby in a sitting position on your lap. Hold the towel (rag) in front of the baby. *Remember to support the infant's head and neck for the first 3 months after birth.*
- *On the baby's stomach.* First place a clean towel (rag) on your lap where the baby's head will be. Position the baby on your lap with the stomach down.

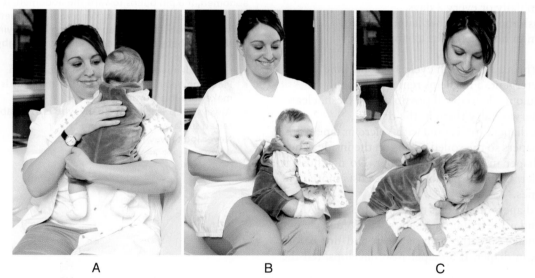

FIGURE 56-16 Burping a baby. **A,** The baby is held over the shoulder. **B,** The baby is supported in the sitting position. **C,** The baby is laid on the stomach.

DIAPERING A BABY

A newborn's first bowel movement is a dark green to black, tarry bowel movement called *meconium*. By day 3 or 4, stools are greenish brown to yellowish brown in color and less sticky. By day 4 or 5:

- *Breast-fed babies*—have yellow and seedy-looking stools. They are soft or runny. Breast-fed babies usually have a bowel movement (BM) with every feeding.
- *Formula-fed babies*—have yellow to brown stools. Formula-fed babies have fewer stools than breast-fed babies and their stools are firmer. They may have 1 or 2 stools a day.

Over time, an elimination pattern develops. Some babies have 1, 2, or 3 stools a day. Stools are usually soft and unformed. Hard, formed stools signal constipation. Watery stools mean diarrhea. Diarrhea is very serious in infants. Their fluid balance is upset quickly (Chapter 32). Tell the nurse at once if you suspect constipation or diarrhea.

Babies wet at least 6 to 8 times a day. Diapers are changed when wet or when stools are present.

Cloth diapers are re-used. With Velcro fasteners, no diaper pins are needed. The danger of sticking the baby or yourself with a diaper pin is avoided. To care for cloth diapers:

- Rinse a soiled cloth diaper. Rinse stools into the toilet.
- Store soiled diapers in a diaper pail.
- Wash them daily or every 2 days.
- Do not wash them with other laundry items.
- Wash them in hot water. Use a baby laundry detergent.
- Put them through the wash cycle a second time without detergent. This helps remove all soap.
- Hang them outside to dry if possible for a fresh, clean smell. Otherwise, dry them in the dryer.

Disposable diapers are secured with Velcro or tape strips. Fold soiled diapers so the soiled area is on the inside. Then discard the diaper in the trash container. Do not flush it down the toilet. Using disposable diapers costs more than using cloth ones.

Changing diapers often helps prevent diaper rash. Moisture, stools, and urine irritate the baby's skin. When changing diapers, make sure the baby is clean and dry before applying a clean diaper. If a diaper rash develops, tell the nurse at once.

See *Delegation Guidelines: Diapering a Baby*.
See *Promoting Safety and Comfort: Diapering a Baby*.
See procedure: *Diapering a Baby*.

DELEGATION GUIDELINES
Diapering a Baby

Diapering a baby is a routine nursing task. Before changing a baby's diaper, you need this information from the nurse and the care plan.

- The size and type of diaper to use (cloth or disposable)
- If you need to give cord care or circumcision care (p. 845)
- What cream or ointment to use
- What observations to report and record:
  - Color and amount of urine—small, medium, large
  - Color, amount, consistency, and odor of stools
  - Condition of the baby's skin and genital area
  - Redness or irritation of the skin or genital area
  - Blood or discharge on the diaper
- When to report observations
- What concerns about the baby to report at once

PROMOTING SAFETY AND COMFORT
Diapering a Baby

Safety
Older babies can tear and pull disposable diapers apart. They can choke or suffocate on diaper material if placed in the nose or mouth. Observe babies closely. Change any torn or damaged diaper at once.

Diaper pins for cloth diapers must point away from the abdomen. If a pin opens toward the abdomen, it can pierce the skin and damage organs. Keep your hand between the pin and the baby's skin when removing or applying a pin.

Keep the baby safe during diapering. The baby may squirm, wiggle, or kick and cry. To prevent falls:

- Gather all needed supplies before you begin.
- Place the baby on a firm surface. If the baby is on a table, make sure it is sturdy.
- Always keep 1 hand on a baby who is on a table or other raised surface.
- Never look away from the baby.

Diapering a Baby

- Knock before entering the baby's room.
- Address the baby and parents by name.
- Introduce yourself by name and title.

- Explain the procedure to the parents before starting and during the procedure.
- Protect the baby's rights during the procedure.
- Handle the baby gently during the procedure.

PRE-PROCEDURE

1 Follow *Delegation Guidelines: Diapering a Baby*. See *Promoting Safety and Comfort: Diapering a Baby*.
2 Practice hand hygiene and get the following supplies.
- Gloves
- Clean diaper
- Waterproof changing pad
- Washcloth and towel or disposable wipes

- Basin of warm water (if needed)
- Baby soap (if needed)
- Laundry bag (if needed)
- Cream or ointment as directed by the nurse
3 Arrange items in your work area.
4 Provide for privacy.

PROCEDURE

5 Practice hand hygiene. Put on gloves.
6 Place the changing pad under the baby.
7 Unfasten the clothing and dirty diaper. Place diaper pins out of the baby's reach if used.
8 Wipe the genital area with the front of the diaper (Fig. 56-17, *A*, p. 844). Wipe from the front to the back (top to bottom).
9 Note the color and amount of urine and stools. Fold the diaper so urine and stools are inside. Set the diaper aside.
10 Clean the genital area from front to back (top to bottom). Use a wet washcloth or disposable wipes (Fig. 56-17, *B*, p. 844). Wash with mild soap and water for a large amount of stools or if the baby has a rash. Rinse thoroughly and pat the area dry. Place a used washcloth and towel in the laundry bag. Discard used wipes.
11 Remove and discard soiled gloves. Practice hand hygiene. Put on clean gloves.
12 Clean the circumcision (p. 845). Follow the nurse's instructions for cord care (p. 845).
13 Apply cream or ointment to the genital area and buttocks. Do not use too much. Caking can occur.

14 Raise the baby's legs. Slide a clean diaper under the buttocks.
15 Fold a cloth diaper as shown in Figure 56-18 (p. 844).
  a *For a boy:* The extra thickness is in the front (see Fig. 56-18, *A*).
  b *For a girl:* The extra thickness is at the back (see Fig. 56-18, *B*).
  c Bring the diaper between the baby's legs.
16 Make sure the diaper is snug around the hips and abdomen.
  a It is loose near the penis if the circumcision has not healed.
  b It is below the umbilicus if the cord stump has not healed.
17 Secure the diaper in place (Fig. 56-19, p. 844). Use the tape strips or Velcro on disposable diapers (see Fig. 56-19, *A*). Make sure the tabs stick in place. Use baby pins or Velcro for cloth diapers. Pins point away from the abdomen (see Fig. 56-19, *B*).
18 Apply a diaper cover or waterproof pants if cloth diapers are worn. Secure the baby's clothing.
19 Put the baby in the crib, infant seat, or other safe place.

POST-PROCEDURE

20 Clean up and store supplies and equipment. (Wear gloves. Change gloves as needed.)
  a Dispose of stools from a cloth diaper in the toilet and flush. Store used cloth diapers in a designated covered pail.
  b Discard disposable items. Put a disposable diaper in the trash.
  c Follow agency procedures to clean and disinfect re-usable equipment. Return supplies and equipment to their proper place.
  d Follow agency policy for used linens.
  e Remove and discard gloves. Practice hand hygiene.

21 Ask the parent what privacy measures to maintain. Follow the parent's preferences.
22 Complete a safety check of the room. (See the inside of the back cover.)
23 Practice hand hygiene.
24 Report and record your care and observations.

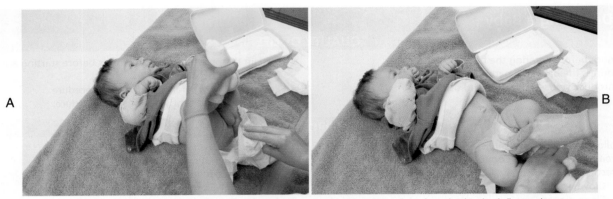

FIGURE 56-17 **A,** The front of the diaper is used to wipe the genital area from front (top) to back (bottom). **B,** A disposable wipe is used to clean the genital area from front (top) to back (bottom).

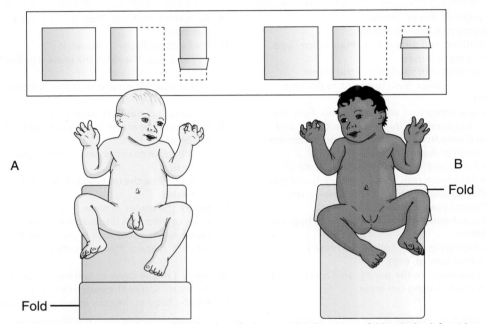

FIGURE 56-18 **A,** A cloth diaper is folded in front for boys. **B,** The diaper has a fold in the back for girls.

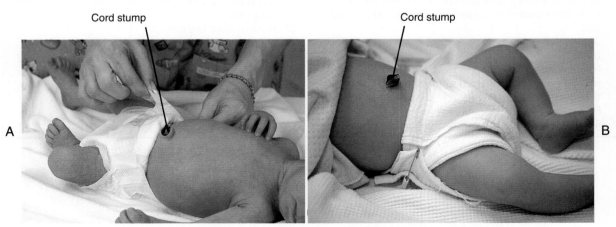

FIGURE 56-19 Securing a diaper. **A,** A disposable diaper is secured in place with tape strips. **B,** Diaper pins secure a cloth diaper. Pins point away from the abdomen. Note: The diapers in A and B are below the cord stump.

UMBILICAL CORD CARE

The *umbilical cord* connects the mother and fetus (unborn baby). It carries blood, oxygen, and nutrients from the mother to the fetus (Fig. 56-20). The cord is not needed after birth. Shortly after delivery, the cord is clamped and cut. A cord stump is left on the baby (see Fig. 56-19). The stump dries up and falls off usually within 3 weeks after birth. Slight bleeding can occur when the cord comes off.

The cord provides a place for microbes to grow. Keep the cord clean and dry. Cord care is done at each diaper change. Cord care is continued for 1 or 2 days after the cord comes off. It involves the following.

- Do not get the stump wet.
- Keep the diaper below the cord as in Figure 56-19. This prevents the diaper from irritating the stump. It also keeps the cord from becoming wet from urine.
- Give sponge baths until the cord falls off. Then the baby can have a tub bath.
- Do not pull the cord off—even if it looks ready to fall off.
- Report the following.
  - Swelling, redness, odor, or drainage from the navel area
  - Bleeding from the navel area
  - Fever
  - Crying when the cord or skin near the cord is touched

See *Promoting Safety and Comfort: Umbilical Cord Care.*

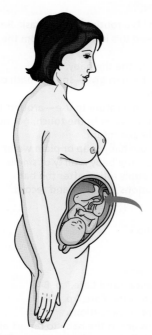

FIGURE 56-20 The umbilical cord connects the mother and fetus.

CIRCUMCISION CARE

Boys are born with foreskin on the penis. The surgical removal of foreskin from the penis is called a *circumcision* (Chapter 24). The procedure is optional. The parents decide whether or not to circumcise.

Circumcision is thought to:

- Allow for easier hygiene.
- Prevent urinary tract infections in infants.
- Lower the risk of cancer of the penis.
- Prevent problems with foreskin retraction. Some foreskin is too tight to be pulled back (retracted) over the penis.
- Decrease the risk of certain sexually transmitted diseases (infections).

The procedure is usually done within 10 days after birth. It is often performed within the first 2 days. Circumcision is a religious ceremony in the Jewish and Islamic faiths.

The tip of the penis is often sore and may look red, swollen, or bruised. However, the entire penis should not be swollen. And the circumcision should not interfere with voiding. Carefully observe for signs of infection. There should be no odor, drainage, or fever. A slight yellowish discharge or crust at the tip of the penis is normal. It does not signal infection. A small amount of bleeding can occur. Excessive bleeding (more than a quarter-sized amount on the diaper) needs to be reported. Report any concerns at once. The area should heal in 7 to 10 days.

Circumcision care involves the following.

- Clean the penis at each diaper change. This is very important after a BM.
- Use mild soap and water or plain water as the nurse directs.
- Apply a petrolatum gauze dressing or petrolatum jelly to the penis as the nurse directs. This protects the penis from urine and stools. It also prevents the penis from sticking to the diaper. A cotton swab is used to apply the petrolatum jelly (Fig. 56-21, p. 846).
- Apply the diaper loosely. This prevents the diaper from irritating the penis.

See *Promoting Safety and Comfort: Circumcision Care,* p. 846.

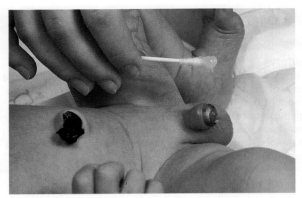

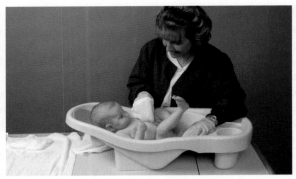

FIGURE 56-22 The baby is given a bath in a baby bathtub.

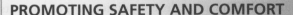

FIGURE 56-21 Petrolatum jelly is applied to the circumcised penis.

PROMOTING SAFETY AND COMFORT

Circumcision Care

Safety

In the uncircumcised baby, foreskin covers the penis (Chapter 24). Foreskin does not retract (pull back) until later in childhood. *Do not retract a baby's foreskin.* Forcing the foreskin to retract can cause pain, tearing, and bleeding. When bathing, gently clean the penis with soap and water.

▌▌ BATHING AN INFANT

Infants do not need a bath every day. Bathing too often can cause dry skin. Bathing 3 times a week is common. Areas with creases need special attention—under the arms, behind the ears, around the neck, and the genital area. Also wash and dry well between the fingers and toes.

Baths comfort and relax babies. They provide a wonderful time to hold, touch, and talk to babies. Stimulation is important for development. Being touched and held helps babies learn safety, security, and love and belonging.

Planning for the bath is important. You cannot leave the baby alone if you forget something. Gather needed equipment, supplies, and the baby's clothes before you start the bath. Everything you need must be within your reach.

There are 2 bath procedures for babies. Sponge baths are given until the cord stump falls off and the umbilicus and circumcision heal. *The cord must not get wet.* A bath in a baby bathtub is given after the cord site and circumcision heal (Fig. 56-22).

See *Focus on Long-Term Care and Home Care: Bathing an Infant.*

See *Delegation Guidelines: Bathing an Infant.*

See *Promoting Safety and Comfort: Bathing an Infant.*

See procedure: *Giving a Baby a Sponge Bath.*

See procedure: *Giving a Baby a Bath in a Baby Bathtub,* p. 849.

FOCUS ON LONG-TERM CARE AND HOME CARE

Bathing an Infant

Home Care

Families have routines. Some babies are bathed in the morning. The baby is more alert and ready to interact at this time. Others bathe in the evening. Evening baths:

- Comfort and relax the baby. This helps some babies sleep longer at night.
- Allow a parent who works during the day to be involved in the bath.

Sometimes 1 parent bathes the baby so the other parent can rest or tend to other children. Follow the family's routine when working in the home.

DELEGATION GUIDELINES

Bathing an Infant

Bathing an infant is a routine nursing task. Before bathing an infant, you need this information from the nurse and the care plan.

- How often to bathe the baby.
- What type of bath to give—sponge bath or a bath in a baby bathtub.
- What water temperature to use—around 100°F (37.8°C). Water should be warm to the touch, not hot or cool.
- When to bathe the infant.
- If you should use baby soap or plain water. Usually soap is not used unless the baby is dirty or smells.
- If you should apply lotion after the bath.
- What observations to report and record:
  - Bruising
  - Rashes
  - Skin irritation
  - Redness
  - Swelling
  - Open skin areas
  - See "Umbilical Cord Care," p. 845
  - See "Circumcision Care," p. 845
- When to report observations.
- What concerns about the baby to report at once.

PROMOTING SAFETY AND COMFORT
Bathing an Infant

Safety
To protect an infant during a bath, follow these safety measures.

- Turn up the thermostat and close windows and doors about 20 minutes before the bath. Room temperature should be 75°F to 80°F for the bath. The room may be too warm for you. Remove a sweater or lab coat or roll up your sleeves before starting the bath.
- Measure bath water temperature with a water thermometer. The nurse tells you what temperature to use (around 100°F [37.8°C]). Test water temperature with the inside of your wrist (Fig. 56-23). The water should feel warm and comfortable. Babies have delicate skin and are easily burned.
- Use a baby bathtub manufactured on or after October 2, 2017. Such tubs meet current safety standards. Follow the manufacturer's instructions for use of the bathtub.

- Never carry a baby in a baby bathtub.
- Never leave the baby alone on a table or in a baby bathtub.
- Always keep 1 hand on the baby if you must look away for a moment.
- Hold the baby securely during the bath. Babies are slippery when they are wet. A wet, squirming baby is hard to hold.
- Keep the baby's face out of the water.

Comfort
Keep the baby warm and comfortable during the bath. For a sponge bath, cover the table or other bathing surface with a towel. You can also wrap the baby in a towel and expose only the body parts being washed. When in a baby bathtub, pour warm water over the baby's body during the bath.

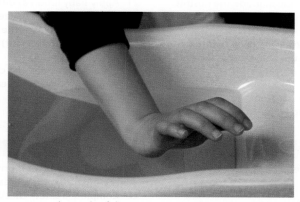

FIGURE 56-23 The inside of the wrist is used to test bath water temperature.

Giving a Baby a Sponge Bath

QUALITY OF LIFE

- Knock before entering the baby's room.
- Address the baby and parents by name.
- Introduce yourself by name and title.

- Explain the procedure to the parents before starting and during the procedure.
- Protect the baby's rights during the procedure.
- Handle the baby gently during the procedure.

PRE-PROCEDURE

1 Follow *Delegation Guidelines: Bathing an Infant.* See *Promoting Safety and Comfort: Bathing an Infant.*
2 Practice hand hygiene and get the following supplies.
   - Baby bathtub
   - Water thermometer
   - Bath towel
   - 2 hand towels
   - Receiving blanket
   - Washcloth
   - Items for diaper changing (see procedure: *Diapering a Baby*, p. 843)
   - Clean clothing for the baby
   - Cotton balls

   - Baby soap (if needed)
   - Baby shampoo
   - Baby lotion
   - Petrolatum gauze or petrolatum jelly (if needed)
   - Laundry bag
   - Gloves
3 Arrange items in your work area.
4 Practice hand hygiene.
5 Identify the baby. Check the identification (ID) bracelet against the assignment sheet. Use 2 identifiers (Chapter 14). Follow agency policy.
6 Provide for privacy.

Continued

Giving a Baby a Sponge Bath—cont'd

PROCEDURE

7. Fill the baby bathtub with 2 to 3 inches of warm water. Water temperature should be around 100°F (37.8°C). Measure water temperature with the water thermometer or use the inside of your wrist. The water should feel warm and comfortable.
8. Put on gloves.
9. Undress the baby. Leave the diaper on.
10. Wash the baby's eye lids (Fig. 56-24).
    a. Dip a cotton ball into the water.
    b. Squeeze out excess water.
    c. Wash 1 eye lid from the inner part to the outer part.
    d. Repeat this step for the other eye with a new cotton ball.
11. Moisten the washcloth and make a mitt (Chapter 24). Clean the outside of the ear and then behind the ear. Repeat this step for the other ear. Be gentle. *Do not use cotton swabs to clean inside the ears.*
12. Rinse and squeeze out the washcloth. Make a mitt with the washcloth.
13. Wash the baby's face (Fig. 56-25). Clean inside the nostrils with the washcloth. Do not use cotton swabs to clean inside the nose. Pat the face dry.
14. Pick up the baby. Hold the baby over the baby bathtub using the football hold. Support the baby's head and neck with your wrist and hand.
15. Wash the baby's head (Fig. 56-26).
    a. Squeeze a small amount of water from the washcloth onto the baby's head. Or bring water to the baby's head using a cupped hand.
    b. Apply a small amount of baby shampoo to the head.
    c. Wash the head with circular motions.
    d. Rinse the head by squeezing water from a washcloth over the baby's head. Or bring water to the baby's head using a cupped hand. Rinse thoroughly. Do not get soap in the baby's eyes.
    e. Use a small hand towel to dry the head.
16. Lay the baby on the table.
17. Remove the diaper. (If the baby is soiled, perform steps 8 through 11 in procedure: *Diapering a Baby* on p. 843.)
18. Wash the front of the body with a washcloth or your hands. Do not get the cord wet. Also wash the arms, hands, fingers, legs, feet, and toes. Wash the genital area and all creases and folds. Rinse thoroughly. Pat dry.
19. Follow the nurse's instructions for cord care. Clean the circumcision.
20. Turn the baby to the prone position. Wash the back and buttocks. Use a washcloth or your hands. Rinse thoroughly. Pat dry.
21. Apply baby lotion as directed by the nurse.
22. Apply petrolatum gauze or petrolatum jelly to the circumcised penis as the nurse directs.
23. Apply cream (ointment) to the genital area and buttocks if directed.
24. Put a clean diaper and clean clothes on the baby.
25. Wrap the baby in the receiving blanket. Put the baby in the crib or other safe area.

POST-PROCEDURE

26. Clean up and store supplies and equipment. (Wear gloves. Change gloves as needed.)
    a. Discard disposable items.
    b. Follow agency procedures to clean and disinfect re-usable equipment. Return supplies and equipment to their proper place.
    c. Follow agency policy for used linens.
    d. Remove and discard gloves. Practice hand hygiene.
27. Ask the parent what privacy measures to maintain. Follow the parent's preferences.
28. Complete a safety check of the room. (See the inside of the back cover.)
29. Practice hand hygiene.
30. Report and record your care and observations.

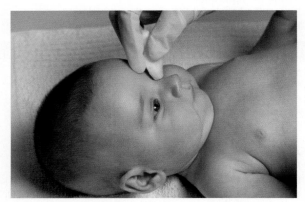

FIGURE 56-24 Wash the baby's eyes with cotton balls. The eye lids are cleaned from the inner to the outer part.

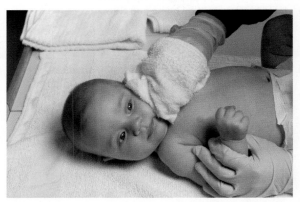

FIGURE 56-25 The baby's face is washed with a mitted washcloth.

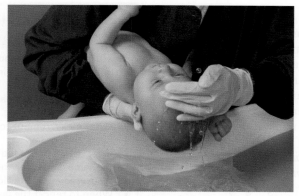

FIGURE 56-26 The baby's head is washed over the baby bathtub.

Giving a Baby a Bath in a Baby Bathtub

QUALITY OF LIFE

- Knock before entering the baby's room.
- Address the baby and parents by name.
- Introduce yourself by name and title.

- Explain the procedure to the parents before beginning and during the procedure.
- Protect the baby's rights during the procedure.
- Handle the baby gently during the procedure.

PROCEDURE

1 Follow steps 1 through 17 in procedure: *Giving a Baby a Sponge Bath* (p. 847).
2 Hold the baby as in Figure 56-27.
  a Place 1 hand under the baby's shoulders. Your thumb should be over the baby's shoulder. Your fingers should be under the arm.
  b Support the buttocks with your other hand. Slide your hand under the thighs. Hold the far thigh with your other hand.
3 Lower the baby into the water feet first.

4 Wash the front of the baby's body. Also wash the arms, hands, fingers, legs, feet, and toes. Wash the genital area and all creases and folds.
5 Wash the baby's back and buttocks. (Hold the baby securely. Keep the baby's face out of the water.)
6 Rinse thoroughly.
7 Lift the baby out of the water and onto a towel.
8 Wrap the baby in the towel. Also cover the baby's head.
9 Pat the baby dry. Dry all creases and folds.
10 Apply baby lotion as directed by the nurse.
11 Follow steps 23 through 30 in procedure: *Giving a Baby a Sponge Bath.*

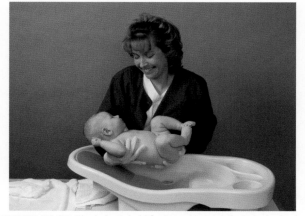

FIGURE 56-27 The baby is held for lowering into the baby bathtub.

NAIL CARE

The baby's fingernails and toenails are kept short. Otherwise, the baby can scratch the self and others. Nails are best cut after a bath or when the baby is sleeping. The sleeping baby is quiet and will not squirm or fuss. Use infant nail clippers and a soft emery board.

- Hold the finger or toe with 1 hand.
- Press the skin under the nail. This moves the skin out of the way to avoid pinching or cutting the skin.
- Trim the nails with an infant nail clipper.
  - *Fingernails:* Clip following the natural shape of the nail.
  - *Toenails:* Clip straight across as for an adult (Chapter 25).
- Smooth rough or sharp edges with a soft emery board.

WEIGHING INFANTS

The infant's birth weight is a baseline for measuring growth. The nurse uses weight measurements in the assessment step of the nursing process. They also are used to measure the amount of breast-milk taken in during breast-feeding. The baby is weighed before and after breast-feeding. The difference in the weights is the amount of milk taken in during breast-feeding. It tells the nurse if the baby is getting enough milk.

See *Focus on Math: Weighing Infants.*
See *Delegation Guidelines: Weighing Infants.*
See *Promoting Safety and Comfort: Weighing Infants.*
See procedure: *Weighing an Infant.*

FOCUS ON MATH

Weighing Infants

 Weight can be measured in pounds or kilograms (Chapter 37). For weighing infants, the following may be used.

- Pounds (lb) and ounces (oz). There are 16 ounces in 1 pound. (NOTE: Ounces used for weight are different than ounces used for liquid measurements [Chapter 32].)
- Kilograms (kg). See Chapter 37 for converting kilograms and pounds.
- Grams (g). There are 1000 grams in 1 kilogram. Grams are often used for "before" and "after" feeding weights.

Know what is used in your agency. Follow agency policy for reporting and recording.

For a "before" and "after" feeding weight, subtract the infant's "before" weight from the "after" weight. The nurse uses the weight difference to calculate the amount of breast-milk taken in.

For example, a baby's "before" feeding weight is 2720 grams. After feeding, the baby weighs 2750 grams. You report a weight change of 30 grams.

*2750 grams (after feeding) – 2720 grams (before feeding)
= 30 grams (weight change)*

DELEGATION GUIDELINES

Weighing Infants

Measuring weight is a routine nursing task. Before weighing an infant, you need this information from the nurse and the care plan.
- When to weigh the baby.
- What scale to use (Fig. 56-28).
- What measurement to use—pounds and ounces, kilograms, grams.
- If the baby is breast-fed or bottle-fed. Breast-fed babies wear the same diaper for "before" and "after" feeding weight measurements. The clothes and blanket are removed.
- When to report the weight measurement.
- What concerns about the baby to report at once.

PROMOTING SAFETY AND COMFORT

Weighing Infants

Safety
You must meet the baby's safety needs. Protect the baby from chills. Keep the room warm and free of drafts. Also protect the baby from falling. Always keep a hand over the baby when measuring weight. Remember to keep 1 hand on the baby if you need to look away.

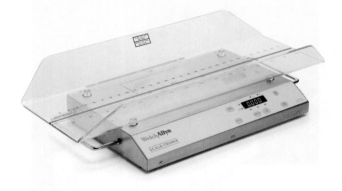

FIGURE 56-28 Digital infant scale. (Courtesy Welch Allyn, Skaneateles Falls, NY.)

Weighing an Infant

QUALITY OF LIFE

- Knock before entering the baby's room.
- Address the baby and parents by name.
- Introduce yourself by name and title.

- Explain the procedure to the parents before beginning and during the procedure.
- Protect the baby's rights during the procedure.
- Handle the baby gently during the procedure.

PRE-PROCEDURE

1 Follow *Delegation Guidelines: Weighing Infants.* See *Promoting Safety and Comfort: Weighing Infants.*
2 Practice hand hygiene and get the following supplies.
   - Baby scale (see Fig. 56-28)
   - Paper for the scale
   - Items for diaper changing (see procedure: *Diapering a Baby,* p. 843)
   - Gloves

3 Arrange items in your work area.
4 Practice hand hygiene.
5 Identify the baby. Check the ID bracelet against the assignment sheet. Use 2 identifiers (Chapter 14). Follow agency policy.
6 Provide for privacy.

PROCEDURE

7 Place the paper on the scale. Adjust the scale to zero (0).
8 Put on gloves.
9 Undress the baby and remove the diaper as directed. (See *Delegation Guidelines: Weighing Infants.*) Clean the genital area. Remove and discard the gloves and practice hand hygiene. Put on clean gloves.

10 Lay the baby on the scale. Keep 1 hand over the baby to prevent falling.
11 Read the digital display or move the weights until the scale is balanced (Chapter 37).
12 Note the measurement.
13 Take the baby off of the scale.
14 Diaper and dress the baby. Lay the baby in the crib.

POST-PROCEDURE

15 Clean up and store supplies and equipment.
   a Discard the paper and soiled diaper.
   b Disinfect the scale following agency policy.
   c Remove and discard gloves. Practice hand hygiene.
16 Ask the parent what privacy measures to maintain. Follow the parent's preferences.

17 Complete a safety check of the room. (See the inside of the back cover.)
18 Practice hand hygiene.
19 Return the scale to its proper place.
20 Report and record your care and observations.

CARE OF THE MOTHER

Postpartum means after *(post)* childbirth *(partum)*. The postpartum period starts with the birth of the baby. It ends 6 weeks later. The mother's body returns to its normal state during this time. The mother adjusts physically and emotionally to childbirth.

The uterus returns almost to its pre-pregnant size. This is called *involution of the uterus.* If the mother does not breast-feed, she can expect a menstrual period within 4 to 6 weeks. Breast-feeding is not an effective method of birth control. Without birth control measures, the mother can get pregnant again.

Lochia

After childbirth, a vaginal discharge called *lochia* occurs. (*Lochia* comes from the Greek word *lochos.* It means childbirth.) Lochia consists of blood and other matter left in the uterus from childbirth. The lochia changes color and decreases in amount during the postpartum period.

- *Lochia rubra*—is dark or bright red *(rubra)* discharge. Mainly blood, it is seen during the first 3 to 4 days.
- *Lochia serosa*—is pinkish-brown *(serosa)* drainage. It lasts until about 10 days after birth.
- *Lochia alba*—is whitish *(alba)* drainage. It continues for 10 to 14 days or more after birth.

Lochia increases with breast-feeding and activity. When standing after lying or sitting, the mother may feel a gush of lochia. A sanitary napkin (sanitary pad) is worn to absorb lochia. Normally lochia smells like menstrual flow. Foul-smelling lochia signals infection.

Good perineal care is important. Sanitary pads are changed often. When wiping after elimination, the mother wipes from front (top) to back (bottom). Sanitary napkins are applied and removed from front to back (top to bottom). Good hand-washing is essential after perineal care, changing sanitary napkins, and elimination. Standard Precautions and the Bloodborne Pathogen Standard are followed.

Episiotomies

Some mothers have episiotomies. An *episiotomy* is an incision *(otomy)* into the perineum. (*Episeion* means pubic region.) The doctor performs this procedure during childbirth. It increases the size of the vaginal opening for the baby. The incision is sutured after delivery. The doctor may order sitz baths for comfort and hygiene (Chapter 43). Like other incisions, complications can develop. These include infection and wound separation *(dehiscence).* Tell the nurse at once if the mother complains of pain, discomfort, or a discharge.

Cesarean Section Delivery

Some mothers deliver by *cesarean section (C-section)*. The baby is delivered through an incision made into the abdominal wall. The doctor performs a C-section when:

- The baby must be delivered to save the baby's or mother's life.
- The baby is too large to pass through the birth canal or is in an abnormal position.
- The mother has a vaginal infection that could be transmitted to the baby.
- A normal vaginal delivery will be difficult for the baby or mother.

The C-section incision needs to heal. See Chapter 41 for wound healing and wound care.

Postpartum Complications

Complications can occur during pregnancy, labor, and delivery. They also can occur in the postpartum period. Report any sign or symptom listed in Box 56-6 at once.

Postpartum Depression. Many women have emotional reactions called "baby blues" after childbirth. Hormone changes, life-style changes, and lack of sleep are causes. Symptoms last for a few days to up to 2 weeks. The mother may:

- Have mood swings.
- Feel sad, anxious, irritable, or over-whelmed.
- Have crying spells.
- Have trouble concentrating.
- Lose her appetite.
- Have problems sleeping.

Postpartum depression is a form of depression (Chapter 53) that occurs after childbirth. Signs and symptoms are more severe and last longer than "baby blues" (over 2 weeks). See Box 56-7. Postpartum depression can interfere with the mother's ability to care for the baby or self. Treatment is needed. Report signs and symptoms of depression at once.

See *Focus on Long-Term Care and Home Care: Postpartum Depression.*

BOX 56-6	Postpartum Complications: Signs and Symptoms

- Temperature of 100.4°F or greater
- Pain: abdominal or perineal
- Discharge:
  - Foul smelling from the vagina
  - From an episiotomy
  - From a C-section incision
- Bleeding from an episiotomy or C-section incision
- Redness, swelling: episiotomy or C-section incision
- Lochia:
  - Red lochia after lochia has changed color to pinkish-brown or white
  - Lochia with large clots
  - Saturating a sanitary napkin within 1 hour of application
- Urination: burning
- Leg pain, tenderness, or swelling
- Sadness or feelings of depression
- Breast pain, tenderness, or swelling

FOCUS ON LONG-TERM CARE AND HOME CARE

Postpartum Depression

Home Care

Rest and self-care are important after childbirth. These measures can help the mother at home.

- Resting as much as possible. Sleeping when the baby sleeps is helpful.
- Performing personal hygiene and grooming measures. Taking a shower and hair care are examples.
- Spending time alone with the person's partner. Or planning time to go out or visit friends.
- Avoiding doing too much. The mother may need help from a supportive partner, family member, or friend. When feeling depressed, someone else may need to help care for the baby.

BOX 56-7	Postpartum Depression: Signs and Symptoms

- Persistent sad, anxious, or empty mood
- Crying more than usual or for no reason
- Feeling irritable, frustrated, guilty, worthless, negative (pessimistic), hopeless, or helpless
- Loss of interest in activities usually enjoyed
- Fatigue that is abnormal
- Restlessness or having trouble sitting still
- Trouble concentrating, remembering, or making decisions
- Sleep problems—sleeping too much or being unable to sleep enough
- Abnormal appetite, weight changes, or both
- Aches or pains, headaches, or digestive problems with no other cause or that do not resolve with treatment
- Trouble forming an emotional attachment (bonding) with the baby
- Doubting the ability to care for the baby
- Thinking about harming oneself or the baby

Modified from National Institute of Mental Health: Perinatal depression, NIH publication No. 30-MH-8116, Bethesda, Md, revised 2023, National Institutes of Health and Office on Women's Health, Postpartum depression, updated October 17, 2023, U.S. Department of Health and Human Services.

FOCUS ON **PRIDE**
The Person, Family, and Yourself

Personal and Professional Responsibility

A newborn may go to the nursery while the mother rests or leave the room for a test or procedure. You must return the baby to the correct parent. Follow agency policy to identify the mother and newborn. You must not rely on the parent to identify the baby. Safe identification is a professional responsibility.

Rights and Respect

A parent's preferences for newborn care may differ from yours. Your opinion must not affect the care you give. Respect parent preferences.

Independence and Social Interaction

Parents must learn to care for their baby. The nurse teaches parents about newborn care. They watch the nurse. Then they try it on their own. Parents gain confidence by giving care independently.

Parents who rely on the staff may not know how to provide care at home. Avoid doing everything for the parents. Tell the nurse if the parents rely on the staff too much.

Delegation and Teamwork

Alarm systems protect the security of newborns. The baby wears an electronic security bracelet. An alarm sounds when the baby is carried toward an exit. Alarms and exits are checked at once. All staff members respond. If a baby is missing, security staff send out a message to the entire agency. Procedures are followed to find the baby. The entire agency works as a team to protect the newborn.

Ethics and Laws

Having a baby is usually a happy time. However, this is not always the case. The health team must monitor closely for signs of mistreatment. A parent may not be interested in the baby. Or the parent may be unwilling to learn how to care for the baby. The baby must be protected from abuse and neglect. Tell the nurse about any concerns at once.

FOCUS ON **PRIDE**: Application

New parents have to adjust to many new things. Explain the health team's role in helping parents adjust. How can you provide support and encouragement?

REVIEW QUESTIONS

Circle the BEST answer.

1 A baby's head and neck are supported for the first
 a 7 to 10 days
 b Month
 c 3 months
 d 6 months

2 Which is *unsafe* when holding a newborn?
 a Holding the infant securely
 b Cuddling the infant
 c Using 2 hands
 d Lifting the infant by the arms

3 Which is *safe?*
 a A crib without bumper pads
 b A crib with a loose crib sheet
 c A crib with a soft blanket and stuffed toys
 d A crib with a drop-side rail

4 Which increases the risk of sudden unexpected infant death?
 a Sleeping on a firm, flat mattress
 b Being exposed to smoke
 c Breast-feeding
 d Pacifier use

5 Which is *safe* for infant sleep?
 a Sleeping in an adult bed with a parent
 b Getting hot during sleep
 c Sleeping in a crib in the same room as a parent
 d Being placed on the stomach for sleep

6 You observe the following. Which is *normal?*
 a The baby looks flushed and is perspiring.
 b The baby has watery stools.
 c The baby's eyes are red and irritated.
 d The baby spits up a small amount when burped.

7 A breast-feeding mother should
 a Nurse the infant every 4 to 6 hours
 b Avoid wearing a bra
 c Clean the breasts with soap and water
 d Stimulate the rooting reflex

8 A breast-fed baby is burped
 a Every 5 minutes
 b After nursing from a breast
 c After 1 ounce of breast-milk
 d After half the formula is taken

9 You are shopping for baby formula. Which should you buy?
 a The one that is on sale
 b The ready-to-feed type
 c The one ordered by the doctor
 d The powdered form

10 When warming a baby bottle
 a Warm the bottle in the microwave
 b Leave the formula out to warm at room temperature
 c Check that the formula is warm on the inside of your wrist
 d Boil the formula in a pan for 5 minutes

11 When bottle-feeding a baby
 a Tilt the bottle so the formula fills the neck of the bottle and the nipple
 b Save remaining formula for the next feeding
 c Burp the baby every 5 minutes
 d Leave the baby alone with the bottle

12 When should an infant's diaper be changed?
 a Whenever the diaper is wet or soiled
 b When it is convenient for the parent
 c Every 6 to 8 hours
 d Before and after each feeding

Continued

13 A newborn's cord has not yet healed. The diaper should be
a Loose over the cord
b Snug over the cord
c Below the cord
d Disposable

14 A circumcision is cleaned
a Once a day
b With an alcohol wipe
c 3 times a day
d At every diaper change

15 A baby had a circumcision. Which should you report at once?
a There is bruising at the tip of the penis.
b There is a slight yellowish crust at the tip of the penis.
c There is blood in the diaper that is larger than quarter-sized.
d The parent applied petrolatum jelly to the area.

16 Which water temperature is safe and comfortable for a baby's bath?
a 80°F
b 90°F
c 100°F
d 120°F

17 When bathing an infant
a Have needed supplies within reach
b Retract the foreskin to rinse the penis
c Leave the baby alone in the tub
d Lower the room temperature to 70°F

18 A baby's circumcision has not yet healed. The cord stump has not fallen off. Which is best for bathing?
a No bathing
b A shower
c A bath in a baby bathtub
d A sponge bath

19 A breast-fed baby needs a "before" and "after" feeding weight. Which will you do?
a Remove the baby's diaper.
b Subtract the "before" weight from the "after" weight.
c Only report and record the "after" weight.
d Keep the baby's clothes on.

20 A mother has a red vaginal discharge the first few days after childbirth. This
a Is a menstrual period
b Signals a postpartum complication
c Is lochia rubra
d Is from her episiotomy

21 A cesarean delivery involves
a A vaginal incision
b A perineal incision
c An abdominal incision
d A normal delivery through the birth canal

22 A month after giving birth, a mother has a persistent sad and irritable mood. It interferes with her ability to care for the baby and perform daily activities. This
a Is normal after childbirth
b Is "baby blues"
c Is not concerning if there are no thoughts of self-harm
d May signal postpartum depression

Answers to Chapter 56 questions are on p. 904.

FOCUS ON PRACTICE

Problem Solving

A mother had a vaginal delivery yesterday. She just finished breast-feeding and stands to lay the baby down. As she stands, she says: "I just felt a gush of blood. Is that normal?" How will you respond? Describe normal and abnormal vaginal discharge after birth.

Assisted Living

- Define the key terms and key abbreviations in this chapter.
- Describe assisted living.
- Describe the usual needs and abilities of assisted living residents.
- Describe assisted living resident rights.
- Identify the services usually offered in assisted living residences.
- Describe common features of assisted living units.
- Describe the requirements for assisted living staff.

- Describe what is included in an assisted living service plan.
- Explain how to safely assist with meals, housekeeping, laundry, and medications.
- Identify the reasons for transferring, discharging, or evicting a person.
- Explain how to promote PRIDE in the person, the family, and yourself.

KEY TERMS

assisted living A housing option for persons who need help with activities of daily living but do not need 24-hour nursing care
medication reminder Reminding the person to take drugs, observing them being taken as prescribed, and recording that they were taken

service plan A written plan listing the services needed, the help needed, and who provides services

KEY ABBREVIATIONS

ADL	Activities of daily living	**RN**	Registered nurse
ALR	Assisted living residence		

Many older people cannot or do not want to live alone. Some need help with self-care or taking drugs but do not require ongoing nursing care. *Assisted living* is a housing option for persons who need help with activities of daily living (ADL) but do not need 24-hour nursing care. Assisted living residences (ALRs) offer a home-like setting that promotes independence, quality of life, security, and social involvement.

ALRs may be part of a retirement community, nursing center, senior citizen housing, or a stand-alone facility. Licensing requirements and residents' rights vary from state to state.

See *Promoting Safety and Comfort: Assisted Living.*

PROMOTING SAFETY AND COMFORT
Assisted Living

Safety
The same infection prevention measures used in other health care settings apply in ALRs. Contact with blood, body fluids, and potentially contaminated items and surfaces is likely. Follow Standard Precautions and the Bloodborne Pathogen Standard. Follow the rules of hand hygiene and the guidelines for glove use in Chapters 17 and 18.

ASSISTED LIVING RESIDENTS

Assisted living residents usually have stable health and do not need 24-hour nursing care. They usually need some help with 1 or more ADL.

- Personal care—bathing, dressing, grooming, elimination, transferring
- Meals—cooking, eating
- Taking drugs
- Housekeeping
- Personal safety
- Transportation

ALR resident requirements vary. For example, an ALR may require that residents be able to walk. Others allow wheelchair use. An ALR may serve residents with mild memory loss but not those with severe memory impairments.

Resident Rights

ALR residents have rights and liberties as United States citizens. They also gain special rights under state laws and rules for ALRs. Such rights are similar to those in Chapter 2. See Box 57-1. If unable to exercise one's rights, family members, legal representatives, or ombudsmen act on the person's behalf.

ALR SERVICES AND LIVING AREAS

Assisted living residences usually offer:

- On-site staff available 24 hours a day for supervision and assistance
- 24-hour security
- Meals
- Personal care—help with ADL
- Housekeeping, laundry, and maintenance
- Arrangements for transportation
- Social, recreational, and spiritual services
- Exercise, health, and wellness programs
- Medication (drug) management or help taking drugs
- Coordination of services given by health care providers outside the ALR

Sometimes an injury or illness requires temporary hospital or skilled nursing care or rehabilitation. The person is able to return to the ALR when needs can be met within the ALR. Additional outside services are arranged if not provided by the ALR. For example, a home health agency provides nursing or therapy services (physical, occupational, speech-language) within the person's apartment.

Some ALRs have special services for persons with memory problems or other disabilities. Many ALRs offer different levels of care and services at varying levels of cost. (Medicare [Chapter 1] does not cover ALR expenses. Usually, assisted living is paid for through personal finances.)

Living areas vary. A small cottage or apartment has a bedroom, bathroom, living area, kitchen, and laundry areas (Fig. 57-1). Some people just want a bedroom and bathroom. Box 57-2 lists some common features of ALRs.

BOX 57-1   Assisted Living Resident Rights

A resident has the right to:
- Not be discriminated against based on race, national origin, religion, gender, sexual orientation, age, disability, marital status, or diagnosis.
- Be treated with dignity, respect, and consideration.
- Be protected from abuse, neglect, and other forms of mistreatment (Chapters 2 and 5).
- Be informed of policies on health care directives. (See "Advance Directives" in Chapter 59.)
- Be informed of policies on the process for voicing grievances.
- Not be photographed without consent, except for the purpose of resident identification.
- The privacy of medical and financial records. Consent is required for the release of records.
- Access to one's own medical record.
- Request or consent to relocation within the ALR. Except for when a change in the resident's condition requires a transfer, the resident can refuse to relocate within the ALR.
- Receive ALR services that support and respect the person's individuality, choices, strengths, and abilities.
- Be informed of rates and charges for services before services are given. The resident is informed of any changes in rates (charges) and services at least 30 days before the change takes effect.
- Receive privacy in:
  - Personal care
  - Correspondence, communication, and visits
  - Financial and personal matters
- Maintain, use, and display personal items. Such items must not pose a safety hazard.
- Take part in or refuse to take part in activities—social, recreational, rehabilitative, religious, political, community.
- Be referred to another health care institution if the ALR does not or cannot provide services needed by the person.
- Choose to access services from another health care provider, institution, or pharmacy.
- Take part in developing a service plan (see "Service Plans"). The resident's family or representative may be involved.
- Have help from others (family, representative) in understanding, protecting, or exercising resident rights.

Modified from Resident Rights, *Arizona Administrative Code (R9-10-810).*

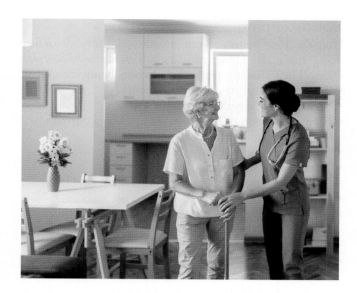

FIGURE 57-1 An assisted living residence provides a home-like setting for persons who need some help with activities of daily living. Staff are available for supervision and assistance. (Copyright © iStock.com/PixelsEffect.)

<table>
<tr><td>BOX 57-2</td><td>Assisted Living Residences: Common Features</td></tr>
</table>

Physical
- Attractive and home-like decor
- An easy-to-understand and easy-to-follow floor plan
- Wide doors, hallways, and bathrooms for walker and wheelchair use
- Elevators in 2-story or higher buildings
- Hand rails in hallways and stairways
- Easy-to-reach cupboards and shelves
- Flooring material for easy walking and easy walker and wheelchair use
- Good general and task lighting
- Clean and odor-free
- Clearly marked exits
- Smoke alarms and a fire sprinkling system

Personal Areas
- Resident doors lock
- 24-hour emergency communication system
- Private bathroom large enough for a walker or wheelchair
- Grab bars/safety bars in bathrooms
- Furnishings—personal and provided
- Access to phone, TV, and Internet
- Kitchen with a refrigerator, sink, and cooking means

Activities
- Daily schedule of activities—within the ALR and the community
- Volunteers or families help residents with activities
- Transportation to appointments, shopping, and activities
- Barber and beauty services

Food
- Menus vary daily
- 3 meals a day and snacks
- Common dining areas
- Meal times vary to meet resident needs
- Special diets and requests available

Modified from Assisted Living Federation of America: Guide to choosing an assisted living community.

STAFF REQUIREMENTS

Staff requirements vary among states. Some require a nursing assistant training and competency evaluation program (NATCEP) for staff assisting with personal care. Staff also may need additional training in these areas.
- The needs, goals, and rights of ALR residents
- Elder abuse and neglect
- Memory and dementia problems
- Using service plans
- Menu planning and food preparation, service, and storage
- Housekeeping
- Assisting with drugs

Criminal background and fingerprint checks are common requirements. The ALR cannot employ a person with a criminal record.

State requirements on registered nurse (RN) staffing in ALRs vary. Some require an RN on staff. Others only require an RN to be available. Some states do not have an RN requirement. If you work in an ALR, you need to know who to go to for guidance and assistance and who to report to. In this chapter, reporting to the nurse is directed.

SERVICE PLANS

Similar to a care plan, a *service plan* is a written plan listing:
- The services needed
- The help needed
- Who provides the services

The plan relates to ADL, activities and social services, dietary needs, taking drugs, and special needs.

For example, the service plan states that you will help the person get dressed. For physical therapy, a physical therapist will visit in the resident's room. And a family member will assist with the person's drugs.

The resident and family (or representative) are encouraged to participate in developing the service plan. The person should receive a copy of the plan. The plan is reviewed periodically and when the person's condition, wants, or service needs change. Services are added or reduced as needed.

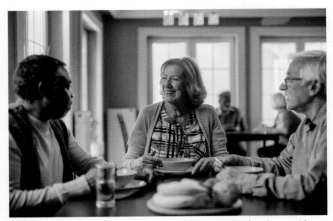

FIGURE 57-2 Some assisted living residents eat with other residents in the dining room. Others dine in their personal living areas. (Copyright © iStock.com/Drazen [Zigic].)

Meals

Three meals a day and snacks are provided. Special dietary needs are met. Menus are posted for residents to see.

Dining options range from cafeteria style to fine dining. Residents eat in the dining room with others (Fig. 57-2). Or they can eat in their rooms if they wish.

Food Safety

Certain measures are needed to handle, prepare, and store food. They protect against infection. See "Foodborne Illness" in Chapter 31. Also practice these safety measures for food preparation and clean-up.

- Follow the safe handling instructions on food labels.
- Scrape and rinse eating and cooking items before washing or placing them in the dishwasher.
- Use liquid detergent and hot water to wash eating and cooking items. Wash the least soiled items first. These are usually glasses, cups, and flatware. Follow with plates, bowls, and serving pieces. Wash cookware last. Rinse well with hot water.
- Place washed items in a drainer to dry. Air-drying is more aseptic than towel drying.
- Use dishwasher soap for a dishwasher.
- Do not wash pots and pans and cast iron, wood, and some plastic items in a dishwasher.
- Clean appliances, counters, tables, and other surfaces after each meal. Use hot, soapy water and paper towels or clean cloths.
- Remove grease spills and splashes. Use a liquid surface cleaner.
- Clean sinks with a sink cleaner.
- Save or discard left-overs.
- Dispose of garbage and other soiled supplies after each meal. Use a garbage disposal for food and liquid garbage but not bones.
- Recycle paper, boxes, cans, and plastic containers according to ALR policy.
- Empty garbage at least once a day. Empty it at once if there is an odor.

Housekeeping

Housekeeping helps prevent infection and provides a neat living space. Your role may include some housekeeping duties. The following measures help keep living areas clean.

- Make beds and straighten bedrooms.
- Wipe up spills right away.
- Use a dust mop or broom to sweep. Use a dustpan to collect dust and crumbs.
- Sweep daily or more often as needed.
- Make sure toilets flush after each use.
- Rinse the sink after washing, shaving, or oral hygiene.
- Clean the tub or shower after each use.
- Remove and dispose of hair from the sink, tub, or shower.
- Hang towels to dry. Or place them in a hamper.
- Follow agency procedures to clean and disinfect bathroom surfaces and items.
  - The toilet bowl, seat, and outside areas of the toilet
  - The floor
  - The tub or shower
  - Towel racks and toilet paper and soap holders
  - The sink and mirror
  - Window sills
  - The wastebasket, laundry hamper, and bath mats
- Mop or vacuum the bathroom floor every day.
- Empty wastebaskets every day. Empty them at once if there is an odor.
- Put out clean towels and washcloths every day.
- Replace toilet paper and facial tissues as needed.
- Open bathroom windows for a short time. Also use air fresheners.
- Dust furniture at least weekly.
- Vacuum floors at least weekly and as needed.

Laundry

Clean linens may be provided. For personal laundry, residents can use a washer, dryer, iron, and ironing board. When assisting with laundry:

- Wear gloves to handle soiled laundry (see *Promoting Safety and Comfort: Assisted Living* on p. 855).
- Separate white, colored, and dark items. Separate sturdy and delicate fabrics. Also separate by the amount of dirt, soiling, or stain.
- Empty pockets.
- Fasten buttons, zippers, snaps, hooks, and other closures.
- Wash very dirty or heavily soiled or stained items separately.
- Follow detergent directions.
- Follow care label directions and the person's preferences for the correct:
  - Wash cycle and water temperature
  - Drying temperature and cycle
- Fold, hang, or iron clothes as the person prefers.
- Clean out a lint screen (filter) in a dryer after use. Remove and discard lint. Check that it is clean before using the dryer.

See *Teamwork and Time Management: Laundry.*

Laundry

Residents may share washers and dryers. If assisting with laundry, remove clothes from washers and dryers promptly. Others may need the machines.

Sometimes laundry is left in a washer or dryer. First, try to find the person who left the laundry. Politely tell the person that the machine is done and that you have laundry to do. Offer to remove the laundry if the other person is busy. If you cannot find that person, do the following.

- *If left in a washer*—Neatly place wet items on a clean surface or in a designated cart or area. Do not place them in the dryer. Some items may need to dry flat, hang to dry, or need certain dryer settings. Or the resident may have drying preferences.
- *If left in a dryer*—Neatly fold and place items on a clean surface. Or lay the items flat.

While laundry is in the washer or dryer, tend to other tasks. Assist with ADL, do housekeeping, prepare meals, and so on. Plan to return promptly to attend to laundry in the washer or dryer.

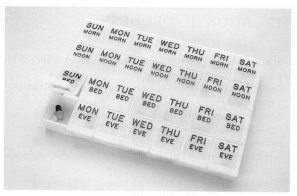

FIGURE 57-3 Pill organizer.

Nursing Services

Some ALRs provide limited nursing services. The nurse assesses each person and monitors health. The nurse guides and assists you with delegated tasks as needed. If a person cannot manage one's own drugs, the nurse gives them.

Medication Assistance

Drugs must be taken as prescribed. The 6 rights of drug administration are:

- The right drug
- The right dose (amount)
- The right route (by mouth, injection, applied to the skin, inhalation, vaginally, or rectally)
- The right time
- The right person
- The right documentation (recording)

Your role depends on your state's laws, ALR policy, and your training and education. *Remember, you do not give drugs (Chapter 3). Also remember that the person has the right to refuse to take prescribed drugs.* Your role may involve:

- Reminding the person to take a drug
- Reading the drug label to the person
- Opening containers if the person cannot do so
- Checking the dosage against the drug label
- Providing water, juice, milk, crackers, applesauce, or other food and fluids
- Making sure the person takes the right drug, the right amount, at the right time, and in the right way (route)
- Recording that the person took or refused to take the drug (right documentation)
- Storing drugs

Self-directed medication management is when residents manage and take their own drugs. The person knows drugs by name, color, or shape. The person knows what drugs to take, the correct doses, and when and how to take them. The person questions changes in the usual drug routine. For example, a pill is not broken in half. Or a pill looks different. Report comments or questions to the nurse.

Pill organizers (Fig. 57-3) have sections for days or times. They are for a week or month. The person, a family member or representative, or a nurse prepares the pill organizer. Drugs are taken on the right day and at the right time.

Some pharmacies offer pre-sorted dose packets. The person's drugs are sorted into packets according to the day and time of day to take the drugs. The person does not need to use pill bottles or pill organizers. Usually a month's supply is provided.

You may need to remind some people. A *medication reminder* means reminding the person to take drugs, observing them being taken as prescribed, and recording that they were taken. Setting clock or phone alarms for when to take drugs is useful for some people.

See *Focus on Communication: Medication Assistance.*

See *Delegation Guidelines: Medication Assistance*, p. 860.

Medication Assistance

To remind a person to take medications, you can say:

- "Ms. Parks, it's time to take your 8 o'clock pills."
- "Mr. Ladd, you need to take your pills in about 10 minutes."
- "Mrs. Young, are you ready to take your medicine?"

To read a drug label to a person, read the following.

- The name of the person on the drug label
- The name of the drug
- How to take the drug (by mouth, with food, with a full glass of water, apply to the skin, rectally, and so on)
- The dosage
- When to take the drug (before meals, with meals, after meals, at bedtime, and so on)
- How often to take the drug
- Warnings and other information on the drug label

DELEGATION GUIDELINES

Medication Assistance

Some agencies use "10 rights of medication assistance." The added 4 are:

- *Right education.* The nurse provides information about the drug.
- *Right to refuse.* The person has the right to refuse any drug. The nurse advises the person about problems that can result if the drug is not taken.
- *Right assessment.* Vital signs may be measured before a drug is given.
- *Right evaluation.* The nurse assesses if the drug had the desired effect or any side effects.

These added rights are nursing responsibilities. The nurse may delegate taking vital signs to you. If so, the nurse may:

- Ask you to report the vital signs before assisting the person.
- Give you guidance about how to proceed. For example, a person takes a drug that affects heart rate. The nurse may tell you that the drug should not be taken if the pulse is less than 60 beats per minute.

A person may refuse to take a drug. If so, report the refusal to the nurse. The nurse will follow the "right to refuse" described above.

Medication Record. A medication record is kept. The record includes:

- The person's name
- Drug name, dose, directions, and route of administration
- Date and time to take the drug
- Date and time help was given
- Signature or initials of the person assisting

Drug Errors. Report any drug error to the nurse. Also complete an incident report. An error means 1 or more of the following.

- Taking another person's drugs
- Taking the wrong drug
- Taking the wrong dose
- Taking an extra dose
- Missing or skipping a dose
- Taking a drug at the wrong time
- Taking a drug by the wrong route
- Not taking a drug when ordered
- Not recording that a drug was taken

Storing Drugs. Drugs are kept in a secure place. This prevents others from taking them. The ALR may keep drugs in a locked area. Some persons store their own drugs. If sharing a room, each person's ability to safely have drugs is assessed. Drugs are in a locked container if safety is a factor.

Drugs must have the original pharmacy label. They are stored as directed on the label. For example, some drugs are refrigerated. Others are kept away from light. The label also has an expiration date. The ALR has procedures for disposing of expired or discontinued drugs.

Activities and Recreation

Residents are encouraged to take part in activity and recreational programs. Social, physical, and community activities promote well-being and independence. An activities director plans, organizes, and conducts the ALR's activity program. ALR and community events and activities are noted on a calendar.

Special Services and Safety Needs

Sometimes emergencies occur. Some people need help getting out of bed or transferring to a wheelchair. Then they can leave the building with little or no help. The ALR and the person agree on how the person's needs will be met.

TRANSFER, DISCHARGE, AND EVICTION

Residents can be transferred, discharged, or evicted. The ALR must tell the person about the action. Most states require advance notice. Reasons are:

- The ALR can no longer meet the person's needs. The ALR cannot provide needed care or safely care for the person.
- The person is a threat to the health and safety of self or others.
- The person fails to pay for services.
- The person fails to comply with ALR policies or rules.
- The person wants to transfer.
- The ALR closes.

FOCUS ON **PRIDE**

The Person, Family, and Yourself

Personal and Professional Responsibility

Moving to an ALR can bring mixed emotions. The person may be happy and excited. Fear, anxiety, and uncertainty are also common. The move may bring the family peace of mind. The person is in a clean, safe setting. Needs are met.

Be professional and caring. Your interactions should assure the resident and family that you will provide safe, dignified care.

Rights and Respect

Federal and state laws protect the person's rights. The person has the right to quality of life, privacy, protection against restraint and abuse, and access to information. The person also has rights regarding the transfer, discharge, or eviction from the ALR. See Box 57-1. Take pride in protecting the person's rights.

Independence and Social Interaction

People choose assisted living for many reasons. Many need some help. Many like the social interaction with other residents. The ALR's activities and services offer other benefits.

To promote independence, assist as needed while allowing as much privacy and personal choice as possible. Follow the resident's service plan.

Delegation and Teamwork

Good teamwork is needed when new residents arrive. The person and family should see that the staff is helpful and works together to meet the person's needs.

Ethics and Laws

How you assist with drugs depends on your state's laws, ALR policy, and your training. There are legal limits to your role. If you act beyond those limits, you could be practicing nursing without a license. You can lose your job and your ability to work as a nursing assistant. Follow the limits for your state and agency.

FOCUS ON **PRIDE**: *Application*

Identify the changes a new ALR resident faces. How might the person respond? Describe positive and negative feelings. How do the following affect the transition?
- The person's attitude
- The family's involvement and support level
- The ALR's appearance
- The ALR staff's conduct

REVIEW QUESTIONS

Circle the BEST answer.

1 Assisted living residences (ALRs) usually provide
- a 24-hour skilled nursing care
- b Help with activities of daily living (ADL)
- c Care that is covered by Medicare
- d Surgical and wound care

2 Which violates a resident's rights within an ALR?
- a A resident is informed of a change in charges 2 months in advance.
- b Staff respect a resident's refusal to take part in an activity.
- c A resident is photographed without consent for a brochure.
- d A resident is allowed to review his own medical record.

3 A service plan in an ALR
- a Lists the person's goals for discharge
- b Identifies what jobs the person will do in the ALR
- c Describes needed services and who provides them
- d Lists service fees and charges

4 Which statement about service plans is *correct?*
- a Service plans are the same for all residents.
- b The resident is not involved in planning.
- c The person's family cannot be involved in planning.
- d The plan changes when the person's needs change.

5 Which statement about ALR dining is *true?*
- a Residents are allowed to eat in their rooms.
- b Residents must cook their own meals.
- c The family provides meals if a special diet is needed.
- d Eating in the dining room is discouraged.

6 When assisting with housekeeping
- a Clean the shower monthly
- b Empty a wastebasket with an odor at once
- c Clean the bathroom only as needed
- d Provide clean washcloths and towels weekly

7 You assist with laundry. Which is *correct?*
- a Care label directions are followed.
- b Hot water is used for all clothing.
- c A heavily soiled item is washed with other items.
- d Gloves are not needed for soiled laundry.

8 Usually ALR nursing assistants are allowed to
- a Give drugs
- b Give medication reminders
- c Refill drugs
- d Prepare pill organizers

9 Drugs are kept
- a In the person's closet
- b In the person's drawer
- c In a secure place
- d With the family

10 A person had a change in condition. The ALR can no longer meet the person's needs. Which is *best?*
- a The person remains at the ALR with the service plan unchanged.
- b The ALR staff give a higher level of care as best as possible.
- c The family is required to provide the needed care.
- d The ALR, person, and family arrange for a transfer.

Answers to Chapter 57 questions are on p. 904.

FOCUS ON **PRACTICE**

Problem Solving

Your state and ALR allow you to give medication reminders. A resident asks you to give an injection. What do you do? Explain what you can and cannot do.

Emergency Care

OBJECTIVES

- Define the key terms and key abbreviations in this chapter.
- Describe the rules of emergency care.
- Identify the signs of cardiac arrest and the emergency care required.
- Describe the emergency care for respiratory arrest.
- Describe the emergency care for poisoning.
- Describe the signs of opioid overdose and the emergency care required.
- Describe the emergency care for heart attack.

- Describe the emergency care for hemorrhage, fainting, and shock.
- Describe the emergency care for stroke.
- Explain how to care for a person during a seizure.
- Describe the emergency care for concussions.
- Describe the emergency care for cold- and heat-related illnesses.
- Describe the emergency care for burns.
- Explain how to promote PRIDE in the person, the family, and yourself.

KEY TERMS

anaphylaxis A life-threatening sensitivity to an antigen

cardiac arrest See "sudden cardiac arrest"

cardiopulmonary resuscitation (CPR) An emergency procedure performed when the heart and breathing stop

convulsion See "seizure"

fainting The sudden loss of consciousness from an inadequate blood supply to the brain; syncope

first aid The emergency care given to an ill or injured person before medical help arrives

frostbite An injury to the body caused by freezing of the skin and underlying tissues

hemorrhage The excessive loss *(rrhage)* of blood *(hemo)* in a short time

hypothermia Abnormally low *(hypo)* body temperature *(thermia)*

respiratory arrest Breathing stops but heart action continues for several minutes

resuscitate To revive from apparent death or unconsciousness using emergency measures

seizure Violent and sudden contractions or tremors of muscle groups caused by abnormal electrical activity in the brain; convulsion

shock Results when tissues and organs do not get enough blood

sudden cardiac arrest (SCA) The heart stops suddenly and without warning; cardiac arrest

syncope See "fainting"

KEY ABBREVIATIONS

AED	Automated external defibrillator	RRS	Rapid Response System
CPR	Cardiopulmonary resuscitation	SCA	Sudden cardiac arrest
EMS	Emergency Medical Services	VF; V-fib	Ventricular fibrillation

Emergencies can occur anywhere. Sometimes you can save a life if you know what to do.

The information in this chapter is basic. First aid and cardiopulmonary resuscitation (CPR) courses provide more training and practice. Most agencies require nursing assistants to be CPR certified. *You need a CPR course for health care providers.* Ask your instructor about courses in your area or on-line.

CPR guidelines are updated as new information becomes available. You are responsible for following current guidelines. Updates can be found on-line at the American Heart Association's website.

EMERGENCY CARE

First aid is the emergency care given to an ill or injured person before medical help arrives. The goals of first aid are to:
- Prevent death.
- Prevent injuries from becoming worse.

In an emergency, the Emergency Medical Services (EMS) system is activated. Emergency personnel (paramedics, emergency medical technicians) give advanced emergency care. They treat, stabilize, and transport persons with life-threatening problems. They have guidelines for care and communicate with doctors in hospital emergency rooms. EMS ambulances have emergency drugs, equipment, and supplies.

To activate the EMS system, do 1 of the following.
- Dial 911.
- Call the local fire or police department.

Each emergency is different. The rules in Box 58-1 apply to any emergency. Hospitals and other agencies have procedures for advanced emergency care. In hospitals, a Rapid Response System (RRS) is activated when a person shows signs of a life-threatening condition. An RRS team may include a doctor, a nurse, and a respiratory therapist. The RRS team brings emergency drugs, supplies, and equipment to the bedside. The goal is to prevent death.

See *Focus on Communication: Emergency Care.*

See *Promoting Safety and Comfort: Emergency Care.*

BOX 58-1 Emergency Care Rules

- Call for help. Or have someone activate the EMS system. *Do not hang up until the operator (dispatcher) has hung up.* Give the following information:
  - Your location—street address and city, cross streets or roads, and landmarks
  - Phone number you are calling from
  - What seems to have happened (for example: heart attack, crash, fire)—police, fire equipment, and ambulances may be needed
  - How many people need help
  - Conditions of victims, obvious injuries, and life-threatening situations
  - What aid is being given
- Wait for help if the scene is not safe enough to approach.
- Know your limits. Do not do more than you are able. Do not perform an unfamiliar procedure. Do what you can under the circumstances.
- Stay calm. This helps the person feel more secure.
- Know where to find emergency supplies.
- Follow Standard Precautions and the Bloodborne Pathogen Standard to the extent possible.
- Check for life-threatening problems. Check for breathing, a pulse, and bleeding.
- Keep the person lying down or as the person was found (unless emergency measures require re-positioning). Moving the person could make an injury worse.
- Move the person only if the setting is unsafe. Examples include:
  - A burning car or building
  - A building that might collapse
  - Stormy conditions with lightning
  - In water
  - Near electrical wires
- Perform necessary emergency measures.
- Do not remove clothes unless you have to. To remove clothing quickly, you may need to tear or cut garments along the seams. (For CPR, remove clothing or move it out of the way. See p. 865.)
- Keep the person warm. Cover the person with a blanket, coats, or sweaters.
- Reassure the person. Explain what is happening and that help was called.
- Do not give the person fluids.
- Keep on-lookers away. They invade privacy and tend to stare, give advice, and comment about the person's condition. This can worry the person.

FOCUS ON COMMUNICATION

Emergency Care

Some illnesses and injuries are life-threatening. You may need to ask questions to find out what happened and the person's condition. For example:
- "Are you okay?"
- "Are you choking?"
- "Tell me what's wrong."
- "Where does it hurt?"
- "Can you point to where it hurts?"
- "Can you move your arms and legs?"

PROMOTING SAFETY AND COMFORT

Emergency Care

Safety

Contact with blood and body fluids is likely. Follow Standard Precautions and the Bloodborne Pathogen Standard to the extent possible.

For an emergency in an agency, call for the nurse at once. You may need to activate the EMS system or the RRS. Or you take the person's vital signs (Chapter 34). Assist as the nurse instructs.

Comfort

Mental comfort is important. Help the person feel safe and secure. Give reassurance. Explain the care you provide. Use a calm approach.

SUDDEN CARDIAC ARREST

Sudden cardiac arrest (SCA) or *cardiac arrest* is when the heart stops suddenly and without warning. Within seconds, breathing stops too. Blood and oxygen are not supplied to the body. Brain and other organ damage occurs within minutes.

SCA is a sudden, unexpected, and dramatic event. It can occur anywhere and at any time—while driving, shoveling snow, playing golf or tennis, watching TV, eating, or sleeping. Common causes include cardiovascular disorders, dysrhythmias (arrhythmias), and congenital heart defects (Chapter 50). Electrical shock, chest trauma, and substance use (Chapter 53) are other causes. The person is at risk for an abnormal heart rhythm called ventricular fibrillation (p. 868). The heart cannot pump blood. A normal rhythm must be restored or the person will die.

Signs of Sudden Cardiac Arrest

There are 3 major signs of SCA.

* *No response.*
* *No breathing or no normal breathing.* The person may have *agonal gasps (agonal respirations)* early during SCA. (*Agonal* means to struggle. Agonal relates to death and dying.) Agonal gasps do not bring enough oxygen into the lungs. Agonal gasps are not normal breathing.
* *No pulse.*

The skin is cool, pale, and gray. The person is not coughing or moving.

To check for SCA:

1 *Check for a response.* In an adult, tap or gently shake the person. Call the person by name, if known. Shout: "Are you okay?" Get help and emergency equipment if there is no response.
2 *Check for breathing and a pulse at the same time.* Do so for 5 to 10 seconds.
   * Look for no breathing or only gasping.
   * In an adult, check the carotid pulse (Fig. 58-1).

CPR

Cardiopulmonary resuscitation (CPR) is an emergency procedure performed when the heart and breathing stop. *Cardio* relates to the heart. *Pulmonary* relates to the lungs. To *resuscitate* means to revive from apparent death or unconsciousness using emergency measures. CPR must be started at once when a person has SCA. CPR provides blood and oxygen to the heart, brain, and other organs until advanced emergency care is given.

CPR involves:

* Giving chest compressions
* Opening the airway and giving breaths
* Defibrillation

See *Focus on Communication: CPR.*
See *Focus on Long-Term Care and Home Care: CPR.*
See *Promoting Safety and Comfort: CPR.*

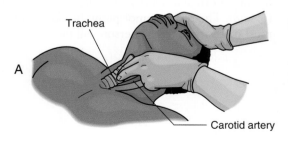
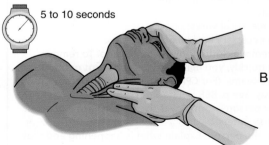

FIGURE 58-1 Checking the carotid pulse. **A,** Place 2 fingers on the trachea. **B,** Move the fingertips down into the groove of the neck to the carotid artery. Feel for a pulse for at least 5 seconds but no more than 10 seconds.

Chest Compressions

Chest compressions force blood through the circulatory system. When pressure is applied to the chest, the sternum compresses the heart (Fig. 58-2). For effective compressions, the person must be supine on a hard, flat surface.

To position the hands for compressions on an adult:

- Expose the chest. Remove clothing or move it out of the way.
- Place the heel of 1 hand (usually the dominant hand) in the center of the bare chest (Fig. 58-3, *A*). The hand is between the nipples on the lower half of the sternum.
- Place the heel of the other hand on top of the heel of the first hand (Fig. 58-3, *B*).

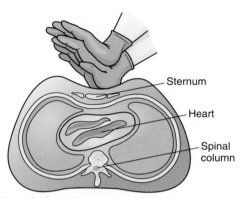

FIGURE 58-2 The heart lies between the sternum and the spinal column. The heart is compressed when pressure is applied to the sternum.

When giving compressions, the arms are straight. The shoulders are directly over the hands. Fingers are interlocked. See Figure 58-4. Press down and release pressure without removing the hands. Releasing pressure allows the chest to recoil—to return to its normal position. Recoil lets the heart fill with blood. Do not lean on the chest.

Compressions are given fast—at a rate of 100 to 120 per minute. The chest is pressed down at least 2 inches for an adult. Compressions are stopped only when necessary and for a short time—less than 10 seconds. Without compressions, blood does not flow to the heart, brain, and other organs.

See *Promoting Safety and Comfort: Chest Compressions.*

PROMOTING SAFETY AND COMFORT

Chest Compressions

Safety

The person must be on a hard, flat surface—floor or back-board. For the person in bed, place a board under the person. Logroll the person so there is no twisting of the spine. Place the arms alongside the body.

In a hospital, the RRS team brings a back-board. The head-board can be removed in some hospital beds for use as a back-board. Other hospital beds have a CPR button that lowers and deflates the mattress for a hard surface.

In a home setting, you may have to move the person to the floor.

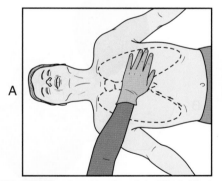
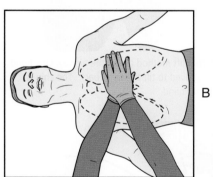

FIGURE 58-3 Hand position for adult CPR. **A,** The heel of the dominant hand is in the center of the chest. It is between the nipples and on the lower half of the sternum. **B,** The heel of the non-dominant hand is on top of the dominant hand.

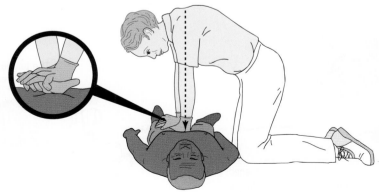

FIGURE 58-4 Giving chest compressions. The arms are straight. The shoulders are over the hands. The fingers are interlocked.

Airway and Breathing

The airway is often obstructed (blocked) during SCA. The tongue falls to the back of the throat and blocks the airway. The airway must be open to give breaths. The head tilt–chin lift method is used to open the airway. See Figure 58-5.

The rescuer breathes air into the person's mouth. To give mouth-to-mouth breaths to an adult (Fig. 58-6):

1. Keep the airway open with the head tilt–chin lift method.
2. Pinch the nostrils shut to keep air from coming out of the nose. Use the fingers on the hand on the person's forehead.
3. Take a normal breath.
4. Place your mouth tightly over the person's mouth. Seal the mouth with your lips.
5. Blow air into the person's mouth. The breath is given over 1 second. *The chest should rise as the lungs fill with air.*
6. Repeat the head tilt–chin lift if the chest did not rise.
7. Remove your mouth from the person's mouth. Take in another breath.
8. Give another breath. Watch for the chest to rise.

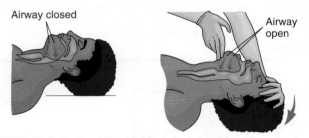

FIGURE 58-5 The head tilt–chin lift method opens the airway. One hand is on the forehead. Pressure is applied to tilt the head back. The chin is lifted with the fingers of the other hand.

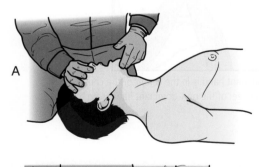

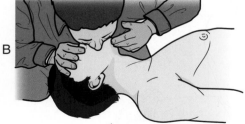

FIGURE 58-6 Mouth-to-mouth breathing. **A,** The airway is opened. The nostrils are pinched shut. **B,** The person's mouth is sealed by the rescuer's mouth.

Masks. A mask or other barrier device is used to give breaths when possible (Fig. 58-7, *A*). The device prevents contact with the person's mouth and blood and body fluids. Place the mask over the person's mouth and nose (Fig. 58-7, *B*). Make a tight seal. Open the airway and blow through the mouth-piece to give breaths.

EMS and hospital staff often use a bag valve mask (Fig. 58-8) to give breaths. The device consists of a hand-held bag attached to a mask. The mask is held securely to the face. The bag is squeezed to give breaths. The bag can be connected to an oxygen source.

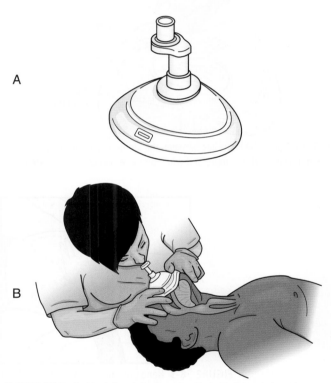

FIGURE 58-7 A, Mask for giving breaths. **B,** A mask is used to give breaths.

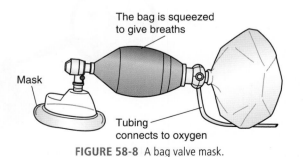

FIGURE 58-8 A bag valve mask.

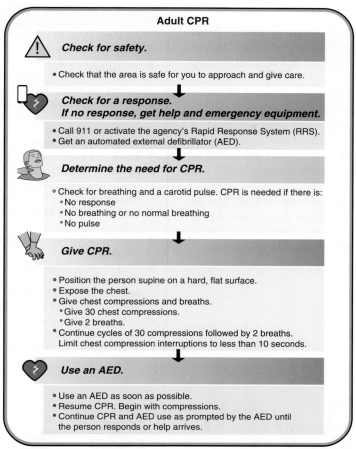

Adult CPR

⚠️ **Check for safety.**

• Check that the area is safe for you to approach and give care.

Check for a response.
If no response, get help and emergency equipment.

• Call 911 or activate the agency's Rapid Response System (RRS).
• Get an automated external defibrillator (AED).

Determine the need for CPR.

• Check for breathing and a carotid pulse. CPR is needed if there is:
  • No response
  • No breathing or no normal breathing
  • No pulse

Give CPR.

• Position the person supine on a hard, flat surface.
• Expose the chest.
• Give chest compressions and breaths.
  • Give 30 chest compressions.
  • Give 2 breaths.
• Continue cycles of 30 compressions followed by 2 breaths. Limit chest compression interruptions to less than 10 seconds.

Use an AED.

• Use an AED as soon as possible.
• Resume CPR. Begin with compressions.
• Continue CPR and AED use as prompted by the AED until the person responds or help arrives.

FIGURE 58-9 Sequence of adult CPR. (NOTE: Follow Standard Precautions and the Bloodborne Pathogen Standard to the extent possible. This includes the use of gloves and a mask or other barrier device.)

Adult CPR Cycle

In an adult, a cycle of CPR involves 30 chest compressions and 2 breaths. Continue cycles of 30 compressions followed by 2 breaths until the person responds or help takes over. CPR is paused briefly to use a defibrillator (p. 868). Then CPR continues with compressions first. See Figure 58-9 for the sequence of CPR for an adult.

CPR is done by 1, 2, or more rescuers (Fig. 58-10). With more rescuers, a team approach promotes effective CPR. For example, with 2 rescuers:

• Rescuer 1 checks for a response. If no response, rescuer 1 tells rescuer 2 to call 911 and get an automated external defibrillator (AED) (p. 868).
• Rescuer 2 leaves to call for help and get an AED.
• Rescuer 1 gives CPR alone until rescuer 2 returns.
• Rescuer 2 returns and uses the AED.
• Rescuer 2 resumes compressions after AED use. (Rescuer 1 needs a break from compressions.)
• Rescuer 1 gives 2 breaths after every 30 compressions.
• Both rescuers continue CPR. They switch roles about every 2 minutes to avoid fatigue and inadequate compressions. They follow the AED's prompts to repeat AED use.

See *Focus on Communication: Adult CPR Cycle.*

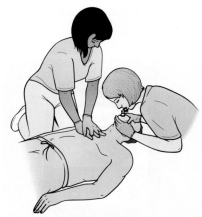

FIGURE 58-10 Two people perform CPR.

FOCUS ON COMMUNICATION

Adult CPR Cycle

Good communication is needed when 2 rescuers give CPR. The rescuer giving compressions counts out loud so the other rescuer is ready to give breaths. Clear communication prevents delays and lessens interruptions in chest compressions.

Defibrillation

Ventricular fibrillation (VF, V-fib) is an abnormal heart rhythm (Fig. 58-11). It causes SCA. Rather than beating in a regular rhythm, the heart quivers and does not pump blood.

A *defibrillator* delivers a shock to the heart. The shock stops the VF (V-fib). This may allow a regular rhythm to return. Defibrillation as soon as possible after the onset of VF (V-fib) increases the chance of survival.

Automated external defibrillators (AEDs) are found in health care agencies and in many public places (Fig. 58-12). Some persons have them at home.

See Box 58-2 for how to use an AED on an adult. Use an AED as soon as possible. You will learn more about AEDs in a CPR certification course.

See *Focus on Children and Older Persons: Defibrillation.*

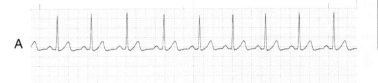
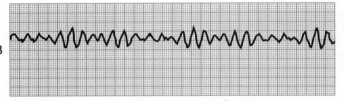

FIGURE 58-11 A, Normal rhythm. **B,** Ventricular fibrillation. (From Ignatavicius DD, Workman ML, Rebar CR: *Medical-surgical nursing: concepts for interprofessional collaborative care,* ed 9, St Louis, 2018, Elsevier.)

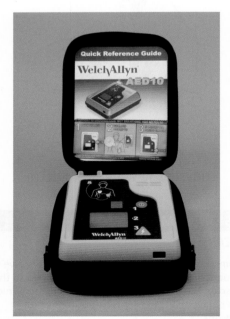

FIGURE 58-12 An automated external defibrillator (AED).

BOX 58-2	Using an AED

Follow these steps to use an AED on an adult.
1 Open the AED case.
2 Turn on the AED (Fig. 58-13, *A*).
3 Apply adult electrode pads to the chest (Fig. 58-13, *B*). Follow the AED's instructions and diagram.
4 Attach the connecting cables to the AED (Fig. 58-13, *C*).
5 Clear away from the person. Make sure no one is touching the person (Fig. 58-13, *D*).
6 Let the AED check the heart rhythm.
7 Make sure everyone is clear of the person if the AED advises a "shock" (see Fig. 58-13, *D*). Loudly tell others not to touch the person. Say: "Everyone, clear!" Look to make sure no one is touching the person.
8 Press the *SHOCK* button if the AED advises a "shock" (Fig. 58-13, *E*).
9 Resume CPR beginning with compressions. Continue cycles of CPR.
10 Repeat steps 5 through 8 when prompted by the AED—after about 2 minutes of CPR. (NOTE: With 2 rescuers, rescuers switch roles at this step to avoid fatigue and inadequate compressions.)
11 Continue CPR and use of the AED until help takes over or the person responds.

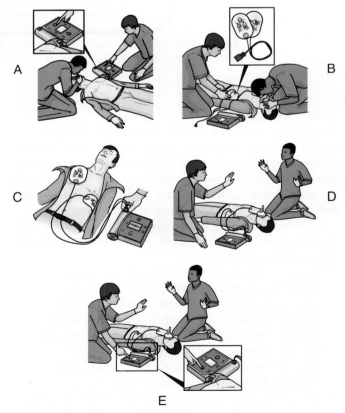

FIGURE 58-13 Using an AED. **A,** The rescuer turns on the AED. **B,** Electrode pads are placed on the chest. **C,** The cables are connected to the AED. **D,** The rescuers "clear" the person. The rescuers make sure no one is touching the person. **E,** The *SHOCK* button is pressed to deliver a shock.

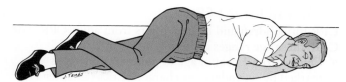

FIGURE 58-15 Recovery position.

Defibrillation

Children

Some AEDs are designed for adults and children. A key or switch is used to lower the shock dosage for a child (Fig. 58-14). Or child pads are applied. Follow the manufacturer's instructions.

For children 8 years old and older, adult pads (adult dose) may be used. A lower shock dosage is used for children younger than 8 years. Use child pads (child dose) if possible. If not, adult pads (adult dose) may be used. Place the pads so they do not over-lap.

For infants, a manual defibrillator is best. Trained staff and EMS use the defibrillator. If one is not available, an AED with child pads (child dose) may be used. If neither is available, adult pads (adult dose) may be used. If needed, place pads on the chest and back so they do not touch.

Recovery Position

The recovery position is used after CPR when the person is breathing and has a pulse (Fig. 58-15). The person may not be responding. The position helps keep the airway open and prevents aspiration.

Logroll the person into the recovery position. Keep the head, neck, and spine straight. A hand supports the head. *Do not use this position if the person might have neck injuries or other trauma.*

Hands-Only CPR

With SCA, survival depends on others nearby. In public, bystanders may worry that they will not do CPR correctly or may cause injury. The "hands-only" method of CPR involves only chest compressions. Breaths are not given. There are only 2 steps.

1 Call 911.
2 Push hard and fast in the center of the chest.

This method is for persons in public who are not trained in CPR. With training and practice, you will learn all of the steps of CPR. As a health care provider, you will use the CPR method learned in your CPR certification course.

See *Focus on Children and Older Persons: Hands-Only CPR.*

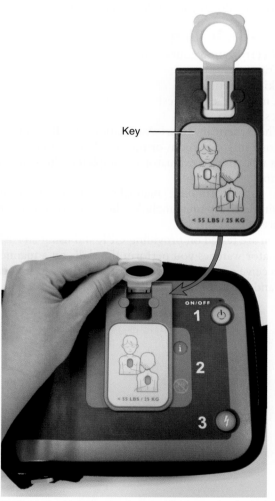

Key

< 55 LBS / 25 KG

ON/OFF

1

2

3

< 55 KG / 25 KG

FIGURE 58-14 On this AED, a key is inserted to lower the shock dosage for a child. Pads are placed on the chest and back so they do not over-lap.

Hands-Only CPR

Children

The hands-only CPR method is intended for adults and adolescents with SCA. In infants and children, SCA caused by heart disease is rare. Usually a respiratory disease or injury causes the heart and breathing to stop. Motor vehicle crashes, drowning, suffocation, burns, smoke inhalation, falls, and poisoning are causes. Sudden infant death syndrome (SIDS) is a leading cause of infant death (Chapter 56).

For infants and children, breaths should be given with CPR. However, if the rescuer is unable or unwilling to deliver breaths, the hands-only method may be used.

Child and Infant CPR

CPR for children and infants differs from adult CPR. For CPR, these age ranges are used.

- *Child*—from 1 year of age to puberty. Puberty is marked by secondary sex characteristics (Chapter 11).
- *Infant*—from birth (outside the delivery room) until 1 year (12 months) of age. Special guidelines are used for newborns.

To check for a response in an infant, tap the infant's foot and shout. Infants cannot answer you. However, shouting should startle a responsive infant.

It may be hard to find a pulse in a child or infant. If you do not feel a pulse within 10 seconds, start CPR. If you feel a pulse, count it. Give CPR if the pulse is less than 60 beats per minute and the child or infant has signs of poor circulation. Such signs include:

- Cold arms and legs
- Unresponsive or decreased level of consciousness
- Weak pulse
- Pale, mottled (blotchy), or bluish skin
  See *Focus on Math: Child and Infant CPR.*

FOCUS ON MATH

Child and Infant CPR

 You count the pulse for at least 5 but no more than 10 seconds. Calculating the number of beats per minute can be done quickly when you count for 6 or 10 seconds.

- If you count for 6 seconds—Multiply the number counted by 10.
- If you count for 10 seconds—Multiply the number counted by 6.

  For example, when checking for a child's pulse you count 4 beats in 6 seconds. Multiply 4 beats (the number of beats in 6 seconds) by 10 to calculate the number of beats per minute.

  4 (number of beats in 6 seconds) × 10 = 40 beats per minute

  You calculate 40 beats per minute. This is less than 60 beats per minute. You give compressions.

As an easier guide, give compressions if the number of beats counted is less than the number of seconds counted. *For example:*

- *Give compressions if you count fewer than 10 beats in 10 seconds.*
- *Give compressions if you count fewer than 9 beats in 9 seconds, and so on.*

All Age-Groups

Some CPR steps are the same for all persons. For *all* age-groups:

- Check that the area is safe for you to approach and give care.
- Check for a response. Get help and emergency equipment if there is no response.
- Check for breathing and a pulse. This takes less than 10 seconds.
- Give CPR for signs of SCA (p. 864).
- Give chest compressions at a rate of 100 to 120 per minute.
- Allow the chest to recoil after each compression. Do not lean on the chest.
- Limit interruptions in chest compressions to less than 10 seconds.
- Give breaths that make the chest rise over 1 second.
- Use an AED as soon as one is available.
  See Table 58-1 for the differences between CPR in adults and adolescents, children, and infants.

CPR Skills Testing

CPR certification courses involve:

- Training
- Skills practice
- A multiple-choice test
- A skills test

The American Heart Association's CPR training may be done in a classroom or on-line. For on-line training, a skills test with an evaluator is completed after the on-line portion.

A current training manual (print or electronic) is required. The manual includes the steps you must perform to pass the skills test.

You are tested on providing CPR and using an AED. An evaluator watches you perform the skills on a mannequin. To receive certification, you must pass the multiple-choice test and the skills test.

TABLE 58-1	CPR: Differences by Age-Group		
CPR Basics	Adults and Adolescents	Children (1 Year to Puberty)	Infants (Birth to 1 Year)
Getting help and an AED	• *If alone with a phone*—Call 911 while giving care. Get an AED if possible. • *If alone without a phone*—Leave the person to call 911 and get an AED before starting CPR. • *If not alone*—Have someone call 911 and get an AED. • *In an agency*—Follow agency procedures to activate the RRS or EMS and get emergency equipment.	• *If alone and the arrest was sudden and witnessed*—Use the guidelines for adults and adolescents. • *If alone and the arrest was not witnessed*—Give 2 minutes of CPR before leaving to call 911 and get an AED. • *If not alone*—Have someone call 911 and get an AED. • *In an agency*—Follow agency procedures to activate the RRS or EMS and get emergency equipment.	
Pulse check	• Carotid artery (neck)	• Carotid artery (neck) or femoral artery (groin) (Chapter 34) • CPR for a pulse less than 60 and poor circulation	• Brachial artery (upper arm) (Fig. 58-16) • CPR for a pulse less than 60 and poor circulation
Hand placement for compressions	• 2 hands on the lower half of the sternum	• 2 hands on the lower half of the sternum • 1 hand may be used if the child is small and the chest is compressed enough (Fig. 58-17)	• *1 rescuer*—2 fingers in the center of the chest just below the nipple line (Fig. 58-18) or the 2-rescuer method • *2 or more rescuers*—2-thumb-encircling hands method in the center of the chest just below the nipple line (Fig. 58-19) • The heel of 1 hand may be used (see Fig. 58-17) to get adequate compression depth
Depth of compressions	• At least 2 inches	• About 2 inches (at least ⅓ of the depth of the chest)	• About 1½ inches (at least ⅓ of the depth of the chest)
Compressions and breaths	• 30 compressions followed by 2 breaths • 100 to 120 compressions per minute	• *1 rescuer*—30 compressions followed by 2 breaths • *2 or more rescuers*—15 compressions followed by 2 breaths • 100 to 120 compressions per minute	
Airway and breathing	• Mouth-to-mouth method or mask	• Mouth-to-mouth method or mask	• Mouth-to-mouth-and-nose method (Fig. 58-20, p. 872) or mask (see Fig. 58-19)

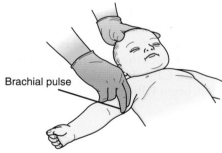

FIGURE 58-16 Locating the infant's brachial pulse.

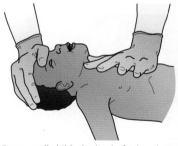

FIGURE 58-17 For a small child, the heel of 1 hand can be used for CPR. The fingers are off of the chest.

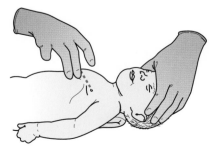

FIGURE 58-18 Locating hand position for infant chest compressions. Imagine a line between the nipples. Find the sternum. For 1-rescuer CPR, you can place 2 fingers on the sternum just below the imaginary line.

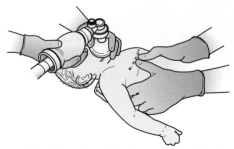

FIGURE 58-19 The 2-thumb-encircling hands method for chest compressions. This method is used when 2 rescuers perform infant CPR. It can also be used when alone.

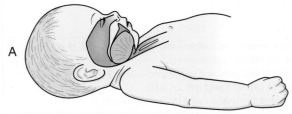

The tongue is at the back of the throat blocking the airway.

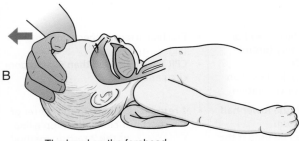

The hand on the forehead is used to tilt the head back.

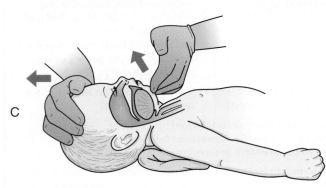

The fingers on the other hand are under the bony part of the jaw (near the chin). The fingers lift the jaw to bring the chin forward.

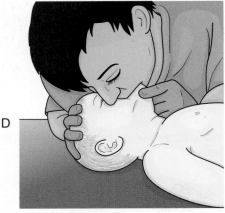

The mouth and nose are covered to give breaths.

FIGURE 58-20 Opening the airway and giving breaths to an infant.

CHOKING

Foreign bodies can obstruct (block) the airway. This is called *choking* or *foreign-body airway obstruction (FBAO)*. Air cannot pass into the lungs. The body does not get enough oxygen. It can lead to cardiac arrest.

Airway obstruction can be mild or severe. With severe airway obstruction, air does not move in and out of the lungs. If the obstruction is not removed, the person will die. Abdominal thrusts are used to relieve severe airway obstruction. See Chapter 14 for emergency care of the choking person.

RESPIRATORY ARREST

Respiratory arrest is when breathing stops but heart action continues for several minutes. If breathing is not restored, cardiac arrest occurs. Respiratory arrest can occur from:

- Blocked airflow—choking (Chapter 14), drowning, suffocation
- Problems affecting nerves, muscles, or areas of the brain that control breathing—amyotrophic lateral sclerosis (ALS), spinal cord injuries, stroke (Chapter 49); drug or alcohol overdose; drug side effects
- Lung disorders and problems—pneumonia, chronic obstructive pulmonary disease (Chapter 50), pulmonary embolism (Chapter 40), chest injuries
- Inhaling harmful substances—smoke, chemicals, fumes

Rescue Breathing

Rescue breaths are given when there is a pulse but no breathing or only agonal gasping. To give rescue breaths:

- Open the airway (p. 866).
- Give 1 breath every 6 seconds for adults.
- Give 1 breath every 2 to 3 seconds for infants and children.
- Give each breath over 1 second. The chest should rise when breaths are given.

Follow the rules in Box 58-1. This includes activating the EMS system. Check the pulse every 2 minutes. If there is no pulse, begin CPR. If the pulse is less than 60 in an infant or child, begin CPR.

POISONING

A *poison* is any substance harmful to the body when ingested (swallowed), inhaled, injected, or absorbed through the skin. See Chapter 14 for measures to prevent poisoning.

Some common signs and symptoms of poisoning are:

- Burns or redness around the mouth and lips
- A chemical odor to the breath
- Burns, stains, or odors on the person, on clothing, or around the person
- Empty drug bottles or spilled drugs
- Vomiting
- *Dyspnea*—difficulty *(dys)* breathing *(pnea)*
- Drowsiness
- Confusion
- Seizures (p. 875)

If you think a person has had contact with a poison, call the Poison Control Center (1-800-222-1222) or 911. Follow the rules in Box 58-1 for basic emergency care. Also follow the directions from the Poison Control Center. Such directions may include:

- *Poison in the eyes*—Rinse the eyes with running water right away. Rinse for at least 15 to 20 minutes. Use room-temperature water. Remove contact lenses, if present.
- *Poison on the skin*—Remove clothing in contact with the poison. Rinse the skin with running water right away. Rinse for at least 15 minutes.
- *Inhaled poison*—Leave the area. Get the person to fresh air at once.
- *Swallowed poison*—Do not have the person try to vomit or give the person anything to cause vomiting. Do not give the person anything to eat or drink unless told to do so by the Poison Control Center.

Call 911 to activate the EMS system if the person stops responding, stops breathing, or has a seizure. Follow the guidelines for CPR and rescue breathing. See p. 876 for emergency care for seizures.

Opioid Overdose

Opioids are a group of pain-relief drugs (Chapter 36). Methadone, oxycodone, hydrocodone, codeine, morphine, and fentanyl are included. Some persons use illicit (illegal) opioid drugs such as illegally made fentanyl and heroin.

An overdose occurs when too much of a drug is taken (Chapter 53). Opioid overdose can slow or stop a person's breathing and cause death. The Centers for Disease Control and Prevention (CDC) reports that overdose deaths are the leading cause of injury-related death in the United States. Most overdose deaths are from opioids.

The CDC lists these signs of opioid overdose.

- Pinpoint pupils—small (constricted) pupils
- Falling asleep or loss of consciousness
- Slow, shallow breathing
- Choking or gurgling sounds
- A limp body
- Pale, blue, or cold skin

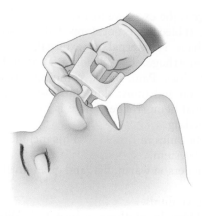

FIGURE 58-21 Naloxone nasal spray is inserted into a nostril. The plunger is pressed to deliver the dose. (From Stein LNM, Hollen CJ: *Concept-based clinical nursing skills: fundamental to advanced competencies*, ed 2, St Louis, 2024, Elsevier.)

If overdose is suspected, do not leave the person alone. Call 911 at once. A reversal drug called *naloxone (Narcan®)* should be given at once, if available. It is safe to use naloxone on a person who has not used opioids.

Naloxone acts quickly (within 2 to 3 minutes) to restore normal breathing to a person whose breathing has slowed or stopped from opioid overdose. Naloxone is available as a nasal spray (Fig. 58-21) or injection. The effects of naloxone last only a short time—30 to 90 minutes. Overdose effects can return. Multiple doses of naloxone may be needed. Be sure that 911 has been called. Most states have laws in place to protect those involved from legal action (arrest, charges) when illicit (illegal) opioid use has occurred.

Try to keep the person awake and breathing. Lay the person on the side to prevent choking. Follow the guidelines for CPR and rescue breathing.

HEART ATTACK

Heart attack (myocardial infarction) occurs when part of the heart muscle dies from the sudden blockage of blood flow in a coronary artery (Chapter 50). Signs and symptoms include:

- Chest pain (not relieved by rest)
- Pain or discomfort in 1 or both arms, the back, neck, jaw, or stomach
- Shortness of breath
- Perspiration (sweating) and cold, clammy skin
- Feeling light-headed
- Nausea and vomiting

If you suspect a heart attack, activate the EMS system at once. Prompt treatment can reduce the amount of heart muscle damage. Have the person sit and rest. Loosen tight clothing. Follow the rules in Box 58-1. Start CPR for cardiac arrest.

HEMORRHAGE

Life and body functions need an adequate blood supply. If a blood vessel is cut or torn, bleeding occurs. The larger the blood vessel, the greater the bleeding and blood loss.

Hemorrhage is the excessive loss (*rrhage*) of blood (*hemo*) in a short time. If bleeding is not stopped, the person will die.

Hemorrhage is internal or external. You cannot see internal hemorrhage. The bleeding is inside body tissues and body cavities. Pain, shock, vomiting blood, coughing up blood, cold and moist skin, and loss of consciousness signal internal hemorrhage. There is little you can do for internal bleeding.

- Follow the rules in Box 58-1. This includes activating the EMS system.
- Keep the person warm, flat, and quiet until help arrives.
- Do not give fluids.

If not hidden by clothing, external bleeding is usually seen. Bleeding from an artery occurs in spurts. There is a steady flow of blood from a vein. To control bleeding:

- Follow the rules in Box 58-1. This includes activating the EMS system.
- Do not remove any objects that have pierced or stabbed the person.
- Place a sterile dressing directly over the wound. Or use any clean material (handkerchief, towel, cloth, or sanitary napkin).
- Apply firm pressure directly over the bleeding site (Fig. 58-22). Do not release pressure until the bleeding stops. If needed, wrap an elastic bandage firmly over the dressing or material.
- Do not remove the dressing or material. If bleeding continues, apply more dressings on top and apply more pressure.
- Bind the wound when bleeding stops. Tape or tie the dressing in place. You can tie the dressing with such things as clothing, a scarf, or a necktie.

See *Promoting Safety and Comfort: Hemorrhage.*

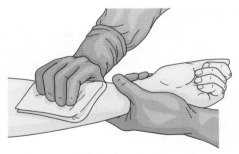

FIGURE 58-22 Direct pressure is applied to the wound to stop bleeding.

PROMOTING SAFETY AND COMFORT

Hemorrhage

Safety
Contact with blood is likely with hemorrhage. Follow Standard Precautions and the Bloodborne Pathogen Standard to the extent possible. Wear gloves if possible. Practice hand hygiene as soon as you can.

FAINTING

Fainting (syncope) is the sudden loss of consciousness from an inadequate blood supply to the brain. Hunger, fatigue, fear, and pain are common causes. Some people faint at the sight of blood or injury. Standing in one position too long and being in a warm, crowded room are other causes. Hemorrhage and other serious problems can cause fainting.

Dizziness, perspiration (sweating), weakness, and vision changes are warning signs. The person looks pale. The pulse is weak. Respirations are shallow if consciousness is lost.

If a person has warning signs of fainting:

- Have the person sit or lie down to prevent fainting.
  - If sitting, the person bends forward and places the head between the knees (Fig. 58-23).
  - If lying down, raise the person's legs.
- Loosen tight clothing (belts, ties, scarves, collars, and so on).

If fainting occurs:

- Activate the EMS system.
- Keep the person lying down. Raise the feet about 12 inches.
- Start CPR for cardiac arrest. Give rescue breathing for respiratory arrest.
- Help the person to a sitting position after recovery from fainting. Do not let the person get up quickly. Observe for warning signs of fainting as the person recovers.

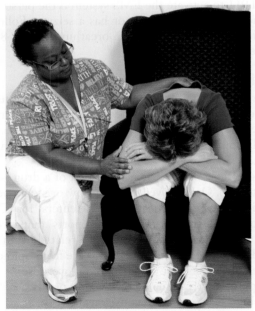

FIGURE 58-23 The person bends forward and lowers the head to prevent fainting.

SHOCK

Shock results when tissues and organs do not get enough blood. Blood loss, allergic reaction, poisoning, heart attack, burns, and severe infection are causes. Signs and symptoms include:

- Low or falling blood pressure
- Rapid and weak pulse
- Rapid respirations
- Cold, moist, and pale skin
- Thirst
- Nausea and vomiting
- Restlessness
- Confusion and loss of consciousness as shock worsens

Shock is possible in any acutely ill or severely injured person. Follow the rules in Box 58-1. Keep the person lying down. If there are no injuries from trauma, raise the feet about 6 to 12 inches. Lower the feet if the position causes pain. Maintain an open airway and control bleeding. Start CPR for cardiac arrest.

Anaphylactic Shock

Some people are allergic or sensitive to foods, insects, chemicals, and drugs. For example, allergies to *penicillin* are common. An *antigen* is a substance that the body reacts to. The body releases chemicals to fight or attack the antigen. The person may react with an area of redness, swelling, or itching. Or the reaction may involve the entire body.

Anaphylaxis is a life-threatening sensitivity to an antigen. (*Ana* means without. *Phylaxis* means protection.) The reaction can occur within seconds.

Signs and symptoms of anaphylaxis include:

- An itchy rash
- Swelling of the face, eyes, or lips
- Flushed or pale skin
- Feeling warm
- Dyspnea or wheezing from airway narrowing or a swollen tongue or throat
- Feeling that there is a "lump" in the throat
- A fast and weak pulse
- Nausea, vomiting, or diarrhea
- A feeling of dread or doom
- Dizziness or fainting
- Signs and symptoms of shock

Anaphylactic shock is an emergency. The EMS system must be activated. Drugs are needed to reverse the allergic reaction. Keep the person lying down and the airway open. Start CPR for cardiac arrest. Give rescue breathing for respiratory arrest.

Some persons carry *epinephrine*—a drug used to treat life-threatening allergic reactions. The person injects the drug into the outer thigh. One dose is given for anaphylaxis. The person may give a second dose if:

- There is no response to the first dose.
- EMS arrival will take longer than 5 to 10 minutes.

STROKE

Stroke (cerebrovascular accident) occurs when the brain is suddenly deprived of its blood supply (Chapter 49). Usually only part of the brain is affected. A stroke may be caused by a thrombus, an embolus, or hemorrhage if a blood vessel in the brain ruptures.

Signs of stroke vary (Chapter 49). They depend on the size and location of brain injury. The National Institute of Neurological Disorders and Stroke lists these major signs.

- Sudden numbness or weakness of the face, arm, or leg, especially on 1 side of the body
- Sudden confusion or trouble speaking or understanding speech
- Sudden trouble seeing in 1 or both eyes
- Sudden trouble walking, dizziness, or loss of balance or coordination
- Sudden, severe headache with no known cause

With stroke, getting treatment quickly can lessen brain damage. The acronym FAST is used as a reminder to check for signs of stroke and act immediately if you suspect stroke. See Box 58-3. The most effective stroke treatments must be given within 3 hours of symptom onset. Activate the EMS system at once. Find out when symptoms began. Tell the EMS staff the time.

While waiting for EMS to arrive, follow the rules in Box 58-1. Keep the person comfortable, warm, and quiet. Give emergency care for seizures if necessary. Start CPR for cardiac arrest. Give rescue breathing for respiratory arrest.

BOX 58-3　Stroke Emergency Care: FAST

F—Face: Ask the person to smile. Does 1 side of the face droop (hang down)?

A—Arms: Ask the person to raise both arms. Does 1 arm drift downward?

S—Speech: Ask the person to repeat a simple phrase. Is speech slurred or strange?

T—Time: If any of these signs are present, call 911 right away.

Modified from Centers for Disease Control and Prevention: Signs and symptoms of stroke, May 15, 2024.

SEIZURES

Seizures (convulsions) are violent and sudden contractions or tremors of muscle groups caused by abnormal electrical activity in the brain. Movements are uncontrolled. The person may lose consciousness. Causes include head injury during birth or from trauma, high fever, brain tumors, poisoning, alcohol use disorder, and nervous system disorders or infections. Lack of blood flow to the brain can also cause seizures.

Epilepsy

Epilepsy is a brain disorder in which clusters of nerve cells sometimes signal abnormally. There are brief changes in the brain's electrical function. The person can have strange sensations, emotions, and behavior. Sometimes there are seizures, muscle spasms, or loss of consciousness.

A single seizure does not mean epilepsy. In epilepsy, seizures recur from a permanent brain injury or defect. Epilepsy can occur with any problem affecting the brain. Such causes include:

- Problems with brain development before birth
- The mother having an injury or infection during pregnancy
- Brain injury during or after birth (Chapter 55)
- Traumatic brain injury (accidents, gunshot wounds, sports injuries, falls, blows to the head)
- Brain tumor
- Infection and inflammation in the brain—such as meningitis and encephalitis
- Stroke
- Dementia

There is no cure at this time. Drugs control seizures in many people. Surgery may be done when drug therapy does not work.

When controlled, epilepsy usually does not affect learning and activities of daily living. Activity and job limits occur in severe cases. For example, a person has seizures at any time. The person may not be allowed to drive. This may limit job choices. Also, the person is at risk for accidents and injuries. Safety measures are needed. They are needed for the home, workplace, transportation, and recreation.

Types of Seizures

Seizures are generalized or focal.

- *Generalized seizures*—affect both sides of the brain. There are 2 types.
  - *Absence (petit mal) seizures*—cause staring and rapid blinking. The seizure lasts a few seconds.
  - *Tonic-clonic (grand mal) seizures*—have 2 phases. In the *tonic* phase, muscles become stiff. The person loses consciousness and falls to the floor. The *clonic* phase follows. Muscles contract and relax. Jerking and shaking movements occur. The person may be incontinent. After the seizure, the person is often tired.
- *Focal (partial) seizures*—affect 1 area of the brain. A body part may twitch or have sensation changes. A strange taste or smell is an example. The person may be confused or unable to respond for a few minutes.

Emergency Care for Seizures

You cannot stop a seizure. However, you can protect the person from injury.

- Follow the rules in Box 58-1.
- Do not leave the person alone.
- Lower the person to the floor. This protects the person from falling.
- Note the time the seizure started.

- Place something soft under the head (Fig. 58-24). This prevents the head from striking the floor. You can use a pillow, a cushion, or a folded blanket, towel, or jacket. Or cradle the person's head in your lap.
- Remove eyeglasses and loosen tight jewelry and clothing around the neck. Ties, scarves, collars, and necklaces are examples.
- Turn the person onto the side. Make sure the head is turned to the side. See Figure 58-24.
- Do not put any object or your fingers between the teeth. Your fingers or the person's teeth or jaw can be injured.
- Do not try to stop the seizure or control movements.
- Move furniture, equipment, and sharp objects out of the way. The person may strike these objects during the seizure.

Monitor the person's breathing during and after a seizure. Gasping or pauses may occur when chest muscles tighten during a seizure. Rescue breathing and CPR usually are not needed. Breathing should return to normal after the seizure.

Note the time the seizure ends. Make sure the mouth is clear of food, fluids, and saliva after the seizure. Do not give food or fluids until the person is fully alert. Also, do not let the person drive after a seizure. See Box 58-4 for when to activate the EMS system.

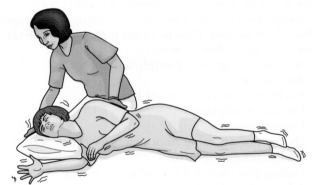

FIGURE 58-24 A pillow protects the person's head during a seizure. The person is turned onto the side.

BOX 58-4	Seizures: Activating EMS

Activate the EMS system for any of the following:

- This is the person's first seizure. (The person has never had a seizure before.)
- The person has trouble breathing after the seizure.
- The person has difficulty awakening after the seizure.
- The seizure lasts longer than 5 minutes.
- The person has another seizure soon after the first seizure.
- The person is or may be injured.
- The seizure happened in water.
- The person has diabetes and loses consciousness.
- The person is pregnant.

Modified from Centers for Disease Control and Prevention: First aid for seizures, *May 15, 2024.*

CONCUSSIONS

Head injuries can be minor or serious and life-threatening. Concussion is the most common brain injury. A concussion results from a bump or blow to the head or jolt to the head or body. The head and brain move quickly back and forth.

Common signs and symptoms after the injury are headache, confusion, and amnesia (memory loss). Memory loss usually involves forgetting the event that caused the injury. Symptoms can occur within minutes to hours after the injury. New symptoms can develop days later. Symptoms can last for days, weeks, or longer and affect:

- *Thinking*—difficulty thinking clearly, concentrating, remembering new information
- *Physical function*—headache, blurred or double vision, nausea and vomiting, dizziness, sensitivity to noise or light, balance problems, feeling tired, no energy
- *Mood*—irritability, sadness, nervousness, anxiety
- *Sleep*—more or less sleep than usual, trouble falling asleep

Some people have repeated concussions. Football players are examples. Long-term effects from repeated concussions include chronic problems with concentration, memory, headaches, and balance.

Emergency Care for Concussions

The following signal the need for emergency care:
- Severe headache or a headache that gets worse or does not go away
- Seizures
- Loss of consciousness; fainting
- Severe dizziness
- Problems with balance or coordination
- Severe nausea or repeated vomiting
- Increasing confusion—trouble recognizing people, places, or things
- Clear, watery fluid coming out of the nose or ears
- Bleeding from the ears
- Numbness, weakness, or tingling in the arms or legs
- Unusual behavior
- Slurred speech
- Large eye pupils or pupils that are not equal in size
- Extreme drowsiness or difficulty being awakened
  Emergency care for a concussion includes the following:
- Follow the rules in Box 58-1. This includes activating the EMS system.
- Start CPR for cardiac arrest. Give rescue breathing for respiratory arrest.
- Place your hands on both sides of the head to keep the head aligned with the spine. Prevent movement.
- Apply firm pressure with a clean cloth to a bleeding area. Be careful not to move the person's head.
- Do not apply direct pressure to the skull if the skull may be fractured. Cover the wound with sterile gauze dressing.
- Do not remove any object from a wound.
- Logroll the person as a unit onto the side if vomiting occurs.
- Apply ice packs to swollen areas.

See *Focus on Children and Older Persons: Emergency Care for Concussions.*

FOCUS ON **CHILDREN AND OLDER PERSONS**

Emergency Care for Concussions

Children

Head injuries are common in young children. In addition to the signs and symptoms already listed, emergency care is needed if the child:
- Will not stop crying.
- Cannot be consoled (comforted).
- Will not nurse or eat.

COLD- AND HEAT-RELATED ILLNESSES

When over-exposed to cold or heat, a person can become seriously ill. The person can die.

Cold-Related Illnesses

Hypothermia and frostbite are 2 cold-related illnesses.

Hypothermia. *Hypothermia* is abnormally low *(hypo)* body temperature *(thermia)*. Prolonged exposure to cold temperatures is the most common cause. Other causes include being cold and wet or being under cold water for too long. A body temperature below 95°F (Fahrenheit) is an emergency.

Persons who spend a lot of time outdoors in cold weather are at risk. So are babies and older persons, especially if in a very cold house or sleeping in a cold room.

Signs and symptoms of hypothermia include:
- Shivering
- Feeling very tired, sleepiness
- Skin color changes: pale with mild hypothermia, cyanosis with moderate hypothermia
- Speech problems: slurring or slowed speech
- Confusion
- Movement problems: moving slowly, trouble walking, being clumsy
- Pulse: weak; rapid with mild hypothermia, slow with moderate hypothermia
- Respirations: shallow; rapid with mild hypothermia, slow with moderate hypothermia
- Losing consciousness

Hypothermia requires emergency care. Activate the EMS system. While waiting for help to arrive:
- Move the person to a warmer place, if possible.
- Remove any wet clothing the person is wearing. Apply dry clothing.
- Wrap the person in warm blankets, towels, or coats. The CDC also suggests the use of body heat from another person or an electric blanket, if available.
- Warm the person gradually. Do not quickly warm the person in a hot bath (shower).
- Give the person something warm to drink. Do not give the person alcohol.
- Do not rub the person's arms or legs.
- Start CPR for cardiac arrest. Give rescue breathing for respiratory arrest.

Frostbite. *Frostbite* is an injury to the body caused by freezing of the skin and underlying tissues. The nose, ears, cheeks, chin, fingers, and toes are the most common sites for frostbite. Damage can be permanent. Severe cases may require amputation (Chapter 49).

Signs and symptoms of frostbite include:
- White or grayish-yellow skin
- Skin that feels unusually firm or waxy
- Numbness
  Emergency care of frostbite includes:
- Seeking medical care.
- Getting into a warm room as soon as possible.
- Removing wet clothing. Applying dry clothing and covering the person to prevent hypothermia.
- Not walking on toes or feet with frostbite.
- Putting the affected part in warm water (not hot water).
- Using body heat to warm the part. For example, warming fingers in the underarm.
- Not rubbing or massaging the part.
- Not using a heating pad, heat lamp, stove, fireplace, or other heat source to warm the part. Affected areas are numb and unable to sense heat. The area is easily burned.

Heat-Related Illnesses

Sweating is the body's way of cooling itself. When sweating is not enough for cooling, body temperature can rise to dangerous levels. Brain and other organ damage can occur.

Staying out in the heat too long is a common cause. Exercising and working outside during hot, humid weather are other causes. Persons at risk include infants, young children, and older persons. Other risk factors include obesity, fever, dehydration, heart disease, mental health disorders, poor circulation, prescription drug use, and alcohol use.

See Table 58-2 for the heat-related illnesses, signs and symptoms, and emergency care.

TABLE 58-2	Heat-Related Illnesses	
Heat-Related Illness	**Signs and Symptoms**	**Emergency Care**
Sunburn	• Painful, red, and warm skin • Blisters	• Move out of the sun. • Apply cool cloths to sunburned areas. Or bathe or shower in cool water. • Apply moisturizing lotion to sunburned areas. • Do not break the blisters.

Heat cramps	• Heavy sweating during exercise
	• Muscle pain
	• Muscle spasms
		• Stop physical activity.
		• Move to a cool place.
		• Drink water or a sports drink.
		• Seek medical help if:
		  • Cramps last longer than 1 hour.
		  • The person is on a low-sodium diet.
		  • The person has heart problems.

Heat exhaustion	• Heavy sweating
	• Cold, pale, and clammy skin
	• Pulse: fast and weak
	• Nausea or vomiting
	• Muscle cramps
	• Tiredness
	• Weakness
	• Dizziness
	• Headache
	• Fainting
		• Move to a cool place.
		• Loosen clothing.
		• Apply cool, wet cloths to the head, neck, underarms, and groin. Or bathe or shower in cool water.
		• Give sips of water.
		• Seek medical care. Get help especially if:
		  • The person is vomiting.
		  • Symptoms worsen or last longer than 1 hour.

Heat stroke	• Body temperature of 103°F or higher
	• Hot, red, dry, or damp skin
	• Pulse: strong and fast
	• Headache
	• Dizziness
	• Nausea
	• Confusion
	• Loss of consciousness
		• Activate the EMS system at once.
		• Move the person to a cool place.
		• Remove excess clothing.
		• Cool the person.
		  • Bathe or shower in cool water.
		  • Apply cool, wet cloths to the head, neck, underarms, and groin.
		• Do not give the person anything to drink.

Modified from Centers for Disease Control and Prevention: Symptoms of heat-related illness, *February 15, 2024.*

BURNS

Burns can severely disable a person. They can also cause death. Most burns occur in the home. Infants, children, and older persons are at risk. Common causes of burns and fires are:

- Scalds from steam or hot liquids
- Playing with matches or lighters
- Electrical injuries
- Cooking accidents (barbecues, microwave ovens, stoves, ovens)
- Falling asleep while smoking
- Fireplaces
- Space heaters
- No smoke alarms or non-functioning smoke alarms
- Sunburns
- Fireworks
- Chemicals

Types of Burns

The skin has 2 layers—the epidermis and dermis. Burns are described as:

- *Superficial (first degree) burns*—involve the epidermis only. They are painful, but the burn is not severe. There is redness and swelling.
- *Partial thickness (second degree) burns*—involve the epidermis and part of the dermis. They are very painful. Nerve endings are exposed. There is redness, swelling, and blistering.
- *Full thickness (third degree) burns*—involve the entire epidermis and dermis. Fat, muscle, and bone may be injured or destroyed. Nerve endings are destroyed, causing numbness in the burned area. The burned skin is white or black.

Some burns are severe (Fig. 58-25). Severity depends on burn size and depth, the body part involved, and age.

Burns to the face, hands, feet, groin, buttocks, or over a joint are more serious than burns to an arm or leg. Infants, young children, and older persons are at high risk for complications and death.

Emergency Care for Burns

Emergency care for severe burns includes the following:

- Follow the rules in Box 58-1. This includes activating the EMS system.
- Do not touch the person if the person is in contact with an electrical source. Have the power source turned off. Do not approach the person or try to remove the electrical source with any object until the power source is turned off.
- Remove the person from the fire or burn source.
- Stop the burning process. Put out flames with water or roll the person in a blanket. Or smother flames with a coat, sheet, or towel.
- Apply cold or cool water for 10 to 15 minutes. Water temperature is between 59°F and 77°F (15°C and 25°C [centigrade]). Do not put ice directly on the burn.
- Remove hot clothing that is not sticking to the skin. If you cannot remove hot clothing, cool the clothing with water.
- Remove jewelry and any tight clothing that is not sticking to the skin.
- Provide rescue breathing and CPR as needed.
- Cover burns with sterile, dry dressings. Or use a sheet or any other clean cloth.
- Do not put oil, butter, salve, or ointments on burns.
- Keep blisters intact. Do not break blisters.
- Elevate the burned area above heart level if possible.
- Cover the person with a blanket or coat to prevent heat loss. (The person is at risk for a drop in body temperature.)

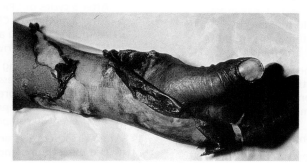

FIGURE 58-25 A severe burn. (From Ignatavicius DD, Workman ML, Rebar, CR: *Medical-surgical nursing: patient-centered collaborative care,* ed 10, St Louis, 2021, Elsevier.)

FOCUS ON PRIDE

The Person, Family, and Yourself

P ersonal and Professional Responsibility

Practicing CPR skills improves confidence. Never practice CPR on another person. Serious damage can be done. Practice on a mannequin. Take pride in learning CPR. Your training can save a life.

R ights and Respect

Protect the right to privacy. Do not expose the person unnecessarily. The person may be in a lounge, dining area, or public place. Do what you can to provide privacy. As always, treat the person with dignity and respect.

I ndependence and Social Interaction

Quality of life and independence are important. In an emergency, choices may be few. However, they are given when possible. For example, the person has the right to choose a hospital.

The EMS staff has guidelines if a person refuses care. For example, the person must be competent and able to legally make medical decisions. The person must also be informed of the risks, benefits, and alternatives to recommended care.

D elegation and Teamwork

On-lookers can threaten privacy and confidentiality. Your main concern is the person's illness or injuries. You cannot give care and manage on-lookers. Ask someone else to deal with on-lookers. If someone else is giving care, keep on-lookers away from the person. Work together to protect the person's privacy.

E thics and Laws

People are curious. They want to know what happened, the extent of injuries or illness, and if the person will be okay. Do not discuss the situation. Do not offer ideas of what is wrong. Information about care, treatment, and condition is confidential. Keep the person's information private. It is the right thing to do.

FOCUS ON PRIDE: Application

Emergencies are stressful. A calm, professional approach helps the person and family feel more secure. Describe professional conduct in an emergency. Explain how you will prepare yourself to respond.

REVIEW QUESTIONS

Circle the BEST answer.

1 When giving first aid, your goal is to
   a Avoid hospital care
   b Prevent death and prevent injuries from becoming worse
   c Keep bystanders informed of the situation
   d Give emergency care alone

2 When giving first aid, you should
   a Know your own limits
   b Move the person away from on-lookers
   c Give the person fluids
   d Keep the person cool

3 The signs of sudden cardiac arrest are
   a Restlessness, rapid breathing, and a weak pulse
   b Confusion, hemiplegia, and slurred speech
   c No response, no normal breathing, and no pulse
   d Dizziness, pale skin, and slow breathing

4 A person is not responsive. To check for breathing
   a Use the head tilt–chin lift method to open the airway
   b Look for no breathing or agonal gasping
   c Look, listen, and feel for air moving in and out of the lungs
   d Take 10 to 15 seconds to listen for breathing

5 Which pulse is checked for an unresponsive adult?
   a The carotid pulse
   b The apical pulse
   c The brachial pulse
   d The femoral pulse

6 Which hand placement is correct for adult chest compressions?
   a 1 hand in the center of the chest
   b 2 hands below the sternum
   c 2 hands on the lower half of the sternum
   d 2 fingers on the lower half of the sternum

7 Which compression rate is used for CPR?
   a 30 compressions per minute
   b 100 to 120 compressions per minute
   c 15 compressions per minute
   d 60 to 100 compressions per minute

8 For adult CPR
   a Give 2 breaths after every 15 compressions
   b Give 2 breaths after every 30 compressions
   c Give 1 breath after every 5 compressions
   d Give 2 breaths when you are tired from giving compressions

9 Two rescuers are giving adult CPR. When should the AED be used?
   a After 5 cycles of CPR
   b After 2 minutes of CPR
   c As soon as the AED arrives
   d When EMS staff arrives

10 Two rescuers are giving a child CPR. Breaths are given
   a After every compression
   b After every 5 compressions
   c After every 15 compressions
   d After every 30 compressions

11 When 2 rescuers give an infant CPR
   a Use the 2-thumb-encircling hands method for compressions
   b Give 30 compressions followed by 2 breaths
   c Check for a carotid pulse
   d Give CPR if the heart rate is less than 100 beats per minute

12 Rescue breathing for an adult involves
   a Giving each breath over 2 seconds
   b Watching the abdomen rise with each breath
   c Giving a breath every 2 to 3 seconds
   d Giving a breath every 6 seconds

13 A person swallowed a chemical. You should
 a Have the person drink a glass of water
 b Have the person try to vomit
 c Call the Poison Control Center
 d Contact the chemical's manufacturer

14 A person is unconscious and has slow, shallow breathing. An opioid overdose is suspected. Which action is *correct*?
 a Let the person sleep off the effects.
 b Call 911 and give naloxone, if available.
 c Leave to avoid legal trouble.
 d Give hands-only CPR.

15 Which statement about heart attack is *true*?
 a It is the same as cardiac arrest.
 b It can cause cardiac arrest.
 c Symptoms resolve with rest.
 d It is a severe response to an antigen.

16 Which statement about hemorrhage is *correct*?
 a External bleeding is usually not seen.
 b Internal bleeding is not as serious as external bleeding.
 c Vomiting blood signals internal bleeding.
 d If an object has pierced the body, you should remove it.

17 A person is hemorrhaging from the forearm. Your *first* action is to
 a Lower the arm
 b Apply pressure to the brachial artery
 c Tape a dressing in place
 d Apply direct pressure to the wound

18 A person is about to faint. What should you do?
 a Have the person sit or lie down.
 b Take the person outside for fresh air.
 c Have the person stand very still.
 d Raise the head if the person is lying down.

19 Which signals shock?
 a High blood pressure
 b Slow pulse
 c Slow and deep respirations
 d Cold, moist, and pale skin

20 A person is severely injured but is conscious and breathing. Signs of shock are present. Which action is *best*?
 a Wait to see if the person improves before calling for help.
 b Give CPR and use an AED right away.
 c Activate the EMS system and keep the person lying down.
 d Use pillows to raise the person's head and upper body.

21 Emergency care for stroke involves
 a Asking when the person's symptoms began
 b Giving the person sips of water
 c Controlling bleeding
 d Positioning the person bent forward with the head lowered

22 A person is having a tonic-clonic (grand mal) seizure. You should
 a Place an object between the person's teeth
 b Loosen tight jewelry and clothing around the neck
 c Try to stop the person's movements
 d Place the person's head on a firm surface

23 After falling down stairs, a person is confused and has a severe headache. You should
 a Place the person in the recovery position
 b Give the person a pain-relief drug
 c Prevent movement of the head and neck
 d Help the person to bed to lie down

24 Which emergency measure is *correct*?
 a Use a hot bath for hypothermia.
 b Massage fingers with frostbite.
 c Give cold water to drink for a heat stroke.
 d Apply cool, wet cloths for heat exhaustion.

25 While waiting for help to arrive, cover a severe burn with
 a A sterile, dry dressing or clean cloth
 b Butter or oil
 c Salve or an ointment
 d Nothing

Answers to Chapter 58 questions are on p. 904.

FOCUS ON PRACTICE

Problem Solving

You are at a local park on a day off of work. You see an adult suddenly collapse. There are others in the park. Describe the steps you will take to:
- Determine if help and CPR are needed.
- Call for help and get emergency equipment.
- Give CPR.
- Use an AED.

KEY TERMS

advance directive A legal document stating a person's wishes about health care when that person is unable to make decisions
autopsy The examination of the body after death
end-of-life care The support and care given during the time surrounding death
palliative care Care that relieves or reduces the intensity of uncomfortable symptoms without producing a cure

post-mortem care Care of the body after *(post)* death *(mortem)*
rigor mortis The stiffness or rigidity *(rigor)* of skeletal muscles that occurs after death *(mortis)*
terminal illness An illness or injury from which the person will not likely recover; death is expected

KEY ABBREVIATIONS

CPR	Cardiopulmonary resuscitation		OBRA	Omnibus Budget Reconciliation Act of 1987
DNR	Do Not Resuscitate		POLST	Physician Orders for Life-Sustaining Treatment
ID	Identification			

*E*nd-of-life care describes the support and care given during the time surrounding death. For some, death is sudden. For others, the process is gradual and death is expected. End-of-life care may involve days, weeks, or months.

Your feelings about death affect the care you give. You will help meet the dying person's physical, psychological, social, and spiritual needs. Therefore you must understand the dying process. Then you can approach the person and family with caring, kindness, and respect.

TERMINAL ILLNESS

Many illnesses have no cure. The body cannot function after some injuries. An illness or injury from which the person will not likely recover is a *terminal illness*. Death is expected.

A person may have days, months, weeks, or years to live. Doctors cannot predict the exact amount of time. People expected to live for a short time have lived for years. Others have died earlier than expected.

Types of Care

Terminally ill persons may need palliative care or hospice care. The person may opt for palliative care and then change to hospice care.

- *Palliative care. Palliate* means to soothe or relieve. *Palliative care* relieves or reduces the intensity of uncomfortable symptoms without producing a cure. The focus is on comfort. The intent is to improve quality of life and provide family support. Palliative care can be given along with disease treatment.
- *Hospice care.* The focus is on the physical, emotional, social, and spiritual needs of dying persons and their families (Chapter 1). Often the person has less than 6 months to live. Cure or life-saving measures are not concerns. Pain relief and comfort are stressed. The goal is to improve quality of life. Follow-up care and support groups for survivors are hospice services. Hospice also supports the health team in dealing with a person's death.

ATTITUDES ABOUT DEATH

Experiences, culture, religion, and age influence attitudes about death. Many people fear death. Others look forward to and accept death. Beliefs and attitudes about death often change as a person grows older and with changing needs.

Many adults and children have not been present when someone dies. Some have not attended a visitation (wake) or funeral. They have not seen the process of dying and death. Therefore it may be frightening, morbid, and a mystery.

Cultural and Spiritual Needs

Practices and attitudes about death differ among cultures. In some cultures, dying people are cared for at home by the family. Some families prepare the body for burial.

Attitudes about death are often closely related to spirituality and religion (Chapter 7). Often people's spiritual beliefs are strengthened at the end of life. Meeting spiritual needs can provide comfort for the dying person and family.

People have different beliefs about what occurs after death. Some believe in life after death. Others do not. To them, death is the end of life. *Reincarnation* is the belief that the spirit or soul is reborn in another human body or in another form of life.

Many cultures and religions have practices, rites, and rituals during the dying process and at the time of death and after. Prayers, blessings, readings, and music are common sources of comfort. So are visits from a cleric, family, and friends.

See *Focus on Communication: Cultural and Spiritual Needs.*

FOCUS ON COMMUNICATION

Cultural and Spiritual Needs

Your cultural or religious practices and beliefs may differ from those of patients and residents. Do not judge the person by your standards. Do not make negative comments or insult the person's beliefs. Respect the person as a whole. This includes the person's beliefs and customs.

Age

Infants and toddlers do not understand death. They know or sense that something has changed. They sense a caregiver's absence or a different caregiver. They also sense changes in when and how their needs are met. They may feel a sense of loss.

Between about 3 and 6 years old, children understand more. They know when family members or pets die. They notice dead birds or bugs. Some children think death is temporary. (The person will come back to life.) Such ideas come from fairy tales, cartoons, movies, video games, and TV. Children this age often blame themselves when someone or something dies. Answers to questions about death often cause fear and confusion. Children who are told the person is "sleeping" may be afraid to go to sleep.

School-age children learn that death is final. They do not think they will die. Death happens to others, especially adults. It can be avoided. Children relate death to punishment and body mutilation. It also involves witches, ghosts, goblins, and monsters. Understanding increases as children grow older and have more experiences with death.

Adults may fear pain and suffering, dying alone, and the invasion of privacy. They also may fear loneliness and separation from loved ones. Worries about the care and support of those left behind are common. Adults often resent death because it affects plans, hopes, dreams, and ambitions.

Older persons know death will occur. Many have lost family and friends. Some welcome death as freedom from pain, suffering, and disability. Like younger adults, many still have worries and fears.

THE STAGES OF DYING

Dr. Elisabeth Kübler-Ross described 5 stages of dying. They also are called the "stages of grief." *Grief* is the person's response to loss.

- *Stage 1: Denial.* The person refuses to believe that death will occur soon. "No, not me" is a common response. The person believes a mistake was made. Information about the illness or injury is not heard. The person cannot deal with any problem or decision about the matter. This stage can last for a few hours, days, or much longer. Some people remain in denial.
- *Stage 2: Anger.* The person thinks "Why me?" There is anger and rage. Dying persons may envy and resent those with life and health. Family, friends, and the health team are often targets of anger. While it may be hard, do not take anger personally. Control any urge to attack back or avoid the person.
- *Stage 3: Bargaining.* Anger has passed. The person now says: "Yes, me but...." The person may bargain with God or a higher power for more time. Promises are made in exchange for more time. The person may want to see a child marry, see a grandchild, have another Christmas, or live for a special event. Usually more promises are made as the person makes "just one more" request. Bargaining is usually private and spiritual.
- *Stage 4: Depression.* The person thinks "Yes, me" and is very sad. The person mourns lost things and the future loss of life. The person may cry or say little. Sometimes the person talks about people and things that will be left behind.
- *Stage 5: Acceptance.* The person is calm, at peace, and accepts death. The person has said what needs to be said. Unfinished business is complete. This stage may last for many months or years. Reaching the acceptance stage does not mean death is near.

Dying persons do not always pass through each stage. A person may stay in one stage. Some move back and forth between stages. For example, a person moves from acceptance back to bargaining and then moves forward to acceptance.

COMFORT NEEDS

End-of-life care involves physical, mental and emotional, and spiritual comfort. Comfort goals are to:

- Prevent or relieve suffering to the extent possible.
- Respect and follow end-of-life wishes.

Dying persons may want family and friends present. They may want to talk about fears, worries, and anxieties. Some want to be alone. Often they need to talk during the night. The setting is quiet, distractions are few, and there is more time to think.

Listening and the use of touch can be meaningful and comforting.

- *Listening.* The person may need to talk and share worries and concerns. Let the person express feelings and emotions. Do not worry about saying the wrong thing or finding comforting words. You do not need to say anything. Being there is what counts.
- *Touch.* Touch shows care and concern when words cannot. Sometimes the person does not want to talk but needs you nearby. Do not feel that you must talk. Silence, along with touch, is a powerful and meaningful way to communicate.

Some people want to see a spiritual leader. Or they want to take part in religious practices. Provide privacy during prayer and spiritual times. Be courteous to the spiritual leader. The person has the right to have religious items nearby—medals, pictures, statues, writings, and so on. Handle them with care and respect.

See *Focus on Communication: Comfort Needs.*
See *Focus on Children and Older Persons: Comfort Needs.*

FOCUS ON **COMMUNICATION**

Comfort Needs

Knowing what to say to the dying person is hard for many health team members. Unless you have been near death yourself, do not say: "I understand what you are going through." The statement is a communication barrier. Instead, you can say:

- "Would you like to talk? I have time to listen."
- "You seem sad. Can I help?"
- "Can I sit with you for a while?"

FOCUS ON **CHILDREN AND OLDER PERSONS**

Comfort Needs

Older Persons
Persons with advanced Alzheimer's disease cannot share their concerns, discomforts, or problems. It can be hard to provide emotional and spiritual comfort. Focus on the person's senses—hearing, touch, sight—to promote comfort. Comforting touch or massage can be soothing. So can soft music or sounds from nature—birds chirping, gentle breezes, ocean waves, and so on.

Physical Needs

Dying may take a few minutes, hours, days, or weeks. Body processes slow. The person is weak. Levels of consciousness change. The person is independent to the extent possible. As the person weakens, basic needs are met by others. Every effort is made to promote physical and psychological comfort. The person is allowed to die in peace and with dignity.

Pain. Pain can range from none to severe. Report signs and symptoms of pain at once (Chapter 36). Some persons cannot tell you about pain. Watch for signs of pain or discomfort.

- Restlessness
- Agitation
- Frowning, grimacing
- Sighing
- Moaning
- Whimpering, crying
- Tense muscles
- Rapid pulse

Skin care, personal and oral hygiene, back massages, and good alignment promote comfort. So do frequent position changes and supportive devices. Turn the person slowly and gently. Follow the care plan to prevent and control pain. The nurse can give pain-relief drugs.

Breathing Problems. Shortness of breath and difficulty breathing *(dyspnea)* are common end-of-life problems. Semi-Fowler's position and oxygen (Chapter 44) are helpful. An open window for fresh air may be helpful. So might a fan circulating air.

Noisy breathing—the *death rattle*—is common as death nears. This is from mucus collecting in the airway. These measures may help.

- The side-lying position
- Suctioning to remove secretions
- Drugs to reduce the amount of mucus

Vision, Hearing, and Speech. Vision blurs and gradually fails. The person turns toward light. A darkened room may frighten the person. The eyes may be half-open. Secretions may collect in the eye corners.

Because of failing vision, explain who you are and what you are doing to the person or in the room. The room should be lit to meet the person's needs. Avoid bright lights and glares.

Good eye care is needed (Chapter 24). If the eyes stay open, a nurse may apply a protective ointment. Then the eyes are covered with moist pads to prevent injury.

Hearing is one of the last functions lost. Many people hear until the moment of death. Even unconscious persons may hear. Always assume that the person can hear. Speak in a normal voice. Give reassurance and explain care. Offer words of comfort. Avoid upsetting topics. Do not talk about the person.

Speech becomes harder. It may be hard to understand the person. Sometimes the person cannot speak. Anticipate needs. Do not ask questions with long answers. Ask a few "yes" or "no" questions. Despite speech problems, you must talk to the person.

Mouth, Nose, and Skin.
Oral hygiene promotes comfort. Give routine mouth care if the person can eat and drink. Give frequent oral hygiene as death nears and when taking oral fluids is difficult. Suctioning (Chapter 45) is needed if mucus collects in the mouth and the person cannot swallow. A lip balm may be used for dry lips.

Crusting and irritation of the nostrils can occur. Nasal secretions, an oxygen cannula, and a naso-gastric tube are common causes. Carefully clean the nose. Apply lubricant as directed by the nurse and the care plan.

Circulation fails. Body temperature changes as death nears. The skin is cool, pale, and mottled (blotchy). Sweating increases. Skin care, bathing, and preventing pressure injuries are necessary. Linens and gowns are changed as needed. Although the skin feels cool, only light bed coverings are needed. Blankets may cause warmth and restlessness. However, observe for signs of cold—shivering, hunching shoulders, and pulling covers. Prevent drafts and provide more blankets.

Nutrition.
Nausea, vomiting, and loss of appetite are common at the end of life. Drugs for nausea and vomiting are ordered.

You may need to feed the person. Favorite foods may help loss of appetite. So may small, frequent meals.

As death nears, loss of appetite is common. The person may choose not to eat or drink. Do not force the person to eat or drink. Tell the nurse.

Elimination.
Urinary and fecal incontinence may occur. Use incontinence products or waterproof under-pads as directed. Give perineal care as needed. Constipation and urinary retention are common. A catheter may be needed. Follow the care plan for catheter care and bowel elimination.

The Person's Room.
Provide a comfortable and pleasant room. Remove unnecessary equipment. Some equipment is upsetting to see (suction machines, drainage containers). If possible, keep such items out of the person's sight.

Mementos, pictures, cards, flowers, and religious items provide comfort. The person and family arrange the room as they wish. This helps meet love, belonging, and esteem needs. The room should reflect the person's choices.

Mental and Emotional Needs
Mental and emotional needs are very personal. Some persons are calm and at peace. Others are anxious or depressed or have specific fears and concerns. Examples include:
- Severe pain
- When and how death will occur
- What will happen to loved ones
- Dying alone

Simple measures may be soothing—touch, holding a hand, back massage, soft lighting, music at a low volume.

THE FAMILY
The family usually gathers at the bedside to comfort the person and each other. This is a hard time for the family. It may be hard to find comforting words. Be available, courteous, and considerate. These actions show that you care.

Sometimes the family keeps a *vigil*. That is, someone is always with the person even at night. They watch over or pray for the person. Provide for the family's comfort.

Respect the right to privacy. The person and family need time together. However, do not neglect care because the family is present. Most agencies let family members help give care. Or you can suggest that they take a beverage or meal break.

The family may be very tired, sad, and tearful. Watching a loved one die is very painful. So is dealing with the eventual loss of that person. The family goes through stages like the dying person. They need support, understanding, courtesy, and respect. A spiritual leader may provide comfort. Communicate this request to the nurse at once.

ADVANCE CARE PLANNING
The *Patient Self-Determination Act* and the *Omnibus Budget Reconciliation Act of 1987 (OBRA)* give persons the right to accept or refuse treatment. This right includes personal choice in end-of-life decisions. *Advance care planning* allows persons to make end-of-life wishes known beforehand. In the event that a person can no longer communicate for oneself, the person's preferences are known.

Advance Directives
An *advance directive* is a legal document stating a person's wishes about health care when that person is unable to make decisions. Advance directives include living wills and a durable power of attorney for health care. See Box 59-1 (p. 886). A person may have one or both types.

Advance directives are completed by the individual. Once established, a person can make changes at any time. States have different forms and requirements for advance directive documents.

Agencies must inform all persons of the right to advance directives on admission. The medical record documents whether or not the person has made them.

See *Focus on Surveys: Advance Directives*.

> ### FOCUS ON SURVEYS
> #### Advance Directives
>
> Advance directives are a focus of surveys. Nursing staff must know the person's current wishes. Surveyors review medical records and perform interviews to check that advance directives are current. The health team must regularly review the advance directive with the person or the person's representative to be sure that it reflects the person's current wishes.

Medical Orders

Medical orders are written by health care providers. An order gives specific instructions for care. *Do Not Resuscitate (DNR)* orders and *Physician Orders for Life-Sustaining Treatment (POLST)* are 2 types that direct end-of-life care. See Box 59-1. Such orders are intended for persons who are terminally ill or of very old age and frail.

A person's refusal of life-sustaining measures does not mean refusal of all care. Comfort measures are still provided. Other treatments, as desired by the person or as made known through advance directives, are able to be given.

You may not agree with the person's end-of-life decisions. However, you must follow the person's or family's wishes and the doctor's orders. These may be against your personal values. If so, talk to the nurse. You may need an assignment change.

BOX 59-1	Advance Care Planning: Advance Directives and Medical Orders

Living will—a legal document about measures that support or maintain life *(life-sustaining measures)*. Resuscitation, ventilation, tube feeding, and dialysis are examples. A living will directs what care a person wants and does not want in the event that the person cannot communicate about such decisions.

Durable Power of Attorney for Health Care—a legal document designating another person (a *health care proxy*) to make decisions in the event that the person is unable to do so. Usually the proxy is a family member, friend, or lawyer. The proxy should be aware of the person's end-of-life wishes. A proxy is called a *surrogate* or *agent* in some states.

Do Not Resuscitate (DNR) Order—a doctor's order not to resuscitate a person. The order is written after consulting with the person and family. The family and doctor make the decision if the person is not mentally able to do so. Also called a "No Code" order, a DNR order means that cardiopulmonary resuscitation (CPR) or rescue breathing will not be done in the event of cardiac or respiratory arrest (Chapter 58). The order is in effect within a care setting. Some states have DNR forms that are valid outside of a care setting.

Physician Orders for Life-Sustaining Treatment (POLST)—a medical order intended for persons who are seriously ill or frail (known to be nearing the end of life). More specific than a DNR order, the form directs whether or not to:
- Perform CPR.
- Transfer the person to a hospital and what treatments to perform there—all possible life-sustaining treatments, select treatments, or comfort-focused treatments.
- Use enteral nutrition (Chapter 33).

POLST is a "portable medical order." The order is valid at home and in all care settings. States have different names for POLST. *Medical Orders for Life-Sustaining Treatment (MOLST)* is another common name.

SIGNS OF DEATH

In the weeks or days before death, the dying process may involve:
- Restlessness, agitation, anxiety, or depression
- Shortness of breath; pauses in breathing
- Drowsiness
- Weakness
- Confusion
- Constipation or incontinence
- Nausea and loss of appetite

As death nears, the following signs may occur fast or slowly:
- Movement, muscle tone, and sensation are lost. This usually starts in the feet and legs. Mouth muscles relax, the jaw drops. The mouth may stay open. The facial expression is often peaceful.
- Gastro-intestinal functions slow down. Abdominal distention, fecal incontinence, nausea, and vomiting are common.
- Body temperature changes. The person feels cool or cold, looks pale, and perspires heavily.
- Circulation fails. The pulse is fast or slow, weak, and irregular. Blood pressure starts to fall.
- The respiratory system fails. Rapid or slow and shallow respirations are observed. Mucus collects in the airway. Breathing sounds are noisy and gurgling *(death rattle)*.
- Pain decreases as the person loses consciousness. However, some people are conscious until the moment of death.

The signs of death include *no pulse*, *no respirations*, and *no blood pressure*. A doctor determines that death has occurred and pronounces the person dead. If a doctor is not present in a nursing center, a nurse calls the doctor to report the signs of death. The time and place are noted for the death certificate.

Some persons desire to donate tissues or organs when death occurs. Special procedures are followed. You assist as the nurse directs.

■ CARE OF THE BODY AFTER DEATH

Care of the body after *(post)* death *(mortem)* is called *post-mortem care*. You may be asked to assist the nurse. Post-mortem care begins when the person is pronounced dead.

Post-mortem care is done to maintain a good appearance of the body. Discoloration and skin damage are prevented. Valuables and personal items are gathered for the family.

Within 2 to 4 hours after death, rigor mortis develops. *Rigor mortis* is the stiffness or rigidity *(rigor)* of skeletal muscles that occurs after death *(mortis)*. The body is positioned in normal alignment before rigor mortis sets in. The body should appear in a comfortable and natural position when the family sees the body.

In some agencies, the body is prepared only for viewing by the family. The funeral director completes post-mortem care.

Sometimes an autopsy is done. An *autopsy* is the examination of the body after death. It is done to determine the cause of death. Post-mortem care is not done. Doing so could remove or destroy evidence.

Post-mortem care involves bathing soiled areas and positioning the body in good alignment. When moving the body, air in the lungs, stomach, and intestines can be expelled. When air is expelled, sounds are produced. Do not let those sounds alarm or frighten you. They are normal and expected.

See *Delegation Guidelines: Care of the Body After Death*.

See *Promoting Safety and Comfort: Care of the Body After Death*.

See procedure: *Assisting With Post-Mortem Care*.

DELEGATION GUIDELINES
Care of the Body After Death

Parts of post-mortem care may be delegated to you. To assist, you need this information from the nurse.
- If dentures are inserted or placed in a denture cup
- If tubes and dressings are removed or left in place
- If rings are removed or left in place
- If the family wants to view the body
- Special agency policies and procedures

PROMOTING SAFETY AND COMFORT
Care of the Body After Death

Safety

Standard Precautions and the Bloodborne Pathogen Standard are followed. You may have contact with blood or body fluids. Follow the rules of hand hygiene and the guidelines for glove use in Chapters 17 and 18.

Comfort

Respect and dignity must be maintained during post-mortem care. Provide privacy. Keep the body covered as much as possible. Move the body gently. Handle the person's valuables with care. Consider the family and the dignity they would want shown to the person.

Assisting With Post-Mortem Care

PRE-PROCEDURE

1 Follow *Delegation Guidelines: Care of the Body After Death*. See *Promoting Safety and Comfort: Care of the Body After Death*.
2 Practice hand hygiene and get the following supplies.
   - Post-mortem kit (shroud or body bag, gown, identification [ID] tags, gauze squares, safety pins)
   - Disposable bed protectors
   - Wash basin
   - Bath towel and washcloths
   - Denture cup (if needed)
   - Items for shaving facial hair (Chapter 25) as needed
   - Tape
   - Dressings
   - Cotton balls
   - Valuables envelope
   - Gloves
   - Laundry bag
3 Arrange items in the room.
4 Provide for privacy.
5 Raise the bed for body mechanics. Lower the bed rail near you if up.
6 Make sure the bed is flat.

PROCEDURE

7 Put on gloves. (Change gloves as needed.)
8 Position the body supine. Arms and legs are straight. A pillow is under the head and shoulders. Or raise the head of the bed 15 to 20 degrees if this is agency policy.
9 Close the eyes. Gently pull the eyelids over the eyes. Follow the nurse's directions if the eyes do not stay closed. Moist cotton balls may be gently applied over the eyelids.
10 Insert dentures or put them in a labeled denture cup. Follow agency policy.
11 Close the mouth. If necessary, place a rolled towel under the chin to keep the mouth closed.
12 Follow agency policy for rings and jewelry. In some agencies, jewelry is removed except for a wedding ring. List any jewelry that is removed. Place the jewelry and the list in a valuables envelope. Rings that remain in place may be secured with a cotton ball and tape after the family views the body.
13 Remove drainage containers.
14 Remove tubes and catheters with gauze squares as the nurse directs.
15 Remove soiled dressings. Replace them with clean ones.
16 Shave facial hair if agency policy or if desired by the family. Some men normally grow facial hair (beard, mustache). If so, do not shave facial hair.
17 Bathe soiled areas with plain water. Dry thoroughly.
18 Place a disposable bed protector under the buttocks.
19 Remove and discard soiled gloves. Practice hand hygiene. Put on clean gloves.
20 Put a clean gown on the body. Position the body as in step 8.
21 Brush and comb the hair if necessary.
22 Cover the body to the shoulders with a sheet if the family will view the body.
23 Gather belongings. Put them in a bag labeled with the person's name. Be sure to include eyeglasses, hearing aids, and other valuables.
24 Remove supplies, equipment, and linens. Lower the bed. Straighten the room. Provide soft lighting.
25 Remove and discard the gloves. Practice hand hygiene.
26 Let the family view the body. Provide for privacy. Return to the room after they leave.
27 Practice hand hygiene. Put on gloves.
28 Fill out the ID tags. Tie 1 to the ankle or to the right big toe.

Continued

Assisting With Post-Mortem Care—cont'd

PROCEDURE—cont'd

29 Place the body in the body bag or cover it with a sheet. Or apply a shroud (Fig. 59-1). (Raise the bed and have help from co-workers for turning and positioning.)
- Position the shroud under the body.
- Bring the top down over the head.
- Fold the bottom up over the feet.
- Fold the sides over the body.
- Pin or tape the shroud in place.

30 Attach the second ID tag to the shroud, sheet, or body bag.
31 Leave the denture cup with the body.
32 Remove and discard the gloves. Practice hand hygiene.

POST-PROCEDURE

33 Maintain privacy measures. Leaving the privacy curtain, window coverings, and door closed are examples. Follow the nurse's instructions.
34 Clean the unit after the body has been removed if this is your job. Wear gloves for this step.
35 Remove and discard the gloves. Practice hand hygiene.

36 Report the following.
- The time the body was taken by the funeral director
- What was done with jewelry, other valuables, and personal items
- What was done with dentures

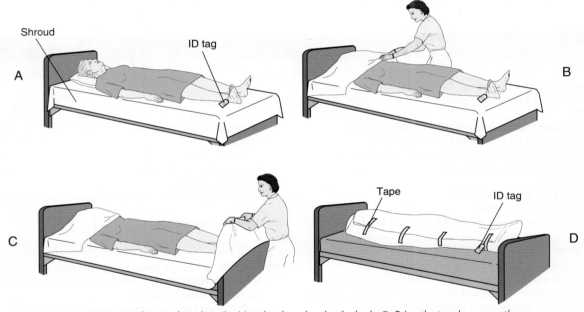

FIGURE 59-1 Applying a shroud. **A,** Position the shroud under the body. **B,** Bring the top down over the head. **C,** Fold the bottom up over the feet. **D,** Fold the sides over the body. Tape or pin the sides together. Attach an ID tag to the outside of the shroud.

CARING FOR THE FAMILY

Courtesy, comfort, and privacy are helpful for the family after a person's death. You can:
- Express sympathy. Be kind and genuine.
- Allow the family time with the person's body. Provide privacy. Do not rush them.
- Provide another private area for the family.
- Provide tissues and offer a beverage.
- Ask if there are other needs.
- Be available.

The Person, Family, and Yourself

Personal and Professional Responsibility

To give quality care to the dying person and family:

- Promote comfort. Report signs of pain at once. Follow the comfort measures in the care plan. Ask about the family's comfort. Offering a drink or a blanket shows concern.
- Provide support to the person and family. Be kind. Show compassion and respect.
- Give the family time alone with the person.

Take pride in supporting the person and family during a difficult time. The family has many emotions during the dying process and after a loved one's death (Fig. 59-2).

Rights and Respect

Understanding the person's needs and desires allows you to give better care. The desire to die in peace and with dignity is respected. The right to privacy and the right to be treated with dignity and respect apply after death.

Independence and Social Interaction

Some days the person can do more and interact more than other days. Consider the person's physical and mental limits. Do not force more. Allow rest. Tell the nurse if you suspect that the family or visitors are tiring the person.

Delegation and Teamwork

Over time, the health team often bonds with the person. This is common in hospice and long-term care. The person's death is difficult for the staff. Sadness and grief may occur.

Tell the nurse if you have trouble coping with a person's death. Support others who need help. A kind word, a hug, or taking time to listen shows concern. Take pride in being a part of a caring and supportive team.

Ethics and Laws

The dying person has rights under OBRA.

- *The right to privacy before and after death.* Proper draping and screening are important.
- *The right to visit others in private.* Moving the dying person to a private room provides privacy. Family can usually stay with the person.
- *The right to confidentiality before and after death.* The final moments and cause of death are confidential. So are statements, conversations, and family reactions.
- *The right to be free from abuse, mistreatment, and neglect.* The person has the right to kind and respectful care before and after death. Report signs of abuse, mistreatment, or neglect at once.
- *Freedom from restraint.* Restraints are used only if ordered by the doctor. Dying persons are often too weak to be dangerous to themselves or others.
- *The right to personal possessions.* The person may want photos and treasured items nearby. Protect the person's property from loss or damage before and after death.
- *The right to a safe and home-like setting.* Everyone must keep the setting safe and home-like. Try to keep equipment and supplies out of view. The room should be free from unpleasant odors and noises. Do your best to keep the room neat and clean.
- *The right to personal choice.* The dying person may refuse treatment. The health team must respect choices to refuse life-sustaining measures.

FOCUS ON **PRIDE**: *Application*

Genuine concern for the dying person is shown in the care you give. How can you show respect at the end of life and with post-mortem care? How can you show care and concern for the grieving family?

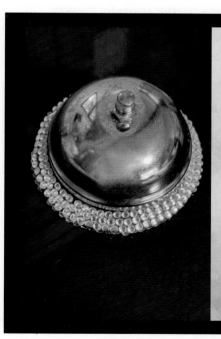

ROGER'S BELL

Mom neared the end of her travail,
she suffered much...so thin, so frail.
I worried a lot; "What if she fell?"
Then I remembered "Roger's Bell!"
I put the bell beside her bed.
"Just ring it anytime," I said,
"and I'll be there to help you stand,
or rub your back, or hold your hand."
I'd tell Mom most every night
to ring that bell if things weren't right.
And once or twice she rang the bell,
she did it for me, I could tell.
The final weeks were Carol's hell...
yet she ignored the nightstand bell.

The bell was quiet the day she died,
when friends she barely knew had cried.
I went to the nightstand...said a prayer,
picked up the bell...Do I dare?
"Why have it there beside your bed,
when now I need your help instead?"
She answered, "If you're sad and lonely too,
ring the bell and I'll be there with you!"
– Now Mom doesn't need my steady hand,
– she marches on...leading the band.
Her ordeal is over, her task complete,
and she watches over me, till again we meet.

–Bob Pinkerton

FIGURE 59-2 Having esophageal cancer, Linda Pinkerton Davis's husband, Roger, had lost his ability to speak. Linda gave Roger a nightstand bell to allow him to ring for help. Roger passed away. Later, the bell was decorated and given to Linda's mom, Carol, who had cancer. Carol's husband wrote this poem for his four daughters after their mother died. (Bell photo courtesy Becky MacMillan; "Roger's Bell" poem printed with permission from the late Robert Pinkerton, July 2017.)

REVIEW QUESTIONS

Circle the BEST answer.

1 Which is *true?*
   a Death from terminal illness is sudden.
   b Doctors know when death will occur.
   c An illness is terminal when recovery is not likely.
   d All severe injuries end in death.

2 Which statement is *true?*
   a Attitudes about death change as a person ages.
   b Culture does not influence attitudes about death.
   c Young children understand death well.
   d A family member's death does not affect a toddler.

3 Which shows respect for the person's spiritual needs at the end of life?
   a Interrupting a time of prayer to refill the person's water mug
   b Providing privacy when a spiritual leader is present
   c Moving a religious item from the bedside stand without asking
   d Arguing with the person about beliefs

4 After a grandparent's death, a 5-year-old asks: "When will Grandpa be back?" The child's response
   a Is age-appropriate
   b Signals denial
   c Signals delayed intellectual development
   d Signals poor parenting

5 A person tries to gain more time during the stage of
   a Anger
   b Bargaining
   c Depression
   d Acceptance

6 A person near the end of life talks about fears. Which response is *best?*
   a Tell the person not to worry.
   b Leave if the conversation makes you uncomfortable.
   c Talk about yourself to distract the person.
   d Sit beside the person and listen.

7 A person near the end of life is restless and moaning. Which action is *best?*
   a Turn the lights off and leave the room.
   b Remind the person to be still and quiet.
   c Provide comfort measures and tell the nurse.
   d Restrain the person to prevent injury.

8 When caring for the dying person, you should
   a Anticipate needs
   b Do most of the talking
   c Ask questions with long answers
   d Speak in a loud voice

9 As death nears, the last sense lost is usually
   a Sight
   b Taste
   c Smell
   d Hearing

10 The dying person's care includes the following. Which should you question?
   a Skin care
   b Oral hygiene
   c Active range-of-motion exercises
   d Suctioning secretions

11 A person is near death. You should
   a Make sure the person eats
   b Offer your opinion on end-of-life decisions
   c Position the person for comfort and good alignment
   d Tell the family what to expect while at the bedside

12 A DNR order means that
   a CPR will not be done
   b A representative will make decisions for the person
   c Life-prolonging measures will be carried out
   d Comfort measures will not be given

13 Which signals approaching death?
   a Increased alertness
   b Slow and shallow respirations
   c Increased blood pressure
   d Warm and dry skin

14 The signs of death are
   a Convulsions and incontinence
   b No pulse, respirations, or blood pressure
   c Loss of consciousness and pale skin
   d Closed eyes and no muscle movements

15 Post-mortem care is done
   a After rigor mortis sets in
   b When the funeral director arrives for the body
   c After the family has viewed the body
   d After the doctor pronounces the person dead

Answers to Chapter 59 questions are on p. 904.

FOCUS ON PRACTICE

Problem Solving

A person is nearing the end of life. You want to provide mouth care. The family arrives. Is this a good time to give care? What will you say to the family?

Getting a Job

OBJECTIVES

- Define the key terms and key abbreviations in this chapter.
- Identify the sources for jobs and places to work.
- Describe what employers look for when hiring staff.
- Describe the qualities and traits needed to work in home care settings.
- Describe how to prove completion of a nursing assistant training and competency evaluation program (NATCEP).
- Explain how to complete a job application.
- Describe in-person, phone, and video interviews.

- Explain how to prepare and dress for an interview.
- Identify common interview questions.
- Explain how to conduct yourself during an interview.
- Describe the questions you cannot be asked during an interview or on a job application.
- Explain what to do after an interview.
- Explain how to accept or decline a job offer.
- Explain how to promote PRIDE in the person, the family, and yourself.

KEY TERMS

discrimination Unjust treatment based on personal qualities

job application An agency's official form listing questions that require factual answers from the person seeking employment; employment form

job interview When an employer asks a job applicant questions about the applicant's education and career

reasonable accommodation To assist or change a position or workplace to allow an employee to do a job despite having a disability

KEY ABBREVIATIONS

EEOC U.S. Equal Employment Opportunity Commission
NATCEP Nursing assistant training and competency evaluation program

OBRA Omnibus Budget Reconciliation Act of 1987

Successfully completing a nursing assistant training and competency evaluation program (NATCEP) is a step toward employment. This chapter will help you find a job in a professional and efficient manner.

SOURCES OF JOBS

There are easy ways to learn about jobs and places to work.

- The Internet—job sites and social media sites
- Newspaper ads
- Local and state employment services
- Agencies you would like to work at
- People you know—instructor, family, and friends
- Your school's or college's job placement counselors
- Job fairs
- Your clinical experience site

Your clinical experience site is an important source. The staff observe students as future employees. They look for good work ethics. They watch how students treat patients or residents, their instructor, other students, and staff. They look for the qualities and traits of a nursing assistant described in Chapter 6. If your clinical agency is not hiring, the staff may suggest other places to apply.

WHAT EMPLOYERS LOOK FOR

If you owned a business, who would you hire? Your answer helps you better understand the agency's point of view. Agencies want staff who:

- Are dependable
- Have needed job skills and training
- Have values and attitudes that fit with the agency
- Have a professional appearance

To function well, you need good work ethics. Review Chapter 6 and the *Focus on PRIDE* boxes at the end of each chapter to help you develop positive attitudes and work practices.

You must be at work on time and when scheduled. Undependable people cause everyone problems. Other staff have extra work. Fewer staff give care. Quality of care suffers. You want co-workers to work when scheduled. Otherwise, you have extra work. You have less time to spend with patients or residents. Likewise, co-workers expect you to work when scheduled.

See *Focus on Long-Term Care and Home Care: What Employers Look For.*

FOCUS ON LONG-TERM CARE AND HOME CARE

What Employers Look For

Long-Term Care

To work in long-term care, you must complete a state-approved NATCEP. This is a requirement of the *Omnibus Budget Reconciliation Act of 1987 (OBRA)*. The agency requests proof of training. The nursing assistant registry is checked. Nursing centers cannot hire persons convicted of abuse, neglect, or mistreatment. This also is an OBRA requirement.

Home Care

Besides the qualities and traits already described and those in Chapter 6, home care requires:

* *The ability to work alone.* Usually a nurse is not with you. If problems occur, you can reach the nurse by phone. You must provide skillful and safe care.
* *Self-discipline.* You must arrive at homes on time. Plan how to complete personal care and housekeeping tasks. Avoid temptations. This includes watching TV, talking on the phone, visiting, and having a cup of coffee.
* *Honesty.* You might need to shop for the person. Be honest and thrifty with the person's money. Accurately report what you bought, the cost with receipts, amount spent, and amount returned.
* *Respect for the person's property.* You will handle valuables and personal property in home care settings. You will use furnishings, appliances, linens, and household items for care and housekeeping. Treat personal and family property with respect. Prevent damage. Read the manufacturer's instructions before using an appliance. Clean the appliance after use.

Job Skills and Training

The agency checks the nursing assistant registry and requests proof of successful NATCEP completion. An agency will accept 1 or more of the following.

* A certificate of course completion from your training program
* A high school, college, or technical school transcript
* An official grade report (report card)

Give the agency a *copy* of your certificate, transcript, or grade report. Never give the original to anyone. Keep originals in a safe place for future use. Some agencies want a transcript sent directly from the school or college.

JOB APPLICATIONS

A *job application (employment form)* is an agency's official form listing questions that require factual answers from the person seeking employment (Fig. 60-1). Personal information (legal name, address, phone number), work history, education, qualifications, and references are examples. The same information is required of all applicants.

You get a job application from the *personnel office (human resources office)* or on-line through an agency's website. For a paper application, use a pen with black ink to complete the form. You can complete the application at the agency or take it home to return by mail or in person. You must be well groomed and behave pleasantly when seeking or returning a job application. It may be your first chance to make a good impression.

On-line job applications require an electronic device—computer, tablet, phone. Follow the agency's website instructions for completing an on-line application.

Completing a Job Application

To complete a job application, see Box 60-1, p. 895. The application may be your first chance to impress the agency. A neat, readable, and complete application gives a good image. A sloppy or incomplete one does not.

A job application is easier to complete if you keep a file of your education and work history. The file should contain:

* A copy of your high school diploma or general equivalency diploma (GED).
* A copy of any grade reports, college degrees, certificates, or military training.
* A copy of your nursing assistant training program certificate of completion.
* NATCEP test results. (See "Competency Evaluation" in Chapter 3.)
* Nursing assistant registry information for each state in which you are certified (licensed, registered).
* Copies of communications with your state's nursing assistant registry agency.
* Copies of court records for criminal convictions.
* A copy of your Social Security card.
* Names, addresses, and phone numbers of references.
* Names, addresses, and phone numbers of current and past employers. Include:
  * Your job title
  * Dates employment started and ended
  * Your supervisor's name
  * Hourly salary
* Proof of in-services attended and continuing education units (CEUs).

When requesting a job application, also ask for the agency's nursing assistant job description (Chapter 3).

EMPLOYMENT APPLICATION

All information listed on this application will be considered and handled as personal and confidential. Please print or write legibly.

AN EQUAL OPPORTUNITY EMPLOYER

This employer provides equal opportunity to all persons without regard to disability, race, color, religion, gender, age, or national origin.

Name

Date of Application

Address

City

State

Zip

Home Phone

Cell Phone

Social Security Number

GENERAL INFORMATION

Position applied for:

Available to work: ☐ Full-time ☐ Part-time ☐ Temporary   Date available to start work:

Will transportation be a problem for you? ☐ No ☐ Yes

Do you have the legal right to work in the United States? ☐ No ☐ Yes

Were you given a job description? ☐ No ☐ Yes

Do you understand the functions of the job? ☐ No ☐ Yes

Can you perform the functions of the job with or without reasonable accommodation? ☐ No ☐ Yes

Have you ever been convicted of a felony? ☐ No ☐ Yes

If yes, explain:

EDUCATION

	Name and Address of School	Major/Degree(s)	Number of Years Completed	Did You Graduate?
High School				
Community College				
4-Year Institution				
Vocational				
Other (specify)				

Describe specialized training, skills, seminars, courses, in-services, continuing education, or extra-curricular activities:

FIGURE 60-1 A sample job application.

Continued

EMPLOYMENT RECORD

Beginning with your current employer, please list your work experience over the last ten years. You may include pertinent volunteer activities.

Name and Address of Employer

Start Date   End Date

Phone

Job Title   Supervisor   Phone   Start Salary   End Salary

Duties

Reason for Leaving

Name and Address of Employer

Start Date   End Date

Phone

Job Title   Supervisor   Phone   Start Salary   End Salary

Duties

Reason for Leaving

Name and Address of Employer

Start Date   End Date

Phone

Job Title   Supervisor   Phone   Start Salary   End Salary

Duties

Reason for Leaving

REFERENCES

Only include persons familiar with your work ability. Do not include family.

Name and Title   Address   Phone

Name and Title   Address   Phone

Name and Title   Address   Phone

Name and Title   Address   Phone

SIGNATURE

I certify that the information provided on this application is true and complete. I understand that any false information or omissions may result in rejection of my application or job loss at any time during employment. I authorize verification of my education and past employment. I release all persons, schools, and past employers from liability for supplying such information.

I understand that the employer will conduct a criminal background check.

I understand that the use of illegal drugs is prohibited during employment. I am willing to submit to drug testing before and during employment.

Signature   Date

FIGURE 60-1, cont'd

BOX 60-1	Guidelines for Completing a Job Application

- Read and follow the directions. They may ask you to print using black ink. Following directions on the job application gives insight about your ability to follow directions on the job.
- Write neatly. Writing must be readable. A messy application gives a bad image. Readable writing gives the correct information. The agency cannot contact you if unable to read your phone number. You may miss getting the job.
- Complete the entire form. If an item does not apply to you, write "N/A" for non-applicable. Or draw a line through the space. This shows that you read the section. It also shows that you did not skip the item on purpose.
- Give information about employment gaps. If you did not work for a time, the agency wonders why. Providing this information shows you are honest. Some reasons are an illness, school, raising children, or caring for a family member.
- Tell why you left a job, if asked. Be brief but honest. People leave jobs for one that pays better. Some leave for career advancement. Others leave for reasons given for employment gaps. If fired from a job, give an honest but positive answer. Do not talk badly about the former agency.

- Give references. List the names, titles, addresses, and phone numbers of at least 4 non-family references. Have this information with you before completing an application. (Always ask references if an agency can contact them.) You may get the job faster if the agency can check references quickly. The agency should not have to wait for missing or incomplete information. This wastes your time and the agency's time. Also, the agency wonders if you are hiding something with incomplete reference information.
- Be prepared to provide the following:
  - Social Security number
  - Proof of the legal right to work in the United States
  - Proof of successful NATCEP completion
  - Identification—driver's license or government-issued ID card
- Report any felony convictions as directed. Write "no" or "none" as appropriate. Criminal background and fingerprint checks are common requirements (Chapter 3).
- Give honest answers. Lying on an application is fraud. It is grounds for being fired.
- Complete a final review of your application. Make sure you have provided all required information.

THE JOB INTERVIEW

A *job interview* is when an employer asks a job applicant questions about the applicant's education and career. The agency gets to know and evaluate you. You learn about the agency.

The interview may be when you complete the job application. Some agencies review applications before scheduling interviews. An interview may be conducted by 1 person or 2 or more people.

When an interview is scheduled, write down the interviewer's name and the interview date and time. If you need directions to the agency, ask for them when the interview is scheduled.

When expecting a call from the agency, answer your phone. Do not let your phone go to voice mail. If the caller has to leave a message, you need an appropriate and professional greeting. Sometimes an agency will contact you through a text or e-mail message. Return messages within 24 hours.

Types of Interviews

Interviews may be in-person, by phone, or by video. You need good communication skills. (See Chapters 7 and 8.)

- *In-person interview.* You and the interviewer meet in the same room face-to-face. Appropriate dress and body language are needed.
- *Phone interview.* A phone interview may be used to decide if an in-person interview will follow. If distance is a factor, a phone interview may work for the agency and you.
- *Video interview.* You use a computer or other electronic device at home or another site. Appropriate dress and body language are needed.

For phone and video interviews:

- Use a quiet room. Turn off music, TV, and other devices. Do not use a room where phones ring, people are talking, or pets are present.
- Be ready to answer the phone or turn on the electronic device at the scheduled time.
- Have your electronic device charged. Consider plugging into a power source to prevent the device from turning off.
- Speak clearly and slowly. Do not shout.
- Listen carefully. Let the interviewer finish speaking before you answer.
- Smile. Smile even for a phone interview. Attitude and facial expression affect your voice tone.

Preparing for the Interview

Box 60-2 (p. 896) lists common interview questions. Prepare and practice your answers ahead of time. Also prepare a list of your skills for the interviewer.

You must present a good image. You need to be neat, clean, and well-groomed. How you dress is important. Follow the guidelines in Box 60-3 (p. 896).

Show that you are dependable. No matter the type of interview, be on time. For an in-person interview, do a practice run (dry run). Go to the agency some day before the interview. Note how long it takes to get there and where to park. Also find the personnel office. A practice run gives an idea of the time needed from your home to the personnel office.

BOX 60-2 Common Interview Questions

What the Interviewer May Ask

- Tell me about yourself.
- Tell me about your career goals.
- What are you doing to reach these goals?
- Describe what *professional* behavior means to you.
- Tell me about your last job. Why did you leave?
- What did you like the most about your last job? The least?
- What would your supervisor and co-workers tell me about you? Your dependability? Your skills? Your ability to work with others?
- Which functions are hard for you? How do you handle this difficulty?
- How do you set priorities?
- How have your experiences prepared you for this job?
- What would you like to change about your last job?
- How do you handle problems with patients, residents, families, and co-workers?
- Why do you want to work here?
- Why should this agency hire you?

What to Ask the Interviewer

- What employee qualities and traits are important to you?
- What do you like about nursing assistants who work here? Are there any challenges?
- What nursing care pattern is used here (Chapter 1)? How are work assignments made?

What to Ask the Interviewer—cont'd

- Who will I work with?
- Are there any job functions that are a priority or an area of focus for quality?
- When are performance evaluations done? Who does them? How are they done?
- What performance factors are evaluated?
- How does the supervisor handle problems?
- What are the most common reasons that nursing assistants lose their jobs here? What are common reasons for resigning? (To *resign* means to leave a job.)
- Do you expect changes in this job in the next year? In the next 5 years?
- How much will I make an hour?
- What hours will I work?
- What uniforms are required?
- What benefits do you offer?
  - Health and dental insurance?
  - Continuing education?
  - Vacation time?
- Do you have a new employee orientation program (Chapter 3)? How long is it?
- May I have a tour of the agency and the unit I will work on? Can I meet the nurse manager and unit staff?

BOX 60-3 Grooming and Dressing for an Interview

- Bathe and brush your teeth. Wash your hair. Men should shave facial hair or groom beards and mustaches.
- Use deodorant or antiperspirant.
- Make sure your hands and fingernails are clean.
- Apply make-up in a simple, attractive manner (if worn).
- Style your hair in a neat and attractive way.
- Wear clothing that looks professional. Slacks (pants) and a shirt or blouse are common (Fig. 60-2). A long-sleeved shirt with a simple pattern or single color (white, light blue, black) is best. A jacket or tie is optional. A simple dress or skirt of an appropriate length may be worn.
- Do not wear jeans, shorts, yoga pants, tank tops, halter tops, or other casual clothing. Also do not wear distracting colors or prints. Do not wear lacy, sheer, tight, or low-cut garments.
- Iron clothing. Sew on loose buttons and mend garments.
- Wear clothing that covers tattoos (body art).
- Wear socks, hose, or tights. Hose should be free of runs and snags.
- Make sure shoes are clean and in good repair.
- Avoid heavy perfumes, colognes, and after-shave lotions. A light fragrance is okay.
- Wear only simple jewelry that complements your clothes. Avoid adornments in body piercings. For multiple ear piercings, wear only 1 set of earrings.
- Brush your teeth again before leaving for the interview. Do not smoke or chew gum before the interview. You must have fresh breath.
- Stop in the restroom when you arrive at the agency. Check your hair, make-up, clothes, and hands.

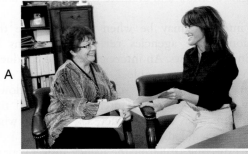
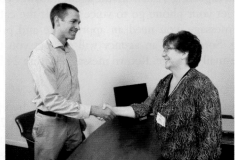

FIGURE 60-2 Dress for an interview. **A,** This applicant wears slacks and a black blouse. **B,** This applicant wears slacks and a blue shirt.

Arriving at the Agency. When you arrive at the agency, turn off your phone and other devices. Tell the receptionist your name, why you are there, and the interviewer's name. Then sit quietly in the waiting area. Do not smoke, chew gum, or use your phone or other devices for calls, e-mails, text messages, or other reasons.

While waiting, review your answers to the common interview questions. Waiting may be part of the interview. The interviewer may ask staff about how you acted while waiting. Smile and be polite and friendly.

During the Interview

Politely greet and address the interviewer as Miss, Mrs., Ms., Mr., or Doctor. For an in-person interview, give a firm hand-shake. Stand until asked to sit. Sit with good posture and in a professional way. If offered a beverage, you may accept. Be sure to thank the person.

Good eye contact is needed for in-person and video interviews. Look directly at the interviewer to answer or ask questions. Poor eye contact sends negative information— shy, insecure, dishonest, or lacking interest.

Watch your body language (Chapter 7)—facial expressions, gestures, posture, and body movements. What you say is important. However, your body tells a great deal. Avoid distracting habits—slumping; biting nails; playing with jewelry, clothing, or your hair; crossing your arms; and crossing and swinging the legs back and forth. Focus on the interview. Do not touch or read things on the person's desk.

Give complete and honest answers. Speak clearly and with confidence. Avoid short and long answers. "Yes" and "no" answers give little information. Briefly explain "yes" and "no" responses.

The interviewer will ask about your skills. Share your skills list. An agency-required skill may not be on your list. Explain that you are willing to learn if your state allows nursing assistants to perform the skill.

Review the job description with the interviewer. Ask questions. Advise the interviewer of functions you cannot perform because of training, legal, ethical, or religious reasons. Honesty now prevents problems later.

Find the right job for you. An employer wants to hire staff who will be happy in the job and the agency. Box 60-2 lists some questions for you to ask at the end of the interview. The interviewer's answers will help you decide if the job is right for you.

The interview usually lasts 15 to 20 minutes. You may be offered a job at this time. Or you are told when to expect a call or letter. Follow-up is acceptable. Ask when you can check on your application. Always thank the interviewer. Say: "I look forward to hearing from you." Shake the person's hand after an in-person interview.

See *Focus on Long-Term Care and Home Care: During the Interview*.

FOCUS ON LONG-TERM CARE AND HOME CARE

During the Interview

Home Care

You need to ask more questions when interviewing with a home care agency.

- What part of the community does the agency serve?
- What neighborhoods will you go to?
- How far will you have to travel between homes?
- Do you use your own car or an agency car?
- How are you paid for mileage and tolls?
- Will you use public transportation? If yes, who pays for bus or train fares? If the agency pays, are you given fare money beforehand or repaid later?

Questions You Cannot Be Asked. The U.S. Equal Employment Opportunity Commission (EEOC) is a government agency. To guard against discrimination in hiring, the EEOC has guidelines for questions that cannot be asked during an interview or on a job application. *Discrimination* involves unjust treatment based on personal qualities. Age, race, biological sex, gender identity, sexuality, pregnancy, religion, and disability are examples. See Box 60-4 (p. 898).

See *Focus on Communication: Questions You Cannot Be Asked*.

FOCUS ON COMMUNICATION

Questions You Cannot Be Asked

If asked a question listed in Box 60-4, you have the right to decline to answer. Decline politely. You can say: "I'm sorry, but the EEOC does not allow that question during an interview. What else can I answer for you?"

BOX 60-4	Interview Questions Not Allowed by the EEOC

- *Age.* Generally, you cannot be asked your age, your birth date, or any question that refers to your age. However, employers are required to show that federal and state child labor laws are followed. You must be at least 16 years old. There are restrictions on the operation of mechanical lifts for workers under age 18. See Chapter 21.
- *Color, race, or national origin.* This includes questions related to your place of birth or that of your parents; language spoken; or how you learned to read, write, or speak a language.
- *Religion or spiritual beliefs.* You cannot be asked about your religion, religious practices, church, priest or pastor, or religious holidays observed.
- *Gender or sexuality.* No questions are allowed about gender identity or your sexuality.
- *Pregnancy or plans for pregnancy.* You cannot be asked if you are pregnant or planning to get pregnant or about your pregnancy history.
- *Marital status.* You cannot be asked if you are married, single, divorced, separated, engaged, or widowed.
- *Children.* You cannot be asked if you have children, how many children or their ages, or who will care for children while you are at work.
- *Arrest record.* Employers must be cautious. Arrests are not proof of criminal conduct. You can be asked about criminal convictions.
- *Finances.* You cannot be asked about credit cards or bank accounts or if you own your home or car.
- *Disabilities.* You cannot be asked if you have disabilities or what they are. This includes physical or mental conditions that cause disabilities. However, you can be asked if you can perform the job with reasonable accommodation. *Reasonable accommodation* means to assist or change a position or workplace to allow an employee to do a job despite having a disability.
- *Medical history.* You cannot be asked about your medical history. However, you may have to take a medical exam or have some tests done after a job offer is made.
- *Citizenship.* You cannot be asked if you are a U.S. citizen. You cannot be asked to provide proof of citizenship. However, if hired, you can be asked to provide proof of the legal right to work in the United States.

After the Interview

A thank-you letter or note is advised within 24 hours after the interview (Fig. 60-3). Write neatly and clearly. Use a computer or other electronic device if your writing is hard to read. The thank-you note should include:
- The date
- The interviewer's formal name with Miss, Ms., Mrs., Mr., or Dr.
- A statement thanking the person for the interview
- Comments about the interview, the agency, and your eagerness to hear about the job
- Your signature, using your first and last names

December 12

Dear [Interviewer's name],

Thank you for the interview yesterday. I enjoyed meeting you and learning more about the nursing center. I was impressed by the friendliness of the staff and would enjoy working in that environment.

Again, thank you. I look forward to hearing from you soon.

Sincerely,
[Your full name]

FIGURE 60-3 Sample thank-you note written after a job interview.

ACCEPTING OR DECLINING A JOB OFFER

You can apply to many places and have many interviews. Think about all offers before accepting one. You might have more questions about an agency. Ask them before accepting a job. To help you decide, discuss the offer with a family member, friend, co-worker, or your instructor.

When you accept a job, agree on a starting date, pay rate, and work hours. Ask where to report on your first day. Ask for all information in writing. That way you and the agency have the same understanding of the job offer. Use the written offer later if questions arise. Also ask for the employee handbook and other agency information. Read everything before you start working.

Accept the best job for you. To decline a job offer, thank the person for offering you a job. If asked why you are refusing, give a positive response. For example: "Thank you for offering me a job. I'm going to accept a job closer to my home."

Sometimes a job is not offered. You may not hear from the agency. Or the agency calls, writes, or e-mails saying that you will not be offered the job. If this happens, thank the person for letting you know. Ask that the agency keep your application active. For example: "Thank you for letting me know. Please keep me in mind for other openings."

DRUG TESTING

State laws vary about drug testing. Drug testing may be part of the application process. If so, review the job application before signing it. The application usually states 1 of the following (see Fig. 60-1).
- Drug testing is part of the application screening process for new staff.
- A job offer depends on passing a drug test.

FOCUS ON **PRIDE**

The Person, Family, and Yourself

Personal and Professional Responsibility

Agencies invest much time and money in new staff. Frequently changing jobs can reflect poorly on you. Before applying, find out about the agency. This helps you decide if the agency is a good fit for you. Also, your interest in the agency can make a good impression during an interview.

Rights and Respect

You have the right to protection from discrimination. Application and interview questions must relate to your ability to do the job. See Box 60-4 for questions that are not allowed.

Job-related questions are allowed if asked to all applicants. These questions are allowed.

- What languages do you read, write, and speak fluently?
- Can you perform the duties of this job? Do you need any special accommodations to perform the job?
- Have you ever been convicted of a crime?

Know your rights. Plan how to respond if you suspect a question violates your rights.

Independence and Social Interaction

Some agencies perform social media background checks. State laws vary about what information can be accessed—public or private. Employers must focus only on information related to the job. Show good judgment when using social media (Chapter 5). Be professional. Agencies may view postings on social media sites.

Delegation and Teamwork

Non–health care work experiences, education, and training are important. They give employers information about your dependability, teamwork, and work quality. Draw from your experiences. Give examples of your positive work ethics.

Ethics and Laws

Agencies watch for safe and ethical conduct. They must act when conduct is unsafe or unethical. Background checks, drug testing, and interview questions help agencies decide if an applicant will meet safety and ethical standards.

Poor conduct outside of work can affect your job. Take pride in making good choices inside and outside the workplace.

FOCUS ON **PRIDE**: *Application*

Being prepared for an interview is helpful. You may be nervous about what questions will be asked, how you will answer, and if you will make a good impression. Describe how you will prepare yourself for a job interview.

REVIEW QUESTIONS

Circle the BEST answer.

1 When should you ask questions about your job description?
   a After completing the job application
   b Before completing the job application
   c When your interview is scheduled
   d During the interview

2 Lying on a job application is
   a Negligence
   b Fraud
   c Libel
   d Defamation

3 When completing a job application
   a Use pencil
   b Leave spaces blank that do not apply to you
   c Give information about employment gaps
   d List family members as references

4 For an interview, you show you are dependable when you
   a Are on time
   b Smile
   c Are well groomed
   d Shake the interviewer's hand

5 What should you wear to a job interview?
   a A uniform
   b Party clothes
   c Slacks and a shirt or blouse
   d Whatever is most comfortable

6 For a phone interview you should
   a Shout answers so they are heard
   b Take another call during the interview
   c Have the interviewer leave a message
   d Use a quiet room

7 Which is poor behavior during a job interview?
   a Crossing your arms and legs
   b Good eye contact with the interviewer
   c Shaking hands with the interviewer
   d Asking the interviewer questions

8 Which is the *best* response to an interview question?
   a Brief explanations
   b "Yes" or "no"
   c Long answers
   d A written response

9 An interviewer asks the following. Which should you decline to answer?
   a Tell me about yourself.
   b Are you married?
   c Have you ever been convicted of a crime?
   d What are your career goals?

10 After an interview
   a Ask if the agency plans to hire you
   b Ask to be paid for your time at the interview
   c Write a thank-you note
   d Do not apply to any other agencies

Continued

11 When accepting a job offer, avoid discussing
   a Starting date
   b Personal finances
   c Pay rate
   d Work hours

12 An agency requires a criminal background check and drug testing as part of the application process. These
   a Are done for workplace safety
   b Cannot legally be required
   c Can be refused if you pay a fee
   d Are only done on select applicants

Answers to Chapter 60 questions are on p. 904.

Answers to Chapter 60 questions are on p. 904.

FOCUS ON PRACTICE

Problem Solving

You are asked the following questions at a job interview. How will you respond to each?

- Why did you decide to become a nursing assistant?
- What are your strengths and weaknesses?
- Describe a problem in your clinical training. How did you resolve it?
- Give an example of when you had to prioritize. How did you decide what to do first, second, and so on?

Review Question Answers

CHAPTER 1: HEALTH CARE AGENCIES
1 a
2 c
3 c
4 d
5 b
6 b
7 a
8 b
9 c
10 b
11 d
12 a
13 b
14 a
15 d
16 c
17 c
18 b
19 d
20 d

CHAPTER 2: THE PERSON'S RIGHTS
1 a
2 b
3 b
4 c
5 d
6 c
7 d
8 b
9 a
10 a
11 c
12 d
13 c
14 b
15 d
16 a
17 d
18 c
19 b
20 a
21 d
22 b

CHAPTER 3: THE NURSING ASSISTANT
1 c
2 d
3 b
4 c
5 d
6 a
7 c
8 a
9 b
10 c
11 a
12 c
13 b
14 d
15 d
16 a

CHAPTER 4: DELEGATION
1 b
2 c
3 a
4 c
5 d
6 b
7 d
8 a
9 d
10 c
11 a
12 b

CHAPTER 5: ETHICS AND LAWS
1 b
2 c
3 d
4 a
5 b
6 d
7 c
8 a
9 d
10 c
11 b
12 a
13 a
14 b
15 d
16 d
17 c
18 a
19 c
20 b
21 d
22 a

CHAPTER 6: STUDENT AND WORK ETHICS
1 b
2 d
3 c
4 a
5 d
6 b
7 a
8 c
9 d
10 a
11 c
12 b
13 c
14 a
15 b
16 d
17 a
18 c
19 d
20 b

CHAPTER 7: THE PERSON AND FAMILY
1 c
2 d
3 b
4 a
5 a
6 c
7 d
8 a
9 b
10 d
11 b
12 d
13 a
14 c
15 a
16 a
17 b
18 d
19 c
20 c
21 a
22 c
23 d
24 b

CHAPTER 8: HEALTH TEAM COMMUNICATIONS
1 d
2 c
3 b
4 b
5 a
6 d
7 c
8 a
9 b
10 c
11 a
12 d
13 a
14 b
15 c
16 d
17 a
18 c

CHAPTER 9: MEDICAL TERMINOLOGY
1 c
2 b
3 a
4 c
5 b
6 c
7 d
8 d
9 b
10 d
11 b
12 a
13 c
14 a
15 a
16 c
17 d
18 b
19 d
20 b
21 a
22 c

CHAPTER 10: BODY STRUCTURE AND FUNCTION
1 a
2 b
3 a
4 c
5 c
6 a
7 d
8 b
9 c
10 d
11 d
12 c
13 b
14 a
15 b
16 b
17 b
18 c
19 d
20 a
21 a
22 b

CHAPTER 11: GROWTH AND DEVELOPMENT
1 b
2 d
3 b
4 a
5 c
6 b
7 b
8 a
9 c
10 c
11 c
12 d
13 b
14 a
15 d
16 a
17 b
18 c
19 a
20 d

CHAPTER 12: THE OLDER PERSON
1 a
2 a
3 b
4 d
5 a
6 d
7 b
8 c
9 a
10 c
11 d
12 d
13 a
14 d
15 b
16 a
17 c
18 c
19 b
20 d
21 c
22 a

CHAPTER 13: THE PERSON'S UNIT
1 d
2 c
3 b
4 d
5 d
6 c
7 c
8 a
9 a
10 b
11 b
12 a
13 c
14 a
15 d
16 c

CHAPTER 14: SAFETY
1 a
2 d
3 c
4 b
5 a
6 c
7 d
8 b
9 c
10 c
11 b
12 d
13 a
14 c
15 b
16 a
17 b
18 a
19 b
20 d
21 b
22 d
23 a
24 c
25 a
26 c
27 b
28 d

CHAPTER 15: PREVENTING FALLS
1 a
2 c
3 c
4 b
5 a
6 c
7 d
8 b
9 c
10 b
11 a
12 c
13 c
14 d
15 d

CHAPTER 16: RESTRAINT ALTERNATIVES AND RESTRAINTS
1 b
2 c
3 d
4 b
5 c
6 a
7 a
8 b
9 d
10 c
11 a
12 b
13 a
14 c
15 d

CHAPTER 17: PREVENTING INFECTION
1 a
2 c
3 b
4 c
5 d
6 a
7 c
8 b
9 a
10 b
11 d
12 d
13 a
14 b
15 d
16 c
17 d
18 a
19 c
20 a
21 b
22 d
23 c
24 d
25 b

CHAPTER 18: ISOLATION PRECAUTIONS
1 a
2 b
3 a
4 c
5 c
6 d
7 b
8 d
9 c
10 d
11 a
12 b
13 c
14 d

CHAPTER 19: SAFE HANDLING AND POSITIONING
1 d
2 c
3 a
4 b
5 a
6 d
7 b
8 b
9 c
10 a
11 d
12 a
13 c
14 d
15 b
16 b
17 c
18 a

CHAPTER 20: MOVING THE PERSON
1 c
2 d
3 a
4 d
5 b
6 c
7 c
8 a
9 d
10 b
11 a
12 c
13 b
14 d
15 c

CHAPTER 21: TRANSFERRING THE PERSON
1 b
2 a
3 c
4 b
5 a
6 c
7 a
8 d
9 c
10 a
11 c
12 b
13 c
14 d

CHAPTER 22: BEDMAKING
1 c
2 d
3 b
4 a
5 d
6 a
7 b
8 d
9 a
10 c
11 c
12 b

CHAPTER 23: ORAL HYGIENE
1 c
2 d
3 b
4 d
5 a
6 d
7 a
8 c
9 c
10 a
11 b
12 c

CHAPTER 24: DAILY HYGIENE AND BATHING
1 c
2 b
3 a
4 b
5 b
6 d
7 c
8 a
9 d
10 c
11 d
12 a
13 d
14 a
15 b
16 c
17 b
18 a

CHAPTER 25: GROOMING
1 d
2 b
3 b
4 c
5 a
6 d
7 d
8 a
9 c
10 c
11 b
12 d
13 a
14 c
15 a

CHAPTER 26: CHANGING GARMENTS
1 d
2 d
3 b
4 a
5 c
6 d
7 a
8 c

CHAPTER 27: URINARY NEEDS
1 c
2 d
3 a
4 a
5 b
6 b
7 d
8 a
9 d
10 c
11 b
12 c
13 d
14 a
15 c

CHAPTER 28: URINARY CATHETERS
1 c
2 d
3 a
4 a
5 c
6 b
7 d
8 c
9 a
10 b
11 a
12 d

CHAPTER 29: BOWEL NEEDS
1 b
2 a
3 d
4 b
5 c
6 d
7 c
8 a
9 b
10 d
11 b
12 b
13 d
14 a
15 b

CHAPTER 30: NUTRITION
1 b
2 b
3 a
4 c
5 d
6 a
7 c
8 b
9 a
10 a
11 b
12 a
13 d
14 d
15 c
16 c

CHAPTER 31: MEETING NUTRITION NEEDS
1 b
2 c
3 d
4 d
5 a
6 a
7 b
8 c
9 a
10 b
11 a
12 c
13 d
14 d
15 c

CHAPTER 32: FLUID NEEDS
1 c
2 d
3 a
4 b
5 a
6 d
7 c
8 b
9 c
10 d
11 b
12 a

CHAPTER 33: NUTRITIONAL SUPPORT AND IV THERAPY
1 c
2 a
3 a
4 b
5 d
6 a
7 a
8 c
9 c
10 d
11 b
12 a
13 b
14 d
15 c
16 b
17 b
18 a

CHAPTER 34: VITAL SIGNS
1 a
2 d
3 b
4 a
5 c
6 a
7 d
8 c
9 b
10 d
11 c
12 c
13 a
14 d
15 c
16 d
17 b
18 b

CHAPTER 35: EXERCISE AND ACTIVITY
1 a
2 b
3 d
4 a
5 b
6 c
7 c
8 a
9 d
10 c
11 a
12 b
13 a
14 c
15 d
16 d
17 b
18 a
19 c
20 a

CHAPTER 36: COMFORT, REST, AND SLEEP
1 c
2 a
3 d
4 b
5 c
6 d
7 a
8 b
9 c
10 d
11 c
12 d
13 b
14 a

CHAPTER 37: ADMISSIONS, TRANSFERS, AND DISCHARGES
1 c
2 b
3 b
4 a
5 d
6 a
7 c
8 c
9 a
10 d

CHAPTER 38: ASSISTING WITH THE PHYSICAL EXAMINATION
1 b
2 c
3 b
4 c
5 d
6 a

CHAPTER 39: COLLECTING AND TESTING SPECIMENS
1 c
2 d
3 b
4 a
5 a
6 c
7 d
8 b
9 c
10 b
11 a
12 b
13 c
14 a
15 d

CHAPTER 40: THE PERSON HAVING SURGERY
1 c
2 b
3 b
4 a
5 a
6 d
7 c
8 a
9 b
10 d
11 b
12 a
13 c
14 a
15 d
16 b
17 d
18 a
19 c
20 b

CHAPTER 41: WOUND CARE
1 a
2 c
3 b
4 d
5 a
6 d
7 c
8 b
9 a
10 b
11 c
12 d
13 b
14 b
15 c

CHAPTER 42: PRESSURE INJURIES
1 b
2 d
3 d
4 a
5 d
6 c
7 b
8 c
9 c
10 a
11 b
12 d
13 a
14 a
15 b
16 c
17 d
18 b
19 c
20 d
21 c
22 a

CHAPTER 43: HEAT AND COLD APPLICATIONS
1 d
2 b
3 b
4 a
5 b
6 a
7 b
8 c
9 a
10 b
11 d
12 c
13 a
14 a

CHAPTER 44: OXYGEN NEEDS
1 a
2 c
3 c
4 b
5 b
6 d
7 c
8 d
9 a
10 b
11 b
12 d
13 c
14 d
15 a
16 a
17 c
18 d

CHAPTER 45: RESPIRATORY SUPPORT AND THERAPIES
1 c
2 c
3 a
4 d
5 b
6 b
7 a
8 d
9 c
10 a
11 b
12 c
13 b
14 b

CHAPTER 46: REHABILITATION NEEDS
1 d
2 c
3 d
4 b
5 a
6 c
7 a
8 a
9 c
10 c

CHAPTER 47: HEARING, SPEECH, AND VISION PROBLEMS
1 b
2 c
3 d
4 b
5 a
6 d
7 c
8 a
9 d
10 a
11 b
12 a
13 c
14 b
15 c
16 a
17 d
18 d
19 c
20 b

CHAPTER 48: CANCER, IMMUNE SYSTEM, AND SKIN DISORDERS
1 b
2 c
3 a
4 b
5 d
6 d
7 c
8 d
9 b
10 c
11 b
12 a
13 c
14 c
15 d
16 a
17 b
18 c

CHAPTER 49: NERVOUS SYSTEM AND MUSCULO-SKELETAL DISORDERS
1 a
2 b
3 d
4 c
5 a
6 b
7 a
8 a
9 c
10 b
11 c
12 a
13 d
14 b
15 a
16 b
17 d
18 d
19 a
20 c

CHAPTER 50: CARDIOVASCULAR, RESPIRATORY, AND LYMPHATIC DISORDERS
1 a
2 d
3 b
4 b
5 c
6 a
7 d
8 b
9 c
10 a
11 d
12 a
13 c
14 c
15 a
16 b
17 b
18 a
19 d
20 d

CHAPTER 51:
DIGESTIVE AND ENDOCRINE DISORDERS

1 b
2 a
3 d
4 a
5 c
6 b
7 c
8 d
9 c
10 b
11 a
12 a
13 b
14 b
15 d
16 c
17 d
18 a
19 c
20 b

CHAPTER 52:
URINARY AND REPRODUCTIVE DISORDERS

1 d
2 a
3 b
4 a
5 c
6 b
7 c
8 d
9 c
10 a

CHAPTER 53:
MENTAL HEALTH DISORDERS

1 b
2 c
3 a
4 b
5 d
6 c
7 c
8 a
9 a
10 c
11 d
12 b
13 a
14 b
15 c
16 a
17 d
18 c
19 d
20 a
21 b
22 d

CHAPTER 54:
CONFUSION AND DEMENTIA

1 b
2 a
3 d
4 c
5 d
6 b
7 b
8 a
9 c
10 c
11 a
12 b
13 d
14 c
15 b
16 d
17 c
18 b
19 a
20 d
21 a
22 c

CHAPTER 55:
INTELLECTUAL AND DEVELOPMENTAL DISABILITIES

1 b
2 a
3 c
4 a
5 d
6 d
7 c
8 b
9 d
10 a
11 b
12 a
13 c
14 b
15 d

CHAPTER 56:
CARING FOR MOTHERS AND BABIES

1 c
2 d
3 a
4 b
5 c
6 d
7 d
8 b
9 b
10 c
11 a
12 a
13 c
14 d
15 c
16 c
17 a
18 d
19 b
20 c
21 c
22 d

CHAPTER 57:
ASSISTED LIVING

1 b
2 c
3 c
4 d
5 a
6 b
7 a
8 b
9 c
10 d

CHAPTER 58:
EMERGENCY CARE

1 b
2 a
3 c
4 b
5 a
6 c
7 b
8 b
9 c
10 c
11 a
12 d
13 c
14 b
15 b
16 c
17 d
18 a
19 d
20 c
21 a
22 b
23 c
24 d
25 a

CHAPTER 59:
END-OF-LIFE CARE

1 c
2 a
3 b
4 a
5 b
6 d
7 c
8 a
9 d
10 c
11 c
12 a
13 b
14 b
15 d

CHAPTER 60:
GETTING A JOB

1 d
2 b
3 c
4 a
5 c
6 d
7 a
8 a
9 b
10 c
11 b
12 a

Appendix A

National Nurse Aide Assessment Program (NNAAP®) Written Examination Content Outline

The NNAAP® written examination is comprised of 70 multiple-choice items; 10 of these items are pretest (non-scored) items on which statistical information will be collected.

I. Physical Care Skills
A Activities of Daily Living — 13 questions
1. Hygiene, Dressing, and Grooming
2. Nutrition and Hydration
3. Elimination
4. Rest/Sleep/Comfort

B Basic Nursing Skills — 21 questions
1. Infection Control
2. Safety/Prevention/Emergency
3. Technical Procedures
4. Data Collection and Reporting

C Self Care/Independence — 4 questions

II. Psychosocial Care Skills
A Emotional and Mental Health Needs — 5 questions

B Spiritual and Cultural Needs — 1 question

III. Role of the Nurse Aide
A Communication — 4 questions
B Client Rights — 5 questions
C Legal and Ethical Behavior — 3 questions
D Member of the Health Care Team — 4 questions

National Nurse Aide Assessment Program (NNAAP®) Skills Evaluation

List of Skills
1. Hand hygiene (hand washing)
2. Applies one knee-high elastic stocking
3. Assists to ambulate using transfer belt
4. Assists with use of bedpan
5. Cleans upper or lower denture
6. Counts and records radial pulse
7. Counts and records respirations
8. Donning and removing PPE (gown and gloves)
9. Dresses client with affected (weak) right arm
10. Feeds client who cannot feed self
11. Gives modified bed bath (face and one arm, hand, and underarm)
12. Measures and records electronic blood pressure (state specific)
13. Measures and records urinary output
14. Measures and records weight of ambulatory client
15. Performs modified passive range of motion (PROM) for one knee and one ankle
16. Performs modified passive range of motion (PROM) for one shoulder
17. Positions on side
18. Provides catheter care for female
19. Provides foot care on one foot
20. Provides mouth care
21. Provides perineal care (peri-care) for female
22. Transfers from bed to wheelchair using transfer belt
23. Measures and records manual blood pressure (state specific)

Appendix B

Minimum Data Set: Selected Pages

Resident _____ Identifier _____ Date _____

Section GG - Functional Abilities - Admission

GG0130. Self-Care (Assessment period is the first 3 days of the stay)
Complete column 1 when A0310A = 01 or when A0310B = 01.
When A0310B = 01, the stay begins on A2400B. When A0310B = 99, the stay begins on A1600.

Code the resident's usual performance at the start of the stay (admission) for each activity using the 6-point scale. If activity was not attempted at the start of the stay (admission), code the reason.

Coding:

Safety and **Quality of Performance** - If helper assistance is required because resident's performance is unsafe or of poor quality, score according to amount of assistance provided.
Activities may be completed with or without assistive devices.
- 06. **Independent** - Resident completes the activity by themself with no assistance from a helper.
- 05. **Setup or clean-up assistance** - Helper sets up or cleans up; resident completes activity. Helper assists only prior to or following the activity.
- 04. **Supervision or touching assistance** - Helper provides verbal cues and/or touching/steadying and/or contact guard assistance as resident completes activity. Assistance may be provided throughout the activity or intermittently.
- 03. **Partial/moderate assistance** - Helper does LESS THAN HALF the effort. Helper lifts, holds, or supports trunk or limbs, but provides less than half the effort.
- 02. **Substantial/maximal assistance** - Helper does MORE THAN HALF the effort. Helper lifts or holds trunk or limbs and provides more than half the effort.
- 01. **Dependent** - Helper does ALL of the effort. Resident does none of the effort to complete the activity. Or, the assistance of 2 or more helpers is required for the resident to complete the activity.

If activity was not attempted, code reason:
- 07. **Resident refused**
- 09. **Not applicable** - Not attempted and the resident did not perform this activity prior to the current illness, exacerbation, or injury.
- 10. **Not attempted due to environmental limitations** (e.g., lack of equipment, weather constraints)
- 88. **Not attempted due to medical condition or safety concerns**

1. Admission Performance		

Enter Codes in Boxes
↓

☐☐	**A.**	**Eating:** The ability to use suitable utensils to bring food and/or liquid to the mouth and swallow food and/or liquid once the meal is placed before the resident.
☐☐	**B.**	**Oral hygiene:** The ability to use suitable items to clean teeth. Dentures (if applicable): The ability to insert and remove dentures into and from the mouth, and manage denture soaking and rinsing with use of equipment.
☐☐	**C.**	**Toileting hygiene:** The ability to maintain perineal hygiene, adjust clothes before and after voiding or having a bowel movement. If managing an ostomy, include wiping the opening but not managing equipment.
☐☐	**E.**	**Shower/bathe self:** The ability to bathe self, including washing, rinsing, and drying self (excludes washing of back and hair). Does not include transferring in/out of tub/shower.
☐☐	**F.**	**Upper body dressing:** The ability to dress and undress above the waist; including fasteners, if applicable.
☐☐	**G.**	**Lower body dressing:** The ability to dress and undress below the waist, including fasteners; does not include footwear.
☐☐	**H.**	**Putting on/taking off footwear:** The ability to put on and take off socks and shoes or other footwear that is appropriate for safe mobility; including fasteners, if applicable.
☐☐	**I.**	**Personal hygiene:** The ability to maintain personal hygiene, including combing hair, shaving, applying makeup, washing/drying face and hands (excludes baths, showers, and oral hygiene).

Resident _____ Identifier _____ Date _____

Section GG - Functional Abilities - Admission

GG0170. Mobility (Assessment period is the first 3 days of the stay)
Complete column 1 when A0310A = 01 or when A0310B = 01.
When A0310B = 01, the stay begins on A2400B. When A0310B = 99, the stay begins on A1600.

Code the resident's usual performance at the start of the stay (admission) for each activity using the 6-point scale. If activity was not attempted at the start of the stay (admission), code the reason.

Coding:
Safety and **Quality of Performance** - If helper assistance is required because resident's performance is unsafe or of poor quality, score according to amount of assistance provided.
Activities may be completed with or without assistive devices.
06. **Independent** - Resident completes the activity by themself with no assistance from a helper.
05. **Setup or clean-up assistance** - Helper sets up or cleans up; resident completes activity. Helper assists only prior to or following the activity.
04. **Supervision or touching assistance** - Helper provides verbal cues and/or touching/steadying and/or contact guard assistance as resident completes activity. Assistance may be provided throughout the activity or intermittently.
03. **Partial/moderate assistance** - Helper does LESS THAN HALF the effort. Helper lifts, holds, or supports trunk or limbs, but provides less than half the effort.
02. **Substantial/maximal assistance** - Helper does MORE THAN HALF the effort. Helper lifts or holds trunk or limbs and provides more than half the effort.
01. **Dependent** - Helper does ALL of the effort. Resident does none of the effort to complete the activity. Or, the assistance of 2 or more helpers is required for the resident to complete the activity.

If activity was not attempted, code reason:
07. **Resident refused**
09. **Not applicable** - Not attempted and the resident did not perform this activity prior to the current illness, exacerbation, or injury.
10. **Not attempted due to environmental limitations** (e.g., lack of equipment, weather constraints)
88. **Not attempted due to medical condition or safety concerns**

1. Admission Performance

Enter Codes in Boxes
↓

[ ][ ] **A. Roll left and right:** The ability to roll from lying on back to left and right side, and return to lying on back on the bed.

[ ][ ] **B. Sit to lying:** The ability to move from sitting on side of bed to lying flat on the bed.

[ ][ ] **C. Lying to sitting on side of bed:** The ability to move from lying on the back to sitting on the side of the bed and with no back support.

[ ][ ] **D. Sit to stand:** The ability to come to a standing position from sitting in a chair, wheelchair, or on the side of the bed.

[ ][ ] **E. Chair/bed-to-chair transfer:** The ability to transfer to and from a bed to a chair (or wheelchair).

[ ][ ] **F. Toilet transfer:** The ability to get on and off a toilet or commode.

[ ][ ] **FF. Tub/shower transfer:** The ability to get in and out of a tub/shower.

[ ][ ] **G. Car transfer:** The ability to transfer in and out of a car or van on the passenger side. Does not include the ability to open/close door or fasten seat belt.

[ ][ ] **I. Walk 10 feet:** Once standing, the ability to walk at least 10 feet in a room, corridor, or similar space. If admission performance is coded 07, 09, 10, or 88 → Skip to GG0170M, 1 step (curb)

[ ][ ] **J. Walk 50 feet with two turns:** Once standing, the ability to walk at least 50 feet and make two turns.

[ ][ ] **K. Walk 150 feet:** Once standing, the ability to walk at least 150 feet in a corridor or similar space.

From Centers for Medicare & Medicaid Services: MDS 3.0, https://www.cms.gov/Medicare/Quality-Initiatives-Patient-Assessment-Instruments/NursingHomeQualityInits/MDS30RAIManual.
NOTE: The Centers for Medicare & Medicaid Services (CMS) updates the Minimum Data Set (MDS). The most current version can be found on-line on the CMS's website.

Appendix C

Care Area Assessment (CAA): Sample Page

Resident _____ Identifier _____ Date _____

Section V - Care Area Assessment (CAA) Summary

V0200. CAAs and Care Planning

1. Check column A if Care Area is triggered.
2. For each triggered Care Area, indicate whether a new care plan, care plan revision, or continuation of current care plan is necessary to address the problem(s) identified in your assessment of the care area. The Care Planning Decision column must be completed within 7 days of completing the RAI (MDS and CAA(s)). Check column B if the triggered care area is addressed in the care plan.
3. Indicate in the Location and Date of CAA Documentation column where information related to the CAA can be found. CAA documentation should include information on the complicating factors, risks, and any referrals for this resident for this care area.

A. CAA Results

Care Area	A. Care Area Triggered	B. Care Planning Decision	Location and Date of CAA documentation
	↓ Check all that apply↓		
01. Delirium	☐	☐	
02. Cognitive Loss/Dementia	☐	☐	
03. Visual Function	☐	☐	
04. Communication	☐	☐	
05. ADL Functional/Rehabilitation Potential	☐	☐	
06. Urinary Incontinence and Indwelling Catheter	☐	☐	
07. Psychosocial Well-Being	☐	☐	
08. Mood State	☐	☐	
09. Behavioral Symptoms	☐	☐	
10. Activities	☐	☐	
11. Falls	☐	☐	
12. Nutritional Status	☐	☐	
13. Feeding Tube	☐	☐	
14. Dehydration/Fluid Maintenance	☐	☐	
15. Dental Care	☐	☐	
16. Pressure Ulcer	☐	☐	
17. Psychotropic Drug Use	☐	☐	
18. Physical Restraints	☐	☐	
19. Pain	☐	☐	
20. Return to Community Referral	☐	☐	

B. Signature of RN Coordinator for CAA Process and Date Signed

1. Signature

2. Date

☐☐ - ☐☐ - ☐☐☐☐
Month   Day   Year

C. Signature of Person Completing Care Plan Decision and Date Signed

1. Signature

2. Date

☐☐ - ☐☐ - ☐☐☐☐
Month   Day   Year

From Centers for Medicare & Medicaid Services: MDS 3.0, https://www.cms.gov/Medicare/Quality-Initiatives-Patient-Assessment-Instruments/NursingHomeQualityInits/MDS30RAIManual.
NOTE: The Centers for Medicare & Medicaid Services (CMS) updates the Care Area Assessment (CAA). The most current version can be found on-line on the CMS's website.

Infant and Child Safety
Home Safety*
The following home safety measures can protect infants and children from harm.

Kitchen
- Knives, forks, scissors, and other sharp tools are kept in a drawer with a childproof latch.
- The stove has a lock and knob protectors.
- A dishwasher lock is installed.
- Childproof latches are installed on all cabinet doors.
- Chairs and step stools are away from the stove.
- When cooking, pot handles on the stove are turned inward or placed on back burners where children cannot reach them.
- Tablecloths and placemats are not used. Infants and children can pull things off the table and onto themselves.
- Glass objects and appliances with sharp blades are stored out of reach.
- The garbage can is behind a cabinet door with a childproof latch.
- Appliances are unplugged when not in use, with cords out of reach.
- Matches and lighters are stored in a locked cabinet.
- Cleaning supplies, bug sprays, dishwasher detergent, and dishwashing liquids are in the original containers and in a locked cabinet. A cabinet under the sink is not a safe storage area.
- Bottles containing alcohol are in the original containers and in a locked cabinet.
- Plastic garbage bags and sandwich bags are out of reach.
- Refrigerator magnets and other small objects are out of reach.
- There is a working fire extinguisher. Family members know how to use it.

Bathroom
- The thermostat on the hot water heater is set below 120°F (49°C).
- Razors, nail clippers, and other sharp items are stored in a locked cabinet.
- Drug bottles are closed tightly with child-resistant caps and stored in the original containers and in a locked cabinet.
- Childproof latches are installed on all drawers and cabinets.
- Toilets are closed and have toilet-lid locks.
- Sinks, tubs, and basins are empty when not in use.
- Outlets have ground fault circuit interrupters. These protect against electrical injuries if an electrical appliance gets wet.
- Hair dryers, curling irons, and electric razors are unplugged when not in use.
- There are slip-resistant strips on the floors of showers and bathtubs.
- There are anti-slip pads under rugs to hold them securely to the floor.
- Cosmetics and cleaners are stored in the original containers and in a locked cabinet.
- Bottles of mouthwash, perfumes, hair dyes, hair sprays, nail polishes, and nail polish removers are stored in the original containers and in a locked cabinet.

Stairways
- Hardware-mounted safety gates are at the top and bottom of every stairway. Gates meet current safety standards.
- Stairways are clear of tripping hazards such as loose carpeting or toys.
- Banisters and railings have guards if a child can fit through the rails.
- The railings and banisters are secure.
- The door to the basement steps is kept locked.
- There is enough light in the stairway.
- Children are supervised around stairs.

*Home Safety modified and adapted from kidshealth.org: *First Aid & Safety*.

Doors, Windows, Walls, and Floors

- Doors have finger-pinch guards.
- Rubber tips are removed from door stops or 1-piece door stops are installed.
- Doorknob covers or childproof locks are used on doors leading outside and to non-childproof areas.
- Glass doors have decorative markers so they are not mistaken for open doors.
- Sliding doors have childproof locks.
- Safety bars or window guards are installed on upper-story windows. A window guard is not used on a window that is an emergency exit.
- Window stops are present to limit how far the window opens.
- Window blind and curtain cords are kept out of reach. The U.S. Consumer Product Safety Commission (CPSC) recommends cordless window coverings.
- Cribs, playpens, beds, or other furniture are not placed near a window.
- Windows are opened from the top down.
- Walls are in good condition with no peeling or cracking paint.
- Mirrors and frames are hung securely.
- Rugs are secured to floors, fitted with anti-slip pads underneath, or removed.
- Floors are free of clutter.

Furniture

- Bookshelves and other furniture are secured to the wall or floor to prevent tipping.
- Children are not allowed to climb on furniture. This includes using shelves as steps.
- Toys or things that attract children are not placed on the top of furniture.
- Protective padding is placed on corners of coffee tables, furniture, and countertops with sharp edges.
- Baby equipment has not been recalled.
- Flatscreen TVs are mounted securely on the wall. Older, heavy TVs are on low, stable furniture.
- Stops are on all removable drawers to prevent them from falling out.

Child's Bedroom and Clothing

- The changing table has a safety belt.
- Painted cribs, bassinets, and high chairs made before 1978 are not used. (Paint was lead-based before 1978.)
- The crib meets federal safety standards. See "Cribs" (p. 915) and Chapter 56.
- There are no pillows, stuffed animals, bumper pads, or soft bedding in the crib.
- Infants are not put to sleep on an adult or child's bed, water bed, couch, pillow, or other soft surface. Death from entrapment and suffocation are risks.
- Strings or ribbons have been removed from hanging mobiles and crib toys.
- Electric cords (including baby monitor cords) are at least 3 feet away from the crib or bed.
- Dressers are secured to walls or floors with drawers closed.
- Lids on toy chests and toy storage containers have a lid support to prevent slamming shut. Toy chests do not lock.
- Night-lights do not touch any fabric such as bedspreads or curtains.
- Sleepwear is flame-retardant.
- Drawstrings are removed from clothing.
- Children are not allowed to wear necklaces, strings, cords, ribbons, or other such items around the neck.
- Bibs are removed before naptime and bedtime.
- Clothing fits well. Clothing is not loose and does not touch or drag the floor.

Garage and Laundry Area

- Gardening, automotive, and lawn care tools and supplies are stored safely away from children.
- Hazardous automotive, pool, and gardening products are in a locked area.
- Recycling containers storing glass and metal are out of reach.
- Garbage cans are securely covered.
- Cleaning products are in the original containers and stored in a locked cabinet.
- Buckets used for cleaning are out of reach.
- Laundry detergent pods are in the original container and in a locked cabinet away from children.
- Washer and dryer doors are kept closed.
- Laundry chutes are locked with childproof locks.

Outdoors, Backyard, and Pool

- Walkways and outdoor stairways are well lit. They are clear of toys, objects, or things blocking a clear path.
- Sidewalks and outdoor stairways are without cracks and missing pieces.
- Playground equipment is safe with no loose parts, splinters, sharp edges, or rust.
- The surface beneath playground equipment is cushioned with material such as sand, mulch, wood chips, or approved rubber surfacing mats to absorb the shock of a fall.
- Outdoor toys are in a secure, dry place when not used.
- Toys are kept away from pools, spas, hot tubs, or whirlpools. Children playing with such toys could fall into the water.
- Toys are removed from pools after swimming.
- Climb-proof fencing is at least 5 feet high on all sides of the pool. The fence has a self-closing gate with a childproof lock.
- The ladder is removed from an above-ground pool when not in use.
- Door, window, and pool alarms are on. They alert you if a child wanders into an unsafe area.
- Inflatable flotation devices are not relied on to keep a child afloat. Children near water must be constantly supervised.
- Buckets, pails, containers, and wading pools are empty and upside down when not in use.

Vehicle Safety

- Children are not left alone in any vehicle even if the windows are down. They can develop heat-related illness, suffocate, and die from high temperatures within minutes.
- Seat-belt laws are followed. Seat belts are worn properly.
- Car seat safety measures are followed. (See p. 915.)
- Children younger than 13 years old sit in the back seat. Serious injuries and death can occur from an air bag hitting a child in the front seat. If a child must ride in front, the air bag is turned off and the seat is moved back as far as possible.
- Vehicle doors and the trunk are locked. Keys are kept out of children's sight and reach.
- Trunk access is kept closed.
- Children are not allowed to play in vehicles.
- Children do not ride as passengers on tractors, mowers, mini-bikes, or all-terrain vehicles.
- Children under age 17 do not ride all-terrain vehicles. A helmet and eye protection are worn. Three-wheeled all-terrain vehicles are never used.

Electrical

- Un-used outlets are covered.
- Electrical items are unplugged when not in use.
- Major electrical appliances are grounded.
- Cord holders keep cords fastened against walls.
- There are no potential electrical fire hazards such as over-loaded electrical sockets and electrical wires running under carpets.
- Equipment with old or frayed cords and damaged extension cords are removed.
- Computers, TVs, and stereo equipment are against walls. This prevents children from touching cords.
- Electronic toys are checked for signs of danger. Toys that spark, feel hot, or smell unusual are repaired or discarded.

Heating and Cooling Elements

- Radiators and baseboard heaters are covered with childproof screens.
- Gas fireplaces are secured with a valve cover or key.
- Working fireplaces have a screen and other barriers in place when in use.
- Chimneys have been cleaned recently.
- Electric space heaters are at least 3 feet from beds, curtains, or anything flammable.

Emergency Equipment and Numbers

- A list of emergency phone numbers is stored in or kept near each phone in the home.
- Fire extinguishers are on every floor and in the kitchen, the basement, the garage, and any workshop area.
- Upper floors of the home have an emergency ladder.
- Smoke alarms are on each floor of the home, outside each sleeping area, and inside each bedroom.
- Smoke alarms are tested monthly and batteries changed every 6 months.
- The home has a carbon monoxide alarm. (See Chapter 14.)

Firearm Safety

- Guns are stored in a securely locked case, safe, or gun vault out of children's reach. All firearms are stored unloaded and in the uncocked position.
- Ammunition is stored in a separate place and in a securely locked container out of reach.
- Keys for gun storage, ammunition, and gun-cleaning supplies are kept where children cannot find them.
- Trigger locks or other childproof devices are used.
- Gun safety is practiced. Adults have taken a firearm safety course to use the firearm safely and correctly.
- Children are taught that guns are not toys, they are not to touch or play with guns, and they should tell an adult if they find one.
- Gun-cleaning supplies are locked up. Cleaning supplies are often poisonous.

Other Safety Measures

- Infants and children are supervised at all times.
- Infants and children are supervised by an adult when in the bathtub or near water. Siblings do not supervise.
- Medication (drug) bottles, loose pills, coins, scissors, magnets, and any other small or sharp objects are out of reach.
- Smoking is not allowed in the home.
- Testing has been done for lead, radon, asbestos, mercury, mold, and carbon monoxide when such substances may be present.
- There are no potentially poisonous houseplants.
- Children are supervised around dogs and other pets.

Nursery Equipment Safety*

Nursery equipment must be safe, in good repair, and used properly. Use the following guidelines to check nursery equipment in an agency or home setting.

Carriers

- The carrier has:
  - Straps that prevent the baby from falling or crawling out
  - A firm, padded head support
  - Durable fabric with strong stitching or large, heavy fasteners to prevent slipping
- The carrier fits the baby's size.
  - The baby does not exceed the weight limit.
  - There is enough depth to support the baby's back.
  - Leg openings are small enough to prevent the baby from slipping out but large enough to prevent chafing.
- A framed carrier has a kickstand that locks in the open position. The folding mechanism is free of areas that could pinch the baby's fingers. There is padding on the metal frame around the baby's face.
- Follow these safety measures when using carriers.
  - Never use a framed carrier before an infant is 4 to 5 months old. Do not use it as an infant seat. It can tip over without warning.
  - Use restraining straps at all times if the carrier has them.
  - If you need to lean over, bend from the knees rather than the waist to prevent the baby from falling out of the carrier.
  - Check the carrier often for loose fasteners or ripped seams.

Infant Seats

- The seat has a wide, sturdy base for stability.
- The base has a slip-resistant surface.
- Locking mechanisms are secure. Push down on the unit to make sure it is sturdy.
- Supporting devices lock securely.
- The safety belt is secure and the fabric is washable.
- Follow these safety measures when using infant seats.
  - Supervise the baby. Do not leave the baby in the seat without a responsible adult nearby.
  - Never place the baby in an infant seat on a table or other raised surface.
  - Use the safety belt every time you place the baby in the seat.
  - Do not place the seat on soft surfaces such as beds or sofas. The seat may tip over and the baby can suffocate.
  - Stop using the seat when the baby reaches the manufacturer's height or weight limit.
  - Move the baby to a safe sleep surface if the baby falls asleep (Chapter 56).
  - Never use the seat to transport the baby in a vehicle.

Baby Bathtubs

- The bathtub has slip-resistant backing to keep it from moving.
- There are no rough edges that can scratch the baby.
- The tub stays firm in the center when filled with water.
- Bath rings, baby flotation devices, and bath seats are avoided. The baby can drown if the device tips.
- Foam cushions are avoided. Pieces can be torn off and swallowed.
- Follow these bathing safety measures.
  - Always check the water temperature before putting the baby in the bathtub. Water that is too hot can burn babies.
  - Only adults should give babies baths. Baths can be dangerous. Babies can drown in less than 1 inch of water.
  - Always keep 1 hand on the baby while in the water.
  - Always take the baby with you if you step away from the bathtub.
  - Gather bathing supplies ahead of time, including shampoo, soap, washcloth, towel, clean clothes, a clean diaper, and wipes.
  - Always empty the bathtub and turn it upside down when it is not being used. A plug at the bottom of the tub makes draining easier.

---

*Nursery Equipment Safety modified and adapted from kidshealth.org: *Choosing Safe Baby Products*.

Changing Tables

- The table is sturdy. The base is wide enough to prevent tipping.
- The table has safety straps to prevent falls.
- The table has drawers or shelves that are easy to reach without leaving the baby unattended. Supplies are within your reach but out of the baby's reach.
- A flat changing surface is surrounded on all 4 sides by a guard-rail that is at least 2 inches high. The surface is lower in the middle than on the sides to keep the baby from rolling.
- Follow these safety measures.
  - Use the safety belt when you change the baby.
  - Never leave the baby unattended, even if you think the baby is secure.
  - Always keep 1 hand on the baby.
  - Stop using the changing table when the baby reaches the manufacturer's age or weight limit. Age 2 or 30 pounds is common.

Gates

- The gate has a pressure bar or other fastener that will resist forces exerted by a child.
- A hardware-mounted gate is used at the top of stairs. Pressure-mounted or free-standing gates can fall if the child pushes hard enough.
- The gate has a straight top edge with rigid bars or a tight mesh screen.
- There is less than 2 inches between the floor and the gate bottom to prevent a child from going underneath.
- Rigid vertical slats or rods are no more than 2⅜ inches apart to prevent head entrapment between the slats.
- There are no sharp edges or pieces that could cut a child's hand. Wooden gates are smooth to prevent splinters.
- There are no openings to use for climbing.
- The gate should be at least three-quarters (¾) of the child's height.
- Accordion-style gates are not used. They can trap a child's head.
- Follow these safety measures when using gates.
  - Keep large toys away from the gate. A child can use the toy to climb over.
  - Pressure-mounted and free-standing gates may be used for doors between rooms unless there are stairs between the rooms. Place the pressure bar away from the child.
  - Gates that swing out are never to be used at the top of stairways.
  - Stop using the gate if the child can open or climb over it.

Playpens

- Playpens have top rails that automatically lock when lifted into the normal-use position.
- The locks for lowering a side are out of the baby's reach.
- The sides are at least 20 inches high, measured from the floor of the playpen.
- Playpen mesh has small weave (less than ¼-inch openings).
  - The mesh has no tears, holes, or loose threads.
  - The mesh is securely attached and checked regularly for breaks and tears.
- A wooden playpen has slats spaced no more than 2⅜ inches apart.
- The playpen has well-protected hinges and supports.
- There is padding on the tops of the rails.
- The bottom of the playpen has a 1-inch firm mattress or pad.
- Follow these safety measures when using playpens.
  - Never leave a baby in a mesh playpen with the side lowered. Entrapment between the mesh side and floor board is a risk.
  - Never use soft bedding or pillows.
  - Do not replace the mattress or pad. The new mattress may not fit the playpen well.
  - Check all padded parts regularly for tears. Cover or repair tears.
  - Do not place the playpen near windows. Cords on window coverings can strangle the baby.
  - Do not use a playpen with large diamond-shaped openings. Entrapment is a risk.
  - Never tie or string toys from the sides of the playpen.
  - Stop using the playpen when the child can easily climb out—when the child is 34 inches tall or weighs 30 pounds.

Strollers

- There is a wide base to prevent tipping.
- The device has a reliable restraining belt. A 5-point harness is safest.
- Brakes securely lock the wheels.
- The shopping basket is low on the back. It is located in front of the rear wheels.
- The leg openings are small enough to prevent an infant from slipping through.
- When used in the reclined position, the leg openings can be closed.
- No stroller parts can pinch a child's fingers or are a choking hazard.
- The stroller steers in a straight line when pushed with 1 hand.
- Handlebars are at waist level or slightly lower.
- Follow these safety measures.
  - Never exceed age, weight, and height limits.
  - Position newborns almost flat. Newborns cannot support the head and neck.
  - Never leave a child unattended.
  - Always use the safety harness.
  - Avoid using a pillow or blanket as a mattress.
  - Apply the brakes when not moving.
  - Never hang purses or diaper bags on the handles.
  - Fold and unfold the stroller away from children to avoid pinching fingers.

Walkers

- Walkers are not used. Walkers are a leading cause of injury in babies. Injury risks include:
  - Falling over objects or down stairs.
  - Rolling into dangerous objects or areas. Hot stoves, heaters, and pools are examples.
  - Reaching higher than normal and touching dangerous items. Stovetops, kitchen knives, and hot coffee cups are examples.

Toys

- Small toys are kept away from children. Make sure toys are too large to fit into the child's mouth. Objects should have a diameter of 1¾ inches or more. This includes marbles, balls, and games with balls.
- Battery cases on battery-operated toys are secured with screws.
- Toys are strong and durable. They do not have:
  - Sharp ends, small parts, and small ends that can extend into the back of a baby's mouth
  - Strings longer than 7 inches
  - Parts that can pinch fingers
- Riding toys are stable and secure to prevent tipping.
- Safety gear is worn for bicycles, skateboards, scooters, in-line skates, and other devices with wheels. A helmet and knee pads, elbow pads, and wrist guards are examples.
- Follow these safety measures for toys.
  - Follow manufacturers' age recommendations.
  - Read all warning labels.
  - Make sure toys have not been recalled for safety reasons.
  - Do not give an infant or toddler painted toys made before 1978. The paint may contain lead.
  - Never give balloons or latex gloves to children younger than 8 years.
  - Never give a baby vending machine toys. They often contain small parts.
  - Check toys and play equipment for cracks, chips, breaks, sharp edges, loose parts, and other damage.
  - Check carnival toys carefully. They are not required to meet safety standards.
  - Keep older children's toys away from infants and younger children.

Cribs

- Side rails are fixed and not adjustable. The U.S. Consumer Product Safety Commission (CPSC) banned the sale of drop-side cribs.
- Slats are spaced no more than 2⅜ inches apart.
- No slats are missing, loose, or cracked.
- The mattress is firm and fits snugly.
- The mattress pad fits tightly and the plastic mattress packaging is removed.
- Crib corner posts are either flush with the top of the head-board and foot-board or are over 16 inches.
- The crib meets federal safety standards for strength, durability, and testing. The crib has not been recalled by the manufacturer.
- Follow these safety measures when using cribs.
  - Always place a baby on the back to sleep.
  - Remove a baby's bib when in the crib.
  - Check that all screws and hardware are present and tight.
  - Never place soft bedding or soft toys in the crib.
  - Bumper pads are not used.
  - Remove a mobile from the crib when 1 of the following occurs.
    - The child can push on the hands and knees.
    - The child reaches 5 months of age.
  - Do not hang toys by strings.
  - Use flame-retardant sheets and sleepwear.
  - Never place a crib near a window or drapes. A baby can become entangled in window covering cords.

Child Safety Seats (Car Seats)

- The car seat is federally approved and fits the child's height and weight.
- Parts and manufacturer labels—including the manufacturer's name, model number, and date made—are intact.
- The seat has not been in a motor vehicle accident.
- The seat is less than 6 years old. Check the manufacturer's recommended expiration date.
- Follow these safety measures for using car seats.
  - Do not use a car seat that does not have the manufacturer's instructions.
  - Infants and toddlers ride rear-facing until they have reached the weight and height limits recommended by the manufacturer.
  - Children in forward-facing seats are harnessed in until they reach the weight or height limit for that seat.
  - A booster seat is used for children who have outgrown the forward-facing harness seat.
  - Children use a booster seat until the vehicle's lap-and-shoulder belt fits properly. This usually occurs when the child has reached 4 feet, 9 inches in height—between 8 and 12 years of age.
  - Follow the car seat guidelines in Chapter 56.

Appendix E

Personal Safety

General Measures

- Know the area where you are going. Ask questions about the area.
- Make a "dry run" of the area. Know the way in advance. The shortest way is not always the safest.
- Let someone know where you are at all times. Tell someone when you leave and when you arrive at your destination. If you do not call when expected, the person knows something is wrong.
- Make it known that you do not carry drugs, needles, or syringes.
- Do not wear expensive jewelry or carry large amounts of money or valuables. Leave them at home. If someone wants what you have, give it. The only thing of value is you.
- Carry wallets, purses, and backpacks safely.
  - Wallets—Carry wallets in an inside coat pocket or side pant pocket. Do not carry wallets in a rear pocket.
  - Purses—Keep a firm grip on a purse. Keep it close to your body. A purse that zips closed is best.
  - Backpacks—Keep the backpack zipped and secure with a padlock.
- Do not display money or other targets of theft. Phones and other hand-held electronic devices are examples.
- Keep your phone accessible but not visible to others.
- Keep your phone charged.
- Carry a whistle or other alarm.
- Avoid ATMs (automated teller machines) at night.
- Be careful when getting on elevators and when entering stairways.
- Do not approach a stranger or someone acting in a strange way. Report the matter at once.
- Be careful what you share on social media. For example, others know your location if you share it.

Home Settings

- Keep doors and windows to the home locked at all times. This includes doors into the garage or the door from the garage into the house.
- Do not open doors to strangers. Ask for identification.
- Do not let a stranger into the home to use a phone or bathroom. Offer to call the police if the person needs help.
- Do not give personal information to callers or people at the door.

Car Safety

- Have plenty of gas in your car.
- Keep your car in good working order.
- Keep these in your car—local map, flashlight with working batteries, flares, a fire extinguisher, first aid kit.
- Raise the hood and use the flares if the car breaks down. Stay in the car. Call the police if you have a phone. If someone stops by to help, ask the person to call the police.
- Lock your car. Sometimes you may want to leave it unlocked. If you need to get in the car fast, you do not want to fumble with keys. Use your judgment. Do not leave anything in the car if you leave it unlocked.
- Have your car key ready so you can get into the car quickly. Do not fumble for keys on the way to or at the car.
- Check under the car as you approach it. A person hiding under the car can grab your ankle or leg. Leave at once if someone is under the car. The person under the car may be working with someone who is waiting to attack you while you are being held or injured at the leg or ankle.
- Check the back seat before getting into the car. Make sure no one is in the car. Leave at once if someone is in the car.
- Lock car doors when you get in the car. Keep windows rolled up.
- Do not open the car door or window to talk to a person approaching your car.
- Do not get out of the car to remove something from the windshield.
- Keep purses, backpacks, and other valuables under the seat or near your side. Do not leave them on the seat. They are easy targets for smash-and-grab robbers.
- Do not hitchhike or pick up hitchhikers.
- Practice safety at a gas pump.
  - Take your wallet or purse with you to the pump. If you must keep your wallet, purse, or backpack in the car, keep all windows up and lock all doors. Keep your wallet, purse, and belongings out-of-sight. Called "sliders" by police, thieves can open the car door (or reach in a window) away from where you are standing and grab purses and other valuables.
  - Keep the car key in your hand. "Smart keys" only need to sense that the key is in the car. The car can simply be started with a foot on the brake and pushing the "start" button.
  - Protect children in the car. Lock all doors and keep the door closest to you open.

Parking Your Car

- Check for places to park. Choose a well-lit area. In a parking garage, park near entrances, exits, and on the lower level. Try to get close to the attendant if possible. The closest space to your destination is not always the safest for parking.
- Park so you can leave quickly and easily. Park at street corners so no one can park in front of you. In parking lots, back in. You see more from the front windshield than from the back window.

Walking

- Do not wear headphones or earbuds. You cannot hear cars, buses, trains, and people around you.
- Use well-lit and busy streets. Avoid vacant lots, alleys, wooded areas, and construction sites. The shortest way is not always the safest.
- Walk near the curb. Stay away from doorways, shrubs, and bushes.
- Carry a phone. Know your location, and keep phone calls simple.
- Switch directions or cross the street if you think someone is following you. If the person follows you, move quickly to an open store, restaurant, or other public place. Ask for help. If nearby, go to a police or fire station.

Public Transportation

- Carry money for bus, train, or taxi fares. Have money in your pocket to avoid fumbling with a purse or wallet.
- Stand with others and near the ticket booth.
- Sit near the driver or conductor.
- Keep your phone accessible.

If You Are Threatened or Attacked

- Run away if possible.
- Scream for help as loud and as long as you can. Keep screaming.
- Use your car keys or house key as a weapon. Hold them in your strong hand. Have 1 key extended. Hold the key firmly. If you are attacked, go for the person's face. Slash the person's face with the key. Do not use poking motions. Do not try for a certain target because you might miss.
- Remember, you have 2 arms, 2 hands, 2 feet, and 2 knees. You can attack from more than 1 direction at once. Do not be shy—your attacker will not be. Push, pull, yank, and so on. You can attack a man's or woman's genitals. Use your thumbs as weapons. Go for the eyes and push hard.

Glossary

A

abbreviation A shortened form of a word or phrase

abduction Moving a body part away from the mid-line of the body

abrasion A partial-thickness wound caused by the scraping away or rubbing of the skin from friction or trauma

abuse
- The willful infliction of injury, unreasonable confinement, intimidation, or punishment that results in physical harm, pain, or mental anguish
- Depriving the person (or the person's caregiver) of the goods or services needed to attain or maintain well-being

accountable To answer to one's self and others about one's choices, decisions, and actions

acetone See "ketone"

acid reflux See "heartburn"

activities of daily living (ADL) The activities usually done during a normal day in a person's life

acute illness An illness of rapid onset and short duration; the person is expected to recover

acute pain Pain that is sharp or severe; felt suddenly from injury, disease, trauma, or surgery

addiction A chronic disease involving substance-seeking behaviors and use that is compulsive and hard to control despite the harmful effects

adduction Moving a body part toward the mid-line of the body

admission The official entry of a person into a health care setting

adolescence The time between puberty and adulthood; a time of rapid growth and physical, sexual, emotional, and social changes

advance directive A legal document stating a person's wishes about health care when that person is unable to make decisions

advocate Someone who acts or speaks on behalf of another person

afebrile Without (*a*) a fever (*febrile*)

affected side The side of the body with weakness from illness or injury; weak side

allergy A sensitivity to a substance that causes the body to react with signs and symptoms

alopecia Hair loss

AM care See "early morning care"

ambulation The act of walking

amputation The removal of all or part of an extremity

analysis Interpreting data and identifying problems; see "nursing process"

anaphylaxis A life-threatening sensitivity to an antigen

anemia A decrease in the amount of healthy red blood cells (*an* means lack of; *emia* means blood condition)

anesthesia The loss (*an*) of all sensation (*esthesia*), especially pain, produced by a drug

anorexia The loss of appetite

anterior At or toward the front of the body or body part; ventral

antibiotic A drug that kills bacteria

anticoagulant A drug that prevents or slows down (*anti*) blood clotting (*coagulate*)

antiseptic A substance applied to living tissue that prevents or stops the growth or action of microbes

anxiety A feeling of worry, nervousness, or fear about an event or situation

aphasia The total or partial loss (*a*) of the ability to use or understand language (*phasia*)

apical-radial pulse Taking the apical and radial pulses at the same time

apnea The lack or absence (*a*) of breathing (*pnea*)

arrhythmia See "dysrhythmia"

arterial ulcer An open wound on the lower legs or feet caused by poor arterial blood flow; ischemic ulcer

artery A blood vessel that carries blood away from the heart

arthritis Joint (*arthr*) inflammation (*itis*)

arthroplasty The surgical replacement (*plasty*) of a joint (*arthro*)

asepsis The absence (*a*) of disease-producing microbes; *sepsis* means infection

aspiration Breathing fluid, food, vomitus, or an object into the lungs

assault Intentionally attempting or threatening to touch a person's body without the person's consent

assessment Collecting information about the person; see "nursing process"

assisted living A housing option for persons who need help with activities of daily living but do not need 24-hour nursing care

assisted living residence (ALR) Provides housing, personal care, support services, health care, and social activities in a home-like setting to persons needing some help with daily activities

atelectasis The collapse of a portion of a lung

atrophy The decrease in size or wasting away of tissue

autopsy The examination of the body after death

avoidable pressure injury A pressure injury that develops from the improper use of the nursing process

avulsion A wound that occurs when skin or tissue is torn away

B

bariatrics The field of medicine focused on the treatment and control of obesity

base of support The area on which an object rests

bath blanket A covering used for privacy and warmth during bathing, hygiene, and other care measures

battery Touching a person's body without consent

bedfast Confined to bed

bed mobility How a person moves to and from a lying position, turns from side to side, and re-positions in a bed or other sleeping furniture

bed rail A device that serves as a guard or barrier along the side of the bed; side rail

bed rest Restricting a person to bed and limiting activity for health reasons

benign tumor A tumor that does not spread to other body parts

biohazardous waste Items contaminated with blood or other potentially infectious materials (OPIM); regulated medical waste, infectious waste

biopsy A procedure in which a piece of tissue is removed for testing

Biot's respirations Rapid and deep respirations followed by 10 to 30 seconds of apnea

birth defect A problem that develops during pregnancy, often during the first 3 months; it may involve a body structure or function

blanch To become white

blindness The absence of sight

bloodborne pathogens Microbes that are present in blood and can cause infection

blood pressure (BP) The amount of force exerted against the walls of an artery by the blood

body alignment The way the head, trunk, arms, and legs align with one another; posture

body language Messages sent through facial expressions, gestures, posture, hand and body movements, gait, eye contact, and appearance

body mechanics Using the body in an efficient and careful way

body temperature The amount of heat in the body that is a balance between the amount of heat produced and the amount lost by the body

bony prominence An area where the bone sticks out or projects from the flat surface of the body; pressure point

boundary crossing A brief act or behavior of being over-involved with the person; the intent of the act or behavior is to meet the person's needs

boundary sign An act, behavior, or thought that warns of a boundary crossing or boundary violation

boundary violation An act or behavior that meets your needs, not the person's

bradycardia A slow (*brady*) heart rate (*cardia*); less than 60 beats per minute

bradypnea Slow (*brady*) breathing (*pnea*); respirations are fewer than 12 per minute

braille A touch reading and writing system that uses raised dots for each letter of the alphabet; the first 10 letters also represent the numbers 0 through 9

breast-feeding Feeding a baby milk from the mother's breasts; nursing

Broca's aphasia See "expressive aphasia"

bullying Repeated, unwanted, aggressive behavior among school-age children and adolescents that involves a real or perceived power imbalance

burnout A job stress resulting in being physically or mentally exhausted, having doubts about your abilities, and having doubts about the value of your work

C

calorie The fuel or energy value of food

cancer See "malignant tumor"

capillary A very tiny blood vessel; nutrients, oxygen, and other substances pass from the capillaries into the cells

cardiac arrest See "sudden cardiac arrest"

cardiopulmonary resuscitation (CPR) An emergency procedure performed when the heart and breathing stop

care plan See "nursing care plan"

carrier A human (or animal) that is a reservoir for microbes but does not develop the infection

catheter A tube used to drain or inject fluid through a body opening

catheterization The process of inserting a catheter

cell The basic unit of body structure

certification Official recognition by a state that standards or requirements have been met

cerumen Earwax

chain of command The order of authority in an agency

chairfast Confined to a chair

chart See "medical record"

chemical restraint A drug or drug dosage that:
- Controls behavior or restricts movement and is not standard treatment for the person's condition
- Is used for discipline or convenience and is not required to treat medical symptoms

Cheyne-Stokes respirations Respirations gradually increase in rate and depth and then become shallow and slow; breathing may stop (*apnea*) for 10 to 20 seconds

child abuse and neglect The intentional harm or mistreatment of a child under 18 years old that:
- Involves any recent act or failure to act on the part of a parent or caregiver
- Results in death, serious physical or emotional harm, sexual abuse, or exploitation
- Presents a likely or immediate risk for harm

cholesterol A soft, waxy substance found in the bloodstream and all body cells

chronic illness A long-term health condition that may not have a cure; it can be controlled and complications prevented with proper treatment

chronic pain Pain that continues for a long time (longer than 12 weeks, occurs off and on, or is persistent [constant])

chronic wound A wound that does not heal easily and within about 3 months

circadian rhythm Daily rhythm based on a 24-hour cycle that involves behavior, sleep, eating, and waking patterns; the day-night cycle or body rhythm

circulatory ulcer An open sore on the lower legs or feet caused by decreased blood flow through the arteries or veins; vascular ulcer

circumcised The fold of skin (foreskin) covering the glans of the penis was surgically removed

circumcision The surgical removal of foreskin from the penis

civil law Laws concerned with relationships between people

clean technique See "medical asepsis"

closed fracture The bone is broken but the skin is intact; simple fracture

code of ethics Rules, or standards of conduct, for group members to follow

cognitive function Involves memory, thinking, reasoning, ability to understand, judgment, and behavior

colostomy A surgically created opening (*stomy*) between the colon (*colo*) and the body's surface

coma A prolonged state of unconsciousness

comatose Being unable to respond to stimuli; unconscious

comfort A state of well-being; the person has no physical or emotional pain and is calm and at ease

communicable disease A disease caused by a pathogen that can spread to others; contagious disease

communication The exchange of information—a message sent is received and correctly interpreted by the intended person

compound fracture See "open fracture"

compress A soft pad applied over a body area

compulsion An over-whelming urge to repeat certain rituals, acts, or behaviors

condom catheter A soft sheath that slides over the penis and is used to drain urine

confidentiality Trusting others with personal and private information

conflict A clash between opposing interests or ideas

confusion A state of being disoriented to person, time, place, situation, or identity

congenital To be born with

consent Permission

constipation The passage of a hard, dry stool

constrict To narrow

contagious disease See "communicable disease"

contamination The process of becoming unclean

contracture Decreased motion and stiffness of a joint caused by shortening (contracting) of a muscle

convulsion See "seizure"

coping Strategies to manage stress and reduce negative emotions caused by stress

courtesy A polite, considerate, or helpful comment or act

crime An act that violates a criminal law

criminal law Laws concerned with offenses against the public and society in general

cross-contamination Passing microbes from 1 person to another by contaminated hands, equipment, or supplies

culture The characteristics of a group of people—language, values, beliefs, habits, likes, dislikes, customs—passed from 1 generation to the next

cyanosis Bluish (*cyano*) color; bluish color (*cyano*) to the skin, lips, mucous membranes, and nail beds

D

dandruff Excessive amounts of dry, white flakes from the scalp

deafness Hearing loss in which it is impossible for the person to understand speech through hearing alone

deconditioning The loss of muscle strength from inactivity

deep Below the surface

defamation Injuring a person's name and reputation by making false statements to a third person

defecation The process of excreting feces from the rectum through the anus; bowel movement

defense mechanism An unconscious reaction that blocks unpleasant or threatening feelings

dehydration A decrease in the amount of water in the body

delegate To authorize or direct a nursing assistant to perform a nursing task

delegated nursing task
- A nursing task that is beyond the nursing assistant's usual work assignment
- Using the delegation process, the nurse transfers responsibility for completion of the task to the nursing assistant

delegation
- The process a nurse uses to direct a nursing assistant to perform a nursing task
- Allowing a nursing assistant to perform a nursing task that is beyond the nursing assistant's usual role and not routinely done by the nursing assistant

delirium A state of sudden, severe confusion and rapid changes in brain function

delusion A false belief

delusion of grandeur An exaggerated belief about one's importance, fame, wealth, power, or talents

delusion of persecution A false belief that one is being mistreated, abused, or harassed

dementia The loss of cognitive function that interferes with daily life and activities

denture A removable replacement for missing teeth

detoxification The process of removing a toxic substance from the body

development Changes in mental, emotional, and social function

developmental disability A life-long condition that begins during the developmental period and impairs physical or intellectual function or both

developmental task A skill that must be completed during a stage of development for development to continue diabetic foot ulcer An open wound on the foot caused by complications from diabetes

dialysis The process of removing waste products from the blood

diaphoresis Profuse (excessive) sweating

diarrhea The frequent passage of liquid stools

diastole The period of heart muscle relaxation; the heart is at rest

diastolic pressure The pressure in the arteries when the heart is at rest

digestion The process that breaks down food physically and chemically so it can be absorbed for use by the cells

dignity Having value and worth as a person

dilate To expand or open wider

disability Any lost, absent, or impaired physical or mental function

disaster A harmful event that can affect the agency, patient or resident population, community, or larger geographic area

discharge The official departure of a person from a health care setting

discomfort See "pain"

discrimination Unjust treatment based on personal qualities

disinfectant A liquid chemical that can kill many or all pathogens except spores

disinfection The process of killing pathogens

distal The part farthest from the center or from the point of attachment

distraction To focus the person's attention on something unrelated to pain

dorsal See "posterior"

dorsal recumbent position The back-lying or supine position; the supine position with the legs together (dorsal means the back of something; recumbent means to lie down); horizontal recumbent position

dorsiflexion Bending the toes and foot up at the ankle

drawsheet A small sheet placed over the middle of the bottom sheet to keep the mattress and bottom linens clean

drug addiction A strong urge or craving to use a substance; the person cannot stop using it; tolerance develops

drug diversion Stealing drugs for personal use, sale, or distribution to others

dysphagia Difficulty (dys) swallowing (phagia)

dyspnea Difficult, labored, or painful (dys) breathing (pnea)

dysrhythmia An abnormal (dys) heart rhythm (rhythmia); arrhythmia

dysuria Painful or difficult (dys) urination (uria); burning on urination

E

early morning care Routine care given before breakfast; AM care

edema The swelling of body tissues with water

ejaculation The release of semen

elder abuse Any intentional act, or failure to act, by a caregiver or other trusted person that causes harm or risk of harm to an older adult

elective surgery Surgery done by choice to improve life or well-being

electrical shock When electrical current passes through the body

electrolytes Minerals dissolved in water

electronic health record (EHR) An electronic version of a person's medical record; electronic medical record

electronic medical record (EMR) See "electronic health record"

elopement When a patient or resident leaves the agency without staff knowledge

embolus A blood clot (thrombus) that travels through the vascular system until it lodges in a blood vessel

emergency surgery Surgery done at once to save life or function

emesis See "vomitus"

end-of-life care The support and care given during the time surrounding death

end-of-shift report A report that the nurse gives at the end of the shift to the on-coming shift; change-of-shift report

endorsement A state recognizes the certificate, license, or registration issued by another state; reciprocity or equivalency

enema The introduction of fluid into the rectum and lower colon

enteral nutrition Giving nutrients into the gastro-intestinal (GI) tract (enteral) through a feeding tube

entrapment Getting caught, trapped, or entangled in spaces created by the bed rails, the mattress, the bed frame, the head-board, or the foot-board

enuresis Lack of bladder control when past the usual age of toilet training

epidermal stripping Removing the epidermis (outer skin layer) as tape is removed from the skin

episiotomy Incision (otomy) into the perineum

equivalency See "endorsement"

erectile dysfunction (ED) The inability of the male to have or maintain an erection; impotence

ergonomics The science of designing a job to fit the worker; ergo means work, nomos means law

erythema Redness

eschar Thick, leathery dead tissue that may be loose or adhered to the skin; it is often black or brown

esteem The worth, value, or opinion one has of a person

ethics Knowledge of what is right conduct and wrong conduct

eupnea Normal (eu) breathing (pnea)

evaluation To measure if goals in the planning step were met; see "nursing process"

evening care Care given in the evening at bedtime; PM care

excoriation Damage to the epidermis (top skin layer) caused by scratching

exploitation To take advantage of for personal gain

expressive aphasia Difficulty expressing or sending out thoughts through speech or writing; Broca's aphasia

extension Straightening a body part

external rotation Turning the joint outward

F

fainting The sudden loss of consciousness from an inadequate blood supply to the brain; syncope

false imprisonment Unlawful restraint or restriction of a person's freedom of movement

febrile With a fever

fecal impaction The prolonged retention and buildup of feces in the rectum

fecal incontinence The inability to control the passage of feces and flatus through the anus

feces The semi-solid mass of waste products in the colon that is expelled through the anus; stool or stools

fever Elevated body temperature

first aid The emergency care given to an ill or injured person before medical help arrives

flashback Reliving a trauma over and over in thoughts during the day and in nightmares during sleep

flatulence The excessive formation of gas or air in the stomach and intestines

flatus Gas or air passed through the anus

flexion Bending a body part

flow rate The number of drops per minute (gtt/min) or milliliters per hour (mL/hr)

Foley catheter See "indwelling catheter"

footdrop The foot falls down at the ankle; permanent plantar flexion

Fowler's position A semi-sitting position; the head of the bed is raised between 45 and 60 degrees

fracture A broken bone

fraud Saying or doing something to trick, fool, or deceive a person

friction The rubbing of 1 surface against another

frostbite An injury to the body caused by freezing of the skin and underlying tissues

full visual privacy Having the means to be completely free from public view while in bed

functional incontinence The person has bladder control but cannot use the toilet in time

G

gait belt See "transfer belt"

gangrene A condition in which there is death of tissue

garment An item of clothing

gastrostomy tube A feeding tube inserted through a surgically created opening (*stomy*) in the stomach (*gastro*)

gavage The process of giving a tube feeding

gender identity A person's sense or feelings of being male, female, a combination of male and female, or neither male nor female

general anesthesia A treatment with certain drugs that produces a deep sleep and the absence of all sensation, especially pain

genupectoral position See "knee-chest position" (*genu* means knee; *pectoral* refers to the chest)

geriatrics The field of medicine concerned with the problems and diseases of old age and older persons; the care of aging people

gerontology The study of the aging process

global aphasia Difficulty expressing or sending out thoughts and difficulty understanding language; mixed aphasia

glucometer A device for measuring (*meter*) blood glucose (*gluco*); glucose meter

glucosuria Sugar (*glucose*) in the urine (*uria*)

gossip To spread rumors or talk about the private matters of others

graduate A measuring container for fluid

gravity A natural force that pulls things downward

groin Where a thigh and the abdomen meet

ground That which carries leaking electricity to the earth and away from an electrical item

growth The physical changes that are measured and that occur in a steady, orderly manner

guided imagery Creating and focusing on a relaxing image

H

hallucination Seeing, hearing, smelling, feeling, or tasting something that is not real

harassment To trouble, torment, offend, or worry a person by one's behavior or comments

hazard Anything in the person's setting that could cause injury or illness

hazardous chemical Any chemical that is a physical hazard or a health hazard

healthcare-associated infection (HAI) An infection that develops in a person cared for in any setting where health care is given; the infection is related to receiving health care

health system A coordinated network of health care agencies and services

health team The many health care workers whose skills and knowledge focus on the person's total care; interdisciplinary health care team

hearing loss Not being able to hear the range of sounds associated with normal hearing

heartburn A burning sensation in the chest or throat; acid reflux

hematoma A swelling (*oma*) that contains blood (*hemat*)

hematuria Blood (*hemat*) in the urine (*uria*)

hemiparesis Partial paralysis (*paresis*) on 1 side (*hemi*) of the body

hemiplegia Paralysis (*plegia*) on 1 side (*hemi*) of the body

hemoglobin The substance in red blood cells that carries oxygen and gives blood its red color

hemoptysis Bloody (*hemo*) sputum (*ptysis* means to spit)

hemorrhage The excessive loss (*rrhage*) of blood (*hemo*) in a short time

hemothorax Blood (*hemo*) in the pleural space (*thorax*)

high-Fowler's position A variation of Fowler's position; the head of the bed is raised 60 to 90 degrees

hirsutism Excessive body hair

holism A concept that considers the whole person; the whole person has physical, psychological, social, and spiritual parts that are woven together and cannot be separated

horizontal recumbent position See "dorsal recumbent position"

hormone A chemical substance secreted by the endocrine glands into the bloodstream

hospice A health care agency or program that promotes comfort and quality of life for the dying person and the person's family

hospital bed system The bed frame and its parts—mattress, bed rails, head- and foot-boards, and bed attachments

hygiene The cleanliness practices that promote health and prevent disease

hyperextension Excessive straightening of a body part

hyperglycemia High (*hyper*) sugar (*glyc*) in the blood (*emia*)

hypertension High blood pressure

hyperventilation Breathing (*ventilation*) is rapid (*hyper*) and deeper than normal

hypoglycemia Low (*hypo*) sugar (*glyc*) in the blood (*emia*)

hypotension Low blood pressure

hypothermia Abnormally low (*hypo*) body temperature (*thermia*)

hypoventilation Breathing (*ventilation*) is slow (*hypo*), shallow, and sometimes irregular

hypoxemia A reduced amount (*hypo*) of oxygen (*ox*) in the blood (*emia*)

hypoxia Cells do not have enough (*hypo*) oxygen (*oxia*)

I

ileostomy A surgically created opening (*stomy*) between the ileum (small intestine [*ileo*]) and the body's surface

immobility The inability to move

immunity Protection against a disease or condition; the person will not get or be affected by the disease

implementation To carry out nursing interventions in the care plan; see "nursing process"

incident Any event that has harmed or could harm a patient, resident, visitor, or staff member; adverse event

incident report Documentation of the details about a harmful or potentially harmful event

incision A cut produced surgically by a sharp instrument; it creates an opening into an organ or body space

indwelling catheter A catheter left in the bladder so urine drains constantly into a drainage bag; retention or Foley catheter

infancy The first year of life

infection A disease state resulting from the invasion and growth of microbes in the body

infection control Practices and procedures that prevent the spread of infection

inferior Below another structure

infestation Being in or on a host

informed consent The process by which a person receives and understands information about a treatment or procedure and is able to decide to receive or refuse the treatment or procedure

inherited That which is passed down from parents to children

insomnia A chronic condition in which the person cannot sleep or stay asleep all night

intact skin Skin that is not broken

intake The amount of fluid taken in; input

intellectual disability A life-long condition that begins during the developmental period and limits intellectual function and adaptive behavior

internal rotation Turning the joint inward

intimate partner violence (IPV) Abuse or aggression that occurs in a romantic relationship

intravenous (IV) therapy Giving fluids through a needle or catheter inserted into a vein; IV and IV infusion

intubation Inserting an artificial airway

invasion of privacy Violating a person's right not to have his or her name, photo, or private affairs exposed or made public without giving consent

involuntary seclusion Separating a person from others against the person's will, keeping the person to a certain area, or keeping the person away from his or her room without consent

ischemic ulcer See "arterial ulcer"

J

jaundice Yellowish color of the skin or whites of the eyes

jejunostomy tube A feeding tube inserted into a surgically created opening (*stomy*) in the *jejunum* of the small intestine

job application An agency's official form listing questions that require factual answers from the person seeking employment; employment form

job description A document that describes what an agency expects you to do

job interview When an employer asks a job applicant questions about the applicant's education and career

joint The point at which 2 or more bones meet to allow movement

K

ketone A substance appearing in urine from the rapid breakdown of fat for energy; acetone, ketone body

ketone body See "ketone"

knee-chest position The person kneels and rests the body on the knees and chest; the head is turned to 1 side, the arms are above the head or flexed at the elbows, the back is straight, and the body is flexed about 90 degrees at the hips; genupectoral position

Kussmaul respirations Very deep and rapid respirations

L

laceration A wound with torn tissues and jagged edges caused by trauma

laryngeal mirror An instrument used to examine the mouth, teeth, and throat

lateral Away from the mid-line; at the side of the body or body part

lateral position The person lies on 1 side or the other; side-lying position

lateral transfer When a person moves between 2 horizontal surfaces

law A rule of conduct made by a government body

libel Making false statements in print, in writing (including e-mail and text messages), through pictures or drawings, through broadcast (radio, TV, video), posted on-line on websites, or through video sites and social media sites

lice See "pediculosis"

licensed practical nurse (LPN) A nurse who has completed a practical nursing program and has passed a licensing test; called *licensed vocational nurse (LVN)* in California and Texas

licensed vocational nurse (LVN) See "licensed practical nurse (LPN)"

lithotomy position The person lies on the back with the hips at the edge of the exam table, the knees are flexed, the hips are externally rotated, and the feet are in stirrups

local anesthesia The loss of sensation, produced by a drug, in a small area

lochia The vaginal discharge that occurs after childbirth

logrolling Turning the person as a unit, in alignment, with 1 motion

low vision Impaired vision that cannot be corrected with eyeglasses, contact lenses, drugs, or surgery; vision changes interfere with every-day activities

lymphedema A buildup of lymph in the tissues causing edema (swelling)

M

malignant tumor A tumor that invades and destroys nearby tissues and can spread to other body parts; cancer

malpractice Negligence by a professional person

mechanical ventilation Using a machine to move air into and out of the lungs

meconium A newborn's first bowel movement; it is a dark green to black, tarry bowel movement

medial At or near the middle or mid-line of the body or body part

medical asepsis Practices used to reduce the number of microbes and prevent their spread from 1 person or place to another person or place; clean technique

medical record The legal account of a person's condition and response to treatment and care; chart

medication reminder Reminding the person to take drugs, observing them being taken as prescribed, and recording that they were taken

melena A black, tarry stool

menarche The first menstruation and the start of menstrual cycles

menopause The time when menstruation stops and menstrual cycles end; there has been at least 1 year without a menstrual period

menstruation The process in which the lining of the uterus (endometrium) breaks up and is discharged from the body through the vagina

mental health Involves a person's emotional, psychological, and social well-being

mental health disorder A serious illness that can affect a person's thinking, mood, behavior, function, and ability to relate to others; psychiatric disorder

metabolism How the body uses nutrients to provide energy and maintain body functions

metastasis The spread of cancer to other body parts

microbe See "microorganism"

microorganism A small (*micro*) living thing (*organism*) seen only with a microscope; microbe

milestone A behavior or skill that occurs in a stage of development

misappropriation The dishonest use of property

mite A very small spider-like organism

mixed aphasia See "global aphasia"

mixed incontinence The combination of stress incontinence and urge incontinence

mobility A person's ability to move

mole A brown, tan, or black spot on the skin that is flat or raised and round or oval

morning care Care given after breakfast; hygiene measures are more thorough at this time

mouth care See "oral hygiene"

musculo-skeletal disorders (MSDs) Injuries and disorders of the muscles, tendons, ligaments, joints, and cartilage

N

nasal speculum An instrument (*speculum*) used to examine the inside of the nose (*nasal*)

naso-enteral tube A feeding tube inserted through the nose (*naso*) into the small bowel (*enteral*)

naso-gastric (NG) tube A feeding tube inserted through the nose (*naso*) into the stomach (*gastro*)

need Something necessary or desired for maintaining life and mental well-being

neglect When a caregiver or responsible person fails to:
- Protect a vulnerable person from harm
- Provide food, water, clothing, shelter, health care, or basic activities of daily living to a vulnerable person

negligence An unintentional wrong in which a person did not act in a reasonable and careful manner and a person or the person's property was harmed

nocturia Frequent urination (*uria*) at night (*noc*)

non-pathogen A microbe that does not usually cause an infection

nonverbal communication Communication that does not use words

normal flora Microbes that live and grow in a certain area

nursing See "breast-feeding"

nursing assistant A person who has passed a nursing assistant training and competency evaluation program (NATCEP); performs delegated nursing tasks under the supervision of a licensed nurse

nursing care plan A written guide about the person's nursing care; care plan

nursing intervention An action or measure taken by the nursing team to help the person reach a goal; nursing action, nursing measure, nursing task

nursing process The method nurses use to plan and deliver nursing care; it includes assessment, analysis, planning, implementation, and evaluation

nursing task Nursing care or a nursing function, procedure, skill, or activity

nursing team Those who provide nursing care—RNs, LPNs/LVNs, and nursing assistants

nutrient A substance that is ingested, digested, absorbed, and used by the body

nutrition The processes involved in the ingestion, digestion, absorption, and use of food and fluids by the body

O

obesity Having a weight that is higher than what is healthy for a given height

objective data Information that is seen, heard, felt, or smelled by an observer; signs

observation Using the sense of sight, hearing, touch, and smell to collect information

obsession A frequent, upsetting, and unwanted thought, idea, or image

obstetrics The field of medicine concerned with the care of women during pregnancy, labor, and childbirth and for 6 to 8 weeks after birth

occupied In use

oliguria Scant amount *(olig)* of urine *(uria);* less than 500 mL in 24 hours

ombudsman Someone who supports or promotes the needs and interests of another person

open fracture The broken bone has pierced the skin; compound fracture

ophthalmoscope A lighted instrument *(scope)* used to examine the internal eye *(ophthalmo)* structures

opposition Touching an opposite finger with the thumb

optimal level of function A person's desired level of ability

oral hygiene The practices that promote healthy tissues and structures of the mouth; mouth care

organ Groups of tissue that function together

orthopnea Breathing *(pnea)* deeply and comfortably only when sitting *(ortho)*

orthopneic position Sitting up *(ortho)* and leaning over a table to breathe *(pneic)*

orthostatic hypotension See "postural hypotension"

orthotic A device used to support a muscle, promote a certain motion, or correct a deformity; *ortho* means to straighten

ostomy A surgically created opening that connects an internal organ to the body's surface; see "colostomy" and "ileostomy"

otoscope A lighted instrument *(scope)* used to examine the external ear *(oto)* and the eardrum (tympanic membrane)

output The amount of fluid lost

over-flow incontinence Small amounts of urine leak from a full bladder

oxygen concentration The amount (percent [%]) of hemoglobin containing oxygen

P

pack A commercial application for heat or cold therapy

pain To ache, hurt, or be sore; discomfort

palliative care Care that relieves or reduces the intensity of uncomfortable symptoms without producing a cure

panic An intense and sudden feeling of fear, anxiety, or dread

paralysis Loss of muscle function

paranoia A disorder *(para)* of the mind *(noia);* false beliefs (delusions) and suspicion about a person or situation

paraphrasing Re-stating the person's message in your own words

paraplegia Paralysis in the legs and lower trunk

parenteral nutrition Giving nutrients through a catheter inserted into a vein; *para* means beyond; *enteral* relates to the bowel

paresis Weak or impaired muscle function without complete paralysis; partial paralysis

patent Open and unblocked

pathogen A microbe that is harmful and can cause an infection

pediatrics The field of medicine concerned with the growth, development, and care of children—newborns to teenagers

pediculosis Infestation with wingless insects that feed on blood; lice

pediculosis capitis Infestation of the scalp *(capitis)* with lice

pediculosis corporis Infestation of the body *(corporis)* with lice

pediculosis pubis Infestation of the pubic *(pubis)* hair with lice

peer A person of the same age-group and background

penetrating wound A wound caused by an object that breaks the skin and enters a body area, organ, or cavity

percussion hammer An instrument used to tap body parts to test reflexes *(percussion* means to strike hard); reflex hammer

percutaneous endoscopic gastrostomy (PEG) tube A feeding tube inserted into the stomach *(gastro)* through a small incision *(stomy)* made through *(per)* the skin *(cutaneous);* a lighted instrument *(scope)* is used to see inside a body cavity or organ *(endo)*

pericare See "perineal care"

perineal care Cleaning the genital and anal areas; pericare

peristalsis The alternating contraction and relaxation of muscles that moves food through the digestive system

personal protective equipment (PPE) The clothing or equipment worn by staff for protection against a hazard

personality The set of attitudes, values, behaviors, and traits of a person

person's unit The space, furniture, and equipment used by the person in the agency

phantom pain Pain that seems to come from a body part that is no longer there

phobia An intense fear of something that has little or no real danger

physical restraint Any manual method or physical or mechanical device, material, or equipment that:
- Is attached to or near a person's body
- Cannot be removed easily by the person
- Restricts freedom of movement or normal access to the body

pivot To turn one's body from a set standing position

planning Setting priorities and goals; see "nursing process"

plantar flexion Bending the foot down at the ankle

plaque A thin film that sticks to the teeth; it contains saliva, microbes, and other substances

pleural effusion The escape and collection of fluid *(effusion)* in the pleural space

PM care See "evening care"

pneumonia Inflammation and infection of lung tissue

pneumothorax Air *(pneumo)* in the pleural space *(thorax)*

poison Any substance harmful to the body when ingested, inhaled, injected, or absorbed through the skin

pollutant A harmful chemical or substance in the air or water

polyuria Abnormally large amounts *(poly)* of urine *(uria)*

position change alarm Any physical or electronic device that monitors a person's movement and alerts staff of movement

posterior At or toward the back of the body or body part; dorsal

post-mortem care Care of the body after *(post)* death *(mortem)*

post-operative After *(post)* surgery; post-op

postpartum After *(post)* childbirth *(partum)*

postural hypotension Abnormally low *(hypo)* blood pressure when the person suddenly stands up *(postural)*; orthostatic hypotension

posture See "body alignment"

preceptor An experienced staff member who mentors a new employee at the start of a job

prefix A word element at the beginning of a word; it changes the meaning of the word

prenatal care The health care a woman receives while pregnant

pre-operative Before *(pre)* surgery; pre-op

presbycusis Decreased hearing ability due to aging; age-related hearing loss

presbyopia The gradual loss of the ability to focus on close-up objects that occurs with aging

pressure injury Localized damage to the skin and underlying soft tissue; the injury is usually over a bony prominence or related to a medical or other device and results from pressure or pressure in combination with shear

pressure point See "bony prominence"

primary caregiver The person mainly responsible for providing or assisting with a child's basic needs

priority The most important thing at the time

professional boundary That which separates helpful actions and behaviors from those that are not helpful

professionalism Following laws, being ethical, having good work ethics, and having the skills to do your work

professional sexual misconduct A violation of professional interactions with an act, behavior, or comment that is sexual in nature

progress note Describes the care given and the person's response and progress

pronation Turning the joint downward

prone position The person lies on the abdomen with the head turned to 1 side

prosthesis An artificial replacement for a missing body part

protected health information Identifying information and information about the person's health care that is maintained or sent in any form (paper, electronic, oral)

proximal The part nearest to the center or to the point of attachment

psychiatric disorder See "mental health disorder"

psychiatry The field of medicine concerned with mental health disorders

psychosis A condition that affects the mind and causes a loss of contact with reality

puberty The period when reproductive organs begin to function and secondary sex characteristics appear

pulse The beat of the heart felt at an artery as a wave of blood passes through the artery

pulse deficit The difference between the apical and radial pulse rates

pulse oximetry Measures *(metry)* the oxygen *(oxi)* concentration in arterial blood

pulse rate The number of heartbeats or pulses in 1 minute

puncture wound A wound caused by piercing from a pointed object

purulent drainage Thick green, yellow, or brown drainage

pyuria Pus *(py)* in the urine *(uria)*

Q

quadriplegia Paralysis in the arms, legs, and trunk; tetraplegia

R

radiating pain Pain felt at the site of tissue damage and that spreads to other areas

range of motion (ROM) The movement of a joint to the extent possible without causing pain

reasonable accommodation To assist or change a position or workplace to allow an employee to do a job despite having a disability

receptive aphasia Difficulty understanding language; Wernicke's aphasia

reciprocity See "endorsement"

recording The written account of care and observations; charting, documentation

referred pain Pain from a body part that is felt in another body part

reflex The body's response to a stimulus that does not require conscious thought; an involuntary movement

reflex incontinence Urine is lost at predictable intervals when a specific amount of urine is in the bladder

regional anesthesia The loss of sensation, produced by a drug, in a large area

registered nurse (RN) A nurse who has completed a 2-, 3-, or 4-year nursing program and has passed a licensing test

regulations Rules made by government agencies

regurgitation The backward flow of stomach contents into the mouth

rehabilitation The process of restoring a person's highest possible level of physical, psychological, social, and economic function

relaxation To be free from mental and physical stress

religion An organized system of spiritual beliefs and practices

reporting The oral account of care and observations

representative Someone with the legal right to act on the patient's or resident's behalf when the person cannot do so alone

respiration The process of supplying cells with oxygen and removing carbon dioxide from them; breathing air into (inhalation) and out of (exhalation) the lungs

respiratory arrest When breathing stops; breathing stops but heart action continues for several minutes

respiratory depression Slow, weak respirations

rest To be calm, at ease, and relaxed with no anxiety or stress

restorative aide A nursing assistant with special training in restorative nursing and rehabilitation skills

restorative nursing care Nursing care that helps persons regain health and strength for safe and independent living

restraint The restriction of voluntary movement or the control of behavior

restraint alternative Measures used instead of restraint to manage a potentially harmful situation

resuscitate To revive from apparent death or unconsciousness using emergency measures

retention catheter See "indwelling catheter"

rigor mortis The stiffness or rigidity (*rigor*) of skeletal muscles that occurs after death (*mortis*)

risk factor Something that increases the chance of illness or injury

root A word element that contains the basic meaning of the word

rotation Turning the joint

routine nursing task A nursing task that is part of a nursing assistant's usual work assignment

S

sanguineous drainage Bloody (*sanguis*) drainage

scabies A skin disorder caused by a female mite

seclusion Confining a person to a room or area and preventing the person from leaving

sedation A state of quiet, calmness, or sleep produced by a drug

seizure Violent and sudden contractions or tremors of muscle groups caused by abnormal electrical activity in the brain; convulsion

self-actualization Experiencing one's potential

self-esteem Thinking well of oneself and seeing oneself as useful and having value

self-neglect When a person's behaviors and way of living threaten the person's own health, safety, and well-being

semi-Fowler's position A variation of Fowler's position; the head of the bed is raised 30 degrees

semi-prone position The person lies on the side of the abdomen

serosanguineous drainage Thin, watery drainage (*sero*) that is blood-tinged (*sanguineous*)

serous drainage Clear, watery fluid (*serum*)

service plan A written plan listing the services needed, the help needed, and who provides services

sex Physical interactions between people involving the body and reproductive organs

sexuality The physical, emotional, social, cultural, and spiritual factors that affect a person's feelings, attitudes, and behaviors about one's gender identity and sexual behavior

sexual orientation A person's emotional, romantic, or physical attraction to males, females, both, or neither

shear When layers of the skin rub against each other; when the skin remains in place and underlying tissues move and stretch, tearing underlying capillaries and blood vessels and causing tissue damage

shearing When the skin sticks to a surface while muscles slide in the direction the body is moving

shock Results when tissues and organs do not get enough blood

side-lying position See "lateral position"

signs See "objective data"

simple fracture See "closed fracture"

skin breakdown Changes or damage to intact skin

skin tear A break or rip in the outer layers of the skin; the epidermis (top skin layer) separates from the underlying tissues

slander Making false statements through the spoken word, sounds, sign language, or gestures

sleep A state of reduced consciousness, reduced voluntary muscle activity, and lowered metabolism

sleep apnea Pauses (*a*) in breathing (*pnea*) that occur during sleep

sleep deprivation The amount and quality of sleep are not adequate, causing reduced function and alertness

sleepwalking When the person leaves the bed and walks about while sleeping

slough Dead tissue that is shed from the skin; it is usually light colored, soft, and moist; may be stringy at times

spastic Uncontrolled contractions of skeletal muscles

sphygmomanometer A cuff and measuring device used to measure blood pressure

spore A bacterium protected by a hard shell

sputum Mucus from the respiratory system that is expectorated (expelled) through the mouth

stage A period of time (age range) in which a person learns certain skills

standard of care The skills, care, and judgments required by a health team member under similar conditions

stasis ulcer See "venous ulcer"

sterile The absence of *all* microbes

sterile field A work area free of *all* pathogens and non-pathogens (including spores)

sterile technique See "surgical asepsis"

sterilization The process of destroying *all* microbes

stethoscope An instrument used to listen to the sounds produced by the heart, lungs, and other body organs

stimulus Anything that causes a body part to respond

stoma A surgically created opening seen on the body's surface; see "colostomy" and "ileostomy"

stomatitis Inflammation (*itis*) of the mouth (*stomat*)

stool Excreted feces

straight catheter A catheter that drains the bladder and then is removed

stress The response or change in the body caused by any emotional, psychological, physical, social, or economic factor

stress incontinence When urine leaks during exercise and certain movements that cause pressure on the bladder

stressor The event or factor that causes stress

subjective data Things a person tells you about that you cannot observe through your senses; symptoms

suction The process of withdrawing or sucking up fluid (secretions)

sudden cardiac arrest (SCA) The heart stops suddenly and without warning; cardiac arrest

suffix A word element at the end of a word; it changes the meaning of the word

suffocation When breathing stops from the lack of oxygen; asphyxia

suicidal ideation Thinking about, considering, or planning suicide

suicide To end one's life on purpose

suicide contagion Exposure to suicide or suicidal behaviors within one's family, one's peer group, or through media reports of suicide

sundowning Signs, symptoms, and behaviors of dementia increase during hours of darkness

superficial On the surface

superior Above another structure

supination Turning the joint upward

supine position The back-lying or dorsal recumbent position

suppository A cone-shaped, solid drug that is inserted into a body opening; it melts at body temperature

supra-pubic catheter A catheter surgically inserted into the bladder through an incision above (*supra*) the pubis bone (*pubic*)

surgical asepsis Practices used to remove *all* microbes; sterile technique

surgical site infection (SSI) An infection that occurs after surgery in the body part where the surgery took place

survey The formal review of an agency through the collection of facts and observations

surveyor A person who collects information by observing and asking questions

symptoms See "subjective data"

syncope A brief loss of consciousness; fainting

system Organs that work together to perform certain functions

systole The period of heart muscle contraction; the heart is pumping blood

systolic pressure The pressure in the arteries when the heart contracts

T

tachycardia A rapid (*tachy*) heart rate (*cardia*); more than 100 beats per minute

tachypnea Rapid (*tachy*) breathing (*pnea*); respirations are more than 20 per minute

tartar Hardened plaque

teamwork Staff members work together as a group; everyone does their part to give safe and effective care

teen dating violence (TDV) Physical violence, sexual violence, psychological aggression, or stalking that occurs in an adolescent romantic relationship

terminal illness An illness or injury from which the person will not likely recover; death is expected

tetraplegia See "quadriplegia"

thermometer A device used to measure (*meter*) temperature (*thermo*)

thrombus A blood clot

tinnitus A ringing, roaring, hissing, or buzzing sound in the ears or head

tissue A group of cells with similar functions

tolerance Needing more of a drug for the same effect

tort A wrong committed against a person or the person's property

tracheostomy A surgically created opening (*stomy*) in the neck into the trachea (*tracheo*)

transfer How a person moves to and from a surface; moving the person to another health care setting; moving the person to a new room within the agency

transfer belt A device applied around the waist and used to support a person who is unsteady or disabled; gait belt

transient incontinence Temporary or occasional incontinence that is reversed when the cause is treated

treatment The care provided to maintain or restore health, improve function, or relieve symptoms

tumor A new growth of abnormal cells that is benign or malignant

tuning fork An instrument vibrated to test hearing

U

ulcer A shallow or deep crater-like sore of the skin or mucous membrane

umbilical cord The structure that connects the mother and fetus (unborn baby); it carries blood, oxygen, and nutrients from the mother to the fetus

unaffected side The side of the body opposite the affected side; strong side

unavoidable pressure injury A pressure injury that occurs despite efforts to prevent one through proper use of the nursing process

uncircumcised Foreskin covers the head of the penis

unconscious Being unaware of one's setting and being unable to react or respond to people, places, or things

under-garment An item of clothing worn next to the skin under clothing

urge incontinence The loss of urine in response to a sudden, urgent need to void; the person cannot get to a toilet in time

urgent surgery Surgery needed for health; it can be delayed for a few days

urinary diversion A surgically created pathway for urine to leave the body

urinary frequency Voiding at frequent intervals

urinary incontinence (UI) The involuntary loss or leakage of urine

urinary retention Not being able to completely empty the bladder

urinary urgency The need to void at once

urination The process of emptying urine from the bladder; voiding

urostomy A surgically created opening (*stomy*) that connects to the urinary tract (*uro*)

V

vaccination Giving a vaccine to produce immunity against an infectious disease

vaccine A preparation containing dead or weakened microbes

vaginal speculum An instrument (*speculum*) used to open the vagina (*vaginal*) to examine it and the cervix

vascular ulcer See "circulatory ulcer"

vector An animal or insect that transmits disease

vehicle Any substance that transmits microbes

vein A blood vessel that returns blood to the heart

venous ulcer An open sore on the lower legs or feet caused by poor venous blood flow; stasis ulcer

ventral See "anterior"

verbal communication Communication that uses written or spoken words

vertigo Dizziness

vital signs Measurements of body function—temperature, pulse, respirations, and blood pressure; pulse oximetry and pain are included in some agencies

voiding See "urination"

vomitus Food and fluids expelled from the stomach through the mouth; emesis

vulnerable adult A person 18 years old or older who has a disability or condition that causes the person to be at risk for harm

W

waterproof under-pad An absorbent pad with a quilted top layer and a waterproof bottom layer

Wernicke's aphasia See "receptive aphasia"

will A legal document of how a person wants property distributed after death

withdrawal syndrome The physical and mental response after stopping or severely reducing the use of a substance that was used regularly

word element A part of a word

work ethics Behavior in the workplace

workplace violence Violent acts (including assault or threat of assault) directed toward persons at work or while on duty

wound Damage to the skin or mucous membrane

Key Abbreviations

AD	Alzheimer's disease; autonomic dysreflexia
ADA	American Dental Association; Americans With Disabilities Act of 1990
ADHD	Attention-deficit/hyperactivity disorder
ADL	Activities of daily living
ADU	Accessory dwelling unit
AE	Anti-embolism; anti-embolic
AED	Automated external defibrillator
AFO	Ankle-foot orthosis
AIDS	Acquired immunodeficiency syndrome
ALR	Assisted living residence
ALS	Amyotrophic lateral sclerosis
AMD	Age-related macular degeneration
ANA	American Nurses Association
APRN	Advanced practice registered nurse
ASC	Ambulatory surgery center
ASD	Autism spectrum disorder
ASL	American Sign Language
AUD	Alcohol use disorder
BiPAP	Bilevel positive airway pressure
BM	Bowel movement
BMI	Body mass index
BON	Board of nursing
BP	Blood pressure
BPD	Borderline personality disorder
BPH	Benign prostatic hyperplasia
C	Centigrade
CAA	Care Area Assessment
CAD	Coronary artery disease
CAUTI	Catheter-associated urinary tract infection
CBC	Complete blood count
CBT	Cognitive behavioral therapy
CCRC	Continuing care retirement community
CDC	Centers for Disease Control and Prevention
C. diff	Clostridioides difficile; Clostridium difficile
CHF	Congestive heart failure
CKD	Chronic kidney disease
cm	Centimeter
CMS	Centers for Medicare & Medicaid Services
CNA	Certified nursing assistant; certified nurse aide
CNS	Central nervous system
CO	Carbon monoxide
CO$_2$	Carbon dioxide
COPD	Chronic obstructive pulmonary disease
CP	Cerebral palsy
CPAP	Continuous positive airway pressure
CPR	Cardiopulmonary resuscitation
CPSC	Consumer Product Safety Commission
C-section	Cesarean section
CVA	Cerebrovascular accident

DNR	Do Not Resuscitate
DOB	Date of birth
DON	Director of nursing
DS	Down syndrome
EBP	Enhanced Barrier Precautions
ECG; EKG	Electrocardiogram
ECHO	Elder Cottage Housing Opportunity
E. coli	Escherichia coli
ED	Erectile dysfunction
EEOC	U.S. Equal Employment Opportunity Commission
EHR	Electronic health record
EMR	Electronic medical record
EMS	Emergency Medical Services
EPA	Environmental Protection Agency
EPHI; ePHI	Electronic protected health information
ET	Endotracheal
F	Fahrenheit
FAS	Fetal alcohol syndrome
FASDs	Fetal alcohol spectrum disorders
FBAO	Foreign-body airway obstruction
FDA	Food and Drug Administration
Fragile X	Fragile X syndrome
ft	Foot; feet
GAD	Generalized anxiety disorder
GERD	Gastro-esophageal reflux disease
GI	Gastro-intestinal
gtt	Drops
gtt/min	Drops per minute
HAI	Healthcare-associated infection
HBV	Hepatitis B virus
HCS	Hazard Communication Standard
Hg	Mercury
HHS	U.S. Department of Health & Human Services
HIPAA	Health Insurance Portability and Accountability Act of 1996
HIV	Human immunodeficiency virus
HPV	Human papilloma viruses
IBD	Inflammatory bowel disease
ICD	Implantable cardioverter defibrillator
ID	Identification
IDD	Intellectual and developmental disability
in	Inch; inches
I&O	Intake and output
IPV	Intimate partner violence
IQ	Intelligence quotient
ISTAP	International Skin Tear Advisory Panel
IV	Intravenous

JA	Juvenile arthritis
lb	Pound; pounds
L/min	Liters per minute
LNA	Licensed nursing assistant
LPN	Licensed practical nurse
LVN	Licensed vocational nurse
MDRO	Multidrug-resistant organism
MDS	Minimum Data Set
mg	Milligram
MI	Myocardial infarction
mL	Milliliter
mL/hr	Milliliters per hour
mm	Millimeter
mm Hg	Millimeters of mercury
MRN	Medical record number
MRSA	Methicillin-resistant *Staphylococcus aureus*
MS	Multiple sclerosis
MSD	Musculo-skeletal disorder
NATCEP	Nursing assistant training and competency evaluation program
NCSBN	National Council of State Boards of Nursing
NFPA	National Fire Protection Association
NG	Naso-gastric
NIA	National Institute on Aging
NPO	*Nil per os;* nothing by mouth
NPIAP	National Pressure Injury Advisory Panel
O₂	Oxygen
OAB	Over-active bladder
OASIS	Outcome and Assessment Information Set
OBRA	Omnibus Budget Reconciliation Act of 1987
OCD	Obsessive-compulsive disorder
OPIM	Other potentially infectious materials
OR	Operating room
OSHA	Occupational Safety and Health Administration
oz	Ounce
PACU	Post-anesthesia care unit
PASS	*Pull* the safety pin, *aim* low, *squeeze* the lever, *sweep* back and forth
PEG	Percutaneous endoscopic gastrostomy
PHI	Protected health information
PID	Pelvic inflammatory disease
PNS	Peripheral nervous system
POLST	Physician Orders for Life-Sustaining Treatment
post-op	Post-operative
PPE	Personal protective equipment
PPS	Prospective Payment Systems
pre-op	Pre-operative
PROM	Passive range of motion
PTSD	Post-traumatic stress disorder

RA	Rheumatoid arthritis
RACE	Rescue, alarm, confine, extinguish or evacuate
RBC	Red blood cell
RN	Registered nurse
RNA	Registered nurse aide
ROM	Range-of-motion; range of motion
RRS	Rapid Response System
RT	Respiratory therapist
SB	Spina bifida
SCA	Sudden cardiac arrest
SCD	Sequential compression device
SDS	Safety data sheet
SIDS	Sudden infant death syndrome
SNF	Skilled nursing facility
SpO₂	Saturation of peripheral oxygen (oxygen concentration)
SRNA	State registered nurse aide
SSE	Soapsuds enema
SSI	Surgical site infection
STD	Sexually transmitted disease
STI	Sexually transmitted infection
STNA	State tested nurse aide
SUD	Substance use disorder
SUID	Sudden unexpected infant death
TB	Tuberculosis
TBI	Traumatic brain injury
TDV	Teen dating violence
TED	Thrombo-embolic deterrent
TH	Thyroid hormone
TIA	Transient ischemic attack
TJC	The Joint Commission
TPN	Total parenteral nutrition
TPR	Temperature, pulse, and respirations
TURP	Transurethral resection of the prostate
U/A; UA	Urinalysis
UI	Urinary incontinence
USDA	U.S. Department of Agriculture
UTI	Urinary tract infection
VF; V-fib	Ventricular fibrillation
VRE	Vancomycin-resistant *Enterococcus*
WBC	White blood cell
WHO	World Health Organization

Index

Page numbers followed by b, t, and f indicate boxes,
tables, and figures, respectively.

932